PHARMACOLOGY AND PHARMACOTHERAPEUTICS

TWENTY FIRST EDITION

R. S. SATOSKAR

M.B.B.S., B.Sc. (Med.), Ph.D. (Sheffield)

Formerly, Professor and Head, Department of Pharmacology, Seth G.S. Medical College; T.N. Medical College; L.T.M. Medical College and Associate in Clinical Medicine, K.E.M. Hospital, Mumbai.

S. D. BHANDARKAR

M.D., F.R.C.P. (Edin), F.R.C.P. (Glasgow)

Formerly, Hon. Professor and Head, Department of Endocrinology, and Associate in Clinical Pharmacology, Seth G.S. Medical College and K.E.M. Hospital, Mumbai.

NIRMALA N. REGE

M.D., Ph.D., D.N.B. (Clin. Pharm)

Professor, Department of Pharmacology and Therapeutics, Seth G.S.Medical College and K.E.M.Hospital, Mumbai

with editorial assistance of

R. R. SATOSKAR

M.S.

Professor, Seth G. S. Medical College and K. E. M. Hospital, Mumbai.

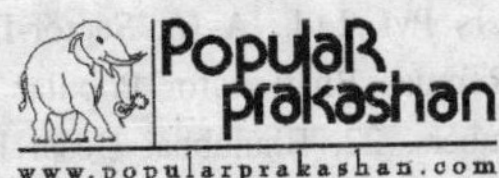

POPULAR PRAKASHAN PRIVATE LIMITED
301, Mahalaxmi Chambers, 22, Bhulabhai Desai Road, Mumbai 400026

First Edition, 1969
Russian Edition, 1985
Twentieth Edition, 2007
Reprinted 2007
Reprinted 2008
Reprinted May 2008
Reprinted July 2008
Twenty First Edition, 2009
Reprinted May 2010

(4275)

ISBN 978-81-7991-527-1

Cover inputs : Mahendra Ghanekar

PRINTED IN INDIA

By Saurabh Printers Pvt. Ltd., A-16, Sector-IV, Noida 201301
and published by Ramdas Bhatkal for Popular Prakashan Pvt. Ltd.
301, Mahalaxmi Chambers, 22, Bhulabhai Desai Road, Mumbai 400026

Contents

Dosage Note

Pharmacology and drug therapy, like medicine is an everchanging science. As new information gets accumulated, changes in drug therapy are inevitable. The authors and publishers of this book have taken special care to provide drug information and dosage schedules, that are generally in accord with the accepted standards at the time of publication. However, it may be noted that in view of the possibility of human error or advances in medicinal sciences, such therapeutic approaches are liable to change. Neither the authors nor the publishers nor any other party who has been involved in the publication of this work warrants that the information contained herein is in every respect accurate and complete. We urge the readers to confirm the information with other sources and refer to the manufacturers recommendation for all dosages, especially for the new drugs and for those used infrequently in clinical practice.

Preface to the Twenty First Edition

Like the earlier editions, the 21st edition has undergone substantial revision. Apart from re-organization of the text material, many new advances in basic and applied pharmacology, along with new figures and tables, have been added. It is hoped the readers will find this edition as useful as its predecessors.

In recent times, for various reasons, the introduction of new molecules by drug companies has slowed down. In fact, quite a few 'new' drugs introduced hurriedly had to be withdrawn from the market because of unacceptable toxicity. This emphasizes the need for vigilance on the part of doctors in accepting cleverly promoted 'new' drugs.

The last decade has witnessed the introduction of many therapeutic biopharmaceuticals. Most of them are prohibitively expensive and beyond the reach of the common man in developing countries. It is frustrating to be unable to offer them to the needy patients as they cannot afford them, nor can the government bear their cost because of financial constraints!

On the other hand, the development of new drugs for tropical diseases still remains a neglected area although there is a great need for them globally. The solution to this problem is not in sight.

We would like to thank Dr. Rakhi Tripathi, Associate Professor of Pharmacology, Seth G.S. Medical College, Mumbai and Dr. Vinod Shetty, a postgraduate student in pharmacology, Seth G.S. Medical College, Mumbai, for their help in preparing this edition. We wish to thank the many authors and publishers who have allowed us to reproduce some of the tables and diagrams in this edition. Finally, we thank Mr. Harsha Bhatkal, Director, Popular Prakashan Pvt. Ltd., and his staff, especially Mrs. Shivani Ganesh, Mrs. Jyoti Nagap and Mrs. Kalpana Deshmukh for their help in bringing out this edition. As always, we welcome constructive criticism and suggestions from our readers.

Mumbai
May 2009

R. S. Satoskar
S. D. Bhandarkar
Nirmala N. Rege

Preface to the First Edition

Pharmacology has undergone a phenomenal growth during the last twenty years and drug therapy now forms a major aspect of therapeutics. So far, pharmacology was traditionally associated with the study of drugs in dogs, cats and rats, while therapeutics or clinical application was regarded as an entirely independent and a mystical skill. Now it is generally agreed that the major object of teaching pharmacology to the medical students is to provide a rational basis for choosing and using drugs skilfully to relieve patients' ailments. This is becoming more and more important as the practising doctor is now confronted with so called "newer drugs" at such a great pace that even a full-time pharmacologist sometimes finds it difficult to keep abreast of their merits and demerits. It is highly desirable, therefore, that students of pharmacology should be educated to develop a critical outlook towards various drugs, as they are introduced. This means that book on pharmacology meant for medical students should not only give detailed account of various pharmacological actions but should also furnish a critical appraisal of their present day use in therapeutics. We have attempted in this book to combine these two important aspects. In addition, an outline of experimental evaluation of drugs in animals and man is also provided. While doing this, it was thought essential to give the relevant information from other disciplines like physiology, pathology and clinical medicine. This, though a repetition to a certain extent, is no doubt useful to understand the basis of rational therapeutics. After all, pharmacology is in some respects a bridge between basic medical sciences on one hand and clinical medicine on the other. Most of the presently available text books, except a few classics written by many authors, fail to achieve this goal. It is a common experience of those who teach pharmacology in this country to find it difficult to recommend one single book to the undergraduate medical students. Many books which give excellent information about pharmacological actions treat the therapeutics very cursorily while others that give delightful therapeutics probably assume that students know most of the basic pharmacology. It is not practicable to recommend routinely the classical multi-author books to undergraduate students, as they have many other subjects to go through, which are equally important and advanced. This book is written to fill up this gap between a big book and a concise, less informative work, so that students will get all the necessary information by reading one book. While doing this, obviously we have to restrict the size of the book, less it would be unwieldy and defeat the very purpose for which it is written. In order to achieve this, history and chemistry are reduced considerably while diagrams are included strictly to facilitate the understanding of the subject. The coverage is given according to the importance of the subject in therapeutics. Wherever multiple drugs of similar type are available, only the important prototype is discussed in detail, while others have received only a brief mention.

Although the book is written mainly for undergraduate medical students, it will also prove useful to post-graduates and practising doctors. The therapeutics part includes many details so that the book would continue to be useful even after passing pharmacology and is expected to serve as a pharmacotherapeutic reference work. The big multi-author books on this subject are no doubt excellent and authoritative but are not easily accessible to practising doctors at the time of emergency. In such circumstances this book should find its use.

The book is not written 'with an eye on examination' but it is the hope of the authors that by reading this book students would develop an attitude of thinking towards newer drugs which are many times made to appear like "therapeutic marvels". It is not expected that undergraduate students should 'cram' this book and try to remember everything that is given. It is neither possible nor necessary. They are expected to learn the basic pharmacology of the drugs in common clinical use and their rational application in therapeutics. However, the authors will feel rewarded, if students can grasp the ideology and spirit behind presentation of this book.

Drug therapy related to tropical problems is emphasized; this topic is often dismissed summarily in other works of this size. Proprietary names are included wherever necessary so that their pharmacological identity is recognised by the reader. No detailed reference list is given as this would have added many more pages. Instead, the books, reviews, symposia and monographs referred to are enlisted at the end of the book. The enthusiastic reader may refer to these for a more extensive reference list. Preparations included in the Indian Pharmacopoeia are marked as I.P. and those included in British Pharmacopoeia are listed in a separate list at the end.

It is not possible to present a book of such a size without generous help of others and the authors are deeply grateful to their many colleagues at Seth G.S. Medical College and Lokmanya Tilak Municipal Medical College, Bombay. Particularly, the help rendered by Drs. B. S. Kulkarni, S. M. Chittal, S. V. Gokhale, M. G. Wagh, C. H. Kewalramani, Mr. N. K. Dadkar, Mr. V. S. Jathar, Dr. S. M. Karandikar and Miss P. Mirwankar is gratefully acknowledged. We also would like to express our grateful thanks to many authors and publishers who promptly conceded our requests and granted permission to reproduce certain tables and diagrams, as indicated in the text. We are greatly indebted to Dr. A. F. Golwalla, Hon. Professor of Medicine, Seth G. S. Medical College and K.E.M. Hospital, Bombay for his encouragement and permission to reproduce E.C.G. records. Finally, our thanks are due to Popular Prakashan and Popular Press (Bom.) Pvt. Ltd., who as publishers and printers respectively are responsible for delivering this book in your hand expeditiously.

Bombay,
November, 1968

R. S. Satoskar
A. K. Kale
S. D. Bhandarkar

Some Abbreviations used in the text

ACD : Anaemia of chronic disease
AChE : Acetylcholinesterase
AD: Alcohol dehydrogenase
ADHD : Attention deficit hyperactivity disorder
ANC : Acid neutralizing capacity
ANF/P : Atrial natriuretic factor/peptide
APP : Acute phase proteins
ARDS : Adult respiratory distress syndrome
ATA : Atmosphere absolute
AUC : Area under curve
AVP : Arginine vasopressin
BMD : Bone mineral density
BMI : Body mass index
BNP : (human) B type natriuretic peptide
BPH: Benign prostatic hypertrophy
CDK : Cyclin-dependent kinases
CFS : Chronic fatigue syndrome
CLDII : Continuous, low dose, insulin infusion
CMRNG : Chromosomally mediated resistant *N.gonorrhoeae*
CPDA: Citrate-phosphate-dextrose-adenine
CPPD: Calcium pyrophosphate dihydrate
DES: Daytime excessive sleepiness
DUB: Dysfunctional uterine bleeding
DVT: Deep vein thrombosis
EAA: Excitatory amino acids
EDRF: Endothelium derived relaxing factor
EGFR: Epidermal growth factor receptor
EPR: Extrapyramidal reaction
ET: Endothelin
FAD: Flavin adenine dinucleotide
$FADH_2$: Reduced flavine adenine dinucleotide
FMN: Flavin mononucleotide
GERD : Gastroesophageal reflux disease
GLUT: Glucose transporter
GM-CSF : Granulocyte/macrophage colony stimulating factor
GPCR : G-protein-coupled receptors
GRA : Glucocorticoid-remediable aldosteronism
HRT : Hormone replacement therapy
HVA : Homovanillic acid
IBD : Inflammatory bowel disease
IBS : Irritable bowel syndrome
IGF: Insulin like growth factor
IL : Interleukin
ILA : Insulin like activity
IRI : Immunoreactive insulin
IRMA : Immunoradiometric acid
IRS : Insulin receptor substrate
LES : Lower esophageal sphincter
LTP : Long term potentiation
LVEF : Left ventricular ejection fraction
MAC : Mycobacterial avium complex
MAC : Minimum alveolar concentration
MAP : Muscle action potential
MDI : Metered dose inhaler
MDR : Multi drug resistant
MHPG : 3 methoxy-4-hydroxy phenol glycol
MIC : Minimum inhibitory concentration
MND : Motor neurone disease
MRP : Multidrug resistance associated protein
NAD : Nicotnamide adenine dinucleotide
NADH : Reduced nicotinamide adenine dinucleotide
NADP : Nicotinamide adenine dinucleotide phosphate
NADPH : Reduced nicotinamide adenine dinucleotide phosphate
NANC : Non-adrenergic, non-cholinergic
NAP : Nerve action potential
NARES : Non-allergic, non-infectious rhinitis with eosinophilia
NEP : Neutral endopeptidase
NGU : Non gonococcal urethritis
NK: Natural killer
NK : Neurokinins
NMDA : N-methyl-D-aspartate
OTC : Over-the-counter
PAOP : Pulmonary artery occlusive pressure
PAT : Paroxysmal atrial tachycardia
PDE : Phospodiasterase
POMC : Pro-opio-melanocortin
PPD : Purified protein derivative
PPNG : Penicillinase producing *N. gonorrhoeae*
PRA : Plasma renin activity
PUFA : Polyunsaturated fatty acids
PVT : Paroxysmal ventricular tachycardia
RIMA : Reversible inhibitor of MAO
RPCFT : Reiter protein complement fixation test
SAM : s-adenosyl methionine
SNpc : Substatia nigra pars compacta
SNRI : Serotonin norepinephrine reuptake inhibitor
SR : Sarcoplasmic reticulum
SSKI : Saturated solution of potassium iodide
SSRI : Selective serotonin reuptake inhibitors
TDM : Therapeutic drug monitoring
TI : Therapeutic index
TSS : Toxic shock syndrome
TSST-1 : Toxic shock syndrome toxin-1
UDPG : Uridine diphospho- glucose
VMA : Vanilylmandelic acid
VMR : Vasomotor rhinitis
VREF : Vancomycin resistant enterococcus faecium

"Good health is not just the absence of disease. It is the positive dynamic energy state in which internal organs work in perfect harmony and concord; and external behaviour is smooth and relaxed."

Swami Vivekananda

Section I
General Pharmacology

General Considerations and Pharmacokinetics

1

The word **Pharmacology** is derived from Greek words *Pharmacon* (an active principle) and *logos* (a discourse or treatise). Illness has been man's heritage from the beginning of his existence, and the search for remedies to combat it is perhaps equally old. The world's oldest known pharmacological or therapeutic writings come from India and China. The earliest Indian records are the *vedas*. Although there are medical descriptions in *Rigveda* (3000 B.C.), it was *Charaka,* and later *Sushruta* and *Vagbhata,* who described various medicinal preparations included in *Ayurveda,* the science of life. Initially, these consisted mostly of herbal drugs and minerals. Thus, *Charaka* described about 300 herbal drugs and classified them according to their effects, mostly on symptoms, into 50 groups. The original Ayurvedic materia medica was later superseded to some extent by the alchemic or chemical substances at about the beginning of Christian era. The Chinese materia medica 'Pan Tsao' was probably written in 2735 B.C. and contained many plant and metallic preparations and a few animal products. The earliest sources of Western medicine come from Egypt and the two kingdoms of Assyria and Babylonia. The 'Papyri' were the first written account of medical experiences from Egypt, and date back to 1900 B.C. The papyrus discovered by Eber in 1872 AD mentions about 700 herbal remedies, including opium. A Babylonian clay tablet (700 B.C.) mentions about 300 drugs.

Modern medicine is considered to date from Hippocrates, a Greek physician (450 B.C.), who for the first time introduced the concept of disease as a pathologic process and tried to organize the science of medicine on the basis of observation, analysis and deduction. Hippocratic practice did not include extensive use of drugs, probably because he did not believe in shotgun or magical remedies, but instead recommended judicious use of simple and efficacious drugs.

Till the beginning of the 19th century, the treatment of diseases included such obnoxious remedies as flesh, excreta and blood of various animals along with metal and plant preparations. James Gregory (1753-1821) was responsible for popularizing heroic symptomatic treatment consisting of blood letting, large doses of emetics and drastic purgatives, often with disastrous results. Such treatment without any rational basis was called *Allopathy* (meaning the other suffering), a term which is still wrongly applied to the system of modern scientific medicine, as opposed to *Homeopathy* (meaning similar suffering). The concept of Homeopathy was first introduced in the early 19th century by Hannemann who thought that "like cures like, and that dilution potentiates the action of drugs." Homeopathy outlines the therapy for various ailments with drugs in very high dilutions. The claims are, however, difficult to understand in the light of present concept of diseases, nor can they be substantiated by various scientific methods applied to the study of modern medicine.

Pharmacology is the science that deals with drugs. Development of modern pharmacology as a science is fairly recent and probably started taking shape following the introduction of experimental procedures in animals by Francois Magendie (1783-1855) and Claude Bernard (1813-1878). Spectacular developments in physiology, biochemistry, organic chemistry and molecular biology have greatly accelerated the advances in pharmacology. In turn, pharmacology has helped to elucidate many basic physiological and pathological mechanisms in health and disease.

With increasing knowledge about the pathophysiology of diseases, their drug therapy has now become more rational — based on logical thinking supported by comprehensive and objective information.This approach reasons out why a particular drug is selected for a given patient. For this, knowledge of the mode of action of a drug, its effects on various body systems and the probable adverse effects is important. **The object of pharmacology** is mainly to provide such scientific data, using which one can choose a drug treatment of proven efficacy and safety from the various options available, to suit the patient.

The word **drug** is derived from the French word *drogue,* a dry herb. A drug is defined as any substance used for the purpose of diagnosis, prevention, relief or cure of a disease in man or animals. According to WHO "A drug is any substance or product that is used or intended to be used to modify or explore physiological systems or pathological states for the benefit of the recipient."

Pharmacology consists of detailed study of drugs, particularly their actions on living animals, organs and tissues. The actions may be beneficial or harmful. It includes such allied topics as :

Pharmacognosy, the science of identification of drugs from natural sources.

Pharmacy, the science of identification, selection, preservation, standardization, compounding and dispensing of medicinal substances.

Clinical pharmacy involves cooperation of the pharmacist with the physician in educating the patient about compliance and counselling him on how to take the medication, and monitoring for errors in drug therapy.

Pharmacokinetics, the study of the absorption, distribution, metabolism and excretion of drugs, and their relationship to pharmacologic response (what the body does to the drug).

Pharmacodynamics, the quantitative study of the biological and therapeutic effects of drugs (what the drug does to the body). Such studies elucidate the mechanism of drug action (Fig. 1.1).

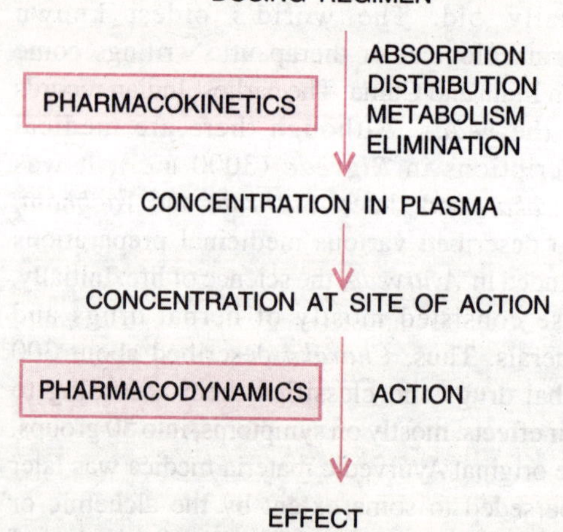

Fig. 1.1: Pharmacokinetics and Pharmacodynamics

Therapeutics which means *to care for, to tend to or to nurse*, and is a branch of medicine concerned with the cure of disease or relief of symptoms; it includes drug treatment.

Toxicology, the science of poisons which includes detection and measurement of poisons as well as treatment of poisoning. Poisons are substances that cause harmful, dangerous or fatal symptoms in animals and human beings; many drugs in large doses act as poisons.

Chemotherapy, concerned with the effect of drugs upon microorganisms and parasites, living and multiplying in a living organism. It now includes the drug treatment of cancer as well.

Pharmacoepidemiology, the study of the use and effects of drugs in large number of people. It helps to gain further insight into the efficacy and safety of new drugs after they are released for community use. Such studies are essentially observational, case-control and cohort studies.

Pharmacoeconomics, the analysis of the cost of drug therapy to the health care system and the society. It examines the quantitative relations between the cost and the benefit (cost-benefit-analysis) of the individual health care measures.

Pharmacovigilance, the process of identifying and responding to the issues of drug safety through the detection of drug effects, usually adverse. It is related to the surveillance of drugs once they are released for use in the community and relies on voluntary reporting, prescription monitoring, medical records and statistical studies in the population.

Pharmacogenetics, the study of inherited variation mediated through single gene, in drug metabolism and response in humans.

Pharmacogenomics, the science that examines the heritable variations in genes that dictate the drug response of humans (see later in this Chapter), microbes (antimicrobials) and tumours (anticancer drugs); and explores the ways these variations can be used to predict whether a patient will have a good response to a drug, a bad response, or no response. This may help in the development of more target-specific and safer drugs.

Pharmacopoeia, an official code containing a selected list of the established drugs and medicinal preparations with descriptions of their physical properties and tests for their identity, purity and potency. Pharmacopoeia defines the standards which these preparations must meet, and may mention their average doses for an adult. Examples are the Indian Pharmacopoeia (IP), the British Pharmacopoeia (BP), the United States Pharmacopoeia (USP) and the European Pharmacopoeia.

A **formulary** provides to the subscriber information about the available drugs, based on original and reputed drug information sources as well as experts' recommendations. **WHO Model Formulary** serves as a resource for countries to develop their own national formularies. **British National Formulary** (BNF) is published by the British Medical Association and Royal Pharmaceutical Society of Great Britain.

British Pharmaceutical Codex is published by Royal Pharmaceutical Society of Great Britain. It gives information about drugs, other pharmaceutical substances and formulated products. Further, it provides standards for identification and purity for a range of substances and materials for which standards are not provided by the BP.

Martindale the Extra Pharmacopoeia is a voluminous database, "published periodically by The Pharmaceutical Press by direction of the Council of the Royal Pharmaceutical Society of Great Britain and prepared in the Society's Department of Pharmaceutical Sciences." It aims to, "provide unbiased concise reports on the actions and uses of most of the world's drugs and medicines to aid the practicing pharmacists and physicians." It also contains, "referenced reviews of important or contentious topics to back up (our) editorial text and has a wide coverage of proprietary names." It is an excellent reference work for the students, teachers and practitioners of pharmacology and medicine.

The Nature and Sources of Drugs

The various sources of drugs are:

I **Mineral:** e.g., Liquid paraffin, Magnesium sulfate, Magnesium trisilicate and Kaolin.

II **Animal:** e.g., Insulin, Thyroid extract, Heparin, Gonadotropins, and Antitoxic sera.

III **Plant:** e.g., Morphine, Digoxin, Quinine, atroine and reserpine.

IV **Micro-organisms:** Bacteria and Fungi, isolated from soil, are important sources of antibacterial substances, e.g., penicillin.

V **Synthetic:** e.g., Analgesics, Hypnotics, Anticancer drugs and Antimicrobials.

VI **Genetic engineering** (DNA recombinant technology), e.g., Insulin and Growth hormone; genes.

VII **Hybridoma technique:** e.g., Monoclonal antibodies.

Majority of the drugs currently used in therapeutics are synthetic.

Plant products: Plants contain mixtures of several chemical constituents (Table 1.1), which vary from plant to plant. Some of them *(active principles)* are responsible for pharmacological effects e.g. the alkaloids morphine in opium and atropine in *Atropa belladonna* respectively; the glycoside digoxin in *Digitalis purpurea*; and the fixed oil castor oil in *Ricinus communis* and *phytoestrogens*. The other phytochemicals in plants are adjuvants and enhance pharmacological effects; or they impart stability to active principles or improve their pharmacokinetics.

Gene based therapy: The developments in biotechnology, including recombinant DNA technology, have made it possible to synthesize short nucleotide sequences (genes). These are

Table 1.1: Plant constituents

Active principle	Nature and source	Examples and uses
Alkaloids	Water-soluble salts of water-insoluble nitrogenous compounds.	Morphine, Atropine, Emetine, Vincristine.
Glycosides	Ether-like combinations of sugar with other organic structures. Acid hydrolysis separates sugar from non-sugar moiety (*aglycone* or *genin*)	Digoxin.
Fixed oils	Edible/non-edible glycerides of oleic, palmitic and stearic acids	Olive, peanut and coconut oils, and castor oil.
Volatile oils (Essential or flavouring oils)	Terpenes or their polymers. Volatile and possess aroma.	Peppermint oil: diluent, solvent and flavoring agent. Ginger, Asafoetida and Eucalyptus oil: carminative. Thymol: antiseptic. Oil of wintergreen, and Turpentine: counterirritant. Oil of clove: toothache relief.
Mineral oils	Hydrocarbons derived from petroleum. No food value	Liquid paraffin: lubricant laxative.
Resins	Oxidized or polymerized volatile oils	
Oleoresins	Mixture of volatile oils and resins	
Gums	Secretory products of plants. Form thick, mucilaginous colloids with water	Gum acacia and gum tragacanth: suspending and emulsifying agents.
Tannins	Non-nitrogenous constituents	Astringent (precipitate proteins) and protective to mucous membranes.
Miscellaneous	Antibacterial substances, Flavonoids, Retinoids, Phytoestrogens, Sterols.	Varied.

responsible for the *in-vivo* synthesis of proteins critical in certain metabolic pathways. They can be introduced into human beings for therapeutic purposes. The object of gene therapy is to introduce functional genetic material into mammalian cells to replace or supplement the activity of defective genes.

A variety of diseases are due to inherited deficiencies of single genes; examples are thalassemia, phenylketonuria and cystic fibrosis. In these conditions, the deficiency of a single gene causes serious metabolic disturbances because of either deficiency or faulty chemical composition of the protein product of the abnormal gene; or accumulation of precursors which cannot be metabolised further because of the enzyme deficiency. In such cases, the metabolic abnormality can be corrected if the synthetic gene is delivered to the target tissue(s).

In contrast, the purpose of gene therapy in acquired diseases such as cancer is to add new molecular function(s) capable of altering the course of the disease, or to block an existing function, rather than correct an underlying deficiency.

Finally, gene-transfer-mediated vaccination is applicable to both infectious and non-infectious diseases. Gene based therapy is in its infancy and many technological and ethical problems remain to be solved.

Stem cell therapy: Isolation and trans-differentiation of stem cells (either embryonic or adult pleuripotent cells) recently have been used as a therapeutic approach for regeneration and proliferation of functional cells in the body in myocardial infarction and other conditions. This approach has great potential in therapeutics but much remains to be done.

Routes of Drug Administration and Dosage Forms

Drugs may be applied locally, or may be administered orally and by injection.

Local application : Dusting powder, paste, lotion, drops, ointment or plaster exert action at the site of application. Drugs may also be administered locally in the following forms: **bougie** for urethra, **pessary** for vagina and **suppository** for the vagina and rectum.

Drugs used as aqueous solutions for local effects on mucous membranes are likely to be absorbed and may produce adverse systemic effects. In case of corneal application, the drug may penetrate into the anterior chamber and affect the ciliary muscle e.g. cocaine. Similarly, during irrigation or spraying of the nose, a compound may find its way into the middle ear through the eustachian tube. Lipoid pneumonia following aspiration of an oily solution into the respiratory tract has been reported.

Enemata : Administration of a medicament in a liquid form into the rectum is called enema. Enemata are of two types :

- ***Evacuant enema***: e.g. soap water enema. The aim is to remove the faecal matter and the flatus. The water stimulates the rectum by distension while soap acts as a lubricant/softner. The quantity of fluid administered is about 600 ml. An enema is useful in treating selected cases of constipation. It is also administered before surgical operations, delivery and radiological investigation of the GI tract.
- ***Retention enema***: The fluid containing the drug is retained in the rectum for local action as with prednisolone enema for ulcerative colitis; or it may act systemically after absorption through the mucous membrane. The quantity of fluid administered is usually 100-120 ml.

Oral or Enteral route: This is the most commonly employed route for drug administration. Its advantages are that it is safe, convenient and economical, and the complications of parenteral therapy are avoided. However, it has the following disadvantages :

- The onset of drug action is tardy.
- Irritant and unpalatable drugs cannot be administered by this route.
- The absorption of certain drugs can be irregular or negligible e.g. aminoglycosides.
- The route may not be useful in the presence of vomiting and diarrhoea.

• The route cannot be employed in an unconscious or uncooperative patient nor in an emergency; and

• Drugs likely to be destroyed by digestive juices cannot be administered orally e.g. insulin and enzymes for systemic action. Further, although a drug like testosterone is absorbed, much of it is inactivated in the intestinal wall and the liver (first pass metabolism) and little reaches the systemic circulation.

Tablets, pills or capsules are sometimes made more acceptable by various types of coating such as synthetic resins, gums, sugars, plasticizers, polyhydric alcohols, waxes, colouring agents and flavouring agents.

Certain precautions should be taken during oral administration of drugs. Capsules and tablets should be washed down with a glass of water with the patient in upright posture, either sitting or standing, as this enhances the passage into the stomach and permits rapid dissolution. Giving drugs orally to a recumbent patient should be avoided, if possible, especially in the case of drugs which can damage the esophageal mucosa e.g. tetracyclines, iron salts, slow release potassium preparations and alendronate.

Enteric coated pills and tablets: Sometimes, pills and tablets are coated with cellulose-acetate-phthalate, gluten and anionic co-polymers of methacrylic acid and its esters. These substances resist the acid juice of the stomach but permit disintegration in the intestinal alkaline juices. Enteric coating is done:

• ***To prevent gastric irritation and alteration of the drug in the stomach.***

• ***To achieve the desired concentration of the drug in the small intestine;*** and

• ***To retard the absorption of the drug.***

If the coating is very hard, a tablet or a pill may pass out without being dissolved in the GI tract (Fig.1.A and 1.B; see art plate).

The above conventional oral dosage forms serve only the purpose of introducing specific amounts of drug into the body. They do little to maintain uniform body drug concentration. Further, in order to produce a therapeutic concentration at the site of action one has to administer much larger quantities of the drug which obviously can cause adverse reactions. These dosage forms may have additional disadvantages such as necessity for frequent dosing, problems related to concomitant food intake and patient compliance, particularly during long term therapy.

Controlled release (CR) or *time release preparations* (Timsules, Spansules) release the active drug over an extended period of time. Such preparations have the particles of drug covered with coatings which dissolve at different time intervals. The coating which dissolves early releases an amount of the drug which establishes its action quickly; the coating which dissolves more slowly ensures a slow release of the remainder of the drug, thus providing uniform medication over a prolonged period (see later).

Parenteral routes: Routes of administration other than the alimentary tract (the enteron) are called parenteral.

The **advantages** of the parenteral routes are:

• They can be employed in an unconscious or an uncooperative patient.

• They can be employed in cases of vomiting and diarrhoea and in patients unable to swallow.

• Drugs which might irritate the stomach or which are not absorbed orally can be administered.

• They avoid drug modification by the alimentary juices and liver enzymes; and

• Rapid action and accuracy of dose are ensured.

The **disadvantages** are that they are:

• Inconvenient for use, self medication being difficult.

• Less safe and liable to cause infection if proper care is not exercised.

• Likely to injure important structures such as nerves and arteries; and

• More expensive.

The parenteral routes are :

I **Inhalation:** Drugs may be administered by this route, using:

• ***Pressurised, metered dose aerosols,*** e.g.,

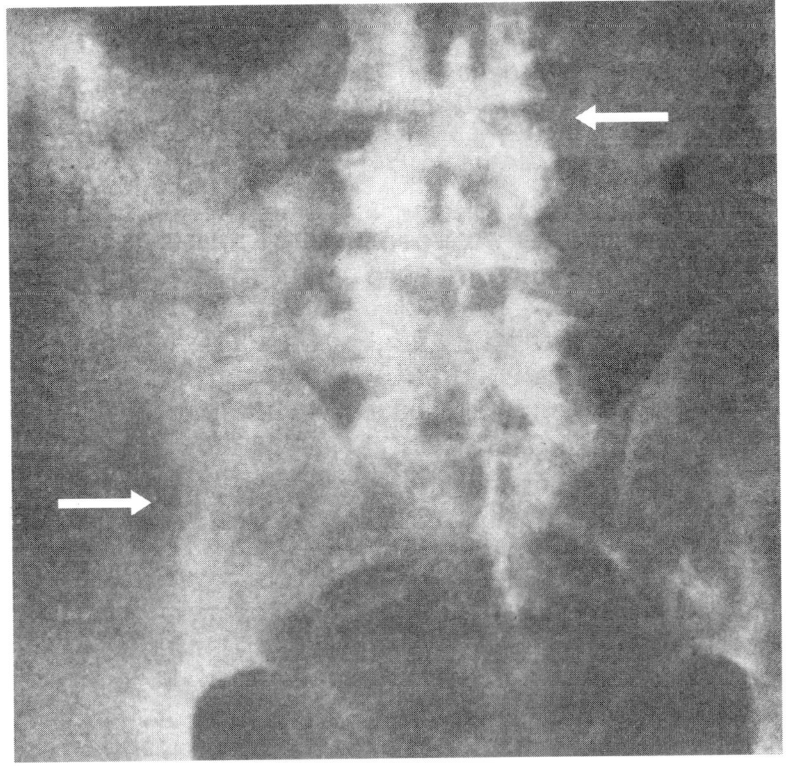

Fig. 1A: Abdominal plain x-ray showing the presence of unabsorbed hard coated tablets of a drug in the colon.

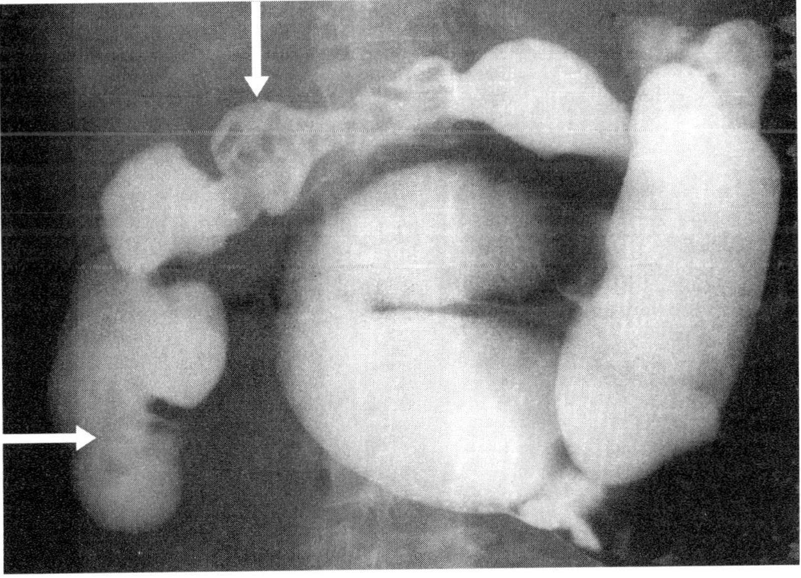

Fig. 1B: Abdominal x-ray barium enema of the same patient.

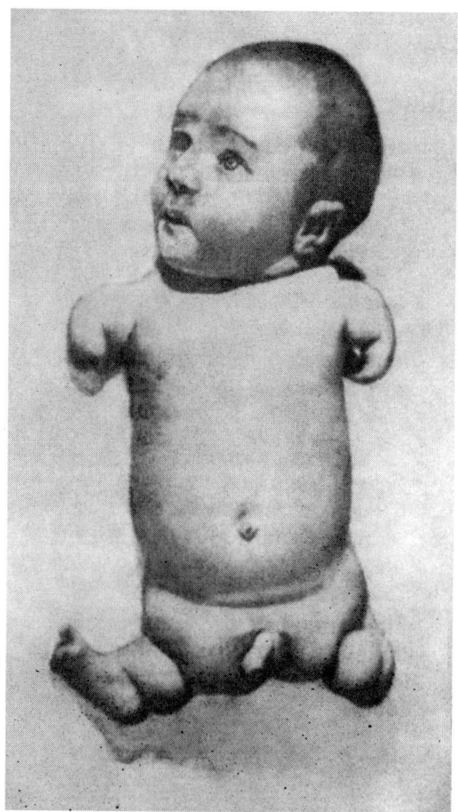

Fig. 2.10 : Limb abnormalities (Seal limbs) following thalidomide administration in the mother. (With courtesy of Dr. R. A. Pfeiffer from the Univ - Kinderkilinic. Munster. Direktor : Prof. Dr. H. Mai.)

Please see the text, page 47.

salbutamol and beclomethasone in bronchial asthma.

- ***Dry powders from inhalers activated by patient's inhalation,*** e.g., salbutamol; or
- ***Oxygen or compressed air driven nebulised solutions,*** e.g., salbutamol in bronchial asthma.
- ***Gases,*** e.g., general anaesthetics.

Drugs given by this route produce rapid effects. Thus, nicotine, morphine and tetrahydrocanabinol are rapidly absorbed following the inhalation of tobacco, opium or marihuana smoke, respectively. Drugs go directly to the left side of the heart through the pulmonary veins and may produce cardiac toxicity. Further, local irritation may result in an increase in the respiratory tract secretions and bronchospasm.

II Injections :

Intradermal (ID) : This is given into the layers of the skin e.g. BCG vaccine. Only a small quantity can be administered by this route and the injection may be painful. Intradermal injection is also employed for testing drug sensitivity.

Subcutaneous (SC) : Only non-irritant substances can be injected by this route. The commonest drug used by this route is insulin. The drug absorption is slower than with IM route. However, the action is sustained and uniform. Absorption by this route is unreliable in shock. Subcutaneous drug implants can act as 'depot' therapy e.g. sex hormone implants.

In pediatric practice, saline is sometimes injected **SC** in large quantities (**hypodermoclysis**). Drug absorption from the subcutaneous area can be enhanced by the addition of the enzyme hyaluronidase (Chapter 74).

Intramuscular (IM) : In addition to soluble substances, mild irritants, suspensions and colloids can be injected by this route. The rate of absorption is reasonably uniform and the onset of action is rapid. The volume of injection should not exceed 10 ml. *However, IM absorption is not always faster than oral absorption e.g. diazepam, hydrocortisone, digoxin and phenytoin are absorbed more slowly IM than orally.*

Drugs injected IM may cause local pain and even necrosis e.g. quinine and paraldehyde. Care should be taken to see that the injection is not given near a nerve since an irritant solution can damage the nerve, causing severe pain and even paresis of the muscles supplied by it. Finally, *IM injection should not be made into the buttock until the child starts to walk, as the gluteus maximus is very tiny till the child starts to walk; the lateral aspect of the thigh should be used.*

Intravenous (IV) : Drugs given directly into a vein produce very rapid action, and the desired blood concentration can be obtained rapidly with a well defined dose. Titration of the dose is possible. A drug may be injected (a) as a bolus e.g. Furosemide; (b) over 5-10 minutes, diluted in 10-20 ml of isotonic glucose or saline e.g. aminophylline or (c) in an infusion in 50-100 ml. or larger in volume. An infusion is employed (i) to slow the administration of the drug to avoid toxicity e.g., morphine; (ii) to maintain a constant plasma level of the drug e.g. insulin or dopamine; and (iii) to administer large volumes either rapidly or over prolonged periods of time e.g. fluids in shock or dehydration.

The **disadvantages** are : Once the drug is administered by this route, its action cannot be halted. Local irritation can lead to phlebitis (Chapter 37). Self medication is difficult and extravasation of certain substances may cause severe irritation and even sloughing (Table 1.2).

The following precautions should be observed during IV therapy :

- Before injecting, ensure that the needle is in the vein. Irritating solutions should be administered by piggybacking into a running IV drip or through a central line. If they are administered through a peripheral vein, the IV site should be rotated at regular intervals. If extravasation occurs, attempts to aspirate the extravasated substance through the cannula should be made before removing the cannula.
- The injection should be given slowly in case of certain drugs such as iron and aminophylline, as a sudden high blood concentration may be dangerous; and
- Only the minimum quantity required to elicit a particular effect should be injected.

Table 1.2: Irritants on IV administration

- Acidic, alkaline or hypertonic solutions.
- Potassium and calcium solutions.
- Parenteral nutrient solutions.
- Aminophylline.
- Iron.
- Cancer chemotherapy agents.
- Quinine, thiopental, phenytoin, diazepam, tetracycline, nitroglycerine, ethyl alcohol, radiocontrast media, propylene glycol, vasopressors.

Possible damage due to vasopressors may be reduced by local infiltration of phentolamine.

Intra-arterial drug administration produces a sudden high concentration in arterial blood and hence, may be harmful locally or damaging to tissues supplied by the artery. This route is used in diagnostic studies, such as angiograms, and in embolization therapy. Certain antimalignancy compounds are administered by regional intra arterial erfusion in localized malignancies.

Intrathecal administration involves introduction of drugs such as spinal anaesthetics into the subarachnoid space. The drugs act directly on the CNS. This route also is convenient for producing high local concentrations in the subarachnoid space e.g. certain antibiotics and antimalignancy drugs. Strict aseptic precautions must be observed.

Lignocaine is now used **extradurally** to produce anaesthesia for pelvic surgery. The **epidural** use of morphine for analgesia is described in Chapter 10.

Intraperitoneal: This route has been sometimes used in infants for giving fluids like glucose saline, as the peritoneum offers a large surface for absorption. It is also used for peritoneal dialysis.

Intraosseous cannulation: Drugs injected into the bone marrow of the iliac crest or the tibia (using a special gadget) are rapidly absorbed into the circulation. Adrenaline injected in this manner is of great help in adults in severe shock, and those with sudden cardiac arrest, and no immediate access to a vein. In infants and children, drugs such as adrenaline and dopamine have been used in this manner for resuscitation in acute, life-threatening situations when standard venous access methods have failed.

Intra-articular and Intra-lesional: Certain drugs are administered directly into a joint for the treatment of local conditions. This ensures a high local concentration of the drug e.g. hydrocortisone acetate in the treatment of rheumatoid arthritis. However, utmost aseptic precautions must be taken during this procedure to avoid infection. Glucocorticoids and local anaesthetics have been administered intra-lesionally into painful and tender spots.

Intracavernosal and Transurethral : See Chapter 67

III Transcutaneous:

Iontophoresis : In this procedure, galvanic current allows the penetration of drugs applied to the skin into the deeper tissues. *Anode iontophoresis* is used for compounds bearing positive charge and *cathode iontophoresis* for the negatively charged compounds. The force of repulsion between similar charges drives the drug ion into the deeper tissues. Salicylates have been used by this method.

Inunction: Certain drugs when rubbed into the skin (inunction) can get absorbed and produce systemic effects e.g. nitroglycerin ointment in angina pectoris. Certain potent glucocorticoids when applied to skin lesions for local effects may get absorbed and cause systemic adverse effects.

Jet injection (Dermojet) : This method involves the transcutaneous introduction of a drug (eg. insulin) by means of a high velocity jet produced through a micro-fine orifice. This method does not require the use of a needle.

Adhesive units: A transdermal therapeutic system in the form of an adhesive unit is available to deliver drugs slowly, producing prolonged systemic effect e.g. scopolamine for prevention of motion sickness. Similarly, Estraderm-TTS is a self-adhesive, releasing predetermined quantities of estradiol per 24 hours, for a period of 3-4 days.

It must be emphasized that percutaneous absorption of topically applied drugs is significantly greater in infants and children, particularly in prematures and if the skin is burnt or excoriated. This can enhance drug toxicity.

IV **Trans-mucosal :**

Sublingual administration: A tablet containing a medicament is placed under the tongue and is allowed to dissolve in the mouth. The active agent thus gets absorbed through the buccal mucous membrane directly into the systemic circulation. Drugs commonly administered by sublingual route are nitroglycerin in angina pectoris and buprenorphine as an analgesic. Some other drugs which may be administered sublingually are nifedipine, diazepam, lorazepam, domperidone, ondansetrone and ergotamine. For advantages of this route, see Table 1.3.

Table 1.3: Advantages of sublingual route

- Can be employed in patients who are vomiting.
- Rapid onset of action.
- Quick termination of the drug effect on spitting the tablet.
- Avoidance of degradation of the drug in the stomach; and
- Avoidance of its rapid inactivation in the intestinal wall and the liver (first pass)

Trans-nasal route, e.g., DAVP, a synthetic analogue of vasopressin, the hormone of the posterior pituitary gland, is administered by this route. The other drugs administered by this route are GnRH and calcitonin. A toxic substance should not be administered by this route, as it may directly reach the brain along with lymphatic channels. Also see Status epilepticus in (Chapter 9).

Trans-rectal route : The rectum has rich blood and lymph supply, and drugs can cross the rectal mucosa like the other lipid membranes; thus, unionized and lipid soluble substances are readily absorbed. The portion absorbed from the upper rectal mucosa is carried by the superior haemorrhoidal vein into the portal circulation whereas that absorbed from the lower rectum enters directly into the systemic circulation via the middle and inferior haemorrhoidal veins. The advantages of this route are that gastric irritation is avoided and by using a suitable solvent the duration of action can be controlled. Moreover, it is often convenient to use drugs rectally in the long term care of geriatric and terminally ill patients. Administration of a rectal suppository or a capsule is a simple procedure which can be undertaken by unskilled persons and by the patient himself. Examples of drugs that can be given rectally are indomethacin in rheumatoid arthritis, aminophylline for bronchospasm, and diazepam for status epilepticus.

Endotracheal route: In patients who have an indwelling endotracheal tube, certain drugs (adrenaline, atropine, diazepam, naloxone and lignocaine) can be administered by this route for an immediate effect. The drug is diluted in 5-10 ml of isotonic saline before administration.

For optimal drug effect, **computerized, miniature, syringe pumps** are now available for:

- ***Continuous administration of insulin and nitroglycerine; and***
- ***Intermittent, pulsed administration of GnRH.***

A drug may exert different effects when given by different routes. Thus, *oral* magnesium sulfate acts as saline laxative. When *injected*, it is a depressant of the CNS and acts as an anticonvulsant. On the other hand, hypertonic magnesium sulfate, given as a *retention enema*, can be used to reduce cerebral edema.

Absorption and Bioavailability

Absorption is the process by which drugs

enter the systemic circulation. Absorption of a drug from various sites, its movement among various body compartments and its distribution within the cell are all determined by the properties of a series of biological membranes in the body.

Molecules, including drug molecules, cross a biological membrane by:

(1) **Simple or passive diffusion** which may be either lipid diffusion or aqueous diffusion.

- ***Lipid diffusion:*** Drug molecules that reach the lipid bilayer of the cell membrane dissolve in the latter, and are rapidly transported across it to the other side of the membrane, down the concentration gradient. *No input of energy is required.* Hydrophobic lipid substances such as O_2, N_2 and unionized lipid soluble drugs are absorbed in this manner. Lipid/aqueous partition coefficient of a drug decides the rate of absorption. In case of weak acids and weak bases, the absorption is dependent upon the pH of the medium. Small, uncharged hydrophilic molecules such as CO_2 are absorbed in this manner.
- ***Aqueous diffusion:*** Most biological membranes are relatively permeable to water. In the epithelial membrane of the gut, the cells are joined by tight epithelial junctions, and water passes *through* the cells rather than between them; this bulk transport of water carries with it water-soluble substances of small molecular weight (less than 700) such as urea and alcohol.

In contrast, water is transported by ***filtration*** *between* the cells of the capillary endothelium except in the CNS. In the CNS, tight junctions create a blood-brain barrier.

(2) **Transport by transmembrane transporters :** These are proteins located across the mucosal cells of the intestine, renal tubules and hepatocytes, and in the capillary endothelium of vital organs. They pick up an endogenous substance or a drug at one face of the cell and release it at another. They may be:

(i) ***Solute carriers (SLC)*** which are either *facilitatory* transporters for nonionic solutes or ion-coupled *secondary active* transporters for neurotransmitter reuptake (Chapter 16); or

(ii) ***ATP binding cassettes (ABC)*** which are the active transporters.

Transmembrane transport occurs :

- ***By facilitated diffusion*** in which an SLC spanning the cell membrane moves molecules *down the chemical/concentration gradient*; OR moves cations into a negatively charged area, or anions into a positively charged area *(i.e. down the electrical gradient*). Examples are transport of glucose and amino acids into cells. Or:
- ***By active transport*** *which requires input of energy:*

(a) Where a ***carrier protein*** moves molecules uphill *against the chemical or electrical gradient* e.g. is iodide transport into the thyroid follicular cells against concentration gradient. Active, carrier mediated transport is also important in the case of molecules whose movement across a membrane would otherwise be unacceptably slow e.g. endogenous hormones, metabolites, neurotransmitters and nutrients, and drugs which structurally resemble them e.g. folic acid antagonists and hormonal analogues.

(b) ***Via ion channels*** in the cell membrane (Chapter 2). Examples are inorganic ions such Na^+, K^+, Ca^{++} and Cl^-; and the ionized fraction of ionizable drugs.

(c) ***By endocytosis***, comprising:

(i) *Receptor mediated endocytosis* e.g. insulin and LDL.

(ii) *Pinocytosis (cell drinking)* where endogenous substances (e.g. immunoglobulins in the small intestine of the neonate) as well as large, highly charged *drug molecules are engulfed* by the cell membrane e.g. lipid droplets.

(3) **Phagocytosis (cell eating)** where *microscopically visible particulate matter is engulfed* by the cell membrane e.g. cell debris.

Majority of the drugs, being lipid soluble, are absorbed by passive diffusion; a few by other modes. As a rule, drugs which are neither lipid soluble nor water soluble e.g. barium sulfate, are not absorbed from the gut.

Information regarding the rate of absorption is necessary :

- ***To determine the frequency of administration.***
- ***To ascertain the duration of effective action;*** and
- ***To predict the onset of desired or undesired effects of the drug.***

The time between the administration of a drug and the development of response is known as the **biological lag.** The route of administration determines the biological lag.

Drugs given orally may be inactive systemically for the following reasons:

- ***Enzymatic degradation*** of polypeptides within the lumen of the gastrointestinal tract e.g. insulin, adrenocorticotropic hormone (ACTH).
- ***Poor absorption*** from the GI tract e.g. aminoglycoside antibiotics; or
- ***Inactivation by first pass metabolism.***

Bioavailability of a drug (availability of biologically active drug) is defined as the amount or percentage of drug that is absorbed from a given dosage form and reaches the systemic circulation following non-vascular administration. When the drug is given IV, the bioavailability is 100%.

Drug formulations are considered to be *pharmaceutically equivalent* if they contain the same active ingredients, and are identical in strength, concentration and dosage forms. The pharmaceutically equivalent drug formulations are considered to be *bioequivalent* when the rates and extent of bioavailability of the active ingredients in the two formulations do not differ significantly when tested by standard procedures. Such substances are likely to be *therapeutically equivalent.*

Factors affecting drug absorption and its bioavailability: These are listed in Table 1.4. Oral absorption mostly occurs in the upper GI tract.

Table 1.4 : Factors affecting oral drug absorption and its bioavailability

Drug related

- Physical properties of the drug.
- Nature of the dosage form.

Patient related

- Physiological factors.
- Pharmacogenetic factors
- Disease states.

I **Physical properties:**

- ***Physical state*** : Liquids are absorbed better than solids and crystalloids are absorbed better than colloids.
- ***Lipid or water solubility*** : Drugs in aqueous solution mix more readily than those in oily solution with the aqueous phase at the absorption site, and hence are absorbed faster. However, at the cell surface, the lipid soluble drugs penetrate into the cell more rapidly than the water soluble drugs. Bile salts emulsify the fat soluble vitamins A and D in the small intestine and assist their absorption.

II **Dosage forms:**

- ***Particle size***: The particle size of *sparingly soluble drugs* can affect their absorption. A tablet that contains large aggregates of the active compound may not disintegrate even on prolonged contact with gastric and intestinal juices and hence, may be poorly absorbed. Small particle size is important for absorption of corticosteroids, antibiotics like chloramphenicol and griseofulvin, certain oral anticoagulants and spironolactone. Thus, the dosage of the active drug can be reduced without lowering efficacy simply by reducing the particle size. On the other hand, in case of an anthelmintic such as bephenium hydroxynaphthoate, the particle size should be large enough to reduce its absorption. Particle size is of no consequence in the case of freely water soluble drugs. Drugs given in an emulsified state are absorbed better e.g. vitamins A and D.
- ***Disintegration time and dissolution rate*** : The effect of the physical factors is commonly evaluated by determining :

(i) The disintegration time which measures

the rate of break up of the tablet or the capsule into the drug granules; and

(ii) The dissolution rate which is the rate at which the drug goes into solution.

The disintegration time of a tablet is a poor measure of the bioavailability of the contained drug. This is because, in addition to disintegration time and particle size, other factors such as crystalline form (polymorphism), saturation solubility and solvation can modify the bioavailability of a drug. The dissolution rate is perhaps a better parameter.

• ***Formulation***: Usually, substances like lactose, sucrose, starch and calcium phosphate or lactate are used as inert diluents in formulating powders or tablets. Such fillers may not be totally inert but may affect the absorption as well as stability of the medicament. Thus, calcium and magnesium ions reduce the absorption of tetracyclines, while calcium phosphate used as a diluent for calciferol has caused calcium toxicity, when given in large doses. Replacement of calcium phosphate by lactose made a marked difference in the efficacy of à reformulated phenytoin preparation. *The method of formulation can markedly influence the drug absorption and thus determine its bioavailability.* A faulty formulation can render a useful drug therapeutically useless. The study of the influence of formulation on the therapeutic activity of drugs is known as **biopharmaceutics.**

III **Physiological factors :**

• ***Ionization***: The mucosal lining of the GI tract is impermeable to ionized form of weak organic acids and weak organic bases. At the body pH, most drugs exist in two forms: (1) an unionized component, predominantly lipid soluble; and (2) an ionized, water soluble component. The unionized fraction can cross the cell membrane rapidly. The amount of the drug which crosses the gut wall is determined by the gradient of its concentration between the lumen of the gut and the portal venous blood. If the plasma concentration of a drug present in a free, unionized form is rapidly reduced by binding with plasma proteins, its absorption from the gut lumen is enhanced.

• ***pH of the GI fluid and the blood* : Weakly acidic drugs** are rapidly absorbed from the stomach as they exist in the acidic medium of the stomach in an unionized form. They act rapidly on oral administration e.g.,salicylates and barbiturates. However, most of the weakly acidic drugs are also absorbed from the duodenum because of their solubility in the alkaline medium and the large absorbing surface area.

Weakly basic drugs are not absorbed until they reach the alkaline environment of the small intestine. The alkaline environment, in which the drugs exist in an unionized form, facilitates their absorption. Their actions are delayed when administered orally e.g. pethidine and ephedrine.

At the pH values found in the intestine, the **strongly acidic or basic drugs** are highly ionized and hence, they are poorly absorbed. Aminogycosides are strong bases and hence, their absorption from GI tract is poor.

• ***GI transit time***: The presence of food, and the volume, viscosity and tonicity of the gastric contents can influence drug absorption by altering the gastric emptying time. Rapid absorption occurs if the drug is given on empty stomach. Table 1.5 shows the effect of food on the absorption of drugs from the GI tract.

Table 1.5: The effect of food on drug absorption

Food aids the absorption of
Chloroquine, carbamazepine, griseofulvin, lithium carbonate, nitrofurantoin, riboflavine, spironolactone.

Food interferes with the absorption of
Ampicillin, aspirin, captopril, digoxin, isoniazid, levodopa, penicillin G, rifampicin, tetracycline.

Increased peristaltic activity, as in diarrhoea, reduces the drug absorption. Anticholinergic drugs, which prolong gastric emptying time, also impair absorption of drugs. Structural changes in the GI mucous membrane result in malabsorption syndrome. Gastrointestinal mucosal edema significantly depresses the absorption of drugs such as hydrochlorothiazide in patients with congestive heart failure.

- ***Enterohepatic cycling*:** This increases the bioavailability of a drug, e.g., morphine.
- ***Area of the absorbing surface and local circulation*:** Drugs are absorbed better from the small intestine than from the stomach because of the larger surface area of the former. Reduction in the absorbing surface following major GI resection, reduces the drug absorption. Increased vascularity can increase absorption.
- ***First pass elimination*** : The bioavailability of certain drugs is reduced by rapid metabolic degradation during the first passage through the gut wall (isoprenaline) or the liver (propranolol). The other examples are opioids, beta-adrenergic blockers, progesterone, isosorbide dinitrate and nortryptiline.
- ***Presence of other agents*:** Vitamin C enhances the absorption of oral iron, while phytates retard it. The absorption of fat-soluble vitamins is reduced in the presence of liquid paraffin, whereas cholesterol absorption is reduced by sitosterol. Calcium, present in milk and in antacids, forms insoluble complexes with the tetracyclines and reduces absorption.

IV **Pharmacogenetic factors:** See later.

V **Disease states:** Absorption and first pass metabolism may be affected in conditions like malabsorption, thyrotoxicosis, achlorhydria, cirrhosis of the liver and biliary obstruction.

The only valid tests of bioavailability of a drug preparation are:

- ***The levels of the drug in biological fluids such as plasma, urine and saliva;*** and
- ***An objectively measureable parameter of its therapeutic efficacy, e.g. heart rate and BP.***

Single dose bioavailability test involves an analysis of plasma or serum concentration of the drug at various time intervals after its oral administration and plotting a serum concentration time curve (Fig.1.2). The area under such a curve (AUC) provides information about the amount of drug absorbed along with the rate of absorption and the time required to achieve the maximum concentration (Tmax). The bioavailability 'F' is determined by comparing

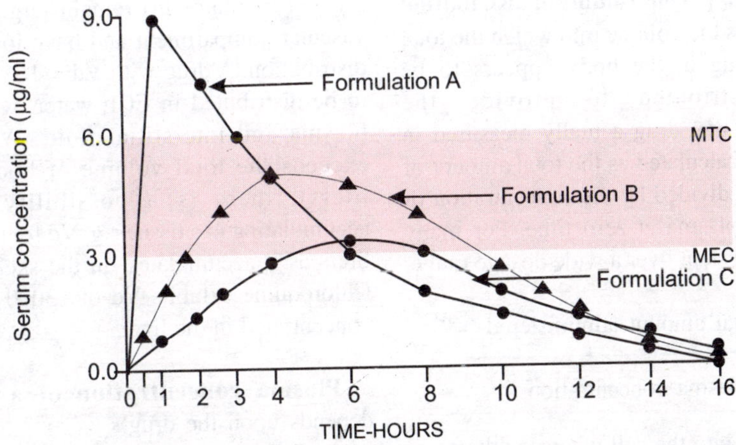

Fig. 1.2: The plasma drug level curves following oral administration of three formulations of the same basic drug. MTC = minimum toxic concentration, MEC= minimum effective concentration. The pink area indicates the therapeutic range. For formulation A and B, the areas under the curves are identical. However, formulation A would produce quick onset and short duration of action compared to formulation B whose effect would last much longer. Formulation C gives inadequate plasma levels and is, therefore, likely to be therapeutically ineffective.

the AUC after oral administration of a drug with the AUC after IV administration of the same dose of the drug.

$$F = \frac{\text{AUC after oral dose}}{\text{AUC after IV dose}} \times 100$$

Therapeutically, bioavailability is more important in the case of drugs with a narrow therapeutic index e.g. digoxin and aminophylline.

Distribution of a Drug

After absorption, a drug enters or passes through the several body fluid compartments depending upon its physicochemical properties (Table 1.6). They are:

- ***Plasma.***
- ***Interstitial fluid compartment.***
- ***Transcellular fluid compartment,*** e.g., fluids in the GI tract, bronchi, CSF.
- ***Intracellular fluid compartment.***

Every drug is distributed in the body depending upon its physicochemical properties (Table 1.6). The **apparent volume of distribution** (Vd) is defined as the volume into which the total amount of a drug in the body appears to be uniformly distributed to provide the concentration of that drug actually measured in the plasma. It is calculated as the total amount of drug in the body divided by the concentration of the drug in the plasma at zero time. For many drugs, (Vd) is constant over a wide dosage range.

$$Vd\ (L) = \frac{\text{Total amount administered}}{\text{Plasma concentration}}$$

Some drugs pass into the cell whereas others are distributed extracellularly. However, a drug can penetrate into and exist in more than one compartment. The rate of passsage of a drug through a membrane is dependent upon the pH of the body compartment and the dissociation constant (pK) of the drug. pK is the pH at which the nonionized and ionized drug concentrations are equal. Nonionized, lipid soluble drugs (the vast majority) readily cross membranes and are distributed throughout the body; they have large volumes of distribution. On the other hand, drugs which are highly protein bound (e.g. warfarin) or ionized (gentamicin) remain largely within the vascular compartment and have low volumes of distribution. A drug with Vd = 16 litres is likely to be distributed in ECF water, which includes plasma and interstitial fluid. Where the Vd exceeds the total volume of body water (42 liters), there is a possibility of a drug accumulating in a tissue e.g. Vd for digoxin is 420 liters as it accumulates in the skeletal muscles. Chloroquine exhibits Vd of 13000 liters as it is concentrated in the liver.

Table 1.6: Distribution of drugs in different body compartments

Body compartment	Types of drugs
• ***Total body water***	Small, water soluble molecules such as alcohol and antipyrine.
• ***Extracellular space***	Large water soluble molecules such as mannitol.
• ***Intravascular space***	Very large, strongly protein-bound molecules such as heparin.
• ***Body fat***	Highly lipid soluble molecules such as DDT and thiopentone.
• ***Bones***	Fluoride and lead.

Plasma concentration of a drug: This depends upon the drug's

- ***Rate of absorption.***
- ***Distribution.***
- ***Metabolism;*** and
- ***Excretion.***

After absorption, the drug circulates in the blood either in the *free* form or *bound* to plasma

Table 1.7: Effects of protein binding on drugs

- Assists enteral absorption of a drug.
- Acts as a temporary store for it and thereby prolongs its action.
- Causes prolonged, low levels of *free* drug.
- Delays its metabolic degradation.
- Delays its excretion; and
- Diminishes its penetration into the CNS.

proteins either albumin or alpha-acid-glycoprotein.Albumin is the main binding protein for many endogenous substances and drugs. The *fraction* bound to protein usually falls as the total concentration of the drug increases and the binding sites become saturated.

Table 1.7 lists the effects of protein binding on drugs. Binding of drugs to plasma proteins assists absorption. Diffusion across the intestinal wall continues as long as the concentration within the gut exceeds that of the unbound fraction in the portal capillaries.

Protein binding acts as a temporary 'store' of a drug and tends to prevent large fluctuations in concentration of unbound drug in the body fluids.

Protein binding reduces diffusion of the drug into the cell and thereby delays its metabolic degradation e.g. 90 per cent of long-acting sulfonamides and 98 per cent of warfarin circulate in bound form whereas protein binding is negligible with ethosuximide and amoxycillin. Protein binding also reduces the amount of drug available for filtration at the glomeruli and hence delays its excretion. *Clearance* is the volume of plasma cleared of the drug by metabolism and excretion per unit time. Protein binding reduces the drug clearance.

The extent of drug binding depends on the binding protein concentration in the plasma. Thus, in pregnancy, the protein bound fraction of substances such as thyroxine increases due to a rise in the concentration of the specific binding protein in the plasma. Conversely, in hypoproteinaemia, there is a rise in the free fraction due to low plasma albumin levels; the therapeutic dose required may thus be smaller.

Since it is the diffusible portion of the drug which determines its activity, with highly protein bound drugs like long-acting sulfonamides, the concentration may be too low in interstitial fluid, cerebrospinal fluid and tissue cells to combat dangerous infections.

While prescribing a new drug such as an antibiotic claimed to achieve higher and prolonged plasma concentration than a previously available drug, one should ascertain the degree of protein binding. With extensively protein bound drugs, the therapeutic activity may be low.

Administration of drugs which get bound to the same binding sites on plasma proteins may result in a sudden increase in the free concentration of one of them, possibly to a dangerous level. Thus, if a patient, stabilised on the anticoagulant warfarin takes salicylates in addition, a sudden increase in free concentration of warfarin due to its displacement from the binding sites by salicylates may result in haemorrhage (Chapter 3).

Drug storage: The concentration of a drug in certain tissues such as fat and liver after a single dose may persist even when its plasma concentration is reduced to low or undetectable levels. Thus, the hepatic concentration of mepacrine within 4 hours after its oral administration is 200 times that of plasma level. This concentration may reach a very high level on chronic administration. Iodine is similarly concentrated in the thyroid tissue. Membrane transporters are involved in drug targeting to a specific tissue e.g. metformin concentrates in the liver with the help of SLC type influx transporters.

Many lipid soluble drugs are stored in the body fat depots e.g. on IV administration, 70 per cent of the barbiturate thiopentone is taken up by the body fat from which it is released slowly. Because of such storage, repeated exposure to certain chemicals (e.g. DDT) even in small doses may lead to chronic toxicity.

Although termination of drug effects mainly occurs due to biotransformation and excretion, it may also result from redistribution of the drug from its site of action into other tissues or sites.

Placental transfer : The passage of drugs through the placenta into the fetal circulation is determined by the properties of the drug, the properties of the placenta and the altered maternal blood levels due to changing pharmacokinetics of pregnancy. The effect on the fetus is determined by its gestational age (Chapter 77).

Blood-Brain Barrier (BBB): The composition of the CSF and the extracellular (EC) fluid in the brain differs significantly from that of the plasma. A specialized system not only maintains the special brain fluid composition in the face of fluctuating composition of the plasma, but also protects the brain from toxic substances.

Unlike in the capillaries of the peripheral circulation, the endothelial cells of the brain capillaries do not permit bulk passage of water and solutes *between* the endothelial cells which are joined to each other by *tight junctions*. Only what can pass *through* the endothelial cells is allowed to pass (*diffusion barrier*). Epithelial cells of the choroid plexus also have *tight junctions* and constitute the Blood- CSF-Barrier.

These barriers allow free passage of lipid soluble drugs such as diazepam. Ionizable organic molecules (which many drugs are) are largely denied such passage from blood into the brain EC fluid. However, substances can pass freely between CSF in the subarachnoid space and the EC fluid in the brain; hence, drugs such as antibiotics introduced into the CSF can enter the brain EC fluid in adequate concentration. Drugs may penetrate into the brain using uptake transporters for endogenous substances and nutrients. Apart from these anatomical features, functional blood-brain-barrier and blood-CSF-barrier involve membrane transporters such as p-glycoproteins and organic anion transporting polypeptides (OATP) which efflux a large number of structurally diverse drugs and protect the brain from their adverse effects. The metabolites of brain neurotransmitters and organic ions are extruded into the CSF at the level of the choroid plexus by mechanisms that are similar to those in the renal tubules. Membrane transporters in the choroids plexus actively secrete drugs from the CSF into the blood. Drugs and endogenous metabolites, irrespective of their molecular size and lipid solubility, exit with bulk flow of the CSF through the subarachnoid villi into the venous sinuses in the brain.

The classical BBB, however, is absent in certain areas of the brain such as the pineal gland and the area postrema of the fourth ventricle. These areas act as brain sensors for changes in the composition of the plasma.

The BBB becomes less efficient in the presence of inflammatory diseases such as meningitis and encephalitis. Parenterally administered antibiotics can reach therapeutic concentrations in the brain EC fluid. When infection is controlled and the inflammation subsides, the BBB tends to be restored. *As that may happen while viable microorganisms persist in the CSF, drug dosage should not be reduced till the CSF is sterilized.*

Fate of a Drug

The changes that a drug undergoes in the body and its ultimate elimination are considered as the fate of the drug. Alteration of a drug within a living organism is known as **Bio-transformation**.

After absorption, drugs could undergo three possible fates :

- ***Metabolic transformation by enzymes*** which may be microsomal, cytosolic or mitochondrial, and may (1) inactivate an active drug; (2) activate an inactive drug (prodrug); or (3) generate active metabolite(s) of an active drug. (Table 1.8).
- ***Spontaneous change into other***

substances without the intervention of enzymes e.g. the anti-cancer drug mechlorethamine (a prodrug) changes spontaneously into the active ethyleniminium cations at the slightly alkaline pH of the plasma; or similar inactivation of the muscle relaxant atracurium (Hofmann reaction).

- ***Excretion unchanged.***

The metabolism of drugs usually tends to make the less polar, lipid soluble substances more polar and water soluble, thus facilitating their excretion by kidneys. If a drug is already highly polar and water soluble, it is not metabolized and gets excreted as such, eg aminoglycosides.

Majority of the drugs, are metabolized by enzymes resulting in their activation, inactivation or modification (Table 1.8). The reactions which bring about these changes are:

Phase I (Non-synthetic) :

- ***Oxidation***
- ***Reduction***
- ***Hydrolysis***; and

Table 1.8 : Effects of biotransformation on drugs

Effect of Biotransformation	Examples
Inactivation of an active drug	Chloramphenicol by conjugation
Activation of a drug to an active product	*Therapeutcally useful*: l-dopa to dopamine and enalapril to enalaprilat *Toxic*: parathion to paraxone
Generation of active metabolites of an active drug	*More active*: Diazepam to oxazepam *Having a different activity* : Pethidine (CNS depressant) to Norpethidine (CNS stimulant)

Phase II (Synthetic) :

- ***Synthesis*** (conjugation or transfer reactions).

Oxidation, reduction and hydrolysis introduce polar groups such as hydroxyl,amino, sulfhydryland carboxy into drugs which are consequently made water soluble and pharmacologically less active. Thus, metabolism of drugs is essentiallya detoxication process. However, during the initial stages of metabolism of certain drugs, active and even toxic compounds may be produced. Thus, parathion, an insecticide, is quite inactive in itself but is converted in the body to paraxon, the active toxic compound; similarly, imipramine, an antidepressant drug is biotransformed into an active compound desipramine; cyclophosphamide, sulindac and enalapril are activated by oxidation (Table 1.8).

There are many tissues which can metabolise drugs, but by far the most active tissue per unit weight is the liver. *The enzymes which metabolize drugs are distinct from those which function in the intermediary metabolism.* However, they also metabolize the endogenous steroid hormones. These enzymes are located in the liver *microsomes* which form a part of the smooth membrane of the endoplasmic reticulum of the hepatic cells. Among these enzymes are esterases, amidases, glucuronyl transferases and others that catalyze a variety of oxidative and reductive reactions. **Microsomal enzyme systems** are accessible only to substances with a high oil/water partition coefficient. These enzymes alter drugs to make them more water soluble, so that they can be excreted by the kidneys. Animal species vary not only in the kinds of microsomal enzymes they possess but also in their quantitative distribution. Many drugs are metabolised by the cytochrome P450 (CYP450) system of enzymes. CYP450 is so named because it absorbs light maximally at 450 nm. A drug bound to cytochrome P450 may be either oxidised or reduced. There are many isozymes of the enzyme CYP450, each of which is encoded by a separate gene; 50 are functionally active. *Variations in their genes structure explain the differences in the drug metabolism among different individuals and ethnic groups.* The naming of the isozymes follows an orderly pattern e.g. in the name CYP3A4, 3 stands for the family, A for the subfamily, and 4 for the chromosome encoding gene exists. CYP3A4 is involved in the metabolism of a large number of the drugs, followed by CYP2D6.

The ability of the microsomal enzymes to metabolise drugs is poor in premature infants and neonates as compared to adults. Chloramphenicol is conjugated with glucuronic acid in the adult liver and only 10 per cent is excreted unchanged in the urine. The liver of a premature infant is unable to conjugate chloramphenicol to the same extent as in adults and this may result in very high serum concentration of chloramphenicol in the infant, which may prove highly toxic. Undernutrition also depresses the functional capacity of these enzyme systems and this should be borne in mind particularly in countries where undernutrition is common.

Certain agents such as ethanol, barbiturates, on repeated administration, stimulate the synthesis of microsomal CYP450 enzyme system. This is called **enzyme induction.** Once the enzymes are they metabolise drugs which are their substrates, more rapidly. Thus, exposure to the insecticide DDT accelerates the bio-transformation of drugs, leading to their faster elimination. Enzyme induction also occurs to a limited extent in kidney, lung, skin, gut and plasma.

Drugs are also metabolized by enzymes which are of **non-microsomal** origin, present in liver, plasma and tissues including placenta and even by those present in the intestinal micro-organisms (*microfloral enzymes*), e.g. MAO, alcohol dehydrogenase, xanthine oxidase and so on.

In practice, patients may differ in their response to a standard dose of a drug. This is largely due to differences in the rate of drug metabolism among individuals. Factors affecting drug metabolism are listed in Table 1.9. The major factors are: genetic, environmental and disease related.

Table 1.9: Factors affecting drug metabolism

- Animal species and strain.
- Age and sex (see later).
- Genetic determinants.
- Nutritional status.
- Hypothermia.
- Route and duration of administration.
- Environmental determinants such as air pollution.
- Simultaneous administration of other drugs (enzyme induction and inhibition); and
- Presence of disease, hepatic/renal damage.

Oxidation : Microsomal oxidation may involve the introduction of a hydroxyl group into the drug molecule (hydroxylation) e.g. conversion of salicylic acid to gentisic acid; or an alky1 or amino group may be removed e.g. conversion of phenacetin to the active compound p-acetaminophenol (dealkylation) or of amphetamine to benzyl-methyl-ketone (deamination). A drug may be oxidized by more than one mechanism and for the same drug this may differ in different species of animals.

Oxidation can also be catalysed by non-microsomal oxidative enzymes. Thus, ethyl alcohol is oxidized to carbon dioxide and water. Methyl alcohol is oxidized to toxic formic acid and formaldehyde.

A mitochondrial enzyme monoamine oxidase (MAO) causes oxidative deamination of substances like adrenaline, 5-HT and tyramine.

Reduction: Many halogenated compounds and nitrated aromatic compounds are reduced by the microsomal enzymes e.g. halothane and chloramphenicol; drugs like chloral hydrate, disulfiram and nitrites are reduced by non-microsomal enzymes.

Hydrolysis : This is usually carried out by enzymes 'esterases' that hydrolyse (split with addition of water) the esters. These enzymes are microsomal, non-microsomal and microfloral in origin. They are usually of low specificity and exhibit considerable species variation. Drugs like pethidine, procaine, acetylcholine, diacetylmorphine, atropine, neostigmine and phenytoin, are hydrolysed by esterases. Digitalis glycosides are rendered inactive by hydrolysis.

Methanamine mandelate is hydrolysed in the urinary tract, at an acid pH, to formaldehyde and ammonia; formaldehyde exerts an antibacterial action in the urinary tract.

Conjugation or transfer reaction: This is a synthetic process by which a drug or its metabolite is combined with an endogenous substance, resulting in various conjugates such as glucuronides, ethereal sulphates, methylated compounds and amino acid conjugates. Conjugation invariably results in inactivation of the compound. After such inactivation, large molecules are eliminated in the bile whereas smaller molecules are excreted in the urine.

Glucuronides are produced by the combination of a hydroxyl, carboxyl or amino group of drug molecule with glucuronic acid. Ethereal sulphates are produced by the combination of sulphate and hydroxyl or amino group. Compounds like morphine, paraamino benzoic acid (PABA), stilboesterol, salicylic acid and phenol are excreted mainly in the form of glucuronides. A classical example of amino acid conjugation is the combination of benzoic acid with glycine to form hippuric acid.

A drug may be metabolized and inactivated by more than one successive reactions e.g. progesterone is first reduced to pregnanediol which is then conjugated; chloramphenicol is similarly reduced and then conjugated.

The ability of the diseased liver to metabolize drugs diminishes. Drugs like pethidine and morphine which are metabolized in the liver may thus have an unusually prolonged action in hepatic cirrhosis. Reduction in hepatic blood flow in shock and congestive heart failure can cause marked reduction in the metabolic degradation of lignocaine.

Drug Excretion

Drugs, except the volatile general anaesthetics, and metabolites of drugs generated by biotransformation (Phase I and II reactions) are usually excreted by a route other than that of absorption. The important channels are:

Kidneys : The processes which determine the elimination of a drug in the urine are :

- ***Passive glomerular filtration*** : Only the unbound fraction of unionized drugs is filtered at the glomerulus, but they are reabsorbed by diffusion back from the tubular lumen into the cells lining the tubules. Thus, ultimately a very small amount of the drug appears in the urine.

Ionized drugs which are poorly absorbed are excreted almost entirely by glomerular filtration and are not reabsorbed.

- ***Active tabular secretion*** : Many weak acids (anionic substances) and weak bases (cationic substances) are actively secreted by proximal tubules by carrier-mediated systems involving transporters such as p-glycoprotein and the multidrug resistance associated protein type 2 (MRP2). These transporters are also responsible for excretion of conjugated metabolites of drugs (Table 1.10).

Table 1.10: Some drugs secreted by proximal tubule into urine

Cationic (weakly basic)	Anionic (weakly acidic)
Atropine	Acetazolamide
Cimetidine	Antibiotics (penicillin, cephalosporins)
Ethambutol	Ciprofloxacin
Metformin	Diuretics (loop diuretics, thiazides)
Procainamide	Probenecid
Pseudoephedrine	Salicylates.
Quinine	Sufonamides
Trimethoprim	Sulfonylureas

Tubular secretion of weak organic acids such as penicillin can be blocked by probenecid and their half-life can be prolonged. Secretion of weak bases by renal tubules can also be blocked but the blocking agents are too toxic for any therapeutic utility.

- ***Passive renal tubular reabsorption*** : Passive diffusion is a bidirectional process and drugs may diffuse across the tubules in either direction depending upon the drug concentration, lipid solubility and the pH e.g. salicylates.

The pH of the urine influences the excretion of certain weak acids and bases. Thus, weak acids are quickly eliminated in an alkaline urine e.g. barbiturates and salicylates; while weak bases are rapidly excreted in an acidic urine e.g. pethidine and amphetamine. On the other hand, the action of these substances in the body can be prolonged if the urinary pH is not favourable for their excretion. The tubular reabsorption of weak acids is minimum when the urine is alkaline because a large portion of these compounds is ionized in an alkaline medium. Similar is the case with weak bases in acid urine. Elimination of weak acids and bases can thus be accelerated by:

- ***Maintaining a high rate of urine flow*** by the use of diuretics; and
- ***Adjusting the urinary pH.***

In the presence of renal damage, the ability of the kidney to excrete drugs is impaired. This might result in high blood levels and prolonged drug action with normal doses. Great care must, therefore, be exercised when drugs like aminoglycosides or coumarin anticoagulants are used in the presence of impaired renal function. Similarly, potassium salts may produce dangerous hyperkalemia if the kidney function is impaired. Some other drugs, the dose of which must be adjusted in renal failure are:

(a) *Only in severe renal failure* : Co-trimoxazole, carbenicillin, cefotaxime, metronidazole and fluoroquinolones; and

(b) *Even in mild renal failure* : Cephalexin, ethambutol, amphotericin B, acyclovir and flucytosine.

Protein binding reduces the amount of the drug available for filtration at the glomerulus but protein bound drugs may still be available for secretion by the proximal renal tubules, e.g., phenylbutazone. This is because the bound form of the drug is released from its combination with plasma proteins when the plasma concentration of the free form of the drug is lowered.

Since drugs, metabolites and toxins are concentrated in the kidneys during their excretion, this organ is frequently the site of drug-induced toxicity.

Lungs: Volatile general anaesthetics and drugs like paraldehyde and alcohol are partially excreted by the lungs. Their presence can be recognised by the odour they impart to the breath.

Bile: Transport systems similar to those in the kidneys are present in the hepatocytes which actively secrete drugs and their metabolites into the bile. Drugs such as phenolphthalein, doxycycline and cefoperazone appear in high concentrations in the bile. Such drugs may get repeatedly reabsorbed from the intestine and reexcreted in bile, thereby exerting a prolonged action (**enterohepatic circulation**).

Intestines : Transporters such as p-glycoprotein are also present in the enterocytes; hence drugs and their metabolites can be actively secreted from the systemic circulation into the intestinal lumen. Further, drugs can passively diffuse from the blood into the intestinal lumen, depending on their pK and the luminal pH. Laxatives like cascara and senna which act mainly on the large bowel are partly excreted into that area from the blood stream, after their absorption from the small intestine. Heavy metals are also excreted through the intestine and can produce intestinal ulceration.

Skin : Arsenic and heavy metals like mercury are excreted in small quantities through the skin. Arsenic gets incorporated in the hair follicles on prolonged administration. This phenomenon is used for detection of arsenic poisoning.

Saliva and milk : Certain drugs like iodides and metallic salts are excreted in the saliva. Lead compounds deposited as lead sulfide produce blue line on the gums. Excessive salivation is a frequent symptom of chronic, heavy metal poisoning.

Secretion of drugs in milk is discussed in Chapter 77.

Many drug-eliminating mechanisms, such as biliary and renal tubular secretion and biotransformation, are capable of saturation. This is discussed below.

Plasma Half-life and its Significance

Information about the time course of drug absorption, distribution and elimination (Pharmacokinetics) can be expressed in mathematical terms. Pharmacokinetic principles aid in the selection and adjustment of drug dose schedules. *However, they are not a substitute for, but rather a supplement to, clinical monitoring and judgement.*

Drugs are eliminated from the body by :

- ***First order kinetics***; or
- ***Zero order kinetics.***

Elimination of most drugs occurs exponentially ***(first order kinetics)*** i.e. a constant fraction of the drug in the body disappears in each equal interval of time. Thus, following a single IV dose, the plasma concentration of the drug falls exponentially (Fig 1.3a). That is, the drug is removed from the body not at a constant rate but at a rate proportional to its plasma concentration. In the case of an exponentially eliminated drug, a plot of the log of concentration against time gives almost a straight line. The rate of an exponential process may be expressed either in terms of its rate constant (K) which expresses the fractional change per unit of time, or in terms of its half time (t½), the time required for 50% completion of the process **(elimination half-time, plasma half-life or biological half-life)**. With drugs whose elimination is exponential, the biological half-life is independent of the dose, the route of administration and the plasma concentration. It depends on Vd as well as on the metabolism and the renal excretion. However, the actual quantity of the drug removed per unit time is smaller at lower plasma concentrations and larger at higher plasma concentrations. Further it should be

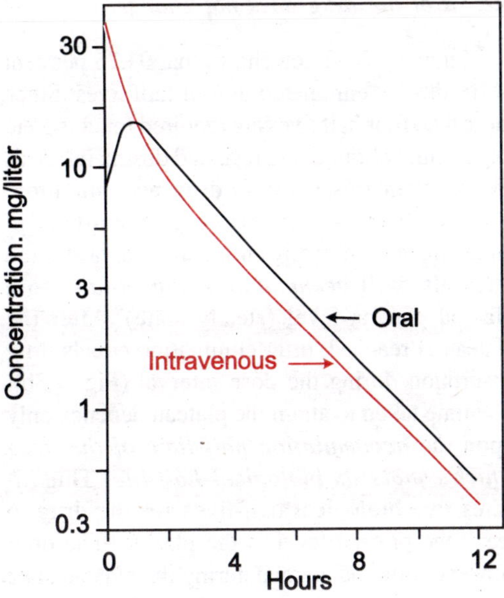

Fig.1.3 (a) : Exponential curves of plasma concentration of a drug following oral and IV administration. The slope is independent of the route of administration (First order kinetics)

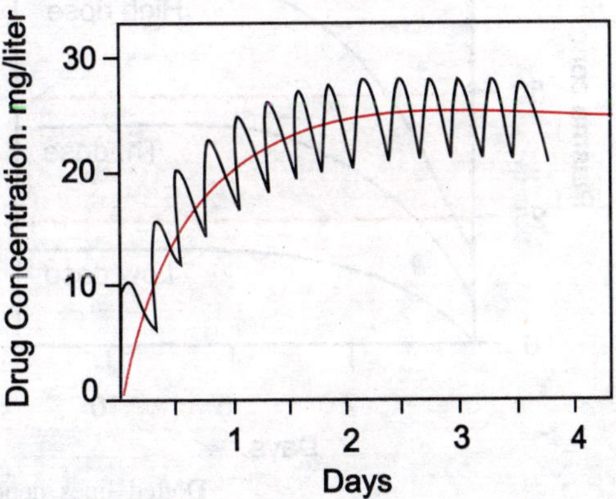

Fig. 1.3 (b) : Rise of drug concentration to a plateau (steady state) level during repeated oral administration of a constant dose. Peaks are the high points of the fluctuations whereas troughs are the low points of the fluctuations.

noted that t½ during long term oral administration of a drug may be different from that after a single IV dose. Reduced clearance of the drug due to disease is expected to prolong biological half-life and the drug effect. *This reciprocal relationship is valid only as long as the Vd of the drug does not change.*

Simple calculation shows that 93.75 per cent of the drug is eliminated in four half lives. Since more than four half lives are required for complete exponential elimination, repeated dosing intervals shorter than this leads to drug accumulation. Under these circumstances a drug administered in equal doses, intermittently, at constant time intervals, will *accumulate exponentially* to a plateau plasma level (steady state). After the plateau is reached, drug elimination equals drug absorption during the dose interval (Fig. 1.3b). The time taken to attain the plateau depends only upon the *accumulation half-time of the drug which equals its biological half-life.* Thus, it takes five biological half-lives for the drug to reach the plateau level in the plasma. The drug concentration maintained during the plateau state is directly proportional to both biological half-life and the quantity of the drug given per unit time (expressed as dose/dosage interval).

When a drug with rapid absorption or short biological half-life is administered repeatedly in the same dose at fixed, long intervals of time, marked fluctuations in the plasma concentration (during plateau state) may occur between the doses. These fluctuations can be reduced by giving the drug at shorter intervals, say by giving half doses at half intervals. Thus, during levodopa therapy, steady plasma levels and a steady clinical response can be maintained only by giving the drug in at least four divided doses per day. Insulin with a very short t½ of a few minutes is best administered by a continuous, IV infusion for maximum efficacy in diabetic coma. On the other hand, with drugs with long half-lives these fluctuations in the plasma concentration at plateau are less marked and hence these drugs may be administered at longer intervals. Thus, for maintenance therapy, digoxin, thyroxine and chlorpropamide may be given once a day to maintain a steady response.

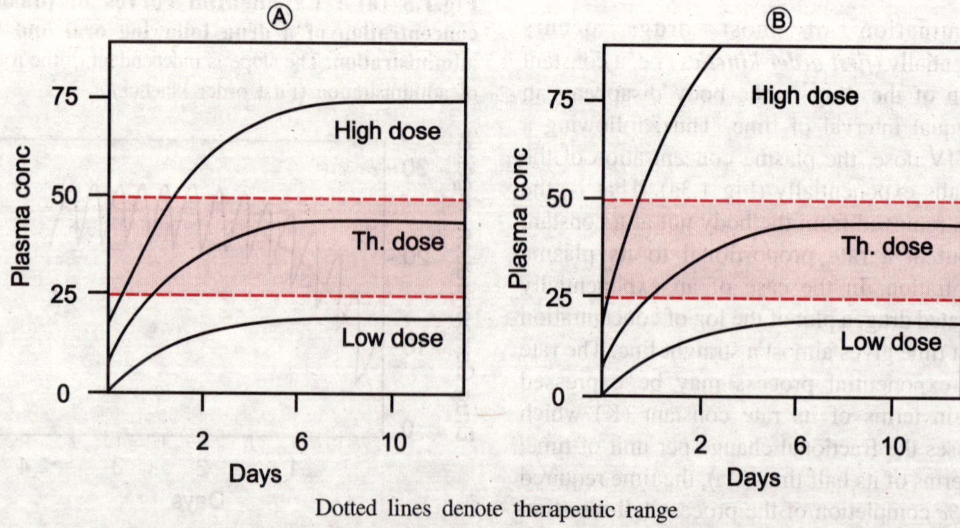

Dotted lines denote therapeutic range

Fig. 1.4 : Comparison of non-saturation and saturation kinetics for drugs, given orally, 12 hourly. Fig. A shows plasma concentration curves of a drug that follows non-saturation kinetics. Note that the steady state plasma concentration is directly proportional to the dose. Fig. B shows curves for a drug that follows saturation kinetics e.g. phenytoin. Note that no steady state is reached with high doses and that even a small increase in the dose results in a disproportionately large (? toxic) plasma concentration.

In the case of some drugs (human growth hormone and propranolol), the pharmacological effects may in fact last much longer than is suggested by their t½. With some drugs (e.g. allopurinol) this may be due to the formation of an active metabolite (e.g. oxypurinol) with a long t½. Such drugs can therefore be given at much longer intervals than their t½ would indicate. Benzylpenicillin, although its t½ is short (30 minutes), is effective in a six hourly dosage regimen. This is so because it is possible to give the drug in such large doses that the lowest concentration achieved in such a regimen is far in excess of the minimum effective concentration, because of a wide margin of safety.

In order to prevent unduly high plasma levels of a drug when its elimination is reduced in a patient with impaired hepatic, renal or cardiovascular function, the maintenance dose must be reduced. This may be achieved either by reducing each individual dose or by lengthening the dosage interval in proportion to the increase in the biological half-life.

With certain drugs such as phenytoin, alcohol, dicoumarol, probenecid, oral propranolol, and large doses of salicylates the elimination is exponential with lower dosage levels, but *when the dose exceeds a certain critical level, the eliminating mechanisms get saturated and then a fixed quantity of the drug is eliminated per unit time.* This is called **dose dependent elimination** or **saturation kinetics** or **zero order kinetics**. With such drugs, an increase in the dose can cause an increase in the biological half-life and a disproportionate increase in the plasma level. This can result in drug toxicity (Fig. 1.4).

For reasons such as differences in the rates of absorption, metabolism and excretion, a given dose of a drug may produce varying plasma levels in different individuals. The concentrations of many drugs at their site(s) of action are in equilibrium with their plasma concentration. Hence, the therapeutic response to some drugs correlates better with plateau plasma levels than with dosage. Plasma concentrations of drugs with low therapeutic index and high rate of adverse drug reactions (Table 1.11) can be a reliable guide to therapy provided they are interpreted in concert with the clinical information.

Table 1.11: Some drugs with low therapeutic index and high rate of ADR

- Digoxin
- Theophylline
- Lithium
- Aminoglycosides
- Antiarrhythmic agents
- Antiepileptic drugs

People differ in the rate at which they metabolize drugs (pharmacogenomics). With drugs such as tricyclic antidepressants and phenytoin, there may be as much as 3-5 fold variation in the plasma concentration achieved in different individuals given similar doses. Further, drug concentration in certain tissues may persist even when the plasma drug concentration is low or undetectable after stopping the drug, thus giving a prolongation of the effect e.g. digoxin in the ventricular muscle.

Methods of Prolonging the Duration of Action of a Drug

The drug action can be prolonged by:

- ***Retarding drug absorption.***
- ***Retarding drug metabolism in the liver.***
- ***Retarding renal excretion of the drug;***
- ***Using compounds which are highly protein bound;*** *and*
- ***Modifying the molecular structure*** eg. Benzodiazepines.

Retarding drug absorption: Oral absorption of a drug can be retarded by administering it on full stomach or by giving it in various coated formulations e.g. *sustained release preparations* of nitroglycerine. Such formulation, however, does not always prolong the action of a drug. (Also, see 'Routes of Drug Administration and Dosage Form' earlier).

Absorption of a drug after **parenteral administration** can be retarded by:

- ***Reduction in the vascularity of the absorbing surface***: This can be achieved by administration of a vasoconstrictor along with the drug, e.g., adrenaline with procaine.
- ***Reduction in the solubility of the drug***: This can be achieved by combining the drug with a compound having poor water solubility or giving the drug in a suspension form. Thus, penicillin is combined with procaine, a compound with poor water solubility.
- ***Administration of the drug in oily solution or in combination with bee's wax***: e.g. pitressin tannate in oil. Mixing of the drug with a water repellent like aluminium monostearate also delays the absorption, as in the case of penicillin with aluminium monostearate.
- ***Combination of the drug with a protein*** from which it is released slowly, e.g., protamine zinc insulin.
- ***Esterification***: Steroidal sex hormones such as testosterone and estrogens, when esterified with carboxylic acids, give compounds such as benzoate, propionate, enanthate and cypionate which are absorbed slowly.
- ***Pegylation*** i.e. combination with polyethylene glycol (PEG).
- ***Depot preparations*** (e.g., DOCA in Addison's disease) ***or of steroid filled silastic capsules*** (e.g., progestogens for contraception).
- ***Long acting dermatological preparations*** such as nitroglycerine ointment and transdermal discs; transdermal patches of estradiol, scopolamine and glucocorticoids.

Retarding drug metabolism : The hepatic microsomal enzyme systems concerned with biotransformation may be inhibited by certain drugs, such as monoamine oxidase inhibitors leading to prolonged drug action. In the case of levodopa, its action can be extended by combining it with a dopa decaroxylase inhibitor which inhibits its metabolism in the blood. However, depression of biotransformation may alter the *milieu interior* of the body by delaying the inactivation of endogenous products like the steroid hormones.

Retarding renal excretion of the drug : Excretion of the drug by glomerular filtration cannot be blocked or slowed without producing harmful effects on the kidney, but the tubular secretion of certain compounds can be blocked by employing compounds which share the same tubular secretory pathway. Thus, probenecid is used to reduce the penicillin excretion.

Increased protein binding of the drug in the plasma: Long-acting sulfonamide sulfamethoxypyridazine is bound to plasma proteins more extensively than short-acting sulfonamide sulfadiazine. Suramin, used in the treatment of trypanosomiasis, is extensively bound to the plasma proteins. Hence, such drugs have prolonged action.

Drugs that are sequestered in the adipose tissue (such as quinestrol, a cyclopentyl ester of estradiol) have a prolonged action.

Special Drug Delivery Systems

Various special drug delivery systems which incorporate drugs in a dosage form that releases the medication at a predetermined site or at a predetermined rate, over an extended period of time from a single application, have been developed. Some of them are :

- ***Devices for slow, prolonged release of a drug for topical action*** such as ocusert, progestasert and drug-eluting stents.
- ***A device for rapid delivery of anti-convulsant lorazepam to the CNS*** (Chapter 9).
- ***Prodrugs.***
- ***Targeted delivery systems*** such as antibody-drug conjugates; and
- ***Liposomes.***

Ocusert, when placed under the eyelid, can deliver a steady flow of pilocarpine round the clock for seven days without causing any discomfort, thus avoiding the need for repeated eye drops. Another device, called **Progestasert,** an intrauterine contraceptive device, produces controlled release of minute quantities of progesterone within the uterus for a year.

Drug-eluting stents (DES) : Such stents consist of a metallic stent backbone covered with a polymer, containing a drug (sirolimus or paclitaxel). The drug is gradually released over the next 14-30 days and modifies the local healing response within the stented artery. They have been used during coraonary angioplasty and stenting, and have reduced the incidence of restenosis markedly. They are expensive.

Prodrug is an inactive chemical compound that, after administration, undergoes biotransformation to the pharmacologically active drug. Such prodrugs may overcome the barriers limiting the usefulness of a drug. These barriers could be in:

- ***The pharmaceutical phase;*** or
- ***The pharmacokinetic phase.***

Thus, propoxyphene napsylate is a tasteless, stable and sparingly soluble derivative of propoxyphene; chloramphenicol palmitate is useful in paediatric practice to reduce the bitter taste of chloramphenicol. Since dopamine does not cross the blood-brain barrier 1-dopa is used to treat Parkinson's disease, to increase the bioavailablity of dopamine inside the CNS. Altering the polarity of ampicillin by esterifying ampicillin to form talampicillin improves the bioavailibility of ampicillin.

Prodrugs may also be used to achieve longer duration of action e.g. esters of antipsychotic phenothiazines like fluphenazine. Another important use of prodrugs is to provide site-specific delivery of drugs. Thus, methenamine is a prodrug for formaldehyde; it is converted to formaldehyde and ammonia at the acidic urinary pH and is used as a urinary tract antiseptic.

Targeted delivery of anti-cancer drugs using *monoclonal antibodies* against cancer cell antigens is one of the innovations in drug delivery systems. These antibodies *'home in* ' on the cancer cells and deliver lethal concentrations of the drug selectively to the cancer tissue.

Liposomes, another vehicle for targeted drug delivery, are concentric, spherical shells of phospholipids in a watery medium, into which drugs are incorporated. They are administered by the IV route. Drugs which have been administered via liposomes are anticancer drugs (daunorubicin and doxorubicin), antifungal drug (amphotericin B) and the antibiotic gentamicin.

Thus, drug administered in a particular dosage form via an appropriate route undergoes all the four pharmacokinetic processes viz. absorption, distribution, metabolism and excretion (Fig 1.1), which are important determinants of the concentration that the drug achieves in the systemic circulation. This concentration, in turn, determines the concentration at the site of action. The pharmacological effects of the drugs are proportional to this target concentration.

Sometimes, for achieving the therapeutic drug concentration, a **loading dose** of the drug is administered, followed by **maintenance doses**. The loading dose is defined as the initial dose that is higher than the subsequent doses, and is administered for achieving the desired plasma concentration rapidly. The subsequent doses are required for maintaining a steady state plasma drug concentration in the therapeutic range.

Pharmacodynamics – Drug Receptor Interaction; Adverse Drug Reactions

2

Pharmacological and biochemical effects of a drug occur when it reaches the site of action in the body. They may be the effects desired by the clinician treating the patient or may be undesirable and sometimes toxic. The site of drug action or *where a drug acts*, and the mechanism of drug action or *how a drug acts*, are the two fundamental and complex problems in pharmacodynamics. Understanding pharmacodynamics is essential as it provides the basis not only for rational selection of drugs but also for their judicious use to produce the maximum benefit with minimum risk.

Site of Drug Action

Generalizing about the site of drug action is easy and a tentative conclusion can be arrived at by the process of elimination; but the precise determination of the specific site and the mechanism of action of the drug is often difficult. A drug may act :

- ***Locally*** i.e. at the point of application e.g. a glucocorticoid ointment for a skin lesion; counterirritants such as methyl salicylate; gastric antacids; or
- ***Systemically*** i.e. after absorption into systemic circulation.

(a) During passage through the body e.g. osmotic diuretics.

(b) By reaching an effective concentration in a *particular tissue* (general anaesthetics in the brain or diuretics in the kidneys); or a *cell type* (anticancer drugs within the cancer cells or antibiotics within microbes).

Methods for localization of site of action of drugs:

- ***Anatomical and physiological*** : These surgical procedures isolate the organ or tissues at different levels by using excision or ablation techniques. Various parts of the CNS or other organs are sequentially exposed, effects of drugs by local application are observed and their disappearance confirmed after ablation, to locate the precise site of action. Such techniques have been used to locate the site of action of emetics and antiemetics.
- ***Biochemical localization*** : The enzyme systems can be isolated in functional condition by means of *in vivo* and *in vitro* technics and the actions of drugs can be conveniently studied e.g. physostigmine and di-isopropyl fluorophosphate (DFP) on cholinesterase.
- ***Pharmacological localization*** : If a drug produces a fall in blood pressure and if this is prevented by prior administration of an antihistaminic it can be concluded that the drug probably acts in the same place and by the same mechanism as histamine. Use of blocking agents may also suggest the probable site of action of drugs e.g. atropine in the investigation of drugs having cholinergic actions.

● ***Tracer technics***: In these procedures, the drug (ligand) is labelled with a radionuclide (tracer). The commonly used radioactive labels are ^{14}C, ^{3}H, and ^{35}S. The tracer technic is potentially the most accurate one in determining the distribution and the site of action of drugs, but it is difficult to differentiate between the drug and its metabolites and this may create difficulties in interpreting the results.

Structure Activity Relationship (SAR)

The activity of a drug is intimately related to its chemical structure. Knowledge about the chemical structure of a drug is useful for :

● ***Synthesis of new compounds with more specific actions and fewer adverse reactions,***

● ***Synthesis of competitive antagonists*** and

● ***Understanding the mechanism of drug action.***

I **Synthesis of new compounds :** New compounds or drug substitutes may be designed for the following purposes :

● ***To increase or decrease the duration of action of the original drug or to get a more potent compound :***

(i) Procaine, a local anesthetic, when administered IV, reduces the cardiac rate and excitability. However, it is rapidly hydrolyzed in the plasma and hence, its cardiac action is too transient. A compound structurally similar to procaine but resistant to hydrolysis, procainamide, has a longer duration of action and is used to treat cardiac arrhythmias.

(ii) Atropine, when instilled into the eye, produces dilatation of the pupil (mydriasis) and also paralyses the accommodation (cycloplegia). However, these effects persists for about a week. The substitute homatropine produces mydriasis and cycloplegia that lasts for 24 hours.

(iii) The diuretics polythiazide and bendroflumethiazide are as effective as the parent compound, chlorothiazide, in much smaller doses.

● ***To restrict the drug action to a particular system of the body***: Chlorpromazine possesses a host of pharmacological actions such as antipsychotic, anticholinergic, sedative and hypotensive. By structural modifications of the chlorpromazine molecule, compounds have been synthesized which have a more potent anti-psychotic effect but negligible sedative and hypotensive properties e.g. trifluoperazine.

● ***To reduce the adverse reactions,and other disadvantages associated with the available drugs:***

(i) Nicotinic acid used in the treatment of pellagra may produce itching and flushing of the skin and sometimes a fall in BP. A related compound nicotinamide has the same efficacy against pellagra but does not produce itching or flushing. (ii) Benzyl penicillin given orally is inactivated by the gastric acid. Staphylococci develop resistance to this penicillin fairly fast. Penicillins have been synthesized which are gastric acid resistant and hence can be given orally e.g. phenoxymethyl pencillin and also those that are penicillinase-resistant, e.g., cloxacillin.

II **Synthesis of competitive antagonists :**

(i) Para-amino benzoic acid (PABA) is an essential growth factor for several micro-organisms. Paramino salicylic acid (PAS) which shows a structural similarity to PABA probably acts by competing with it for the uptake by certain bacteria. Non-availability of PABA ultimately arrests the multiplication of the bacteria.

(ii) The respiratory depressant action of morphine can be antagonized by the structurally similar compound nalorphine (Chapter 10).

III **Understanding the basic chemical groups responsible for drug action :**

(i) Adrenaline stimulates both the alpha and the beta adrenergic receptors. A related compound, isoprenaline, selectively stimulates the beta adrenergic receptors while a very closely similar compound dichloroiso-propylarterenol (DCI) blocks the beta adrenergic receptors (Chapter 16).

(ii) The drug chlorpromazine (a phenothiazine) is a tranquillizer used in psychotic agitational dissorders. A structurally similar compound imipramine (iminodibenzyl derivative), on the other hand, is an antidepressant and is used as a mood elevator.

These examples emphasize the importance of certain chemical groups for the drug action and also give some idea about their mechanism.

Chirality : The word chirality comes from the Greek word 'cheir' meaning the hand. Many commonly used drugs (atenolol, ibuprofen, warfarin) exist as racemates i.e. 50 : 50 mixtures of non-superimposable, right handed and left handed, mirror image stereoisomers (**enantiomers**). The left handed molecules fit only the left handed receptors and the same is true of the right handed molecules (chiral receptors). The two types of molecules may have either the same pharmacological action with different intensities on account of pharmacokinetic differences e.g. verapamil; or entirely different actions e.g. thalidomide in which the l-thalidomide is a potent hypnotic whereas the d-thalidomide is a potent teratogen. This fact, unknown then, accounted for the thalidomide disaster in pregnant women in the 1960s. Several drugs have now been developed as single enantiomers in the interest of selective and uniform pharmacological action and reduced risk of adverse reactions; examples are l-atenolol, s-omeprazol and l-salbutamol. This process is known as chiral switching.

Mechanism of Drug Action

The terms **drug action** and **drug effects** often are used as synonyms. However, the drug action always precedes the drug effects. Drug action is the initial interaction of a drug with cells at the site of action; the resultant physiological and biochemical consequences are the drug effects.

The drug action and drug effects depend upon the drug concentration achieved at the site of action, which is determined by:

- ***Absorption of the drug after oral or parenteral administration.***
- ***First pass metabolism.***
- ***Biotransformation.***
- ***Excretion.***
- ***Tissue affinity***, e.g., ultra short-acting barbiturates are mainly concentrated in the central nervous system; and
- ***Condition of the body or the milieu interior*** e.g. iron is absorbed more rapidly in individuals with iron deficiency anaemia.

A drug may act by virtue of its:

I **Physical properties:**

- ***Colour:*** A pleasant colour may exert a psychological effect, e.g., tincture of cardamom.
- ***Physical mass***: Compounds like agar and psyllium seeds absorb water when administered orally and swell in size. This initiates peristalsis and exerts a laxative effect.
- ***Smell:*** Volatile oils like peppermint oil are used to mask the unpleasant smell of mixtures.
- ***Taste***: Compounds with a bitter taste reflexly increase the flow of hydrochloric acid in the stomach and improve the appetite.
- ***Osmolality***: Osmotic diuretics like mannitol, osmotic purgatives like magnesium sulfate.
- ***Adsorption***: Kaolin and activated charcoal in the treatment of diarrhoea.
- ***Soothing-demulcent***: Syrups as pharyngeal demulcents in the treatment of cough; calamine lotion in eczema.
- ***Reduction in surface tension***: Cationic surfactants like cetrimide for cleaning the skin.
- ***Electrical charge***: Heparin, a strongly acidic compound, exerts its anticoagulant effect by virtue of its negative charge.
- ***Radioactivity***: 131I in the treatment of hyperthyroidism.

- ***Radio-opacity***: Barium sulphate as 'barium meal', organic iodine compounds for the visualisation of the urinary and biliary tracts.

II **Chemical properties:**

- ***Acidity or alkalinity***: Antacids in the treatment of peptic ulcer.
- ***Chelation***: The chelating agent forms a ring structure with the molecules of lead, copper and other metals. This ring structure is non-toxic and water soluble and is excreted in the urine (Chapter 72).

III **Modulating body function regulators:**

These involve

- ***Neurotransmitters (NT) hormones, growth factors:*** Drugs may resemble neurotransmitters, hormones or growth factors, bind to the specialized constituents of cells and mimic or oppose their actions.

Drugs may be used as **replacement** when the production of endogenous substances decreases. Replacement finds an important application in the treatment of hormone deficiencies e.g., insulin in diabetes mellitus, thyroxine in hypothyroidism, and hydrocortisone in Addison's disease.

Drugs may interfere with NT uptake. For example, a neurotransmitter such as noradrenaline is taken up by neurons with the help of membrane transporters of the SLC type (Chapter 1). These transporters can be targets for psychotropic drugs. For example, SERT, the transporter for serotonin, is a target for the antidepressant fluoxetine which inhibits serotonin reuptake and increases its concentration in the synapse.

- ***Enzymes:*** Drugs may act by either increasing the rate of enzymatically mediated chemical reactions (enzyme stimulation) in the body or decreasing such rate (**enzyme inhibition**).

Enzyme stimulation by drugs, which are foreign substances, is unusual; it occurs commonly with endogenous substances such as hormones, e.g. adrenaline stimulates adenylyl cyclase. Apparent enhancement in enzyme activity by drugs is due to enzyme induction (stimulation of synthesis of the enzyme).

Enzyme inhibition occurs commonly with drugs and is either nonspecific, e.g. denaturing by alcohol or heavy metals; or specific, e.g. inhibition of cholinesterase by physostigmine, inhibition of carbonic anhydrase by acetazolamide and that of angiotensin converting enzyme (ACE) by captopril.

- ***Transport processes:*** Various transport processes such as Na^+K^+ ATPase pump, Ca^{++} channels, K^+ channels and Na^+-Ca^{++} exchange regulate the ionic concentrations of the cells and control the cell functions. Drugs may bind to the proteins subserving these transport processes and alter the activity of cells. For example, digitalis binds to and inhibits Na^+- K^+ ATPase pump; verapamil blocks the calcium channel; while minoxidil opens the K^+ channel.
- ***Structural proteins:*** Drugs may also bind to structural proteins of the body. For example, cochicine used to treat gouty arthritis binds to tubulin of inflammatory cells and prevents their chemotaxis. Cyclosprin, an immunosupressant binds to immunophillins.
- ***Other cell constituents such as DNA:*** Many antiviral and anticancer drugs are structural analogs of nucleic acids and compete with them to get incorporated in cellular RNA or DNA, interfering with cellular division and growth, eg. folic acid antagonist methotrexate.

The above mentioned regulators serve as receptors for the drug. For details, see later.

Types of drug effects: Drugs may produce their effects by:

- ***Stimulation;***
- ***Depression;***
- ***Irritation;***
- ***Antimicrobial effects***; and
- ***Modification of the immune status.***

It must be emphasized that a drug produces only a quantitative and not a qualitative change in the function of the target organ.

Stimulation: Increase in the activity of specialized cells is called stimulation. Excessive stimulation may ultimately lead to depression. A drug may specifically stimulate certain portions of a particular system but depress others e.g. morphine stimulates the vagus and the oculomotor nuclei and the CTZ but depresses the respiratory and the cough centres.

Depression: Decrease in the activity of specialized cells is called depression. Quinidine depresses the myocardium while barbiturates depress the central nervous system.

Irritation: The term irritation indicates that a drug produces adverse effects on the growth, nutrition and morphology of living tissues. Irritation is a nonspecific phenomenon that can occur in all the tissues. It produces changes in the cellular structure and can produce inflammation, corrosion and necrosis of cells. The cellular changes produced are:

- ***Astringent effect*** (precipitation of proteins): This may sometimes be beneficial. If the irritant, however, dissolves the precipitated proteins, the tissue damage is more extensive due to deeper penetration of the irritant. This effect is called **corrosive effect**. Many concentrated acids and alkalis exert a corrosive effect.
- ***Dehydration***.
- ***Action on cellular enzymes, usually inhibition*** e.g. gastric cyclooxygenase (COX) by aspirin; and
- ***Cytotoxic action*** (damage to the cell wall or the nucleus) e.g. anticancer drugs.

Heavy metals like mercury and silver are irritants. Mild stimulation may have therapeutic utility e.g. senna and cascara stimulate the mucosal cells of the gut and act as laxatives.

When an irritant agent is applied locally to the skin to relieve deep seated pain, it is referred to as **counterirritant**. Volatile oils like turpentine oil are often used in this fashion. The counterirritant is applied to the skin situated over the organ responsible for pain.

(a) It stimulates the sensory nerve endings in the skin and the afferent impulses are relayed in the cerebrospinal axis to efferent vasomotor fibres supplying the internal organ. Thus, the increased circulation to the skin has its counterpart in the deep integumental structures and viscera innervated from the same segmental level of the central nervous system.

(b) In addition, the sensory impulses emanating from the skin may interfere with the transmission of pain impulses coming from the viscera and may even produce their partial or complete exclusion by occupying the final common sensory pathway (**Gating theory**, Chapter 10). The vasodilatation and blockade of pain impulses may explain the relief of deep seated pain.

Antimicrobial effects : Drugs are used for prevention, arrest and eradication of infections; they act specifically on the causative organisms e.g. antibiotics (Chapter 44).

Modification of immune status: Vaccines, sera and certain other agents (levamisole and corticosteroids) act by altering (enhancing or depressing) the immune status (Chapter 76).

Drug Receptors

The receptors are specific protein macromolecules in the *cell membrane, the cytosol or the nucleus*. Many drugs (ligands) bind to the receptors for the endogenous substances or to enzymes and other constituents, which serve as receptors for the drugs. Such ligand binding initiates biochemical reactions which act as signaling mechanisms for regulating cell function by altering enzyme activity, permeability to ions, conformational features or genetic material in the nucleus. *The term receptors is reserved for these protein macromolecules with functional correlates*, but not for proteins such as binding proteins which have no functional correlates. Numerous receptors for hormones, neurotransmitters and drugs have been identified, purified, cloned and their structure has been determined.

The receptor serves a dual function:

- ***It acts as a recognition molecule for specific ligand(s)*** (molecules which bind to it) from among numerous molecular species present in the fluid that bathes the cell; and

• It ***transmits the signal from the ligand to proteins in the cell membrane and within the cell*** (post-receptor events); such events amplify the original signal by a cascade effect and regulate the function of the cell. The use of **transgenic mice** in whom one of the receptors has been either knocked out or overexpressed have been produced; this has helped in advancing our knowledge of physiology and pathology greatly. The receptor, its cellular target and the intermediary molecules (transporters) if any, are designated as **receptor-effector system.**

Biologically, the receptor is generally inactive till a ligand binds to it; only then it gets 'activated' and triggers the post-receptor events. An exception occurs when the receptor in a target endocrine gland undergoes *constitutive activation* due to a genetic mutation (Chapter 61). In such a case, the target gland overproduces its hormone, and a disease state sets in e.g. an overfunctioning, solitary, thyroid nodule ultimately becomes a toxic nodule (Plummer's disease).

The principal parameters which characterize the interaction between a ligand and a receptor are **selectivity** and **affinity**.

Selectivity of binding of drugs to receptors depends on their physico-chemical structure.

Affinity is a measure of the 'strength' of binding between the drug and its receptor. Affinity is defined by a constant in the binding relationship between the drug and the receptor.

The ability of the drug to elicit a response after its interaction with the receptor is termed as the **intrinsic activity** or the **efficacy** of the drug. The biological response to a drug is also regulated by alteration in the receptor numbers and affinity.

An **agonist** is a drug which initiates pharmacological action after binding to the receptors. It is a drug with high affinity for the receptor and also high intrinsic activity.

An **antagonist** is a drug which also binds to the receptors but does not elicit a pharmacological action; it causes receptor blockade. An antagonist, therefore, has the same affinity for the receptor as the agonist but its intrinsic activity is poor.

Partial agonist is a drug with affinity equal to or less than that of the agonist but less intrinsic activity. Such a drug, no matter how high its concentration, will not produce the full response which the tissue is capable of. Further, a partial agonist, because of its ability to occupy receptors, diminishes the action of an agonist when the two are used simultaneously. In the case of opioids (Chapter 10), which act on several types of receptors, some act as agonists or partial agonists on one type of receptor but as antagonists on another type of receptor, e.g. pentazocine and nalbuphine act as agonists on k receptors but as antagonists on μ receptors. Such drugs are called **agonist-antagonists.**

Sometimes, after combination with a receptor, a drug may produce actions opposite to those produced by a pure agonist (*affinity but*

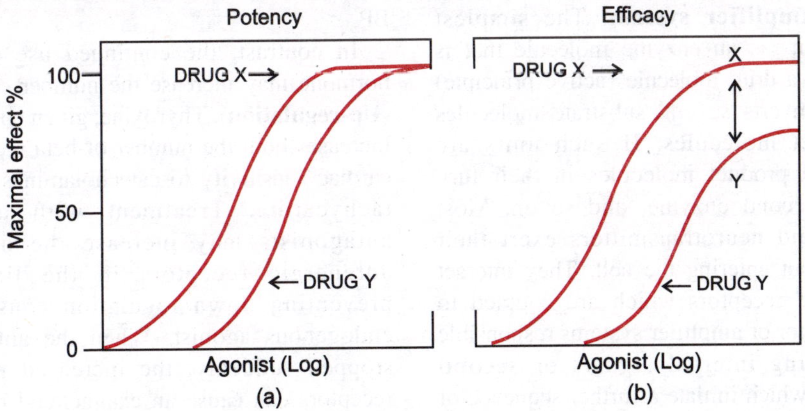

Fig. 2.1 : Relative potency and relative efficacy of two agonist drugs X and Y (See text).

negative efficacy). Thus, betacarbolines through interaction with benzodiazepine receptors produce anxiety, arousal and increase in muscle tone, actions opposite to those produced by diazepam. Such drugs are called **inverse agonists**.

Multiple receptor 'types' and 'subtypes' for a ligand are common. A neurotransmitter may activate several receptor types e.g. dopamine has five receptors, histamine has four, while acetylcholine and adrenaline have five each.

Increasing concentrations of an agonist evoke a progressively increasing tissue response until the maximum response is reached. If another drug that acts on the same receptor system produces quantitatively different maximum response, then its intrinsic activity must differ. Hence, *difference in maximum responses can form the basis for comparing intrinsic activities or efficacy of drugs.* In practice,this means that drug 'X' can produce a therapeutic effect larger than the maximum effect produced by drug 'Y'; e.g., as a diuretic furosemide is more efficacious than hydrochlothiazide (Fig. 2.1b).

The term **potency** of the drug on the other hand means that weight for weight, drug 'X' has a greater effect than drug 'Y'; the maximum effect obtainable is, however, similar; for example prednisolone is more 'potent' than hydrocortisone (Fig. 2.1a).

Some agents are so potent that only a few molecules have to interact with their receptors to induce a massive response. This obviously needs **an amplifier system**. The simplest amplifier unit is an enzyme molecule that is activated by a drug molecule (active principle) and then converts several substrate molecules into product molecules. If such units are coupled, the product molecules in their turn activate a second enzyme, and so on. Most hormones and neurotransmitters exert their effects without entering the cell. They interact with specific receptors which are coupled to various effector or amplifier systems responsible for generating internal signals or **second messengers** which initiate a further sequence of enzyme reactions. In such **amplifier system model**, the active agent needs to activate only a fraction of its receptors to obtain maximal response from the effector system. Thus, there is a **spare capacity** for the specific receptors.

Spare receptors are qualitatively similar to the occupied receptors and are available for action. Thus, adrenaline can elicit the maximum cardiac inotropic response even when 90 per cent of the cardiac $ß_1$ adrenergic receptors are occupied by relatively irreversible antagonists. This indicates that the cardiac tissue possesses a large number of spare $beta_1$ receptors.

Receptor-mediated responses to drugs and hormones often become blunted with time during continued exposure to the durg/hormone. This phenomenon is termed **desensitization, refractoriness** or **tolerance**. Thus, repeated administration of ephedrine and adrenergic agonists in bronchial asthma causes a reduction in therapeutic response. Desensitization is usually reversible.

Downregulation is a process where the actual number of receptors present in the cell/tissue decreases; this occurs more slowly than desensitization and is less rapidly reversible. It involves net degradation of the cell receptors while desenitization usually involves reversible phosphorylation. When the $á_2$ adrenergic agonist clonidine is used to treat hypertension, it causes a reduction in the number of $á_2$ adrenoreceptors. When the drug is withdrawn suddenly, the number of receptors is too small for endogenous agonists to produce their effective stimulation, leading to a sudden rise in BP.

In contrast, the continued use of a drug/hormone may increase the number of receptors (**Up-regulation**). Thyroxine, given continuously, increases both the number of beta receptors and cardiac sensitivity to catecholamines leading to tachycardia. Treatment with adrenergic antagonists may increase the number of adrenergic receptors in the tissues, by preventing down regulation caused by an endogenous agonist. When the antagonist is stopped suddenly, the increased number of receptors can cause an exaggerated response to the physiological concentration of the agonist.

Table 2.1: The main types of receptors

	Type 1	Type 2	Type 3	Type 4
Class	Channel-linked (Ionotropic)	G-protein coupled (GPCR) (Metabotropic)	Kinase linked	Acting on gene transcription
Location	Cell membrane	Cell membrane	Cell membrane	Cytosol and nucleus
Effector	Channel	Enzyme or channel	Enzyme	Gene transcription
Coupling	Direct	G-protein	Direct or indirect	Via DNA
Examples	nAChR $GABA_AR$ Glycine	mAChR Beta adreno R TSH H_2R	Insulin R Growth factor R Cytokine R ANF R	Steroid / thyroid hormone R
Second messenger	None	cAMP, cGMP, Ca^{++}	None	None

R= Receptor. ANF = Atrial Natriuretic Factor. cAMP= cyclic AMP. cGMP= cyclic GMP
N = Nicotinic. M = Muscarinic. H = Histaminic. ACh = Acetylcholine.

Thus, chronic administration of beta-adrenergic blocker, propranolol, is accompanied by increase in the number of beta-adrenergic receptors. Sudden withdrawal of the beta-blockers in a patient with ischemic heart disease makes him more susceptible to the effects of noradrenaline and may precipitate angina. Patients with orthostatic hypotension, who show low concentrations of circulating catecholamines and enhanced responses to noradrenaline and related drugs, have increased number of adrenergic receptors compared to normal subjects.

Types of receptors (Table 2.1) :

- *Type 1* : *Channel-linked* (Ionotropic).
- *Type 2* : *G-protein-coupled* (GPCR) (Metabotropic).
- *Type 3* : *Kinase-linked*; and
- *Type 4* : ***Receptors that regulate gene transcription.***

Ion channels are cell membrane spanning proteins. Agents binding with them open a transmembrane channel and permit ions to cross the membrane phospholipid bilayer. Which ions flow and what voltage changes occur as a consequence depend upon the type of channel. Thus, opening of the nicotinic, acetycholine (ACh) receptor channel permits sodium ions to cross the membrane into the cell and cause depolarization of the membrane. On the other hand, the gamma-aminobutyric acid (GABA) receptor channel allows chloride ions to permeate into the cell, and hyperpolarizes the cell membrane. Many drugs (phenytoin and benzodiazepines) act by modifying the function of receptor channels. Opening of the potassium channels allows potassium ions to leak out of the cell and thus hyperpolarizes the cell membrane e.g. sulfonylurea receptor.

G-proteins or guanine nucleotide binding proteins are a specific class of proteins that are coupled to certain receptors and are involved in the regulation of secondary messengers. GPCR are found on all cell types and are abundant in the brain and the gut. They are either **stimulatory (Gs)** or **inhibitory (Gi)** in action. The G in the name refers to guanosine diphosphate or triphosphate. ACh and GABA can activate ion channels as well as GPCR. A ligand binding to GPCR promotes binding of GTP to G-proteins. The activated G-proteins in turn activate effector systems such as enzymes (adenlyl cyclase and phospholipase) and ion channels (Ca^{++} & K^{+}). The second messengers for such actions are : (a) intracytoplasmic calcium ion concentration; (b) cyclic AMP; and (c) inositol 1, 3, 5-triphosphate (IP_3) and diacylglycerol (DAG) released from the phospholipid in the cell membrane. In some instances, these three are interlinked.

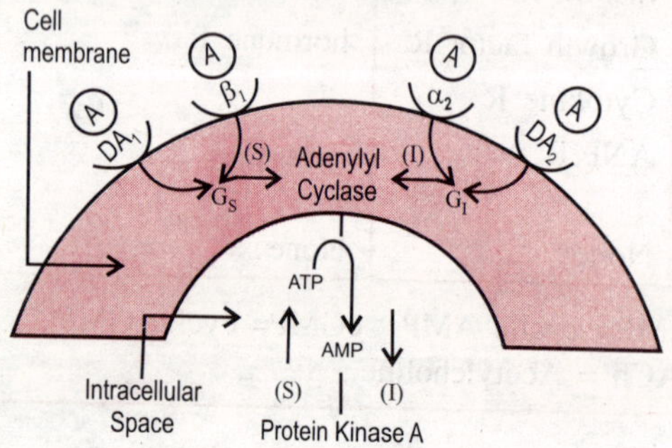

Fig. 2.2: GPCR mechanism for beta1 and alpha2 adrenergic and dopamine A1 and A2 agonist
A = Agonist; S = Stimulation I = Inhibition;
DA = Dopamine receptor
α and β_2 = Adrenergic receptors; G = G protein

The classic examples of GPCR are the adrenergic β_1 and $á_2$ receptors and dopamine receptors (Fig. 2.2). Thus:

(1) The extracellular ligand A binds to a cell-surface G-protein-coupled receptor; which in turn

(2) Activates G-protein located on the cytoplasmic face of the plasma membrane.

(3) The activated G-protein alters the activity of the effector element such as the adenylyl cyclase enzyme (or an ion channel).

(4) Adenylyl cyclase converts intracellular ATP to cyclic AMP, the second messenger.

Many drugs such as opiates act on GPCR either as agonists or as antagonists. Similarly, peptides (eg beta endorphins), acetylcholine (muscarinic actions) and biogenic amines (5-HT) act by binding to GPCR. *Nearly 65% of the prescription drugs are targeted against GPCRs.*

The third family of cell surface receptors are **tyrosine kinases** e.g. insulin and epidermal growth factor receptors. Tyrosine kinases activate themselves by autophosphoryla-tion after the hormone binds to them. The autophosphorylated tyrosine kinase then phosphorylates intracellular proteins on the tyrosine residues.

Receptors for steroids are present in the cytoplasm; *those for thyroid hormones* are present in the nuclear chromatin. These receptors, after activation by hormone binding, act on the genetic material in the nucleus to initiate or inhibit the process of transcription.

It must be emphasized that a given agent may activate more than one type of receptors.

Dose Response Relationship

Wide quantitative variations in drug responses can occur between different species and within the same species under different conditions. Methods have, therefore, been devised to study the phenomenon of variation in pharmacological drug response and to minimize the errors of prediction in therapeutic use of drugs.

Each drug has a characteristic dose response curve for a specified set of conditions,

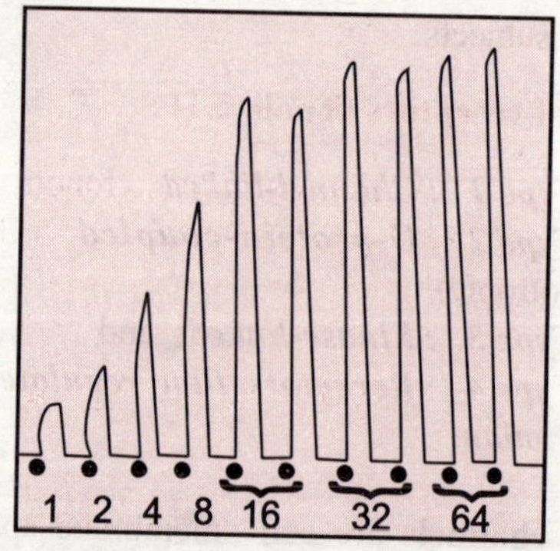

Fig. 2.3 : Effect of graded doses of histamine on isolated guinea-pig ileum.

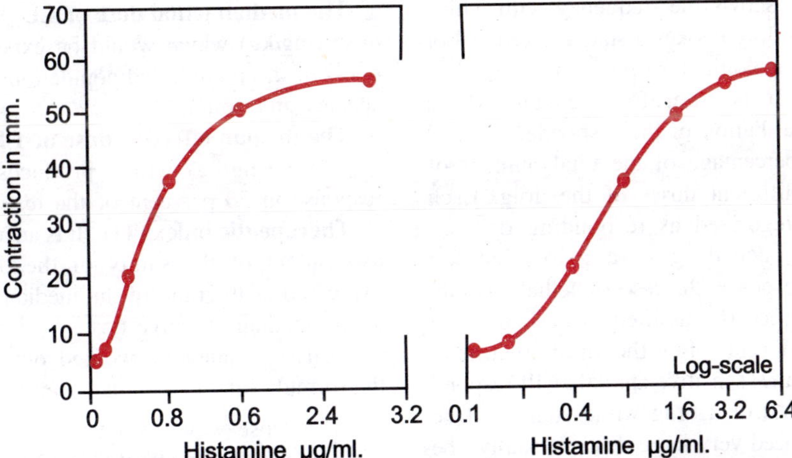

Fig. 2.4 (a) : Dose-response relationship curve from the data in Fig. 2.3

Fig. 2.4 (b) : Same dose-response relationship plotted on logarithmic scale.

but in general, the dose response curve conforms to the S-shaped or sigmoid type, or to segments of the sigmoid. The magnitude of the drug effect is a function of the dose administered. Two basic types of dose effect relationship have been observed.

These are:

- ***Graded or quantitative dose-response relationship;*** and
- ***Quantal or all or none dose-response relationship.***

Graded or quantitative dose-response relationship : This type of relationship relates the size of the response in a single biological unit to the dose of the drug. As the dose administered to a single subject or discrete organ or tissue is increased, the pharmacological response also increases in graded fashion provided the dose has exceeded some critical level called the **threshold dose** (Fig. 2.3). The graded dose-response relation is partially a reflection of the extent of occupancy of the receptors by the drug. Since an entire dose response relationship is determined from one animal, the curve cannot tell us about the degree of biological variation inherent in a population of such animals.

The degree of response produced by increasing doses of a drug eventually reaches a steady level, termed as the **ceiling response**, and the dose with which it is obtained is the **ceiling dose**. If the dose of a drug exceeds the ceiling dose, there is no further increase in the therapeutic effect. In fact, such a dose may provoke different and possibly undesirable responses. The ceiling dose allows us to compare the **therapeutic efficacy** of various pharmacologically active compounds.

Fig. 2.4a shows a 'dose versus response' curve whereas Fig. 2.4 b shows the same data in the form of a 'log-dose versus response' curve. The latter is particularly useful for the comparison of the activity of various compounds.

Quantal or all or none dose-response relationship : In contrast to graded responses, the quantal responses are all or none. The

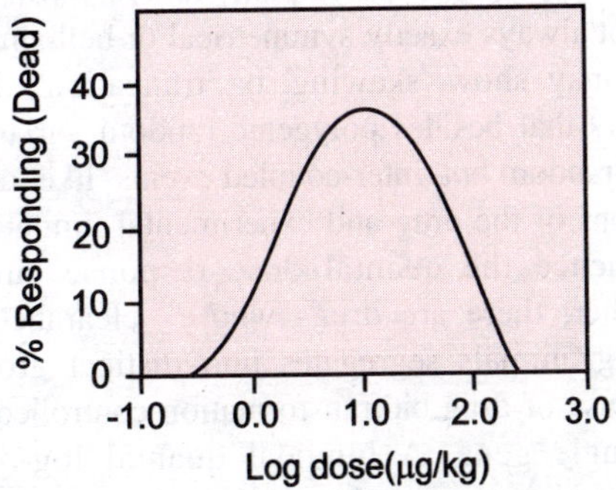

Fig. 2.5: Quantal dose response curve

quantal curve shows the frequency with which any dose of a drug evokes a stated, fixed (all or none) pharmacological response in a subject population. It is, therefore, essentially a frequency distribution of the responders (actual numbers or percentage of the total number of animals) to different doses of the drug. Each animal is categorized as responding or non-responding, according to a prior decided criterion of response. In case of lethal toxicity tests, each animal is classified as dead or alive at a specified time after the drug treatment. Obviously, some sensitive animals will respond to smaller doses of a drug while some will be resistant and need very large doses. Usually, the sensitivity of animals to different doses of a drug is distributed normally with respect to the logarithm of the dose. Thus, for a given drug, if log dose is plotted on the horizontal axis and the per cent responding (dead) to the various dose levels is plotted on the vertical axis, a **Gaussian (normal) distribution** is obtained (Fig. 2.5). The curve represents the distribution of **sensitivity** of a group of animals to the given drug. In this figure about 10 per cent of the animals in a given population are killed at a dose level of log dose '0', while another 10 per cent are not killed until the dose is increased to log dose '2'. Majority of the animals, however, are killed at doses between '0.5' and '1.5' on the log scale. The same data, when plotted as the cumulative number of animals that responded against log dose, would give an S shaped cumulative frequency curve. For a given dose of a drug, a cumulative curve would give the per cent of animals responding to that dose and to all lower doses.

The quantal dose response curve, however, is not always exactly symmetrical or bell-shaped but may show 'skewing' or 'truncation'. This shows that besides polygenic random variation, non-random but inter-coupled events like other actions of the drug and experimental limitations influence the quantal dose response curve. Further, there are drugs whose clearance in living animals segregates into distinct groups because of drug biotransformation controlled by a single gene. A bimodal quantal log-dose response curve may be obtained in such cases.

The median lethal dose or LD_{50} : This is the dose (mg/kg) which would be expected to kill one-half of an unlimited population of the same species and strain.

The median effective dose or ED_{50} : This is the dose (mg/kg) which produces a desired response in 50 per cent of the test population.

Therapeutic index (TI) : It is an approximate assessment of the safety of the drug. It is expressed as the ratio of the median lethal dose to the median effective dose:

As LD_{50} cannot be worked out in humans, the formula for TI in humans can be restated as

$$\text{TI} = \frac{\text{Dose which produces a defined } \textbf{unwanted effect} \text{ (e.g. tachycardia due to salbutamol) in 50\% of the test subjects}}{\text{Dose producing } \textbf{therapeutic effect} \text{ (specified reduction in airway resistance) in 50\% of the test subjects}}$$

The margin of safety is the difference between the therapeutic and the lethal doses.

As the drug metabolism varies from species to species, the TI would also vary in a similar fashion. Therapeutic index supplies reliable information when both the LD_{50} and ED_{50} are determined for the same strain of a given species. ED_{50} can be obtained from either quantal or graded dose response curves.

The larger the TI, the safer is the drug. For safe therapeutic application of a compound, its TI must be more than one. *Such drugs have very little dose-related toxicity*. Thus, penicillin has a very high TI while it is much smaller for digoxin, aminophylline and lidocaine.

In practice, no drug produces only a single effect but has a spectrum of effects. Further, a drug may be selective in one respect but nonselective in another. Thus, although antihistaminics selectively block histamine actions, most of them cause significant sedation. For therapeutic purposes, selectivity of a drug effect is clearly one of its more important properties. The therapeutic index gives only a rough idea about the safety of the preparation. Depending upon its clinical use, a drug may thus have many therapeutic indices. The margin of safety of aspirin when used for headache is far greater than its margin of safety for the relief of arthritic pain or in rheumatic fever. This is because the latter use requires much larger doses.

In clinical practice, there is often a need to use two or more drugs concurrently. The resultant effect may vary depending on the drugs used. There may be :

(1) **Additive effect (Summation) :**

When the total pharmacological action of two or more drugs administered together is equivalent to the sum of their individual pharmacological actions (1+1=2), the phenomenon is termed as an additive effect e.g. combination of aspirin and paracetamol in the treatment of pain and fever.

(2) **Synergism:**

Facilitation of a pharmacological response by the concomitant use of two or more drugs is called drug synergism. The word synergism is derived from the two Greek words, *ergo* (work) and *syn* (with) and indicates a pharmacologic co-operation. This co-operation usually results in a total effect greater than the sum of their independent actions (1+1>2), e.g. codeine and aspirin for pain; hydrochlorothiazide and atenolol for hypertension.

If the synergism results in prolongation of action of one of the drugs, it is termed **time synergism**, e.g. procaine and adrenaline combination increases the duration of action of procaine.

The term **potentiation** is often loosely employed for synergism and should be avoided, as the word 'potentiate' means 'to endow with power', which no drug is really capable of achieving.

(3) **Antagonism :**

The phenomenon of opposing actions of two drugs on the same physiological system is termed as drug antagonism. It can be:

- ***Chemical.***
- ***Competitive (reversible).***
- ***Non-competitive (irreversible);***
- ***Physiological.***

Chemical antagonism: In this case the biological activity of a drug can be reduced or abolished by a chemical reaction with another agent e.g. BAL and arsenic; a cytokine and its antibody.

Competitive or reversible antagonism: When the agonist and the antagonist compete for the same receptors, it is designated as competitive antagonism. The extent to which the antagonist opposes the pharmacological action of the agonist will be decided by the relative numbers of receptors occupied by the two compounds. Competitive antagonism can be overcome by increasing the concentration of the agonist at the receptor site, e.g. acetylcholine and atropine antagonism at muscarinic receptors. If the concentration of acetylcholine at the receptor level is increased by the administration of an anticholinesterase, the blockade produced by atropine can be reversed **(reversible antagonism)**. Similar is the case between noradrenaline and prazosin, an alpha-adrenergic blocking agent.

A competitive antagonist shifts the dose response curve to the right. The maximal response to agonist is, however, not impaired (Fig. 2.6a).

Non-competitive antagonism: In this type of antagonism an antagonist inactivates the receptor (R) so that an effective complex with the agonist cannot be formed, irrespective of the concentration of the agonist. This may happen in various ways: (a) The antagonist might combine with R at the same site, but the combination is so firm that even higher concentration of the agonist cannot displace it (irreversible). (b) The antagonist binds to a different site in such a manner as to prevent the expected characteristic biologic response to the agonist; or (c) The antagonist might itself induce a certain change in R so that the reactivity of the binding site where agonist should interact is reduced or abolished. Examples are, acetylcholine and papaverine on smooth muscle; acetylcholine and decamethonium at the neuromuscular junction.

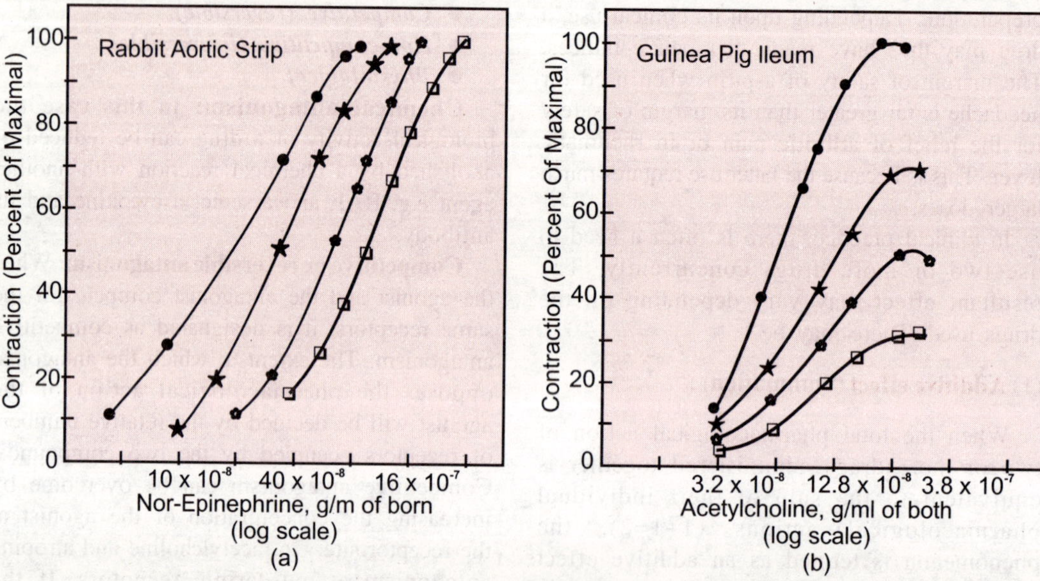

Fig. 2.6: (a) Characteristic of competitive antagonism between noradrenaline and an antagonist. Black dots denote the control curve. Subsequent curves are drawn with increasing concentrations of the antagonist. Note that the curves are almost parallel and maximum response could be obtained with noradrenaline on each occasion. **(b) Characteristic of non-competitive antagonism.** Note the decrease in maximum response to acetylcholine following the increase in antagonist concentration.

Although the agonist curve shifts to the right, the slope is reduced and the maximum response diminishes. The extent of inhibition produced depends on the characteristics of the antagonist itself and the agonist has no influence upon the degree of antagonism or its reversibility (Fig. 2.6b).

Physiological antagonism: This term is sometimes used where a drug reverses the effects of another drug by acting on different receptors, e.g., adrenaline given in histamine reaction. Sometimes the term 'functional antagonism' is used to represent the interaction of two agonists that act independently of each other but happen to cause opposite effects, e.g., acetylcholine and adrenaline.

Importance of drug antagonism:

An understanding of drug antagonism is important in:

- ***Correcting adverse effects of drug***; e.g., chlorpromazine-induced EPR countered by benzhexol.
- ***Treating drug poisoning***; e.g., morphine with naloxone, organophosphorus compounds with atropine; and
- ***Predicting drug combinations which would reduce drug efficacy***, e.g., the penicillin and tetracycline combination is inferior to penicillin alone in pneumococcal meningitis.

Adverse Drugs Reactions (ADR) in Man

An adverse drug reaction is defined as "any response to a drug that is noxious and unintended and that occurs at doses used in man for the prophylaxis, diagnosis or therapy of disease or for modification of physiological function" (WHO). It excludes adverse reactions due to drug overdose (poisoning), drug abuse and therapeutic errors.

The administration of a drug may result in the developement of :

- ***Side effects.***
- ***Untoward effects.***

- ***Toxic effects***; or
- ***Allergic and idiosyncratic effects*** (see later).

Side effects: Side effects are in fact *pharmacological effects produced with therapeutic dose of the drug*, e.g., dryness of mouth with atropine. Side effects which might be troublesome in a particular condition may be useful under other circumstances. Thus, dryness of mouth is undesirable when a person suffering from intestinal colic is given atropine, but it proves useful when atropine is used as a preanaesthetic medication.

Untoward effects: Untoward effects also *develop with therapeutic dose of a drug*, but are undesirable and, if severe, may necessitate the cessation of treatment. Resistant staphylococcal diarrhoea following tetracycline therapy and potassium loss due to diuretic drugs.

Toxic effects : These are seen usually when *a drug is administered repeatedly and/or in large doses*. Drug toxicity is usually the primary attribute of a drug and is dose dependent, e.g., depression of respiration with morphine; and may be associated with organ damage such as hepatotoxicity due to paracetamol.

The term **drug intolerance**, used commonly, literally means 'failure to tolerate' and can be used to describe any type of **Adverse Drug Reaction** (ADR) (Fig. 2.7).

ADR could be either local (irritation, necrosis or thrombophlebitis) or systemic. The basic cause of an ADR may be discernible (pharmaceutical, pharmacokinetic or pharmacodynamic) or may be unknown.

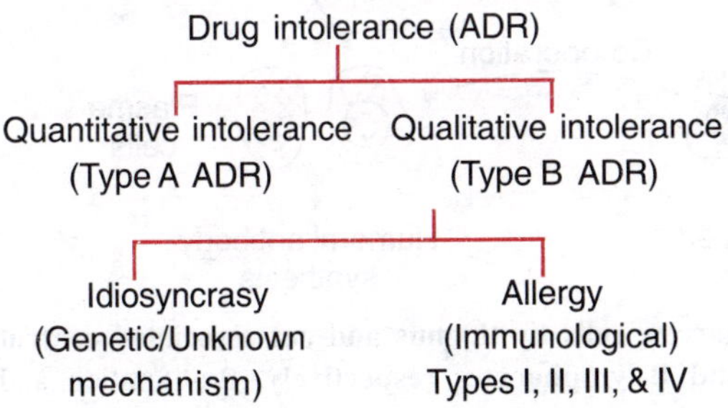

Fig. 2.7 : Classification of drug intolerance

ADRs are generally classified into **Type A** (Augmented); **Type B** (Bizarre); **Type C** (Chronic) and **Type D** (Delayed). The differences between Type A and Type B ADRs are listed in Table 2.2. Type C ADRs (e.g. analgesic nephropathy) are both time and dose related whereas Type D ADRs (e.g. carcino-genesis) are only time related.

Type A ADR: These are also known as augmented/attenuated (**quantitative**) ADR. They are largely predictable on the basis of the known pharmacological actions of a drug and usually are dose related. They comprise a hyper-response to the main action of a drug resulting in excessive effect of the drug (e.g., insulin hypoglycemia); or an effect due to an action of the drugat another site (e.g., anticholinergic effects of phenothiazines).

Type B ADR: These are also known as **qualitative** ADR. The symptoms and signs observed are different from what is expected from the known pharmacological actions of the drug and are not dose-related. Thus, they are bizzare and unpredictable effects. Their mechanism is sometimes known (either genetic or immunological) but may often be unknown.

Table 2.2: Comparison between Type A and Type B ADR

	Type A	Type B
Nature of ADR	Augmented/ attenuated normal response	Totally abnormal, bizarre response
Mechanism	Hyper - or hypo-response	Genetic, immunological/ unknown
Pharmacologically predictable	Largely yes	No
Dose dependent	Yes	No
Incidence and morbidity *	High	Low
Mortality *	Low	High
Treatment	Adjust dose	Stop the drug

* = In the community

Idiosyncrasy: This is a Type B ADR wherein the abnormal response to a drug is either due to a genetic mechanism or is unknown. Thus, in certain circumstances, genetically determined total absence or reduced activity of some enzyme(s) in the body of the recipient is responsible for the observed adverse reaction. Drugs like primaquine, salicyates and sulfonamides produce haemolysis in individuals whose red blood cells lack the enzyme glucose-6-phosphate dehydrogenase. In many cases, however, the cause of this phenomenon is not known e.g. chloramphenicol-induced aplastic anemia. *In general, all unusual, idiosyncratic reactions to drugs should be considered genetically determined until proved otherwise.* As against idiosyncrasy, allergy always has immunological basis.

Drug Allergy

The word **allergy** is derived from Greek words "allos" meaning "altered" and "ergos" meaning energy. Most of the drugs/sera used in therapeutics are capable of causing allergic or hypersensitivity reactions. They may be mild or very severe like anaphylaxis and have immunological basis. They occur in individuals who have been sensitized following the prior administration of the same drug or structurally similar drug.

To understand how drugs cause immunologically mediated reactions it is necessary to study some basic immunological concepts.

The immune system consists of two divisions:

- ***The innate immune system*** an ancient immune recognition system; and
- ***The adaptive immune system***, recently evolved system of immune responses.

Cells of the **innate immune system** include natural killer (NK) cells, macrophages, dendritic cells, neutrophils, basophils, eosinophils, tissue mast cells and epithelial cells. They recognise and destroy foreign antigens and pathogens without prior exposure. It may also take help of the adaptive immune system. The recognition of

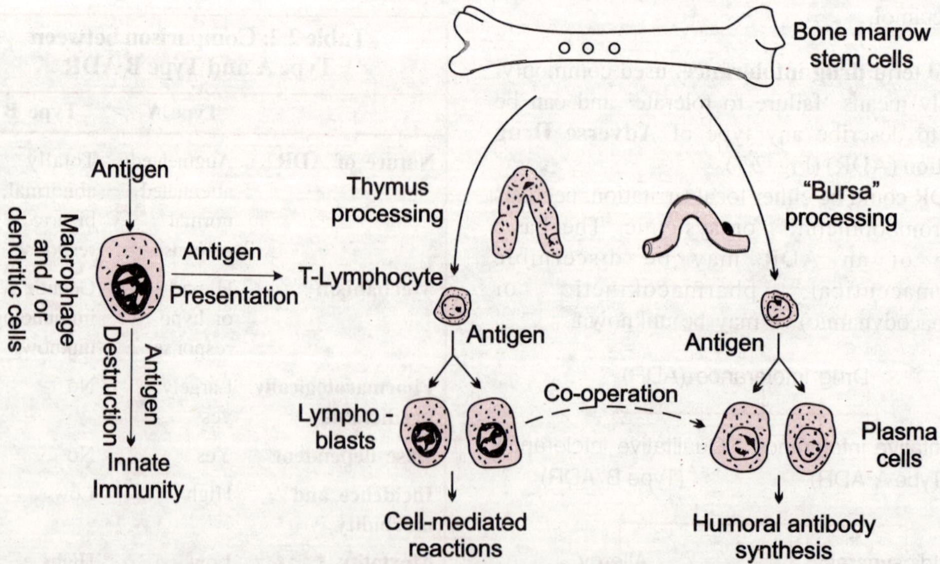

Fig. 2.8 : Innate immunity and processing of bone marrow cells by thymus and gut associated central lymphoid tissue to become immunocompetent T- and B-lymphocytes respectively. Proliferation and transformation to cells of the lymphoblast and plasma cell series occurs on antigenic stimulation. (Modified from Essential Immunology by Ivan Roitt. Courtesy of Blackwell Scientific Publications and Author).

pathogen molecules by the cells leads to activation of the complement cascade, and production of cytokines, and antimicrobial peptides as effector molecules.

In contrast, the **adaptive immune system** is characterized by antigen-specific responses to a foreign antigen or pathogen; unlike **innate (immediate) immunity**, it generally takes several days to develop. An important feature of this system is memory for the antigen so that a subsequent exposure to the same antigen causes a more rapid and more vigorous immune response. The adaptive immune system consists of dual limbs of cellular and humoral immunity (Fig. 2.8). The main effectors of this immunity are lymphocytes which get activated after they recognize a specific antigenic determinant **(epitope)**. These lymphocytes are of two types: **T lymphocytes and B lymphocytes**, with several subtypes of T lymphocytes. T lymphocytes (thymus-derived) are so called because of their origin from lymphocytes which, after they arise in the bone marrow, are processed in the thymus. B lymphocytes are so called because of their relation to the Bursa of Fabricius, a lymphoid organ similar to thymus, present in chicken.

When a foreign antigen enters the animal body, the following responses may occur (Fig. 2.8):

- ***It may be recognized as foreign by the innate immune system and be destroyed.***
- ***The antigen may be taken up by macrophages as well as dendritic cells and presented to a T cell***, which can recognize an epitope on the antigen. The T cell then proliferates into a cluster of T cells identical with the parent T cell (**clone of T cells**). These clones may be of several types: **cytotoxic** (directly destructive of the antigen as well of tissue cells), **helper** (which enhance immune response) and **suppressor** (which inhibit immune response). Each clone has the capacity to recognize and respond to only the parent epitope which led to its generation. The activated T cells secrete a variety of cytokines (Chapter 24) which regulate the inflammatory response as well as T cell function. Further, the cytokines make the activation of B lymphocytes (see below) by antigens more effective.

The various subtypes of T lymphocytes (cytotoxic, helper and suppressor) and their responses collectively constitute **Cell Mediated Immunity** (CMI). Further, as mentioned above the T cells regulate **Humoral Immunity**, primarily a B lymphocyte function, though they themselves do not secrete antibodies.

T cells can also be classified according to the antigens which they carry on their surface.

Those bearing **CD4 antigen** (Cluster Differentiation Molecules) are mainly responsible for the **helper** function and the delayed-type hypersensitivity. Those carrying **CD8 antigen** are responsible for the **cytotoxic** and **suppressor** functions. CD4 bearing T lymphocytes are further subdivided into Th1 and Th2 subtypes. Thl cells enhance CMI but inhibit humoral immunity; Th2 cells have the opposite effect. It has been found that CMI and humoral immunity are mutually exclusive in some situations. For example, *during pregnancy CMI is inhibited whereas humoral immunity is enhanced.* This is beneficial to the continuation of pregnancy as CMI against the foreign antigens of the fetus might otherwise damage it. Likewise, CMI mediated diseases such as rheumatoid arthritis undergo remission during pregnancy. In contrast, infections such as leprosy which are primarily fought by the body through CMI undergo aggravation during pregnancy.

- ***The antigen may be recognized by a specific receptor on the surface of a B lymphocyte***. The B lymphocytes are concerned with the synthesis of circulating antibodies and hence with the humoral immunity. On interacting with a foreign antigen, the B lymphocyte is activated to proliferate into a clone of B lymphocytes, which finally differentiate into **plasma cells**. The plasma cell clone secretes an **antibody** which recognizes and interacts only with the parent epitope which led to its synthesis. Thus, the blood simultaneously

Table 2.3: Biological properties of major immunoglobulin classes

Property	IgG	IgA	IgM	IgD	IgE
Molecular weight	150,000	160,000	900,000	185,000	200,000
Serum concentration (mg%)	1,250	280	120	0.3-30	0.002-0.2
Plasma half life (days)	23	6	5	3	3
Found in	Internal body fluids.	Seromucosal secretions, colostrum, saliva, tears, G I tract	Serum	On lymphocyte surface	On the surface of mast cells and basophils
Physiological role	Main Ab against infection; immunity against microbes in tissues and extravascular spaces	Mucosal immunity	Main intravascular Ab, important role in immunity in circulation	Role in B cell maturation	Immunity against helminthic infection
Injurious	Arthus reaction, serum sickness	Impaired mucosal immunity Autoimmune disorders	Arthus reaction, serum sickness.	Anti D antibodies in Rhesus incompatibility	Local and systemic anaphylatic reaction.

Ab = Antibody. IgG alone crosses the placenta.

contains antibodies of a variety of specificities, made by a variety of plasma cell clones (**polyclonal antibodies**). These antibodies circulate free in the plasma or may be bound to the surface of basophils and mast cells.

Antibodies are molecules (encoded by gens), roduced in response to the presence of foreign substances (**antigens** or **immunogens**; antigens which stimulate IgE production are called **allergens**). The antibodies exist as ß-cell-surface, antigen-recognition molecules or as secreted molecules in the plasma and body secretions. They are globulins, designated as **immunoglobulins** or Ig. Five major groups have been defined in man. They are IgG, IgA, IgM, IgD and IgE. IgG is the main immunoglobulin class (Table 2.3). Apart from their role in body's defence mechanism, certain antibodies (IgE) also have other properties such as fixing to basophils and mast cells (**Homocytotropic or Reaginic antibodies**), which can cause unpleasant and dangerous ADR.

The two important features of the immunological responses are:

- ***Specificity*** which is the ability to recognize and respond to one particular antigen rather than to any other; and
- ***Memory*** which is the ability to recognize and respond more vigorously to an antigen encountered for the second or subsequent time.

Generally, proteins with molecular weight of over 5,000, when administered parenterally, readily stimulate the production of antibodies. Peptides of molecular weight less than 5,000 are less immunogenic. Non-protein compounds such as drugs can become immunogenic after chemical coupling to a carrier protein, and produce antibodies that can react with the drug which thus behaves as a **hapten**. A hapten is a substance which is antigenic in the sense that it reacts with an antibody but itself is incapable of stimulating antibody production unless combined with a carrier protein.

Drug allergy differs from drug toxicity in many ways. The lesion produced by the former is lower in incidence; it is unpredictable; prior exposure to the drug may cause sensitization; the lesion is dose independent and rash, fever, eosinophilia and blood dyscrasias can occur.

When an individual has been sensitized to an antigen, further contact with that antigen can cause tissue-damaging reactions called '**hypersensitivity**' or 'allergic' reactions. These are:

(1) **Type I (Immediate Hypersensitivity) reactions : IgE mediated (a) Allergic reaction and (b) Anaphylaxis.** A single injection of egg albumin into a guinea pig has no obvious effect. However, antibodies to this protein are formed and the animal is sensitized. A repeat injection of egg albumin in such an animal causes a violent reaction called **anaphylaxis**. The animal gets asphyxiated from bronchospasm, the blood pressure falls due to vasodilatation and death occurs within a few minutes.

The antigen reacts with a specific class of antibody, reaginic antibodies (IgE), bound to the surface of mast cells and basophils. Interaction of antigen with IgE antibodies causes degranulation of mast cells and basophils with massive liberation of histamine and other mediators of immediate hyperresponse, leading to anaphylaxis. Mediators released from mast cells and basophils are:

- ***Those that increase vascular permeability and contract smooth muscles***, e.g., histamine, PAF, SRS-A, bradykinin.
- ***Those that are chemotactic for or activate other pro-inflammatory cells***, e.g., leukotriene B4, eosinophil and neutrophil chemotactic factors.
- ***Those that modulate the release of other mediators***, e.g., bradykinin, PAF, prostaglandins; and
- ***Those which cause termination of the inflammatory response.***

Under physiological conditions, mast cell triggering forms a vital part of the acute inflammatory defence reaction.

Different species vary in their response. Thus, anaphylaxis can be readily induced in the guinea pig, much less easily in the rabbit and the least readily in the rat. In humans, death is usually due to laryngeal edema, a feature unique to man, bronchospasm leading to asphyxia, or vasodilatation with circulatory collapse.

A similar systemic reaction can occur in a sensitized human subject following a repeat injection of a drug like penicillin or antitoxic serum. This is the phenomenon of systemic anaphylaxis.

Anaphylactoid reactions (pseudo-allergic) mimicing anaphylactic shock sometimes occur after oral administration of aspirin (Chapter 11) and after IV administration of iodine containing diagnostic contrasts (Chapter 62). They are not immunological in nature.

As compared to systemic anaphylaxis, **local anaphylactic reactions (atopic allergy)** to extrinsic antigens (allergens) such as pollen, animal danders, mites in house dust, and absorbed foodstuffs occur more frequently in man (Chapter 69). Combination of the allergen with cell bound IgE antibody in the bronchial tree, the nasal mucosa or the skin releases mediators of anaphylaxis giving rise to localized reactions such as, asthma, rhinitis (Chapter 26) or urticaria (Chapter 22). The offending antigen can be identified by intradermal prick test. There is a strong familal tendency. The symptoms of atopic allergy are to a certain extent controllable with antihistaminic drugs and other mediator antagonists (see Chapter 22). Courses of antigen injection may desensitize by forming blocking IgG or IgA antibodies, or by turning off IgE production. Figure 2.9 summarises the therapeutic approaches to atopic allergy. The drugs shown

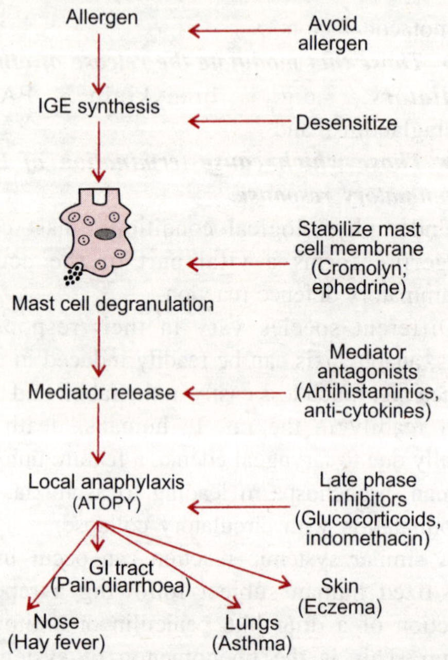

Fig. 2.9 : Atopic allergy and targets for therapy

are discussed in respective chapters.

(2) **Type II (Cytotoxic) reaction:** In this case, the IgG and IgM antibodies bind to an antigen present on the surface of cells and promote their destruction by lysis or phagocytosis by polymorphs and macrophages or by non-adherent lymphoid killer cells (K cells) through an extracellular mechanism. Transfusion reactions, anti-D antibodies in Rhesus incompatibility and antibodies to kidney glomerular basement membrane are examples of this type of reaction.

Drugs such as chloramphenicol can form an antigenic complex with the surface of a formed element of the blood and can evoke the production of humoral antibodies which act as cytotoxic for the cell-drug complex leading to autoimmune hemolysis, agranulocytosis or thrombocytopenia (Chapter 35).

This type also includes the antireceptor subtype, in which an antibody to a receptor on certain cells develops. The antibody may either activate the receptor (LATS in Graves' disease) or block the binding of the ligand (acetylcholine) to the concerned receptor (as in myasthenia gravis).

(3) **Type III (Immune Complex Mediated) reaction:** The union of soluble antigen with **IgG** antibody *in vivo* can form immune complexes which may ultimately cause histamine release, activation of kinin system and aggregation of platelets with formation of microthrombi and further release of vasoactive amines. The attracted polymorphs release tissue-damaging enzymes on contact with the complex. In case of high levels of circulating antibodies, the antigen is precipitated near the site of its entry into the body. The reaction in the skin is characterised by erythema, edema and cellular infiltration, maximal at 3-8 hours (**Arthus reaction**). When the antigen is relatively in excess, soluble complexes formed circulate in the body and are deposited at preferred sites such as the skin, the joints, the renal glomeruli and the choroid plexus. This type of reaction is observed in **serum sickness** following the injection of large quantities of foreign protein e.g. horse serum; in glomerulonephritis associated with systemic lupus erythematosus or infections; and with sulfonamides.

Intrapulmonary Arthus type reactions to exogenous, inhaled antigens is responsible for many hypersensitivity disorders such as farmer's lung; such reactions are often provoked by the local release of antigens from infective organisms. Thus, chemotherapy may cause an abrupt release of microbial antigens, producing dramatic immune complex mediated reactions such as erythema nodosum leprosum in lepromatous leprosy and the Jarisch-Herxheimer reaction in syphilitics treated with pencillin.

(4) **Type IV (Cell Mediated or Delayed Hypersensitivity) reaction:** In this case, T-lymphocytes carrying a specific receptor on their surface are activated by contact with the antigen to release certain active factors. This form of allergic phenomenon is observed in contact dermatitis and in diseases caused by chemicals, dusts, mycobacteria, chlamydia, fungi and helminths, and in the rejection of transplanted tissue. *Inflammatory reactions initiated by mononuclear lymphocytes and not*

by antibody alone are called delayed hypersensitivity reactions. The word *delayed* is used to indicate the secondary cellular response which appears at 48-72 hours after the antigen exposure. In contrast, the *immediate hypersensitivity response* seen within 12 hours of the antigen challenge, is initiated by basophil mediated reactions (Type I) and by preformed antibodies (Types II and III). A typical delayed hypersensitivity response is observed in the Mantoux reaction following the intradermal tuberculin injection, wherein an indurated and erythematous reaction occurs within 48 hours. Histologically, it shows infiltration with mononuclear phagocytes and lymphocytes (granulomatous infiltration). Delayed type of reactions are often observed (a) with drugs that are capable of binding to body constituents and forming new antigens e.g. sulfonamides and penicillin and (b) following insect bites. The phenomenon is also observed following contact with certain plants or food in sensitized individuals.

Desensitisation : This term is used to describe two different processes.

(a) In one case the second dose of antigen fails to evoke any response in a sensitized preparation. This may be due to exhaustion of antibody or of an essential enzyme system activated by the antigen-antibody reaction. Examples are penicillin and insulin allergies.

(b) The second type of desensitization is the one which is carried out in therapeutic practice. In this case, a course of graded injections of an antigen is given to a hypersensitive patient in order to render him less allergic to the antigen. This is believed to be due to formation of blocking antibodies. See Chapter 26 for allergy to plant pollen.

Manifestations of ADR

Drugs can cause ADR related to almost all tissues and organs. Some important ADR are:

I **GI ADR** : Many drugs cause anorexia, nausea, vomiting (e.g. metronidazole, chloroquine), diarrhoea/constipation (e.g. iron salts, morphine). Aspirin and other NSAID can cause gastric ulceration and bleeding.

II **Haemopoietic**: It ranges from anaemia to blood dyscrasias like leucopenia, agranulocytosis, aplastic anaemia and thrombocytopenia. The reduction in clotting factors may lead to haemorrhages (Chapter 35).

III **Hepatocellular** : Drugs can damage the liver:

- ***By direct action***, either themselves or more commonly through their metabolites (e.g. carbon tetrachloride and isoniazid). Such hepatotoxicity is predictable, dose related and can be demonstrated in animals; other organs such as the kidney may also be affected; or
- ***By an immunological reaction***, which renders a constituent of the liver antigenic. This is unpredictable, not dose related and has no animal model. Usually, it is selective and restricted to the liver, although other general allergic manifestations may be present.

The *direct toxicity* may manifest as asymptomatic hepatomegaly, acute hepatic necrosis (tetracycline, halothane), altered hepatic metabolism (chloramphenicol) or as altered bilirubin metabolism (sulfonamides, salicylates). Rarely, acute intermittent porphyria may occur.

As against this, the *hepatotoxic reactions with immunological basis* may cause non-specific hepatitis (isoniazid, pyrazinamide, indomethacin), cholestasis interfering with biliary secretion causing hyperbilirubinemia (certain anabolic steroids) or cholestatic hepatitis (chlorpromazine, chlorpropamide). A serious form of long-lasting cholestasis is the *vanishing bile duct syndrome* in which drugs cause destruction of segments of intrahepatic biliary ductules; examples of drugs causing it are amitryptiline, azathioprine, haloperidol, estradiol, tetracycline and co-trimoxazole. The hepatic effects of potentially hepatotoxic drugs are generally monitored by periodic measurement of SGPT.

In case of some drugs such as methyldopa, chlorpromazine and isoniazid both the mechanisms can operate.

Table 2.4: Drugs causing ototoxicity

- Salicylates
- Aminoglycosides, Macrolides
- Loop diuretics
- Antimalarials (quinine, chloroquine)
- Anticancer drugs (cisplatin, bleomycin)
- Chelating agent (desferrioxamine)
- Ear drops (chloramphenicol, polymyxin, propylene glycol, acetic acid 2%)

IV **Cardiac:** Drugs can cause cardiotoxicity directly. Thus, they may precipitate arrhythmias or even cardiac arrest (e.g. digoxin, quinine, aminophylline, flecainide). Fenfluramin is known to cause valvular fibrosis.

V **Renal:** Drugs can cause albuminuria, hematuria and even tubular necrosis. Nephrotoxicity is either direct or immunologically mediated (Chapter 38).

VI **Abnormalities of taste and smell:** Drugs are known to produce abnormalities of taste and smell sensations: **hypogeusia** is a decrease in taste acuity; **ageusia** is total loss of ability to recognize any taste; **dysgeusia** is distortion of taste sensation; Hyposmia, anosmia and dysosmia represent the corresponding abnormalities of the sense of smell. A patient with hyposmia or anosmia may have decreased ability for perception of the flavour of food. The drugs associated with the above abnormalities are d-penicillamine, pyrazinamide, captopril, methimazole, biguanides, l-dopa and bromocriptine.

VII **Ocular toxicity:** Drugs may cause a variety of ocular injuries, (Chapter 70).

VIII **Ototoxicity:** Some topical preparations and certain drugs given systemically can cause ototoxicity and impair hearing (Table 2.4).

IX **Dermal:** The skin is a common target organ for various allergic and photosensitivity reactions. Anticancer drugs can cause hair loss. Metalloids like arsenic and heavy metals like mercury are secreted in the sweat and can produce skin rashes (Chapter 69).

X **Electrolyte disturbances:** Diuretics like thiazides and furosemide may produce hyponatremia or hypokalemia. NSAID may cause sodium retention and edema.

XI **Endocrine disturbances:** Chlorpromazine may produce menstrual irregularities, galactorrhoea and amenorrhoea. Combination oral contraceptives may arrest lactation in nursing mothers. Glucocorticoids depress the synthesis of ACTH and endogenous cortisol. Abrupt withdrawal of these compounds may, therefore, precipitate acute hypocorticisolism (Addisonian crisis) while vigorous therapy may cause Cushing's syndrome. Amiodarone can cause thyroid disease.

XII **Infertility and sexual impotence:** (Chapters 66 and 67).

XIII **Behavioral and CNS:** Compounds like amphetamine may cause disorientation, confusion and inability to concentrate; glucocorticoids may produce euphoria, restlessness and psychosis; and benzodiazepines may cause *anterograde amnesia* (Chapter 8). For behavioral teratogenicity, see Chapter 77. Ethambutol can cause optic neuritis while dystonic reactions can occur following phenothiazines.

XIV **Carcinogenesis:** Estrogens exacerbate mammary carcinoma in females. Increased risk of developing endometrial cancer has been reported in women receiving prolonged estrogen therapy without concomitant progestogen.

XV **Teratogenicity :** A teratogen is an agent which can cause a *fetal physical malformation* when maternal ad-ministration results in significant exposure during organogenesis (18th to 60th days of fetal life). After that period, during the remainder of pregnancy, exposure to fetotoxic drugs may cause functional disability or an *alteration in growth of the organs/fetus* but no physical defects. The word teratogenicity is derived from the Greek word terataos which means monster. The sedative 'thalidomide', prescribed to pregnant women with morning sickness, was found to produce various types of developmental anomalies in the newborns. The commonest anomalies were 'amelia' or total absence of limbs, and 'phocomelia' or absence of one or more limbs (Fig. 2.10 see art plate).

XVI **Unmasking and exacerbation of disease:** Drugs can exacerbate an already existing disease or unmask a latent condition, e.g. glucocorticoids unmask latent diabetes and may exacerbate an existing peptic ulcer. Isoniazid may unmask latent epilepsy.

XVII **Production of a disease (Iatrogenic disease):** Sometimes, drugs themselves may produce certain pathological syndromes. The diseases produced as a result of therapeutic measures are known as `iatrogenic diseases', the Greek word `iatros' meaning "physician". Thus, glucocorticoid therapy can precipitate hypertension, congestive heart failure and Cushing's syndrome. Glucocorticoids, aspirin and indomethacin may precipitate perforation of duodenal ulcer. Repeated doses of NSAID can cause renal damage.

XVIII **Immunosuppression** (Chapter 76)

XIX **ADR due to drug interaction** : This can occur when two or more drugs are administered concurrently (Chapter 3).

XX **Adverse reactions precipitated by abrupt drug withdrawal:** Abrupt cessation of administration of several groups of drugs after prolonged use can cause :

- ***Exacerbation of underlying disease.***
- ***A typical 'withdrawal syndrome';*** or
- ***Symptoms as a result*** of physiological adaptation e.g. pituitary suppression by glucocorticoids.

The withdrawal syndromes after abrupt stoppage of agents such as alcohol, anticonvulsants and nitrates are described in the respective chapters: With such drugs, the cessation of therapy must be gradual, with small decrements and under close medical supervision. Sometimes, substituting a drug with a longer half life (e.g. methadone in patients taking an opioid; and diazepam in patients taking a short acting benzodiazepine) is helpful.

ADR and p-glycoproteins: Membrane prevent the entry of noxious, naturally occurring substances and drugs into the cells of the vital organs. In species of mice genetically deficient in these cell membrane proteins, the toxicity of vinblastine (an anticancer drug) and ivermectin (an antifilarial drug) is markedly increased. They also serve as protective mechanisms against **xenobiotics**. (chemicals foreign to the body).

Treatment of Acute Drug Poisoning

Table 2.5 outlines the principles of treatment of acute poisoning.

- ***Removal of the poison:*** In a conscious patient, vomiting can be induced by tickling the back of the pharynx. Ipecac syrup (not fluid extract of ipecac which is 14 times more potent) 15-30 ml. (adult dose) followed by 200 ml. of water is useful in inducing vomiting in many cases including infants. Ipecac may be repeated after 20 minutes, if needed. If there is no emesis, gastric lavage should be carried out to remove the ipecac. *Induction of emesis is contraindicated*

(a) If the patient is stuporous, delirious or

Table 2.5 Principles of treatment of acute poisoning

- Supporting measures : attention to "Airway, Breathing, Circulation" (ABC of resuscitation), hydration, nutrition.
- Removal of the poison by emesis / gastric lavage.
- Use of activated charcoal.
- Accelerated elimination of the poison by diuresis, dialysis, hemoperfusion.
- Identification of the poison.
- Specific antidote, if available.
- Patients with altered mental status should receive oxygen, IV glucose and IV thiamine (100 mg).
- Follow up and psychiatric counselling in case of suicidal poisoning.

comatose; is in shock; is getting convulsions; has an inadequate gag reflex; or

(b) If he has ingested a corrosive poison, a CNS stimulant, or a petroleum distillate such as kerosene.

Though salt and water can induce vomiting it may cause hypernatremia. In the hospital, the ingested poison can be removed by gastric lavage.

Absorption of a poison from the GI tract can be reduced in certain cases by using powdered **activated charcoal** (Carbomix) in the dose of 50 g (25 g in children). Activated charcoal adsorbs most of the drugs and poisons except alkalies, arsenic, lithium carbonate, cyanide, mineral acids and ferrous sulfate. *Charcoal should not be administered concurrently with ipecac or a specific antidote as it may adsorb them and render them ineffective.* As most poisons do not dissociate from activated charcoal if it is present in excess, there is no need to remove the charcoal from the GI tract. If activated charcoal is not available universal antidote may be substituted. The composition of the **universal antidote** is 2 parts of powdered charcoal with 1 part of tannic acid and 1 part of magnesium oxide. Activated charcoal is particularly useful for reducing the absorption of alkaloids from the gut.A home made substitute for the *universal antidote* is two parts of burnt toast, one part of strong tea and one part of milk of magnesia.

Repeated oral doses of activated charcoal (50 g initially, followed by 25 g every 4 hours, in adults) enhance the elimination of some drugs which are excreted back into the GI tract after they are absorbed; examples of such drugs are aspirin, carbamazepine, digoxin, barbiturates, phenytoin and theophylline.

Oral administration of **polyethylene glycol** (PEG) may be used for total bowel clearance in case of poisoning (Chapter 41).

● ***Elimination of the poison can be enhanced:***

(a) By increasing the urine output with diuretics like mannitol, furosemide

(b) By adjusting the PH of urine: weakly acidic drugs such as phenobarbitone (Chapter 8) and salicylates (Chapter 11) are excreted faster in an alkaline urine; and

(c) By dialysis or hemoperfusion

Table 2.6 : Antidotes for emergency treatment of certain poisonings

Poison	Antidote
Paracetamol	N-acetylcysteine
Theophylling	Propranold
Mercury, arsenic and copper	BAL
Atropine and other cholinergic antagonists	Neo
Carbon monoxide	Oxygen
Cyanide	Dicobalt edetate; amyl nitrite followed by sodium nitrite, then sodium thiosulfate
Methyl alcohol and ethylene glycol	Ethyl alcohol; 4-Methyl pyrazole
Lead	Calcium disodium edetate; dimercapto-succinic acid
Nitrites	Methylene blue
Opioids	Naloxone
Benzodiazepines	Flumazenil
Organophosphate compounds	Atropine; pralidoxime
Warfarin	Vitamin K_1
Beta-adrenergic stimulants	Propronolol

● ***Administration of specific antidote*** (Table 2.6).

● ***Supportive treatment*** such as maintenance of a patent airway, assisted mechanical ventilation, maintenance of blood pressure by fluids and vasopressor agents, nutrition by intravenous glucose saline and prevention of secondary infection.

Self-medication is often an important cause of drug poisoning. This is particularly true of a commonly used and 'available over the counter' drugs like fever and pain remedies (paracetamol) and vitamin D preparations.

Principles of Drug Prescribing; Factors Modifying the Effects of a Drug; and Drug Interactions 3

Modern therapeutics is not just an art but is more of a science. It is now more and more dominated by evidence-based medicine. Evidence-based medicine is defined by Dr. David Sackett as the "the conscientious, explicit and judicious use of current, best evidence in making decisions about the care of individual patients." Thus, it is essential for the physician, before prescribing any therapy, to examine objectively the available evidence for patient care resulting from systematic research, and to integrate the same with individual clinical expertise.

In practice, the treatment of a sick person includes many aspects, and administration of drugs is one of them. In certain patients, drugs are of the greatest importance while in others they have only a minor role to play.

In all situations, the doctor-patient relationship is of prime importance. "Words have the potential to 'heal' or to 'sicken'. Words that bring expectations are interventions on their own. Words will not 'cure' but they can affect attitudes and emotions, and ultimately body sensations; the right words can lead a patient to optimism, whereas the wrong words can produce despair."

Drug Prescribing

A practitioner who prescribes drugs must know :

- ***Natural course of the disease he is treating.***
- ***Pharmacological actions and toxicity of a drug he uses.***
- ***Reasons for choosing a particular drug.***
- ***Methods of assessing drug efficacy and safety;*** and
- ***The possible interactions when several drugs are administered concurrently.***

Drugs should be prescribed only when:

- ***There is a clear indication for them***; and
- ***The benefit to be expected from them to the patient outweighs the possible harm, immediate or remote.***

Whenever possible, drugs should be prescribed by their official (i.e. **generic** or non-proprietary) names rather than by **proprietary** names. A proprietary name is a trade name applied to a particular formulation by its manufacturer. Drugs sold under non-proprietary or generic names are cheaper than those sold under proprietary names. Life saving drugs may be an exception; this is because sometimes the generic formulations for some reason may not come up to the same standards of quality as branded drug formulations.

New entrants to the drug market are invariably costly; however, many costly preparations sold in the market are neither new nor necessarily better than older, established, inexpensive preparations. In fact, established drugs are often introduced in the market under various brand names, either alone or in various combinations and are sold at a fancy price purely with effective advertisement and modern sales promotion techniques. It should be remembered that real wonder drugs are rarely born and do not require much advertisement; an important principle of economics behind advertisement and sales promotion is *to create a demand where real need does not exist.*

Practitioners, therefore, should always have a critical outlook towards accepting a new remedy. Many times, drugs are marketed without adequate and reliable clinical trials and sometimes with excessive claims regarding their properties and superiority over the established remedies. It is surprising that such products are extensively prescribed even though there is no reliable evidence of their value nor their safety.

How you use a drug is often more important than what drug you use. Proper use requires familiarity with both therapeutic and toxic effects of drugs. This is difficult if one switches from one drug to another frequently. Usually, it is beneficial to be slow in accepting any new agent. In practice, the initial choice of the drug and the dose regimen will depend upon the correct diagnosis, the severity of the disease and the presence of complication/associated disease. In addition, the risk/benefit and cost/efficacy ratios of the drugs selected should be taken into account.

It is unfortunate that doctors often over-prescribe drugs for trivial complaints. The reasons for this are not clear. Although this has some relation to increased demand by patients for drugs, the major fault probably lies with the medical profession. Many busy practitioners find it difficult to keep in touch with the current literature and are easily persuaded by the promotional material from the pharmaceutical industry. Others probably would like to impress their patients by their 'most up-to-date' knowledge about 'the latest drugs', while some may not even bother about what preparation they prescribe and what drugs it contains. Majority of them are not aware of the cost of the preparation they prescribe.

As experience accumulates, physicians find that smaller doses work equally well, and are safer and more economical. It is well known that individuals vary in their response to drugs. The importance of pharmacogenomics is now being increasingly recognized. New drugs are often introduced at a dose that will be effective in about 90% of the target population, because this is known to help market penetration. Doses are also partly determined by an irrational preference for round numbers. A sizeable minority (30%) are likely to be needlessly overdosed by following doses recommended during early marketing period of a new drug. Although such recommended doses are rapidly effective in a high proportion of patients, they may cause increased adverse effects in some. This should be borne in mind while prescribing a drug, especially a recently marketed one. Dose searching should continue even after a drug is marketed; atenolol, a beta blocker, used initially in the dose of 100 mg daily, in the treatment of hypertension has been found to be equally effective in the dose of 50 mg daily. A wise policy is **"Start low, go slow,"** particularly in children and the elderly.

There is no objection to prescribing proven plant preparations. However, while prescribing such heavily promoted **Herbal Remedies**, the physician should keep in mind the following:

- These preparations are difficult to standardize nor can one be sure of their pharmacological activity.
- It is almost impossible to test for the presence of the ingredients mentioned in the package insert/container label.
- The herbal combinations offered and the doses recommended are not supported by any scientific data.
- Tall claims are made about their efficacy without adequate scientific data.
- The DCGI regulations applicable to the modern drugs are not applicable to them. If not processed properly, Ayurvedic herbo-mineral formulations (*bhasmas*) can lead to toxicity. Their safety during pregnancy is unknown.

- Herbal remedies previously thought to be innocuous are known to be potentially toxic. The best example of this is the Chinese herbal teas which are now known to be hepatotoxic. They are not always cheap as claimed.

Some of the so called 'herbal medications' have been found to be adulterated with modern drugs such as glucocorticoids, diclofenac, benzodiazepines, phenytoin, statins and sildenafil. Great care should therefore be taken to ascertain the ingredients before recommending herbal remedies to patients.

Fixed-dose combinations: Their use is sometimes helpful. They may

- ***Be convenient and improve compliance;***
- ***Enhance the efficacy of therapy***, e.g antituberculosis therapy, where they prevent drug resistance; and combined estrogen-progesterone contraceptive pills which demonstrate synergy; or
- ***Reduce drug toxicity,*** e.g. levodopa-carbidopa combination.

However, combinations of drugs such as antimicrobial drugs expose the patient to additional toxicity, and sometimes may even reduce the effectiveness of therapy. Further, it is difficult to adjust the dose of the individual drugs. Combination drug formulations are always expensive. Hence, a combination should not be prescribed unless there is reason to consider that the patient needs all the drugs in the formulation and that the doses are appropriate and will need no individual adjustment.

Often, such combinations:

(1) Contain inadequate dose of the main ingredient.

(2) Contain a second agent of doubtful efficacy e.g. serratiopeptidase added to paracetamol or NSAID.

(3) Have ingredients that may exert only additive effects.

Their usefulness and superiority in a given condition is not supported by adequate scientific evidence. They are, however, sold at a

Table 3.1: Principles of prescription writing

- Write the prescription on your letterhead.
- Write legibly and indelibly.
- Write the patient's name, age and address.
- Do not abbreviate names of drugs/ preparations(s) or instructions about taking the medicines. Write 'Units' not 'u'. Write mcg not mg. When decimals are unavoidable, write, say, 50mcg, not 0.05mg.,
- Write clearly dose (so many tablets/ capsules/ puffs), dosing interval (so many hours), time of the day, relation to meals, and duration of therapy.
- When prescribing a drug 'as required', write the minimum dosing interval and the maximum number of doses per day.
- In case of scheduled drugs, write the quantity of drug to be supplied at a time and how many times the prescribed drugs may be supplied without revalidation.
- Advise the parents/ patients that : no medicine should be added to the infant's feeding bottle; tablets /capsules should be taken in sitting position and washed down with plenty of water; ointments should be used as supplied and not diluted before use; residual ointment after use by one patient should be discarded and not stored for future use; medicines should be stored beyond the reach of chidren.
- Sign the prescription.
- Write date and your registration number.
- Avoid painful IM injections in children whenever possible. Liquid preparations are more suitable for children and old persons.

Some abbreviations used in prescription orders are: od = once a day; /d = per day; bid = twice a day; tid = thrice a day; qid = four times a day; q as in q4hr = 4 hourly; HS = at night; sos = as required e.g. a sleeping pill (Chapter 7).; prn (pro re nata) = an extra dose as required, in addition to the basal orders e.g. an analgesic (Chapter 11).

much higher price than the sum of prices of the ingredients.

Table 3.1 outlines the principles of prescription writing. The drugs prescribed should be the most suitable, the least expensive and easily available. Prescribing "fancy and expensive tonics" to patients who can hardly afford two meals a day is also unethical. It is mandatory to explain to the patient what to expect from the drug(s) prescribed, and their possible ADRs.

It is not enough simply to note the failure of drug therapy and the adverse reactions produced. If one has to make any purposeful decision about the future use of the drug, it is necessary to know more about it. What is the cause of the failure? How useful is the drug usually? Is it commonly used? For what condition is it usually given? What good does it do? Is the risk in its use worth the benefits expected? Can therapy be improved? This consitutes a **therapeutic audit** and would help the doctor in using drugs in future cases more rationally and effectively.

Patient compliance: Except when hospitalized, patients are responsible for taking their own drugs. Often, there is a discrepancy between what is prescribed and what the patient actually takes. The reasons for this are :

- ***Complexity of the regimen (several drugs to be taken several times a day).***
- ***Cost.***
- ***Adverse reactions.***
- ***Poor motivation.***
- ***Length of therapy*** and
- ***Natural disinclination to take injections.***

The drug regimen should be as simple as it can be kept: as few drugs as possible and once or twice a day administration, if permissible. Cost being a major consideration in long-term treatment, only cost-effective drugs should be prescribed; this often means prescribing drugs by their generic names.

The patient's motivation may be improved by personal contact. A sympathetic discussion about the difficulties of drugs prescribed and the possible adverse effects is likely to have a salutary effect on compliance. On the other hand, mere distribution of printed leaflets about drugs prescribed, diet etc. may educate the patient but is less effective in improving patient compliance. Occasionally, it is necessary to take into confidence the patient's care takers, particularly with old or mentally disturbed patients. Finally, a surprise check on urine or plasma level of the drug or its metabolite helps to detect defaulters but may be impracticable.

Drug 'generations': In recent times, newer drugs belonging to an existing group are often promoted as 2nd and 3rd 'generation' drugs, implying that they are universally superior to the older members of the group. This is not always true. The 'older generation' drugs may still be the drugs of choice in selected indications. An example of this truism is: cephalosporins of the first generations are (among cephalosporins) the preferred drugs in Gram positive infections.

Drugs expiration date: Do the drugs become useless after the expiry date mentioned by the manufacturers? No. Drug companies, because of certain legal compulsions and liability concerns, will not advocate such use after the expiry date mentioned on the package which is usually 2-3 years from the date of manufacture. Shelf-life of a drug is the time where a given product, stored under reasonable conditions, is expected to remain stable (> 90% of potency). Most of the drugs remain stable for long time beyond their expiry dates. According to Medical Letter (Volume 44, 93, 2002), " There are virtually no reports of toxicity from degradation products of outdated drugs (except tetracycline). How much of their potency they retain varies with the drug and the storage conditions, especially humidity, but many drugs stored under reasonable conditions retain 90% of their potency for at least 5 years after the expiration date on the label, and sometimes much longer".

Spurious drugs: Spurious drugs present a

serious health problem. In some countries, counterfeit medicines may constitute 20-50 % of the available products. They may comprise low quality manufacture of correct ingredients; wrong/undisclosed ingredients; adulteration; insufficient quantity of ingredients; false labeling; or no active ingredient at all. Examples are glucocorticoids added to herbal medicines for asthma and arthritis; and turmeric dispensed as tetracycline. For detection of counterfeit drugs, one needs a good infrastructure for vigilance and for enforcement of drug regulations.

P-drug (Personal drug) Concept

In practice, the physician usually needs 50-60 drugs routinely to treat common ailments. **P-drugs** are the drugs one chooses for prescribing regularly and with which one becomes familiar. Such a list would spare the physician repeated search for a good drug from among the many available, in day-to-day practice. The various steps involved in choosing P-drugs are outlined in Table 3.2.

Sometimes, although a drug may be very efficacious it may not be suitable in a given patient because of other patient-related factors such as renal/hepatic damage, diabetes mellitus, pregnancy, lactation or drug allergy. The cost of treatment and, especially, the cost/benefit ratio of a drug or a dosage form is also a major selection criterion. Many patients may have to be treated with a less-than-ideal (not the best) drug which has to be accepted because of the unaffordable cost or non-availability of the ideal drug.

Table 3.2: Guidelines for selecting P-drugs

(1) Define the diagnosis (Pathophysiology).
(2) Specify the therapeutic objective(s).
(3) Make an inventory of the effective drug groups.
(4) Choose a group and select the individual drug from the group according to efficacy, safety, suitability and cost.
(5) Prescribe treatment for a standard duration.

(Adapted from: ''Guide to Good Prescribing'', WHO Action Programme on Essential Drugs, 1999).

Personal treatment (**P-treatment**) and P-drugs are not identical. Not every P-treatment includes a P-drug, e.g. life style modifications in obesity. As with P-drugs, the choice of P-treatment is guided by the therapeutic objectives in a given patient, and depends upon efficacy, safety, suitability and cost of the treatment.

With the availability of increasing number of drugs and formulations, and the flood of promotional material, it is desirable to prepare *one's own pocket p-drug formulary*. It should contain not only names of p-drugs but also dosage form, dosage, frequency and duration of administration of the drugs; patient–teaching material about the drugs; and patient monitoring information for doctor's own use. *Of course, one has to keep oneself well informed about the new drugs and their usefulness and limitations, and revise one's P-drug list from time to time.*

Essential Drugs

WHO defines the essential drugs as follows : "Essential drugs are those drugs that satisfy the health care needs of the majority of the population. They should therefore be available at all times in adequate amounts and in appropriate dosage forms, at a price the individual and the community can afford."

The list of such drugs is presented in **two levels.**

(1) The **core list** should indicate the minimum drug needs for a basic health care system, listing the most cost-effective drugs for priority conditions; and

(2) The **complementary** list should consist of

drugs for priority diseases which are cost-effective but not necessarily affordable, or which may need specialized health care facilities, and should include essential drugs for less frequent diseases. The section on reserve anti-infective agents could thus be integrated into the complementary list.

This concept has been advocated for use in hospitals and has many advantages :

- ***It improves the practitioner's knowledge of the drugs he is prescribing and hence the quality of prescribing.***
- ***It reduces the cost of patient care.***

The drugs from such selected lists are made available at all times, even at the remotest places in the country. Obviously, the list will differ according to factors such as local disease pattern, disease incidence, available infrastructure and the financial resources at disposal. Genetic, environmental and demographic factors have also to be taken into account.

Only those drugs which are of proven value, relatively safe and cost-effective are included. Such lists need revision from time to time. Fixed-dose combinations are acceptable only when the dosage of each ingredient meets the requirements of a defined population group, and the combination has advantage over a single compound in therapeutic effects, safety and compliance as e.g. antituberculosis drugs. Many countries have now prepared essential drug lists based on their priorities.

Of course, it is not correct to say that drugs not included in such lists are all 'non-essential' and hence not required. Some of them are indeed useful for special indications under specific circumstances. Many anti-cancer drugs not appearing in the 'Essential Drugs List' are important in special circumstances.

Orphan Drugs

Orphan drugs are drugs meant for the diagnosis, prevention or treatment of rare diseases. They are not easily available because their manufacture is not commercially viable for various reasons which include :

- ***Their limited demand.***
- ***Enormous cost of production.***
- ***Non-patentability of the drug;*** and
- ***The complex and costly procedure*** for establishing the efficacy and safety of the drug, and for the governmental approval process.

Some examples of orphan drugs are: certain anti-cancer and anti-viral drugs; certain chemotherapeutic agents such as pentamidine; and drugs used in the treatment of rare genetic enzyme deficiencies.

Further, one should also remember that some of the older drugs, which had been proven useful for many years and have high cost-effectiveness for routine use, have now become "orphan drugs" because their commercial production is no longer profitable. Thus, drugs such as hydrochlorthiazide, chlorpropamide, reserpine, diloxanide furoate and iodoquinol are not easily available. They have become "the victims of myth (that newer drugs are necessarily superior), master-marketing and fashionable prescribing."

Factors Modifying the Effects of a Drug

Individuals differ both in the degree and the character of the response that a drug may elicit. The doses of official preparation of drugs are, therefore, always expressed in the form of a range which gives the therapeutic effect in majority of subjects. The important factors which influence the effect of a drug are:

I Body weight:

The average dose is mentioned either in terms of mg. per kg. body weight or as the total single dose for an adult weighing between 50-100 kg. The smaller dose should be used in Indians whose average weight is about 50 kg.

Table 3.3: Determination of children's doses from adult doses on the basis of body surface area*

Weight (kg)	Approx. surface area in square meters	Approx. percentage of adult dose **
2	0.15	9
4	0.25	14
6	0.33	19
8	0.40	23
10	0.46	27
15	0.63	36
20	0.80	46
25	0.95	55
30	1.08	62
35	1.20	70
40	1.30	75
45	1.40	81
50	1.51	87
55	1.58	91

* Based on Done, A.K.: "Drugs for Children" in Modell, W. (Ed) Drugs of Choice 1972-73. St. Louis : The C.V. Mosby Co., 1972.

** Based on average adult surface area of 1.73 sq

However, dose expressed in this fashion may not apply in cases of excessively obese individuals or those suffering from edema, dehydration or emaciation. Nutritional factors can sometimes alter drug metabolizing capacity and this should be kept in mind in undernourished patients.

II **Age:**

Children may not react to all drugs in the same manner as young adults. The *pharmacokinetics* changes with age. Thus, gastric emptying is prolonged and gastric pH fluctuates in neonates and infants. Further, the liver capacity to metabolize drugs is low, renal function is less well developed and proportion of body water is higher in the new born. The metabolic clearance of drugs such as chloramphenicol, barbiturates, pethidine, salicylates, sulfonamides, diazepam and aminoglycosides is less in infants than in adults. The *pharmacodynamics* of drugs in children may differ from that in adults as well. Drugs may show *unique effects* in children, not seen in adults. Thus, some substances may disturb the patterns of growth and development that occur only during particular periods of life e.g. tetracyclines and glucocorticoids in children. Metoclopramide and other dopamine antagonists produce acute dystonic reactions more often in children and adolescents than in adults. With few exceptions, drugs are more active and more toxic in the newborn than in older animals. The doses of antidiphtheria serum and antitetanus serum, however, are not modified by age.

The pediatric doses are expressed in terms of body weight (mg/Kg per dose or per day) or in terms of body surface area (mg/M^2per dose or per day) (Table 3.3). *In practice, it is better to rely on a handy reference book than on one's memory or above calculations* (Chapter 77) *during neonatal and pediatric prescribing.* Adult doses should be used in children over 55 kg of weight and in those who have achieved puberty.

Old people also present problems in dosage adjustment and this may vary widely with different people. The hepatic blood flow and metabolism of drugs may diminish in the elderly

Table 3.4: Some drugs to be used with special care in the elderly

- NSAID.
- CNS depressants.
- Psychotropics.
- Antihypertensives and other drugs causing postural hypotension
- Diuretics.
- Anticholinergics and drugs with anti-cholinergic adverse effects.
- Digoxin.
- Drugs causing bone marrow depression; and
- Nephrotoxic drugs.

and the renal function declines with age. Elderly patients are more sensitive to some drug effects. Central depressants such as hypnotics and tranquillizers may produce confusional states or falls in the old people. Plasma half-lives of drugs such as diazepam, pethidine and propranolol are longer in the elderly. Drugs needing special care in old people are listed in Table 3.4.

III Pregnancy and lactation:

Special care should be exercised when drugs are administered during pregnancy and lactation.

- ***Pregnancy***: Drugs which may stimulate the uterine smooth muscle are contraindicated during pregnancy. Further, many drugs administered to the mother are capable of delaying the onset of labour or of crossing the placenta and affecting the fetus (Chapter 77).
- Lactation: See Chapter 77.

IV Diet, Tobacco, Alcohol and Environment:

Medicines are usually taken after a meal to reduce the risk of gastric irritation, nausea and vomiting. Food, however, can have significant effect on the pharmacokinetics of drugs (Table 1.4). Generally, food depresses the rate and the extent of drug absorption. Drugs may be given on empty stomach (i) to prevent mixing with the foodstuffs e.g. the anthelmintics, (ii) to get an immediate action e.g. drugs used against motion sickness, and (iii) to prevent drug inactivation in the stomach, e.g., penicillin V. Tetracyclines form insoluble chelates with aluminium, calcium and magnesium salts, which reduces their absorption. Captopril, digoxin, thyroxine sodium and rifampicin are examples of drugs better absorbed on empty stomach (Chapter 1).

The dose of a hypnotic required to produce sleep during daytime is higher than that required to produce sleep at night. High altitude with low barometric pressure diminishes the capacity of the body to oxidize drugs and this may precipitate drug toxicity.

Polycyclic hydrocarbons present in the cigarette smoke and hydrocarbon pesticides such as DDT induce hepatic microsomal enzymes P450. This accelerates the biodegradation of several drugs and increase the biotransformation of drugs such as theophylline.

Alcohol modifies the response to many drugs e.g. it enhances the effect of CNS depressants. It also induces hepatic enzymes and causes rapid metabolism of certain drugs. On the other hand, hepatic injury due to alcohol can enhance response to drugs.

V Route of administration:

Intravenous doses of the drugs are usually smaller than oral doses, particularly in case of drugs which are incompletely absorbed orally e.g. digoxin. The onset of drug action is quicker with the IV route; this might enhance the chances of drug toxicity.

VI Psychological factors:

The personality of the physician may influence the drug effect considerably, particularly if the drug is intended for use in a psychosomatic disorder. Inert dosage forms called placebos resemble the actual medicament in the physical properties. Placebos are known to produce therapeutic benefit in conditions like angina pectoris and bronchial asthma. The personality of the patient may also modify the drug effect. The dose of chlorpromazine required to produce tranquillization in an otherwise normal individual is 50 to 100 mg/day. However, the same drug has to be administered in the dose of 500 to 1000 mg/day to achieve the quietening effect in highly agitated schizophrenic patients.

VII Genetic factors:

Variations in the genetic constitution determine the genetically mediated differences in drug metabolism and response (pharmacogenomics). The latter are usually due to defective/deficient enzyme systems responsible for inactivating the drug. Often, this results in drug accumulation and toxicity. *Patients with hereditary disorders of intermediary metabolism such as diabetes mellitus rarely show a disturbance in the metabolism of drugs and other foreign compounds*. This is because the microsomal enzyme system, involved in the metabolism of drugs, does not participate to a significant extent in the intermediary metabolism. Some examples of genetic variations are:

- ***Acetylation and hydroxylation of drugs:*** The rate of acetylation of INH, dapsone, hydralazine and some sulfonamides is controlled by an autosomal recessive gene and the dosage of these drugs depends upon the acetylator status of individuals. Similarly, slow hydroxylators are liable to exaggerated responses (excessive beta blockade with metoprolol) and to drug toxicity (lactic acidosis with phenformin).
- ***Plasma cholinesterase* (Pseudo-cholinesterase) :** Some persons inherit a modified type of esterase (atypical pseudocholinesterase) that is less efficient than the normal enzyme in hydrolysing the drug succinylcholine. Such people may develop prolonged respiratory paralysis even with a therapeutic dose of succinylcholine.
- ***Phenytoin hydroxylation:*** Certain individuals are unable to p-hydroxylate diphenylhydantoin and develop marked toxicity, during phenytoin therapy of epilepsy.
- ***Glucuronide conjugation:*** Many drugs and even endogenous compounds like bilirubin are conjugated as glucuronides. In a hereditary disorder termed Crigler-Najjar syndrome, the conjugation of bilirubin is impaired, resulting in a severe nonhemolytic jaundice, kernicterus and cerebral disturbances.
- ***Erythrocyte diaphorase:*** The enzyme erythrocyte NAD-diaphorase protects the erythrocytes by reducing methemoglobin to hemoglobin. Individuals with a hereditary deficiency of this enzyme are likely to develop methemoglobinemia after administration of drugs such as sulfonamides and nitrites.
- ***Glucose-6-phosphate dehydrogenase (G6PD):*** Primaquine and certain other drugs cause hemolysis in individuals with a deficiency of G6PD (Chapter 35).
- ***Miscellaneous:*** These include abnormal drug response in miscellaneous hereditary conditions, such as,

(i) Inherited resistance to coumarin anti-coagulants.

(ii) Chinese patients tend to respond to lower doses of propranolol than do the Western patients although the metabolism of propranolol is significantly faster in the Chinese than in the white group.

About 90% of whites have in their liver a form of alcohol dehydrogenase which metabolizes alcohol *in vitro* more slowly than the corresponding liver enzyme in 90% of orientals. Genetic variations in the activity of aldehyde dehydrogenase among various ethnic groups have also been reported.

(iii) Barbiturates markedly enhance the activity of the hepatic enzyme delta-aminolevulinic acid synthetase leading to a marked rise in the rate of porphobilinogen synthesis. This precipitates an acute attack of porphyria in susceptible individuals.

(iv) Precipitation of severe hyperpyrexia, muscle rigidity, hyperkalemic cardiac arrest and death (malignant hyperthermia, an autosomal dominant condition) by anaesthetics such as halothane, methoxyflurane and cyclopropane.

VIII Metabolic disturbances:

Changes in water-electrolyte and acid-base balance, body temperature and other physiological parameters may modify the effects of drugs e.g.

- Aspirin reduces body temperature only in the presence of pyrexia.
- The vasoconstrictor effect of noradrenaline is reduced in the presence of metabolic acidosis.
- The absorption of iron from the gut is maximum if the individual has an iron deficiency anemia. Hypokalemia can enhance digoxin cardiotoxicity.

IX Presence of disease (Comorbidity) :

Drugs like morphine and chlorpromazine may produce unusually prolonged effect in cirrhotic patients. Antibiotics like streptomycin and kanamycin, excreted mainly by the kidneys may prove toxic if the kidney function is impaired. In myxedema, morphine acts for a much longer time because of the low rate of oxidation. In congestive heart failure, the clearance of lignocaine may diminish by 50%. Pulmonary and GI disease may also alter pharmacokinetics.

X **Cumulation:**

If a drug is excreted slowly, its repeated administration may build up a sufficiently high concentration in the body to produce toxicity e.g. digoxin, emetine and heavy metals. Sometimes, a cumulative effect is desired e.g. with phenytoin in the treatment of epilepsy. Most often, however, it is undesirable. Substances like lead can remain deposited in bones without producing toxic effects. This is called *passive cumulation.* It can produce the toxic manifestations as soon as it is released into the blood.

To avoid cumulation:

(a) One must know if the drug is eliminated slowly or rapidly.

(b) Stop the drug administration at the appearance of the first warning symptom.

(c) Select carefully the form in which the drug is to be administered; and

(d) Check liver and kidney function before and during drug administration, as even an otherwise non-cumulative drug would produce cumulation in the presence of hepatic and renal damage.

XI **Other drugs and chemicals:**

Previous or concurrent therapy with certain drugs may result in stimulation or inhibition of the metabolism of other drugs. Both tobacco smoke and alcohol consumption induce CYP450 liver enzymes. They accelerate the metabolism of a number of drugs, leading to a reduction in their therapeutic effects (see later).

XII **Additive effect (Summation) :** See Chapter 2

XIII **Synergism:** See Chapter 2

XIV **Antagonism:** See Chapter 2

XV **Drug tolerance:**

When a large dose of a drug is required to elicit an effect ordinarily produced by its normal therapeutic dose, the phenomenon is termed as **drug tolerance**. Drug tolerance is of two types.

True tolerance: This is seen on both oral and parenteral administration of a drug and can be subdivided into : (a) Natural and (b) Acquired.

(a) **Natural tolerance:** This is seen in various animal species and also among the various human races. It includes:

- ***Species tolerance***: Certain animal species can tolerate certain drugs in quantities lethal to man, e.g., some rabbits can tolerate large quantities of belladonna. This is attributed to the enzyme atropine esterase in their liver and plasma, which rapidly detoxifies belladonna.
- ***Racial tolerance***: A solution of ephedrine instilled into the conjunctival sac of the Caucasians produces prompt dilatation of the pupil but in Negroes it may not produce any dilatation.

(b) **Acquired tolerance**: This tolerance, unlike the racial or species tolerance, develops only on repeated administration of a drug and may take weeks or months to develop. Many drugs, including opiates, barbiturates, nitrites and xanthines, produce tolerance. Tolerance is sometimes desirable, e.g., barbiturates, when used in the treatment of epilepsy, produce tolerance for their soporific but not for their antiepileptic effect. Generally however, tolerance is undesirable.

- ***Tissue tolerance:*** In this type, the development of tolerance is confined to certain effects or to certain systems, e.g., morphine produces tolerance for its euphoriant effect, but the pupils and the GI tract do not become tolerant. Thus, the same dose of morphine invariably produces pinpoint pupils and constipation but may fail to produce euphoria.
- ***Cross tolerance:*** If an individual initially develops tolerance to a drug belonging to a particular group, he also shows tolerance to other drugs from the same group. This

phenomenon is known as cross tolerance e.g. that between alcohol and the general anaesthetics like ether.

Apparent or pseudotolerance: This is confined to the oral administration of a drug. The feudal kings, much worried about poisons, were often in the habit of taking small doses of arsenic by mouth. This apparently rendered them immune to oral arsenic but poisoning could occur if any other route was chosen. This tolerance is probably due to the *local changes developed by the GI tract which prevent the poison from getting absorbed from the gut.*

Mechanism of development of tolerance:

Tolerance can be :

(a) **Pharmacokinetic (Dispositional)**; or

(b) **Pharmacodynamic (Functional)**

Dispositional tolerance is due to changes in drug absorption, distribution, excretion and metabolism leading to decreased intensity and duration of contact between a given drug and the target tissue. Thus, the barbiturates after repeated administration enhance their own detoxification by stimulating hepatic microsomal enzyme systems. p-Glycoprotein transporters in many tumours pump out the administered anti-cancer drugs and make the tumours resistant to therapy.

Functional tolerance is probably due to changes in the properties and functions of the target tissue, that make them **less sensitive** to a given drug concentration. Thus, it is associated with some cellular changes. With some drugs, this may be related to a decrease in drug receptors **(down-regulation)**. With compounds like morphine, alcohol and barbiturates, it has been demonstrated that the cells of the CNS, which usually develop tolerance to these drugs, become capable of normal physiological functions in the presence of high concentrations of these drugs. The adaptive mechanisms involved are not clearly understood.

Tachyphylaxis: Tolerance to drugs as described above usually takes some time to develop. However, with certain drugs like ephedrine, tyramine, amphetamine and 5-hydroxytryptamine, tolerance may appear within a few minutes in isolated preparations as well as in the intact animals. Thus, if any of these drugs is administered repeatedly, at very short intervals, the pharmacological response elicited decreases progressively. This phenomenon is known as **tachyphylaxis or acute tolerance** (Fig 3.1). Similarly, repeated doses of ephedrine at short intervals, in the treatment of bronchial asthma, may produce diminishing response.

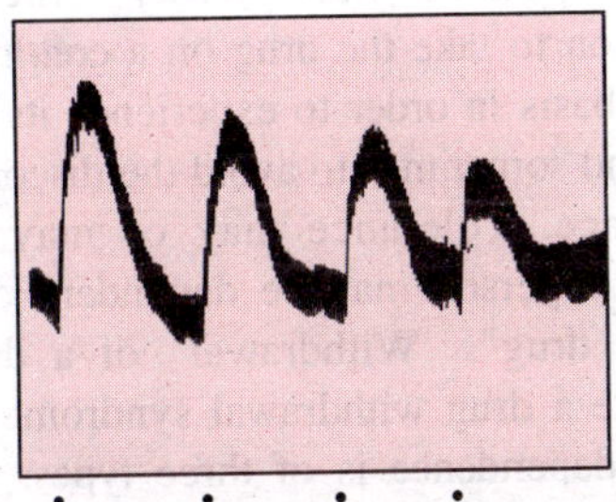

Fig. 3.1 : Effect of repeated doses of tyramine on BP in anaesthetized dog. Black dots denote administration of the same dose. Note the decreasing response.

Various mechanisms are responsible for the appearance of tachyphylaxis. In case of tyramine, it is due to depletion of the noradrenaline stores from the sympathetic nerves. However, with sympathomimetics like ephedrine and amphetamine, tachyphylaxis can occur without appreciable depletion of the noradrenaline stores. Tachyphylaxis probably can occur if the drug dissociates only slowly from its combination with the receptor, thus continuing receptor blockade while losing its intrinsic activity and hence its pharmacological effect. It has been observed that tachyphylaxis or refractoriness with isoprenaline is accompanied by a decline in beta receptor number while receptor affinity for the agonist remains unaltered. Such refractoriness may have therapeutic relevance in human disease. With other drugs, however, tachyphylaxis is probably due to some unidentified 'adaptive response' of the tissue concerned.

XVI Drug dependence:

Repeated administration of certain drugs may induce a habit and dependence. If the habit forming agent is not made available to the habitué, he develops withdrawal symptoms characterized by psychic/physical disturbances like headache, restlessness and emotional upset and/or convulsions and vasomotor collapse. WHO has defined **drug dependence** as "A state, psychic and sometimes also physical, resulting from the interaction between a living organism and a drug, characterized by behavioural and other responses that always include a compulsion to take the drug on a continuous or periodic basis in order to experience its psychic effects and sometimes to avoid the discomfort of its absence. Tolerance may or may not be present. A person may be dependent on more than one drug". Withdrawal of a drug can precipitate a drug withdrawal syndrome.

Drug dependence is of three types:

(a) **Psychic**;

(b) **Physical**; and

(c) **Combined**.

A condition in which a drug produces "a feeling of satisfaction and a psychic drive that require periodic or continuous administration of the drug to produce pleasure or to avoid discomfort," is called **psychic dependence**. In case of **physical dependence**, the body "achieves" an adaptive state that manifests itself by intense physical disturbances when the drug is withdrawn (**withdrawal syndrome**). The term 'addiction' was formerly used to denote the phenomenon involving both psychic and physical dependence on drugs. It is currently called **drug abuse**. Its characteristics include

- ***An overpowering desire (compulsion) to continue taking the drug in spite of knowing its harmful effects.***
- ***A tendency to increase the dose;*** and
- ***A high tendency to withdrawal symptoms.***

Compulsive drug use is commonly but not necessarily associated with the development of tolerance and physical dependence. There are some drugs where tolerance and physical dependence develop after chronic use; but they are not self administered nor used compulsively by man. Table 3.5 lists important drugs known to cause dependence.

Table 3.5: Important drugs known to cause dependence

I **Drugs that cause severe psychic as well as physical dependence :**

- ***Opiate or morphine type*** **:**
  Morphine and its congeners like codeine, dihydromorphinone (Dilaudid) and heroin. Synthetic morphine substitutes such as meperidine (pethidine) and its congeners, methadone and its congeners, morphinan compounds, phenazocine and diphenoxylate (Lomotil)
- ***Alcohol-barbiturate type*** **:**
  Ethyl alcohol, barbiturates, paraldehyde, chloral hydrate, meprobamate, glutethemide, methyprylon, ethinamate, ethchlorvynol, benzodiazepines and methaqualone.
- ***Nicotine*** (tobacco).

II **Drugs that cause definite psychic but mild or questionable physical dependence:**

- ***Opiate antagonist type*** **:**
  Morphine antagonists like nalorphine; morphinan antagonists like levallorphan; and benzazocine antagonists like cyclazocine.
- ***Amphetamine type*:**
  Amphetamine, methamphetamine and phenmetrazine. Piperidines like methylphenidate and pipradol.

III **Drugs that cause only psychic dependence:**
Cocaine, LSD, psilocybin, mescaline, cannabis (marihuana, hashish), caffeine (coffee, tea).

Man has long sought ways of enhancing his pleasure and of easing his discomfort. Various agents are consumed to achieve this goal. Commonly used beverages like tea and coffee stimulate the CNS and are capable of producing drug dependence but this is not necessarily harmful in itself. Tobacco on the other hand is a dependence-producing agent capable of causing physical harm to the user although it produces relatively little stimulation of the CNS. Most of the drugs used by the addicts have predominantly CNS effects. Such drugs as opiates, barbiturates, alcohol and cocaine all produce sense of well-being in the user. This is termed **euphoria** and contributes considerably to the development of dependence. Stimulation of the CNS probably plays an important role. However, when exposed to these drugs under similar environmental influences, all the recipients do not develop dependence. It is not clear why some individuals stop after initial experimentation. Others continue drug use but do not become dependent and still others become compulsive drug users or addicts. But majority of those who develop dependence have some psychological problems. Besides the user's personality, availability of the drug plays an important part in the development of drug dependence. Thus, for the development of drug dependence, both the 'seed' and the 'soil' are required.

A potential addict may start and continue taking a dependence inducing drug:

- ***Following its medicinal use.***
- ***To achieve a sense of relief from stresses and tension of life.***
- ***To satisfy curiosity about drug effects.***
- ***To achieve a sense of belonging, to be 'accepted' by others in the group.***
- ***To express hostility or independence.***
- ***To have pleasurable (euphoric), new, thrilling or even dangerous experiences.***
- ***To gain an improved understanding or creativity***; or
- ***To escape from reality, to have a dreamy state.***

The experience achieved by the individual under the influence of the drug is so impressive that he develops a craving for it and finds it difficult to give it up. These drugs themselves are **powerful reinforcers**. Hence, they are also called **masterful drugs**. Drugs that cause serious disability of functioning normally by inducing psychic/physical dependence are called **Hard Drugs** e.g. cocaine and heroin. Factors which appear to facilitate the initiation of drug abuse are given in Table 3.6.

Table 3.6: Factors which facilitate initiation of drug abuse

- Ready availability of drugs as in case of doctors and medical students.
- General public acceptance of the use of mood modifiers such as alcohol.
- Increasing mobility particularly of youth.
- Peer group pressure.
- An abundance of information about drug effects and sources.
- Lack of adequate publicity given to harmful effects of these agents; and
- Unstable or broken homes, socio-cultural pressures and social ills.

The exact mechanism of drug dependence is not known. Alteration of the cellular metabolism of the CNS is a prime factor in the development of dependence (Chapter 6). Other systems may become tolerant to the drug but *only the CNS is capable of developing physical dependence.* Withdrawal of the drug under these circumstances produces distorted homeostasis leading to the development of a **withdrawal syndrome** or an **abstinence syndrome**. The withdrawal syndrome may vary from a mild to a severe one, sometimes resulting in fatality. All the drugs that cause physical dependence act on the CNS. The symptoms of withdrawal syndrome are usually characterized by rebound effects in those same physiological systems that were initially modified by the drugs. Thus, general CNS depressants, on withdrawal, cause hyper-excitation while withdrawal of central stimulant amphetamine produces weakness, lack of energy, hyperphagia and depression. Withdrawal symptoms due to drugs with long half-lives e.g. phenobarbitone are usually less

Table 3.7: Principles of treatment of drug dependence

- Hospitalization of the patient.
- Gradual or sudden withdrawal of the drug.
- Substitution therapy.
- Psychotherapy and occupational therapy.
- Specific drug therapy, e.g., disulfiram in alcohol addiction.
- Correction of nutritional deficiencies; and
- Community treatment and rehabilitation.

severe but more protracted.

Dug dependence, once developed, is difficult to treat. To achieve any success, complete co-operation of the individual is vital.

Table 3.7 summarises the principles of treatment of dependence. The details are described in the respective chapters.

It is highly desirable that drugs which are likely to be administered over a prolonged period should be screened for their dependence liability in animals.

Drug Interactions

Drug interactions result from the use of two or more drugs. This may lead to enhanced or diminished effect that may be useful or harmful. The **useful drug interaction** is illustrated by synergistic combinations of drugs such as antibiotics or antihypertensives. **Harmful drug interactions** are, unfortunately, more numerous and are discussed below.

A new symptom appearing during treatment with a drug may be due to the disease or the drug. This can be perplexing enough. But, if the patient is receiving several drugs and two or more drugs are capable of causing the same new symptom as the underlying disease, or if two drugs in concert elicit symptoms that would not otherwise appear, the physician is in quandary. In this situation, he may attribute the new symptom wrongly to the disease itself or to idiosyncracy to one of the drugs, instead of recognizing it as a drug interaction. It is known that the incidence of adverse reactions to drugs rises from 4.2% when five or fewer drugs are used to 45% when twenty or more drugs are used. A physician who uses multiple drugs must, therefore, be constantly alert to the possibility of drug interaction. Further, he must be aware of both 'risky drugs' (Table 3.8) and 'vulnerable patients' (Table 3.9) in this respect.

It is absolutely essential that when a patient's clinical condition changes, particularly if he is severely ill or elderly, all drug treatment should be reviewed as a matter of course.

Drug interactions may occur either outside the body or in the body.

I Drug interactions outside the body:

The most glaring examples of this are seen when several drugs are mixed in an IV infusion. One or more of the drugs may get inactive or even precipitate. This is often attributable to changes in the pH of the solutions. The following are some of the examples:

- ***Use of wrong vehicle for infusion :*** No

Table 3.8: Risky drugs

- ***Those that affect a vital process in the body,*** e.g., warfarin, chlorpromazine and morphine.
- ***Those that have a steep dose-response curve,*** e.g., verapamil, levodopa and chrorpropamide.
- ***Those that have saturable kinetics,*** e.g., phenytoin, theophylline and salicylates.
- ***Those that demonstrate dose dependent toxicity,*** e.g., digoxin, lithium, amino-glycosides and methotrexate.
- ***Those where a loss of effect leads to a breakthrough of disease,*** e.g., quinidine, glucocorticoids and antiepileptics; and
- ***Those where the patient depends on the prophylactic action,*** e.g., oral contraceptives and cyclosporin.

Table 3.9 : Vulnerable patients

- Elderly patients receiving many drugs.
- Patients with liver/kidney damage.
- Patients with unstable disease, e.g., epileptics, brittle diabetics, demented patients and those with cardiac disease.
- Patients dependent upon drug treatment for survival, e.g., transplant recipients and patients with Addison's disease; and
- Patients who have more than one prescribing doctor.

drug should ever be added to blood, plasma, amino acid solutions, fat emulsions (which tend to crack), sodium bicarbonate solution, mannitol solution (from which mannitol tends to crystallize) and to heparin infusion. An infusion set should be discarded after administration of blood and not used for other infusion fluids.

Highly acidic solutions (pH may be as low as 3.5) such as dextrose or fructose are unsuitable as vehicles for sodium or potassium salts of weakly acidic drugs such as phenytoin, barbiturates, methicillin and novobiocin, as the latter tend to get precipitated at this pH. Drugs such as benzyl penicillin, ampicillin, heparin and aminophylline are unstable at the pH of these solutions. Dextrose solution is, however, eminently suitable for infusing noradrenaline which is stable at the acidic pH. Isotonic saline is slightly acidic or neutral and is a suitable vehicle for most drugs with the exception of noradrenaline. If noradrenaline has to be infused in isotonic saline, vitamin C should be added to the infusion.

Most antibiotics become unstable and deteriorate in large volumes of fluid. Moreover, erythromycin lactobionate is unstable in electrolyte solutions but may be diluted with 5% dextrose solution. Amphotericin B should be diluted with 5% dextrose solution of a pH recommended by the manufacturer, but not with saline.

- ***Addition of drugs to an infusion:*** Drugs should be added to infusion containers only when constant plasma concentrations are needed or when the administration of a more concentrated solution would be harmful. If a centralized additive service is available, ready-to-use infusions containing the additional drug are to be preferred to making extemporaneous additions in the ward.

No more than one drug should be added to any infusion container and the components should be compatible. Solutions should be mixed thoroughly and checked for absence of particulate matter before use. The container should be labelled with the patient's name and the quantity of the additive and with the date and time of the addition. Infusion should be examined from time to time for cloudiness, crystallization or change of colour; if any sign of deterioration is observed, discontinue the infusion. Barbiturates, phenytoin, phenothiazines, vitamin B complex (± vitamin C), amphotericin, sulfadiazine and furosemide should not be mixed with any other drug in solution.

Beta-lactam antibiotics should not be mixed with any proteinaceous material for fear of forming immunogenic and allergenic conjugates. The following undergo loss of potency when added to large volume infusions e.g. ampicillin in glucose or lactate containing infusions; mustine hydrochloride in isotonic saline; gentamicin-carbenicillin added to the same infusion.

Also see Chapters 1 and 37 for IV infusions.

II **Drug interactions in the body can be:**

(a) **Pharmacokinetic**, one drug affecting the absorption, distribution, transport, metabolism or excretion of another drug; or

(b) **Pharmacodynamic**, one drug altering the pharmacological action of another drug.

Drug absorption:

- Drugs given orally can interact in the gut to form complexes which may not be absorbed. Thus, calcium, magnesium, aluminium and iron salts interfere with absorption of tetracycline and of prednisolone. Sucralfate reduces the

Table 3.10: Drug-induced acceleration of metabolism of drugs

Inducer	Drugs whose metabolism is accelerated (victim drugs)
Barbiturates	Barbiturates, oral Anticoagulants, Steroids (oral contraceptives, testosterone, glucocorticoids), vitamins (D and K), Thyroxine, Phenylbutazone, Phenytoin, Griseofulvin, Chloramphenicol, Theophylline.
Phenytoin	Glucocorticoids, Vitamin D, Theophylline.
Griseofulvin	Warfarin
Rifampicin	Oral contraceptives, Glucocorticoids, Metoprolol, Propranolol.
Carbamazepine	Vitamin D.

Dicophane and gamma benzene hexachloride are powerful inducers of drug-metabolising microsomal enzymes. Hence, research on drug metabolism could be misleading if the animal quarters are sprayed with either of these insecticides. Nicotine is also a powerful enzyme inducer.

bioavailability of phenytoin. Such interactions can be avoided by separating the administration of the two drugs by at least two hours.

- A drug altering the gastric pH can alter the solubility of another agent and thus may influence its absorption e.g. sodium bicarbonate reduces the absorption of tetracycline. Drugs can also affect the absorption by modifying the gut motility and gastric emptying. Anticholinergic drugs and opioids can slow down the absorption of other drugs by delaying gastric emptying.
- Sorbitol accelerates the gastrointestinal absorption of paracetamol.
- A few women taking low dose, combination oral contraceptives may be put to risk of pregnancy by the concurrent administration of a broad spectrum antibiotic (ampicillin or tetracycline but not co-trimoxazole). By reducing the bacterial flora in the intestines, these antibiotics disrupt the deconjugation and hence re-absorption of the steroids secreted into the intestine.

Drug distribution : Some drugs are bound

Table 3.11: Drug-induced inhibition of metabolism of drugs

Inhibitor	Drugs whose metabolism is inhibited (victim drugs)
Allopurinol	Tolbutamide, Methotrexate, Probenecid.
Disulfiram	Alcohol, Tolbutamide, Warfarin, Phenytoin.
Isoniazid	Glucocorticoids, Oral Contraceptives, Carbamazepine, Phenytoin.
Chloramphenicol	Tolbutamide, Probenecid, Phenytoin.
Cimetidine	Warfarin, Diazepam.
Fluoxetine	Warfarin, Phenytoin, some benzodiazepines.
Erythromycin	Amiodarone, Digoxin, Antipsychotics, Warfarin, Theophylline.
Ketoconazole	Cyclosporin, Astemizole, Terfenadine.
Phenylbutazone	Phenytoin, Tolbutamide.
Ethanol	Methanol (beneficial effect)
Valproate	Lamotrigine.
Grape fruit juice*	Cyclosporin, Terfenadine and most Calcium channel blockers.

Many drugs inhibit the p-hydroxylation of phenytoin, increasing the chance of phenytoin toxicity. They include dicumarol, isoniazid, disulfiram, chloramphenicol and methylphenydate.

* Contains psoralen.

strongly to plasma proteins and remain pharmacologically inactive. Certain groups of drugs seem to share a limited number of protein binding sites and can be displaced from them by each other. This results in an increase in the unbound and pharmacologically active form of one of the drugs leading to toxicity. However, this type of drug interaction is clinically significant only with drugs which are extensively (> 90%) protein bound, have a small apparent volume of distribution (V_d) and have effects proportional to their concentration. e.g.

(i) Clofibrate can displace warfarin sodium from the binding sites, leading to a bleeding tendency.

(ii) Salicylates can displace tolbutamide from the binding sites, leading to hypoglycemic coma.

Drug transport : Guanethidine and the related adernergic neruone blocking drugs are actively transported into adrenergic neuron by the same transport system that is responsible for noradrenaline uptake into the neuron. This system is inhibited by the antidepressant imipramine, which interferes with the antihypertensive activity of guanethidine.

Drug metabolism:

- ***Stimulation:*** The synthesis of the drug-metabolizing microsomal enzymes is enhanced (**enzyme induction**) by a number of commonly used drugs, insecticides and polycylic hydrocarbons (Table 3.10). This reduces the efficacy and increases the therapeutic dose of the drugs metabolized by the microsomal enzymes. It should be noted that different inducers are relatively selective for certain families of CYP450 enzymes.
- ***Inhibition***: Inhibition of the metabolism of one drug by another may lead to toxicity of the former. A number of examples of such drug induced inhibition of metabolism of important drugs is known (Table 3.11).

Drug excretion: This can be facilitated or interfered with by certain drug combinations. Thus, the excretion of weakly acidic drugs like sulfonamides, salicylates and barbiturates can be enhanced by making the urine alkaline. Probenecid inhibits the tubular secretion of penicillin, indomethacin and riboflavine. Quinidine, verapamil and amiodarone can double the plasma digoxin concentration.

Receptor site (*Pharmacodynamic interaction*): In this case, drugs acting on the same receptor site or at different active receptors may enhance or decrease the response, e.g., tubocurarine and aminoglycoside antibiotics may accentuate the block at the neuromuscular junction; marked CNS depression is caused by concurrent administration of morphine and barbiturates. Several examples of pharmacodynamic drug interactions are described in respective chapters.

Changes in electrolyte and fluid balance: Drugs that cause potassium depletion may potentiate the effects of digitalis and non-depolarizing muscle relaxants, but antagonize the anti-arrhythmic action of lignocaine, quinidine and procainamide.

Interactions among chemotherapeutic agents: Injudicious combinations of chemotherapeutic agents may prove harmful in therapeutics. (Chapter 49).

Unfortunately, drug interactions are not always predictable from animal studies. Hence, the physician should always be wary about including too many drugs in his prescription so as to minimize this danger. Further, the physician should always enquire about alcohol consumption by the patient. Numerous drug interactions between alcohol and other drugs can occur (Chapter 6).

Many of the drug interactions reported in the literature (especially those which are due to competitive binding to the same plasma protein) may not be clinically significant. *Therefore, one should be careful in distinguishing between drug interactions which are clinically significant and those which are not.*

Drug Discovery; New Drug Development; and Drug Assay 4

A new drug is defined as a new substance of chemical, biological or biotechnological origin for which adequate data is not available for the regulatory authority to judge its efficacy and safety for the proposed claim.

Until recently new drug development has been a slow and expensive process. Drugs were discovered largely by trial and error, and often by chance. In the 20th century, drug development involved sequential screening of synthetic chemicals or extracts of biological material in isolated animal organs, followed by their testing in whole animals. Many drugs were found and evaluated with these methods. In late 1950s, radioligand binding assays were developed, which enabled the scientists to study the interaction of compounds with receptors and then select the ones with the best fit for studying their biological activity. In the late 20th century, combinatorial chemistry changed the scenario. This new technique involves computer based molecular modeling of compounds and can produce a large number of compounds with best fit to the receptor. Advances in cell biology and receptor technology have been helpful in developing screening systems. It involves automated, micro techniques to screen as many as 50,000 compounds in a day. One of the popular techniques today is High Content Screening (HCS), in which *in vitro* or cell-based assays are used to screen large numbers of compounds for their effects on cellular or subcellular targets. New areas have been developed to collect, store and interpret the information generated this way *viz.* bioinformatics, chemoinformatics and functional genomics. Thus, with the help of Computer-Aided Drug Design (CADD) and HCS, 'hits and leads' are found out. A "Hit" is a molecule with confirmed structure, confirmed activity in primary throughput screening and a good profile in secondary assay; whereas a "Lead" is a hit series with proven structure activity relationship both *in vitro* and *in vivo*. The leads are then tested by the classical pharmacological methods to determine their efficacy and safety and finally in humans by clinical pharmacological studies.

Prior to any clinical evaluation, the investigator should obtain reasonably clear answers to three important questions :

- ***Is the data from animal studies adequate?***
- ***What is the probable risk involved in giving the drug to humans? Is it worth the risk?***
- ***Is there any need for a new drug in the disease under consideration and if so does the new remedy seem promising?***

Animal Toxicity Studies

In order to assess the safety of a drug,

various toxicity studies are carried out in animals such as mice, rats, guinea pigs, dogs, and monkeys, under varying conditions of drug administration. The tests include:

- ***Systemic toxicity studies*** (i) with a single dose; and (ii) with repeated doses.
- ***Local toxicity studies***
- ***Specialized toxicity studies*** including tests for male fertility; female reproduction and fetal developmental toxicity; allergenicity/hypersensitivity; genotoxicity and carcinogenicity.

I Systemic toxicity studies:

(a) ***Single dose toxicity studies:*** In these studies a drug is tested for the effects of a single dose. Graded doses are given in 2 rodent species (mice and rats of both sexes), using the same route as that intended for humans. One additional route is used in one of the species to ensure systemic absorption of the drug. Animals are observed for mortality for up to 14 days (72 hours if the administration is parenteral). Detailed observations are made of the effects of the drug on important physiological functions and body weight. Microscopic examination of grossly affected organ is carried out. LD_{10} and LD_{50} should preferably be estimated.

The main object of a single dose study is to determine minimum lethal dose (MLD), maximum tolerated dose (MTD) and if possible, the target organ of toxicity.

(b) ***Repeated dose toxicity studies:*** These studies are also carried out in at least 2 species, of which one should be non-rodent. After the initial dose-ranging studies for MTD, the *final systemic toxicity study (FSTS)* is carried out. Three doses are selected: (1) the highest dose having observable toxicity; (2) mid-dose causing some symptoms but no gross toxicity or death; and (3) the lowest free of toxicity and comparable to the intended therapeutic dose or its multiple. A control group treated with vehicle is a must for comparison. Selected doses are administered depending on the duration of intended use in humans and the phase of the proposed clinical trial. The route of drug administration should be the same as that proposed for human use.

Parameters for safety include cage side observations for eye changes, loss of fur, behavioural and physiological observations, body weight changes, food/ water intake, blood chemistry, hematology and examination of organs. The sites of injections are inspected for gross and microscopic changes. ECG recording and fundoscopy are done in non-rodent species. Sometimes, 'high-dose reversal study' is included wherein animals are studied after stopping the treatment or after recovery from signs of toxicity.

II **Local toxicity studies:** The drug is applied to an appropriate site, e.g. skin, vagina or cornea to determine local effects in suitable species (guinea pigs or rabbits). If the drug gets absorbed from the site of application, appropriate systemic toxicity studies will also be required.

III Specialized toxicity studies:

(a) ***Male fertility studies*** detect effects of a drug on structure and functions of male reproductive organs.

(b) ***Female reproduction and fetal developmental toxicity studies*** include observations on the mating behaviour, progress of gestation, parturition, health during pregnancy and in post-partum period. Ability of the drug to induce fetal malformations and / or death in utero (i.e. **teratogenicity**) when given throughout organogenesis is looked for. **Perinatal toxicity study** is undertaken if the drug is to be given to pregnant or nursing mothers for long periods or where possibility of adverse effects on fetal development is high; the drug is administered throughout the last trimester. These studies are carried out in one rodent species (preferably rat) and one non-rodent species (rabbit).

(c) ***Allerginicity/hypersensitivity tests*** are carried out in guinea pigs to determine the minimum irritant dose and the effect of a challenge after sensitization.

(d) ***Genotoxicity tests:*** Certain drugs are known to produce genetic abnormalities. As genes are bearers of hereditary information, abnormal genes may produce various types of overt and covert abnormalities in the subsequent generations. These are *in vivo* and *in vitro* tests conducted to detect genetic damage, if any.

(e) ***Carcinogenicity studies*** detect the ability of a drug to induce malignancy. They are performed for all drugs that are expected to be used clinically for more than 6 months, as well as for those which are intended to be used frequently in an intermittent manner.

Generation of pharmacokinetic data during the toxicity studies (**toxicokinetic data**) helps to relate doses and systemic exposures achieved with toxicological findings.

Although animal studies provide analogies and serve as useful experimental models, the administration of a biologically active agent to human beings is associated with an element of risk which cannot be predicted by even the most careful and exhaustive animal studies. Hence, the drug has to be carefully evaluated by human experiments for its safety and efficacy before it is accepted for therapeutic use.

A new drug with a completely novel structure and with novel pharmacological action is born rarely. It is often discovered by chance observation (serendipity) as in the case of penicillin, antidiabetic sulfonylureas and thiazide diuretics. Most of the new drugs prepared are related to, or are very similar to, already known drugs. Obviously, the benefit offered by such imitative, **me-too** agents to the patient is generally small, and sometimes the new drug may even be worse than the well tried parent compound. The clinical studies with such imitative drugs are justifiable only if the other established drugs are far from ideal and if animal studies indicate distinct advantages over the parent compound in clearly defined terms. Effectiveness of the drug in very small doses, in itself, is not a justification for human studies, when the toxic effects are known to run parallel with 'higher potency'. Such a preparation would be difficult to dispense and difficulties in regulating its dosage may be enormous. A clinical trial is justified if the new drug is shown to be more efficacious or at least potentially less toxic without significant reduction in its therapeutic efficacy.

A drug with a completely new structure and/ or a new mode of action, if found reasonably safe in animal studies, certainly deserves to be studied clinically. Human pharmacological studies with such a compound with particular reference to its mode of action and its actions on various systems of the body may eventually lead to formulation of a new potentially useful structure. A new compound with a related but widely different chemical structure is likely to produce more novel actions than a closely related imitative compound and hence, it certainly deserves clinical studies.

Interpretation of animal data:

No tests on animals, however meticulous and prolonged, can ever prove with absolute certainty the *efficacy* or *safety* of a new drug in man. Animal pharmacological studies would only indicate the probable beneficial and toxic effects that may be expected during human trials; one must weigh the probable benefits against possible harm that could occur. Almost every drug with biological activity will produce some adverse effects. Drugs that are claimed to be absolutely harmless are also likely to be therapeutically useless.

Although animal studies can eliminate obvious toxicity, certain serious adverse reactions such as allergy, neuropsychological toxicity and blood dyscrasias are difficult to detect in animals. It is known that pharmacokinetics and pharmacodynamics of a drug differ both qualitatively and quantitatively in different species. A drug found highly effective in animals may be totally ineffective in humans because of differences in genomic profiles. Thus, penicillin, a potent and reasonably safe antibiotic used in humans, can produce fatal toxicity in guinea pigs even in small doses. Further, the animals used in toxicity studies are not necessarily suffering from the disease for which the drug would be used in humans. Hence, such studies should be carried out in many species and, if possible, in both healthy and diseased animals. In toxicological experiments, high doses of the drug should be used to bring out the possible toxic effects, and subacute and chronic toxicity studies in animals must always precede the chronic administration of the drug in man. Such studies in animals help the physician to understand and treat the effects of over-dosage of drugs in man.

Subjective responses like nausea, headache, tinnitus, weakness and loss of libido due to a new drug are difficult to discover by animal studies. Some of these effects, if severe, could considerably reduce the therapeutic utility of the new drug.

The relative usefulness of animal studies would be decided by *the relevance of animal tests to the human condition*, where the drug would be used. Thus, the animal studies regarding a potential diuretic or hypotensive or an antibacterial drug will provide more useful information than those regarding drugs supposed to be effective in human mental diseases, since similar conditions cannot be experimentally produced in animals.

While deciding the dose to be administered for the first time in humans, it should be remembered that dose in smaller animals tends to be larger (on mg/kg basis) than that in larger animals, and dosage schedule based on weight basis in animals, should never be applied to human studies. If possible, the pharmacological actions of a new drug in humans should be controlled by measuring blood levels guided by similar estimations done in different species of animals. It has been suggested that during the first cautious trial in humans, about $1/10^{th}$ to $1/5^{th}$ of the predicted effective dose should be administered and then increased gradually.

Clinical Evaluation

The first evaluation of a new drug in humans should be carried out by a clinical investigator who has the requisite 'know how', necessary facilities and time to undertake such work. Such a clinical investigator who has an adequate background in interpreting animal studies and who studies drugs cautiously and critically in humans, with continuing analysis of the result achieved is called a Clinical Pharmacologist. Unimaginative screening of drugs in man is not clinical pharmacology. **Clinical Pharmacology**, therefore, involves the study of various aspects of drug action (pharmacodynamics) and metabolism (pharmacokinetics) in humans, both in health and in disease and, therefore, is a discipline which is a part of medicine as a whole. The Clinical Pharmacologist should be a combination of a pharma¬cologist and a clinician. Clinical Pharmacologists can be clinicians working in the disciplines of medicine, therapeutics, cardiology, anaesthesiology or surgery, and having interest in pharmacology. Obviously, one should restrict such work to the field of one's specialization where one has the requisite experience and full knowledge of the ever increasing advances in the subject. This is essential because the safety and effectiveness of new drugs solely depend on his strict, unbiased and uncompromising adherence to the highest scientific standards. More than the equipment and finances, it is the honesty and calibre of the investigator involved that matters the most.

It is essential to have information about the chemical and pharmaceutical properties (such as solubility and stability) of a new product before it is tested clinically.

Prior, informed consent of the subjects (both volunteers and patients) undergoing the clinical studies with a new drug should always be obtained. Further, the study should be approved by the institutional ethics committee and statutory authority. Healthy subjects with **risk factors** for an ADR e.g. age less than five years, old age, reproductive age in women, history/family history of drug allergy and so on, should be *generally* excluded from the drug trials. "A risk factor is a personal attribute (age and gender), an aspect of behaviour or lifestyle, environmental exposure, or inborn/inherited characteristic, which, on the basis of *epidemiologic evidence*, is known to be associated with a health-related condition considered important to prevent".

Phase 1 **(Human pharmacology):** The first clinical evaluation in normal, healthy humans is undertaken to find out :

- ***The safety and tolerability*** of the drug and the dosage range.
- ***Any ADRs that may occur.***
- ***Pharmacodynamic effects*** that it may produce; and
- ***Pharmacokinetic parameters.***

Such studies are carried out at limited centres by competent investigators. The aim is to obtain precise information from the smallest number of healthy volunteers in the minimum possible time. Both subjective and objective evaluation is done along with relevant laboratory studies.

Once the safety is proved in volunteer studies, further studies are carried out in pathological states which the new drug is expected to modify. The prime requisites for such an evaluation are:

- ***Uniformity of subjects with respect to age, sex, nutritional status etc.***
- ***Precise diagnosis in the case of patients.***
- ***A clear index of response relevant to the therapeutic objective,*** e.g., in the trials of lipid lowering drugs the end-point that matters is the reduction in the incidence of stroke and coronary events; mere demonstration of lowering of one or the other plasma lipids does not carry the same conviction.

The clinical investigator must decide how far it is ethical to withhold a known treatment for the sake of trial with a new drug and whether any additional ancillary therapy is needed. If other known drugs are also to be administered simultaneously for some reasons, it is necessary to watch for drug interactions.

In certain fields like endocrinology or infectious diseases, where the etiopathology is precisely known, the clinicopharmacological studies with the new compound could be precise, quantitative and predictable e.g. penicillin in pneumonia and thyroxine in hypothyroidism. But often such knowledge about the disease is not available and the natural history of the disease is such that the correct assessment of a new drug becomes difficult as in atherosclerosis, psychiatric disorders and rheumatoid arthritis. Clinical assessment is also difficult in case of drugs expected to produce subjective relief of symptoms such as pain, anorexia and sleeplessness. Hence, controlled clinical trials are absolutely necessary to prove or disprove the therapeutic usefulness of the drug as well as for comparing it with the previously established drug. Further evaluation is carried out in Phase 2 and Phase 3 studies.

Phase 2 **(Therapeutic exploration):** Further evaluation is carried out in patients to get more data on efficacy, metabolic activity and ADRs, and to determine final dose and dosage form of the drug.

Phase 3 **(Therapeutic confirmation)** : studies follow and include **controlled clinical trials.** A controlled clinical trial may be defined as one where a new drug therapy is compared with the previously established therapy or placebo therapy, under standardized conditions. It is designed to ensure that the comparisons made are as precise, as informative and as convincing as possible. Such studies are mainly conducted in two ways:

- ***Where drug is given to one group and results are compared with those in the other group (parallel design);*** and
- ***Where the drug therapy is alternated with control therapy (crossover design)*** either with an inert substitute or with the previously established drug, in the same patient.

In the first method, patients are allocated to various groups. In order to balance the groups and to avoid any bias, allocation should be carried out by **randomization** by a person who is completely unaware of the therapy allotted to an individual group. One of the groups gets the new treatment while the other receives control therapy in a similar form and in similar way as the drug under evaluation.

When both the evaluating clinician and the subject are unaware of the nature of the drug being administered, the procedure is called a **double blind controlled trial.** It effectively reduces the influence of extratherapeutic factors. In case any laboratory investigations are involved, the specimens should be submitted to the laboratory under a code number. The treatments are decoded only after the trial is over.

In the second method, the patient acts as his own control. This reduces the chances of erroneous results due to individual variation amongst the patients. Allocation of the patient to new therapy first or to control treatment first is decided by *randomization* and the evaluating clinician should not know the sequence of drug administration before completion of the trial. As in the first method such a study can be made a double blind controlled trial.

Finally, the results of such controlled trials at a few centres are confirmed by broad **multicentric clinical trials** at many centres before the drug is recommended for general use.

Phase 4 including Postmarketing Surveillance : Since ADRs continue to occur even after a new drug is released for general use in the community, careful **pharmacovigilance** must continue to avoid tragedies like that which occured following the use of thalidomide. For this purpose, pharmacovigilance centres (Chapter 1) are established in various parts of the country, to whom the various ADR observed in practice are reported by the physicians. In turn, these centres will alert the doctors about any unusual and previously unknown ADR with the drug. It is during this phase, that astute observation by practising doctors leads not only to early detection of adverse reactions but also to recognition of unanticipated additional benefits which result in additional, secondary uses for drugs e.g. ocular beta blockers for glaucoma and minoxidil for baldness.

Table 4.1 summarises the objectives of the animal studies and the clinical trial.

Table 4.1: Objectives of animal studies and clinical trial of a new drug

The objectives of animal studi(are to evaluate:

- Activity.
- Toxicity.
- Selectivity and specificity.
- Mechanism of action.
- Drug metabolism.

The objectives of a clinical trial are to establish:

- Safety (in Phases 1, 2, 3 and 4).
- Efficacy (in Phase 2).
- Therapeutic confirmation in a double blind controlled trial, especially vis-a-vis the established therapy (in Phase 3).
- Drug metabolism in humans (in Phases 1, 2 and 3).
- Safety, quality of life, unpredicted adverse reactions and new therapeutic applications during wide use in the community (Phase 4).

Role of Placebo:

Placebo is a Latin term which means "I may please you". The placebo effect is an effect attributable to a medicament as a procedure, and is not due to any specific pharmacodynamic property of the substance for the condition being treated. Placebo effect may be defined as "how the patient's perception of treatment influences his/her response". Placebos are used:

- ***During the clinical trial, to eliminate the possibility that the benefit of the drug is solely due to chance;*** and
- ***As therapeutic agents*** that work psychologically.

A placebo preparation is usually an inert substance like starch or lactose. However, occasionally it may be a drug that is active but in a different situation. In fact, even when an active drug is used, its placebo effect often comforts the patient much before the drug is effective. It is well known that the patient as well as his relatives get some immediate relief as soon as the doctor's medicine is administered, irrespective of its drug content. This is because of their faith in the doctor that things will go well in his hands.

Placebos can often produce relief of subjective symptoms associated with psychological disturbances. This includes relief from anxiety, headache, pain, insomnia and breathlessness. Hence, placebos are often employed in the treatment of certain diseases where the psychic element is suspected to be responsible for subjective symptoms. Objective responses such as increase or decrease in neutrophils and eosinophils may sometimes be seen with placebos.

When administered for its therapeutic effects, the placebo preparation :

- ***Must appear to be relevant to the illness.***
- ***Must be harmless***; and
- ***Should preferably conform to the patient's expectations.***

To be effective, the 'potency' of the preparation must be shown by some signs such as strong taste, a colourful capsule or a tablet of odd shape and sometimes even by obvious but harmless side effect like coloured urine.

During clinical trials, placebos are used to eliminate the effect of bias of the physician and the patient, particularly in evaluating a drug claimed to be effective in conditions such as bronchial asthma, angina pectoris, pain and psychiatric disorders. In such cases the placebo should be indistinguishable from the active medicament in physical properties like colour, smell, taste and dosage form.

Placebo effect may be modified by:

- ***Personality of the physician:*** Reassurance and optimistic outlook often achieve a better effect. "The doctor himself must inspire confidence. It is difficult to define this quality. It does not lie so much in what is said as in the doctor's shape and bearing, and in those instinctive signs whereby one animal unknowingly conveys its mood to another. Some have it and some do not. In this respect, the hospital specialist is in an easier position than the GP because he is backed by a temple of healing, which is clearly nearer the seat of power than a wayside shrine. Since few doctors are good enough actors to simulate the confidence they do not have, it often happens that one who is kind and credulous is a better healer than another who is informed and critical. Placebo reactions go faster when both parties have faith and in this respect knowledge is an inhibitor. It follows that anyone who wants to know whether a cure was due to a drug, and therefore, reproducible, would have to observe the ceremony conducted by sceptics",.
- ***Personality of the patient:*** Some individuals are amenable to suggestions. Such people are termed *placebo reactors*, and since a placebo acts by suggestion, they derive benefit from the use of placebos. Neurotics are great placebo reactors while depressed or psychotic subjects are usually resistant. Individuals who are of conservative, suspicious, or sceptical nature are not likely to benefit from placebos. Such negative reactors, on the contrary, may become worse as per their 'own expectations'. A strong negative reactor may even take a pride in saying that he or she is "allergic to all drugs".
- ***Form of administration:*** It is not surprising that the greatest placebo effect (as high as 81%) is achieved with injections. This may perhaps explain the preference for the use of injections by the practitioners! Colour, taste, presence or absence of stress are other factors which modify placebo effect.

Like active drugs, placebos can produce certain adverse subjective reactions such as drowsiness, headache, dryness of mouth, fatigue, insomnia, constipation, impotence, difficulty in concentrating and a 'drugged feeling'. An abstinence syndrome, which responds to injection of normal saline, has been described after prolonged placebo therapy.

Much of the routine treatment such as vitamins, tranquillisers and tonics, prescribed by the doctors often acts as a placebo for themselves too! Many physicians cannot "bear to think they are doing nothing; so they, like their patients, are willing to believe. They persuade themselves or are persuaded of the virtues of their treatment".

Interpretation of clinical results: After the completion of the clinical trial, the results are subjected to statistical analysis. If the difference between the two groups of treatment is so large that the probability of its occurrence simply by chance is less than 5 times in 100 ($p<0.05$), then the new drug is said to have produced a significant effect. It is necessary, however, to rule out all other possible explanations for such difference, before the verdict is accepted.

Various statistical designs have been suggested to ensure that the results obtained are as precise as possible without interference by other biological factors and individual bias; and there is no doubt that such statistical safeguards are essential. However, elaborate statistics cannot validate a poorly designed and executed clinical trial. Further, in a given study it is more important to know whether a new drug is significantly better than the older one or placebo in terms of its 'clinical effect' and not merely statistically. In fact, an effect whose reality is revealed only after elaborate statistics is hardly likely to be clinically important. **Statistical significance** and **Therapeutic significance** of results are not necessarily equivalent. Many times statistics would show 'a statistically significant difference', but it cannot tell whether such difference really matters in therapeutics. Thus, a drug may lower the plasma cholesterol concentration statistically but may not prevent myocardial infarction.

Most of the new drugs are not 'wonder drugs' and need proper clinical assessment. Unfortunately, because of various factors the quality of many clinical trials is far from satisfactory. As pointed out by the Lancet, there is no doubt that a prior design of the trial is important but "It is clearly not worth devoting such energy to trial design if the trained observer is not both trained and observing. After all, the controlled trial requires as much in 'clinical observation' as it does in design. No one should play at clinical trials". As pointed out by Parkhouse, "a good trial of a poor drug is a great deal better than no trial at all. It is infinitely better than a poor trial of a poor drug". Even the use of double blind technique does not guarantee valid results in an otherwise poorly designed and executed study.

Drug Assay

Assay is the estimation of the amount or the activity of an active principle in a unit quantity of the preparation. It can be:

- ***Chemical.***
- ***Biological;*** or
- ***Immunological.***

I **Chemical assay:** In this assay, the mass concentration of the active principle is estimated by means of a chemical method, e.g. the salicylates, sulfonamides, and many others. It is the most commonly used procedure. The useful techniques are spectrophotometry, fluorometry, gas chromatography, mass spectrometry and high pressure liquid chromatography.

II **Bioassay:** Bioassay is a measure of the concentration of the specific active ingredient in a sample of biological material and is performed by determining the amount of the unknown sample required to produce a defined effect on a suitable test animal or organ under standard conditions. Thus, bioassays can be performed on whole animals either singly or in groups and on isolated tissues or even cells.

Indications for bioassay:

(a) When the chemical composition is not known but the substance has a specific biological action e.g. long acting thyroid stimulator (LATS).

(b) When the chemical assay method is too complex or insensitive e.g. adrenaline and histamine can be bioassayed in microgram quantities.

(c) When drugs differ in composition but have the same pharmacological action e.g. the digitalis glycosides obtained from various sources; or

(d) When the active principle is unknown, cannot be isolated easily, e.g. peptide hormones.

Sensitivity and specificity make the bioassay a very important tool in pharmacology. In fact, it has proved an economic and convincing way of examining the presence of a number of endogenous compounds of physiological, pharmacological and toxicological importance such as hypothalamic factors, serotonin, prostaglandins, encephalins and EDRF.

International Unit (IU): Internationally agreed-upon standards are necessary to compare the *potency* (Chapter 2) of the various biologically assayed compounds in terms of their activity.

If it is not possible to purify chemically the substance to be bioassayed, a stable standard solution has to be employed for comparison. Standards for sera are held at the State Serum Institute, Copenhagen, the National Institute for Medical Research at Mill Hill, UK. and by the WHO. An International Unit is defined as a particular quantity of the standard preparation (one IU of tetanus antitoxin is 0.1547 mg. of a preparation held in Copenhagen).

Principles of bioassay

- The specific effect produced by the active principle to be bioassayed must be the same in all animal species.
- A certain quantity of a drug produces the same degree of pharmacological response in the same animal or animals of the same species, provided the other conditions remain constant e.g. adrenaline will always elicit the same degree of rise in BP when given in the same dose, in the same animal and under identical conditions.
- The reference standard must owe its activity to the principle for which the sample is being bioassayed.
- The activity assayed should be the activity of interest.
- Problems of individual variation must be minimized or taken into account.

It must be remembered that the bioassay may measure a different aspect of the same substance as compared to the chemical assay as in the case of testosterone and its metabolites.

Types of bioassay:

Indirect assays: If the potency of the sample is estimated by comparing the log dose response curve of the sample with a similar curve of the standard, the method is referred to as an indirect assay.

Ergot preparations, when injected in the white leghorn cock, produce vasoconstriction and this results in a bluish discoloration of the comb. The colour intensity varies with the dose and this effect may be employed for bioassay of crude ergot preparations by the indirect method.

Direct assay on several animals: In this method, the dose of the sample required to elicit a particular pharmacological effect (ED_{50} or LD_{50}) is measured e.g. death in guinea pigs. This dose is known as the 'tolerance' or 'threshold dose'. The ratio of the threshold dose of the sample to the threshold dose of the standard gives the relative potency of the sample in terms of the standard. To employ this method, the drug must produce clear-cut pharmacological effects, e.g. digitalis bioassay in guinea pigs.

Direct comparison on same tissues: In this method, the concentration of the unknown is determined by:

- ***Interpolation*** wherein a log dose response curve (Chapter 2) is plotted initially by using at least 4 submaximal concentrations of the standard. The concentration of the unknown is then read off the graph (Fig 2.4).
- ***Matching:*** A constant dose of the sample is bracketted by varying the dose of the standard, till an exact matching between the sample dose and a particular dose of the standard is achieved. This method, however, is rather inaccurate and it is difficult to estimate the margin of error; examples are histamine bioassay on the guinea pig ileum, posterior pituitary assay on the rat uterus.
- ***The four point assay*** which incorporates the principles of interpolation and matching and hence, is the most accurate of the three methods.

To avoid the influence of extraneous factors such as bias, inherent activity of the animal etc., on the bioassay, various techniques like cross-over designs (subjecting the 'control' and the 'sample' animal groups to the sample drug and the standard drug respectively) are employed. The results obtained are subjected to statistical analysis and the margin of error is calculated. Allowance must be made for this error when expressing the potency of the sample.

To be useful, the bioassay procedures must satisfy the following requirements:

- ***High sensitivity.***
- ***Specificity***, e.g. the ileum of the guinea pig contracts with both acetylcholine and histamine. The tissue, therefore, has to be atropinised for the bioassay of histamine.
- ***Reproducibility:*** The pharmacological response with the same dose should remain the same under identical conditions.
- ***Accuracy.***
- ***Stability:*** The animal or the tissue should remain 'bioassay fit' for a sufficiently long time.
- ***Easy availability of the animals.***

Table 4.2 lists some bioassays in animals, cells and micro-organisms.

Interestingly, clinical trials for assessing drug effects in humans involve similar principles as bioassays in animals.

Table 4.2: Certain important bioassays

- ***Whole animal:***

(a) Vasopressin : (i) Anaesthetized rat, rise in B.P. and (ii) Hydrated rat, reduction in the urine output.

(b) Estrogens : Ovariectomised female rat, vaginal cornification.

(c) Vitamin D : Rat, alleviation of the rachitic state.

(d) Insulin: Mice, hypoglycemic convulsions or death.

(e) d-tubocurarine: Rabbit, head drop due to paralytic relaxation of the skeletal muscles of the neck.

- ***Isolated tissue:***

(a) Acetylcholine: Frog, rectus muscle, contraction.

(b) Histamine: Guinea pig ileum, contraction.

(c) Adrenaline: Rat uterus in diestrus, relaxation.

(d) Oxytocin: Rat uterus estrogen primed, contraction.

(e) 5-HT : Gastric fundus contraction.

- ***Cells dispersed in a suitable medium:*** e.g. plasma LH can be measured by its ability to stimulate testosterone synthesis *in vitro* by isolated Leydig cells of the testes. Such an assay is the most advanced type of bioassay used in research.
- ***Micro-organisms***: Vitamin B_{12} : growth of *Euglena gracilis.*

Biostandardization: Comparison and adjustment of the strength of the sample with that of the standard under controlled condi¬tions is termed as biostandardization. This is necessary to regulate the doses of crude extract.

III **Immunoassay:** Many immunological methods have been developed to estimate hormones and drugs. One of the widely used method is radioimmunoassay (RIA). Unlike the bioassay *in vivo* or *in vitro*, the radio-immunoassay is a physico-chemical assay and depends upon the reaction between an antigen (say hormonal) and its specific antibody in the test tube. The antibodies used are generally obtained from the sera of animals, such as rabbits, which have been previously immunized by repeated injections of the hormone (antigen). Such antibodies raised in animals are polyclonal. Monoclonal antibodies prepared by the hybridoma technique give superior immunoassays. The principle of the radio-immunoassay can be summarized by a set of competing reactions in a mixture containing radiolabelled hormone, antibody and unlabelled hormone (either standard or unknown).

Radioiodine labelled hormone H* exists as 'unbound' i.e. free (F) or 'bound' (B) to the antibody. This binding of the labelled hormone is competitively inhibited by the unlabelled hormone H. Hence, the per cent binding of labelled hormone or alternatively B/F ratio diminishes progressively as the concentration of the unlabelled hormone increases. (Fig. 4.1).

Labelled hormone H* (Free)	+	Specific antibody Ab	→ ←	(H*Ab) (Bound)
		+		
		Unlabelled hormone		
		H		
		↑↓		
		(H.Ab)		

Fig. 4.1 : Radioimmunoassay, principles

A standard curve is obtained by plotting B/F ratios against known concentrations of unlabelled hormone in a set of standards prepared for the assay. The biological material (plasma) containing an unknown quantity of the unlabelled hormone is allowed to react with the mixture of labelled hormone and the antibody under the same set of conditions as the standards. The B/F ratio is obtained and the concentration of the unlabelled hormone in the plasma is read off the standard curve (Fig. 4.2). Using this principle, plasma concentration of various hormones, other biological substances and drugs can be measured easily and accurately.

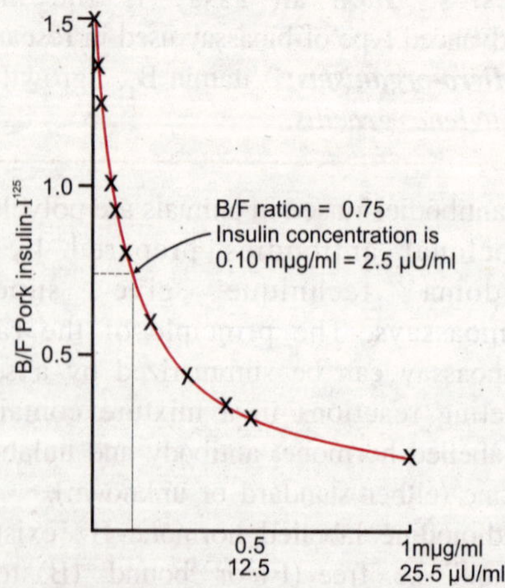

Fig 4.2 : A standard curve for radio-immunoassay of insulin (Reproduced, with permission, from Diabetes Mellitus: Theory and Practice, by M. Ellenberg & H. Rifkin, 1970, McGraw-Hill Book Co., N.Y.)

Table 4.3: Symbols for fractions of a gramme

Fraction	Prefix of g.	Symbol
10^{-3}	milli	mg
10^{-6}	micro	µg
10^{-9}	nano	ng
10^{-12}	pico	pg
10^{-15}	femto	fg
10^{-18}	atto	ag

It is possible to measure minute quantities of circulating hormones and other biologically active substances by the radio-immunoassay and certain symbols are commonly used to express the small quantities (Table 4.3).

Immunologic methods measure all the immunologically active components, some of which may be less active biologically e.g. insulin (Chpater 63) or LH (Chapter 65). Further, the reliability of the results depends largely on the specificity of the antiserum (antibody). When the results of such an assay differ from those obtained by the biological assay, the latter should not be ignored.

Radio-receptor assays embodying the principles of both bioassay and radioimmunoassay are more sensitive and more specific than the radioimmunoassays.

Labelled antibody (instead of labelled antigen) is used in **immunoradiometric assays** (IRMA). They are more specific and more sensitive than RIAs. Such assays are commonly used to measure protein hormones (e.g. TSH, Chapter 62) in the serum.

Enzyme Linked Immunosorbent Assays (ELISA), in which enzymes such as alkaline phosphatase and penicillinase are used in place of radioactive iodine to label the ligands, are widely used to assay hormones (e.g. hCG, Chapter 63) and other substances.

More sensitive and specific methods of measuring hormones in the biological materials (chemilluminescence assay and fluoroimmunoassay) are also now available.

SECTION II
Drugs Acting on the Central Nervous System

General Considerations 5

Anatomically, the nervous system in higher animals can be divided into:

- ***The central nervous system*** (CNS); and
- ***The peripheral nervous system*** consisting of somatic and autonomic nerve fibres.

The CNS is not only concerned with the regulation of specialized functions like circulation, digestion and respiration but it also is responsible for the psychic processes such as feeling, attitude, thoughts and memory. The ability to think logically, to learn from past experiences and to communicate appropriately are the unique qualities of man and can be attributed to the development of the highly specialized CNS.

Both the CNS and peripheral nervous system are analogous to an elaborate system of telegraphy wherein numerous wires and connections in theform of neurons and synapses bring in information from both internal and external sources. This information is received, 'decoded', decisions are made by various centres in CNS and instructions are sent out to various peripheral tissues to produce appropriate responses such as:

- ***Psychic***, as manifested by change in emotions, thought and attitude.
- ***Somatic***, as demonstrated by various types of body movements; and
- ***Autonomic***, as indicated by changes in respiration, circulation and visceral functions.

The major anatomical divisions of the CNS are the cerebrum, the cerebellum, the brain stem and the spinal cord. Functionally, it consists of billions of neurons organized to form several neuronal systems with nuclei and their tracts, each concerned with certain specialized functions such as motor activity, perception and regulation of various body functions. These systems, however, are interdependent and a disturbance in one may produce repercussions in other systems as well. Further, one area may modify or control more than one function.

When the CNS is exposed to the action of depressant drugs, the recently acquired or phylogenetically newer functions such as fine control of movements, association and memory are affected before those controlling respiration and circulation which are primitive and basic. The depression thus starts from the cortex and proceeding through the diencephalon, the midbrain and the spinal cord, affects the vital medullary centres last. This *irregularly descending paralysis* is a built-in safety mechanism which conserves the functions essential for life at the cost of more sophisticated and dispensable functions. The recovery from the depressant effect occurs in the reverse order.

The physiological functions attributed to various parts of the CNS are shown in Table 5.1. There is no absolute control of a particular function vested in a given area of the CNS and the ultimate modulation of a function is the result of interaction among several components.

Table 5.1 : Functions of various parts of central nervous system

Part of CNS	Functions attributed
Cerebral cortex	Higher functions like judgement, memory, fine voluntary movements, fine pain, tactile discrimination and temperature, special senses like vision, smell and hearing. It also acts as an important coordinator and exerts inhibitory control over lower centres.
Frontal lobes	Thinking, integration of emotional behaviour.
Limbic system	Integrates emotional state with motor and visceral activities.
Basal ganglia	Extrapyramidal control of skeletal muscle tone, co-ordination of posture. Lesions produce tremors and rigidity in flexion.
Thalamus	Relay centre for sensory pathways to cortex. Conscious appreciation of pain, temperature and crude touch sensations. Exerts regulatory control over visceral functions.
Hypothalamus	Control of the autonomic nervous system, control of adenohypophysis. Important centre for integration of eating, drinking, sexual behaviour, temperature regulation, sleep, circadian rhythms and other vegetative functions.
Cerebellum	Control of vestibular function and body posture.
Reticular formation	Sleep-wakefulness cycle, control of blood pressure, respiration, swallowing, vomiting; transmission of crude pain, voluntary muscle tone and posture; control of upper motor neurons.
Spinal cord	Reflex movements, control of muscle tone (particularly the red muscles) and the upper and the lower motor neurons through pre-synaptic and post-synaptic inhibition.

The limbic system consists of the hippocampus, the amygdaloid complex, the septum, the hypothalamus, the olfactory and pyriform lobes, the basal ganglia, and a part of the thalamus; this is also sometimes called the visceral brain.

The reticular formation is a hetero¬genous mass of cell bodies enmeshed in a network of dendrites and axons located in the central core of the medulla, pons and midbrain. It is a diffuse multisynaptic system. Caudally it is continuous with the spinal gray matter while rostrally it disappears into subcortical nuclei, particularly of the thalamus. The reticular formation is intimately concerned with transmission of crude pain and other sensations, state of consciousness, control of muscle tone and posture and such vital functions as respiration and circulation.

A complex, interrelated group of pathways coursing through the reticular formation have been termed as **reticular activating system**. All the sensory information courses through the reticular formation. The latter arouses the cerebral cortex. It is essential for the regulation of sleep and wakefulness and for coordination of gaze and eye movements. It has the major monoamine containing neurons in the brain.

Drugs act on the CNS :

- ***Directly*** on neurons and modify the neuronal functions.
- ***Reflexly*** by sending afferent impulses to the CNS via the chemoreceptors, baroreceptors and peripheral nerves, thereby eliciting psychic, somatic or visceral responses; and
- ***By affecting the nutrition and oxygen supply of the CNS*** by altering its blood supply or affecting its metabolism e.g. by causing hypoglycemia or ammonia intoxication.

To reach the CNS, a drug must have a high lipid solubility (high oil/water partition coefficient) or a specialized transport mechanism. Ionized drugs normally cannot penetrate into the CNS. Hence the existence of a 'blood-brain barrier' has been postulated.

The condition of the meninges, however, can alter to a certain extent the penetrability of drugs into the CNS. Thus, in the presence of meningeal inflammation (meningitis) considerable amount of penicillin can cross the blood-brain barrier, which is not so in a healthy individual.

Types of drug action: Drugs may either stimulate or depress the CNS. Excessive stimulation of the CNS may produce convulsions, which could be cortical, medullary or spinal in origin. In therapeutic doses, the stimulant action is usually selective (confined to specific areas of the CNS) whereas toxic doses may cause convulsions. Excessive CNS stimulation is followed by its depression.

Suppression of inhibitory areas in the CNS may result in an apparent stimulation. Thus, ethyl alcohol eliminates the inhibitory control exerted by the higher cortical centres and leads to garrulousness and hilarity.

Depression or inhibition of the CNS may be achieved through more than one mechanism. The CNS contains a number of inhibitory and excitatory chemical transmitters. Inhibition achieved as a result of hyperpolarization of the postsynaptic membrane by the active release of an inhibitory transmitter is termed the **postsynaptic** inhibition, while inhibition achieved by reduction in the quantum of the excitatory transmitter released in the synaptic cleft is termed **presynaptic** inhibition. An example of postsynaptic inhibition is that exerted by the Renshaw cells of the spinal cord on the lower motor neurons. Renshaw cells probably exert this inhibitory control by the release of an inhibitory neurohumoral transmitter.

Depression could be **non-selective** (general) or **selective** (localized), restricted to certain areas within the CNS. Thus, depressants like general anaesthetics and barbiturates are non-selective in action, while drugs like phenytoin sodium and chlorpromazine exert more selective actions. However, a specific depressant may produce un¬usual excitation under certain circumstances. Thus, barbiturates may induce anxiety and apprehension when employed in the presence of pain, and tranquillizers like chlorpromazine may unmask epilepsy.

The action of the selective CNS depressants may also be modified by the internal environment; the amount of a general anaesthetic required to anaesthetize a highly excited subject is more than that required in a normal person. Although selectivity of action may be remarkable, a drug normally affects several CNS functions to varying degrees, which could cause unwanted side effects.

Neurochemical transmission in the nervous system: Because communication within the mammalian nervous system is almost exclusively, through chemical messengers, neurosecretion is a fundamental property of all neurons. A *neurosecretion* is a chemical released at the nerve terminals; those released into the blood circulation are called *neurohormones* e.g. hypothalamic hormones released into the hypothalamopituitary portal circulation. There are three processes occurring in connection with impulse transmission within the nervous system:

- ***Neurotransmission.***
- ***Neuromediation;*** and
- ***Neuromodulation.***

Neurotransmission is the process by which an impulse is transmitted across a synapse between two neurons. **Neurotransmitters (NT)** are released into the synaptic cleft and either stimulate or inhibit the post-synaptic neuron. A substance must satisfy certain criteria in order to be accepted as a NT:

- It must be present in the neurons and presynaptic nerve endings and should have a discrete rather than a uniform pattern of distribution.
- It must be released from the presynaptic nerve terminals.
- Local concentration of the substance should be related to the function of the neuronal structure, and fluctuations in its concentration should take place in response to the functional changes in the neuron.
- Enzymatic mechanisms capable of synthesizing and degrading the the substance should be present within the neurons.
- Clearly demonstrable effects should be obtained by increasing or decreasing the local

concentration of such substance in the CNS. When applied to the post-synaptic cell body, the substance should mimic the action of the synaptically released chemical transmitter; and

- Known blocking agents of this substance should produce demonstrable effects by prevening the access of the transmitter to the specific receptor site.

Neuromediation implies the elicitation of the post-synaptic responses to the released NTs through second messangers (neuromediators) such as cAMP, cGMP and inositol phosphate (Chapter 2).

Neuromodulation is a less clearly defined process than neuro- transmission and is thought to occur at pre- and post-synaptic levels to regulate the release of NTs, modulate the post-synaptic excitability or induce long-term changes by affecting gene transcription. Neuromodulators arise from neurons as well as from the non-neuronal cells. They are not stored or released like the NTs. They act with a longer latency of action, and have a longer duration of action. Examples are adenosine, prostaglandins and nitric oxide.

CNS neurotransmitters: The CNS has both **excitatory** and **inhibitory** chemical transmitters. They are :

- ***Amines.***
- ***Amino acids;*** and
- ***Peptides.***

Some of these NTs are listed in Table 5.2. Of these, GABA and glycine are inhibitory transmitters whereas dopamine is selectively either stimulatory or inhibitory at different synaptic sites. Many drugs which modify the functions of the CNS affect the concentration of one or more of them in the central as well as the peripheral nervous system. The bodies of the nerve cells in the CNS are densely covered by synapses and it is probable that they have more than one transmitter acting on their surface. For details, see Chapters 16 and 23.

Several endogenous peptides have been discovered in the brain, e.g. angiotensin, endorphins, vasopressin, endocrine peptides and gut peptides. They regulate neuronal function by themselves or in concert with other NT.

Gamma amino butyric acid (GABA): This is a major inhibitory amino acid NT in the brain; its synthesis from glutamate is catalysed by the enzyme glutamic acid decarboxylase. It binds to either GABA-A or GABA-B receptor following its release from the presynaptic vesicles. GABA-A receptor is part of a complex that surrounds and regulates a chloride ion channel (ionotropic receptor). Most GABA receptors are composed of á, ß and γ subunits. Receptors composed of á and ß subunits produce functional GABA-A receptors that respond to barbiturates but not to benzodiazepines. Co-assembly with γ subunits is necessary for assembly of benzodiazepine receptors. In the absence of GABA, benzodiazepines have no effect on GABA-A receptor function. GABA-B receptor is a metabotropic receptor; its activation by the drug baclofen causes muscle relaxation.

Glutamate and aspartate (Excitatory Amino Acids, EAA): These amino acids, present in high concentration in various parts of the brain, are believed to play an important role as excitatory NT throughout the CNS. Glutamate released from the presynaptic terminals binds to several glutamate receptor subtypes; their activation increases the conductance of Na^+ and Ca^{++} into the cells, leading to depolarization (**ionotropic glutamate receptors**); or it stimulates phoshphatidyl inositol turnover (**metabotropic glutamate receptors**). Two ionotropic glutamate receptors are (a) N-methyl-D-aspartate (NMDA) receptors; and (b) non-NMDA (a-amino-3 hydroxy–5-methyl-4-isoxazole propionic acid, AMPA) receptors. Non-NMDA receptors mediate the fast excitatory neurotransmission associated with excitatory postsynaptic potentials at glutamatergic synapses. The activation of NMDA receptors is associated with long term potentiation (LTP), a prolonged increase in the size of a postsynaptic response to a presynaptic stimulus. EAA are believed to be involved in brain processes such as learning, memory and thinking; and their concentration is

Table 5.2: Some neurotransmitters found in the nervous system

Name	Distribution	Effects
• Amines		
Acetylcholine (ACh)	Widely distributed in almost all regions of CNS, predominantly in cerebral cortex, ascending reticular system, cerebellum and spinal cord.	Both excitatory and inhibitory in nature. Central effects can be blocked by atropine.
Noradrenaline (NA)	High concentration in the hypothalamus, limbic system and reticular formation in the brain stem.	Both excitation and inhibition in the brain stem.
Dopamine (DA)	Mainly in the basal ganglia, to some extent in the median eminence of hypothalamus, adenohypophysis and frontal cortex.	Predominantly inhibitory action. Deficiency causes extrapyramidal disturbances.
5-Hydroxytryptamine (5-HT, serotonin)	Similar to noradrenaline. Extends into the cerebral cortex, raphe nucleus and hippocampal areas.	Both excitatory and inhibitory effects.
Histamine (H)	Distribution similar to noradrenaline and 5-HT but irregular.	Mainly inhibitory effects. Functions uncertain.
• Amino acids		
L-glutamic acid and aspartic acid (EAA)	Widely distributed in CNS and spinal cord	Excitatory effects.
Gamma-aminobutyric acid (GABA), glycine	GABA in CNS; glycine mainly in the spinal cord and brain stem.	Inhibitory effects in brain and spinal cord.
• Peptides		
Substance P	Hypothalamus, thalamus, basal ganglia; the dorsal column and dorsal roots of the spinal cord; enteric nervous system (ENS)	Excitatory
Cholecystokinin	Brain (cortex, hippocampus, limbic system and hypothalamus), pancreas	Inhibits eating and stimulates oxytocin release.

decreased in patients with Huntington's chorea and Alzheimer's disease. Very high concentrations of glutamate can cause neuronal cell death.

Regulation of neurotransmitter (NT) release: NT-containing vesicles are localised at specialised release sites or active zones on the presynaptic membrane, in a state of readiness to release the NT which acts on the receptor. Neurons communicate with each other through the release of NTs. NT release is influenced by many factors which allow the strength of synaptic transmission to be constantly modulated. Normally, highly localised Ca^{++} influx acts as a stimulus to the rapid release of the NT. In this respect, **presynaptic receptors** play an important role (Fig 5.1). Activation of the presynaptic receptors closes a feedback loop which results in either enhancement or inhibition of the NT release. These receptors are called **autoreceptors.**

Presynaptic receptors are of several types, including members of both G protein linked (**metabotropic**) and multiunit ion channel (**ionotropic**) types. Activation of both types can

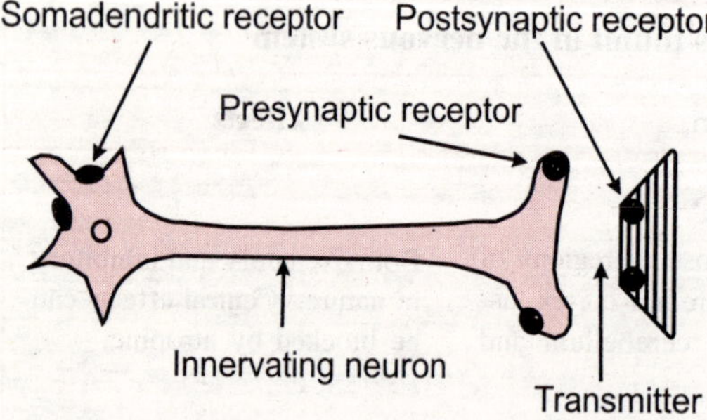

Fig. 5.1 : Pre and Postsynaptic receptors

regulate NT release in different situations. Activation of the G protein linked receptors usually leads to a reduction in evoked NT release, thereby closing a negative feedback loop. Activation of the ionotropic receptors can enhance the release of NT as a result of their ability to raise the concentration of calcium ions in the terminals directly. Many transmitters use several of these mechanisms.

The presynaptic terminals may also have receptors responding to NTs released from other neurons. Activation of these receptors, **hetero-receptors**, can also influence the NT release. Presynaptic receptors are thus important from the neurophysiological point of view and as potential targets for therapeutic agents.

Neurotrophic factors: These neuropeptides, produced by neurons, astrocytes, microglia, and inflammatory/immune cells, assist in repairing tissue damage.

Basis of drug action: Treatable conditions due to neurotransmitter disorders could be due to either "too much" or "too little" neurotransmitter. Drugs may:

- ***Modify the synthesis, storage, release or metabolism of the inhibitory or excitatory neurochemical transmitters.*** Thus, monoamine oxidase inhibitors act as antidepressants by inhibiting the degradation of noradrena¬line by the enzyme monoamine oxidase.
- ***Act by modifying ionic fluxes across the cell membrane***, e.g. phenytoin sodium.
- ***Specifically act as antagonists*** by acting at post-synaptic receptors, directly or by antagonizing the effects of endogenous neurotransmitters, e.g. chlorpromazine.
- ***Act as neuromodulators***; or
- ***Modify the energy supply of the CNS.*** This may be achieved by local inhibition of the synthesis of high energy phosphate bonds (barbiturates), by inhibition of action of certain enzymes involved in cellular respiration and energy processes or by altering the availability of the substrate for energy production.

Under certain circumstances, the central and the peripheral effects of a drug may be antagonistic. Atropine in small doses stimulates the central vagal nucleus and induces bradycardia while the therapeutic doses usually induce tachycardia by peripheral cholinergic blockade.

Methods of investigation: In a broad screening programme, initially, overall drug effects like CNS stimulation and depression are investigated in small animals. The tests used for this purpose include the effect of drugs on consciousness, righting reflex and the motor response as gauged by the patellar reflex. A variety of drugs may evoke a similar response with a particular test. For example, all the CNS depressants are capable of producing a loss of righting reflex, when administered in a sufficiently large dose, and such a loss can also be produced by the peripherally acting skeletal muscle relaxants like d-tubocurarine. Following these preliminary investigations, specialized properties like analgesic, hypnotic and anticonvulsant effects are studied with the help of more sophisticated techniques. The properties of cellular response to drugs can be studied electrophysiologically by recordings from a single cell and highly localized drug administration (Microiontophoresis). However, in many cases, the complexity of the system and lack of experimental analogy to human pathological conditions preclude clear conclusions. Certain latitude, therefore, must be allowed for critical correction of current concepts, even those which at the moment may appear quite adequate and sound.

Aliphatic Alcohols

6

Consumption of alcohol in one form or another is increasing all over the world, sometimes for its medical use but often for its pleasurable, stress relieving and blissful effects on the mind/mood. In doing so, alcohol has become the major drug of abuse. Aliphatic alcohols are hydroxy (OH) derivatives of the aliphatic hydrocarbons. They contain one, two or more OH groups and are designated as

- ***Monohydroxy*** e.g. ethyl, methyl, propyl alcohols.
- ***Dihydroxy***, also called as glycols due to the sweet taste, e.g. ethylene glycol, propylene glycol.
- ***Trihydroxy***, e.g. glycerol or glycerine.
- ***Polyhydroxy*** e.g. mannitol, sorbitol.

Only ethyl alcohol is commonly consumed. Glycerol is released during the digestion of fat.

ETHYL ALCOHOL (Ethanol): This is the main constituent of alcoholic beverages and is obtained by fermentation of sugars by yeast. The alcohol is separated by simple distillation. It is a colourless, volatile and inflammable liquid. Neutral spirit contains 90-95% alcohol by volume. Wines containing more than 16% of alcohol are prepared by fortification with neutral spirit. The alcohol content of various beverages varies between 4-55% by volume. Stronger preparations are called spirits. Beer contains 4-6% (v/v) of alcohol.

Pharmacological actions : Applied locally, it evaporates quickly, has a cooling and refreshing effect, and is used for reducing the temperature in fevers. Eau-de-cologne and after-shave lotion are other examples of cosmetic preparations used for their cooling effect. In concentrations of 40-50%, it has a rubifacient and mild irritant action. Higher concentrations denature proteins by partial precipitation and dehydration; in such concentrations it acts as an astringent and germicidal. Alcohol in the concentration of 70% by weight acts as an antiseptic; the action is seen only against vegetative forms of organisms; spores are resistant (Chapter 66). Concentrated alcohol, if injected, produces tissue destruction.

Gastrointestinal tract : Taken orally, it gives a local feeling of warmth and increases the salivary secretion probably by reflex action. It has an irritant action on the gastric mucousa and enjoys reputation as an appetizer; 50 ml. of 7-10% alcohol increases the gastric secretion, by releasing histamine and gastrin from the gastric antrum, in addition to its psychic and local irritant effects. Concentrations above 15% inhibit both gastric motility and secretion, and this effect may persist for many hours. Concentrations above 20% reduce the enzymatic activity of the gastric and the intestinal juices. Concentrations of 40% and over have a direct toxic effect on gastric mucosa and may precipitate gastritis, giving rise to pain, nausea, vomiting and other symptoms. Many chronic alcoholics suffer from gastritis and chronic achlorhydria. *The irritant effect of alcohol on the gastric mucosa is accentuated by aspirin and other NSAIDs* (Chapter 11) *which inhibit the local synthesis of prostaglandins (PG).* Alcohol is frequently the cause with gastro-esophageal reflux disease (GERD) and even esophageal cancer.

Central nervous system: Ethanol is primarily a CNS depressant and acts by enhancing the inhibitory GABA-A receptor activity and inhibiting the excitatory NMDA receptors, the normal agonist of which is the excitatory glutamate. It also affects the functioning of the other receptors such as those for dopamine, 5-HT_3, noradrenaline and endorphin. Although it was thought that alcohol acts by dissolving the cell membrane lipid, it is now believed that proteins are the primary site of its actions.

(a) The pleasurable (**euphoric**) effects are mediated by a dopaminergic pathway that projects from the ventral, tegmental area to the hypothalamic nucleus accumbens. It is believed that other pleasure-giving activities such as eating, sex and consumption of other substances of abuse (e.g. opium, cannabis) also act through this *central dopamine reward system.*

Craving defined as the conscious desire to drink alcohol has been linked to dopaminergic, 5-HTergic and opioid systems that mediate the reinforcement and to the GABAergic, glutamatergic and noradrenergic systems that mediate the withdrawal.

(b) Long term exposure to alcohol brings about adaptive changes in the neuronal systems including downregulation of the inhibitory neuronal GABA receptors and upregulation of the excitatory glutamatergic receptors, thus increasing the central noradrenaline activity.

(c) Sudden withdrawal of alcohol causes excitation and hyperactivity of the CNS.

Normally, man exercises inhibitions in order to live a disciplined life as desired by the society. Alcohol removes these inhibitions and thus diminishes such processes as hesitation, caution and self-criticism. The pattern of behaviour then depends on the environment and the basic personality of the individual. Initially, it produces euphoria (feeling of well-being). Later, under its influence, mood swings and uncontrolled emotional outbursts are common; the individual may do silly and harmless antics but sometimes he can become vicious and anti-social, or reckless. Alcohol is thus incriminated in one out of five crimes of violence.

This initial effect is due to a depression of the reticular activating system. The cortex is thus released from the integrating control or inhibitions required for purposeful activity.

Alcohol reduces visual acuity and interferes with muscular co-ordination even in small doses. It impairs the ability of the brain to co-ordinate motor activity such as typing, standing and hand steadiness. It lengthens the reaction time for both visual and auditory stimuli; in a mildly intoxicated person the reaction time may be lengthened by 10-15 per cent. Hence, *even moderate drinking is considered dangerous to public and individual safety.* This is more so if the individual is already taking some other CNS depressants like a sedative or a tranquillizer.

Although it is not an analgesic, it alters the patient's reaction to pain from one of concern to one of relative detachment.

With increasing consumption, there occur difficulty in speech, unsteadiness of gait and complete loss of self control.

Large quantities ultimately cause unconsciousness. Respiration becomes slow and stertorous, the face becomes pale and cyanotic and the BP falls. Death occurs due to medullary depression, mainly the respiratory centre. Some of the CNS effects of alcoholic beverages consumed in large quantities are probably due to substances (ethyl acetate, isoamyl alcohol and butanol) other than ethanol present in these beverages. In epileptics, alcohol may precipitate convulsions. *Chronic alcohol abuse causes shrinking of the brain by its neurotoxic action.*

Cardiovascular system : Epidemiological evidence has been touted as suggesting that drinking wine may have a cardioprotective effect due to elevation of HDL cholesterol level and inhibition of platelet activation. However, *there is no substantive evidence that alcohol reduces the incidence of coronary heart disease.* Usefulness of alcohol as a coronary vasodilator has been overrated. Alcohol may relieve anginal pain but that is more likely due its central action. The false sense of well being induced by alcohol may prompt the patient to ignore the warning given by the chest pain, and then he is likely to get into further trouble.

Regular consumption of alcohol may be associated with hypertension. *Even small amounts of alcohol depress the myocardial function in patients with preexisting heart disease.* Alcohol affects the conduction system of the heart and may precipitate arrhythmias. Further, alcoholism is an important causative factor in cardiomyopathy and stroke.

In view of the above, *it is not justifiable to advise/encourage abstainers to start consuming alcohol as a protective against the development of CHD; nor to prescribe it as a coronary vasodilator in patients with preexisting CHD.*

Alcohol in moderate amounts dilates skin vessels by depressing the vasomotor centre, resulting in flushing and feeling of warmth. This effect prevents normal cutaneous vasoconstriction on exposure to cold. Hence, it may be harmful to take alcohol for warming up in cold weather as the body would lose more heat.

Taken in concentrated form (Brandy 20-30 ml.) alcohol probably stimulates the vital medullary centres reflexly by irritating the pharyngeal mucosa, resulting in a slight rise in BP, tachycardia and an increase in the cardiac output. Hence, it is used as a household remedy for fainting attacks.

Liver : Ethanol causes dose-related hepatotoxicity. The common effects are fatty infiltration and hepatomegaly. This results in:

- ***Impaired gluconeogenesis.***
- ***Glycogen depletion.***
- ***Reduced synthesis of albumin and transferrin.***
- ***Diminished fatty acid oxidation***; and
- ***Increased synthesis of VLDL, with consequent hypertriglyceridemia.***

Acute alcohol ingestion inhibits the hepatic microsomal CYP450 enzyme systems whereas **chronic ingestion induces** them with resultant increase in the rate of metabolism of many drugs such as phenobarbitone, warfarin and steroids. However, alcohol itself is metabolically degraded by alcohol-inducible CYP450 system to a trivial extent. It is primarily metabolized by cytosolic and mitochondrial oxidative enzymes.

Clinically, hypoglycemia and hepatomegaly are the two important manifestations. Hypoglycemia is liable to occur in people who ingest large quantities of alcohol but eat poorly, particularly if they are on insulin or sulfonylurea drugs. If severe, it can cause irreversible brain damage. The hepatomegaly may be:

- ***Simple hepatomegaly with normal hepatic architecture;*** or
- ***Due to fatty degeneration, alcoholic hepatitis, cirrhosis or hepatoma.***

Alcoholic damage is a direct effect of alcohol on the liver and it is doubtful if a high protein diet protects the liver from the ravages of alcohol. However, it takes many years of heavy drinking to produce cirrhosis. Elevated serum level of gamma glutamyl transpeptidase (GGTP) is the most sensitive index of alcoholic liver disease.

Kidney: Alcohol causes diuresis due to decreased tubular reabsorption of water following inhibition of ADH release. It increases the excretion of magnesium and calcium.

Skeletal muscle: Ethanol causes a decrease in muscle strength and irreversible damage to muscle tissue.

Teratogenic effects: Drinking during pregnancy can cause fetal damage. The fetus has been described to have "characteristic facial appearance, microcephaly, growth retardation, mental deficiency and an increase in the frequency of major abnormalities" **(the fetal alcohol syndrome)**. *Even moderate alcohol consumption during pregnancy increases the risk of spontaneous abortion and low birth weight.*

Miscellaneous: Alcohol has an erroneous reputation as a sexual stimulant (aphrodisiac). The feeling of false confidence produced by the loss of inhibitory control is probably responsible for that. But as Shakespeare correctly noted in 'Macbeth', "Lechery, Sir, it provoketh and unprovoketh; it provoketh the desire, but it taketh away the performance". In fact, it significantly depresses the sexual responsiveness. Further, in men, chronic alcohol ingestion causes reduction in plasma testosterone levels, impotence, sterility and gynecomastia. It may also produce prostatic congestion causing acute urinary retention.

Chronic alcohol use is associated with various types of anemia, macrocytic anemia being common. It may also cause leucopenia, decrease in T cells, mutagenesis and decrease in IgG production. Chronic alcoholics may also suffer from hyperlipidemia, hyperuricemia, hypomagnesemia and pancreatitis.

By stimulating ACTH secretion, chronic ingestion of large doses can lead to 'pseudo Cushing's syndrome'.

Absorption, fate and excretion: Ethyl alcohol is absorbed very rapidly from the stomach, duodenum and small intestine, 50% within 15 minutes and 100% within 1-2 hours. The absorption is delayed by the presence of food in the stomach. After ingestion, alcohol is partly metabolized by gastric and hepatic alcohol dehydrogenase (AD) enzyme. By inhibiting this enzyme, aspirin increases the bioavailability of alcohol. It is distributed throughout body water and is stored in all tissues; it diffuses back into the blood when blood level falls.

In the lungs, alcohol passes from blood to breath, which smells of alcohol. The ratio of concentrations of alcohol in blood and alveolar air is constant and is about 2,100:1. Because of this high ratio, it is difficult to wash out blood alcohol by artificial ventilation in case of acute alcohol poisoning.

Over 90 per cent of alcohol is metabolized in the liver by the non-microsomal, cytosolic enzymes. The rest is mostly excreted by the kidneys and lungs. Alcohol dehydrogenase (AD) oxidises alcohol to acetaldehyde which is converted to acetate by aldehyde dehydrogenase. The last is oxidized to carbon dioxide and water by liver and other tissues.

$$CH_3CH_2OH + NAD \xrightarrow{(1)} CH_3CHO + NADH + H^+$$

$$CH_3CHO \xrightarrow{(2)} \text{Acetate} \xrightarrow{(3)} CO_2 + H_2O + \text{Energy}$$

(1) = Alcohol dehydrogenase

(2) = Aldehyde dehydrogenase

(3) = Enters Kreb's cycle as acetyl Coenzyme A

Fig. 6.1 : Metabolism of ethyl alcohol

At very low concentrations, alcohol is metabolized by First Order Kinetics (Chapter 1); at higher concentrations (>10 mg/dl) it is metabolized at a constant rate which is independent of blood alcohol concentration (Zero Order Kinetics) but is proportional to the body weight and probably to liver weight. As NAD is consumed during the metabolic degradation of alcohol, the limited availability of hepatic NAD sets the upper limit on the rate of alcohol metabolism, and changes the first order kinetics to zero order kinetics.

Is alcohol a food? One gramme of alcohol gives 7.1 calories in the form of acetate. Although it can spare carbohydrates, alcohol is not a food, because it has no protein, vitamin or any other nutrients ('empty calories'). Chronic alcoholics who do not eat properly suffer from nutritional deficiencies.

Therapeutic uses of ethyl alcohol : It is a solvent for various active ingredients. It is sometimes used :

- ***In the symptomatic treatment of fever*** because of its cooling effect on skin.
- ***In the prevention of bed sores*** as it hardens the skin.
- ***As an antiseptic*** (70%)
- ***As an appetizer*** *(10%).*
- ***In methyl alcohol poisoning*** (see later).
- ***To wash out phenol in cases of accidental skin contamination;*** and
- ***By local injection to destroy a nerve*** as in trigeminal neuralgia.

Acute Alcohol Intoxication

Chemical analysis of blood and urine can

Table 6.1: Correlation of blood alcohol levels (BAL) with behavioural changes

Blood concentration mg. per 100 ml.	Behavioural changes	Interpretation
<50	Not significant	Not under the influence of alcohol but may affect the reaction time.
50-100	Feeling of exaltation, talkativeness	Possibly under the influence
100-200	Emotionally unstable, motor incoordination, nystagmus	Probably under the influence
200-300	Staggering, loss of self control	Definitely under the influence
300-400	Stupor-dead drunk	Grossly intoxicated
400-500	Coma, anaesthetic effect	
>500	Respiratory arrest and death	

give some idea about the degree of intoxication in an individual who has ingested alcohol (Table 6.1). *However, it is difficult to associate a particular blood alcohol concentration with a specific degree of impairment. Consumption of alcohol before driving is hazardous.*

After death, the degradation of alcohol ceases and the brain and blood levels of alcohol remain constant for sometime. Hence, post-mortem samples of blood can give reliable estimates about the degree of intoxication at the time of death. Approximately 600 ml. of pure alcohol can produce a fatal effect in an individual of 70 kg. body weight. Coma in an acute alcoholic bout may be due to the CNS depressant effect of alcohol, head injury or severe hypoglycemia which is especially likely to occur in fasting individuals. Hypomagnesemia is common. Some individuals may develop severe acute hepatitis. Death due to acute alcohol poisoning is, however, uncommon.

The treatment consists of:

- ***General nursing care.***
- ***Maintenance of vital functions.***
- ***IV thiamine*** 100 mg (bolus); and
- ***IV glucose*** 50%, 50 ml, for hypoglycemia.
- ***IV magnesium sulfate*** 2-4 g over 1-2 hours.

If the acutely intoxicated patient is not comatose but only rowdy, careful use of a sedative is indicated.

Chronic Alcoholism

"At risk" (heavy) drinking is defined by National Institute on Alcohol Abuse and Alcoholism (NIAAA) as consuming greater than 14 drinks per week or more than 4 drinks per occasion for men, and greater than 7 drinks per week or more than 3 drinks per occasion for women. A 'drink' is that amount of any alcoholic beverage which contains 12 g of alcohol.

Although all those who drink alcohol are not addicts, repeated ingestion can lead to dependence. In addicts, the feeling of well being depends on a continuous availability of alcohol and there may be such an *intense craving* that the desire to drink remains the major interest in life.

Alcohol addicts are liable to suffer from **neuropsychiatric syndromes** such as Korsakoff's psychosis, hallucinosis, suicidal tendencies and Wernicke's encephalopathy. Generally, there are associated changes due to **nutritional deficiencies** such as polyneuritis

Table 6.2 : Alcohol withdrawal syndrome

8 hours : Tremulousness, anxiety, irritability, nausea and vomiting (Tremulous syndrome).
24 hours : Hyperexcitability, insomnia, disordered perception and convulsions (Seizure syndrome).
2-5 days : Tremor, hallucinations, disorientation and ANS overactivity (Delirium tremens).

due to thiamine deficiency and anemia. Chronic alcoholics may also suffer from other organ damage leading to hepatic cirrhosis, chronic pancreatitis and cardio-myopathy. Apart from history and the obvious physical and mental degeneration, alcohol addiction can be diagnosed by demonstration of ethanol in breath, blood or urine.

Sudden withdrawal of alcohol leads to *withdrawal syndrome* (Table 6.2). **Delirium tremens,** though rare, is the most severe component of the abstinence syndrome which develops some days after sudden withdrawal of alcohol in chronic alcoholics. The symptoms consist of restlessness, insomnia, tremors, hallucinations generally involving great fear, delirium and even convulsions.

The treatment of withdrawal syndrome is outlined in Table 6.3.

Table 6.3: Symptomatic treatment of alcohol withdrawal syndrome

- Maintenance of nutrition and electrolyte balance.
- IV thiamine (100 mg).
- IV glucose for hypoglycemia.
- Diazepam IV **to treat** seizures and delirium.
- Alpha-adrenergic agonist Clonidine 0.1-0.4 mg qid, or beta-blocker Atenolol (orally) 50-100 mg daily, to combat autonomic hyperactivity; Haloperidol for agitation.
- Carbamazepine, to **prevent** seizures

Benzodiazepines, particularly the long acting ones such as diazepam, are considered the treatment of choice. Abatement of symptoms occurs within two days of therapy. Lorazepam and oxazepam are preferred in the elderly and those with liver failure (Chapter 8).

Carbamazepine, an antiepileptic drug (Chapter 9), is an effective alternative in treating mild to moderate withdrawal symptoms. It prevents seizures and does not cause respiratory depression nor impair memory. It reduces emotional distress and allows faster return to work. It is relatively safe and non-addictive.

Alcohol dependence, treatment: This can be divided into:

(a) Detoxification; and
(b) Rehabilitation.

Detoxification aims at providing safe withdrawal to make the patient alcohol-free. **Rehabilitation** includes (a) Psychotherapy; and (b) Institutional therapy.

The drugs that help in preventing relapses and support complete abstinence during rehabilitation are classified as:

I **Aversion drugs,** e.g., Disulfiram, Citrated Calcium cyanamide (CCC).
II **Opioid antagonists,** e.g., Naltrexone, Nalmephene.
III **Dopaminergic antagonists,** e.g., Tiapride.
IV **NMDA receptor antagonist: e.g.,** Acamprosate; and
V **Supporting drugs,** e.g., Lithium, Carbamazepine, Topiramate and Selective 5-HT reuptake inhibitors.

DISULFIRAM (Tetraethylthiuram disul-phide. Antabuse) : Therapy is initiated after ensuring that alcohol has not been consumed for at least 12 hours. Treatment is initiated with 500 mg as a single daily dose for 1-2 weeks, followed by 125-250 mg OD as the maintenance dose; treatment may be continued for upto 1 year.

After a week's therapy, even a small amount of alcohol produces toxic reactions, such as flushing, perspiration, palpitation, marked nausea, vomiting and fall of BP. The patient realises that while on this drug he cannot tolerate even small amounts of alcohol and abstains from drinking. *Severe reactions can occur even with the first dose and hence, this treatment should be carried out in a hospital.* Cases in which disulfiram has produced a violent reaction and even death following alcohol ingestion have been reported. However, the drug hardly improves the success rate of continued abstinence nor does it delay the resumption of drinking.

Mechanism of action: The drug inhibits aldehyde dehydrogenase and blocks the oxidation of acetaldehyde (Fig. 6.1). This raises the blood level of acetaldehyde which acts directly on the cardiovascular system. In addition, disulfiram also inhibits dopamine beta oxidase and thus interferes with the synthesis of NA which gets depleted.

Given orally, it is slowly and incompletely absorbed from the gut and is metabolized slowly.

Adverse reactions: It can cause drowsiness, nausea, headache, cramps, fatiguability, a metallic taste in the mouth and acidosis.

Drug Interactions: *Disulfiram inhibits metabolic degradation of warfarin, theophylline, benzodiazepines, carbamazepine, tricyclic antidepressants and phenytoin. The first and the last interactions can be hazardous.*

Contraindications to disulfiram:

- ***Hepatic and circulatory diseases.***
- ***Uncontrolled diabetes mellitus.***
- ***In alcoholics with obvious personality-changes.***

A general anaesthetic should not be administered simultaneously with disulfiram as this can cause marked fall in BP and collapse.

Carbimide (citrated calcium cynamide) has similar properties, but a shorter duration of action. It is claimed to have fewer adverse effects than disulfiram.

NALTREXONE : Naltrexone and the other mu opioid antagonists (Chapter 10) block alcohol induced release of dopamine in the nucleus accumbens and helps to maintain abstinence. Naltrexone, 50 mg once daily, reduces alcohol consumption and craving for alcohol. It has to be given for as long as 12 weeks or more. Once-a-month injection of naltrexone (Vivitrol) is available.

Nalmephene, an analogue of naloxone with a longer duration of action, is claimed to be less hepatotoxic.

ACAMPROSATE: This drug, an analogue of GABA, given orally, acts as an agonist at the GABA receptors, and as an antagonist at the NMDA receptors. It reduces voluntary alcohol consumption, and excitement and craving that occur in alcohol withdrawal and early abstinence. It is largely excreted by the kidneys. Adverse effects are usually mild and include diarrhoea and headache. The usual dose is 2-3 g/day in divided doses. It can be given along with disulfiram. It is as effective as naltrexone and can be combined with it.

LITHIUM: Oral lithium acts as a mood stabiliser and reduces alcohol consumption. It may be used to treat alcohol withdrawal (Chapter 13).

Among all the above mentioned drugs for the treatment of alcohol dependence, the evidence for efficacy is strongest for naltrexone and acamprosate. In all alcoholics, the possibility of an underlying psychiatric disorder such as schizophrenia, anxiety disorder, panic disorder or depression must be considered and treated.

- ***Psychotherapy***: Alcohol dependence is often reversible if treated during early stages, if the addict realizes that his drinking has become a problem to him. An addict is a sick person sometimes with a feeling of guilt. One way to overcome this guilt is to convince the addict that he is a sick person. Outright condemnation of his drinking can do harm. Psychotherapy by a sympathetic doctor can often give rewarding results. Complete co-operation by the patient is very essential and he should be explained that indulgence in even small quantities of alcohol again would lead to a relapse.

• ***Institutional therapy***: Psychotherapy and drug therapy can be reinforced by institutional therapy (**Alcoholics Anonymous**, AA) where the patient can see for himself the ex-alcoholics who have become abstainers and are living a happy life. This can help to boost the patient's morale. A religious and spiritual approach is also helpful.

Certain abnormalities of personality develop in very chronic cases which make the treatment far more difficult. Thus, in Korsakoff's psychosis there is a marked impairment of memory, disorientation in space, impaired physical capacity and diminution of will power. The results of aversion therapy with drugs are generally disappointing in such cases.

Drug interactions: Numerous drug interactions between alcohol and other drugs have been described (Table 6.4). *This should be borne in mind while prescribing these drugs to alcoholics.*

Table 6.4 : Interactions of ethyl alcohol with other drugs

- CNS depressants such as opioids, hypnotics, tranquillizers, antihistaminics, reserpine, methyldopa and clonidine can cause *severe CNS depression* in the presence of alcohol.
- Vasodilators (hydralazine and nitroglycerine) can cause additive *orthostatic hypotension.* On the other hand, heavy consumption of alcohol is known to cause transient hypertension.
- Alcohol *potentiates* the adverse effects (GI bleeding) of aspirin and other NSAID, sulfonylureas (hypoglycemia) and oral anticoagulants (bleeding).
- Isoniazid can cause *hepatic toxicity* in chronic alcoholics because of increased conversion to a toxic metabolite.
- Chlorpropamide, metronidazole and its analogues, griseofulvin, tolbutamide, cephalosporins and phenylbutazone can cause a mild *disulfiram - like reaction* (see below) in alcohol users.

METHYL ALCOHOL (Methanol): This is used as a solvent and is added in a 5% concentration to denature ethyl alcohol. After ingestion, absorption and distribution are similar to those of ethyl alcohol; the rate of metabolism, however, is very slow. It is mainly oxidized to formaldehyde and subsequently to formic acid, which is toxic. The latter reaction is folate dependent and causes folate depletion.

Pharmacological actions: Methyl alcohol poisoning usually results from ingestion of methylated spirit or adulterated wines. Initial symptoms resemble those of ethyl alcohol ingestion. The later symptoms are due to:

- ***CNS depression.***
- ***Acidosis*** following the production of formic and other organic acids.
- ***Toxic effects of formaldehyde and formic acid*** on the retinal cells.

The symptoms may be delayed, particularly if ethanol is also consumed simultaneously. Usually, headache, vertigo, nausea, vomiting severe abdominal pain, dyspnoea and motor restlessness occur. Bradycardia has a bad prognostic significance. Coma can develop very rapidly, followed by death. Death is usually preceded by blindness. *However, total blindness could occur with as little as 15 ml. of methyl alcohol while ingestion of 30 ml. is fatal.* Many deaths have been reported following the ingestion of methylated spirit (adulterated brew) for its ethyl alcohol like effects.

Treatment of toxicity: This is summarised in Table 6.5. It is directed mainly correcting the acidosis. The development of blindness, though not due to acidosis, is enhanced by acidosis. *Methyl alcohol is oxidised slowly and hence, acidosis can recur even after adequate initial alkali administration.* It is necessary, therefore, to observe the patient closely for several days. Treatment of metabolic acidosis is discussed in Chapter 36. Hypokalemia, if present, needs correction; so also the maintenance of adequate nutrition and water and electrolyte balance. The patient's eyes should be protected from strong light. Folinic acid accelerates the metabolic degradation of formate.

Table 6.5: Treatment of methanol poisoning

- Hospitalization, nursing care
- Gastric lavage, activated charcoal
- Treatment of acidosis/ hypoglycemia
- Inhibition of methanol metabolism
  - (a) Ethyl alcohol 10% IV; 0.6 g/kg loading dose, followed by 10 g/hour infusion, in adults
  - (b) Use of 4 - methyl pyrazole
- Promote metabolic degradation of formate:
  - (a) Folinic acid 1mg/kg (Max. 50 mg) IV, together with folic acid 1mg/kg IV, 4 hourly for 6 doses.
  - (b) 4-methyl pyrazole
- Hemodialysis in severe case
- Maintnance of nutrition

The infusion of ethyl alcohol has been recommended on the basis that it slows down the oxidation of methyl alcohol by competing for the same metabolic pathway. Ethanol administration can be life saving if, for some reasons, alkali therapy is delayed.

ETHYLENE GLYCOL (EG) : This compound is used as an antifreeze in automobile radiators and such products are the usual cause of EG poisoning. Further, the therapeutic misuse of industrial glycerol, which is contaminated with EG, causes fatal nephrotoxicity. Ingestion of about 100 ml of EG, if untreated, can be fatal. Fig. 6.2 shows the steps of the hepatic metabolism of EG. These reactions produce dihydronicotinamide adenine nucleotide (reduced NAD i.e. NADH) from nicotinamide adenine nucleotide (NAD) and hence favour the development of lactic acidosis. EG causes CNS depression and narcosis; oxalate and other intermediates are nephrotoxic and can cause acute renal failure.

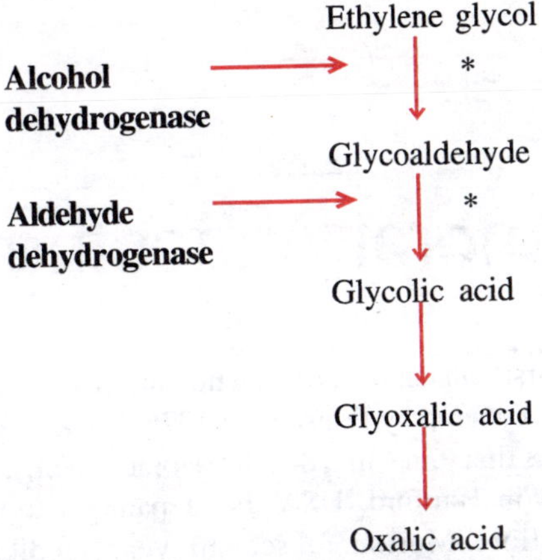

Fig 6.2 : Hepatic metabolism of ethylene glycol
* = NAD is reduced to NADH during these steps

Treatment of EG poisoning is similar to that of methanol poisoning (Table 6.5). Additionally, pyridoxine should be administered IV in the dose of 100 mg daily, to promote the conversion of glyoxalate to glycine. Diuretics, urinary alkalinization and early hemodialysis (which removes EG from the blood) may be helpful.

4-METHYL PYRAZOLE (Fomepizole): is an inhibitor of alcohol dehydrogenase and is useful in the treatment of poisoning with methyl alcohol and EG. The inhibitory effect of the drug is rapid and prolonged. It is well tolerated and causes hardly any toxicity. Methyl alcohol and EG are rapidly cleared by the kidneys if the renal function is normal. Its use appears to be more effective than the use of ethyl alcohol. It is administered in the dose of 100 mg diluted in 250 ml of isotonic saline and infused slowly over 45 minutes.

General Anaesthetics 7

The first inhalation anaesthetic, nitrous oxide, was discovered by Priestley in 1776. It was used for the first time in 1844 by Horace Wells, a dentist in Hartford, USA, for a painless tooth extraction. Morton, a second year medical student, in 1846 successfully showed the use of ether as a general anaesthetic in the first classic demonstration held in the operating room of the Massachusetts General Hospital, Boston, USA. Since then, anaesthesiology has progressed considerably and many safer agents are now available for use.

General anaesthetics are the agents which bring about loss of all modalities of sensation, particularly pain, and a reversible loss of consciousness. **Local anaesthetics** abolish the pain sensation in localized areas without affecting consciousness.

The general anaesthetic agents can be classified as :

I **Inhalation general anaesthetics:**

- ***Volatile liquids***: Chloroform; Diethyl ether; Ethyl chloride; Trichloroethylene; Halothane; Enflurane; Isoflurane.
- ***Gases***: Cyclopropane; Nitrous oxide. Chloroform and Cyclopropane are no more used.

II **Nonvolatile general anaesthetics (Intravenous anaesthetics) :**

- ***Ultra short acting barbiturates :*** Thiopental sodium; Methohexital.
- ***Non-barbiturates***:
  (i) Benzodiazepine: Midazolam, Diazepam
  (ii) Phencyclidine derivative : Ketamine
  (iii) Steroid : Pregnenolone.
  (iv) Etomidate, Propofol.

Site and Mechanism of action : Although the general anaesthetics are capable of depressing all the functional elements of the CNS including the spinal cord, their clinical effects vary, depending upon their chemical structure, and their ability to localize within CNS and interact with target sites e.g. specific cortical areas exhibit different sensitivities to inhalational and IV anaesthetics. Inhibition of motor response to pain, such as that caused by surgical incision, is primarily mediated by the spinal cord. By inhibiting the spinal cord activity, the general anaesthetics decrease the transmission of noxious stimuli ascending from the spinal cord to the brain, and thereby decrease supra-spinal arousal. They also modify the descending signals and cause immobilization. Above the spinal cord, general anaesthetics globally depress blood flow and glucose metabolism and selectively alter neuro-transmission in multiple supra-spinal regions, making those areas electrically silent. Their behavioural and physiological effects, including hypnosis and amnesia, are mediated by the brain. The reticular activating system, thalamus, pons, amygdala and hippocampus are involved in cognition, memory, learning, sleep and attentiveness.

Although there is no definitive evidence for specific targets for general anaesthetics, it is postulated that they affect these areas. Tuberomamillary nucleus, a GABA modulated region of hypothalamus that is linked with the sleep states, is also implicated in the sedative actions of some anaesthetic agents.

Till recently, it was felt that there existed a single unifying mechanism of action for all the structurally unrelated anaesthetic agents. This contention was consistent with the observation by Overton and Meyer that there is a close correlation between the potency of an anaesthetic agent and its lipid solubility. This led to the theory that they act nonspecifically on hydrophobic lipid component of cells. However, *current evidence suggests that molecular targets for anaesthetic agents are primarily proteins of the neuronal ion channels. The major channels associated with nicotinic receptors, 5-HT$_3$, GABA-A; glycine and glutamate receptors are the binding sites for anaesthetic agents.* Though the specific receptors vary from anaesthetic to anaesthetic (e.g. nicotinic receptors or NMDA for nitrous oxide; GABA-A for most IV anaesthetics; and NMDA for ketamine), *in general, these agents inhibit the release of the pre-synaptic excitatory neurotransmitters. They also alter the post-synaptic responsiveness to the released neurotransmitters by increasing the activity of the inhibitory ion channels in the post-synaptic receptors and by enhancing inhibitory neurotransmission within the CNS.* Specific behavioral effects of an anaesthetic are attributable to the selectivity of ion channel it is acting on.

Inhalation General Anaesthetics

The factors which control the transfer of an inhalation anaesthetic agent from the alveoli to the blood, and from there into the tissues are :

- ***Its solubility in blood.***
- ***Its density*** : The lighter the gas, the faster does it diffuse into and out of the tissues.
- ***Its partial pressure*** in the anaesthetic mixture (solubility in blood is proportional to the partial pressure), in the arterial and mixed venous blood, and in the tissues; and
- ***The rate of blood flow through the lungs and the tissues.***

The highly soluble anaesthetic agents such as diethyl ether show slow induction, slow recovery and slow change of depth of anaesthesia.

The general anaesthetics have a low margin of safety and the therapeutic indices vary from 2 to 4. It is also difficult to estimate the dose accurately. The anaesthesiologists describe the measure of potency of inhalation anaesthetic agents in terms of Minimum Alveolar Concentration (MAC) of the anaesthetic, at one atmospheric pressure, that produces ablation of movement in response to the surgical incision. Usually, 0.5 to 2 MAC are required for adequate anaesthesia. The MAC required for halothane and enflurane are 0.75 and 1.68, respectively, while that for nitrous oxide is 105. Thus, nitrous oxide is a poor anesthetic, when used alone.

Methods of administration of general anaesthetics:

- ***Open method***: This is a simple method of administering a volatile anaesthetic. A simple mask like Schimmelbusch mask covered with six to ten layers of gauze, which does not fit the contour of the face is held on the face and an anaesthetic like ether, or ethyl chloride is poured on it in drops. The anaesthetic vapour, diluted with air, is inhaled through the gap between the mask and the face. The method does not need any anaesthesia apparatus. There is no rebreathing. This is also called an 'open drop' procedure.
- ***Semi-open method***: This method is similar to open method but the dilution with air is prevented by using either a well-fitting mask like Ogston's mask or layers of gauze between face and the mask. A small carbon dioxide build-up occurs with this method.
- ***Semi-closed method*** : This method allows some rebreathing of the anaesthetic drug with the help of a reservoir but in addition, part

of the volume of each succeeding inspiration is a new portion from an anaesthetic mixture. This method involves accumulation and rebreathing of carbon dioxide.

- ***Closed method*** : This method essentially employs the chemical agent soda lime to reabsorb the carbon dioxide present in the expired air. It requires the use of a complicated apparatus but is particularly useful when the anaesthetic agent is potentially explosive.

Stages of Anaesthesia : Guedel, in 1920, referring mainly to the anaesthetic ether, outlined the four stages of general anaesthesia and divided the third stage of surgical anaesthesia into four planes (Fig. 7.1). These stages can be distinctly discerned with the majority of the volatile general anaesthetics. The stages are:

- ***Stage I: Stage of analgesia.***
- ***Stage II: Stage of delirium.***
- ***Stage III: Stage of surgical anaesthesia.***
- ***Stage IV: Stage of respiratory paralysis.***

I Stage of Analgesia:

This stage stretches from the beginning of inhalation of anaesthetic to loss of consciousness. The gradual depression of the cortical entres which develops during this phase is manifested as a sensation of remoteness, falling, suffocation or as visual or auditory aberrations. A feeling of warmth is experienced by some individuals.

Analgesia is produced before consciousness is lost. Minor surgical procedures such as incision of an abscess, dental extraction and obstetrical manoeuvres can be carried out successfully during this stage; However, it is difficult to maintain it for a long time. The patient rapidly passes into the second stage, the stage of delirium.

II Stage of Delirium or Excitement :

This stage extends from the loss of consciousness to the beginning of surgical anaesthesia. It may be associated with excitement, shouting, increased muscular activity, breath holding, tachypnoea and hyperventilation. Some of these manifestations are due to release of the lower centres from the inhibitory control of higher centres as a result of cortical depression. The pupils may dilate and marked hypertension and tachycardia may develop, due to release of adrenaline. Struggling, increased tone of the skeletal

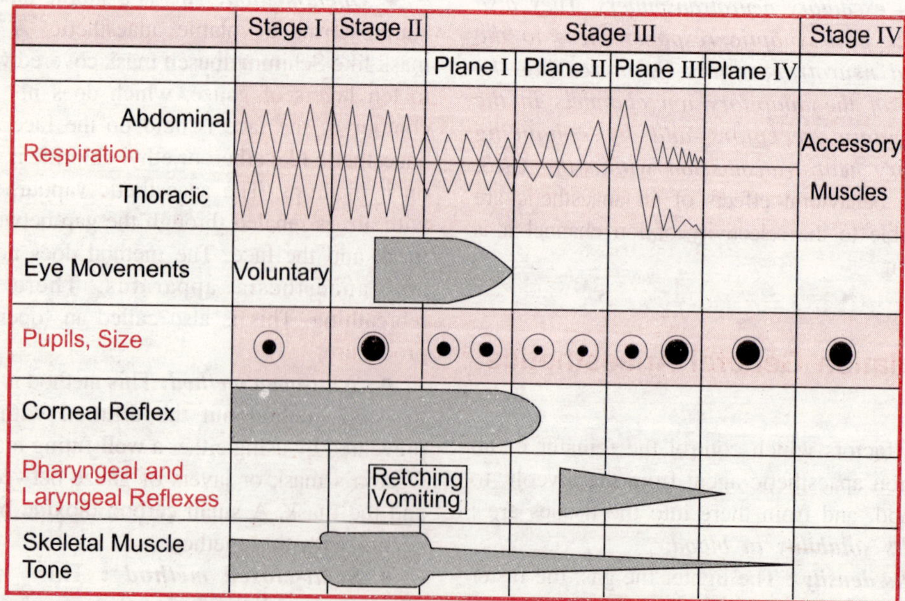

Fig. 7.1 : The signs and stages of ether anaesthesia

muscles, retching and vomiting are the undesirable features of this stage. They can be minimised by proper pre-anaesthetic medication.

III Stage of Surgical Anaesthesia:

As more drug gets in, deep breathing starts and the patient passes into the third stage. It is characterized by a gradual loss of reflexes, regular respiration and relaxation of the skeletal muscles. Reflex activity is lost. This stage is usually employed for surgical intervention and is divided into four planes (Fig. 7.1).

Plane i : The pupils *dilate progressively with the depth of anaesthesia.* The respiration is full, regular, deep and of thoracoabdominal character. The blood pressure and the pulse rate are normal. The skeletal muscles are incompletely relaxed. The lid reflex, swallowing, retching and vomiting get abolished. The corneal reflex is present but the conjunctival reflex is lost. The loss of pharyngeal reflex in the middle of this plane enables the anaesthesiologist to pass a pharyngeal airway.

Plane ii : The respiratory excursions are regular but the amplitude is diminished. Muscular relaxation is adequate. Reflexes arising from the larynx are also abolished and endotracheal intubation can be performed.

Plane iii : This is characterised by the beginning of asynchrony between the thoracic and the abdominal respiratory movements. The blood pressure begins to fall, the intercostal muscles are gradually paralysed and the respiration assumes an increasingly abdominal character. *The pupillary light reflex and the corneal reflex are lost.* The muscular relaxation is essentially complete.

Plane iv : The paralysis of the intercostal muscles is complete, the pupils are dilated, do not respond to light, the muscles are flaccid and the blood pressure is low. The secretions are completely abolished.

IV Stage of Respiratory Paralysis:

This stage is characterised by severe depression of the vital medullary centres. Eventually respiratory arrest with the paralysis of accessory muscles and diaphragm supervenes. This is accompanied by vasomotor collapse and cardiac arrest.

The stages described here may differ considerably with different anaesthetic agents. Halothane produces hypotension much more readily than ether. Pupillary dilatation is a progressive and reliable sign with ether while it is insignificant with halothane. With ether the skin becomes pale, cold and wet in preparalytic stage while with halothane, it is warm and dry until the development of marked hypotension. Preanaesthetic medication with the opioid analgesics, atropine and the use of skeletal muscle relaxants also modifies the signs of the anaesthesia and may interfere with the proper assessment of the depth of anaesthesia.

In modern anaesthetic practice, the stages are never discerned separately because a combination of agents (balanced anaesthesia) is used. Every effort is made to achieve a rapid and smooth induction, avoiding the stage of delirium with the help of IV inducing agents such as thiopental.

Inadequate anaesthesia is indicated by :

- ***Signs of ANS overactivity***, such as tachycardia, rise of BP, sweating and lacrimation.
- ***Grimacing***; or
- ***Other muscle activity.***

Surgical anaesthesia is indicated by :

- ***Loss of eyelash (lid) reflex;*** and
- ***Development of rhythmic respiration.***

Deep anaesthesia is suggested by :

- ***Depression of respiration.***
- ***Marked hypotension;*** and
- ***Asystole.***

Associated blood loss and hypoxia can aggravate the situation. They must be avoided.

With agents such as halothane, hypotension can be used as an index of dosage.

Volatile Liquid Anaesthetics

The volatile general anaesthetics which are

liquid at room temperature are all extremely potent but relatively soluble in blood, cell water and fat; hence, both induction and recovery with these agents are slower than that with the gaseous general anaesthetics.

C_2H_5 — O — C_2H_5

F, Br; F—C—C—Cl; F, H

Fig 7.2 : Ether Halothane

DIETHYL ETHER : Ether is a colourless, volatile liquid with a pungent odour and with the boiling point 35^{0}C. Anaesthetic ether contains 96-98 per cent diethyl ether. Ether vapour is irritating. Ether, when exposed to air, moisture or light may form ether peroxides or acetic aldehyde, which are irritant. To avoid this conversion, ether is marketed in sealed containers or amber coloured bottles covered with black paper.

Ether is inflammable and mixtures of ether with air, nitrous oxide or oxygen may explode over the entire range of anaesthetically useful concentrations.

A concentration of 10-15 per cent of ether in the inspired air is usually required for induction while a concentration of 4 to 5 per cent ensures a satisfactory maintenance of anaesthesia in plane iii; with a concentration of more than 7 per cent respiratory failure may develop.

Ether rubbed into the skin produces local vasodilatation with a sense of warmth and pain (rubefacient action). It dissolves the sebaceous secretion and, in the form of etheral soap, is used as a cleansing agent. It is also used as a solvent.

Absorption, fate and excretion: Only a minor portion of ether is oxidized within the body; 85 to 90 per cent is eliminated through lungs and the remainder through the skin, urine, milk and sweat. Ether crosses the placental barrier and reaches comparable concentrations in the foetal blood.

Advantages of ether:

- Can be administered without complicated apparatus and air can be used as a diluent and source of oxygen.
- Can be used during an emergency without pre-anaesthetic medication.
- Has a wide margin of safety.
- Excellent analgesic.
- Curarimimetic and hence causes satisfactory muscle relaxation.
- Reflex stimulant of respiration and bronchodilator.
- Less likely to precipitate cardiac arrhythmias.
- Little hepato-/nephro-toxicity.
- Can be used during delivery; and
- Economical

Disadvantages of ether:

- Inflammable and explosive, and therefore potentially hazardous; cautery cannot be used.
- Induction is slow and may be stormy; and recovery slow.
- Irritant and may cause nausea/vomiting. Increase in salivary and bronchial secretion may cause cough/laryngeal spasm.
- Rarely may cause cardiac arrest.
- May cause convulsion, especially in children; and
- Exhibits cross tolerance with ethyl alcohol.

HALOTHANE (Fluothane): It is a fluorinated volatile anaesthetic with structural similarity to chloroform. It is a heavy, colourless liquid with a characteristic sweet, fruity odour and is supplied for anaesthesia in amber-coloured bottles. It boils at 50^{0}C.

Halothane readily attacks most of the metals including stainless steel, brass and copper and may also affect the rubber elements of the anaesthetic equipment.

Halothane produces loss of consciousness in a concentration of 2 to 3 per cent in oxygen vapour and the anaesthesia can be maintained by using 1 to 2 per cent of halothane vapour with oxygen and nitrous oxide. A special apparatus is necessary to achieve a precise control of concentration.

Absorption, fate and excretion: About 60-80% of halothane is eliminated unchanged through lungs in the first 24 hours. About 20% appears to be retained in the body and is probably metabolized.

Advantages:

- Non-inflammable and non-irritant to the respiratory tract; hence not unpleasant for induction. It has a fruity odour.
- Inhibits pharyngeal and laryngeal reflexes, making tracheal intubation easy. It does not cause laryngospasm, bronchospasm or coughing but in fact causes bronchodilatation.
- Potent anaesthetic with speedy induction and recovery.
- Postoperative vomiting infrequent.
- Can induce controlled hypotension and a bloodless field; to be used only by experts for this purpose.

Disadvantages:

- Special apparatus is necessary.
- Muscular relaxation inadequate for abdominal surgery, unless combined with a muscle relaxant.
- Poor analgesic.
- Depresses respiration.
- Can raise intracranial tension due to cerebral vasodilatation.
- Causes hypotension by direct depression of myocardium, and may cause cardiac arrhythmias. This is a major drawback.
- Postoperative recovery of mental function slow. Shivering during recovery is common.
- Hepatocellular microsomal enzyme induction can occur; rarely, it causes allergic hepatic necrosis due to the toxic metabolite trifluoroacetyl chloride.
- Can cause malignant hyperthermia in susceptible individuals.

ENFLURANE (Ethrane) : This halogenated volatile liquid anaesthetic is chemically 2-chloro 1, 1, 2-trifluoroethyl difluoromethyl ether. It is non-inflammable, with mild, sweet odour and boils at 57°C. Chemically it is very stable. About 80% of enflurane is excreted unchanged by lungs and only 2-5% is metabolized by liver.

Anaesthesia produced by enflurane resembles closely that produced by halothane, except that the muscular relaxation is better and tachypnoea is uncommon. It causes hypotension and it potentiates the activity of nondepolarizing muscle relaxants. Further, it depresses myocardial contraction force and sensitizes the heart to the actions of catecholamines. There is no bradycardia and there is less tendency to tachycardia and cardiac arrhythmias. Like halothane, it causes bronchodilatation.

The compound could produce seizures and involuntary motor activity during deep anaesthesia. Hence, it is relatively contraindicated in patients with epilepsy and brain lesions. Liver damage is rare and in this respect enflurane appears to be superior to halothane.

ISOFLURANE: This is a liquid related to enflurane with uptake and excretion more rapid than halothane. Its pharmacological properties are similar to those of halothane but it is less liable to cause sensitization of the heart to catecholamines. The drug is metabolized only to the extent of 0.2%.

Advantages of isoflurane:

- Physically stable and non-inflammable.
- Rapid induction and recovery of anaesthesia.
- Bronchodilator.
- Good muscle relaxant.
- Potent coronary vasodilator. Does not affect renal blood flow.
- Less likely to sensitize the myocardium to adrenaline; and
- Hepatotoxicity rare.

Isoflurane is considered by many as the "near ideal" anaesthetic. It is the preferred agent in neurosurgery.

Disadvantages of isoflurane:

- Pungent and respiratory irritant.
- Causes peripheral arterial vasodilatation

and can cause coronary steal; and

- It does not protect against local ischemia.

Desflurane has properties similar to those of isoflurane; it has rapid onset of action and rapid recovery. It may cause cough, salivation and bronchospasm. Hence, it is not preferred for induction of anaesthesia. **Sevoflurane** is non-irritating to the respiratory tract and can be used for induction of anaesthesia in children as it is pleasant to inhale.

ETHYL CHLORIDE: Ethyl chloride is a nonirritating, highly volatile and inflammable liquid with a boiling point of 12^{0}C. The vapour has a characteristic but not unpleasant odour. When sprayed on the skin, it rapidly evaporates and thus cools the skin. This produces transient paralysis of cutaneous sensory nerve endings and local anaesthesia. If ethyl chloride spray is used as a local anaesthetic, the skin should be prepared with petrolatum to prevent sloughing. The spray may produce local oedema. As the local anaesthetic effect lasts from a few seconds to a minute, only very minor operations such as incision of an abscess can be carried out.

Though ethyl chloride induces anaesthesia quickly, the maintenance of a steady depth of anaesthesia is extremely difficult and the margin of safety is narrow. It is now rarely used.

TRICHLOROETHYLENE: Trichloroethyl-ene is a clear, colourless liquid with a characteristic odour. It boils at 80^{0}C. It is non-irritant and non-inflammable. It is usually coloured blue to distinguish it from chloroform.

Trichloroethylene is a potent analgesic with a rapid onset of action. However, muscular relaxation with this agent is inadequate. It may produce tachypnoea and even apnoea, and sensitizes the myocardium to adrenaline.The agent breaks down in the presence of soda lime to highly toxic product dichloroethylene and hence cannot be used in closed circuit. Its use is restricted as a supplement to nitrous oxide - oxygen combination to obtain a greater degree of analgesia. It has been used as a self-medication analgesic during labour in the form of intermittent inhalation.

The drug may cause nausea, vomiting and headache. Tachypnoea and cardiac dysrhythmias are dose related. It is contraindicated in raised CSF pressure.

Gaseous Anaesthetics

NITROUS OXIDE: Nitrous oxide is a colourless, inorganic gas with a sweet taste. The oxygen in the nitrous oxide molecule is not available for tissue respiration as nitrous oxide does not undergo significant decomposition in the body.

Nitrous oxide, if administered along with air, produces a stage of excitement and delirium and also produces amnesia. Hence the name "laughing gas". It is commonly used together with oxygen and ether (Gas-Oxygen-Ether or G-O-E technique).

Nitrous oxide produces analgesia when inhaled in the concentration of 35 to 40 per cent with air. Loss of consciousness occurs with the concentration of 65 to 70 per cent and plane i of surgical anaesthesia can be reached with an 80 : 20 mixture of nitrous oxide and oxygen. A further increase in the concentration of the anaesthetic agent produces hypoxia.

Nitrous oxide has no serious, deleterious effects on circulation, respiration, liver and kidneys, and it is probably the safest anaesthetic agent.

Absorption, fate and excretion : Nitrous oxide is not altered within the body and is carried in the form of a physical solution in the blood. It is rapidly eliminated through lungs within 2 to 5 minutes after its withdrawal.

Advantages:

- Non-inflammable and non-irritant.
- Rapid induction and recovery.
- Analgesic in subanaesthetic concentration; and
- Nausea and vomiting are uncommon.

Disadvantages :

- Not a potent anaesthetic agent by itself; must be supplemented with either a pre-anaesthetic agent or ether or a muscle relaxant.
- Excitement may be violent.
- CO_2 accumulation and hypoxia may develop during prolonged use.
- A special apparatus is required.
- *An increase in spontaneous abortions has been reported in the wives of male dentists and in female chairside, dentists' assistants.*
- Any closed gas-filled space tends to expand during administration of nitrous oxide. It is therefore, contraindicated in patients with collections of air in the pleural, pericardial or peritoneal cavities; intestinal obstruction; occlusion of the middle ear; chronic obstructive airway disease; or emphysema. It is also contraindicated in patients who have recently undergone pneumoencephalography.

Therapeutic uses: It may be used for tooth extraction, obstetric analgesia; and during painful procedures such as changing dressings in burns patients, cleaning and debridement of wounds and cauterization.

Other uses: Measurement of coronary/cerebral blood flow by Fick's principle.

Since modern surgery makes increasing use of electronic devices, inflammable and/or explosive anaesthetics like cyclopropane, ethyl chloride and ether are now considered obsolete in many advanced countries. *Open ether, however, is still being used in many developing countries and is considered as a safe anaesthetic despite its inflammable and explosive nature, particularly when a qualified anaesthetist and anaesthetic equipment are not available.*

Non-Volatile General Anaesthetics

Ultra short acting barbiturates: The ultra short acting barbiturates administered IV to produce general anaesthesia are the thiobarbiturates (thiopental, thiamytal and thiobarbitone) and the. methylated oxy-barbiturates (hexobarbitone and methohexitone) (Chapter 8). The compound employed most commonly is thiopental.

THIOPENTAL: Thiopental sodium is readily soluble in water but the solution deteriorates on keeping. The clinically used solution is intensely alkaline with a pH varying from 10.5 to 11. High alkalinity causes local irritation and venous thrombosis. Given IV, it rapidly induces hypnosis and anaesthesia without analgesia.

Anaesthetic action: The induction is very quick and pleasant. The subject passes through the stages of hypnosis and deep sleep to anaesthesia. Consciousness is lost first, then the reflex activity and muscle tone and lastly, the vital medullary centres are depressed. Pupils react to light and remain contracted in light hypnosis. There may be nystagmus or divergent strabismus. The corneal reflex remains active until deep anaesthesia is achieved. Cerebral blood flow and cerebral metabolic rate are reduced and there is a marked reduction of intracranial tension.

A fairly reliable sign of an adequate induction by thiopental is the absence of the eyelid reflex. Presence of swallowing, phonation and reflex movements of eyes during anaesthesia also indicate need for further injection.

Though the reflexes return in 10-30 minutes, the patient remains disoriented for several hours after stoppage and hence, must not be left alone.

Absorption, fate and excretion of thiobarbiturates: The very short duration of action is attributed to its high lipid solubility. With successive doses, body fat depots get saturated with the drug. The rapid metabolism of the drug by liver may also contribute to its short duration of action. Slow release of the stored drug back into the plasma is responsible for the continuation of drowsiness observed after the cessation of anaesthesia. Thiobarbiturates readily cross the placental barrier and appear in breast milk.

Therapeutic uses:

- ***For induction*** of general anaesthesia.
- ***As anaesthetic agent*** for operations of short duration e.g. fracture reduction, dilatation and curettage, laryngoscopy and bronchoscopy.
- ***As an anaesthetic*** in patients with history of malignant hyperthermia.
- ***As anticonvulsant*** in the emergency treatment of intractable convulsions.

Advantages of IV thiopental:

- Non-explosive and non-irritant; easy to administer.
- Rapid and smooth induction, and rapid recovery after small doses.
- Quiet respiration; no cardiac arrhythmias; and
- Nausea, vomiting, excitement and post-operative complications infrequent.

Disadvantages of IV thiopental:

- Conducting anaesthesia and judging its depth are difficult as the usual stages of anaesthesia are not discernible.
- Pharyngeal and laryngeal reflexes persist, permitting occurrence of coughing, apnoea, laryngospasm and bronchospasm. Hence, *equipment for controlled ventilation must be available.*
- Depression of respiratory center which becomes less sensitive to CO_2.
- Depresses myocardium and vasomotor center; hypotension and cardiac arrhythmias can occur. *Must never be given to a patient who is sitting* such as in a dental chair.
- Poor analgesic and muscle relaxant.
- Highly irritant if extravasated; nerve palsy and limb gangrene reported.
- Relaxes gastroesophageal sphincter, causing silent regurgitation; and
- *Can precipitate acute attack in acute intermittent porphyria.*

Barbiturate anaesthesia is to be used with great caution in the presence of hepatic and/or renal damage, in shock, in airway obstruction, in individuals with a past history of bronchial asthma and severe cardiovascular disease.

Preparations:

(i) Thiopental sodium 0.5 to 1.0 g. powder. It is used as a freshly prepared, 2.5% solution for IV anaesthesia.

(ii) Methohexitone (Brevital) : Twice as potent as thiopental and claimed to be shorter acting. It is used as 1 per cent solution and may be less irritant to veins but as damaging to the arteries as thiopental.

MIDAZOLAM (Hypnovel): This short acting benzodiazepine (Chapter 8) is used either IM as a premedication or IV for sedation for endoscopic procedures and for induction of anaesthesia. The IV dose is 2.5 to 7.5 mg; the usual IM dose is 5 mg. With IV administration of midazolam, the same precautions are required as with IV diazepam. It is water soluble and less irritant to the veins than diazepam (Chapter 8). It has also been used by subcutaneous infusion (by means of a syringe pump) as an anticonvulsant. It is a relatively safe drug.

KETAMINE (Ketalar) : This non-barbiturate general anaesthetic agent is related to phencyclidine. It acts as an anatagonist at NMDA receptors. It probably acts on the cerebral cortex, particularly the limbic system. It has analgesic property in subnarcotic doses, and light anaesthesia usually does not cause depression of the protective pharyngeal and laryngeal reflexes. It is a potent bronchodilator.

Given IV it is quick acting although the onset of action is slower than that of thiopental. Following a single dose, it induces a state of **dissociative anaesthesia** characterized by complete analgesia combined with amnesia; the patient can open his eyes and can obey instructions. Respiratory support in not needed. Analgesia lasts for about 40 minutes whereas anaesthesia lasts for about 15 minutes only. The pattern of sleep is different from that which occurs with barbiturates.

Anaesthesia can be induced by both IM (5-10 mg/kg) and IV (1-2 mg/kg) routes. A dose of

0.5 mg/kg IM or IV produces adequate *analgesia* which can be maintained by 0.25 mg/kg.

The drug increases the BP, heart rate and cardiac output by raising the blood levels of NA and can be used in patients in shock. However, it should be avoided in patients with ischemic heart disease.

Disadvantages of ketamine:

- It sometimes causes nystagmus, involuntary movements and hypertonus.
- It may cause delirium, hallucinations and colourful dreams during induction and recovery, especially in adults. Diazepam or midazolam given rapidly abolishes these disturbances.
- Rarely, laryngospasm may occur; salivation may be troublesome.
- Muscular relaxation is inadequate.
- It increases intraocular and intracranial pressures.
- *It is a drug of abuse (Day Rape Drug).*

Therapeutic uses: The drug is advocated as an inducing agent and for maintenance of anaesthesia during short-lasting diagnostic procedures like cardiac catheterization and bronchoscopy. It has been used in adults for such short procedures as the dressing of burns, forceps delivery, breech extraction, manual removal of the placenta and dental work. It can be used in children.

It is not used:

- In patients suffering from hypertension, cardiac decompensation or a cerebrovascular accident.
- For surgery of the pharynx, larynx or bronchi.
- In abdominal surgery, as it relieves visceral pain poorly.
- In thyrotoxic patients, in whom it may cause rise in blood pressure.
- In pregnant women at term, because of its oxytocic activity. *However, it may be used during caesarian section* as it causes less fetal and neonatal depression.
- During operations on the eye, as it causes a rise in the intra-ocular pressure; and
- In the presence of psychiatric disorders such as acute psychosis and schizophrenia.

Barbiturates and diazepam are chemically incompatible with ketamine. They should never be administered from the same syringe or via the same infusion set.

ETOMIDATE (Hypnomidate) : This drug, a carboxylated imidazole, has potent hypnotic and anaesthetic properties. A single IV dose of 300 mcg/kg produces loss of consciousness within 10 seconds and a state of anaesthesia, followed by sleep. Recovery is rapid and complete. Cardiovascular and respiratory changes are minimal. In fact, cardiovascular stability during and after induction is considered to be a major advantage of etomidate; hence it is preferred in patients prone to hemodynamic instability. The drug, however commonly causes nausea and vomiting. Further, it inhibits certain adrenocortical enzymes, resulting in suppression of adrenocortical stress response. Rarely, it causes involuntary movements. It is primarily used for induction.

PROPOFOL (Diprivan) : This intravenous anaesthetic causes rapid induction and rapid recovery with small hangover effect. It is generally used for induction and maintenance of general anaesthesia. In equianaesthetic doses, it produces a slightly greater degree of respiratory depression than thiopental. It causes dose-dependent cortical depression and is an anticonvulsant. It is largely (88%) metabolized by the liver. Its advantages are :

- It has specific anti-emetic action and is less likely to cause bronchospasm.
- It has no effect on the hypoxic, pulmonary vascular reflexes.
- Because of quick recovery from anaesthesia, it may be preferred to thiopental for day-care surgery.
- It is safe during pregnancy.

It is used by IV infusion for maintenance of anaesthesia.

Steroids: Various steroids such as althesin introduced earlier have now been withdrawn because of their unacceptable adverse effects. **Pregnenolone** (Etanolol) is a naturally occurring metabolite of 17-alpha-hydroxy progesterone and is 3 times as potent as propofol. It is not used in practice.

Neuroleptanalgesia

Neuroleptics (antipsychotics) are a group of drugs which induce a state of apathy and mental detachment in which the patient is mildly sedated and uncaring about his surroundings. These compounds are used in the treatment of major psychoses and are discussed in detail in Chapter 13. **Neuroleptanalgesia** is a method of IV anaesthesia which combines the use of a **neuroleptic drug with an opioid analgesic** drug. Such a combination produces a state which differs from the classical general anesthesia in that the subject is conscious and is able to co-operate during the operative procedure. The most favoured combination is that of the neuroleptic droperidol and the analgesic fentanyl.

DROPERIDOL (Droleptan) : This is a butyrophenone derivative like haloperidol. Its pharmacological actions are similar to those of chlorpromazine (Chapter 13); but it is short acting (2-3 hours) and more potent than haloperidol. Apart from typical behavioural effect of calming, droperidol also has antiemetic and alpha-adrenergic blocking (adrenolytic) actions. Like all neuroleptic drugs it can produce extrapyramidal reactions.

FENTANYL (Sublimaze) : This drug belongs to the group of 4-acylanilino piperidines. It is a morphine-like opioid analgesic (Chapter 10) used exclusively as a supplementary analgesic in inducing general anaesthesia. Like morphine, it suppresses the respiratory and cough centres and causes nausea, vomiting and miosis. It is 100 times more potent than morphine. However, its action is of shorter duration. Given IM or IV, it rapidly produces profound analgesia lasting for about 30 minutes. These actions can be antagonized by naloxone.

In clinical practice, the **combination** usually preferred contains **droperidol** 2.5 mg. and **fentanyl citrate** 50 mcg. in 1 ml (Thalamonal, Innovar). Given IV, it causes complete analgesia, without marked hypnosis, sufficient for surgical procedures. The onset of anaesthesia is slow. Major advantages of this procedure are:

- ***Smooth onset and rapid post-anaesthetic recovery.***
- ***Less danger of hypotension and other circulatory disturbances.***
- ***Suppression of vomi-ting and coughing.***
- ***Continued analgesia in postoperative period.***
- ***Availability of patient's co-operation during the operative procedures*** such as eye, oral and orthopaedic surgery, angiocardiography, myelography and bronchoscopy.

Since the combination does not disturb the cardiovascular dynamics, it is claimed to be very useful in old people and in 'poor risk' cases. Further, the combination can be used to induce anaesthesia which can then be continued with other general anaesthetic agents like nitrous oxide-oxygen mixture and muscle relaxants.

Adverse reactions : They are due to toxicity of individual drugs. They include hallucinations, mental depression, extrapyramidal disturbances due to droperidol and respiratory depression due to fentanyl. The latter may be marked and assisted, controlled ventilation is necessary. As compared to droperidol, fentanyl has a shorter duration of analgesic action (30 minutes) and supplementary doses of fentanyl (1 mcg/kg) may be needed after 20 minutes.

Fentanyl and **alfentanil** (Rapifen) are sometimes used as IV analgesics in short operations because of their brief duration of action. **Remifentanil,** a synthetic opioid, has rapid onset of action and is metabolized rapidly in the plasma and tissues. As a result, its duration of action is extremely short.

Pre-Anaesthetic Medication

Pre-anaesthetic medication is the term applied to the use of drugs prior to the administration of an anaesthetic agent, with the object of making anaesthesia safer and more agreeable to the patient. The reasons for such medication are:

- ***For sedation, to reduce anxiety and apprehension*** without producing much drowsiness.
- ***To obtain an additive or synergistic effect so that induction could be smooth and rapid*** and the dose of the general anaesthetic could be reduced.
- ***To counteract certain adverse effects of the anaesthetic drug used*** such as salivation, bradycardia and vomiting.
- ***To relieve pre- and post-operative pain.***
- ***To suppress respiratory secretions and to reduce reflex excitability.***

There is no single drug which can achieve all these objectives and hence usually a combination of drugs is used. It must be emphasized, however, that factors other than drugs can favourably affect preoperative psychological preparation and a preoperative visit by the anaesthesiologist and a sympathetic discussion with the patient about the events of the next day in itself have a high therapeutic value.

The drugs commonly used for preanaesthetic medication are :

(1) **Opioid analgesics** such as morphine (10-15 mg. IM), pethidine (50-100 mg. IM) and buprenorphine (300 mcg. IM), are commonly employed for their sedative and analgesic properties. Buprenorphine has longer duration of action than morphine and pethidine (Chapter 10). They also reduce the amount of general anaesthetic required.

Disadvantages are:

- They may depress respiration and may cause respiratory arrest. Further, drugs like morphine increase the tone of smooth muscle such as bronchial muscles. In emphysema or in kyphoscoliosis where the pulmonary reserve is already low, use of opioids may precipitate pulmonary insufficiency.
- They may cause vasomotor depression, and may decrease the ability of circulation to respond to stress. They often delay the awakening as their clinical effect lasts for 4-6 hours.
- Morphine may induce vomiting, antidiuresis and can interfere with pupillary reactions.
- Pethidine by its vagolytic action may produce tachycardia.
- Both these drugs are histamine liberators.

(2) **Sedatives and tranquillizers:** Benzodiazepines (diazepam, nitrazepam) are preferred because of their safety, muscle relaxant property and less respiratory depression (Chapter 8). They also provide amnesia. Diazepam in doses of 5 to 20 mg. has been most widely used. It is active orally and can also be given parenterally, though its action is less predictable by this route. Other tranquilli-zer compounds used belong to phenothiazine and butyrophenone groups. They exhibit similar properties. Phenothiazines possess sedative, antiarrhythmic, antiemetic and anti-histaminic properties. They, however, can potentiate the effects of barbiturates and mor-phine and may cause respiratory depression and hypotension. Phenothiazines comm-only employed are promethazine and trimeprazine (Vallergan). They can be given orally as well as parenterally (Chapter 13).

Dexmedetomidine: This imidazole derivative causes analgesia and sedation with very little respiratory depression by its central and peripheral α_2 adrenergic receptor agonist action. Its main adverse effects are hypotension and bradycardia. It is used IV for short term sedation of critically ill adults and as anaesthetic adjunct.

(3) **Antimuscarinic drugs:** Atropine (600 mcg. IM) is generally combined with morphine to block the vagal actions so as to reduce

salivary and respiratory secretions and to prevent parasympa-thetically induced reflex hypotension and bradycardia. It may thus lessen the possibility of cardiac arrhythmias during the induction stage. Due to blockade of cardiac vagal action, atropine may produce tachycardia.

It causes initial vagal stimulation by its central action; use of atropine in combination with neostigmine to reverse the neuro-muscular blockade by the muscle relaxant d-tubocurarine, therefore, may cause cardiac arrest. Synthetic anti-muscarinics such as glycopyrrolate (Pyrolate), a long acting quaternary amine, can be used instead of atropine for this purpose and are sometimes preferred because of their less central actions and less tendency to cause excessive tachycardia (Chapter 19).

(4) **Antiemetics:** The commonly used phenothiazines such as **promethazine** and **trimeprazine** have antiemetic properties and thus may help to prevent the post-operative nausea and vomiting. This advantage should, however, be weighed against the possible hypotension following these drugs. Other drugs used are **cyclizine**, 50 mg., **trimethobenzamide** 200 mg and **benzquinamide** 25-50 mg.

(5) **Other drugs:** In addition to the use of above mentioned drugs, proper pre-evaluation and specific premedication are needed in patients with special problems such as chronic lung disease, emphysema, ischemic heart disease, diabetes mellitus, hypertension, undernutrition and in debilitated and old people. Antibiotic prophylaxis may be needed (Chapter 49).

The risk of stopping longterm medication before surgery is often greater than the risk of continuing it during surgery. This applies particularly to glucocorticoids, analgesics, antiparkinsonian drugs, anti-glaucoma drugs, and thyroid or antithyroid drugs. On the other hand, it is advisable to discontinue combined oral contraceptive pills 4 weeks before major surgery; monoamine-oxidase inhibitors 2 weeks before surgery; and lithium 2 days before surgery.

Drugs Administered During Anaesthesia

These are:

- ***Skeletal muscle relaxants*** like succinyl choline and curarimimetics to achieve good muscle relaxation (Chapter 21).
- ***A very short acting ganglion blocking agent*** like trimethaphan camphor sulfonate or sodium nitroprusside to produce controlled hypotension (Chapter 29).
- ***Drugs administered to counter the anaesthetic complications*** e.g. vasopressor agents (such as methoxamine or phenylephrine) to correct hypotension, anti-arrhythmics to correct cardiac arrhythmias, anti-convulsants and respiratory stimulants.

The prophylactic administration of supplementary glucocorticoids to patients receiving steroid therapy or those with a history of such therapy within two years prior to surgery is necessary to avoid serious hypotension and shock during surgery. Antibiotics like streptomycin and neomycin have neuromuscular blocking action and hence, can produce skeletal muscle paralysis when instilled into pleural or peritoneal cavities during anaesthesia; these drugs can also potentiate the actions of skeletal muscle relaxants like d-tubocurarine. Patients on beta-adrenergic blockers tend to develop hypotension more often following certain anaesthetic agents.

Malignant hyperthermia is a serious but rare complication of general anaesthesia (see Chapter 21).

Sedatives, Hypnotics and Pharmacotherapy of Sleep Disorders

8

Physiologically, sleep is regarded as absence of wakefulness, where the responses to environmental stimuli are greatly reduced. But, in fact, it is an active state, related to definite anatomic structures as well to specific biogenic amines. Yet, its exact mechanism is not known. The determinants of natural sleep are many but the most important regulator is probably a "central pacemaker" (or the biological clock) in the suprachiasmatic nuclei of the hypothalamus. The normal circadian rhythm is related to production of melatonin by the pineal gland. We all need sleep. It is believed that restoration of natural balance among the neuronal centres in the brain takes place chiefly during sleep, and the association between sleep and growth in the early years of life is generally accepted.

Based on electrophysiological studies (EEG, electromyogram and electro-oculogram), sleep has been classified into two types:

- ***Non Rapid Eye Movement sleep (NREM);*** and
- ***Rapid Eye Movement sleep (REM).***

While falling asleep, one passes sequentially through stages 1, 2, 3 and 4 of NREM sleep.

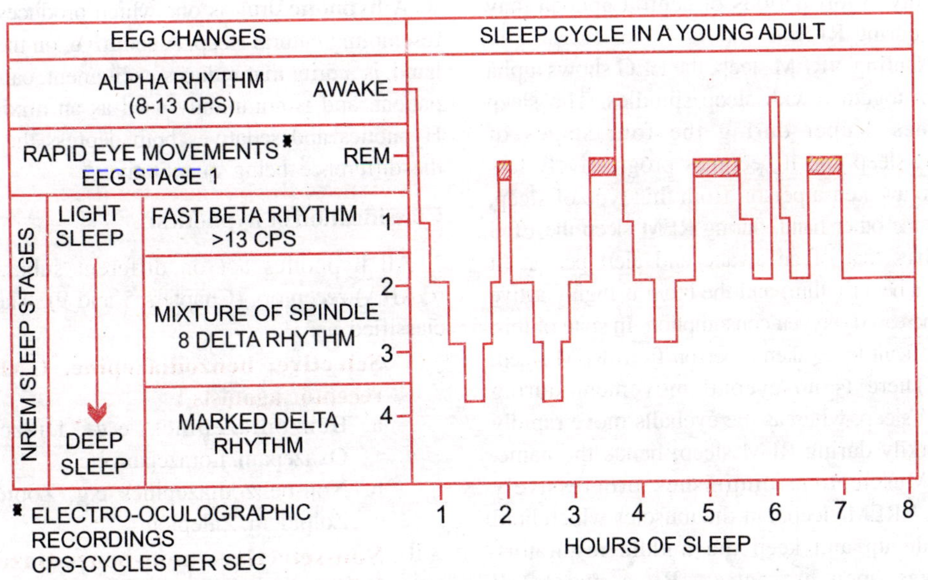

Fig. 8.1: Sleep cycle and EEG changes in a normal young adult. Shaded areas denote REM sleep.

After about 90-120 minutes of NREM sleep, REM sleep occurs, lasting for 5-30 minutes. The NREM-REM cycle repeats 4-5 times during the night, with progressive lengthening of the REM bouts until one awakens from REM (not NREM) sleep in the morning.

There are important differences between NREM and REM sleep. They are :

- NREM sleep is very peaceful with preponderance of the parasympathetic activity and diminution of the metabolic rate, heart rate, cardiac output and peripheral vascular resistance. Dreaming is infrequent and the dreams are rarely recalled on awakening.

On the other hand, the sympathetic activity predominates during REM sleep. The sleep is not so restful; 75% of the dreams occur in this type of sleep; the dreams tend to be more vivid, bizzare and often sexual, with erections occuring in the males. Dreams are accompanied by appropriate cardiovascular responses to the perceived dream activities such as running or escaping. As a result, the heart rate, BP, cardiac output, peripheral vascular resistance, small airway resistance and metabolic rate rise markedly. Short periods of central apnoea may occur during REM.

- During NREM sleep, the EEG shows alpha rhythm together with sleep spindles. The sleep becomes deeper during the four stages of NREM sleep and it becomes progressively less easy to awaken a person from this type of sleep.

On the other hand, during REM sleep the EEG resembles that of an awake and alert person (it shows a beta rhythm) and the brain is highly active with increased oxygen consumption. In spite of this, it is difficult to awaken a person from REM sleep.

- There is no eyeball movement during NREM sleep, whereas the eyeballs move rapidly and jerkily during REM sleep; hence the name.
- Muscle tone diminishes progressively during NREM sleep, but the muscles which hold the chin up and keep the middle respiratory passages open are active. By contrast, *all* voluntary muscles except extraoccular muscles are profoundly flaccid during REM sleep.
- Growth hormone secretion occurs during stages 3 and 4 of NREM sleep, but none during REM sleep.

REM sleep normally occupies about 25% of the sleeping time; this pattern is altered by various diseases, sleep disorders and drugs. The notion that sleep is a uniformly quiescent and peaceful state, and therefore devoid of stress, is not correct. Both NREM and REM types of sleep expose a person to different types of stress. For example, relative hypotension during stage 4 of NREM sleep accounts for some of the ischemic cerebro-vascular strokes during sleep. On the other hand, the extreme hypotonia of the small muscles that hold the middle respiratory passages open can lead to *obstructive sleep apnoea,* with possible disastrous consequences, during REM sleep. Further, the rise in the cardiovascular parameters due to catecholamine secretion during REM sleep can lead to hypertensive-hypoxic cardiovascular events.

A normal person spends about one-third of his life in sleep. Adequate sleep is a necessity of life. In practice, many individuals complain of lack of sleep, **insomnia**.

A **hypnotic** drug is one which produces sleep resembling natural sleep. A **sedative**, on the other hand, is a drug that reduces excitement, calms the patient, and is commonly used as an **anxiolytic**. Hypnotics and sedatives both depress the CNS, the difference being quantitative.

Classification of hypnotics:

All hypnotics act on different subunits of (GABA) receptors (Chapters 5 and 9). They are classified as:

I **Selective, benzodiazepine, GABA-A receptor agonists :**

a. Benzodiazepines e.g. Diazepam, Oxazepam, Lorazepam etc.

b. Non-benzodiazepines e.g. Zopiclone, Zolpidem, Zaleplon.

II **Non-selective, non-benzodiazepine GABA-A receptor agonist :**

a. Barbiturates e.g. Phenobarbitone, Pentobarbitone.

b. Non-barbiturates e.g. Chloral hydrate, Paraldehyde.

III **Miscellaneous** e.g. Antihistaminics Diphenhydramine, Promethazine.

Drugs like morphine and pethidine, besides acting as opioid analgesics, also possess hypnotic property. Hence, they are grouped as *Anodyne hypnotics.* However, they should not be used as hypnotics in the absence of severe pain (Chapter 10).

Benzodiazepines

BENZODIAZEPINES (BDZ): These compounds have largely replaced the barbiturates as hypnotics (see later) (Chapters 7 and 13).

Fig. 8.2 : 1,4 - Benzodiazepine nucleus **Diazepam**

Mechanism of action: BDZ bind selectively to the α subunit of the GABA-A receptors surrounding the chloride channels in the CNS, a site distinct from that to which barbiturates bind, and designated as *benzodiazepine receptors* (**BDZ receptors**). They modulate the effects of GABA, thereby increasing the frequency of chloride channel opening, and increasing the chloride ion concentration in the neuron. This causes hyperpolarization of the neuronal membrane, making it more difficult for the excitatory neurotransmitters to depolarize the cell. They enhance the effectiveness of GABA by lowering the concentration of GABA required for opening the chloride channels (Fig 8.3).

Although all the BDZ have similar pharmacological properties, they differ in their selectivity and vary in their clinical usefulness owing to the existence of multiple BDZ receptor subtypes in the CNS. For example, the antispasticity effect appears to involve the GABA-A receptors in the brain stem and the spinal cord, whereas the sedative and anticonvulsant actions are localized to the limbic system.

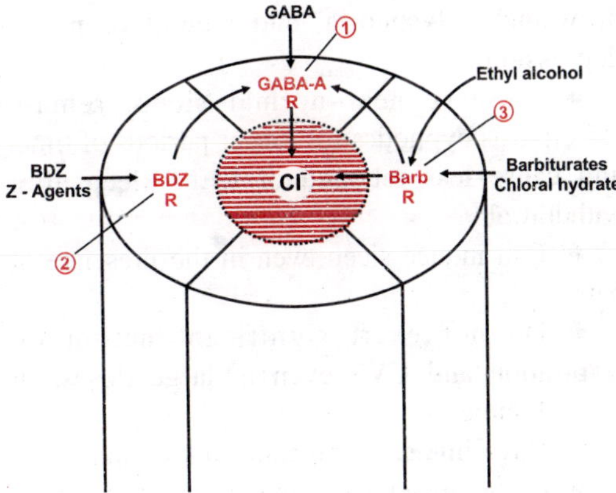

Fig. 8.3: $GABA_A$ - BDZ - Barbiturate receptor complex

R : Receptor site, Z-agents : Zolpidem etc.

Note : Selective BDZ-$GABA_A$ receptor agonist acts through $GABA_A$ receptor. Barbiturates in therapeutic doses directly open chloride channel.

Pharmacological actions: Benzodiazepines act as

- ***Anxiolytics.*** (Chapter 13)
- ***Hypnotics.***
- ***Anticonvulsants***; and
- ***Muscle relaxants.***

Sedative-hypnotic action: In small doses, BDZ produce relief from anxiety and in larger doses, they induce sleep. All benzodiazepines are qualitatively similar in their effects on the important sleep parameters. Thus, they decrease the time to onset of sleep, prolong stage 2 of sleep, and shorten stages 3 and 4 and REM sleep. The total sleep time is increased.

Clinically, BDZ are preferred as hypnotics because they:

- Induce sleep which is more refreshing and with fewer hangover symptoms such as drowsiness, dysphoria, and mental or motor depression.

- Preserve near–normal sleep, remain effective as hypnotics for longer periods of time, and cause less rebound of REM sleep after withdrawal.
- Can induce sleep even in the presence of pain.
- Do not exert significant action on respiration and CVS even in large doses, in normal subjects.
- Have higher therapeutic index; and
- Cause fewer drug interactions and have less potential than barbiturates for drug abuse.

All can induce **anterograde amnesia**, where there is impairment of memory for events after the drug.

Muscle relaxant and anti-convulsant actions: They have a central muscle relaxant action (Chapter 21). They increase the seizure threshold and act as anticonvulsants.

Anaesthetic action: (Chapter 7)

Miscellaneous actions: They may lower the BP and decrease the respiratory rate.

Absorption, fate and excretion: The various BDZ differ from each other in their pharmacokinetic characteristics. Given orally, diazepam and cholrazepate are most rapidly and completely absorbed from the proximal small intestine; prazepam and oxazepam are the least rapidly absorbed; flurazepam and lorazepam fall in between these two groups. The absorption of chlordiazepoxide and diazepam given IM is slow, incomplete and erratic. *The only BDZ with reliable absorption from the IM site are lorazepam and midazolam.* Rectal route for diazepam is generally used in the convulsing patient.

The duration of action following a single dose depends upon the rate and extent of drug distribution and of metabolic degradation. BDZ are metabolized by hepatic microsomal CYP450 enzymes, and hepatic damage prolongs their action. The t½ is prolonged in subjects over 60 years` age and in infants due to reduced hepatic clearance; hence, dosage should be reduced under such conditions. Depending on their elimination t½, they can be grouped as shown in Table 8.1.

Some of the BDZ are biotransformed to clinically active metabolites, some of them with longer half-life than the parent compound. Thus, desmethyldiazepam (t½ 36-200 hours), a major metabolite, plays an important role in the clinical effects of cholrdiazepoxide, diazepam, prazepam, chlorazepate and medazepam. Clorazepate and prazepam are in fact pro-drugs and reach the systemic circulation only as desmethyldiazepam. Flurazepam is converted to the active metabolite desalkylflurazepam. *Multiple dose therapy with such drugs leads to accumulation of the long half-life, active metabolites, resulting in prolongation of the effect,* and may cause unwanted daytime sedation. However, it should be noted that the clinical drug effects do not necessarily increase in direct proportion to plasma concentration because of development of tolerance.

Because of long half-life, clinically important amounts of chlordiazepoxide, diazepam or desmehtyl-diazepam may persist in the blood and in the body for many days/weeks after termination of prolonged therapy. This could be beneficial in anxiety state as it prevents the rapid return of anxiety and delays the development of withdrawal symptoms.

BDZ with short t½ such as oxazepam, lorazepam, temazepam are preferred hypnotics when residual daytime effect is undesirable. Oxazepam and lorazepam lack active metabolites and are preferred in the elderly.

Preparations and doses: See Table 8.1.

Adverse reactions: Benzodiazepines in general are well tolerated. The common side effects are due to dose related depression of CNS: drowsiness, lethargy and ataxia. They also cause impairment of visual-motor coordination, behavioural changes, daytime sedation, and anterograde amnesia.

The drugs may occasionally produce personality changes and may cause a paradoxical increase in hostility, irritability and anxiety especially in the elderly. They should be

Table 8.1: Benzodiazepine derivatives and oral doses

Name	Bed time hypnotic single dose mg Δ	Total ** daily anxiolytic dose mg
I *Effective half-life more than 24 hrs :		
Chlordiazepoxide (Librium)	—	30-100
Diazepam *** (Valium, Calmpose)	5 - 15	10 - 30
Flurazepam (Dalmane)	15 - 30	15 - 30
Chlorazepate (Tranxene)	3.75 - 15	7.5 - 22.5
II Effective half-life 5-24 hrs :		
Nitrazepam (Nitravate, Hypnotex)	5 - 10	5 - 10
Lorazepam (Larpose)	0.5 - 2	1 - 4
Oxazepam (Serapax)	15 - 30	45 - 60
Temazepam	15 - 30	10 - 30
III Effective half-life less than 5 hrs :		
Alprazolam (Alprax)	-	0.75-1.50
Triazolam (Halcion)	0.25	-

* These compounds are metabolised to clinically important active metabolites with elimination half-life values ranging between 36 and 200 hrs.

** In divided doses.

*** For IV use, inject 5 mg directly and slowly.

Δ Use half the dose in old people.

used cautiously in the presence of respiratory, liver and cardiac diseases.

Rarely, BDZ cause leucopenia allergy, photosensitization, vertigo, headache, impaired sexual function and menstrual irregularities.

Patients develop tolerance to the sedative (but not to the anxiolytic) action, as well as physical and psychic dependence. **Withdrawal symptoms** include insomnia, agitation and rarely convulsions. The withdrawal symptoms are more intense following the discontinuation of shorter acting BDZ than of longer acting BDZ. The treatment is similar to that of barbiturate dependence (see later).

Administration of BDZ to the mother before delivery can cause apnoeic spells, reluctance to feed, hypotonia and hypothermia in the newborn (**floppy baby syndrome**).

Drug interactions : They may produce bizarre interactions with alcohol, MAO inhibitors, barbiturates and amitriptyline. H_2 receptor blockers like cimetidine and the antituberculous drug INH retard the elimination of diazepam by inhibiting the hepatic microsomal enzymes. However, serious drug interactions are rare.

Therapeutics uses :

- ***As hypnotics*** (see later)
- ***In anxiety states and neuroses*** (Chapter 13).
- ***During withdrawal of alcohol*** (Chapter 6)
- ***As anticonvulsants*** (Chapter 9).
- ***As anaesthetic medication*:** Short half-life midazolam may be used IV in anaesthesia (Chapter 7).

FLUMAZENIL (Anexate), an imidazo-benzodiazepine, binds competitively to BDZ receptors and antagonises many of the actions of BDZ. It does not block the pharmacologic effects of GABA or all GABA-mimetics but it *specifically* antagonizes the actions of BDZ. Given alone, it has minimal effect on the CNS. The drug can cause withdrawal syndrome in patients dependent on BDZ. Clinically, it can rapidly reverse the effects of BDZ. Flumazenil infusion can facilitate the return of consciousness within 5-15 minutes in patients with BDZ poisoning.

Given orally, it is rapidly absorbed and has a high hepatic clearance. It is metabolized in the liver and little is excreted unchanged. It is given IV initially in the dose of 0.2 mg over 15 seconds, and then repeated in the dose of 0.1

mg every minute to a total dose of not more than 1 mg. It is also given by IV infusion. The duration of action of a single dose is 30-60 minutes.

Therapeutics uses:

- ***In BDZ poisoning,*** and
- ***For reversal of sedative effect of a BDZ administered during general anaesthesia, a diagnostic or therapeutic procedure.***

It is contraindicated in patient with raised intracranial pressure as after severe head injury.

Non-benzodiazepine, Benzodiazepine-receptor Agonists

Non-benzodiazepines like **zopiclone, zolpidem, zaleplon** and **efzopiclone (Z agents)** are the newer sedative hypnotic agents which have varied chemical structures (Table 8.2). They bind selectively to a subset of BDZ receptors. Their characteristic features are:

- As sedative-hypnotics, they are as effective as benzodiazepines and provide normal architecture of sleep.
- Sleep stages are not significantly changed with usual hypnotic doses.
- They have anti-convulsant and muscle relaxant effects.
- They have fewer adverse effects on memory and cognitive function.
- Next-day hangover effects are minimal. Zaleplon is perhaps the best (even with middle-of-night use) because of its ultra-short t½.
- They are less liable to cause tolerance, dependence and rebound insomnia than the BDZ.
- They are metabolized in the liver. Zopiclone has active metabolites.

However, habituation, drug abuse and withdrawal symptoms have been reported even with these drugs.

Zaleplon is effective in reducing sleep latency and therefore used in insomnia with difficulty in falling asleep. But it does not decrease premature awakening nor increase total sleep time. Zopiclone, with longer t½ can be used for intiating and maintaining sleep. Zolpidem also decreases nocturnal arousal. **Efzopiclone** (Lunestra) is the S-isomer of zopiclone and has similar actions. Its plasma t½ is 6 hours.

These drugs, however, are not superior to BDZ, which are equal to them in efficacy and

Table 8.2: Comparison of zopiclone, zolpidem and zaleplon

Property	Zopiclone	Zolpidem	Zaleplon
Structure	Cyclopyrrolone	Imidazopyridine	Pyrazolopyrimidine
Elimination half-life (h)	4-5	1.5-2.4	1-1.5
Bioavailability	80 %	70 %	30 %
Memory effects	+	+	+/–
Cognitive effects	+	+	+/–
Negative effects on memory and cognition next day	+	+	+/–
Common adverse effect	Metallic after-taste	Headache	Headache

± = Very mild effect; + = Mild effect

safety; and are cheaper. Hence, BDZ are preferred for routine use.

Barbiturates

BARBITURATES are the derivatives of barbituric acid which is a condensation product of urea with malonic acid. Barbituric acid itself is devoid of any hypnotic activity (Fig. 8.4).

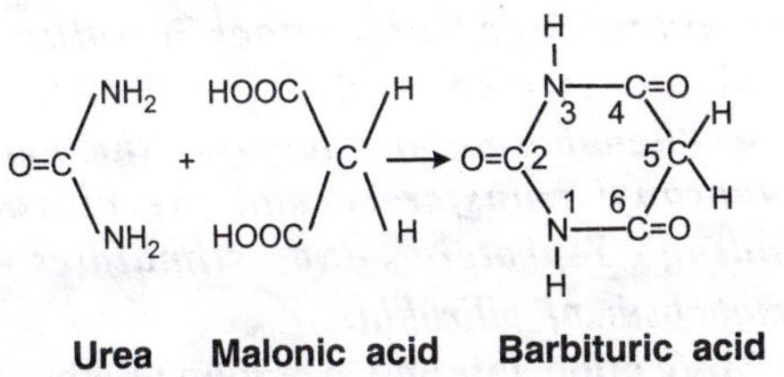

Urea Malonic acid Barbituric acid

Fig. 8.4 : Synthesis of barbituric acid

Barbiturates are sparingly soluble in water; however, their sodium salts form alkaline solutions in water. Conventionally, they are divided according to their duration of action as:

I **Long acting** (8 hours or more) e.g. Phenobarbitone.

II **Intermediate acting** (4 to 8 hours) e.g. Amylobarbitone, Butobarbitone, and Pentobarbitone.

III **Short acting** (less than 4 hours) e.g. Secobarbitone (quinalbarbitone).

IV **Ultra short acting:** Replacement of the oxygen attached to C2 by sulphur enhances markedly the lipid solubility of the compounds. Because of rapid onset and short duration of action, they are used for IV anaesthesia, e. g., Thiopentone (Chapter 7).

Mechanism of action: Barbiturates cause reversible depression of all excitable tissues, the CNS being exquisitely sensitive. They bind to beta subunit of the inhibitory GABA-A receptor, a site distinct from the site at which benzodiazepines bind (Fig. 8.3). At lower doses, they enhance the action of GABA whereas in therapeutic doses they open the chloride channels directly. They also inhibit the exitatory AMPA-glutamate receptors.

Pharmacological actions: Barbiturates act at multiple sites in the CNS and are **less selective** than BDZ.

Central Nervous System: Barbiturates can cause varying depth of depression of the CNS from a mild sedation through hypnosis to general anaesthesia. Thus, they depress the CNS in a dose-dependent manner, acting at multiple sites.

- ***Sedation and hypnosis*:** Phenobarbitone given in small doses acts as a daytime sedative. Larger doses produce sleep. The sleep resembles natural sleep with characteristic sleep EEG pattern of high voltage and low frequency. However, they

(a) Cause more reduction in duration of REM sleep and number of cycles than BDZ

(b) Exhibit hangover (residual sedation and headache on waking) more than with BDZ.

(c) Cannot induce sleep in presence of pain, whereas BDZ can; and

(d) Cause rebound increase in REM sleep on sudden withdrawal; this can lead to increased dreaming and nightmares during the withdrawal period, especially in addicts. Further,

(e) Hypnotic doses of barbiturates produce motor incoordination.

Barbiturates reduce anxiety but may cause distortion of judgement. They also impair vigilance and attention to external stimuli.

In old people and children, however, barbiturates may occasionally produce dysphoria or excitement and a state of confusion.

- ***Anaesthetic effect*:** Thiobarbiturates IV produce general anaesthesia (Chapter 7).
- ***Anticonvulsant and antiepileptic effect*:** Barbiturates administered in anaesthetic doses inhibit or abolish drug induced convulsions and those due to epilepsy and tetanus. Phenobarbitone and mephobarbitone have a selective antiepileptic action in the *prevention* of grand mal epileptic seizures (Chapter 9).
- ***Respiration*:** Respiration is normally maintained as a result of :

(i) *A neurogenic drive* originating in the reticular activating system.

(ii) *A chemical drive* depending upon the concentration of carbon dioxide and pH of the arterial blood which directly modify the activity of the medullary respiratory centre; and

(iii) *A hypoxic drive* mediated through the carotid and the aortic body chemoreceptors.

Barbiturates cause dose-dependent depression of the respiration centre. Increase in the dose of barbiturates initially results in abolition of the 'neurogenic drive' followed by a decrease in the chemical drive. With toxic doses, the respiration is maintained mainly by the 'hypoxic drive'. A further increase in the barbiturate concentration abolishes the hypoxic drive and also causes a direct paralysis of the medullary centre.

- ***Spinal cord*:** Both the polysynaptic and the monosynaptic reflexes of the spinal cord are depressed by barbiturates.

Cardiovascular system: Hypnotic doses may cause a slight fall in BP and a decrease in heart rate as occurs during natural sleep. Toxic doses produce a sustained hypotension as a result of (i) direct depression of the myocardium and the vasomotor centre, (ii) hypoxia and (iii) probably, blockade of sympathetic ganglia.

Gastrointestinal tract: They do not affect the motility of the gut significantly.

Kidney: Barbiturate anaesthesia results in reduction of urinary output as a result of decrease in the GFR, and stimulation of secretion of ADH. Acute barbiturate poisoning is often associated with oliguria largely due to severe hypotension.

Liver: In patients intolerant of barbiturates, hepatic involvement may occur along with dermatitis and damage to other parenchymatous organs.

Barbiturates exert various actions on certain liver enzymes :

- ***On acute administration***, barbiturates combine with various subtypes of CYP450 enzymes and competitively inhibit the metabolism of drugs and endogenous steroids.
- ***Chronic administration causes induction of hepatic microsomal enzymes*** (Chapters 1, 3) leading to inactivation of certain drugs, including barbiturates themselves. This may explain the phenomenon of tolerance to barbiturates.
- ***They induce delta-amino-levulinic acid (ALA) synthetase, a mitochondrial enzyme, and aldehyde dehydrogenase, a cytoplasmic enzyme.*** Increase in ALA synthetase results in an increase in ALA and porphobilinogen synthesis. *In patients suffering from acute intermittent porphyria, barbiturates may precipitate a severe attack resulting in paralysis and even death.*
- ***Phenobarbitone increases the hepatic glucuronyl transferase and the bilirubin-binding Y-protein and stimulates the metabolism of bilirubin.***

Absorption, fate and excretion : Barbiturates are weak acids and maximum absorption occurs from the stomach where the barbiturates exist in an unionized form. Given orally, sodium salts are uniformly and rapidly absorbed but because of their extreme alkalinity, they may cause epigastric distress. Satisfactory absorption also occurs from the intestine and the rectum. Following absorption, a fraction of the drug in blood is reversibly bound to plasma albumin. The barbiturates are distributed in all tissues and body fluids. They readily cross the placental barrier and small amounts may be secreted in milk. No harmful effects on the suckling infant are known.

The factors which affect the distribution and fate of barbiturates are their

- ***Lipid solubility.***
- ***Degree of protein binding, and***
- ***Extent of ionization.***

The short acting barbiturates are highly soluble in lipids. Hence, these compounds have a rapid onset of action. They are more rapidly metabolized, but at the same time tend to get completely reabsorbed by the kidney tubules.

Barbiturates exist in the plasma in an ionized and a non-ionized form. An increase in pH (alkalinization) of blood and urine increases the ionization of the barbiturates causing an efflux of barbiturates from the tissues such as brain into the plasma. The ionized form does not cross the biological membranes and is excreted in urine.

All barbiturates are metabolized in the liver. The inactive metabolites are conjugated with glucuronic acid and are excreted in the urine. In the case of phenobarbitone, however, 25-30% of the dose is excreted unchanged.

Preparations and dosage:

(i) Phenobarbitone as an antiepileptic: See Chapter 9.

(ii) Amylobarbitone (Amytal) 50 mg tablets. Hypnotic dose 50-200 mg at bedtime.

(iii) Butobarbitone (Soneryl) 100 mg tablets. Hypnotic dose 100-200 mg at bedtime.

(iv) Secobarbitone (Seconal) 100 mg tablets. Hypnotic dose 100 mg at bedtime.

(v) Thiopental sodium as an IV anaesthetic: See Chapter 7.

Adverse reactions:

- ***Intolerance***: They may cause excitement (with hypnotic doses) headache, nausea, vomiting, diarrhoea and lassitude. Occasionally, barbiturates themselves may produce paroxysmal pain.
- ***Allergic reactions*** include urticaria, angioneurotic edema, other skin reactions, agranulocytosis and thrombocytopenic purpura.
- ***Anemia***: Prolonged phenobarbitone therapy may produce megaloblastic anemia which responds to folic acid (Chapter 34).
- ***Depression of fetal respiration***: Barbiturates, if administered to a woman during labour, may depress the foetal respiration.
- ***Porphyria*** : Barbiturate administration may precipitate an attack of acute intermittent hepatic porphyria.
- ***Drug automatism*** : If a barbiturate is being employed as a hypnotic, because of confusion and amnesia, a patient may repeatedly take the barbiturate at night and poison himself. This phenomenon is known as *drug automatism*.
- ***Tolerance*** : Repeated administration of barbiturates causes tolerance to their sedative and hypnotic actions. It can be attributed to : (i) increased hepatic inactivation and (ii) adaptation of the neuronal tissue to the drug. Barbiturate addicts often show cross tolerance to other general CNS depressants such as general anaesthetics. *However, tolerance to the hypnotic effect of barbiturates fails to modify their lethal dose significantly.* Acquired barbiturate tolerance usually disappears completely within 1 to 2 weeks of abstinence.
- ***Drug dependence*** : Repeated ingestion of barbiturates causes drug dependence.The manifestations of chronic barbiturate intoxication are thick slurred speech, ataxia, impaired reflexes, hypotonia, nystagmus and difficulty in accommodation. The nutrition is usually unimpaired. Barbiturate withdrawal symptoms are summarised in Table 8.3.

Table 8.3 : Barbiturate withdrawal symptoms

- **First 12-16 hours:** An apparent improvement may occur.
- **After 16 hours:** Anxiety, restlessness, tremors, abdominal cramps, nausea, vomiting, orthostatic hypotension and prostration.
- **2nd-3rd day:** Convulsions on withdrawal of short acting barbiturates.
- **4th-7th day:** Convulsions on withdrawal of long acting barbiturates. Also, visual hallucinations, disorientation and delirium may occur, and may be accompanied by cardiovascular collapse.
- **8th day:** Withdrawal symptoms, if mild, clear up; if severe, they may last for many weeks.

The treatment of barbiturate dependence is purely symptomatic. Generally the withdrawal should be gradual, over 10 days to 3 weeks, depending upon the severity of the dependence. If desired, replacement could be made with a hypnotic such as chlordiazepoxide 50 mg., or diazepam 10 mg.

Drug interactions : See Table 8.4.

Table 8.4: Important drug interactions of barbiturates

- Severe CNS depression: other CNS depressants (alcohol, benzodiazepines and antihistaminics) and monoamine oxidase inhibitors.
- Hepatic microsomal enzyme induction with diminished efficacy of other drugs: See Chapter 3.

Therapeutic uses of barbiturates:

- ***As hypnotics*** : They have now been largely replaced by benzodiazepines.
- ***As anticonvulsants*** : Barbiturates have been used to control convulsions in eclampsia and status epilepticus. They have now been replaced by benzodiazepines. For the use of phenobarbitone in epilepsy, see Chapter 9.
- ***General anaesthesia*** : See Chapter 7.
- ***Psychiatric uses*** : Amylobarbitone, pentobarbitone and thiopentone are employed by IV route to produce a state of deep sedation in which the cortical inhibitions are abolished. This may bring forth the suppressed psychic disturbances; the patient becomes more communicative and amenable to suggestions. This procedure of **narcoanalysis**, amytal interview (lie detection test) may be useful.
- ***Neonatal Jaundice*** : Phenobarbitone stimulates the liver to produce glucuronyl transferase, the enzyme essential for metabolism of bilirubin. It is, therefore, used to treat certain types of neonatal jaundice.

Acute barbiturate poisoning : Acute barbiturate poisoning causes depression of the CNS, particularly the respiration, and a peripheral circulatory collapse. The frequent and often fatal complications are respiratory (atelectasis, pulmonary edema and bronchopneumonia) or renal (acute renal shutdown).

Treatment of acute barbiturate poisoning: The severity of barbiturate poisoning is assessed by clinical signs prior to treatment and correlates well with plasma levels of barbiturate. Presence of reflexes, response to painful stimuli and maintenance of BP and of respiration without external assistance indicate a fair prognosis, while cases showing deep coma with absent reflexes, respiratory depression and cardiovascular collapse have a high mortality.

Table 8.5: Principles of management of acute barbiturate poisoning

- Hospitalization
- Attention to *airway*, *breathing* and *circulation* (ABC).
- Gastric lavage.
- Forced alkaline diuresis; adequate fluids IV; electrolyte balance.
- Peritoneal dialysis, hemodialysis, hemoperfusion
- Nursing care, nutrition.
- Prophylactic antibiotics.

Table 8.5 summarises the principles of management of acute barbiturate poisoning.

- ***Gastric lavage***: *If the patient is conscious* and less than four hours have elapsed since ingestion, vomiting may be induced with syrup of ipecac or concentrated salt solution. *If the patient is unconscious*, simple aspiration of the gastric contents is helpful if carried out *within four hours* of barbiturate ingestion. In comatose patients, endotracheal intubation should precede gastric intubation to prevent aspiration.
- ***Endotracheal intubation***: Adequate ventilation is important. If the respiration is not much affected, oxygen can be given by a nasal catheter. Endotracheal intubation is performed when spontaneous respiration is inadequate and also to remove secretions. If assisted ventilation is required for more than 24 hours, tracheostomy is usually performed. Frequent turning of the patient, tracheal suction and encouraging the patient to cough on awakening help to minimize respiratory complications. Frequent monitoring of blood gases and blood pH is helpful. Respiratory physiotherapy minimizes lung complications.

• ***Forced diuresis***: Hypotension and release of ADH reduce the urinary output in barbiturate intoxication. *Barbiturate excretion can be enhanced by increasing the urinary flow by using diuretics* like mannitol and furosemide.

Mannitol, an osmotic diuretic, is given IV, initially in the dose of 100-120 ml. of 25 per cent solution. Subsequently, a sustained infusion of 5 per cent mannitol alternately in a litre of normal saline and a litre of 5 per cent dextrose is administered at the rate of 500 ml. per hour for next 3 hours. The infusion is thereafter adjusted depending upon urine output and the state of hydration. Potassium chloride (10 to 20 mEq.) is added to each litre according to serum chemistry, and alkalinization with sodium bicarbonate may be conveniently carried out through the drip. An average urine volume of 10-12 litres in 24 hours (a flow rate of 8-10 ml. per minute) is considered as satisfactory diuresis. The dose of mannitol should not be more than 20 g. per hour. Forced diuresis is terminated on awakening.

Alternatively, **furosemide** (Lasix) is used in the dose of 20 mg. along with 500 ml. of 1.2 per cent sodium bicarbonate and one litre of 5 per cent dextrose IV in the first hour. The urine flow should be above 5 ml. per minute at the end of the hour. If it is not, furosemide should be given IV in large doses (upto 500 mg. per 24 hours); it is essential to monitor the serum chemistry, central venous pressure and urine output.

Forced diuresis is most useful in poisoning due to phenobarbitone, barbitone and allobarbitone, but not in poisoning due to other barbiturates which are more protein bound, have a large volume of distribution and are less ionized at the achievable urine pH. Shock, cardiac failure and renal impairment are absolute contraindications to forced diuresis.

It must be noted that forced diuresis is a potentially dangerous procedure and should only be considered for those patients who have taken phenobarbitone in such doses that they are unlikely to survive with supportive therapy alone. Forced diuresis must not be used as a substitute for the intensive supportive therapy as outlined above as most of the deaths are because of failure to maintain adequate tissue oxygenation.

• ***Intravenous fluids*** : Fluids must be given in sufficient quantity as an adjuvant to forced diuresis, in order to prevent dehydration and for maintaining the blood volume. Normal saline with dextrose is employed for this purpose. If hypotension does not respond to replacement by fluids (Chapter 31), vasopressor agents like dopamine may be used. Overloading of the circulation should be avoided.

• ***Alkalinization of the urine*** : This increases the excretion of long acting barbiturates, such as phenobarbitone; it has no significant effect on the renal elimination of short acting barbiturates. Sodium bicarbonate 3.75g. (45 mEq) as 50ml of a 7.5% solution may be added to every litre of fluid intended for IV administration. The urinary pH should be maintained between 7.5 and 8.5.

• ***Prophylactic antibiotics***: These should not be used routinely but may be necessary in those requiring tracheostomy or catheterization of urinary bladder.

• ***Dialysis and hemoperfusion***: Elimination of barbiturates from the body can be hastened by peritoneal dialysis, charcoal hemoperfusion and hemodialysis. All are more effective in removing long acting barbiturates than in removing short acting ones. In general, peritoneal dialysis is more suitable than forced diuresis in patients who have severe renal impairment and in those in whom the cardiac status precludes vigorous fluid administration.

Table 8.6: Indications for hemodialysis in acute barbiturate poisoning

- Shock.
- Progressive deterioration with conservative therapy.
- Ingestion of a potentially lethal dose.
- Potentially lethal blood barbiturate levels, and
- In patients in whom peritoneal dialysis is ineffective or contraindicated.

Hemodialysis is about forty times more effective than forced diuresis in promoting barbiturate elimination. Indications for hemodialysis are outlined in Table 8.6. Charcoal hemoperfusion is now considered superior to peritoneal dialysis and hemodialysis in this therapy.

Alcohols

ETHANOL : Taken at bedtime, ethyl alcohol may act as a mild sedative. However, it cannot be recommended as a hypnotic as small doses may produce excitement; further the diuresis induced by it may interrupt sleep. In addition, there is the danger of drug dependence.

CHLORAL HYDRATE AND TRICHLOROETHANOL: Oral chloral hydrate and its active metabolite trichloroethanol act as hypnotics. Its mechanism of action is similar to that of barbiturates. In small doses, it causes sedation. A slightly larger dose (0.5-1 g) at bed time results in normal sleep. Sleep is induced within 1 hour and lasts for 4 to 5 hours. From the practical point of view, it is a rapidly effective, reasonably safe, and cheap hypnotic drug.

Absorption, fate and excretion: Chloral hydrate is satisfactorily absorbed from the GI tract including the rectum. A part of it is oxidized to trichloroacetic acid in the liver and the kidney, the reaction being catalysed by the enzyme alcohol dehydrogenase. The remainder is reduced to trichloroethanol which is conjugated with glucuronic acid and excreted in the urine as urochloralic acid.

Adverse reactions: The common adverse reactions are allergic skin rash and epigastric pain.

It has an unpleasant taste, and may produce nausea and vomiting due to gastric irritation. *It should be given well diluted*, preferably in fruit juice, after a meal. Hangover may occur. In therapeutic doses, it may sometimes produce delirium and excitement in the presence of pain.

Toxic doses (more than 5 g.) cause loss of reflexes and depression of the vasomotor and respiratory centres. Large doses cause cardiac, hepatic and renal damage. Tolerance and drug dependence occur rarely and abrupt withdrawal of the drug may result in delirium, mania and convulsions. Chloral hydrate produces an additive effect with ethyl alcohol.

Preparations and dosage:

(i) Chloral hydrate: Dose 0.5 to 2.0 g. In children, 30-50 mg/kg. as syrup to a maximum of 1g. Infants may be given 50 to 75 mg. per dose.

(ii) Trichloroethyl phosphate (Triclofos, Trichloryl) : This sodium salt of the phosphoric acid ester of trichloroethanol is supplied as a syrup containing 0.5 g./5 ml. and 0.5 g. tablet.

Therapeutic uses: Though it is now rarely used as a hypnotic, its relative safety makes it a useful alternative to a benzodiazepine in the elderly and in children; further, its low cost makes it attractive for use in public hospitals. It is recommended only for short term use as its effectiveness is likely to wane after 2 weeks.

The drug should be avoided in the presence of marked hepatic, cardiac or renal damage, peptic ulcer, oesophagitis or gastritis.

Aldehydes

PARALDEHYDE : Paraldehyde is a colourless and inflammable liquid with a characteristic odour and an acidic taste. It has hypnotic and anticonvulsant properties. Oral paraldehyde induces sleep within 15 to 30 minutes, which lasts for 6 to 8 hours. Hangover is uncommon. Therapeutic doses of paraldehyde have no deleterious effects on the respiratory and the vasomotor centres. However, it crosses the placental barrier and may delay the establishment of breathing in the newborn. The drug is mainly metabolized in the liver. About 11-28 per cent is excreted unchanged through the lung.

Adverse reactions : Paraldehyde is irritant to

the mucosa and given IM, it may cause tissue necrosis and nerve damage. The drug decomposes to acetic acid and acetaldehyde in the presence of light and heat; and death may result from administration of old paraldehyde. *Hence, paraldehyde stored for more than 6 months should not be used.*

It may produce excitement and delirium in the presence of pain. It is excreted in breath and imparts an unpleasant odour to it.

Tolerance and addiction to paraldehyde are rare. Alcoholics exhibit cross tolerance to paraldehyde. *It can dissolve plastics and hence should not be injected with a plastic syringe.*

Preparation and dosage:

(i) Inj. paraldehyde 5 to 10 ml. administered deep IM in the buttock. When the larger dose is being administered, it is divided between two sites to minimize local irritation. The drug does not support the growth of micro-organisms and may be used as such in an emergency. The dose in children is 0.2 ml/kg.

(ii) It can also be given rectally in the dose of 15-30 ml. after suitable dilution with three parts of a vegetable oil.

Therapeutic uses: ***It is used IM as an anticonvulsant*** in status epilepticus, tetanus and eclampsia. Its IV use is not recommended as it may cause violent coughing and pulmonary edema. The drug should not be administered per rectum in patients with inflammatory lesions of the bowel. It should be avoided in the presence of severe impairment of hepatic and pulmonary function.

It is now rarely used as a hypnotic.

Miscellaneous

In addition to the drugs described above, which have a primary hypnotic action, various other drugs have hypnotic action as their prominent side effect. These are listed in Table 8.7. Antihistaminics **diphenhydramine** and **promethazine** are sometimes preferred as hypnotics in pediatric practice. Scopolamine may be preferred as a mild sedative with a peripheral parasympathetic blocking action. Amitryptiline is useful in treating depressed patients. (Chapter 13).

Table 8.7: Drugs with sedation as a prominent side effect

- **Certain antipsychotics,** e.g., chlorpromazine.
- **Certain antidepressants,** e.g., amitryptiline.
- **Certain antihistaminics,** e.g., diphenhydramine, promethazine.
- **Certain anticholinergics,** e.g., scopolamine; and
- **Certain antiepileptics,** e.g., primidone.

Some drugs used as hypnotics (barbiturates, phenothiazine antihistaminics and chlorpromazine) may cause insomnia as an idiosyncratic reaction.

Dexmedetomidine : See Chapter 7.

Older sedative-hypnotics such as ethinamate, glutethimide, methyprylon, meprobamate and inorganic bromides are now rarely used.

Methaqualone, once used as a hypnotic, is extensively misused as a drug of abuse. It has no therapeutic application.

Pharmacotherapy of Insomnia and Other Sleep Disorders

Ability to go to sleep is a very personal attribute and people are either 'good sleepers' or 'poor sleepers'. The latter, on the whole, take longer to fall asleep, sleep less, awaken more, have less REM and stage 4 NREM sleep, and have higher physiological arousal (heart rate, body temperature) than good sleepers. At the extreme end of the spectrum of poor sleepers is the person who sleeps through the whole night in several cat naps instead of sleeping continuously. Reduced total sleep time without any subjective or objective consequences suggests that the subject may be a physiologically short sleeper. As with all other things in life, most people learn to live with their own sleeping pattern.

Insomnia is said to be present when an individual *complains* of inability to fall or stay asleep, of reduction in the total sleep period, of sleep disturbed by nightmares or of sleep that does not refresh. *Transient* (no more than three nights) and *short-term (acute) insomnia* (less than about 3 weeks) may occur in the absence of disease and is then due to stress caused by reactions to life changes, environmental factors, grief, job demands, travelling through time zones etc. Other than this, acute insomnia may be due to physical discomfort such as pain, dyspnoea, fever, nocturnal myoclonus or psychiatric causes such as anxiety. It may occasionally be induced by drugs (see later).

Chronic insomnia by definition lasts for at least 3 weeks and needs detailed evaluation. A two week sleep diary and an interview with the sleep-partner may be useful. Between 30-60% of the patients with chronic insomnia have a recognizable psychiatric illness such as chronic anxiety, depression or psychosis. Chronic insomnia is a complex process and rarely benefits from hypnotics alone. Persistent insomnia is both a risk factor in and a precursor of mood disorders; it is associated with increased risk of automobile accidents, increased alcohol consumption and daytime sleepiness.

If insomnia is due to pain, fever, dyspnoea or myalgia, appropriate treatment should be prescribed. It is imperative to ascertain whether any organic disease is responsible for insomnia and attempts should be made to treat it. *Sudden fearful awakening with palpitation and sweating should arouse the suspicion of an associated major disorder such as angina, hypoglycemia or severe anxiety state.* The presence of dyspnoea in such a patient may indicate early heart failure which should be ruled out.

Table 8.8: Non-pharmacological measures for treating insomnia

The patient is advised to :

- Avoid day-time naps.
- Take moderate exercise in the morning or afternoon; it has been shown to increase stage 4 NREM sleep.
- Avoid the consumption of alcohol, tobacco and caffeinated beverages close to bedtime.
- Establish a regular bedtime hour and condition himself to go to bed only when feeling sleepy; he should not remain in bed if he cannot sleep soon.
- Use the bed for sleeping and sex, not for eating, reading or television watching.
- Avoid all complex mental activity prior to bedtime.

Further :

- He may need a change in the mattress.
- The elderly should restrict fluids in the evening to decrease nocturia.
- Some fill up for the stomach such as a glass of warm milk is useful. Milk contains tryptophan, and d-tryptophan is known to reduce the time to onset of sleep in volunteers.
- Training in relaxation, yoga or meditation can be helpful.

Insomnia due to mental disturbances needs psychiatric evaluation. Difficulty in staying asleep is a frequent complaint of depressed patients. This is associated with marked decrease in stage 4 of NREM sleep. It is not benefited by hypnotics, and treatment of depression is of prime importance (Chapter 13).

Rational therapy of insomnia depends upon the accurate diagnosis, and its precipitating and perpetuating factors. These can be easily identified in subjects with acute insomnia.

In cases with 'primary' insomnia, certain simple, **non-pharmacological measures** (Table 8.8) may help the subjects to establish good sleep habits. If these measures fail to rapidly restore the normal sleeping pattern, there should be no hesitation in using `hypnotic' drugs.

Pharmacologically, it is impossible to clearly separate sedative, antianxiety and hypnotic drugs. It would appear that with most drugs belonging to these classes, the desired effect can be produced by an appropriately adjusted dose.

In therapeutic doses, most 'hypnotic' drugs have similar actions; they

- ***Decrease the latent period of sleep.***
- ***Increase the total sleep time.***
- ***Decrease the awake time and the awakenings.***
- ***Increase the duration of stage 2 sleep;*** and
- ***Reduce the period of REM sleep.***

There are more similarities than differences among the hypnotic drugs. The differences are, however, of practical importance. They are :

(a) Rapidity of action.

(b) Duration of action.

(c) Differences in the degree of suppression of REM sleep; and

(d) Adverse reactions, especially liability to produce respiratory depression, dependence and impairment of cognitive function.

Table 8.9 outlines the principles of drug therapy of insomnia.Transient insomnia can be helped by a short course for 2-3 nights.

Although claims have been made for superiority of one drug over another based on differential actions on the sleep stages, clinical criteria of efficacy in alleviating a particular sleeping problem (difficulty in falling asleep, frequent awakenings, short duration of sleep or ''unrefreshing'' sleep) are more useful.

If an elderly person has difficulty in falling asleep (sleep onset insomnia), a drug that is rapidly effective and short acting such as a short acting BDZ should be administered 20-30 minutes before the usual bedtime. For persons with difficulty in maintenance of sleep, longer acting drugs like lorazepam or temazepam may be preferred. Long half-life BDZ such as diazepam and flurazepam are preferred when day-time sedation is also desired.

Many antidepressant drugs are powerful in suppressing the signs of REM sleep. Since in patients with duodenal ulcer, marked increase in gastric acid secretion frequently occurs during REM sleep and episodes of nocturnal angina are associated with REM sleep, its suppression may be useful in such patients. *In such cases, treatment once started should not be withdrawn suddenly for fear of 'rebound' reaction, which could worsen the condition.* Sudden withdrawal of REM suppressants causes a sharp increase in the REM sleep. Such a 'rebound' in an anxious patient is often associated with increased dreaming, nightmares, restlessness, insomnia and even fits. In its most severe form, the withdrawal state is one of delirium tremens with terror and marked insomnia. Some patients may, therefore, continue the hypnotic to avoid these reactions,

Table 8.9 Principles of drug therapy of insomnia

Transient insomnia :

- A hypnotic with short duration of action
- Use the lowest dose for 2-3 nights

Short term insomnia :

- Counselling
- A hypnotic 30 minutes prior to retiring to bed
- Use lowest effective dose
- After getting 1-2 night's acceptable sleep, skip a dose
- Use intermittently (2-4 times a week) for a short time, not more than 3 weeks at a time
- Discontinue gradually.
- Be alert to rebound insomnia after stopping.

Chronic insomnia :

- Psychotherapy and behavioural therapy
- Chronotherapy
- Treatment of associated depression or psychosis
- Hypnotics as adjuvants, use every 3rd night
- Discontinue gradually after 3-6 months

thus leading to drug dependence. Eventually, a chronic state of intoxication ensues with tremor and confusion during day and insomnia at night.

Whichever hypnotic is chosen, it should be used initially in a small dose and increased only if absolutely necessary. Once a good night's sleep is obtained, attempts should be made to omit the drug for a few nights. The drug should be used to condition the patient to sleep better and should not be allowed to make a slave out of him. He should be explained that he can now sleep well without the drug and that an occasional night of imperfect sleep will not harm.

Unlike the drugs mentioned above, antipsychotic phenothiazines are poor hypnotics. It is, therefore, rational to prescribe a conventional hypnotic to treat uncorrected insomnia in a patient on antipsychotics.

The important drawback of all hypnotics is the 'hangover'. All of them impair performance the next day. Even smaller amounts used as daytime sedative can impair social judgement and performance. Patients should be warned not only about the possible interactions of hypnotics with alcohol and other drugs, but also about the possibility of impaired performance such as car driving the next day.

Rarely, these drugs can cause

(a) severe hypersensitivity reactions including anaphylaxis and/or angioedema; and

(b) hazardous sleep-related activities such as sleep driving, telephoning while asleep, and preparing and eating food while asleep.

It is unlikely that a potent hypnotic will not cause a hangover and will be free from dependence liability. However, the newer benzodiazepines with short t½ such as lorazepam and the non-benzodiazepines are safer.

Often, a patient taking hypnotics also takes other drugs simultaneously. Such combinations can be sometimes dangerous. Thus, MAO inhibitors taken to relieve mental depression may lead to slow inactivation of other depressant drugs, giving rise to serious toxicity in otherwise nontoxic doses (Chapter 13).

Sedatives and hypnotics are indicated in various situations in children but they should not be employed as a substitute for other important measures such as discussion with the parents about their children's behavioural problems and the importance of change in parental attitudes. Chloral hydrate 60 mg 2-3 times a day is a good daytime sedative in infants. For sleep problems in adults, chloral hydrate in doses of 500 mg. is highly effective and safe. Routine use of hypnotics for things like tics, nightmares, breath-holding attacks, masturbation, aggressiveness, fears and school phobias, and head banging is not considered justifiable. The more rational approach in all such cases is to discuss the psychological problem with the mother.

Sleepwalking, night terrors and nightmares are designated as **parasomnias.**

Sleepwalking and night terrors are the mild and severe manifestations of the same disorder occurring about 1-3 hours after the onset of sleep, when stage 3 and 4 sleep is more prevalent. The disorders are idiopathic when they begin in childhood and benefit from (a) safety precautions and (b) the use of drugs like diazepam and flurazepam which suppress stages 3 and 4 of sleep. An organic cause such as a brain tumour must be ruled out in adult patients.

Nightmares, commonly known as bad dreams, occur during REM sleep. They may occur in normal children and in children with fever. The best way to handle them is to avoid terrifying stories, movies and frightening TV programmes. *When they occur for the first time in adult life, depression is an important cause, and such depressed patients may be at increased risk for suicide. They are treated with REM suppressants such as tricyclic antidepressants.*

Often, a clinician is tempted to prescribe a hypnotic readily under pressure from patients, relatives, nursing staff or himself. In the long run, this attitude may cause more harm to the patient than good. It is useful to remember that :

- Detailed history must be taken to rule out

causes such as severe anxiety or depression; and consumption of drugs (Table 8.10), excessive tea, coffee and colas.

- Periodic loss of sleep in itself is not harmful and therefore, does not require treatment with drugs. Professionals like doctors, nurses and seamen who also lose sleep on and off remain resilient and healthy.
- The clinician should not have a negative approach to what lies behind the presented symptom of sleeplessness, and hypnotics must not be prescribed readily *'on demand'*.
- One should be critical in repeating the *'sleeping pill'* prescription and try to avoid its continuation.
- No hypnotic is safe, all can cause harm and none is effective in helping patients with problems underlying their insomnia; moreover some of these drugs lose their effectiveness on repeated administration. Special caution is necessary in patients with respiratory diseases, suicidal tendencies and history of drug dependence. The risk of falls and fractures increases especially in the elderly patients using hypnotics and other psychotherapeutic agents.
- The difficulties of stopping the hypnotic in chronic hypnotic users could be enormous and can cause depression.
- Effectiveness and safety are still the main considerations in prescribing hypnotic drugs.
- Chronic insomnia usually needs long term strategy for its management, with combination of drugs and cognitive behavioural therapy.
- *Hynotics should not be used in patients with sleep apnoea.*

It is important to remember that drugs themselves can cause insomnia. (Table 8.10).

Table 8.10: Drug induced insomnia

- CNS stimulants: ephedrine, amphetamine, methylphenidate, caffeine, nicotine
- Anorexiants
- Nasal decongestants
- Bupropion
- Antidepressants: MAO inhibitors, SSRI
- Levodopa
- Amantadine
- Chloroquine
- Metronidazole
- Fluoroquinolones
- Diuretics
- Systemic glucocorticoids

The commonest causes of *insomnia in the elderly* are age-related changes in the sleep cycle and daytime napping. One should also look for medical illnesses, depression, anxiety, dementia and loss of family support. The patient should understand that improvement rather than total relief of insomnia is an achievable goal. Because of reduced body water, renal and heptic function and increase in body fat, the pharmacological profile of hypnotics may be altered in the elderly, with prolongation of their half life (Chapter 1). The following points are important while treating insomnia in this age group:

(a) Restriction of fluids in the evening.

(b) Smaller than usual doses of *short acting* BDZ which are the hypnotics of choice

(c) If BDZ are not tolerated, use zolpidem and zaleplon.

(d) Avoid sedative antihistaminics as they are liable to cause delirium and anticholinergic side effects.

(e) Look for any psychosocial problem such as loneliness, anxiety and depression causing the sleep disturbance.

Drugs Effective in Seizure Disorders

9

Drugs used in the treatment of seizure disorders can be divided into :

I Drugs which are used to abolish seizures (anticonvulsants) and

II Drugs which are administered prophylactically to prevent seizures.

These drugs can be classified as :

- ***Centrally acting*** e.g. General anaesthetics, Diazepam, Praldehyde, Barbiturates (Chapters 7 and 8) and specific antiepileptic drugs.
- ***Acting mainly on the spinal cord*** e.g. Mephenesin (Chapter 20).
- ***Peripheral skeletal muscle relaxants*** e.g. d-Tubocurarine and Succinylcholine (Chapter 21).

Experimentally, drugs with a potential antiepileptic activity are assessed against seizures induced in mice by injecting medullary stimulants or by applying a maximal electrical shock. The chemical commonly used to produce seizures is pentylenetetrazol (leptazol). Drugs which antagonize leptazol seizures are generally useful in petit mal. Drugs likely to be effective in grand mal epilepsy usually confer protection against electrically induced seizures.

A model for human focal epilepsy is that produced in animals by "Kindling". This consists of delivery of brief localized trains of electrical stimuli to an area of the brain, repeatedly, at about 24 hour intervals. After a time, generalized motor seizures are regularly elicited during such electrical stimulation. Eventually, spontaneous, recurring seizures start occurring; such 'kindled' animals are very sensitive to a variety of chemical and sensory convulsive stimuli.

Types of Epilepsy

Epilepsy is a collective term for a group of chronic seizures having in common sudden and transient episodes (**seizures**) of disturbance of consciousness and/or a characteristic body movement (**convulsion**), and sometimes autonomic hyperactivity. The seizure nearly always correlates with an abnormal electrical brain discharge.

A seizure may also occur due to a systemic disorder such as hypoglycemia or hypocalcemia, or an intracranial/severe systemic infection. In these cases, an **aura** (see later) is absent and the seizures are self-limited. Further, unlike in the case of the epileptic seizures, there generally is no environmental or physiological trigger such as strong emotions, intense exercise,flashing lights or loud music immediately preceding the seizure. These seizure are called **Non Epileptic Seizure (NES).** Their main treatment comprises that of the cause.

In practice, the drug treatment of epilepsy is guided by the nature of seizures. Table 9.1 shows the currently used classification of seizures, based on history, clinical findings, EEG recording and imaging studies. Thus, the seizures can be divided into two broad groups. (1) **generalized seizures**; and (2) **partial seizures**.

The drugs used for all partial seizures are generally the same; whereas in the case of the generalized seizures, they depend upon the type of seizure in the different subgroups.

Table 9.1: Types of seizures

I Primarily generalized seizures
Generalized tonin-clonic seizures (Grand mal)
Tonic seizures
Atonic seizures
Absence seizures (Petit mal)
Myoclonic seizures
Infantile spasms
II Partial seizures
Simple partial seizures
Complex partial seizures
Secondary generalized seizures

I **Primarily generalized seizures.** These are due to (a) mutations in Con channels; (b) changes in the neuronal network.

- ***Tonic-Clonic seizures*** are generalized from their onset and are accompanied by a generalized abnormality in the EEG (**grand mal or major epilepsy**). They are characterized by sudden loss of consciousness without any warning (aura), followed by generalized tonic, and finally clonic convulsive movements. This is followed by a period of headache, drowsiness, confusion and sleep. The attack may be accompanied by tongue biting, frothing at the mouth and incontinence.
- ***Tonic seizure*** **:** As above but without clonic phase.
- ***Atonic seizure*** (Drop attack) : Such a seizure consists of sudden loss of postural tone, without accompanying tonic or clonic movements. The head may drop for a few seconds or the child may drop to the floor without any apparent cause. Such seizures reflect diffuse brain damage and may be a manifestation of secondary generalized epilepsy.
- ***Absence seizure (Petit mal)*** **:** It consists of sudden cessation of ongoing conscious activity *without convulsive movement and without loss of postural control*. The patient appears to go blank for a few seconds to one minute, and there may be accompanying fluttering of eyelids or small chewing movements. Awareness of the surroundings is regained quickly at the end of an attack, and the patient may not even know that one has occurred. The EEG is diagnostic with diffuse, bilaterally synchronous 3 per second wave and spike discharges. Absence seizures almost always begin in childhood and are idiopathic in origin. The child may outgrow these seizures. Some children have additional generalized tonic-clonic seizures.

Typical idiopathic absence seizures respond well to drug treatment. In children with underlying brain disease, absence seizures may co-exist with other types of generalized seizures and then are resistant to drug treatment.

- ***Myoclonic seizure*** **:** This is a sudden, brief, repetitive muscle contraction involving a body part or the whole body. In the latter case, there is violent fall without loss of consciousness. Myoclonic seizures may occur by themselves or coexist with other seizures. They may be idiopathic-genetic or due to a metabolic or CNS disease. The EEG changes are characteristic.
- ***Infantile spasms***

II **Partial seizures** are focal i.e. originate in a localized area of the brain with a focus of EEG abnormality and may or may not become generalized. They are subdivided into *simple partial seizures, complex seizures* and *secondary generalized seizures.* In adults, the commonest form of epilepsy is partial epilepsy; wherein the commonest associated lesion is hippocampal sclerosis; whether it is the cause of the result of partial epilepsy is debatable.

- ***Simple partial seizures*** **:** A wide range of clinical phenomena also known as **auras** may occur depending on the site of the brain lesion.

(a) ***Motor*** **:** This begins as recurrent

contractions of a part of the body and may spread to involve contiguous areas. These are the visible manifestations.

(b) ***A variety of subjective symptoms*** may be experienced by the patient : sensory (numbness or parasthesiae limited to one part of the body); olfactory; gustatory; auditory; vertiginous; autonomic; or psychic such as deja-vu and dreamy state or unwarranted fear or anger.

The patient is conscious and is aware of the event which lasts for a few seconds to a few minutes. These seizures are associated with a highly localized abnormal discharge; but the latter spreads widely into the limbic system.

- ***Complex partial seizures*** **:** These consist of an aura (unusual smell, sudden intense emotional feelings), followed by loss of contact with the environment. There may be repetitive motor activity such as lip smacking, swallowing or aimless wandering or unconscious performance of highly skilled activities such as car-driving (**automatism**). There is amnesia for the entire period of the seizure. Only 70-80% of the complex partial seizures arise from the temporal lobe. *Hence, although the terms psychomotor, temporal and limbic have been used synonymously, all such seizures are not the same.* Focal slowing or sharp wave activity or both, on the EEG, provides confirmation.
- ***Secondarily generalized seizures*** **:** These start as simple partial seizures and develop into one of the generalized seizures listed above. Such a seizure may be followed by postictal neurological deficit (**Todd's paralysis**). When the spread of the motor phenomena is orderly, the seizure is called Jacksonian seizure.

Status epilepticus (SE) : Prolonged seizures (more than 5-10 minutes) or repetitive seizures (of any variety) without recovery of consciousness between attacks comprise SE. When tonic-clonic seizures go into SE, the situation can be life threatening and is a medical emergency (see later).

The above description applies to a classification of the 'seizures'. The classification of 'epilepsies', on the other hand, must also take into account age of onset, genetic factors, EEG findings, associated neurologic defects, imaging results, response to treatment and prognosis. Defining a specific **epilepsy syndrome** may be more helpful in selecting the drug treatment and judging the prognosis than taking into consideration only the seizure characteristics.

In about 10% of persons with true seizures, multiple EEG studies reveal no abnormalities. *Therefore, a normal EEG does not rule out a seizure disorder in a person with a diagnostic clinical picture.*

Neurophysiology: John Hughlings Jackson postulated about a century ago that epileptic seizures were caused by "occasional, sudden, excessive, rapid, local discharges from the grey matter". Modern electrophysiology has confirmed this. Depending on the neurotransmitter released, the brain neurons are grouped as **excitatory** and **inhibitory**. The primary inhibitory transmitter in the brain is GABA whereas the excitatory transmitter is mostly the amino acid glutamate. GABA acts on the GABA receptors, and glutamate acts through the N-methyl-D aspartate (NMDA) and non-NMDA receptors (Chapter 5). Activation of these receptors modifies various voltage-gated Na^+, K^+, Ca^{++} and Cl^- ion channels and excites or inhibits the neuron. An action potential is an *all or none* phenomenon; once the threshold is reached, the action potential fires. This cellular event is associated with influx of Na^+ into and efflux of K^+ out of the neuronal cell. Normally, the neurons fire action potentials singly or in short runs; and the excitability is kept under control by powerful inhibitory influences.

Pathophysiology of epilepsy involves two, importantly related events: (i) **hyper-excitability;** and (ii) **hypersynchrony.** Hyperexcitability is the abnormal responsiveness of the neurons to an excitatory input, leading to multiple discharges. Chronic hyperexcitbility can result from a number of mechanisms. Hypersynchrony refers to the recruitment of a large number of nearby neurons to an abnormal firing mode.Thus, epilepsy is a network phenomenon involving the participation of many neurons firing simultaneously. The characteristic patho-physiologic event in a seizure is believed to be paroxysmal depolarization shift (PDS) of neuronal membrane potential and associated burst discharge. Excitatory neurotransmitters, are thought to be involved in the initiation and spread of the seizure discharge, and the inhibitory transmitter GABA is believed to be responsible for its termination.

The normal brain contains billions of neurons which 'fire' asynchronously (i.e. at different times). Inhibitory feedback loops in the normal brain regulate the frequency of firing of individual neurons and prevent synchronization. When such inhibitory feedback is defective, a large number of cells in a given area of the brain fire at the same time (i.e. they synchronize) and produce a self-regenerating electrical impulse. Such an area constitutes an **epileptic focus**. Such foci may be cortical or subcortical. They may discharge intermittently, only to be shown up on the gross surface EEG but not cause symptoms because their spread is blocked by the inhibitory mechanisms in the surrounding brain tissue. Factors which themselves cannot initiate seizures may trigger off the abnormal focus or permit the spread of activity to the normal brain. Such factors include hyperventilation, alkalosis, hypoglycemia, overhydration, hypocalcemia, overeating, and emotional stress. Spread of the abnormal electrical activity to the normal brain tissue causes a generalized seizure.

The clinical type of seizure is independent of the brain pathology but is determined by the site of the abnormal focus. The response to treatment correlates best with the site of the epileptogenic focus.

Antiepileptic Drugs (AED)

AED can be classified according to their mechanism of action as shown in Table 9.2.

Table 9.2: AED classified according to their mechanism of action

- **Those that decrease the neuronal excitability by delaying the recovery from inactivation of Na^+channels:** Phenytoin, Carbamazepine, Lamotrigine, Topiramate.
- **Those which decrease the low threshold calcium currents (T-current) in the thalamic neurons:** Ethosuximide.
- **Those that act similarly to both phenytoin and ethosuximide as mentioned above:** Valproic acid, Zonisamide.
- **Those which enhance inhibition through GABA:**
  - (a) Acting through GABA-related receptors: Barbiturates, Benzodiazepines.
  - (b) By releasing GABA from neuronal endings: Gabapentin.
  - (c) By inhibiting GABA transaminase: Vigabatrine.
  - (d) By inhibiting GABA reuptake : Tiagabine.
- **Those that inhibit excitatory neurotrammitters:** Lamotrigine; and
- **Miscellaneous:** Levetiracetam, Acetazolamide.

I Hydantoin derivatives:

DIPHENYLHYDANTOIN (Phenytoin sodium, Dilantin, Eptoin): This drug, introduced by Merritt and Putnam in 1938, is still an important drug in the treatment of epilepsy with the exception of petit mal and myoclonic seizures. It is structurally related to barbiturates.

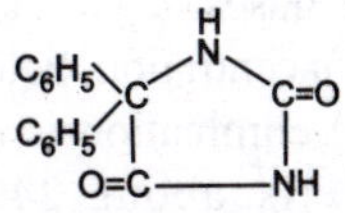

H
N
C_6H_5 C C=O
C_6H_5
O=C NH

Fig. 9.1 : Diphenylhydantion

Mechanism of action: The drug slows the recovery of voltage-dependent sodium-ion channels (**stabilizing effect**) on all neuronal membranes including the peripheral nerves as well as on all non-excitable and excitable membranes. It inhibits the spread of seizure discharges in the brain and shortens the duration of after-discharge.

It reduces the neuronal Na+ concentration leading to a reduction in paroxysmal depolarization shift (PDS). It also decreases post tetanic potentiation (PTP) which is responsible for the spread of the seizure activity. The PTP is an enhancement of synaptic transmission following repeated tetanic, high frequency stimulation of the presynaptic fibres. In patients in whom it is effective, the generalized abnormality in EEG disappears but the abnormal focal electrical activity persists.

High concentrations of phenytoin also augment brain level of GABA, 5-HT and homovanillic acid. This may contribute to its toxicity.

Pharmacological actions:

CNS actions : It exerts a selective antiepileptic action (see above) without causing drowsiness. The onset of action is slow even on IV injection but the action persists for a considerable time after cessation of therapy.

Cardiovascular actions : It has a cell membrane stabilizing effect (Chapter 27).

Absorption, fate and excretion: Phenytoin is slowly and variably absorbed from the gut, with plasma peak level at 3-12 hours after ingestion. In plasma, it is 70-95% albumin bound and is metabolized mainly by parahydroxylation in the liver. The drug is concentrated in bile and is reabsorbed from the intestine as parahydroxyphenol. In individuals deficient in the liver parahydroxylase, toxicity can occur even with small doses.

At plasma concentration below 10 mcg/ml, (sub-therapeutic) elimination is exponential and the plasma t½ is about 24 hours. As it approaches the therapeutic concentration of 20 mcg/ml, its metabolism becomes saturated; it then exhibits dose dependent (Zero order) elimination and the plasma concentration rises disproportionately to the dose increment; the elimination t½ increases. Hence, *the dose increments must be smaller with increasing dosage*. About 94 per cent of a single dose is excreted in urine within 48 hours. On chronic medication, the drug disappears from the plasma within 3 days after stopping the treatment.

It induces hepatic microsomal enzymes.

Adverse reactions: Within the therapeutic range of plasma phenytoin level (10-20 mcg/ml) the drug is usually well tolerated.

With higher plasma levels(> 20 mcg/ml), the half-life increases to 35 hours or longer. When this happens, even a slight increase in the dose can cause increased toxicity. However, the toxicity disappears equally quickly on reducing the daily dose. Death due to phenytoin is rare.

- ***Intolerance***: Urticarial, scarlatiniform and measles-like skin rashes may occur. The skin reactions may be accompanied by lymphadenopathy, hepatomegaly and jaundice.
- ***Central nervous system***: Mild toxicity consists of drowsiness, fatigue, headache and confusion. Larger doses can cause *a vestibulocerebellar syndrome* characterised by vertigo, ataxia, nystagmus and dysarthria. Ocular pain with blurring of vision, delusions, hallucinations and other psychotic episodes are sometimes encountered. Rarely, cognitive impairment, behavioural changes may occur.

Peripheral neuropathy has been reported particularly in old people. These effects are dose related and usually disappear following dose reduction. Ataxia, however, may occasionally persist for long periods after drug withdrawal.

- ***Gastrointestinal tract***: Alkalinity of the drug causes nausea and vomiting which can be prevented by taking the daily dose in divided portions, after meals, with plenty of water.
- ***Face and gums***: Hyperplasia and hypertrophy of the gums with edema and bleeding occur in approximately 15 per cent of patients. It is not related to the dose of phenytoin. Scrupulous dental hygiene but not vitamin C can prevent the gingival hyperplasia. In most cases, the gums return to normal within a year after discontinuation of the drug.

Long term phenytoin therapy sometimes causes hypertrophy of the facial subcutaneous tissue, hypertrichosis and coarsening of facial features (**phenytoin facies**) which may be disfiguring.

- ***Endocrine effects***: Hypertrichosis is seen especially in children. Less commonly, hyperglycemia and osteomalacia have been observed. Rarely, hyperglycemic, hyperosmolar, nonketotic coma complicates IV phenytoin therapy, due to inhibition of insulin secretion.
- ***Enzyme induction :*** Phenytoin is a potent inducer of hepatic microsomal enzymes. *It accelarates its own metabolism and that of other drugs* such as vitamin D, folate, glucocorticoids, gonadal steroids, thyroxine, OC pills and doxycycline thereby reducing their therapeutic efficacy. Thus, it may cause osteomalacia and megaloblastic anemia.
- ***Teratogenicity***: Hydantoins, administered during the first trimester of pregnancy, can cause **fetal hydantoin syndrome**. It comprises midline hypoplasia, ptosis, wide mouth, inner epicanthic folds, short neck, mild webbing of the neck, short phalanges and hypoplastic nails. Some children may develop congenital heart defects, microcephaly and mental subnormality.
- ***Miscellaneous***: Rarely, blood dyscrasias including aplastic anemia and agranulocytosis, may occur. Appearance of LE cells and methaemoglobinaemia can also occur.

Table 9.3 : Drug interactions of phenytoin

- Isoniazid, cimetidine, cotrimoxazole and coumarin anticoagulants *inhibit phenytoin metabolism,* leading to rise in phenytoin plasma level and toxicity.
- Folic acid, during its chronic administration, *reduces the effectiveness of phenytoin.*
- Phenytoin *competes with drugs* such as sulfonamides, salicylates and vitamin B_{12} for binding to plasma proteins.
- Rifampian and ethanol decrease plasma phenytoin because of *hepatic enzyme induction.*

Rapid IV administration can cause cardiovascular collapse and/or severe CNS depression.

Drug interactions : See Table 9.3.

Preparations and dosage : Phenytoin sodium tablets 50 and 100 mg. and IV preparation 50 mg/ml. IV dose should not exceed 25-50 mg. per minute. *It should not be given IM because of its poor absorption from this site.*

Bioavailability of phenytoin may differ with different brands and the patients should be advised to use the same brand all the time.

Fosphenytoin sodium, a prodrug of phenytoin, can be given IV more rapidly; it causes fewer reactions; it can also be given IM. Its dose is expressed in phenytoin equivalents (PE).

Therapeutic uses:

- ***Grand mal***: It abolishes grand mal seizures in nearly 60% of the patients and reduces their severity and frequency in another 15 to 20%.
- ***Partial seizures:*** Phenytoin is preferred to phenobarbitone in this type of seizures. The drug often controls but does not completely abolish the seizure activity. It is also occasionally useful in infantile spasm.
- ***Status epileptieus grand mal*** (see later).
- ***Cardiac arrhythmias***: Chapter 27.
- ***Miscellaneous*** : It has been used with some success in certain types of neuralgia, including trigeminal neuralgia, in diabetic neuropathy with dysasthesias (Chapter 11) and in chorea.

II **Barbiturates :**

PHENOBARBITONE (Gardenal) : Phenobarbitone is discussed in Chapter 8. It is concentrated in the epileptic focus. Its antiepileptic activity is similar to that of diphenylhydantoin but in addition it raises the seizure threshold. It has a different mechanism of action (Chapter 8). Hence, it can be combined with phenytoin in the treatment of resistant cases of grand mal, focal cortical seizures and hypsarrhythmia. The daily dose for anticonvulsant activity varies from 60 to 180 mg. given in divided doses or as a single dose at night.

The main advantages of phenobarbitone are:

- ***It is well tolerated by most patients.***
- ***Its half life is long, permitting single-dose-a-day therapy, with better compliance.***
- ***Therapeutic drug monitoring is usually not necessary.***
- ***It is cost-effective.***

Phenobarbitone is of limited value in temporal lobe epilepsy and may aggravate petit mal seizures. It may produce excitement or hyperactivity in children and in old people. Because of its long half life, it takes 2-3 weeks to reach a steady therapeutic plasma level.

Adverse reactions : Drowsiness, lethargy and depression are common. However, they tend to abate after a few weeks of treatment Nystagmus and ataxia are seen with larger doses. Other long term adverse effects include memory loss, irritability and hematologic changes. Sometimes, connective tissue abnormalities such as frozen shoulder and Dupuytren's contractures may occur. It is also teratogenic (Chapter 8).

Convulsions following phenobarbitone withdrawal are difficult to control with phenytoin. Hence, while switching over from phenobarbitone to phenytoin, the dose of phenobarbitone must be reduced gradually and that of phenytoin increased slowly, till the latter drug fully takes over.

Therapeutic uses:

- ***Grand mal epilepsy.***
- ***Status epilepticus grand mal.***

Mephobarbitone and **primidone** (Mysoline) are prodrugs and their antiepileptic effect is due to their active metabolite phenobarbitone. Primidone is also used in the treatment of essential tremor resistant to propranol.

III Iminostilbenes :

CARBAMAZEPINE (Tegretol, Mazetol) is a tricyclic (iminostilbene) compound with structural resemblance to the antidepressant drug imipramine.

CH=CH
N
CONH$_2$

Fig. 9.2 : Carbamazepine

Pharmacological actions : Its mechanism of action is similar to that of phenytoin. It is claimed to cause less cognitive impairment than phenytoin.

Carbamazepine is also useful in the treatment of **trigeminal neuralgia**, a condition characterised by paroxysms of intense stabbing pain within the distribution of trigeminal nerve, without sensory loss or other evidence of organic disease of the nerve. This condition, because of its paroxysmal nature, tendency to relapse and partial response to phenytoin has been regarded as a type of epilepsy. Carbamazepine is remarkably specific for trigeminal neuralgia and probably for the related syndrome of *glossopharyngeal neuralgia.*

It is also effective in the **deafferentiation pain** in diabetic neuropathy, cancer and multiple sclerosis.

Absorption, fate and excretion: Oral absorption is slow; overall bioavailability however, approaches 90%. It is metabolized by the liver (98%). Children metabolize the drug faster than adults. The plasma half-life, initially 24-36 hours, falls to around 12 hours on chronic dosing because of autoinduction. It is a potent hepatic microsomal enzyme inducer and accelerates its own metabolism as well as that of many other lipid soluble drugs.

Adverse reactions: Generally, these appear within the first week of treatment and include nausea, anorexia, giddiness, vomiting, ataxia, mental confusion and skin rash. Diplopia and blurred vision may occur, making driving dangerous. The rare but serious toxic effects reported include obstructive jaundice, peripheral neuritis, agranulocytosis, thrombocytopenia and aplastic anaemia. Long term use of carbamazepine may cause fluid retention and insidious development of sluggishness, both mental and physical. The loss of physical and mental drive can be so gradual that the patient and the family may wrongly attribute it to the normal process of ageing. It is a minor teratogen.

Drug interactions : See Table 9.4.

Table 9.4 : Drug interactions of carbamazepine

- Induction of hepatic metabolism of oral contraceptive steroids, vitamin D, theophylline, warfarin.
- Inhibition of carbamazepine metabolism by erythromycin, isoniazid, verapamil.

Preparations and dosage : It is available as 100, 200 and 400 mg. tablets and as 400 mg controlled release (CR) tablets. The initial dose is 100 mg. bid, gradually increased to 600-1200 mg. per day in divided doses in temporal lobe epilepsy and to 400-800 mg. in neuralgias.

Therapeutic uses:

- ***Grand mal and partial seizures*** where it is used singly or in combination.
- ***Trigeminal neuralgia*** : see above.
- ***Deafferentition pain*** in various disorders (Chapters 10, 11).
- ***Diabetes insipidus of pituitary origin***, where it stimulates ADH release (Chapter 38).
- ***As an alternative to lithium carbonate*** in the management of manic-depressive psychosis and as an adjunct in the treatment of drug resistant schizophrenia (Chapter 13).
- ***In the treatment of alcohol withdrawal syndrome*** (Chapter 6).

Oxcarbazepine, a prodrug, has similar activity and therapeutic uses as carbamazepine but it is more expensive. It is less toxic and is a selective inducer of cytochrome isoenzyme that metabolizes estrogens.

IV Succinimides :

ETHOSUXIMIDE (Zarontin) : This is the most frequently used succinimide.

H
N
O O
CH_3
C_2H_5

Fig. 9.3 : Ethosuximide

Mechanism of action: The drug reduces the low threshold calcium currents (T currents) in the thalamic neurons which are responsible for the generation of the absence seizures.

Pharmacological actions : It is effective only in petit mal epilepsy. It does not induce liver enzymes and monitoring of blood levels is not required.

Absorption, fate and excretion: It is completely absorbed from the GI tract and is present in the plasma mostly in the free form. About 20% is excreted unchanged in the urine and the rest is metabolized by the liver.

Adverse reactions : These comprise anorexia, nausea, vomiting, drowsiness, dizziness and occasionally parkinsonism. Skin rashes, blood dyscrasias SLE and psychic disturbances may rarely occur. It can unmask grand mal epilepsy.

Preparations and dosage : It is available as 250 mg. capsules and as a syrup (250 mg. per 5 ml.). The usual starting dose is 250 mg. per day in children. It is increased by 250 mg. increments at weekly intervals till the seizures are controlled. A daily dose of 750-1000 mg. (generally given in a single dose) is usually not exceeded.

Therapeutic uses : It is the drug of choice in petit mal epilepsy. Additional drug(s) may be needed to control associated or unmasked grand mal epilepsy.

V Valproic acid :

SODIUM VALPROATE (Epilex, Epilim): Chemically sodium valproate is sodium dipropyl acetate (Fig 9.4).

$CH_3-CH_2-CH_2$
$CH-COONa$
$CH_3-CH_2-CH_2$

Fig. 9.4 : Sodium valproate

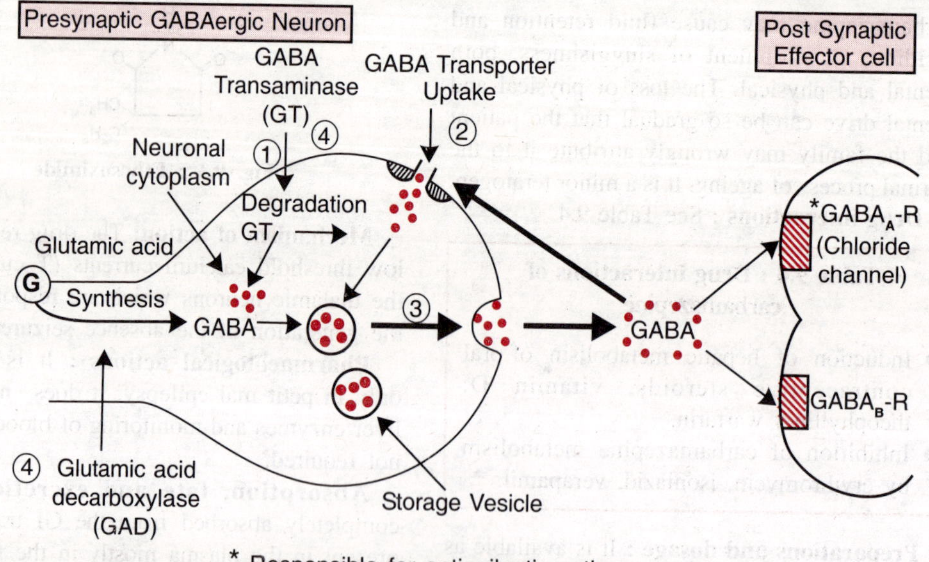

Fig. 9.5: Antiepileptic drugs acting on GABA metabolism :
(1) Vigabatrin inhibits GT
(2) Tiagabine blocks GABA reuptake
(3) Gabapentin promotes GABA release.
(4) Valproate inhibits GT and stimulate GAD

Mechanism of action: This is a broad spectrum antiepileptic which probably acts at multiple sites. Its actions are similar to that of both ethosuximide and phenytoin. Thus, the drug inhibits the T type Ca^{++} current and also delays the recovery of the inactivated Na^+ channels. In addition, it inhibits GABA transaminase, thus increasing the GABA activity. (Fig. 9.5)

Pharmacological actions: In petit mal, it is as effective as ethosuximide. However, it is more liable to cause GI adverse effects than ethosuximide.

In patients who have both petit mal and grand mal seizures, sodium valproate may be the drug of choice as it is able to control both types of seizures. It has also been used successfully in myoclonic seizures and with variable success in akinetic seizures and infantile spasms. It is not particularly effective in cortical focal epilepsy nor in temporal lobe epilepsy. It is claimed that it does not alter the patient's behaviour, alertness and cognitive function, and therefore does not impair learning ability and performance. *Valproate is well tolerated by the elderly and is the drug of choice in them.*

Absorption, fate and excretion: Sodium valproate is rapidly and almost completely absorbed after oral administration. Eighty to 95% of plasma valproate is protein bound. More than 90% is metabolized in the liver.

Adverse reactions: The main adverse reactions are nausea and vomiting. It increases appetite and may cause weight gain. Dose related hair loss may occur. Hypoalbuminemia is common. Hepatotoxicity with death has been reported during treatment with this drug, especially in children under two years of age. *It is advisable to do baseline hepatic function studies before starting sodium valproate.* The other infrequent adverse effects are sedation, ataxia, incoordination, thrombocytopenia and pancreatitis. Sodium valproate inhibits platelet aggregation, although this is unlikely to be of clinical significance unless the patient is also on other drugs that affect coagulation.

Valproate does not cause hepatic microsomal enzyme induction; infact it is an inhibitor of these enzymes. It increases plasma lamotrigine levels and can enhance its toxicity.

It is teratogenic, and spina bifida is associated with its use during pregnancy.

Preparations and dosage : Sodium valproate 100 and 200 mg tablets; syrup 200 mg / 5 ml. Therapy is initiated with the daily dose of 10 mg/kg in two divided doses in adults and in children. This is increased by 5 to 10 mg/kg/day at weekly intervals upto 20-30 mg/kg/day. Doses as high as 60 mg/kg/day have been used.

Therapeutic uses:

- ***Petit mal.***
- ***Combined grand mal and petit mal.***
- ***Myoclonic epilepsy.***
- ***Partial epilepsy;*** and
- ***Manic depressive psychosis*** (Chapter 13)

VI GABA transaminase inhibitor :

VIGABATRIN (r-vinyl GABA, Sabril) : This drug acts as a GABA transaminase inhibitor (Fig. 9.6), thereby leading to increased concentration of brain GABA. It is not metabolized but is excreted unchanged in the urine. At present, its use is restricted to epilepsy not satisfactorily controlled by other drugs. The adverse effects are weight gain, drowsiness, depression, memory disturbances, diplopia and constriction of visual fields. *Hence, visual field testing is mandatory.* Attacks of acute behavioral changes in some patients is a major disadvantage and the drug should be avoided in patients with mental illness. Vigabatrine is particularly useful in infantile spasm. *It worsens absence seizures and myoclonic seizures.*

VII GABA re-uptake inhibitor:

TIAGABINE: This nipecotic acid analogue, acts by selectively inhibiting the neuronal and astrocytic re-uptake of GABA, leading to an increase in synaptic GABA concentration. Given orally, it is almost completely absorbed. Food delays its absorption. The drug is extensively metabolized in the liver and has a half-life of 7 to 9 hours. Common adverse reactions include headache, dizziness, somnolence and tremor.

The drug is mainly used as an "add on" drug for the treatment of partial seizures, with or without secondary generalisation in adolescents and adults. `It is usually administered in a dose of 4 to 12 mg tid.

VIII GABA agonists:

GABAPENTIN (Neurotin): This is a GABA molecule bound to a lipophilic cyclohexane ring. It increases the release of GABA by binding to calcium channels. It also reduces the release of glutamate.

Absorption, fate and excretion: The drug is well absorbed orally, is not metabolized and is excreted unchanged in the urine. It has a plasma half life of 5-9 hours. Concurrent use of gabapentin does not affect the blood levels of other antiepileptic drugs.

Adverse reactions : It usually causes mild to moderate somnolence, dizziness, ataxia and fatigue.

Therapeutic uses : Gabapentin is not useful as a monotherapy but is effective, when used in combination with other drugs, in partial seizures, resistant to other drug therapy. It is administered in the dose of 900 to 1800 mg per day, in three divided doses.

Pregabalin: This drug, is related chemically to gabapentin, and has similar mechanism of action. It is excreted unchanged in the urine. The adverse effects include dizziness, somnolence and ataxia. It does not affect the CYP450 systems nor interacts with the other antiepileptic drugs. It is used as an add-on drug in the treatment of partial-onset epilepsy. It is also recommended in painful diabetic neuropathy.

Both the drugs are also used in the treatment of migraine, deafferentiation pain such as post-herpetic neuralgia, and in bipolar disorders.

IX Benzodiazepines :

Benzodiazepines, in general, are anti-convulsants but not antiepileptics. Clonazepam and diazepam are believed to act by increasing the effectiveness of the inhibitory neuro-transmitter GABA. (Chapter 13).

Table 9.5 : Drugs commonly employed in the treatment of epilepsy

Drug	Steady State (days)	Serum Half-Life Hours		Dose * mgs/day	Dose Interval	Therapeutic plasma conc. (mcg/ml)
		Adults	Children			
Phenytoin sodium**	7-8	24	20	100-400	od	10-20
Phenobarbitone**	>21	120-140	72-96	60-180	od	10-40
Carbamazepine**	3-4	12	8	200-1500	bid, tid	4-12
Ethosuximide	7-10	55	30	500-1500	bid, tid	40-100
Valproate†	1-4	15	11	500-2000	bid, tid	50-100

od = once daily * In adults ** Hepatic microsomal enzyme inducers.

† Hepatic microsomal enzyme inhibitor. Plasma valproate levels are not a useful index of therapeutic efficacy.

DIAZEPAM : When given IV or rectally, it can be life saving in status epilepticus and is the treatment of choice in this condition as well as in non-epileptic seizures. Because of its high lipid solubility and good penetration into the brain, it has a very rapid onset of action (within seconds on IV administration).

Midazolam and **lozazepam** are used as anticonvulsants in status epilepticus.

Benzodiazepines are not a good choice for the long term treatment of epilepsy because:

(a) Tolerance and drug dependence can develop.

(b) Dose related adverse effects such as drowsiness and ataxia can occur; and

(c) Status epilepticus on abrupt cessation of these drugs is difficult to treat.

CLONAZEPAM (Rivotril): This drug is useful in the treatment of petit mal, myoclonic seizures and infantile spasms. In petit mal, it is used in patients who do not respond to ethosuximide and sodium valproate and not as the primary drug. Tolerance develops and breakthrough seizures may occur after 1 to 2 months of therapy. It has also been used as an adjunct to phenobarbitone and phenytoin in the treatment of resistant grand mal.

The serious adverse effects are mainly neurological and comprise drowsiness, ataxia, personality changes, slurred speech, tremor, vertigo and confusion. These are dose-related. Skin eruption, anemia, leucopenia and thrombocytopenia have been reported. It is liable to cause respiratory depression and to increase the salivary and bronchial secretions. The other adverse effects involve the cardiovascular, the gastrointestinal and the genitourinary systems. Tolerance is known to occur during chronic administration, and psychic and physical dependence have been reported.

Clonazepam is available as 0.5 mg tablets and as 1 mg/ml ampoules for IV injection.

Therapy is initiated in adults and in children over 10 years of age with oral administration of 0.5 mg twice a day; the dose is gradually increased to maximum of 4-8 mg per day.

CLOBAZAM (Frisium): This drug has actions and disadvantages similar to those of diazepam. It is used as an adjunct in treatment of epilepsy. Clobazam is useful in short courses in patients in whom seizures occur in clusters; to prevent exacerbations around menstruation in catamanial epilepsy; and to ensure seizure control for important occasions like examinations and marriage.

X **Miscellaneous:**

LAMOTRIGINE (Lamictal): This phenyl-triazine compound acts by delaying the recovery of the inactivated Na^+ channels. Possibly, it also inhibits the release of the excitatory amino acid glutamate in the brain. Reduction of excess glutamate has a stabilising effect on neuronal membranes. Given orally, lamotrigine is almost completely absorbed and is eliminated mainly by hepatic metabolism.

It is used as an add-on drug in patients with partial and secondarily generalised seizures, resistant to other drugs. Because of its membrane stabilising action, it is used in the treatment of deafferentiation pain. The drug can cause skin rash, nausea, vomiting, diplopia, ataxia, Stevens-Johnson syndrome and DIC. It is used in the dose of 50 mg bid, increased gradually to 200 mg per day.

TOPIRAMATE (Topamax) : This drug probably acts in a fashion similar to that of phenytoin. In addition, it also has some GABA receptor enhancing and glutamate receptor inhibiting activity. It has been used in the treatment of refractory partial seizures in combination with other antiepileptic drugs. The adverse effects are mainly neuropsychological viz. dizziness, drowsiness, psychomotor slowing, difficulty in concentrating, confusion, ataxia, depression, acute myopia and raised intracranial tension. It is used in chronic alcoholism as an anti-craving drug.

LEVETIRACETAM : This broad spectrum drug, a pyrolidone derivative, is structurally related to the older nootropic drug piracetam. However, it differs considerably from it in properties. It is effective in the *kindling* animal model but has no effect on the maximal electroshock or pentylenetetrazole induced seizures.

Given orally, it is absorbed rapidly and completely. It is excreted (70-80%) unchanged in the urine. Its plasma t½ is 7.6 hours. Adverse reactions are mild and include drowsiness, asthenia and dizziness. Rare, important side effects are emotional lability, agitation and nervousness. Hence, it is wise to monitor carefully patients prone to psychiatric disturbances. It is currently used as a add-on drug to treat myoclonic seizures and refractory partial seizures.

Zonisamide: This sulfonamide derivative inhibits T type Ca^{++} currents and also the recovery of the inactivated Na^+ channels. Given orally, it has a long t ½ and is mainly excreted in the urine. It is used as an add-on drug in refractory seizures. The adverse reactions are somnolence, ataxia, anorexia, and fatigue; rarely, renal calculi develop.

Acetazolamide (Diamox): The anti-epileptic activity of this drug is correlated with its carbonic anhydrase inhibitory activity (Chapter 38). As an adjunct, it is occasionally effective in resistant petit mal and in patients with grand mal who show increased frequency of seizures during menstruation.

General Principles of Management of Epilepsy

Seizures are a symptom of an underlying disorder: genetic, traumatic, metabolic, inflammatory, drug induced or due to drug withdrawal. Although treatment of the cause can cure seizures, this is not possible in many cases.

Epilepsy should be considered as an illness and not a social stigma. As long as an epileptic is willing to be careful and to take the treatment continuously under proper supervision, he should be given a fair chance in finding a job for himself. Occupations involving driving of vehicles and working with machines, near water or at heights are not suitable for epileptics. Likewise, swimming is a forbidden sport. Within these limits, a well controlled epileptic may be a good employee if he knows his limitations.

The population incidence of epilepsy is 1-2%. Marriage of an epileptic is a difficult issue. About 65-70% of epileptics are found to have an underlying brain lesion (*secondary* epilepsy), and *idiopathic* epilepsy accounts for the remaining cases. *Secondary epilepsy is not heritable* and marriage between two persons with secondary epilepsy has no genetic implications. When a person with idiopathic epilepsy marries a non-epileptic, the chance of transmission to an offspring is about 2%. When two persons with idiopathic epilepsy marry, the chance is about 60-70%. When two persons with the same, documented, *genetic* epileptic disorder marry, the chances of transmission are very high.

The rational management of epilepsy needs an accurate evaluation of the epileptic syndrome and, if possible, of the specific underlying cause. *Currently, there is no drug cure for epilepsy*. The aim of antiepileptic drug therapy in the past was complete control of seizures. That sometimes meant unbearable side effects and/or psychosocial difficulties, with a lot of hardship. The current aim, therefore, is the best possible control while still permitting the patient to lead as full a life as his/her capabilities permit. Antiepileptic drugs must be continued even if they prevent the seizures only partly as repeated major seizures can damage the brain.

Drugs, used judiciously and continuously, abolish seizures completely in 60-80 per cent of the patients and reduce their frequency in another 10-20 per cent. This is usually achieved without producing intolerable adverse effects. Patients can be restored to a full working life, making social rehabilitation possible. Occasionally, these drugs will suppress the abnormal electrical activity and after therapy for years, may produce complete clinical cure in some cases. This is especially true in patients with petit mal epilepsy. To achieve best results with drugs, the following must be carefully observed:

- Proper initial evaluation is necessary to rule out other neurological events (e.g. syncope) that might be mistaken for seizures; to ascertain if a single seizure was precipitated by a reversible abnormality (eg., hypoglycemia); and to determine if a structural (eg. brain tumour) or a metabolic (e.g., hypoxia or hypocalcemia due to primary hypoparathyroidism) cause underlies chronic seizure disorder.
- An AED is advised if the patient has had two or more seizures. A patient who gives history of a single seizure is treated with medication if there are one or more risk factors for recurrence of seizures such as the presence of structural lesions, abnormal EEG, partial seizures or a family history of seizures; otherwise the patient is only observed and not prescribed drugs. The initial choice of the drug depends upon the type of epileptic seizure, and not on whether it is idiopathic or secondary.
- The drug therapy should be simple. Treatment should be started with the least toxic and the most established primary antiepileptic drug appropriate for the particular seizure.
- Changes in therapy should be made after careful weighing of pros and cons and not every time a new drug appears in the market.
- The patient, or in case of children, the parents, should be educated regarding the duration of treatment and the need for compliance, to keep a seizure record and to attend the follow-up clinic regularly.
- Therapy should always be started with a single drug (**monotherapy**) in small dose, increasing it gradually till the maximum benefit is obtained *without an increase in adverse effects*. Repeated EEG evaluation and determination of the plasma level of the drug (phenytoin and carbamazepine) may help in difficult cases.
- The mild toxic effects can be managed by reducing the dose by 25-30% and waiting for tolerance to develop.Most antiepileptic drugs may give rise to skin rash during the first weeks of therapy. The drug need not be stopped for that reason. Gabapentin, valproate and levetiracetam are claimed to cause skin rash rarely.
- Monotherapy results in satisfactory control of seizures, i.e., 70% reduction, in 60% of

patients. If adequate control is not achieved by a single drug in maximum tolerated doses and if compliance and absence of precipitating factors are confirmed, *another drug is substituted.* If this fails, combined therapy should be started.

- Adequate trial (for 2-3 months) should be given to an antiepileptic drug before rejecting it in favour of another one. While changing from one drug to another, the first drug must be tapered off slowly while the second one is introduced in gradually increasing doses.
- Patients with focal epilepsy due to an underlying structural lesion, and those with multiple seizure types are most likely to require multi-drug therapy (**resistant epilepsy**). In them, the intial combination should be from among the older drugs such as phenytoin, carbamazepine, phenobarbitone and valproate. If resistance persists,then a newer drug such as gabapentine, lamotrigine or topiramate is added.
- When a drug combination is used, each drug should be prescribed separately and fixed-dose drug combinations should be avoided.
- It has been customary to prescribe the AED 2-3 times a day. Patients often tend to forget one or more of the doses, leading to poor seizure control. With phenobarbitone, phenytoin, primidone and ethosuximide, sustained therapeutic plasma levels can be achieved by giving the entire daily dose once a day. This is likely to elicit better compliance. Sodium valproate is best prescribed on a twice a day basis and carbamazepine, 2-4 times a day. Young children require frequent doses as they metabolise AED more rapidly than adults.
- When experience shows that in a given patient the frequency or likelihood of attacks increases under stressful circumstances e.g. examination or social events, it is advisable to increase the dose, often to the limit of tolerance, well in advance of the event, and to reduce it gradually afterwards. Trauma, including that of surgery, also increases the drug requirement.
- *Sudden cessation of an antiepileptic drug can precipitate status epilepticus. The patient should be warned about this.*
- Epileptic seizures that initially respond to drug therapy sometimes escape from control. In the case of phenobarbitone, primidone, phenytoin and carbamazepine, the escape may be due to hepatic enzyme induction.
- Most patients will need treatment for their lifetime, except in petit mal. However, an attempt may be made to discontinue the drug in those individuals with idiopathic grand mal epilepsy who have remained seizure free for 3-4 years. Patients with focal seizures are more likely to have a recurrence of seizures. The drug should be tapered off slowly over weeks or months. The risk of recurrence is about 25% in patients without risk factors such as abnormal EEG, structural lesions and resistant seizures. About 80% recurrences occur within 4 months of initiation of tapering.
- Routine periodic determination of the blood level of an AED (Therapeutic Drug Monitoring, TDM) is not necessary. Clinical monitoring by recording the seizure frequency and ADR is more important than TDM. TDM is not useful with valproic acid, and rarely required with phenobarbitone and ethosuximide.With other drugs, it has been usefully employed as a help : (a) in adjusting the dose of a drug during the intitial days of its use; (b) in detecting non-compliance; and (c) to attribute toxicity to a (particular) drug and adjust its dose.
- *The patient should be advised to avoid using OTC formulations as some of them may*

Table 9.6: Some drugs which induce seizures

- Central stimulants: Ephedrine, Amphetamine, Terbutaline; Aminophylline; Cocaine
- Some tricyclic antidepressants
- Phenothiazines (antipsychotics and antihistaminics), Haloperidol
- Alcohol withdrawal
- Anaesthetic agents such as Ether, Halothane and Ketamine
- Antibacterials: Penicillin, INH, Imipenem
- Methotrexate, Cyclosporine
- Lignocaine

contain drugs which lower seizure threshold and precipitate seizures (Table 9.6).

Table 9.6 lists some drugs which can induce seizures.

Epilepsy and Pregnancy

Well over 90% of women taking AED give birth to healthy babies, and pregnancy need not be terminated in well controlled epileptics. However, women with epilepsy have almost twice the rate of complications such as toxemia, intrapartum hemorrhage and premature labour, regardless of the drug used. The major fetal malformations such as cardiac defects, cleft palate, neural tube defects and spina bifida occur in almost 2% of pregnancies in epileptics; they are probably drug-related. The use of two or more AED increases the frequency to 10%. Minor malformations such as nail hypoplasia, low set ears and prominent lips also occur with higher than normal frequency in infants born of mothers on antiepileptics. Almost all AED promote hemorrhagic diathesis in the neonate.

Sudden cessation of AED is liable to precipitate status epilepticus and consequently abortion. Hence, AED should not be stopped abruptly during pregnancy. Their dose should be reduced to a minimum. *Women on AED should receive folic acid supplements 5 mg/day starting before the conception, and the drug continued throughout the pregnancy.*

The newborn of mothers who have received an AED during pregnancy should be examined carefully for congenital abnormalities and they should receive vitamin K at birth, in order to prevent bleeding due to deficiency of vitamin K dependent clotting factors. Further, phytomenadione (not menadione) 20 mg/day should be given to the mother in the last month of pregnancy (see Chapter 77).

AED can be used safely during breast feeding (Chapter 77).

Drug Therapy of Epilepsy

Drugs used in the treatment of epilepsy may be clinically classified into:

- ***Those that are effective in petit mal***: ethosuximide, sodium valproate, clonazepam and acetazolamide.
- ***Those that are effective in all other varieties***: phenobarbitone, iphenylhydantoin, primidone, carbamazepine, valproate and oxcarbazepine; and
- ***Newer add - on drugs.***

Table 9.7 lists the factors which determine the selection of the antiepileptic drug.

Table 9.7 : Factors determining the selection of the AED

- Type of epilepsy syndrome.
- Tolerability of the drug.
- Convenience of the drug schedule.
- Cost of therapy.

I GRAND MAL:

During an epileptic attack: If a known epileptic person is under close observation, it may be possible to recognize an attack early enough to avert a fall. More often, by the time a fit is noticed, tonic or clonic phase has already started.

When flaccidity of the muscle supervenes after the clonic phase is over, the patient can be choked by his own saliva and by his tongue falling back into the pharynx. This can be prevented by turning the patient into a semiprone, head-low position and by inserting a pharyngeal airway. The patient is then watched till he recovers consciousness. *A child, unless it is known to be an epileptic, should be admitted to a hospital at this stage, as meningitis is a common cause of convulsions in childhood.*

Prevention of attacks : An epileptic should be advised to use hard pillow to prevent being smothered, if an attack occurs during sleep.

Phenobarbitone should be started in the dose of 30 mg. twice or thrice a day and the dose should be increased gradually, until seizures are controlled or a total daily dose of 200 mg. is reached. If seizures continue at this dosage level, change over to phenytoin sodium. With higher doses, phenobarbitone has a high incidence of sedation and cognitive impairment. *Some authorities, therefore, recommend phenytoin or carbamazepine as the principal agents to treat grand mal and simple partial seizures.* Because of its long shelf life, inexpensive phenobarbitone monotherapy at night is still a useful first line drug in adults. The fewer side effects as compared with phenytoin is an advantage. "The drug has gone out of fashion not so much because of its limitations but because its virtues are no longer promoted."

When phenytoin is used in the maintenance dose (300-400 mg/day) from the outset, therapeutically effective plasma levels are achieved only after 7-10 days. When the need to control seizures is more urgent, therapeutic plasma levels can be reached within 12-24 hours by giving a loading dose of 1 g. before commencing the daily maintenance dosage schedule. The maximum tolerated maintenance dose of this drug for an adult is 600 mg. per day.

There is considerable variation in the bioavailability of phenytoin sodium from the many marketed formulations. This might account for the sudden appearance of toxicity or of loss of seizure control on changing the proprietary preparation without changing the dose.

Phenytoin can occasionally cause adverse cosmetic effects, which makes carbamazepine the drug of choice particularly in young women. Carbamazepine is started in adults in the dose of 200 mg twice daily and the dosage gradually increased to 600 -1200 mg per day.

Once seizures are under control, the drug or drug combination must be continued for a least 3-4 years after the last seizure episode. Patients must be warned against sudden cessation of drug treatment. Drug treatment is not effective in preventing mental deterioration. This is, however, rare in well controlled epileptics.

Epilepsy during drowsiness is a condition where fits occur when the patient is drowsy but not asleep. Anticonvulsants like phenobarbitone which produce drowsiness increase the frequency of attacks in this condition and must be avoided.

Phenobarbitone is the drug of choice for grand mal epilepsy in children under the age of 5 years, as they do not seem to tolerate phenytoin as well as older children and adults do. However, phenobarbitone is known to cause behavioral disturbances in children.

II ATONIC SEIZURES: These are resistant to almost all drugs; valproate, benzodiazepines and lamotrigine have been used with some success. A ketogenic diet may be helpful.

III PETIT MAL : It is essential to confirm the diagnosis of petit mal by an EEG as the specific drugs are effective only in patients with typical EEG changes. It is also essential to inquire about concomitant grand mal attacks as anti-petit mal drugs are liable to aggravate grand mal.

Ethosuximide and valproate are equally effective in this condition. Ethosuximide is started in the dose of 250 mg. three times a day, increasing the dose upto 1500 mg. per day, if necessary. If the patient cannot tolerate ethosuximide or it fails to control the seizures, sodium valproate may be used.

Sodium valproate as a single drug is the drug of choice if tonic-clonic seizures are also present or emerge during therapy with ethosuximide. If valproate is not available or is not tolerated phenobarbitone may be added to ethosuximide; this combination is preferred in children below three years in whom valproate is known to cause a higher incidence of fatal hepatotoxicity.

Drug treatment of petit mal can be withdrawn 3-4 years after cessation of attacks. It is rare for this variety of epilepsy to recur.

IV MYOCLONIC SEIZURES : These are often refractory to treatment. Sodium valproate seems to be the drug of choice; other drugs used are clonazepam and levetiracetam.

V INFANTILE SPASMS: The treatment is disappointing. The drugs used are benzodiazepines, glucocorticoids and vigabatrine. Though they may control the seizures, they do not improve the mental retardation. A ketogenic diet may be helpful.

VI PARTIAL SEIZURES : The drug treatment of this condition is similar to that of grand mal epilepsy. The seizures are often refractory to drug therapy. Carbamazepine and phenytoin are the preferred drugs in this condition. Phenobarbitone is rarely effective.

VII POST-TRAUMATIC SEIZURES : Head injury predisposes to the development of seizures and is a common cause of them. There is some clinical evidence that prophylactic treatment with phenobarbitone or/and phenytoin may help such patients.

VIII FEBRILE SEIZURES : Febrile convulsions are not associated with, nor do they cause, mental retardation, affect IQ, poor scholastic performance or behavioral problems; hence, *routine prophylactic administration of antiepileptic drugs is not warranted.*

Brief febrile seizures need only treatment of the fever (tepid sponging or bathing, and paracetamol) in an otherwise normal child. If a febrile convulsion lasts longer than 15 minutes, rectal administration of diazepam in solution (10 mg per 2 ml) in the same dose as in status epilepticus is rapidly effective.

Chronic prophylactic therapy should be started in a child with a febrile convulsion if :

- ***The first seizure occurs before the age of 18 months.***
- ***The convulsion was focal or prolonged (longer than 15 minutes).***

Table 9.8: Choice of AED

Type of seizure	Drug/s of choice	Alternative/s-1	Alternative/s-2
Grand mal (clonic-tonic)	Phenobarbitone* Carbamazepine	Phenytoin Sodium valproate	Lamotrigine Topiramate
Simple partial	Carbamazepine Phenytoin	Sodium valproate Phenobarbitone	Lamotrigine Newer antiepileptics[1]
Complex partial	Carbamazepine Phenytoin	Sodium valproate Phenobarbitone	Lamotrigine Newer antiepileptics[1]
Partial with secondarily generalized clonic-tonic	Phenytoin Carbamazepine	Sodium valproate Phenobarbitone	Newer antiepileptics[1]
Petit mal	Sodium valproate Ethosuximide	Lamotrigine	
Petit mal with tonic-clonic seizures	Sodium valproate	Phenobarbitone + Ethosuximide	
Myoclonic	Sodium valproate	Lamotrigine	Topiramate; Clonazepam

* In developing countries, because of low cost. [1].For patients resistant to established drugs.

- ***The patient has any neurological abnormality.***
- ***Any sib or either parent of the patient has epilepsy;*** or
- ***The febrile convulsions are recurrent.***

When indicated, therapy is initiated with phenobarbitone, 3-4 mg/kg/day. *Phenytoin is not well tolerated by small children and valproate is more toxic at this age.*

The child should be treated for 2 years or for 1 year after the last seizure, whichever is longer.

IX ECLAMPTIC SEIZURES : See Chapter 29.

Table 9.8 summarises the choice of antiepileptic drugs.

X STATUS EPILEPTICUS (SE) : This term is used to indicate either a convulsive seizure lasting for more than 15 minutes; or rapidly recurring seizures without return of full consciousness between seizures. Such patients need emergency IV medication if death or permanent brain damage, especially hippocampal sclerosis (which can occur in 30-60 minutes in untreated patients), is to be prevented. Table 9.9 summarises the principles of management of grand mal status epilepticus. SE can occur in epileptics but may also occur in patients with other disorders such as brain tumours or meningitis as well in alcoholics.

The IV administration of anticonvulsant drugs requires the availability of cardio-pulmonary resuscitative support equipment.

Diazepam IV *is the treatment of choice* for controlling the seizures. It may be given in the dose of 10 mg. IV, slowly (over 5 minutes) in adults, 5 mg. for children over 7 years of age and 2.5 mg. for those between 1-7 years of age. The dose may be repeated twice more at 15 minute intervals. The dose may be further repeated every 2 to 4 hours, if necessary. Hypotension and respiratory depression should be watched for, especially in patients who have received barbiturates earlier. Rarely, cardiac arrest has been reported after IV diazepam.

Table 9.9: Management of tonic-clonic SE

- Hospitalize
- Ensure adequate airway
- Prevent aspiration and physical injury.
- Maintain BP.
- Obtain appropriate blood samples (glucose, calcium, poison screen if available).
- Establish IV line with normal saline.
- Give 50 ml of 50% glucose and 100 mg of thiamine IV, only if hypoglycemia is documented.
- Give sodium bicarbonate IV if the arterial blood pH is less than 7.2.
- Give an anticonvulsant, eg., diazepam, followed by an antiepileptic such as phenytoin.
- Institute long term antiepileptic therapy.

The IV administration of anticonvulsant drugs requires the availability of cardio-pulmonary resuscitative support equipment.

If IV administration is not possible, diazepam may be given rectally : 10 mg in adults and children over 3 years, and 5 mg in children 1-3 years and in elderly patients; it may be repeated, if necessary, after 5 minutes. **Midazolam** (buccal or IV, 10 mg)/**lorazepam IV** is an alternative to diazepam. Lorazepam has also been administered by squirting it intranasally, using an atomizing pump. It reaches the brain rapidly along the perineural pathways of olfactory and trigeminal nerves bypassing the BBB, and acts within minutes. As diazepam has short lasting effect, it should be immediately followed by **IV phenytoin sodium** (15-20 mg/kg) at not more than 50 mg/min. (not more than 25 mg/min. in elderly patients). Phenytoin should not be administered diluted in glucose solution.

If seizures persist, (a) inject 200 mg of **phenobarbitone IV** at not more than 100 mg/minute; or (b) intubate the patient and then inject phenobarbitone (10 - mg/kg) IV at a similar rate. If seizures still persist, induce **general**

Table 9.10: Points to remember while treating SE

- During prolonged SE, cerebral seizure activity may continue even after convulsions have stopped.
- Do not inject 50% glucose IV routinely; hyperglycemia can damage cerebral neurons.
- Diazepam is an anticonvulsant, not an antiepileptic. Do not inject diazepam if convulsions have stopped.
- **IV Lorazepam** 4-8 mg (2 mg/min) is almost as rapid acting as but much longer acting (12-24 hours) than diazepam IV (3-4 hours). Midazolam has 3-4 hours of action.
- Phenytoin is incompatible with glucose-containing solutions; is contraindicated in patients having 2nd or 3rd degree heart block; should be injected IV at not more than 25 mg/min is elderly patients.
- Phenobarbitone has rapid and prolonged antiepileptic action; it is concentrated in the epileptic focus. It is indicated when phenytoin is contraindicated or has failed to control convulsions.
- BP normally rises at the onset of SE. Do not allow systolic BP to fall below high normal level during the course of treatment as otherwise cerebral ischemic damage may occur.
- Muscle relaxants stop convulsions but do not abolish cerebral seizure activity. Do not use them unless EEG monitoring is available.
- Refractory SE is always due to a serious underlying disease.

anaesthesia with a short acting barbiturate in consultation with an anaesthetist. **IV lidocaine** may be used in resistant cases but it must be remembered that lidocaine itself can induce seizures; it should be used only after adequate amounts of anti-epileptic drugs (phenytoin and/or phenobarbital) have been injected. Where facilities for intubation/resuscitation are not available, **IM phenobarbitone** (200 mg, repeated as necessary) or **paraldehyde deep IM** (5 ml into each buttock, in an adult) may be useful. Alternatively, **paraldehyde may be given rectally** as follows : 0.2 ml/kg mixed with a threefold volume of a vegetable oil (maximum single dose 10 ml) every 4-6 hours upto 48 hours. Further management for the next 24 to 48 hours is that of an unconscious patient.

Patients in SE are liable to develop hyperpyrexia. It should be looked for and treated immediately.

Between convulsions, a soft object, large enough not to be swallowed, such as a folded napkin, should be inserted between jaws to prevent tongue biting during convulsions.

Immediately on recovery, the patient should be put on the oral antiepileptic drug therapy. Table 9.10 lists 'The Points to Remember' in the treatment of status epilepticus.

Emergency management of convulsions due to other disorders such as withdrawal of sedatives (including barbiturates), tetanus, eclampsia, cerebral hemorrhage, poisoning from convulsive agents and during administration of local anaesthetics is similar to that of SE. Diazepam or lorazepam is the drug of choice; paraldehyde IM may also be used. Phenytoin is not useful. The same is true of convulsions occurring during the withdrawal of CNS depressant agents in addicts.

AED in non-epileptic disorders: These drugs have been used in many non-epileptic disorders. The most successful uses are: **carbamazepine** in trigeminal neuralgia, bipolar disorder and restless leg syndrome; **gabapentine** in neuropathic pain syndromes, migraine/tension headache, spasticity, and social phobia; **lamotrigine** in neuropathic pain syndromes; **primidone** in essential tremor; **topiramate** in migraine/tension headache, essential tremor and binge disorder; **vigabatrine** in spasticity; **valproate** in migraine/tension headache and bipolar disorder; **phenytoin** in digoxin-induced ventricular tachycardia; and **phenobarbitone** in neonatal hyperbilirubinemia.

Opioid Analgesics and Antagonists

10

Pain is an unpleasant sensory and emotional experience, associated with actual or potential tissue damage or described in terms of such damage. It is a subjective experience which cannot be objectively defined or quantified satisfactorily. Pain acts as a warning signal against disturbances either in the body or in the external environment of an individual and thus has a protective function. However, on many occasions pain seems pointless, only contributing to the discomfort in the subject. As a symptom, pain demands instant relief and in practice its dramatic relief highly impresses a layman.

Pain receptors are distributed throughout the body. Clinically, pain can be considered as:

- ***Superficial or cutaneous pain.***
- ***Deep non-visceral pain from muscles, joints, ligaments and bones.***
- ***Visceral pain.***
- ***Referred pain;***
- ***Deafferentiation or neuropathic pain;*** and
- ***Psychogenic or functional pain.***

Pain arising from the skin and from the deep non-visceral structures like muscles, bones and joints is also termed as **somatic pain**. It is usually well defined and is generally caused by an inflammatory reaction in the tissues; it may be accompanied by contraction of the surrounding skeletal muscles as in patients with rheumatoid arthritis. However, other causes such as direct irritation of a nerve as in trigeminal neuralgia, herpes zoster, increased pulsation of the intracranial arteries as in migraine, or vascular insufficiency as in thromboangitis obliterans are also incriminated in the genesis of somatic pain.

Pain arising from the skin and superficial mucous membrane or nerves is felt as pricking, if brief, and stinging, smarting or burning if prolonged. The sensation of 'pinprick' elicits a reflex withdrawal reaction of a part or all of the organism.

Deep nonvisceral (skeletomusular) pain usually has a dull character and it may be accompanied by a sickening sensation due to an autonomic response. Sometimes, it spreads to other areas and may even occur as referred pain. BP and pulse, however, are not much affected, unless the pain is acute and severe.

Visceral pain, unlike the somatic pain, is diffuse, less easily localized and often 'referred'. It is dull-aching or colicky in character and is often accompanied by sweating, nausea, fall in BP and even shock. In addition, muscle rigidity and hyperaesthesia are common accompaniments. In practice, visceral pain may be due to spasm (renal or biliary colic), ischemia (myocardial infarction), inflammation (appendicitis, pancreatitis) or stimulation of the sensory nerve endings (peptic ulcer).

Deep pain, whether visceral or somatic in origin, may be misinterpreted as coming from some part of the body other than the actual site of stimulation. This is called **referred pain.** Thus, cardiac pain is commonly referred to the left arm and diaphragmatic pain to the shoulder. Usually, the pain is referred to a cutaneous area which receives its nerve supply from the same spinal segment as the affected viscus.

Although various theories have been proposed to explain the pain mechanism none can explain all its aspects. The assimilation of sensory pain at the level of consciousness depends on various factors such as the nature of sensory receptors, the intensity of the impulses transmitted to the CNS, their integration and finally their modulation by other sensory information. The conscious appreciation of pain appears to depend upon the widespread activity of the entire cortex; and *individuals differ widely in their reactions to similar painful experiences.*

Deafferentiation pain is caused by partial damage to axons and nerve membranes, which become very sensitive to mechanical and chemical stimuli. Such pain may either be of burning, superficial (dysasthetic) type; or of stabbing (lancinating) character. It has a peculiarly unpleasant quality about it and may not respond to opioids nor to NSAID (see later).

Psychogenic or **functional pain** is usually a vague pain which follows no definite anatomical pattern of distribution. Such pain is usually continuous from day to day and involves more than one part of the body. It however, does not disturb sleep. Psychogenic pain is often preceded by a phase of exhaustion while organic pain brings about exhaustion. There is a psychic element in all types of pain.

Pain pathways: Painful stimuli may primarily be physical stimuli such as pressure or heat, or they may be chemical stimuli from the products of inflammation.

A variety of naturally occurring compounds can elicit pain response in experimental animals, e.g. histamine, acetylcholine, bradykinin, PGs, 5-HT and substance P. These substances are present in venoms and products of inflammation.

It appears that tactile sensation is transmitted by large diameter (L), fast conducting nerve fibres, and pain via small diameter (S), slow conducting (C) nerve fibres. Such an impulse, on reaching the spinal cord, activates the first transmission cell and also the collateral cells in the substantia gelatinosa (SG). Anatomically, these nerve fibres are carried in the dorsal nerve roots and end in the SG at the apex of the dorsal gray horn and in the intermediate gray matter in the spinal cord. The SG cells inhibit the passage of signals and thus decrease the output reaching the higher centres. If, however, pain stimulus is more intense, then the SG cells are inhibited, releasing the dorsal horn cell from inhibition, resulting in higher output reaching the higher centres, leading to perception of pain. This **gate control** mechanism allows the sensory input to be decreased or augmented depending on the relative activity of L fibres and S fibres.

The secondary axons which arise from the dorsal horn travel through the opposite spinothalamic tract; the latter terminates in the thalamus that project to the post central gyrus which is mainly responsible for localization of pain sensation. Although the thalamus is responsible for perception of pain, the cerebral cortex is essential for its discriminative, exact and meaningful interpretation and for some of its emotional components. The other intermingled fibres which form an ascending multisynaptic pathway terminate in the thalamus and from there project to frontal and limbic systems, and the hypothalamus. This system is concerned with the emotional concomitants of pain.

Higher centres, through their central inhibitory and facilitatory mechanisms, exert modulating influence on the gating mechanism. Thus, clinically the sensation of pain has several components including the emotional reaction.

Analgesics are drugs which relieve pain without causing loss of consciousness.

Experimental evaluation of analgesics: Analgesics can be evaluated in various ways :

(a) Prevention or relief of artificially induced pain in experimental animals.

(b) Relief of experimental pain in human

volunteers induced by radiant heat, ischemia induced with sphygmomanometer cuff or intraperitoneal bradykinin and

(c) Relief of pathological or incisional pain, post-puerperal pain, post-operative pain and pain due to malignancy.

Evaluation of analgesics against pathological pain is preferred to that against experimentally induced pain. It is usually desirable to compare the effects of several doses of several drugs in the same patient, before drawing conclusions. Because of the subjective component of pain, use of a cross over double blind technique using a placebo or a standard drug is essential in evaluating analgesics in man.

Classification: Analgesics are classified into:

(I) Opioid and
(II) Non-opioid.

I Opioid analgesics:

The word **opiates** refers to the products obtained from the opium poppy. In this context, the term **opioid** (opiate-like) is used to denote all naturally occurring, semi-synthetic and synthetic drugs which have a morphine like action viz relief from pain and depression of the CNS, both reversed by naloxone. These drugs were formerly called 'narcotic' analgesics because some of them (such as morphine) induce sleep. The word narcotic is derived from the Greek prefix 'narco' which means to deaden, or to benumb. The term 'narcotic' is no longer applied to opioids but is restricted in the legal sense to drugs capable of producing dependance.

The opioids are further subclassified as :

(a) **Agonists** such as morphine and compounds which resemble it in most of their actions, viz, derivatives of morphine; codeine and its derivatives; synthetic compounds such as pethidine, methadone, propoxyphene, levorphanol and tramadol.

(b) **Partial agonists** e.g. buprenorphine and meptazinol. They have partial agonist action only on the mu receptors (see later).

(c) **Mixed agonist-antagonists** which act as agonists at one type of opioid receptors and as competitive antagonists at another type of receptors, e.g., nalbuphine, pentazocine, and butorphanol. Patients who have received repeated doses of a morphine-like drug to the point of physical dependence may experience an opioid withdrawal reaction when given a mixed agonist-antagonist.

Peptides with strong opiate-like analgesic and mu receptor binding activity are now known to be present in the CNS and other tissues. In the CNS, they act as *endogenous analgesics*, as neuro-transmitters and as behaviour modulators. They are:

- ***Beta-endorphin***, a potent analgesic, is derived in the pituitary from a larger, parent molecule, pro-opio-melanocortin (POMC). It is released along with ACTH and is believed to be a pain modulator in the CNS.
- ***Enkephalins***, derived from pro-enkephalin, are more widespread; they are found in the pituitary, brain, GI tract, spinal cord, pancreas and adrenal medulla.
- ***Dynorphins*** A and B, derivatives of pro-dynorphin, have been found to be widely distributed in the CNS.
- ***Nociceptin/orphanin*** FQ is a peptide with behavioural and pain modulating effects that are complex and distinct from those of the three above mentioned peptides; and
- ***Endomorphins 1 and 2***, tetrapeptides with high, selective affinity for mu receptors.

Although these peptides have affinity for more than one receptor type, beta-endorphin has high affinity for mu-receptors, enkephalins for delta-receptors and dynorphin for k receptors. Opioids may also act by releasing these peptides.

Milk and milk products contain opioid peptides such as beta-casomorphins, which are released from casein in the intestine during digestion of milk. They may modulate GI function on local release.

Opioid antagonists, by themselves, produce

few effects unless an opioid agonist has been administered previously e.g. naloxone. However, when endogenous opioids are activated as in shock or stress, an opioid antagonist does produce visible effects.

II **Non-opioid analgesics** which do not interact with opioid receptors and relieve pain without depression of the CNS e.g. salicylates and related compounds (Chapter 11).

Mechanism of action of opioids : The opioid drugs produce their effects by binding to opioid receptors which are widely distributed in the CNS and other tissues. In the CNS, the opioid receptors are localized to:

(1) The periaquiductal grey matter of the brain stem, and the thalamus.

(2) The area postrema which has the CTZ and the solitary nuclei which receive visceral sensory fibres from the vagus and glossopharyngeal nerves.

(3) The amygdalae which may be responsible for the influences of the opioids on the emotional reactions; and

(4) The spinal cord substantia gelatinosa, the first site in the CNS which integrates the sensory information.

Table 10.1: Pharmacological effects associated with opioid receptor types

Receptor type	Effects
Mu	Supraspinal/spinal analgesia, euphoria, respiratory depression, sedation, miosis, decreased GI motility, smooth muscle spasm, physical dependence, release of prolactin and growth hormone, nausea and vomiting, feeding
Kappa	Supraspinal/spinal analgesia, sedation, miosis and decreased GI motility (of lesser degree), less physical dependence, dysphoria, psychomimetic effects, diuresis, feeding
Delta	Supraspinal/ spinal analgesia, less respiratory depression, decreased GI motility, release of growth hormone, feeding
Nocciceptin /Orphanin FQ	Drug reward and reinforcement, Stress responsiveness, learning and memory

Table 10.2 : Selectivity of common opioid analgesic drugs for different receptors

Compound	Receptor type: Mu	Receptor type: Kappa
Pure agonists		
Morphine	+++	+
Methadone	+++	0
Codeine	+	+
Partial agonists		
Buprenorphine*	(+++)	?
Butorphanol	(++)/-	+++
Agonist/antagonists		
Pentazocine	(+)/–	++
Nalbuphine	–	++

+ = agonist, (+) = partial agonist,
– = antagonist, 0 = no action
* Antagonist of Mu receptors in high doses.

The **opioid receptors** have been classified into mu (mu_1, mu_2), delta ($delta_1$, $delta_2$), kappa (k_1, k_2, k_3) and nociceptin (orphanin) types. Opioid receptors are a part of the family of G-protein coupled receptors, and act to open K^+ channels and prevent the opening of Ca^{++} channels on the presynaptic neurons. They thereby inhibit the release of the neurotransmitters from nociceptive nerve terminals. The pharmacological effects associated with these receptor subtypes and the selectivity of the various opioid drugs for these receptors are summarized in Tables 10.1 and 10.2.

The vast majority of opioid drugs used as analgesics are agonists at mu receptors. Similarly the opioid antagonists naloxone and naltrexone, show a high selectivity for mu receptors. Drugs with mixed agonist-antagonist properties bind to more than one receptor class at the usual clinical doses.

Opioid receptors are also present in the peripheral nerves where they probably respond to peripherally applied opioids and locally released endogenous peptides during inflammation.

Opium Alkaloids

Opium is the milky exudate obtained by incising the unripe seed capsule of the poppy plant *Papaver somniferum.* The poppy seeds, however, are devoid of pharmacological activity and are in fact used in food preparations. On drying, the exudate forms a gummy, brownish mass. The pharmacologically active alkaloids of opium (Table 10.3) are divided chemically into:

- ***Phenanthrene group***; and
- ***Benzyl isoquinoline group***.

The benzyl isoquinoline alkaloids are devoid of analgesic activity but act as smooth muscle relaxants. They are described later.

Table 10.3: Opium alkaloids

	Name	Percentage
Phenanthrene series	Morphine	9 to 14
	Codeine	0.5 to 2
	Thebaine	0.2 to 1
Benzyl isoquinoline series	Papaverine	0.8 to 1
	Noscapine	3 to 10
	Narcine	0.2 to 0.4

MORPHINE is the most important alkaloid of opium and is used as sulfate or hydrochloride; both salts are soluble in water.

Pharmacological actions: Morphine acts

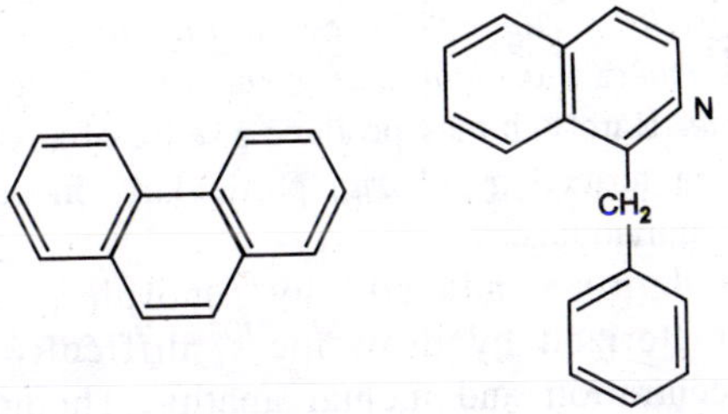

N

CH_2

Fig. 10.1 Phenanthrene Benzylisoquinoline

predominantly on *mu receptors* situated both in the CNS and other tissues such as GI tract. Opioids and endogenous opioid-like peptides have been shown to modify the release of acetylcholine, NA, DA and substance P.

Central nervous system:

- ***Analgesia***: Morphine, by acting on μ_1 receptors, produces relief of pain in a dose that usually does not cause motor incoordination. Other modalities such as touch, vibration and hearing are not obtunded. *In subanaesthetic doses*, morphine and its analogues have little effect on pinprick sensation and the withdrawal reflex, though pain arising from the tissues is well suppressed. *In moderate doses*, morphine is effective in relieving continuous, dull pain. *Larger doses*, relieve sharp intermittent pain caused by trauma and by visceral pathology. *Morphine, pethidine, methadone and the other agonists do not have a ceiling dose as far as their analgesic effect is concerned;* the dose can be increased to a level just short of causing toxicity (as in the treatment of terminal cancer).

Morphine raises the pain threshold, reducing the perception of pain. This action may be assisted by the feeling of well-being produced by morphine (μ_1 receptors). Morphine modifies the emotional reaction to pain. Thus, it may not completely abolish pain perception but the latter is no longer a source of concern to the patient.

- ***Euphoria, sedation and hypnosis***: With therapeutic doses, morphine produces a sense of emotional well-being termed euphoria (μ_1 receptors). Euphoria eliminates the normal fear, panic, withdrawal and flight response to pain and aids the analgesic action of morphine. *The ability* *to produce euphoria even in the absence of pain makes morphine one of the worst drugs of abuse.* Rarely, it may produce a sense of anxiety or fear termed *dysphoria,* particularly in pain-free individuals.

Sedation induced by morphine is characterized by drowsiness, difficulty in concentration and mental apathy. Thoughts may lack a logical sequence and imagination becomes extravagant, producing vivid and colourful daydreams. Larger doses induce sleep with EEG changes similar to those observed during natural sleep.

Morphine depresses the respiratory and cough centers and stimulates the vagal and oculomotor centers and the CTZ.

- ***Respiration***: Therapeutic doses of morphine depress all phases of respiratory activity. It acts by:

(i) Direct depressant action on the respiratory centre (μ_2 receptors); and

(ii) Reducing its sensitivity to increased plasma CO_2 concentration.

Retention of CO_2 brought about by initial respiratory depression by morphine increases the rate and depth of respiration to the pre-drug value. At a later stage, the hypoxic drive tends to maintain the minute volume despite diminished sensitivity of the respiratory centre to accumulated CO_2. The respiratory rate and minute volume, therefore, are not adequate monitors of respiratory depression caused by morphine. Bronchoconstriction as a result of histamine released by morphine and indifference to breathing as a result of psychological action of morphine, further enhance respiratory difficulties.

With toxic doses, breathing is entirely maintained by the 'hypoxic drive' mediated through the carotid and the aortic body chemoreceptors, and this may result in *Cheyne-Stokes respiration.* Inhalation of pure oxygen at this stage abolishes the hypoxic drive and produces apnoea. Hence, in such cases controlled assisted ventilation and moderate concentrations of oxygen are indicated.

- ***Cough suppression***: Morphine depresses the cough reflex as a result of direct depression of the cough centre.

- ***Pupils***: In humans, morphine produces characteristic pin-point pupils. The miosis is due to an action on the Edinger-Westphal nucleus of the oculomotor nerve.

- ***Nausea and emesis***: Morphine produces vomiting by stimulation of the CTZ in the area postrema of the medulla. Morphine-induced vomiting is abolished by nalorphine and by prochlorperazine (5-10 mg 4-8 hourly), metoclopramide (10 mg 4-8 hourly) and haloperidol (1-2 mg daily) but not by antihistaminics.

In large doses, it depresses the vomiting centre. Thus in case of morphine poisoning, vomiting is absent and emetics are ineffective.

- ***Vagus stimulation***: Morphine stimulates the medullary vagal nucleus and may cause bradycardia.

- ***Spinal cord***: Morphine increases the reflex excitability of the spinal cord. This action is, however, usually masked by the depression of the higher centres in the CNS. Therapeutic doses of morphine may produce a significant increase in the CSF pressure.

- ***Miscellaneous***: Morphine produces a release of ADH with resultant decrease in the urinary output. Administration of morphine reduces the efficacy of diuretics in patients with CHF. Morphine in large doses lowers the body temperature by central action.

Gastrointestinal tract: Morphine induces spasm of the smooth muscle of the gut, the ileocolic and the anal sphincters, and reduces the propulsive peristaltic movements (μ_2 receptors). Spasmogenic action of morphine is particularly evident in the duodenum and the large intestine. There is a reduction in the secretion of saliva, gastric acid and the intestinal secretions. Dessication of the faeces, abolition of the peristaltic movements, spasm of the sphincters, particularly the anal sphincter, and inattention to normal sensory stimuli from a loaded rectum as a result of the psychological effect of morphine, all lead to constipation. Atropine partially antagonizes the spasmogenic action of morphine on the human colon but fails to initiate the propulsive movement. Patients on long-term administration of morphine should receive a high fibre diet and a laxative such as senna regularly. Lubiprostone (Chapter 41) may be helpful in these patients.

Morphine increases the intrabiliary pressure by producing a spasm of the sphincter of Oddi. Hence, although it may relieve the biliary colic because of its analgesic action, the underlying disease is exacerbated. Atropine partially antagonizes this action.

In mice, morphine produces a severe spasm of the anal sphincter resulting in erection of the tail. This test, termed *Straub's test,* was formerly employed to detect morphine in biological fluids.

Other smooth muscles : Morphine produces:

- ***An increase in the tone of the ureters and the detrusor muscle of the bladder.*** The vesical sphincter is contracted. These effects are augmented by inattention to stimuli arising from the bladder and may result in urinary retention.
- ***An increase in the tone of the bronchi and the bronchioles.***

Except in large doses, it has no significant effect on the normal human uterus at full term.

Cardiovascular system: Therapeutic doses of morphine have negligible effect on the myocardium, the BP or the heart rate. Morphine produces dilatation of the peripheral blood vessels, particularly the cutaneous blood vessels. This may reduce the pre-load on the heart (see later). Pruritus, sweating and flushing often accompany the cutaneous capillary dilatation. Toxic doses may produce hypotension.

Neuroendocrine system: Morphine acts in the hypothalamus and inhibits the release of GnRH and CRH. It thus decreases the plasma concentration of FSH, LH and ACTH (Chapter 61). The plasma prolactin increases.

Immune system: Opioids suppress the various immune functions and increase the susceptibility to infection in experimental animals, both by a direct action and an indirect action mediated by the CNS.

Absorption, fate and excretion : Given orally, morphine is adequately absorbed but extensively metabolized during first pass through the liver; hence its bioavailability on oral administration is about 20-40%. Sustained-release preparations have a longer duration of action. The drug can also be given rectally. Given subcutaneously, it produces analgesic effect within 15 to 20 minutes with peak effect at 60 to 90 minutes; it persists for 3 to 5 hours. Given IV, it produces an immediate effect.

Morphine circulates in the plasma partly protein-bound and partly in the free form. It enters the brain rapidly. It crosses the placental barrier readily and is also secreted in milk. It is metabolized by the liver and the kidney. Morphine is conjugated with glucuronic acid to form both active and inactive products; morphine - 6 - glucuronide is more potent than morphine. In adults the plasma t½ of morphine is about 2 hours whereas that of the glucuronide is longer.

Approximately 90 per cent of the administered dose is eliminated in urine within 24 hours, mainly in conjugated form. Biliary excretion of this form accounts for approximately 7 to 10 per cent of the dose.

Preparations and dosage:

(i) Tincture opium is a hydro-alcoholic solution containing 10 per cent opium and 1 per cent morphine W/V. Dose: 0.3 to 2.0 ml.

(ii) Chlorodyne: This is a chloroform and morphine tincture containing 0.229 per cent of morphine hydrochloride. Dose : 0.3 to 0.6 ml.

(iii) Morphine solutions (2-20 mg/ml) for oral use. Dose in adults is 10-30 mg. Larger doses (up to 200 mg) are needed in patients with terminal cancer. Orally, it is only about one sixth as effective as parenteral administration.

(iv) Morphine hydrochloride or sulfate injection. Dose: 10-20 mg SC or IM.; 2.5-5 mg IV over 5 minutes. It has also been used by a continuous, low dose, IV infusion and by epidural and intrathecal administration. If given by IV infusion, 10 mg are infused over the first 1 hour and 10 mg over the next 4 hours.

(v) Controlled release tablets (10, 30 and 60 mg) of morphine sulfate for prolonged action.

(vi) Transdermal patches.

Adverse reactions:

- ***Intolerance***: These reactions include allergic skin rashes, pruritus and contact dermatitis. It is a histamine liberator. Anaphylactoid reaction with fall in BP has been reported after morphine injection.
- ***CNS:*** By its pharmacological actions, morphine can produce a variety of adverse effects like dysphoria, mental clouding, vertigo, nausea and vomiting, headache, fatigue and paraesthesiae. Morphine may occasionally produce tremors and delirium.
- ***Respiratory depression*** can occur even in small doses (see earlier).
- ***Constipation*** following morphine may be dangerous in old people as it may precipitate intestinal obstruction. It may also cause abdominal distension and increased biliary pressure.
- ***Hypotension*** : Morphine occasionally produces hypotension as a result of peripheral vasodilatation, more so in patients with reduced blood volume.
- ***Urinary retention*** : Morphine may produce urinary retention in old people with prostatic hypertrophy.
- ***On the foetus*** : Morphine administered to the mother during labour can depress fetal respiration. This asphyxia can be reversed by injection of 0.1 to 0.2 mg. of nalorphine or 0.05 to 0.1 mg. of levallorphan in the umbilical vein of the newborn.
- ***Tolerance***: Repeated administration of morphine results in the development of tolerance. With intermittent use of morphine, however, tolerance to analgesic and sedative effects does not develop. Tolerance also develops to the respiratory depressant, analgesic, sedative and euphoriant effects of morphine as well as to urinary retention, *but the pupils and the gastrointestinal tract do not share this tolerance.* A morphine addict thus has characteristically pinpoint pupils and is habitually constipated.

Tolerance to morphine is attributed primarily to the ability of the cells of the central nervous system to withstand large doses of the drug.

Persons tolerant to morphine exhibit cross tolerance to other opioid analgesics and even to compounds like barbiturates and alcohol.

- ***Drug dependence***: This is a major drawback of morphine therapy. Opium has been in use as a drug of abuse for several centuries and has precipitated wars. Dependence on morphine and morphine-like drugs results mainly from their euphoriant effects. In addition, these drugs produce a variety of sensations such as a 'turning in the stomach', a feeling of warmth in the epigastrium and other parts of the body due to flushing; and sensations in the lower abdomen described by addicts as akin to sexual orgasm, and known as "kick" or "thrill".

Morphine addicts are usually malnourished and debilitated. Even though they do not suffer from motor incoordination and are capable of performing complex motor and intellectual tasks, the productivity and the utility of these individuals to the society usually suffer. As the drug is commonly self injected, the incidence of injection abscesses, tetanus, AIDS and serum hepatitis is high among the addicts.

Table 10.4 : Manifestations of opiate withdrawal

Abstinence period	Manifestations
6-12 hours	Intense craving for the drug, lethargy and weakness.
12 hours	Yawning, lacrimation, perspiration, rhinorrhoea, tremors and anorexia.
48 hours	Peak of the withdrawal syndrome. Fever, rise in BP, increase in heart rate, dilatation of the previously constricted pupils and intestinal cramps.
7-10 days	Symptoms clear up but the patient may complain of restlessness, insomnia, weakness, and back and leg pains for several weeks.

Manifestations of withdrawal syndrome (**opiate withdrawal syndrome**) are summarised in Table 10.4.

In order to prevent morphine dependence, morphine should not be prescribed readily for chronic pain except in cases of terminal cancer pain. At the same time, however, it is not justifiable to withhold morphine from an advanced case of malignancy with excruciating pain. Such patients rarely develop psychological dependence on morphine.

The mechanism of opiate withdrawal syndrome is not known but the involvement of the neurotransmitter noradrenaline is suspected.

The treatment of morphine dependence, in principle, is similar to that of alcohol or barbiturate dependence. The results, however, are unsatisfactory because of the severity of withdrawal syndrome and the high relapse rate. Gradual withdrawal of morphine with substitution of another opioid analgesic to decrease the severity of withdrawal syndrome is usually advocated. Methadone orally is often used for replacement as it has a longer duration of action than morphine. One milligram of methadone will substitute for 4 mg of morphine. Once the patient is stabilized on methadone, its dose is gradually reduced by 20 per cent daily and the drug can be completely stopped from 6th to 10th day.

Acute opiate withdrawal symptoms and signs can be controlled to a certain extent by drugs like chlorpromazine, propranolol and clonidine which counter the noradrenergic overactivity.

• ***Acute morphine poisoning***: Acute morphine poisoning may occur from clinical overdosage, accidental overingestion in an addict or from suicidal or homicidal intention. It is difficult to define the lethal doses of morphine. A dose of 60 mg. is usually toxic but rarely fatal in a normal adult who is not in pain. Doses of 250 mg. are usually fatal. Larger doses are generally required to produce toxicity in individuals with pain, whereas in addicts, the toxic as well as the fatal doses are much higher.

Morphine poisoning is characterised by respiratory depression, pinpoint pupils, cyanosis, reduced body temperature and urinary output, hypotension, shock and coma. Convulsions may occur in infants. Death is usually due to respiratory depression, or shock and pulmonary edema.

If a toxic dose of morphine has been ingested, even late gastric lavage is justified as the spasmogenic action of morphine frequently delays its absorption.

Naloxone and **nalorphine** are the specific morphine-antagonists. They produce dramatic reversal of morphine-induced respiratory depression. Naloxone is usually preferred because of its specific antagonistic and negligible agonistic action (see later). Opioid antagonists should be administered with caution in treating acute morphine poisoning in addicts as they may produce a severe withdrawal syndrome. *The duration of action of opioid antagonists is shorter than that of opioids and the patient has to be carefully monitored to prevent relapse into coma.*

Drug interactions: CNS depressants, phenothiazines, monoamine oxidase inhibitors and tricyclic antidepressants enhance the sedative effects of morphine and increase the respiratory depression.

Therapeutic uses of morphine:

• ***For relief of pain :*** Morphine is one of the most potent analgesics, employed to alleviate severe pain in conditions such as acute myocardial infarction, fractures of long bones, burns, terminal stage of malignancy, pulmonary embolism, acute pericarditis, and spontaneous pneumothorax. For relief of sudden excruciating pain, morphine is usually administered IV; prompt relief of pain minimises shock. Morphine SC is not advocated in the presence of shock, as its absorption is hampered. Repeated SC administration of morphine under these conditions may result in a sudden absorption of toxic quantities into the systemic circulation after the correction of hypotension.

Morphine can be used for relief of pain in

renal and biliary colic. However, for this purpose it is *always combined with atropine* which produces smooth muscle relaxation and thus helps to relieve spasm.

Parenteral morphine has been used to reduce post-operative pain; thoughtless use for this purpose should be avoided as it can produce respiratory depression, urinary retention and constipation; it reduces coughing and may mask the signs of recovery and of complications.

Since opiate receptors are located within the spinal cord, *intrathecal and epidural* morphine produces analgesia. Such analgesia is essentially segmental in distribution, the pain relief being remarkable for its specificity without any interference with motor function or autonomic changes. The typical adverse effects of systemic opiates are rare. Such analgesia can last upto a few days. Because of greater safety and ease of administration, most investigators prefer the epidural route to intrathecal route. It has been used in the prevention and treatment of labour pain, and in the treatment of cancer pain.

Not all types of pain respond to opioids. For example, the deafferentiation pain is relatively resistant. It needs treatment with an anti-depressant if it is dysasthetic, and with either phenytoin or carbamazepine if it is stabbing or lancinating (Chapter 11).

- ***In acute left ventricular failure*:** Morphine is valuable in the treatment of acute left ventricular failure and pulmonary edema. It acts by reducing apprehension and the effort of breathing. Morphine-induced peripheral vasodilatation results in shunting of the blood from the pulmonary arteries to the dilated peripheral vasculature and this in turn reduces central venous pressure, pulmonary artery blood flow and pulmonary artery pressure. Thus, it reduces the cardiac work load, and relieves dyspnea, provided oxygenation is maintained.
- ***Sedation and sleep*:** Morphine is a valuable sedative in the presence of severe pain. As it does not affect the uterine motility, it has been used as a sedative in threatened abortion.

Although morphine has been used routinely for sedating patients with internal bleeding such as haematemesis, a tranquillizing drug like diazepam is safer for this purpose.

- ***As preanaesthetic medication*:** See Chapter 7.
- ***To control diarrhoea*:** Tincture opium (0.5 to 1 ml) and paregoric are now rarely used for symptomatic relief of severe diarrhoea.
- ***As an anaesthetic*:** Morphine IV, it has been used, alone or in combination with other drugs, to produce general anaesthesia especially in subjects who are considered as bad anaesthetic risks.

Precautions with morphine therapy:

- ***COPD*:** Morphine should be administered with caution to persons with diminished respiratory reserve e.g., individuals with emphysema, kyphoscoliosis and chronic obstructive pulmonary disease (COPD). Such patients are already on the verge of hypoxia which they avert by increasing their respiratory rate. Opioids decrease ciliary activity, depress cough reflex, cause bronchospasm and depress respiration, all of which can precipitate respiratory failure in such individuals. Deaths have been reported in patients with COPD following therapeutic doses of morphine.
- ***Myxoedema* :** The lower BMR and reduced rate of metabolic disposal of drugs make such patients more sensitive to opioids and sedatives, and frank coma may be precipitated by even their conventional therapeutic doses. Patients with hypopituitarism and Addison's disease are also more sensitive.
- ***Old people and infants*** are more prone to develop respiratory depression with morphine.
- ***Head injuries:*** Morphine should be avoided in such cases as it produces an increase in the CSF pressure, stimulates the spinal cord and produces respiratory depression, vomiting and miosis. Miosis and mental clouding produced by morphine may interfere with the diagnosis.
- ***Acute abdomen:*** In this condition, morphine relieves pain symptomatically without modifying the underlying pathological process.

It does not alter the physical signs such as abdominal rigidity. It may, therefore, facilitate clinical evaluation and permit diagnostic procedures. Its use does not mask the diagnosis; and it may be helpful *provided the pain is not forgotten.* However, morphine-induced vomiting and its spasmogenic action on the GI and biliary tracts are its drawbacks.

- ***Shock:*** Morphine IV may produce hypotension if administered during hypovolemic shock. Restoration of blood volume is more important in that condition.
- ***Severe impairment of liver and/or kidney function:*** Cumulative toxicity can occur.

Other phenanthrene alkaloids of opium:

CODEINE: Codeine, by itself, is a much less potent analgesic than morphine (weak agonist). It does not produce significant depression of respiration and has a low dependence liability. In toxic doses, it may produce excitement and convulsions. It enhances the analgesic effect of aspirin and is often combined with it. Unlike morphine, it is much better absorbed when given orally, with the bioavailability of about 50%. About 10% codeine is converted to morphine in the liver and this may explain its analgesic property. It is used most commonly as an antitussive; this action may involve different receptors that bind codeine itself. Codeine phosphate is available for oral and IM use. Its main disadvantage is constipation.

Therapeutic uses:

- ***As an analgesic,*** 30-60 mg t.i.d.
- ***As an antitussive,*** for suppression of dry cough (Chapter 25); and
- ***As an antidiarrhoeal agent.*** (Chapter 40).

Dihydrocodeine and **oxycodone** are other drugs used orally for similar purposes as codeine (Chapter 25).

TRAMADOL (Tramazac) : This synthetic codeine derivative is a weak agonist of the μ receptors and also exerts a part of its analgesic action by inhibiting noradrenaline and serotonin uptake. It is rapidly absorbed and is metabolized in the liver to an active compound with analgesic action. Its t½ is 6 hours. It has a low addiction potential. It is as effective as pethidine in mild to moderate pain but causes less respiratory depression. It can be used in labour pains. The drug causes dizziness, sedation, and nausea. It is expensive.

Benzylisoquinoline alkaloids of opium :

PAPAVERINE: Papaverine is devoid of opioid and analgesic activities. It is a smooth muscle relaxant and causes vasodilation. Intracavernosal injection of papaverine causes penile erection and was used for symptomatic treatment of erectile dysfunction. This procedure, however, can cause complications (Chapter 67).

NOSCAPINE : This alkaloid has significant antitussive action in therapeutic doses, without other disadvantages of morphine. It is a potent releaser of histamine and large doses can cause bronchospasm and hypotension. Its use in the therapy of cough is described in Chapter 25.

Semisynthetic Derivatives of Natural Opium Alkaloids

Codeine derivatives are mainly antitussive (see above). Only the derivatives of morphine are described below.

HEROIN (Diacetylmorphine, Diamorphine) : It is a more potent analgesic than morphine, produces greater euphoria and consequently has a higher dependence liability. It is rarely employed therapeutically because of this drawback but it is extensively used (as *brown sugar*) as a drug of abuse.

The newborn children of mothers who are heroin addicts have been known to develop a 'withdrawal syndrome' a few hours after birth. The treatment of heroin dependence is similar to that of morphine dependence; one mg. of methadone can substitute for 2 mg. of heroin.

Dihydroxymorphinone (Dilaudid), **oxymorphone** (Numorphan) and **methyldihydromorphinone** (Metopon) in the doses of 1.5 mg., 1.5 mg., and 3.5 mg. respectively are effective analgesics with 4-5 hours of duration of action. Their toxicity is similar to that of morphine.

APOMORPHINE: This drug is obtained by the acid-catalyzed rearrangement of morphine. It stimulates CTZ and acts as potent emetic. The emesis is due to activation of dopaminergic (DA) receptors which in turn stimulate the emetic centre. The effect is blocked by neuroleptics like chlorpromazine but not by antihistaminic agents. The drug acts on both pre- and post-synaptic DA receptors and thus produces a variety of behavioural, neuropharmacological and endocrine effects. It also produces, in threshold doses, an increase in exploratory activity and discontinuous sniffing in rats. Larger doses cause purposeless behaviour characterized by continuous sniffing, grooming, biting and licking, described as **stereotyped behaviour syndrome**. In cats and dogs, it causes side to side head movements and incessant running around the cage. These effects due to direct stimulation of DA receptors located in the neostriatum are also blocked by neuroleptics.

Apomorphine is of great pharmacological interest and is used to evaluate the action of psychotropic drugs in experimental animals.

In man, a dose of 0.1 mg/kg SC ordinarily causes vomiting within a few minutes. Adverse reactions include nausea, severe vomiting, dizziness, hypotension and bradycardia.

Synthetic Morphine Substitutes

These are:

I **Pethidine and its congeners**
II **Methadone and its congeners**
III **Morphinan compounds and congeners,** e.g., Levorphanol and Butorphanol
IV **Benzomorphan derivatives,** e.g., Pentazocine.
V **Miscellaneous:** Nalbuphine, Buprenorphine.

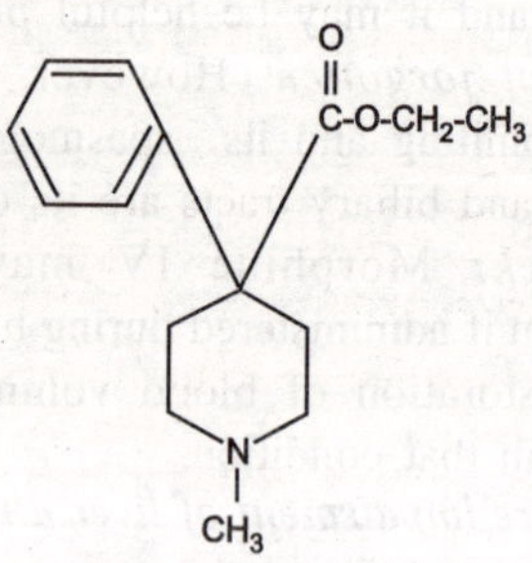

Fig. 10.2 Pethidine

PETHIDINE (Meperidine, Demerol): As the pharmacological actions of this synthetic opioid closely resemble those of morphine, only the salient differences between these two compounds will be pointed out. Thus,

- On weight basis, it is about 1/10th as potent as morphine as an analgesic when given IV but it has a rapid onset and shorter duration of action.
- In equianalgesic doses, pethidine produces as much sedation, euphoria and respiratory depression as morphine. However, unlike morphine, it reduces the tidal volume without significantly affecting the respiratory rate. Therefore, respiratory depression may be missed if respiratory rate alone is watched.
- The incidence of nausea and vomiting following pethidine is higher than with morphine.
- Pethidine is devoid of significant antitussive activity.
- Pethidine exerts a vagolytic action on the isolated intestinal strip but usually produces in vivo spasm of the smooth muscle of the bowel wall and sphincters. It also raises intrabiliary pressure by producing spasm of the sphincter of Oddi. Compared to morphine, it is less spasmogenic and causes less constipation.
- Pethidine occasionally produces hypotension and syncope due to peripheral vasodilatation. Unlike morphine, however, IV

pethidine may produced tachycardia and dryness of the mouth due to its vagolytic effect.

Absorption, fate and excretion: Pethidine is satisfactorily absorbed from the gut with a bioavailability of about 50%; the analgesic effect appears within 10 to 15 minutes. On parenteral administration the action lasts for 2 to 4 hours as compared to 3 to 5 hours with parenteral morphine. Pethidine crosses the placental barrier and is also secreted in milk. It is mainly metabolized by the liver; the metabolic product norpethidine possesses significant excitatory action on the CNS. Norpethidine may accumulate during chronic use. Only a small portion of pethidine is excreted unchanged in the urine. The urinary excretion of the drug is enhanced when the urine is acidic.

Preparations and dosage:

(i) Pethidine hydrochloride tablets. Dose : 25 to 100 mg.

(ii) Pethidine hydrochloride injection 50 mg. per ml. Dose : IM/SC 25 to 100 mg. IV : 25 to 50 mg. to be repeated, if necessary, after 4 hours.

Adverse reactions:

- The adverse effects apart from local irritation on parenteral administration, include sweating, euphoria, dizziness, dry mouth, vomiting, dysphoria, visual disturbances, weakness and palpitation. Anaphylactoid shock following pethidine has been reported. Constipation and urinary retention is less common.
- Pethidine administered to mothers at term produces significant depression of foetal respiration.
- It can produce bronchospasm and drying of secretions. As it also produces respiratory depression, *it is not a suitable drug in patients with bronchial asthma.*
- Pethidine overdosage causes respiratory depression and coma, or tremors, myoclonus and convulsions. Nalorphine can antagonize the respiratory depression and coma but fails to modify the convulsant action of pethidine which is due to norpethidine. Acute pethidine poisoning should be treated on similar lines as acute morphine poisoning.
- ***Tolerance and dependence*** : Tolerance to analgesic and emetic effects develops on prolonged administration. The pethidine addict often shows dilated pupils, tremors, mental confusion, twitchings and occasionally convulsions.

Dependence on pethidine is fairly common. The withdrawal syndrome usually develops within 3 hours after the last dose, reaches a peak by 8 to 12 hours and declines by 4 to 5 days. There is little nausea, vomiting or diarrhoea but the patient may show more excitement than during morphine withdrawal. The treatment of pethidine addiction is similar to that of morphine addiction. Methadone is employed initially as a substitute. One mg. of methadone can substitute for 20 mg. of pethidine.

Drug interactions : Phenytoin increases the biodegradation of pethidine. Cimetidine (but not ranitidine) reduces the clearance of pethidine (but not morphine). Thus, morphine is a safer drug than pethidine to use in patients who are on cimetidine. Its administration to patients receiving imipramine or an MAOI may result in confusion, cerebral excitement and collapse.

Contraindications to the use of pethidine are similar to those for morphine.

Therapeutic uses:

- ***Analgesia***: It is particularly useful when short duration of action is required, as in gastroscopy, cystoscopy or ascending pyelography. Pethidine serves as a morphine substitute for relief of acute visceral pain e.g. in myocardial infarction, *particularly that associated with bradycardia,* and in burns. The precautions to be observed with morphine administration for the treatment of shock also apply to pethidine. *It is not the drug of first choice in severe/prolonged pain.*
- ***Preanaesthetic medication***: Chapter 7.
- ***Obstetrical analgesia***: As pethidine does not interfere with uterine contractility, it is often used in minor procedures like dilatation and curettage.

• ***Epidural and intrathecal analgesia*** (see Chapter 7).

PETHIDINE CONGENERS: These are **piminodine, phenoperidine, fentanyl** (Chapter 7), **alfentanil, remifentanil, anileridine,** and **alphaprodine.** They are used mainly as anaesthetic adjuncts. Buccal transmucosal route can be used for fentanyl. Alphaprodine has a shorter duration of action (one half to two hours) on SC administration and causes emesis less frequently than other opioid analgesics. It is administered orally or parenterally in the dose of 40 to 60 mg. It has been used for relief of pain in the first stage of labour. **Diphenoxylate** and its metabolite difenoxin are used in the treatment of diarrhoea and in therapeutic doses, they do not produce morphine-like subjective effects; large doses, however, cause typical opioid symptoms. **Loperamide**, a piperidine derivative, is used for its selective constipating action (Chapter 40).

METHADONE (Physeptone): Methadone has analgesic potency equivalent to or slightly greater than that of morphine.

Pharmacological actions : These are more or less similar to those of morphine. A single therapeutic dose, however, exerts much less hypnotic activity than an equianalgesic dose of morphine. The drug depresses respiration to the same degree as morphine and has a marked antitussive effect. The actions of the drug on the gastrointestinal tract and the cardiovascular system are similar to those of morphine.

In addition, methadone inhibits the re-uptake of noradrenaline and 5-HT; further, it also blocks the action of NMDA receptors, known modulators of neuropathic pain.

Absorption, fate and excretion : Unlike morphine, methadone is satisfactorily absorbed orally with a bioavailability of about 80%. The analgesic effect occurs within 10 to 15 minutes following parenteral and 20 to 30 minutes after oral medication. It is highly bound to plasma proteins and also to the tissue proteins, including those in the brain. Given IV, it is as potent as morphine and *has a longer duration of action.* Its plasma half-life is 24-36 hrs. It crosses the placental barrier.

Methadone is mainly metabolized in the liver. Less than 10 per cent of the drug is excreted unchanged by the kidneys.

Preparations and dosage:

(i) Methadone hydrochloride, 5 mg. tablets. Dose : 5 to 10 mg.

(ii) Methadone hydrochloride injection, 5 mg. per ml. Dose 5 to 10 mg. by IM/SC injection.

Adverse reactions : They are similar to those of morphine. Methadone may produce irritation on parenteral injection and its repeated administration can result in cumulative toxicity. Methadone shares the respiratory depressant action of morphine. Acute methadone intoxication responds to naloxone.

Tolerance and the withdrawal syndrome develop more slowly and are less intense. The symptoms, however, persist much longer, approximately 10 to 15 days. Codeine is often used as a substitute during treatment of methadone addiction.

Therapeutic uses: The oral effectiveness of methadone, its analgesic potency and lack of marked hypnosis make it a useful drug for the management of chronic pain. Further, it can be used as a substitute for morphine and pethidine for relief of severe visceral pain and it is the drug of choice in the treatment of opioid abstinence syndrome.

As an antitussive, codeine is preferred to methadone owing to the higher addiction liability of the latter.

METHADONE CONGENERS: These are levomethadyl acetate and propoxyphene. **Levomethadyl acetate** exhibits slow onset and prolonged duration of action, contributed partly by its active metabolite. It is used in the long-term management of heroin addicts to prevent protracted withdrawal syndrome, wherein a single dose every 72 hours needs to be prescribed.

d-Propoxyphene (Darvon) has been claimed

to produce less depression of respiration, and fewer GI side effects. In fact, the drug retains only minimal pharmacological properties of opioid analgesics and yet has significant addiction liability. As an analgesic, it is only 1/25-1/50th as potent as morphine and is ½ as potent as codeine. Sixty-five mg of propoxyphene hydrochloride is no more effective than 650 mg of aspirin. It is administered orally in the dose of 65 mg 3-4 times a day. It can cause respiratory depression and has abuse potential. It enhances the anticoagulant effect of warfarin. The drug has little advantage over codeine.

MORPHINAN COMPOUNDS: The compound **levorphanol** is a more potent analgesic than morphine, is better absorbed orally and produces less constipation. It can cause drug dependence. It is administered orally or IM/SC in the dose of 2 to 3 mg.

PENTAZOCINE (Fortral, Fortwin, Talwin): This benzomorphan derivative has potent analgesic (agonist) action at the kappa receptors in the spinal cord and a weak opioid antagonist activity at the mu receptors. Compared to morphine:

- ***It is half as effective as an analgesic and has a shorter duration of action.***
- ***It does not cause euphoria.***
- ***It has lower dependence liability.***
- ***Constipation is uncommon.***
- ***It causes less respiratory depression.***
- ***It raises the systemic and pulmonary arterial blood pressures*** with resulting increase in cardiac load; hence *it is not recommmended in M.I.*

Absorption, fate and excretion: Pentazocine is given orally, rectally and SC, IM and IV. Although it is well absorbed orally, only 20% is bioavailable due to first pass metabolism. It is extensively metabolized by the liver and is excreted as glucuronide. Smokers metabolize 40% more pentazocine than non-smokers.

It is available as 25 mg tablets and as 30 mg (lactate) per ml injection. The oral dose is 25-100 mg every 3-4 hours. The parenteral dose (SC, IM, IV) is 30-60 mg every 3-4 hours, as necessary.

Adverse reactions: These include

- ***CNS:*** Sedation, sweating, dizziness and nausea.
- ***Psychomimetic reactions***, hallucinations and unpleasant dreams. This is an important limitation to its use.
- ***Precipitation of acute withdrawal syndrome*** in a morphine addict because of its antagonist action at μ receptor.
- ***Tolerance and physical dependence*** have been reported, though the incidence is low.

Nalorphine is valueless as an antidote to pentazocine but naloxone is useful.

BUTORPHANOL is a partial agonist, morphinan congener. Its agonist activity (on weight basis) is 4-7 times that of morphine and it is 20 times as potent as pentazocine. It is administered IM or IV in the dose of 2 mg, as well as intranasally.

NALBUPHINE (Nubain): This synthetic compound is chemically related to oxymorphone and the opioid antagonist naloxone. It has both agonist and antagonist properties. As an agonist, it is 3-4 times more potent than pentazocine while its antagonistic property is about 10 times more than that of pentazocine. The adverse effects are similar to those of pentazocine. It probably causes fewer psychotomimetic effects and its adverse hemodynamic effects are less than those of pentazocine. It is administered SC, IM, or IV in the dose of 10-20 mg every 3-6 hours.

MEPTAZINOL: This partial agonist opioid is given orally or by injection. It is 1/10 th as potent as morphine as an analgesic and has a shorter duration of action. It does not cause euphoria and causes less respiratory depression than morphine

BUPRENORPHINE (Buprine, Norphin, Tidigesic): Buprenorphine, a highly lipophilic semisynthetic derivative of thebaine, has mainly partial mu agonist properties. It is a weak antagonist at the kappa receptors and does not precipitate acute withdrawal symptoms in morphine addicts.

Pharmacological actions: As an analgesic, it is more potent than morphine on a weight basis and has a longer duration of action (6 hours). It causes less respiratory depression. It has similar cardiovascular actions as morphine and can be used in MI. It has much less abuse potential than morphine; and naloxone does not precipitate withdrawal syndrome.

When it is given following induction of anaesthesia with nitrous oxide and fentanyl, it reverses the anaesthetic and respiratory depressant effects of fentanyl but prolongs the analgesia.

Absorption, fate and excretion: It is given sublingually, IM or IV as it is inactive orally because of the first pass effect. The drug is highly protein bound and is excreted largely unchanged in the faeces, and in smaller amount in the urine.

Adverse reactions: It can cause respiratory depression similar to morphine at equianalgesic doses. *However, unlike morphine, the action is not readily reversed by naloxone.* Doxapram, a respiratory stimulant, may be useful. Other adverse effects are drowsiness, nausea, vomiting, constipation, miosis, bradycardia and hypotension.

It is available as 0.2 mg tablets, as 0.3 mg/ml injections and as transdermal patches. The dose is 0.2-0.4 mg sublingually every 8 hours and 0.3-0.6 mg IM or slow IV every 6-8 hours.

All partial agonists and mixed agonist/antagonists have a ceiling on their analgesic effect roughly equivalent to that of moderate doses of morphine.

It has been reported that women obtain more benefit than men from Kappa agonists.

Non-analgesic uses of opioids :

- ***Anti-diarrhoeal***: Diphenoxylate, loperamide (Chapter 40).
- ***Central cough suppressant***: Codeine dextro-methorphan (Chapter 25).
- ***Emetic***: Apomorphine (Chapter 40); and
- ***In acute left ventricular failure***: Morphine (Chapter 30).

Opioid Antagonists

Drugs that antagonize the effects of morphine and other opioid analgesics act mainly by **competitive antagonism.** In addition, some of them also exert other actions not related to morphine receptors. They are classified as:

I **Pure antagonists** such as Naloxone, Naltrexone.

II **Partial agonists of Nalorphine-type** e.g. Nalorphine, Levallorphan and Cyclazocine; and

III **Partial agonists of the Morphine-type** e.g. Propiram and Profadol. In man, drugs from this group produce similar agonistic actions as morphine, which are antagonized by nalorphine or naloxone. However, they precipitate withdrawal symptoms in subjects maintained on very potent agonists such as morphine and heroin.

NALOXONE (Narcan): This drug, N-allyl analogue of oxymorphone, a pure antagonist, selectively antagonizes the respiratory depressant action of morphine and other opioids. By itself, it is not a respiratory depressant, analgesic or euphoriant. Given orally, it is only 1/50 as potent as when given parenterally because of its metabolism in the liver. One mg of naloxone given IV completely blocks the effects of 25 mg of heroin. Its duration of action is 3-4 hours. It is almost completely metabolized in the liver.

It is available in 1 ml vials containing 0.4 mg/ml. and is the antagonist of choice in the treatment of opioid poisoning. It is administered as an IV bolus in the dose of 0.8 - 2.0 mg every 2-3 minutes to a total maximum dose of 10 mg.

The IV dose in children is 10 mcg/kg (bolus); if there is no response, inject a 100 mcg/kg (bolus). It is also used to reverse the residual respiratory depressant effects of an opioid analgesic at the end of an operative procedure.

Endogenous opioid peptides, released by stress, may be responsible for hypotension observed in shock. Naloxone, IV, has been reported to correct the hypotension in septicaemic shock, though the effect is short lived.

NALTREXONE (Nalorex) : This is an orally administered, *long acting, pure opioid antagonist.* Naloxone is too short acting and is ineffective by mouth. Naltrexone is well tolerated and has no euphoric effect, does not cause physical dependence and consistently blocks the effects of heroin and other addictive opiates for upto four days.

Naltrexone is available as 50 mg scored tablets. For treating heroin addiction, small doses (25 mg/day) are used initially, followed by 50 mg/day. For better compliance, the total weekly dose (350 mg) may be given on three days of the week (e.g.100 mg on Monday and Wednesday, and 150 mg on Friday). Since naltrexone blocks the euphoric action of opioid agonists, it is given to former addicts to prevent re-addiction. For its use in alcoholism, see Chapter 6.

The drug can cause GI disturbances, nervousness, sleeping difficulty and muscular pain. Rarely, thrombocytopenia and liver function abnormalities may occur.

Methylnaltrexone is used SC to treat morphine-induced severe constipation.

Nalmefene is a pure μ receptor antagonist, more potent than naltrexone.

Fig. 10.3: Morphine **Nalorphine**

NALORPHINE (N-allyl normorphine): Nalorphine, a semi-synthetic congener of morphine (Fig. 10.3). It is used mainly in the treatment of acute morphine poisoning.

By itself it acts as a partial agonist, and produces analgesia and respiratory depression. When administered after morphine, it displaces morphine from the receptor sites (competitive

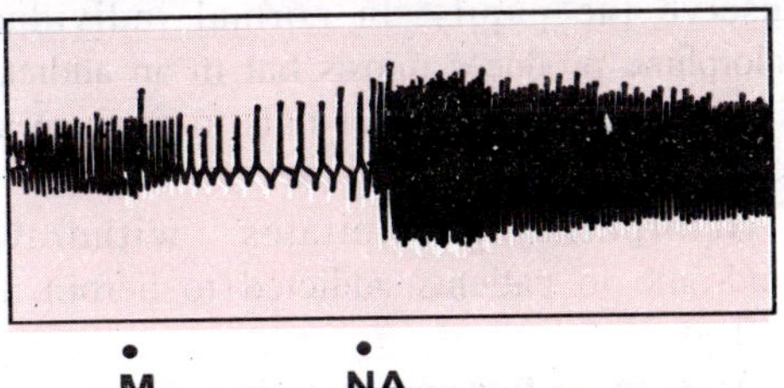

Fig.10.4 : Effect of nalorphine (NA) on morphine (M) depressed respiration in anaesthetized cat.

antagonism) within the CNS, reversing the effects of morphine (Fig. 10.4).

Pharmacological actions:

- ***When administered without prior medication with morphine***, nalorphine in therapeutic doses exerts significant analgesic effect comparable to that of morphine. Nalorphine analgesia is accompanied by drowsiness but a number of patients experience dysphoric symptoms such as anxiety, confusion, and visual hallucinations.

  Nalorphine shares many other pharmacologi-cal actions of morphine. Thus, it has spasmogenic activity, antitussive effect, and in large doses, produces nausea, vomiting and miosis. Large doses also induce respiratory depression. However, unlike morphine, nalorphine does not produce drug dependence.

- ***When administered after morphine or its semisynthetic derivatives***, nalorphine promptly abolishes all the effects produced by them. Nalorphine is also a potent antagonist of codeine, heroin and synthetic morphine substitutes. *However, it is much less effective against pethidine than against the other opioid analgesics.*

• ***When administered to a morphine addict*** in the dose of 1 to 3 mg., nalorphine precipitates the typical morphine withdrawal syndrome within 3 to 15 minutes, reaching a peak by 45 minutes and disappearing within 2 hours. Another test to diagnose an addict is to observe the pupils. In normal individuals nalorphine produces miosis but in an addict, it either dilates the pupils or fails to produce any demonstrable effect.

Nalorphine precipitates withdrawal syndrome in patients addicted to heroin and methadone.

Absorption, fate and excretion : Given orally, it is absorbed poorly but more rapidly than morphine on SC administration. The drug is metabolized in the liver by conjugation.

Preparations and dosage: Nalorphine injection (Lethidrone) 10 mg. per ml., administered SC or IV in the dose of 3 to 10 mg. The dose may be repeated to a total of 40 mg.

Therapeutic uses:

• ***Acute poisoning due to morphine and related compounds.***

• ***Diagnosis of morphine addiction.***

• ***Nalorphine has been administered to morphine addicts along with morphine.*** Withdrawal of the mixture produces a milder withdrawal syndrome than that observed after withdrawal of morphine alone.

Levallorphan : This opioid antagonist is similar to but more potent than nalorphine. It is given IV in the dose of 0.2 mg. It generally fails to reverse pethidine induced respiratory depression.

CYCLAZOCINE : Cyclazocine is a *nalorphine type of opioid antagonist.* The compound itself is a potent analgesic and respiratory depressant but cannot be used clinically because of the high degree of tolerance and dysphoria.

ALVIMOPAN : This drug acts as a *selective opioid-mu receptor antagonist*. Given orally, it is not much absorbed and blocks the GI effects of opioids by binding to GI opioid-mu receptors, without blocking the central analgesic action of opioids. It has been used orally, for treating postoperative ileus after bowel resection. It is given ½ – 5 hours before surgery and continued for 7 days. It helps in achieving early recovery of opioid induced bowel dysfunction without affecting the analgesic action of opioids. It is usually well tolerated. It is not likely to be useful, unless started before ileus develops.

Analgesic-Antipyretics and Nonsteroidal Anti-inflammatory Drugs (NSAIDs)

11

In contrast to the opioid analgesics, the non-opioid analgesics as a group :

- ***Relieve pain without interacting with opioid receptors.***
- ***Reduce elevated body temperature*** (anti-pyretic effect).
- ***Possess anti-inflammatory property*** and are known as **Non Steroidal Anti-inflammatory Drugs** (NSAID).
- ***Have antiplatelet activity*** to varying degrees.
- ***Do not cause sedation and sleep;*** and
- ***Are non-addicting.***

Temperature regulation: Although the **body surface temperature** is ordinarily measured in clinical practice, it is the **body core temperature** which is physiologically important. The rectal temperature (which reflects core temperature closely) is about 0.6° C (1° F) higher than oral temperature and about 1.4° C (2.5° F) higher than axillary temperature. The generally accepted normal limits of rectal temperature in adults are 36.1°C and 37.8° C (97°F and 100° F); the body temperature is higher in infants.

If the core temperature rises by more than a few degrees in man, mental changes occur. It is well known that an individual with high fever is often confused and delirious. The working of many tissue enzymes is also adversely affected and **hyperpyrexia** (core temperature 41°C or 106° F) may result in death. However, core temperature below 40.5° C (105° F) is generally well tolerated by most individuals.

The hypothalamus plays an important role in thermoregulatory mechanisms of the body. It controls the body temperature by two mechanisms :

(i) Cutaneous vasodilatation; and
(ii) Increase in sweat gland activity through sympathetic cholinergic fibres.

Normally, 60 per cent of the body heat loss occurs by radiation, 20 per cent by evaporation of water and the rest by convection and conduction. The commonest manifestation of a change in the core temperature is fever. The increase in temperature is brought about by the hypothalamus which reduces heat loss by peripheral vasoconstriction and increases heat production by inducing shivering. It then regulates the temperature around the new setting.

According to the current hypothesis, bacterial liposaccharides (LPS) activate the mononuclear phagocytes to release **interleukin-1 (IL-1) and tumour necrosis factor (TNF-α)**. These then act on the vascular endothelial cells in the hypothalamus and stimulate the local synthesis of prostaglandins, PGE_2. This causes fever and anorexia. The PG inhibitors reduce fever by inhibiting the synthesis of PG. Thus, IL-1 and TNF-α are now accepted as the **endogenous pyrogens.** IL-1 and TNF-α alpha, along with other cytokines, also play a major role in the manifestations of inflammation.

The role of fever in the defence reaction is not clear, though increased destruction of *T. pallidum* which causes syphilis, at high temperature, has been reported. In practice, as with pain, relief from fever with drugs adds to the comfort of the patient. It also impresses the patient and the relatives favourably about the therapeutic capability of the doctor! Finally **fever** (as caused by infections, inflammatory disorders, malignancies, tissue infarction and trauma) must be distinguished from **heat illnesses** (as due to malignant hyperthermia, heat stroke, atropine overdose and the use of street drugs). Fever is due to an upward resetting of the hypothalamic thermostat; the core temperature rarely exceeds 41^0 C (106^0 F); and the drugs described in this chapter are effective in lowering the body temperature. On the other hand, heat illness is due to failure of the thermoregulatory mechanisms; the body temperature is 106^0 F or higher (hyperpyrexia) and does not respond to the antipyretic drugs. *Heat illness may be fatal and needs urgent lowering of the body temperature with external cooling including immersion in ice water.*

Experimental evaluation of anti-inflammatory activity: Inflammation is the reaction of the living tissues to injury; it comprises systemic response (involving nervous and hormonal adjustments, and proliferation of the lymphoreticular system); and local response (pain, redness, warmth and swelling). The three important aspects of inflammation that render themselves readily to measurement are erythema (local vasodilatation), edema (increased capillary permeability) and formation of granulation tissue. Compounds claimed to possess anti-inflammatory activity can be evaluated either by their ability to reduce one or more of these phenomena in experimentally induced inflammation or by testing their anti-inflammatory activity in experimental arthritis produced in animals.

The commonly employed methods are:

- ***Erythema assays*:** Irradiation of the shaven back skin of a guinea pig with ultra violet light causes erythema. Erythema can also be produced in human beings with certain specific irritants like tetrahydrofurylnicotinate. The anti-inflammatory property of a new agent is assayed by comparing its ability to reduce the erythema with that of a known anti-inflammatory drug.
- ***Edema assays* :** Anti-inflammatory activity of a drug can also be measured by noting the reduction in edema produced by the local injection of substances like formaldehyde, carrageenin, histamine, dextran and ovalbumin. A modification involves the measurement of leakage of a protein bound marker (Evans blue, 131I) from the circulation into the tissues; the results obtained however, vary considerably from laboratory to laboratory.
- ***Granuloma assays*:** The 'Cotton wool pellet' and the 'granuloma pouch' are the most commonly used methods. The former involves SC implantation of weighed cotton wool pellets, impregnated with a 'foreign' material like carrageenin, in rat. This causes localised inflammation. The animals are sacrificed after the drug treatment; the cotton pellets, now encapsulated and heavily infiltrated with connective tissue are removed, dried, weighed and compared with those in control animals not given the drug.

In the granuloma pouch assay, an irritant like croton oil diluted with cotton seed oil or air is injected SC in the rat, usually on its back. After drug treatment the animal is sacrificed, the pouch is dissected, its exudate content is measured and compared with that in control animals.

- ***Experimental arthritis assays*:** Poly-arthritis induced in rats by injection of dead tubercle bacilli suspended in liquid paraffin (Freund's mycobacterial adjuvant) is a frequently used method for measurement of anti-inflammatory activity. Kaolin and talc have also been injected directly into the joints of rats and pigeons to induce arthritis.
- ***Miscellaneous*:** Localised inflammatory reaction can be produced in rats by intrapleural injection of turpentine or by intraperitoneal injection of acetic acid. Ability of the new agent to suppress acute inflammatory reaction to

albumin or horse serum in animals previously sensitised to these antigens (Arthus reaction) can also be studied.

The inflamed paw technique and the adjuvant arthritis model (both in rats) are the most successful methods of predicting anti-inflammatory activity in man. Paw inflammation and edema are produced by intra-plantar injection of napthoylheparamine or carrageenin.

Classification: The analgesic-antipyretic NSAID can be classified as :

I Non-selective COX inhibitors :

1. **Salicylates and their congeners.**
2. **Para-aminophenol derivatives** e.g. Phenacetin, Paracetamol.
3. **Pyrazolone derivatives** e.g. Phenylbutazone and Oxyphenbutazone
4. **Indoles and related drugs** : Indomethacin, Sulindac.
5. **Heterocyclic arylacetic acid derivatives:** Diclofenac, Tolmetin, Ketorolac.
6. **Propionic acid derivatives :** Ibuprofen, Fenoprofen, Naproxen, Ketoprofen and Pirprofen.
7. **Fenamates,** e.g., Flufenamic acid and Mefenamic acid.
8. **Oxicams,** e.g., Piroxicam.

II Selective COX-2 inhibitors: Nimesulide, Nabumetone, Etodolac, Meloxicam, Celecoxib.

General properties of NSAID are given in Table 11.1.

Mechanism of analgesic-antipyretic action: Though these drugs have different chemical structures, they produce qualitatively similar analgesic, antipyretic and anti-inflammatory effects. According to the current unifying concept of NSAID action, during inflammation, pain and fever, arachidonic acid (AA) is liberated from phospholipid fraction of the cell membrane by phospholipase A_2. Arachidonic acid is then converted via cyclo-oxygenase (COX-1 and 2) pathways to prostaglandins (PGs). The steps are (1) oxidation of AA to the endoperoxide PGG_2; (2) its subsequent reduction to the hydroxy-endoperoxide PGH_2; and (3) PGH_2 is then transformed into the primary prostanoids PGE_2, PGF_2, PGD_2, PGI_2 and TXA_2 (Chapter 24).

Table 11.1: General properties of NSAID

- They are weakly acidic compounds with ionization constants ranging from 3.0 to 5.0.
- They have varying degrees of lipid solubility, and are absorbed almost completely orally.
- They are highly albumin bound and have small volumes of distribution; and
- They are metabolized by the liver.

COX-1 and COX-2 both use the same endogenous substrate AA and form "the same products by the same catalytic mechanism. Their major difference lies in the pathophysiological functions:

- ***COX-1 activity is constitutively present in nearly all cell types at a constant level and is involved in tissue homeostasis;*** whereas
- ***COX-2 activity is normally absent from cells (except those of kidneys and brain) but is inducible*** by bacterial liposaccharides, IL-1 and TNF-α in activated leucocytes and other inflammatory cells.

Thus, COX-1 is physiological while COX-2 is usually (but not always) pathological.

PGs sensitize blood vessels to the effects of other inflammatory mediators that increase permeability. PGs particularly PGE and PGI produce hyperalgesia associated with inflammation. They sensitize the chemical receptors of the afferent pain endings to other mediators such as bradykinin and histamine. Further, release of PGs in the CNS may lower the threshold of the central pain circuits. Prostaglandins cause headache and vascular pain when infused IV and are also involved in the pyretic response in man.

Aspirin and aspirin like NSAIDs inhibit COX-1 and 2 and block synthesis of PGs and thus produce beneficial therapeutic effects. A similar mechanism also explains some of their adverse effects e.g. nephrotoxicity (see later). They are effective as analgesics only in pathological states where PGs are synthesized locally. They are ineffective in sharp 'stabbing' pain caused by direct stimulation of sensory nerves.

The quantitative differences in the actions of different PG inhibitors and their propensity to cause adverse reactions may be explained by the differences in the sensitivities of COX (PG synthetase) in different tissues to the various NSAID. For example, the cyclo-oxygenase in the brain is much more sensitive to paracetamol than the cyclo-oxygenase in the blood vesssels. Many NSAID non-selectively inhibit COX-1 and COX-2, while others act more selectively on COX-2. Thus, piroxicam and indomethacin are 10-40 fold selective for COX-1 whereas nabumetone is 15 fold selective for COX-2. Propionic acid derivatives like ibuprofen, fenamates, and aspirin inhibit both COX-1 and COX-2 equally.

In addition to its conversion to PGs via the cyclo-oxygenase pathway, arachidonic acid is converted via lipo-oxygenase pathway to leukotrienes (Chapter 24). Most NSAID do not inhibit the production of leukotrienes; in fact, by blocking the synthesis of PGs, they may make more arachidonic acid available for synthesis of leukotrienes. This might explain the symptoms of hypersensitivity in some subjects following the ingestion of aspirin and other NSAID.

Although inhibition of PG biosynthesis can explain many effects of NSAID, other mechanisms may also play an important role. Thus, indomethacin inhibits phosphodiesterase and increases the intra-cellular concentration of cyclic AMP. Cyclic AMP has been shown to stabilize membranes including lysosomal membranes in polymorphs. This prevents the release of enzymes important in the inflammatory response. Further, the anti-inflammatory drugs which are weak PG inhibitors appear to act by inhibiting the activation of T-lymphocytes which are abundant in the inflamed tissues and release cytokines (Chapter 24); the cytokines play an important role in mediating inflammation. Aspirin has both properties: PG synthesis inhibition and inhibition of T-lymphocyte activation. In addition to acting on cyclooxygenase, diclofenac and indomethacin inhibit the lipoxygenase pathway, thus decreasing the production of leukotrienes by the leucocytes and the synovial cells. NSAID may also unmask T cell suppressing activity, thereby suppressing the production of rheumatoid factors.

Salicylates

Salicylates are esters or salts of salicylic acid e.g. methyl salicylate and sodium salicylate; or alternatively, also occur as salicylate esters of organic acids such as acetyl salicylic acid (**aspirin**), the most commonly used salicylate. A compound which resembles the salicylic acid esters is salicylamide.

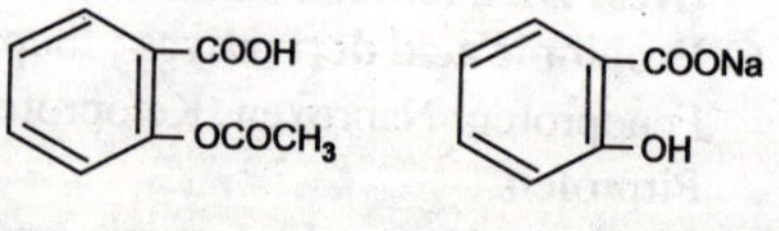

COOH
$OCOCH_3$
COONa
OH

Fig. 11.1 : Aspirin Sodium Salicylate

Pharmacological actions of salicylates:

Local actions: Salicylic acid and methyl salicylate are irritants; salicylic acid also has keratolytic, antiseptic and fungistatic actions (Chapters 60 and 69). The salts of salicylic acid do not irritate the unbroken skin but when ingested, may release free salicylic acid in the stomach causing local irritation.

Central nervous system:

• ***Analgesia***: Aspirin, introduced as an analgesic-antipyretic in 1899, is still an important drug in the therapy of pain and inflammation. *Salicylates, unlike the opioid analgesics, produce relief of pain without hypnosis or impairment of mental activity*. Their analgesic action is predominantly peripheral but a central component cannot be ruled out.

Therapeutically it may be rational to combine aspirin with opioid analgesic like codeine for a synergistic effect.

Aspirin inhibits the biosynthesis of PGs by **irreversible** acetylation and inactivation of COX in contrast to other NSAID which cause its **reversible** inhibition. They are mainly useful for relieving (1) dull aching, throbbing pain of low intensity arising from integumental structures such as muscles and joints; (2) dysmenorrhoea; and (3) toothache. *They are not useful in either deafferentiation pain or in visceral pain.*

In smaller doses, salicylates exert mainly analgesic action. With larger doses, they exert anti-inflammatory activity and relieve vascular congestion and edema.

Salicylates do not affect the emotional reactions (anxiety, fear) to pain. Toxic doses of salicylates produce stimulation of the CNS followed by depression (see later).

- ***Antipyretic action***: In fever, the thermostatic mechanism is set at a higher level even though it is not completely deranged. Salicylates act centrally and reset this mechanism at the normal level and thereby reduce the temperature; they do not lower the body temperature in a normal individual.

Salicylates, paracetamol and other antipyretics act by inhibiting brain PG synthesis and release. They do not reduce heat production but increase dissipation of heat mainly by producing cutaneous vasodilatation. Accompanying sweating assists the reduction of body temperature. They, however, do not affect the pathological process responsible for the inflammation.

- ***Respiration***: Salicylates stimulate respiration as a result of direct and indirect actions.

As a result of their action on the mitochondria (see later), therapeutic doses of salicylates increase the consumption of oxygen primarily by the skeletal muscles; this results in increased production of carbon dioxide which causes direct stimulation of the respiratory centre producing an increase in the depth and to some extent in the rate of respiration.

Salicylates also stimulate the medullary respiratory centre directly. In addition, they stimulate the chemoreceptors. This produces an increase in the rate as well as the depth of respiration leading to hyperventilation, washing out the plasma carbon dioxide and causing respiratory alkalosis. In man, a plasma level of 35 mg % of salicylates is usually associated with hyperventilation and severe dyspnoea occurs when the level approaches 50 mg %.

Acid-base balance and electrolytes: The respiratory alkalosis produced by therapeutic doses of salicylates is countered by excretion of alkaline urine containing bicarbonate along with sodium and potassium. This is termed the stage of *compensated respiratory alkalosis.*

Hypokalemia as a result of urinary loss of potassium is accompanied by water loss through lungs due to hyperventilation, through skin via augmented sweating and through urine as a result of alkalosis. This may lead to dehydration and hypernatremia.

With acute toxic doses of salicylates, hypokalemia is aggravated, the respiratory centre is depressed and *metabolic acidosis* develops. The mechanism of these effects is discussed later.

Gastrointestinal tract: Depending on the dose, they may produce

- ***Dyspepsia, nausea and vomiting*** as a result of gastric irritation; and
- ***Peptic ulceration with GI bleeding***, leading to hematemesis or melena.

The acid pH of the stomach favours the existence of salicylate in non-ionized form. The non-ionized form of salicylates is, however, relatively water insoluble; hence, it tends to adhere to the gastric mucosa thereby producing irritation. Further, local absorption into the mucous cell causes inhibition of COX-1 leading to decreased PGE_2 and PGI_2 synthesis, thus, causing a loss of the protective effect of PGE on the stomach. Salicylates also reduce the motility of the stomach and increase the gastric emptying time. These effects increase the period of contact of salicylate with the gastric mucosa.

Alkalies induce ionization of salicylates,

thereby reducing their gastric absorption and local irritant effect. As the ionized salicylate is more water soluble, it tends to pass more quickly into the intestine and does not adhere to the mucous membrane of the stomach.

To avoid gastric irritation, salicylates may be administered

- ***With plenty of water, after food.***
- ***With milk.***
- ***As soluble or buffered aspirin.***
- ***With an alkali such as sodium bicarbonate;*** or
- ***With misoprostol, a PGE analogue*** (Chapter 42).

Anti-inflammatory and anti-rheumatic effect : Salicylates suppress the clinical signs and improve the clinical picture in acute rheumatic fever and rheumatoid arthritis. Salicylates and other NSAID thus reduce the 'inflammatory component' of the disease by :

- ***Inhibiting PG synthesis in the peripheral tissues.***
- ***Reducing the capillary permeability***, thereby minimising the exudation of fluid and development of inflammatory edema.
- ***Inhibition of neutrophil aggregation and activation.*** Neutrophils injure the tissues by releasing proteases, leukotrienes and cytokines (Chapter 24).

Prostaglandins present in the inflammatory exudate are potent vasodilators and can cause edema, erythema and pain following intradermal injection. It has been suggested that aspirin-like drugs, by inhibiting the synthesis of PG, prevent sensitization of the pain receptors to agents such as histamine, 5-HT and bradykinin, the known chemical mediators of pain and inflammation.

The kinins (e.g. bradykinin) are formed from kininogen by the action of kallikrein and can produce the cardinal signs of inflammation when this system is activated by a variety of stimuli. Aspirin inhibits the formation of activated kallikrein from inactive plasma and leucocytic kallikrein.

The acidic mucopolysaccharides such as hyaluronic acid, chondroitin and mucoitin sulfuric acid constitute the ground substances of the extracellular matrix. Salicylates, other NSAID and the glucocorticoids inhibit the muco-polysaccharide biosynthesis. Such inhibition may reduce edema, tissue swelling and inflammatory response.

Immunological phenomena: Salicylates suppress a variety of antigen-antibody reactions *in vivo* including systemic anaphylaxis induced by egg-white challenge in rabbits, allergic encephalomyelitis in guineapigs and serum sickness in man. They also prevent the release of histamine as a result of antigen-antibody reaction *in vitro*. Salicylates, however, do not interfere significantly with the development of agglutinins following typhoid inoculation in humans. Further, they may reduce the cell-mediated immunity. The amounts of NSAID required to produce the above experimental effects are large and their relative contributions to the clinical antirheumatic activity is not clear.

Blood and platelets: Aspirin inhibits platelet aggregation. *It is unique in that it irreversibly inhibits COX by acetylation.* Platelets play an important role in thrombus formation. The drug by inhibiting cyclo-oxygenase (Chapter 24) suppresses the synthesis of thromboxane A (TXA_2) in the platelets. Daily doses of 75-150 mg almost completely suppress the synthesis for 7-10 days (Chapter 32). *Non-acetylated salicylates such as sodium salicylate do not possess such anti-platelet action.* Other NSAIDs inhibit the enzyme reversibly so that the platelet function is restored when the drug is eliminated.

Salicylates do not affect the normal leucocyte count. However, they reduce the leucocytosis and lower the high ESR observed in acute rheumatic fever. The latter effect is due to a reduction in the plasma fibrinogen content.

Hepatic and renal effects: Salicylates in therapeutic doses do not modify hepatic and renal functions significantly. They can, however, affect renal function in compromised kidneys by inhibiting COX-1. Salicylates increase the secretion of bile by stimulation of the hepatic parenchyma (*choleretic action*) but reduce the total concentration of cholates. Large doses, particularly in children, can cause hepatic damage and even necrosis.

Uricosuric effects: Urate present in the glomerular filtrate is reabsorbed by the proximal tubules of the kidney and the main excretion of urate in urine occurs due to its secretion by the distal tubule. Aspirin exerts *biphasic* action on the excretion of urate.

- ***In small doses*** (1-2 g. per day), aspirin interferes with urate secretion by the distal tubule, thereby elevating the plasma urate level, and block the action of other uricosuric drugs such as probenecid.
- ***Large doses*** (over 5 g. per day) inhibit the reabsorption of urate by the proximal tubule, which can cause uricosuria. The high doses, however, invariably result in adverse effects.

Cardiovascular system: Therapeutic doses of aspirin do not produce any deleterious effects on the cardiovasular system.

Endocrine effects : Salicylates interfere with the binding of thyroid hormones to their binding proteins, especially thyroxine binding albumin. This comes in the way of interpretation of serum thyroxine and tri-iodothyronine values.

Metabolic effects: The uncoupling by salicylates of oxidative phosphorylation (Chapter 62) leads to conversion of a large part of energy derived from oxidation into heat. Large doses of salicylates may, thus, lead to hyperpyrexia, increased protein catabolism leading to aminoaciduria and a negative nitrogen balance.

In ccrtain diabetic individuals salicylates can reduce the blood sugar level and glycosuria. This effect is probably due to an enhanced peripheral utilization of glucose and inhibition of neoglucogenesis induced by salicylates. However, large doses of salicylates produce hyperglycemia and glycosuria in normal individuals.

Salicylates reduce lipogenesis and at the same time inhibit adrenaline induced lipolysis in the fat cells. Toxic doses lead to formation of ketone bodies.

Absorption, fate and excretion: Both salicylic acid and methyl salicylate are absorbed from intact skin, especially when applied in alcohol, petrolatum, lard or lanolin base and systemic poisoning in children has been reported following such local applications. Salicylates are absorbed from the stomach and largely from the upper small intestine. Factors such as particle size, pH of the GI tract, solubility of the salicylate preparation and presence of food in the stomach modify the absorption. Sodium salicylate in a single therapeutic dose is absorbed within 30 minutes, peak plasma level is achieved within 2 hours; approximately 50 per cent of the dose is eliminated in urine within 24 hours.

After absorption, approximately 80 per cent of the salicylate (but only 50% of aspirin) is bound to plasma proteins, mainly albumin. It is rapidly distributed through most of the tissues and achieves a significant concentration in the saliva, milk, spinal, synovial and peritoneal fluids and in the erythrocytes. High salicylate concentrations are observed in the liver, heart and muscle while the brain contains relatively smaller amounts.

Aspirin, even though absorbed as such, is subject to rapid metabolism (50-60%) to salicylate by deacetylation during first pass and is further hydrolysed in the blood and tissues to salicylic acid. Aspirin can be detected in the plasma only for a short time (t/2 15 minutes).

Like phenytoin, aspirin exhibits dose dependent pharmacokinetics:

- ***At lower dose levels*** (300-600 mg individual doses), the plasma level increases in proportion to the dose (*first order kinetics*).
- ***At higher dose levels*** (1-2 g individual doses), the increase in the plasma level is disproportionate and severe toxicity can occur (*zero order kinetics*).

Salicylates are mainly excreted in urine in the form of conjugates with glycine and glucuronic acid. A small portion is oxidised to gentisic acid and excreted in the urine.

An alkaline urine, by ionizing the salicylate to a water soluble and indiffusible form, prevents salicylate back-diffusion in the distal tubule and enhances its excretion. Thus, the concentration of free salicylate in urine varies according to urinary pH. Its excretion is reduced by probenecid, oliguria and kidney failure and is augmented by diuresis and alkaline pH.

Adverse reactions:

● ***Intolerance*:** Salicylate can cause allergic or pseudoallergic reactions. These include skin rashes, urticaria, pruritus, angioneurotic edema, bronchospasm, anaphylaxis-like shock or thrombocytopenic purpura. Aspirin may sometimes cause bronchospasm. Salicylate induced angioedema and anaphylactoid reaction respond to adrenaline. Aspirin can induce idiosyncratic, mild haemolysis in individuals with G-6-PD deficiency.

Salicylic acid and its derivatives are ingredients of a large number of substances including fruits like apples, grapes, oranges, peaches and plums, soaps containing oil of wintergreen, perfumes, beverages (especially birch beer), tooth pastes, gum and lozenges. Individuals with idiosyncrasy to salicylates should also be warned against taking proprietary drug mixtures, which often contain salicylates.

● ***Gastrointestinal tract*:** The commonest side effects of salicylates and other NSAID are dyspepsia, nausea, vomiting, heartburn and ulceration. In subjects taking 3-4 g. of aspirin daily, the actual blood loss may be about 3-6 ml. per day. Occasionally, asprin can cause haematemesis, and prolonged therapy can lead to anemia. The incidence of major GI bleeding due to aspirin is estimated at 15 per 100,000 chronic aspirin users per year. Gastric bleeding is due to (a) local mucosal action; (b) inhibition of platelets; and (c) hypoprothrombinemia.

● ***Haemopoietic system*:** Salicylates but not the newer NSAID in large doses reduce the plasma prothrombin level by interfering with action of vitamin K in the liver. Salicylate induced hypoprothrombinemia can be reversed by administration of vitamin K. Salicylates exert a synergistic effect with the coumarin anticoagulants on prothrombin synthesis and hence, these drugs should be avoided by patients receiving oral anticoagulant drugs. For similar reasons, cautious use of salicylates is also indicated in individuals with hepatic damage and in those who are about to undergo surgery.

● ***Kidneys*:** Discussed later.

● ***Reye's syndrome*:** This serious and often fatal complication occurs a few days after a viral infection, especially influenza and varicella, in children below the age 12 years. There occurs anicteric liver dysfunction due to hepatic mitochondrial injury and a consequent metabolic encephalopathy. There is epidemiological evidence to associate administration of aspirin during the initial viral infection and the subsequent occurrence of this serious disease. *Aspirin should, therefore, be avoided in infants and in children under the age of 12 years, unless specifically indicated e.g. for juvenile rheumatoid arthritis.*

● ***Pregnant women and infants*:** Taken at term, aspirin by inhibiting PG synthesis in the uterus may delay the onset of labour and cause greater blood loss at delivery. The administration of aspirin or indomethacin at term has been reported to cause premature closure of the ductus arteriosus with resultant serious pulmonary hypertension in the newborn. Salicylates readily cross the placental barrier, and may prove toxic to the newborn as its ability to detoxify and excrete salicylates is poor. The toxic manifestations in newborn include hyperpnoea and haemorrhages. Hypoglycemia after prolonged salicylate therapy has also been reported in infants. Repeated use of an NSAID in pregnant women should be avoided. Low dose aspirin is probably safe.

● ***Salicylism*:** High doses of salicylates may produce a condition of mild salicylate intoxication termed salicylism. The syndrome usually develops when the plasma salicylate level exceeds 25 mg. per cent and is characterised by headache, dizziness, vertigo, tinnitus, difficulty in hearing and dimness of vision; drowsiness, lethargy and mental confusion, nausea, vomiting and diarrhoea may also occur. These symptoms may be associated with tachypnoea and respiratory alkalosis. It is reversible on cessation of therapy.

- ***Acute salicylate intoxication***: Acute salicylate intoxication may be due to overzealous therapy in infants or following an accidental ingestion. A serum salicylate level of 50 mg% indicates mild toxicity; levels above 75 mg.% are potentially fatal. The characteristic features of acute intoxication are acidbase and electrolyte disturbances, hyperglycemia, dehydration, hyperpyrexia, GI irritation and occasional haemorrhages. The stimulation of CNS causes restlessness, vertigo, tremor, apprehension, hallucinations and convulsions.

With toxic doses, the respiratory centre is depressed resulting in CO_2 accumulation and true metabolic acidosis. Salicylates induce derangement of the carbohydrate metabolism leading to an accumulation of pyruvic, lactic and acetoacetic acids.

Table 11.2 gives the principles of management of salicylate poisoning. Correction of acidosis and urinary alkalinization should be carried out cautiously using normal saline containing 2 per cent dextrose and 2 per cent sodium bicarbonate, at the rate of 2 litres/hr, with frequent determination of blood pH and plasma bicarbonate, to prevent metabolic alkalosis.

Table 11.2 : Principles of management of salicylate poisoning

- Hospitalization.
- Activated charcoal 50g orally.
- Correct hyperthermia, dehydration (5% dextrose), hypokalemia, acid-base disturbances, ketosis.
- Increase elimination by alkalinization, peritoneal dialysis or hemoperfusion.
- Vitamin K, blood transfusion.
- Exchange transfusion in very small children.

Sedatives like barbiturates are dangerous when the patients show excitement with salicylate intoxication. These agents, by producing respiratory depression, may aggravate metabolic acidosis and precipitate coma.

Preparations and dosage:

(i) Acetyl salicylic acid (Aspirin 300 mg tablets). Dose : 0.3 to 0.6 g. 4-6 hourly (maximum 4g./day) orally, for relief of integumental pain; in the treatment of acute rheumatism, 4 to 8 g. daily in divided doses.

(ii) Soluble aspirin tablet contains aspirin (300 mg.), citric acid (30 mg.) with calcium carbonate (100 mg) and saccharin sodium (3 mg.). When mixed with water, citric acid reacts with calcium carbonate to form calcium citrate solution and this dissolves aspirin forming calcium acetyl salicylate. It is not possible to dispense the latter directly in tablet form, as it is hygroscopic and is rapidly hydrolysed in the presence of moisture. Dose : same as above.

(iii) Buffered aspirin tablets contain aspirin and an antacid like magnesium hydroxide, aluminium hydroxide or aluminum glycinate.

(iv) Sodium salicylate has a characteristic sweetish, saline, unpleasant taste and is soluble in water. It is administered in a mixture form with alkali. It is available as 500 mg tab (Succisalyl forte containing sodium salicylate 500 mg and sodium succinate 300 mg per tab). Dose: for integumental pain 0.5 to 2 g., for acute rheumatic fever, 5 to 10 g., daily in divided doses.

(v) Methyl salicylate (oil of Wintergreen): Methyl salicylate liniment 25 per cent v/v in peanut oil and, methyl salicylate ointment 50 per cent in white bees wax and hydrous wool fat.

(vi) Salicylic acid : Salicylic acid ointment contains 2-6 per cent salicylic acid w/w while Whitfield's ointment contains 6 per cent benzoic acid and 3 per cent salicylic acid.

(vii) Lysine acetyl salicylate (Injisprin, Biospirin): Intravenous infusion of this preparation may be used to treat postoperative pain. It provides pain relief and may reduce the requirement for morphine.

Therapeutic uses of salicylates:

- ***Local application*** : Salicylic acid is used for its keratolytic, fungistatic and mild antiseptic activity. Methyl salicylate is used as a counter irritant (Chapter 69). For local use of 5-aminosalicylic acid in the treatment of inflammatory bowel disease, see Chapter 40.

● ***As analgesic-antipyretic*** : Salicylates are beneficial in a variety of conditions such as arthralgias, myalgias, neuralgias, toothache, headache, backache and dysmenorrhoea. For analgesia, aspirin is used either alone or in combination with an opioid analgesic like codeine. When combined with opioid analgesics such as codeine, it can reduce the dose of the former and fewer adverse effects of both drugs might result. In single doses of 300-1200 mg., aspirin shows graded responses. *Doses higher than 1200 mg. however, simply increase the risk of toxicity and should not ordinarily be prescribed.*

Aspirin and other NSAIDs are valuable in primary dysmenorrhoea. Treatment is started on the first day of the menstrual period and is continued for 2-3 days.

They are also very useful as antipyretics in the symptomatic treatment of fever.

● ***As anti-inflammatory***: Aspirin is commonly used to treat inflammatory conditions such as arthritis and fibromyositis. It can modify or diminish but does not arrest the inflammatory response.

● ***As antirheumatic***: Salicylates, in a sufficiently large dose, produce within 24 to 48 hours dramatic relief of pain and inflammation in **acute rheumatic fever**. There is a significant reduction in swelling, immobility, heat and redness of the joints involved. The fever is reduced, the pulse rate slows down and further joint involvement is prevented. Salicylates, however, cannot prevent or reverse the cardiac complications, chorea, subcutaneous nodules or encephalopathy and fail to shorten the duration of the disease.

In SLE, aspirin may ameliorate arthritis and serositis but the vasculitic component caused by immune complex deposition is not affected.

Aspirin, being a better analgesic, is preferred to sodium salicylate. The adult dose is 4 to 8 g. daily given at intervals, in 1 g. dose. For children the recommended daily dose is 120 mg. per kg. of body weight per day (with a maximum of 8 gm.) given in 4-6 divided doses. A plasma salicylate level of 25 to 40 mg. per cent usually achieves adequate control. Full doses are continued for at least 2 weeks after disappearance of symptoms and signs of inflammation, and the drug is then gradually discontinued over a period of 7 to 10 days. Sudden salicylate discontinuation may produce a relapse. Large doses of salicylates in patients with rheumatic carditis may increase the plasma volume, cardiac output and metabolic rate and this may precipitate congestive heart failure.

Glucocorticoids are useful in cases not responding to salicylates and appear to be more effective in the severely ill patients with high fever, rheumatic pericarditis and concomitant congestive cardiac failure or cardiac arrhythmias. The incidence of relapse after stoppage of corticosteroid therapy is relatively high. Some authorities recommend combined aspirin and glucocorticoid therapy.

Concurrent penicillin therapy is recommended for eradication of streptococcal infection. This is discussed in Chapter 45.

For use of aspirin in rheumatoid arthritis, see Chapter 71.

● ***As antiplatelet agent***: Aspirin is used to prevent platelet aggregation in patients with ischemic heart disease. It blocks COX activity within an hour of administration, inhibiting the platelets for 8-10 days after a single dose of 75-100 mg. (Chapter 32).

● ***Miscellaneous***: PGs have been implicated in the maintenance of patency of ductus arteriosus. Indomethacin has been used in persistent patent ductus arteriosus in the neonate with success. The treatment of **Bartter syndrome** (a rare condition associated with hypokalemia and increased plasma renin and aldosterone levels) with aspirin has been quite successful. Prophylactic doses of aspirin (600-900 mg.), indomethacin or ibuprofen have been shown to prevent symptoms of food intolerance in patients who showed acute GI symptoms after eating specific foodstuffs. Aspirin has also been shown to exert the beneficial effect in radiation induced and other diarrhoeas. These symptoms are probably mediated through prostaglandin release. Taken orally and applied locally, aspirin and other PG inhibitors have been found useful in reducing erythema due to sunburn. NSAID have been used locally in the treatment of ocular inflammatory conditions (see later). PGD_2 release from the mast cells in the tissues causes vasodilatation and hypotension in patients with mastocytosis. Addition of an NSAID to antihistaminic for the treatment of this condition gives better results. *An inverse correlation has recently been reported between the chronic use of aspirin and colorectal cancer.*

Diflunisal is a non-acetylated difluorinated salicylate which has analgesic and antiinflammatory properties. There is some evidence to suggest that it has greater potency, better tolerance and a longer duration of action than aspirin. It is available as 250 mg tablets (Dolobid). The dose is 0.25 - 0.5 g twice a day.

Para-Aminophenol Derivatives

The commonly used drug is paracetamol. Acetanilid and phenacetin are no longer used in therapeutics.

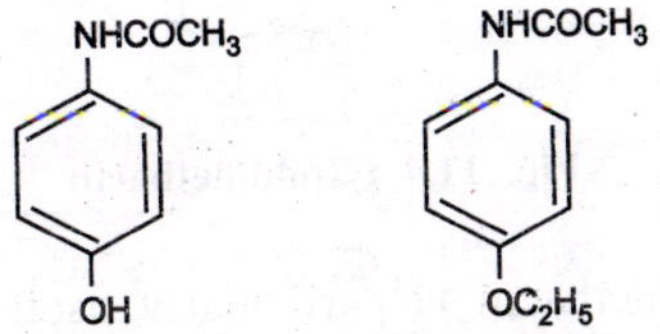

$NHCOCH_3$ … OH $NHCOCH_3$ … OC_2H_5

Fig 11.2: Paracetamol **Phenacetin**

PARACETAMOL (Acetaminophen, Crocin, Calpol): This compound exerts analgesic and antipyretic effects like salicylates. It has weak activity on prostaglandin synthetase (COX) in the inflamed peripheral tissues which have high concentration of peroxides; however, it equals the blocking effect of aspirin on this enzyme in the brain. Therefore, *paracetamol is a potent antipyretic and is equianalgesic with aspirin in therapeutic doses but devoid of significant anti-inflammatory effect.*

Compared to salicylates, it does not produce GI irritation, acid-base imbalance, electrolyte disturbances, nor does it affect blood clotting. Hence, it is preferred to aspirin as an analgesic, antipyretic for routine use and for treating osteoarthritic pain.

Absorption, fate and excretion: Paracetamol is rapidly absorbed orally and peak plasma levels are reached within ½ to 1 hour. It is metabolized in the liver and the metabolites excreted in urine as conjugation products of glucuronic and sulfuric acids. The ability of infant liver for glucuronidation of paracetamol is poor and this may result in enhanced toxicity in neonates.

Adverse reactions: At recommended therapeutic doses (500-1000 mg) in healthy subjects, paracetamol is generally well tolerated and causes hardly any side effects.

- ***Hepatic and renal toxicity :*** Large doses (7-10 g) of paracetamol produce extensive hepatocellular damage and renal tubular necrosis, and may cause death. In fact, this is a major problem in acute paracetamol poisoning.

The liver toxicity is due to the toxic metabolite N-acetyl-P-benzoquinoneimine which normally turns harmless by conjugation with glutathione. Depletion of hepatic and renal glutathione potentiates this toxicity whereas treatment with sulfhydryl compounds such as cysteamine, l-methionine and n-acetyl cysteine is beneficial. N-acetyl cysteine may be administered orally as 5% solution in the dose of 140 mg/kg, followed by 70 mg/kg every 4 hours for 3 days. Prior liver damage as in chronic alcoholics may increase the liability to hepatotoxicity.

- Paracetamol may cause fever, neutropenia, thrombocytopenia, nephropathy and skin reactions.
- It may rarely produce anemia as a result of haemolysis. Individuals with G6PD deficiency may exhibit increased sensitivity to this drug. Methemoglobinaemia occurs uncommonly.

Preparation and dosage : (1) Paracetamol (500 mg tablets) is used as an analgesic and antipyretic. Dose: 250 to 500 mg. The total daily dose should not exceed 2.5 g. in adults. It can be used in a liquid dosage form in children. (2) Injection Febrinil (150 mg/ml).

Pyrazolone Derivatives

These are :

- Aminopyrine and antipyrine
- Phenylbutazone and oxyphenbutazone
- Other drugs like phenyldimethyl pyrazolone (analgin, dipyrone).

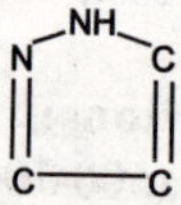

Fig. 11.3 : Pyrazolone ring

Aminopyrine and Antipyrine, though potent analgesic, antipyretic and antiinflammatory agents, are not well tolerated. They are no longer used in therapeutics because of their toxicity.

PHENYLBUTAZONE: This compound initially used as a solvent for aminopyrine injection, is a potent anti-inflammatory drug. The anti-inflammatory activity of phenylbutazone exceeds that of salicylates. However, the drug is poorly tolerated by many patients and causes various GI, hepatic, renal and fatal hematologic toxic effects. It gives rise to various drug interactions. Hence it is now rarely used.

OXYPHENBUTAZONE (Phenabid, Oxyrin): This compound, a metabolic degradation product of phenylbutazone, is claimed to cause less gastric irritation than phenylbutazone. The drug, however, shares all the toxic effects of phenylbutazone.

ANALGIN (Dipyrone, Novalgin): It has potent analgesic and antipyretic actions but no uricosuric effect. It has no advantage over aspirin except that it can be injected. The toxic effects are similar to those of phenylbutazone, and include fatal blood dyscrasias. Hence, it is risky and unjustifiable to use this drug routinely, simply to relieve pain and fever where aspirin or paracetamol would be adequate.

Indoles and Related Drugs

INDOMETHACIN (Indocid): This indole acetic acid derivative is a potent anti-inflammatory agent.

Pharmacological actions: It has antiinflammatory, analgesic and anti-pyretic actions. In patients with rheumatoid arthritis with swollen joints, it brings about a quick reduction in the joint swellings. However, the drug is not superior to aspirin for this purpose.

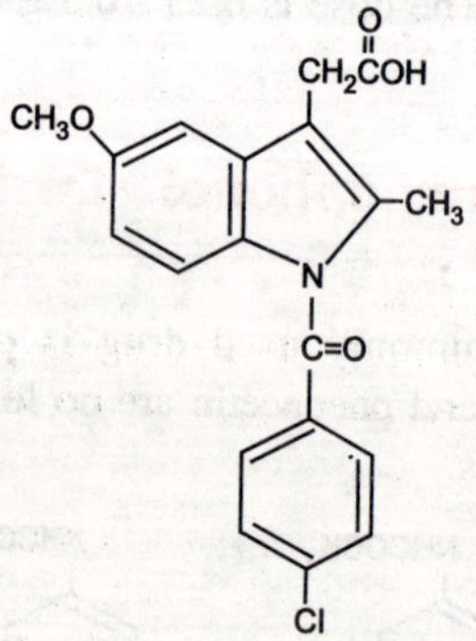

Fig. 11.4 : Indomethacin

Indomethacin is particularly useful in the treatment of acute attacks of gout, where it relieves pain within 2 hours of the first dose. It also acts as an analgesic even in the absence of clinically obvious inflammation e.g. osteo-arthritis, ankylosing spondylitis.

Absorption, fate and excretion : Given orally, it is rapidly and almost completely absorbed, reaching a peak plasma concentration within 1 to 2 hours, is mainly metabolised by the liver, and is rapidly eliminated by the kidneys as glucuronide. Nearly 50-90 per cent of a single dose is excreted in urine within 24 hours. Its action is more prolonged than is suggested by its t½ (2 hours).

Adverse reactions : The reported incidence of adverse effects has ranged from 25 to 50 per cent. Even with the low doses, the incidence is 15-20 per cent. Headache is the most common effect, followed by giddiness, mental confusion, blurring of vision, depression and psychotic disturbances. Some of these effects would make it dangerous for the patient to drive a vehicle. *Such neuropsychiatric adverse reactions are more frequent with indomethacin than with other NSAIDs.*

Less common adverse effects are nausea, vomiting, dyspepsia, diarrhoea, skin rashes and rarely blood dyscrasias. Peptic ulceration associated with bleeding and liver damage have been reported. It may cause sodium retention, edema and transient rise in blood urea and serum creatinine. It may aggravate preexisting kidney disease. It can cause reduction in renal clearance of lithium and thus, a rise in serum lithium level in patients on lithium therapy.

Preparation and dosage: Indomethacin 25 mg. capsules. Total daily dose recommended is 50-150 mg. in divided doses, after food. Indomethacin suppository is also available.

Therapeutic uses: The drug cannot be recommended as the drug of choice in rheumatoid arthritis because of its toxicity. It may be preferred in the treatment of acute gouty attacks and in ankylosing spondylitis *for short term therapy.*

SULINDAC (Clinoril) is a fluorinated derivative of indomethacin. It is a prodrug and has a longer duration of action. Its active metabolite is claimed to be much less nephrotoxic. It is given orally in the dose of 100-200 mg. twice a day.

Heterocyclic Arylacetic Acid Derivatives

DICLOFENAC (Voveran): This drug probably has substantially greater activity than indomethacin, naproxen and other NSAIDs, probably because of its higher COX-2 inhibiting property. Fifty per cent of the sodium salt is metabolized during the first pass through the liver. It is extensively bound to plasma proteins, with a t½ of 1-2 hours. It accumulates in the synovial fluid, which probably is responsible for its longer duration of action than its plasma t½ suggests. Its selectivity for COX-2 also explains the increased cardiovascular risk associated with this drug.

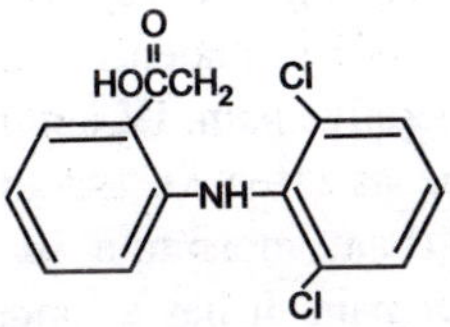

O
HOCCH$_2$ Cl
NH
Cl

Fig. 11.5: Diclofenac

Adverse reactions: The incidence of adverse reactions is about 20%. Commonly, it causes adverse effects similar to those caused by propionic acid derivatives (see below). GI symptoms including bleeding and elevation of liver enzymes occur more frequently than with propionic acid derivatives. Hence, liver enzymes should be evaluated in the first few weeks of long term therapy. Other adverse effects include CNS effects and fluid retention. The drug may cause severe oliguria due to marked reduction in renal blood flow and GFR. Its use is not recommended in children, pregnant women and nursing mothers, and in patients who are likely to be having renal disease, such as diabetic nephropathy.

Therapeutic Uses: It is used mainly in rheumatoid arthritis, severe osteoarthritis and in ankylosing spondylitis. Its dose is 75 - 100 mg orally, daily, in 2-3 divided doses after food; and 75 mg by deep IM injection once or twice a day. Diclofenac is also used as 0.1% eye drops for the inhibition of intraoperative miosis (but it does not possess intrinsic mydriatic activity) and to prevent postoperative inflammation in cataract surgery. For postoperative analgesia, the drug is used rectally as suppositories (Voltarol) in the dose of 75-100 mg per day in divided doses.

Studies confirm that **dipyrone** (analgin) is a major cause of agranulocytosis and that phenylbutazone, diclofenac and indomethacin can cause aplastic anemia. They should be used only when aspirin, ibuprofen and other safer NSAID are ineffective.

KETOROLAC (Ketorol, Ketanov): Ketorolac IM, 20-30 mg (single dose), is a moderately effective analgesic in patients with moderate to severe postoperative pain. IV ketorolac has been reported to be as effective as, and have fewer side effects than, morphine in surgical and chronic cancer pain. It has a longer duration of action (t½ 5 hours). However, even such parenteral administration can cause as much gastric mucosal injury as oral administration. It has less antinflammatory activity. Like other NSAIDs, ketorolac inhibits platelet function. The initial dose of 20-30 mg IM may be followed by 10-15 mg by the same route 6-8 hourly, to a maximum of 80 - 120 mg daily, for upto 2 days. IV doses are similar to IM doses.

Tolmetin (Tolectin) : This drug, a pyrrole acetic acid derivative, resembles ibuprofen in its actions and its toxicity. It is, however, less potent than indomethacin.

Propionic Acid Derivatives

These compounds like **ibuprofen, naproxen, fenoprofen, flurbiprofen** and **ketoprofen** have analgesic-antipyretic and antiinflammatory properties similar to aspirin but are better tolerated orally. The incidence of adverse reactions is lower than that after high doses of aspirin and indomethacin. They can, however, cause many of the adverse reactions produced by aspirin, including gastric irritation and ulceration and liver damage. Further, any patient who is intolerant of aspirin may also suffer a severe reaction following their administration.

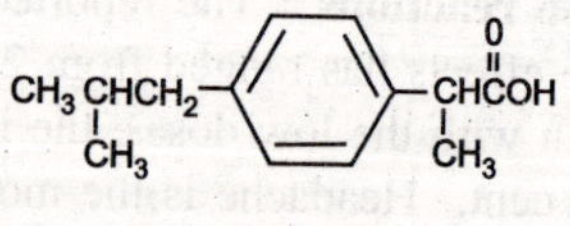

Ibuprofen

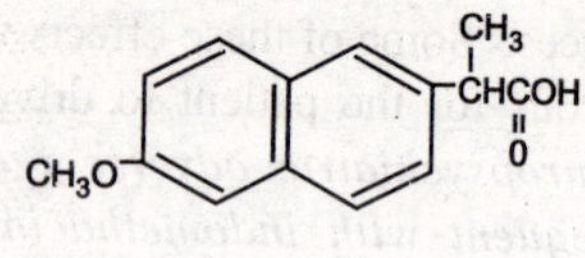

Fig. 11.6: Naproxen

These drugs are highly bound to plasma albumin (92-99%) and, like aspirin, can displace drugs such as hydantoins, sulfonylureas and warfarin. They, however, differ in their pharmacokinetics and hence, in their duration of action following single doses.

Adverse reactions: They may cause GI disturbances such as epigastric pain, nausea, sensation of fullness in the stomach and heartburn. Occult blood loss is less common. Less frequently, they may cause CNS symptoms such as headache, dizziness, blurred vision and tinnitus. In a few cases, fluid retention and edema may occur. Hepatitis, impairment of renal function and thrombocytopenia are rare.

Therapeutic uses: They are particularly useful in patients with RA, osteoarthritis and ankylosing spondylitis, who cannot tolerate aspirin. The pharmacodynamic profiles of various propionic acid derivatives do not differ significantly, and the choice depends upon the relative cost. In general, ibuprofen is the better tolerated drug among the propionic acid derivatives, is cost effective and is a good substitute for aspirin as an antiinflammatory agent. Flurbiprofen is also available as eye drops for eye inflammation.

The use of ibuprofen simultaneously with aspirin reduces its antiinflammatory effect. Further, ibuprofen and other NSAIDs interfere with the antiplatelet action and hence affect the cardioprotective effect of low dose aspirin.

Fenamates

MEFENAMIC ACID (Meftal, Pontstan): This is an anthranilic acid derivative useful in chronic and dull aching pains. Fenamates have shown no clear advantages over other NSAIDs and frequently cause adverse effects such as diarrhoea. Mefenamic acid is a weaker analgesic than aspirin. Adverse reactions include gastric upset, diarrhoea, dizziness, headache, skin rashes and hemolytic anemia. The dose is 500 mg 2-3 times a day.

Therapeutic uses :

- Menstrual bleeding in menorrhagic women may diminish by upto 50% with the use of PG inhibitors such as ibuprofen and mefenamic acid when used during menses.
- Dysmenorrhoea.

Flufenamic acid has similar properties.

Oxicams

PIROXICAM (Feldene, Pirox): This NSAID is structurally different from other agents. Given orally, it is well absorbed and has a *long halflife* of 38-45 hours. Hence, it can be administered once a day. Doses between 10 and 20 mg produce analgesic-antipyretic effect whereas larger doses (20-40 mg) are needed for the anti-inflammatory effect. It commonly causes GI upset, peptic ulceration and CNS disturbances. It has been used to treat RA, ankylosing spondylitis, osteoarthritis and acute gout. It has no advantage except a longer duration of action.

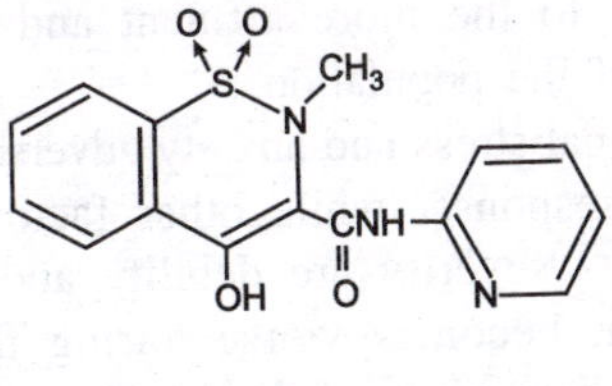

Fig. 11.7: Piroxicam

Table 11.3: Anti-inflammatory doses of non-selective NSAID

Name	Available as	Dose/Frequency
Ibuprofen (Brufen)	200, 400 mg tab	400 - 600 mg tid
Fenoprofen (Fenopron)	300 mg tablets	300-600 mg tid
Ketoprofen (Octofen)	50 mg capsules	50 mg tid
Naproxen (Naprosyn)	250 mg tablets	250-500 mg bid
Flurbiprofen	100 mg tablets	100-150 mg bid
Diclofenac (Voveran)	50 mg tablets	50 mg bid
Indomethacin (Indocid)	25 mg capsules	25-50 mg tid
Sulindac (Clinoril)	100 mg tablets	200 mg bid
Piroxicam (Pirox)	10, 20 mg capsules	10-20 mg od

Tenoxicam, meloxicam and **lornoxicam** are the other oxicams.

The NSAIDs commonly used as antiinflammatory agents are listed in Table 11.3.

Selective COX-2 Inhibitor NSAIDs

Drugs belonging to this group selectively block COX-2 activity more than COX-1 activity, thus interfering less with the protective action of COX-1 in the stomach, blood vessels and kidneys. This group includes **nimesulide, meloxicam, nabumetone, celecoxib, rofecoxib** and **valdecoxib.** The last two are highly selective (Table 11.4).

Given orally, their absorption is complete. They are claimed to be as effective as the nonselective analgesic-antiinflammatory NSAIDs. They have been shown to be effective in the treatment of osteoarthritis and rheumatoid arthritis. Their major advantage is that they cause fewer gastric ulcers and do not inhibit

Table 11.4: Selective COX-2 inhibitors

Drug	Half-life (hours)	Dose (mg)*	Comments
Nabumetone (Relifex)	24	500-1000 od	Prodrug converted to active metabolite
Nimesulide (Nimulid, Nise)	< 5	100 mg tid	Less selective
Meloxicam (Muvera, Mobic)	20	7.5-15 od	Less selective
Celecoxib (Celebrex)	11	200 OD or bid	Highly selective

* Small in osteoarthritis, large in rheumatoid arthritis.

platelet aggregation. In that sense, they are 'stomach friendly'. *However, they have prothrombotic effect, leading to a higher incidence of cardiovascular events.*

Adverse reactions: The most common adverse reactions are nausea, vomiting, dyspepsia, abdominal pain, diarrhoea, skin reactions and edema. These drugs share some of the renal adverse effects of nonselective COX inhibitors and renal toxicity viz. decrease in renal blood flow, edema and dose-related worsening of hypertension has been reported. *Their use should be restricted to patients who do not tolerate ther NSAIDs for some reason.* Studies in animals suggest that inhibiting COX-2 may interfere with wound (ulcer) healing, bone remodeling, ovulation and prenatal renal development. Their use is not recommended in children and women of child–bearing age, and during lactation, as they are excreted in breast milk. Celecoxib is contraindicated in patients allergic to sulfonamides. Life-threatening skin reactions have been reported with valdecoxib.

Nimesulide has been reported to cause nephrotoxicity and hepatotoxicity. The drug was not licensed for use in some developed countries, and it has been banned/withdrawn from others. The use of nimesulide should be avoided, especially in children and old persons.

It is now established that at least three selective COX-2 inhibitors, rofecoxib, valdecoxib and celecoxib, "confer dose-related increased risk of heart attack and stroke." Hence, the first two have been withdrawn by the manufacturers. *Currently, all the selective COX-2 inhibitors are under suspicion regarding their long term toxicity. They have been described as drugs with "marginal efficacy, heightened risk and excessive cost compared with traditional NSAIDs."*

Table 11.5 summarises the effects of commonly used analgesic–antipyretic agents.

Pharmacotherapy of Pain

The boundaries between normal discomfort and pathologic pain are often obscure. The intensity of pain suffered differs enormously with the personality, intelligence and culture of the individual. Tribal people often display a stoic disregard for pain. As a generalisation, pain is complained of more vehemently by people belonging to the more affluent and the elite sections of the population.

Emotional stress and anxiety adversely affect the pain response, while other factors which enhance its severity are debility and fatigue. Pain often becomes worse during the night when the distractions of daytime are absent and

Table 11.5: Effects of commonly used analgesic-antipyretic agents

	Acetylsalicylic acid			Sodium Salicylate	Newer* NSAIDs	Paracetamol
	Low dose	Intermediate dose	High dose			
Antipyretic	0	+	+	+	+	+
Analgesic	0	+	+	+	+	+
Anti-inflammatory	0	0	+	+	+	Minimal
Inhibition of PG synthesis in platelets	+	+	+	0	+	0
Inhibition PG synthesis systemically	0	+	+	±	+	0

Low Dose = 75-300 mg/day; Intermediate dose = 500 mg – 3 g/day; High dose = more than 3 g/day. Anti-inflammatory effect = Relief of fever, pain, redness and swelling. Newer NSAIDs* include indomethacin, ibuprofen, naproxen, diclofenac, piroxicam.

the patient has time to ruminate his ailment. Protracted severe pain can become so dominant a factor in a patient's life that it can eventually lead to both physical and psychological exhaustion. The relief of pain by the use of appropriate drugs forms an important aspect of therapeutic skills in practice. *The management of pain is always multidisciplinary and involves pharmacotherapy, physiotherapy and cognitive behavioral therapy.* The choice of therapy depends upon:

- ***The nature of the painful disease,***
- ***The mechanism by which it produces pain,***
- ***Associated conditions and complications;*** and
- ***The risk of toxicity involved due to the drug so selected.***

An attempt should always be made to find out the probable cause. *Where the cause is obvious, therapy should be directed to treat it.* Thus, pain due to an abscess can be relieved by appropriate chemotherapy and surgery, whereas that due to a bony metastasis can be relieved by local radio-therapy.

In patients in whom, for some reason, *the cause cannot be treated*, immediate relief of pain can be obtained by *modifying the mechanism by which pain is produced* e.g. use of nitrates in angina pectoris, miotics in glaucoma and muscle relaxants in certain musculoskeletal disorders. Mechanism of production of abdominal pain is often obscure and a demonstrable cause is absent. The pain in chronic duodenal ulcer can be relieved promptly by sodium bicarbonate powder. Individuals with "functional dyspepsia", are known to be benefited by 'carminatives' which have been used for ages. It is a common experience that a few seeds of cardamom, fennel or a little ginger can make the stomach comfortable after a sumptuous meal. These agents form the traditional ingredients of many stomachache powders and gripe waters sold in the market. Genuine intestinal or biliary colic, however, needs administration of an anticholinergic drug like atropine or its substitutes.

Opioid and non-opioid analgesics (NSAIDs) are the most commonly employed agents for symptomatic relief of pain. It is important to administer analgesics at the very onset of pain. The longer the pain is allowed to continue untreated, the less effective the analgesics become. This is seen especially in such conditions as migraine. *Severe pain of sudden onset* particularly visceral pain (e.g. MI) can produce shock. In such cases, opioids are indispensable and should not be withheld simply for fear of initiating drug dependence, e.g., in acute MI, fractures and pneumothorax. The opioids, in addition, also induce a state of tranquillity, thus creating an indifference towards residual discomfort. When used with skill and discrimination, the adverse effects are not much bothersome.

In order to give the maximum benefit to the patient, opioid drugs should be administered in full doses, if necessary IV. It should be noted that patients with severe pain are remarkably tolerant to full therapeutic doses of morphine. If morphine is to be administered IV, it should be injected slowly, the dose being 2.5-5 mg. injected over 5 minutes. Pethidine has a shorter duration of action than morphine; this can lead to unsuspected undertreatment. Conditions in which morphine or pethidine is recommended and the frequency of doses suggested make the possibility of drug addiction very remote. However, patients with acute pain treated with opioids for more than 5-7 days are likely to develop tolerance to the analgesic effects, so that if they need relief from pain after additional surgery, the usual doses may not give relief.

In the treatment of severe pain, morphine is not only more **potent** but more **efficacious** *than* aspirin. Further, as the onset of pain relief by NSAIDs is much slower than that by the opioids, the latter may be combined with NSAIDs with advantage.

Starting equianalgesic doses of opioids are given in Table 11.6; the optimum dose for each patient is determined by titration. Table 11.7 lists equipotent oral doses of aspirin and opioids for relief of moderate pain.

Table 11.6: Equianalgesic doses of opioids

Drug	IM Dose mg	Oral Dose mg
Morphine	10	60
Pethidine	75	300
Methadone	10	60
Codeine	-	120
Pentazocine	60	180
Buprenorphine	0.4	0.8*

* Sublingual, not oral

Table 11.7: Equipotent oral doses for relief of moderate pain

Aspirin	600 mg
Codeine	30-60 mg
Pethidine	50 mg
Pentazocine	30 mg
Dextropropoxyphene	65 mg

For the symptomatic relief of dull aching and chronic type of pain, non-opioid, non-addicting analgesics like NSAID are preferred, and aspirin deserves the widespread popularity it enjoys for this purpose. The frequency of adverse effects due to this drug appears to be relatively low when one considers the annual world consumption of aspirin which now runs into several thousands of tons. Clinical studies show no substantial difference in the therapeutic benefits of various NSAID, although the individual preference may vary. Further the duration of action (as in early morning stiffness of rheumatoid arthritis) and the availability in injectable form may determine the choice of NSAID. Table 11.8 gives the plasma half lives of NSAID. In most instances, the selection of NSAID for an individual patient remains more of an art than science.

Because of variation in the response of individuals to different NSAIDs, several NSAID may be tried before one finds the drug which suits a patient most. If used *as an analgesic*, the NSAID should be changed if no response is obtained within a week. If used *as an anti-*

Table 11.8: Plasma half-lives of NSAID

Less than 5 hours	: Aspirin, Diclofenac, Ketoprofen, Flurbiprofen, Indomethacin, Tolmetin, Flufenamic acid.
10-30 hours	: Diflunisal, Fenoprofen, Naproxen, Sulindac, Nabumetone.
More than 50 hours	: Phenylbutazone, Piroxicam, Tenoxicam.

inflammatory agent, the NSAID should be changed if no response is obtained within 3 weeks. Aspirin is effective in many kinds of pain, not merely those related to the musculo-skeletal disorders. It is also anti-inflammatory and anti-pyretic. It can be used over prolonged periods without fear of addiction. Aspirin and other NSAID are also useful in *pain associated with injury to soft tissues* e.g., sprains and postoperative pain. Indomethacin and related compounds are also more toxic and hence their routine use is not justified. The combination of aspirin with codeine is synergistic as these drugs alleviate pain by different mechanisms.

In chronic pain, the abnormal activity of the pain-mediating afferent system continues irrespective of the original cause. Simple blocking of the neural pathways, therefore, may not be helpful. Several mediators of chronic pain have now been demonstrated (cytokines, bradykinin, substance P etc) and countering their effects may be useful.

The cause of **headache** is many times obscure in practice. Migraine can be treated with sumatriptan (Chapter 23). Many headaches are, however, caused by anxiety, tension, fatigue or depression; and use of proper psycho-therapeutic drugs like benzodiazepines or antidepressants can give dramatic results. Realisation of this psychic aspect of pain will prevent other unnecessary therapy including extensive and irrelevant sinus operations. In such cases some minor adjustments in patient's life can be more therapeutic than even drugs. Headaches due to common cold, influenza or other fevers respond to administration of paracetamol or aspirin. Headaches due to sinusitis and eyestrain need specific treatment.

Backache presents similar diagnostic problems as headache. It can be due to many causes. *The commonest causes are faulty posture and lack of exercise.* Mental depression and nervous tension can often produce backache. Failure to recognise this in women may lead to unnecessary correction of normal retroverted uterus or even its removal for no sensible reason. Mild backache of spinal osteoporosis may be relieved by oral calcium, physiotherapy and vitamin D. However, severe pain of ankylosing spondylitis needs treatment with indomethacin; that of an acute vertebral fracture in osteoporosis needs a short period of bed rest followed by physiotherapy, in addition to an NSAID. Severe unremitting pain due to spinal osteoporosis may respond to calcitonin (Chapter 68).

In inflammatory conditions such as RA and gout, *the NSAIDs* can relieve pain without affecting the basic disorder. Other drugs used in RA may induce remission (Chapter 71).

In *single doses*, NSAID have analgesic activity comparable to that of paracetamol. They may, therefore, be used on demand to treat mild or intermittent pain or to supplement regular treatment. In regular *full doses,* they also have an anti-inflammatory effect and are effective in treating continuous or regular pain associated with inflammatory arthritides such as RA and ankylosing spondylitis. They are also useful in the pain of advanced osteoarthritis when paracetamol fails to work; even in such cases much smaller doses are needed to control pain than those required in RA. Drugs such as colchicine are relatively specific in that they act in a single, inflammatory, painful condition viz. acute gouty arthritis (Chapter 71).

Chronic cancer pain: Pain is a common problem in cancer patients and 70% of patients with advanced cancer have it as a major symptom. It can be caused by the cancer itself or by other associated conditions such as osteoarthritis, bedsores or surgery. It may be related to bones, nerve compression, metastases in soft tissues; further, psychological reactions to the illness including depression and a sense of helplessness may worsen the pain. Unremitting pain itself can cause secondary symptoms such as anorexia, disturbed sleep, irritability and impaired concentration. It is, therefore, necessary to assess the causes of pain, as well as its effects, at the very outset in a patient with cancer; further, periodic reassessment of both is necessary so as to be able to offer to the patient treatment appropriate to a given stage.

The therapy consists of drug treatment and alternative methods. An example of the latter is local radiation to a painful bony metastasis. The radiation may be given either by an external beam, or by a radioactive isotope such as 89Strontium. The latter, when injected as 89SrCl, gets incorporated into hydroxyapatite of the bone lattice, preferentially at the sites of active osteogenesis. Thus, it gets deposited near the osteoblastic metastases from the prostate and the breast. Irradiation of the nearby metastases with beta rays from ^{89}Sr alleviates the bone pain. Severe bone marrow toxicity is uncommon.

The drugs used in the treatment of cancer pain can be classified as :

- ***Analgesics***: Non-opioids (paracetamol and NSAID); weak opioids (codeine and dextropropoxyphene); and strong opioids (morphine, buprenorphine, pethidine and methadone); and
- ***Adjuvant analgesics:*** These are a diverse group of drugs that were originally developed for a primary indication other than pain Many of these medications are currently used as primary analgesics in specific circumstances e.g. carbamazepine in trigeminal neuralgia and topical lignocaine in post-herpetic neuralgia. They and others are also used when the standard primary analgesics (opioids and NSAID) have failed to provide adequate pain relief, are not tolerated, or are contraindicated. They are: (a) Antidepressants; (b) Anti-convulsants; (c) Alpha-2 adrenergic agonists-Clonidine, Tizanidine; (d) Glucocorticoids; (e) Local anaesthetics-Transdermal lignocaine, Mexiletine; (f) Topical agents-Capscaicin; (g) NMDA antagonists- Dextromethorphan, Methadone, Amantadine, Ketamine; (h) Cannabinoid-Delta-9-THC; (i) Biphosphanates and Calcitonin; (j) GABA agonists-Baclofen; (k) Neuroimmunomodulatory agents-Thalidomide and its newer analogues.

The analgesics are used in a step ladder fashion, commencing with NSAID, and changing to weak and finally strong opioids as the drugs from the earlier used group cease to be effective. Ibuprofen and other NSAID may be useful in relieving pain of bony metastases and that due to mechanical compression of tissues other than nerves. The opioids (weak/strong) are added sequentially as and when the need arises.

In severe cancer pain, morphine is used by the clock and one does not wait till the pain returns and the patient demands its relief. The oral route is the preferred one; a commonly used dose is 5-30 mg every 4 hours; but much larger doses may be needed. Nausea may be common at the beginning of treatment with morphine and is treated with a drug such as prochlorpromazine (5-10 mg 4-8 hourly), metoclopramide (10 mg 4-8 hourly) or haloperidol (1-2 mg daily). Constipation may be troublesome; physical dependance and tolerance may develop during treatment with morphine; but psychological dependence rarely, if ever, occurs in cancer patients receiving morphine and other strong opioids for chronic pain. Metastases to the liver are not a contraindication to the use of strong opioids; but care should be exercised in patients with concomitant hepatic dysfunction. *In cancer patients, the use of potent analgesics is dictated by the intensity of pain and not by the brevity of prognosis;* no cancer patient should be denied relief of pain. The starting doses of other strong opioids are : buprenorphine (0.2-0.4 mg sublingually); methadone (5-10 mg orally) and pethidine (50-100 mg orally), on a 4 hourly basis. *Being a mixed agonist-antagonist, buprenorphine can reverse the analgesia caused by other strong opioids, and therefore should not be combined with drugs such as morphine.* A self-adhesive skin patch which releases the opioid fentanyl transdermally can be used in patients with difficulty in swallowing. Its effects last for 72 hours.

Patient controlled analgesia: This is an approach where the patient himself injects a programmed dose of an opioid analgesic. This has been shown to causes better pain control. Careful monitoring is however needed to avoid overdosing leading to respiratory depression.

Ziconotide, a synthetic, non-opioid, neuronal calcium channel blocker, by intrathecal infusion, has been reported to help some patients with chronic, severe, refractory pain.

Pain is not simply a perception. It is a complex syndrome, one component of which is the sensation described by the subject as pain. The other component, the emotional and psychological one, contributes considerably to the "suffering", an affective reaction. In fact, the affective reaction can often be of overriding importance. In such cases, analgesics alone may not be adequate and adjuvant drugs as well as non-drug therapy may be more important. The *concurrent* use of a phenothiazine, an anxiolytic or an antidepressant (Chapter 13), may help to relieve the pain by modifying the affective component of the pain complex. Used in combination with analgesics, these drugs help to reduce the doses of the latter as well as relieve the suffering, and improve the quality of life in chronic pain.

Chronic neuropathic (deafferentiation) pain occurs in diabetic neuropathy as well as following herpes zoster. It is due to altered neuronal excitability resulting in abnormal spontaneous discharge. The shooting or stabbing pain occurring in these conditions responds to antiepilepics such as phenytoin, gabapentin, pregabalin (Chapter 9) and carbamazepine, and to duloxetine, a selective serotonin and norepinephrine re-uptake inhibitor (SNRI; Chapter 13). The deep, dull aching pain in these situations may respond to antidepressants like amitriptyline. Pain resistant to amitriptyline may respond to capsaicin derived from chillies (hot peppers). Capsaicin is applied to the concerned skin area as a 0.025 to 0.075% cream. It is believed to act by interfering with pain transmission in the peripheral neurons by depleting and inhibiting the reuptake of substance P in these neurons. Such local application may cause local burning sensation. Further, the chronic constant deep pain of diabetic neuropathy and post-herpetic neuralgia may be relatively resistant. Lignocaine ointment 5%, applied locally, may sometimes relieve pain due to herpetic neuralgia.

Miscellaneous pains: *Obstetric analgesia* is achieved by the use of nitrous oxide (Chapter 7) or pethidine (Chapter 10).

Relief of *postoperative pain* not only increases the patient's comfort but can also remove an impediment to adequate ventilation in major upper abdominal surgery. If an NSAID such as ketorolac or diclofenac does not give adequate relief, buprenorphine (0.2-0.4 mg sublingually every 6-8 hours) may be used.

The use of phenazopyridine to relieve *lower urinary tract pain* is discussed in Chapter 50.

Local treatment of pain: Counterirritants such as methyl salicylate applied as a liniment relieve dull-aching, localised musculo-skeletal pain. Further, counterirritants do not mask underlying internal disease.

Several NSAIDs are marketed as gels/creams/ ointments for topical use, to be applied to the skin over joints and muscles; they may be of some value. They can also be used to treat post-surgical dental pain. *However, they can induce photosensitivity reaction and should not be applied to broken or inflamed skin.*

Eye drops containing diclofenac 0.1%, flurbiprofen 0.03% and suprofen 1% are useful in patients undergoing cataract surgery. When started before surgery, they act synergistically with local mydriatics to prevent miosis. They do not elevate intraocular tension. *They may, however, delay wound healing and interfere with local clotting mechanisms.*

NSAID and renal damage: The relation between analgesic use and renal damage has now been confirmed. Phenacetin was the first drug proven to cause 'analgesic nephropathy'. But, all NSAID can cause acute or chronic renal damage following repeated use, sometimes as short as two weeks. Drugs with a long half life (naproxen and piroxicam) are more likely to cause renal damage than those with shorter half life (ibuprofen). Clinically, the renal injury can present itself in several forms :

- ***Acute renal failure.***
- ***Mild asymptomatic renal impairment.***
- ***Chronic renal impairment due to papillary necrosis or interstitial fibrosis;*** and
- ***Serious hyperkalemia.***

The first three are related to the action of NSAID to inhibit intra-renal PG synthesis by blocking COX-1. Locally produced PGE acts as intra-renal vasodilators to counteract the vasoconstricting effect of angiotensin II and noradrenaline (as in shock); they also influence the tubular transport of ions and water. *The renal perfusion is less dependent on the locally produced PGs in healthy, young persons than in old people and individuals with diseases such as diabetic nephropathy.*

Inhibition of synthesis of PGs within the kidney has several effects:

(a) The protective intrarenal vasodilator effect is lost.

(b) Renal blood flow and GFR are reduced (in people with pre-existing renal impairment).

(c) The natriuretic effect of PGE_2 on the renal medulla is lost with consequent sodium retention.

Hyperkalemia is due to diminished aldosterone synthesis secondary to inhibitio of renin synthesis by NSAID (hyporeninimic hypoaldosteronism). Hyperkalemia is particularly likely to occur in patients with diabetes mellitus, renal disease and in those on potassium sparing diuretics. *The sodium retention caused by NSAID may cause edema and congestive heart failure.*

Mechanisms of NSAID-induced renal damage include :

- ***Analgesic nephropathy***
- ***Allergic type of interstitial nephritis***; and
- ***Urate nephropathy*** (Chapter 38).

Renal toxic effects are often overlooked because the patients may forget to divulge that they are taking an NSAID and the toxic effects are slow in onset. The risk of developing renal damage due to NSAID is increased by the concurrent presence of : old age; hypertension; congestive heart failure; cirrhosis of liver; diabetic nephropathy; gout; renal or renovascular disease; and salt/volume depletion. Finally, NSAID enhance the effects of vasopressin on the kidneys and can diminish excretion of free water.

Studies indicate that ***aspirin, in less than full anti-inflammatory doses, is perhaps safer*** in that its chronic use is less associated with analgesic nephropathy.

The possibility of chronic ingestion of analgesics, especially OTC preparations, should always be borne in mind when dealing with unexplained chronic renal damage.

Central Nervous System Stimulants

12

The stimulants of the CNS are therapeutically not as useful as the CNS depressants as they lack selectivity of action. Further, excessive stimulation of CNS is followed by depression. Some of the CNS stimulants are mainly used as **analeptics.** Analepsis is a Greek word which can be loosely translated as 'picking up those who have been cast down'. Analeptics stimulate the CNS particularly the respiratory centre and, in large doses, they cause generalised convulsions. Thus, these drugs have a wide range of effects of which, stimulation of breathing is only one, and perhaps may not be the dominant one.

Classification : The CNS stimulants are :

I **Those acting directly on the CNS.**

- ***Predominantly cortical stimulants*** like Xanthine alkaloids, Amphetamine, Methylamphetamine, Methylphenidate and Pipradrol.
- ***Predominantly medullary stimulants,*** e.g. Picrotoxin, Pentylenetetrazol, Nikethamide, Amiphenazole, Camphor and Carbon dioxide.
- ***Predominantly spinal stimulants,*** e.g. Strychnine.

II **Those which stimulate the CNS reflexly,** e.g., Lobeline, Ammonia, Veratrum and Nicotine.

The above classification is arbitrary and a CNS stimulant, when administered in a sufficiently large dose, can stimulate the entire CNS.

Stimulants of the Cerebral Cortex

XANTHINE ALKALOIDS : The three naturally occurring xanthine alkaloids, **caffeine, theophylline** and **theobromine,** are purine bases which occur in several plants all over the world. These alkaloids leave behind a yellow residue when heated with nitric acid and hence, the term xanthine derived from the Greek word 'xanthos' meaning yellow. Coffee prepared by grinding the seeds of *Coffea arabica* contains caffeine; tea from leaves of *Thea sinensis* contains caffeine and small amounts of theobromine and theophylline; while cocoa obtained by grinding seeds of *Theobroma cacao* contains caffeine and theobromine. The cola flavoured soft drinks also contain caffeine.

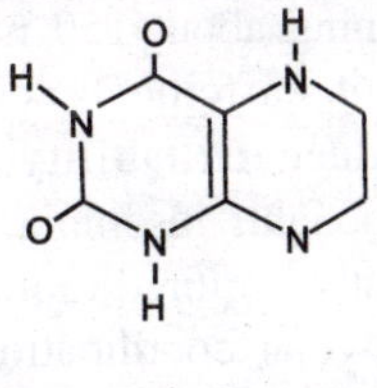

Fig. 12.1 : Xanthine

Mechanism of action: Methyl xanthines act in many ways:

- ***By inhibiting cyclic nucleotide phosphodiesterase*** (PDE), thus preventing the conversion of cyclic AMP to 5' AMP. Following administration of methyl xanthines, tissue concentration of cyclic AMP increases. The catecholamines which also increase the concentra-tion of cyclic AMP by a different mechanism act synergistically with methyl xanthines.

- ***By bringing about changes in distribution of calcium at the intracellular sites;*** and
- ***By blocking adenosine receptors.***

The relative contributions of these mechanisms in producing different pharmacological actions is not established.

Pharmacological actions:

Central nervous system: Of the three xanthine alkaloids, caffeine possesses the most significant action on CNS, followed by theophylline and theobromine. Threshold doses of caffeine mainly act on the cerebral cortex, whereas larger amounts stimulate the medullary centres and toxic doses result in convulsions.

- ***Cerebral cortex*:** Caffeine in small doses produces a more rapid and clearer flow of thoughts, increases mental alertness, and delays fatigue and drowsiness. It stimulates mental activity when it is below normal following fatigue or boredom; it does not raise it above normal. Caffeine also reduces reaction time, improves motor activity and augments conditioned responses. Thus, it improves physical performance. The cortical effects may be produced by ingestion of 1 or 2 cups of coffee, one cup containing about 150 mg. of caffeine. Larger doses of caffeine (exceeding 300 to 500 mg.) produce irritability, nervousness, confusion of thought, insomnia, headache and tremors. Recently acquired motor skills calling for delicate muscular coordination and accurate timing may be affected adversely as a result of nervousness and tremors. Toxic doses may cause focal and generalised convulsions.
- ***Medulla*:** Larger doses of caffeine stimulate the respiratory, vasomotor and vagal centres. Caffeine-induced respiratory stimulation is more marked in individuals breathing 3 to 5 per cent carbon dioxide than in normal individuals; this suggests that the drug probably increases the sensitivity of the respiratory centre to carbon dioxide. The stimulation of vasomotor and vagal centres tends to raise the blood pressure and induces bradycardia, respectively.
- ***Spinal Cord*:** Very large doses of caffeine produce an increase in reflex excitability of the spinal cord, and may lead to clonic convulsions and death in animals. In man, no fatalities after caffeine administration have been reported.

Cardiovascular system: Theophylline has the most prominent action on the CVS.

- ***Heart*:** Xanthines have a direct stimulant action on the myocardium and tend to increase the heart rate, the force of contraction and the myocardial oxygen consumption. The positive chronotropic action on the myocardium is antagonized by central vagal stimulation, particularly with caffeine, and therapeutic doses of caffeine may produce a variable effect on the heart rate. Large doses of caffeine, however usually produce palpitation, tachycardia and occasionally cardiac arrhythmias.

Increase in cardiac output with xanthines may occur even in the absence of tachycardia. The increased force of contraction assures a better emptying of the heart and reduces the central venous pressure. In healthy individuals, the lowering of the venous pressure may outlast the cardiac stimulant effect, resulting in a fall in the cardiac output following an initial rise, but in individuals with congestive heart failure, the lowered venous pressure produces an increase in the cardiac output.

- ***Blood vessels*:** Xanthines tend to produce peripheral vasodilatation by a direct action on vascular smooth muscle and cause a decrease in cardiac preload.

Coronaries : The coronary blood vessels are dilated and the coronary blood flow is increased.

Cerebral blood vessels : Xanthines produce a marked increase in the cerebral vascular resistance and reduce the cerebral blood flow and the CSF pressure. This constriction may be responsible for the relief of migraine headache.

Pulmonary blood vessels : Xanthines produce

relaxation of the pulmonary arterioles and reduce the pulmonary artery pressure.

Blood pressure : The direct cardiac stimulant action of xanthines tends to raise the BP. This action is aided by the stimulant action on the vasomotor centre and is antagonized by the central vagal stimulation and peripheral vasodilation. Changes in BP are, therefore, unpredictable. The combination of peripheral vasodilatation and increased cardiac output, however, raises the pulse pressure and the velocity of blood flow and tends to improve circulation. IV aminophylline (a theophylline derivative) may produce a fall in BP.

Kidneys: The xanthines produce an increase in urinary output. Theophylline is the most potent compound in this respect, followed by theobromine and caffeine (Chapter 38).

Smooth muscle: Xanthines also relax other smooth muscles, particularly the bronchial smooth muscle. Theophylline abolishes bronchospasm produced by histamine, pilocarpine and anaphylactic shock.

Voluntary muscles: Xanthines, particularly caffeine, strengthen the contraction, increase the metabolism and postpone fatigue of skeletal muscles by both central and peripheral actions. Improved contractility of the diaphragm contributes to the therapeutic efficacy of aminophylline in bronchial asthma.

Miscellaneous actions: The xanthines increase the gastric acid secretion. Decaffeinated coffee also has similar effect. The basal metabolic rate is slightly increased by caffeine, probably as a result of increased metabolism of the skeletal muscles. Theophylline also elevates plasma renin activity in man.

Absorption, fate and excretion: The xanthines are readily absorbed on oral, rectal or parenteral administration. After absorption, about 17 per cent of caffeine, 20 per cent of theophylline and 3 per cent of theobromine are bound to plasma proteins. They are metabolized in the liver, mainly by demethylation and oxidation by mixed function oxidase enzymes and xanthine oxidase. Caffeine metabolism varies widely among individuals; its t½ varies from 2 to 12 hours. None of the xanthines is converted into uric acid and hence, beverages containing xanthines are not contraindicated in gout.

Adverse reactions: In the usual doses, caffeine does not cause serious toxicity.

- ***CNS*:** Excessive, prolonged use of the drug may produce confusion, tremors, insomnia and excitement which may progress to mild delirium. The individual may complain of ringing in the ears, headache and may develop tachypnoea, tachycardia, emesis, fever and occasionally extra-systoles or cardiac arrhythmias. *Hence, inquiry into anxiety symptoms, especially in a subject with recurrent headache, should include questions about excessive tea or coffee drinking.* The symptoms can be treated with sedatives.

- ***GI tract*:** The xanthine alkaloids and beverages should be administered with caution in patients with peptic ulcer. Theophylline, in such patients, may produce hyperacidity, nausea, vomiting, epigastric pain and occasionally haematemesis, even when it is given parenterally. GI irritation can be reduced by the administration of theophylline with food.

- ***Miscellaneous*:** Aminophylline, on parenteral administration, may produce dizziness, hypotension, severe precordial pain, and even ventricular fibrillation. Fatalities have been reported following IV use. In children, aminophylline intoxication is characterized by vomiting, severe thirst, dehydration, delirium, convulsions and shock.

- ***Tolerance*:** Tolerance develops after prolonged use of xanthines, mainly to their cortical stimulant, diuretic and peripheral vasodilator effects. It is usually abolished after abstinence from xanthine beverages.

- ***Habituation*:** Habituation to xanthine beverages such as tea, coffee and cola is extremely common. However, it does not seem to be harmful.

Tea, coffee and cola drinks are better avoided in small children as they are thought *to be less tolerant of the stimulant effects of caffeine.*

Preparations and dosage:

(i) Caffeine citrate Dose : 120 to 600 mg. orally.

(ii) Caffeine and sodium benzoate ampoules containing 250 mg. per ml. Dose : 250 to 500 mg.

(iii) Aminophylline : Chapter 26.

(iv) Deriphylline (Chapter 26).

Therapeutic uses of xanthines :

- ***As a CNS stimulant*** : Caffeine in the form of coffee or tea is often employed for relief from fatigue. Theophylline and caffeine are used to treat neonatal apnoea.
- ***Migraine***: Because of its action on the cerebral blood vessels, caffeine is used along with ergotamine tartrate for relief of migraine (Chapter 23).
- ***Acute left ventricular failure***: Aminophylline is an adjuvant in the treatment of paroxysmal nocturnal dyspnoea due to LVF. Aminophylline increases the cardiac output, reduces the pulmonary artery pressure and the cardiac preload, induces bronchodilatation, stimulates the respiratory centre and causes diuresis. When the distinction between dyspnoea due to acute LVF (cardiac asthma) and bronchial asthma is not clear, it is safer to administer IV aminophylline rather than adrenaline (which is dangerous in the former condition) or morphine (which is dangerous in the latter condition). It is administered *slowly* IV in the dose of 500 mg. along with other treatment such as morphine, oxygen and phlebotomy. Its use has now declined because of the availability of more specific preload reducing drugs (Chapter 30).
- ***In bronchial asthma*** (Chapter 26).
- ***As a diuretic*** (Chapter 38).
- ***Strong coffee is used in orthostatic hypotension of autonomic failure*** (Chapter 43).

AMPHETAMINE: Amphetamine and Methylamphetamine are sympathomimetic amines. Their central actions are similar to xanthines but peripherally they produce adrenaline-like actions (Chapter 17).

PIPRADROL AND METHYLPHENIDATE are mild psychomotor stimulants and are discussed in Chapter 13.

Stimulants of the Brain Stem and Medullary Centres

Most drugs belonging to this group (**picrotoxin, pentylenetetrazole, nikethamide** and **camphor**) are no longer used as respiratory stimulants *(analeptics)* because of their toxicity and unproven efficacy. In large doses these drugs produce clonic convulsions followed by tonic convulsions.

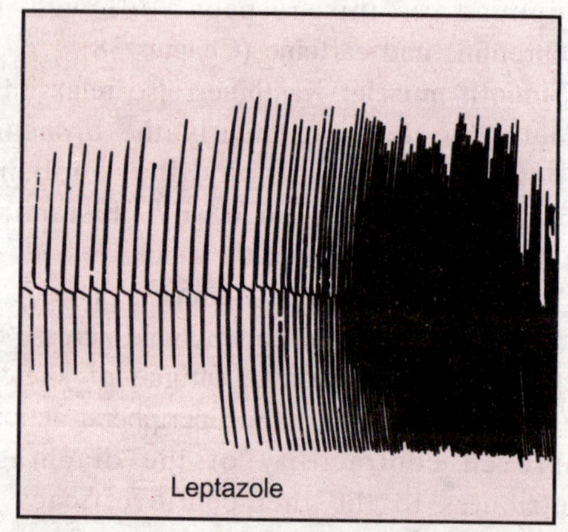

Fig 12.2 : Effect of pentylenetetrazole on respiration in dog under barbiturate anaesthesia.

DOXAPRAM (Dopram): This is a non-specific analeptic used mainly as a respiratory stimulant in the post-anaesthetic period and in patients with hypoventilation. It has a reasonable margin of safety. It is administered by IV drip in the total dose of 0.5-1.5 mg. per kg. at the rate of 5 mg. per minute. It may be repeated after 1 hour. A single IV injection (0.7 mg. per kg.) produces peak action in 1 minute lasting for 5-10 minutes. Doxapram is used to treat opioid induced postoperative respiratory depression. Doxapram has also been usedp as a temporary measure to correct acute respiratory insufficiency in patients with COPD (Chapter 26). Serious adverse reactions include hypertension, tachycardia, arrhythmias, muscle twitchings, tremors, convulsions and vomiting.

MEDROXYPROGESTERONE ACETATE: Like progesterone, medroxyprogesterone acetate has respiratory stimulant action. It is effective by mouth. It has been used with some success in patients with chronic ventilatory failure due to pathological obesity (*Pickwickian syndrome*).

CARBON DIOXIDE : Chapter 73.

Therapeutic uses of analeptics: Analeptics are of limited use in practice. The uses are :

- ***Postoperative respiratory depression*:** Naloxone (Chapter 10) can be used if the depression is caused by opioid analgesics. Unless the dose is carefully titrated, it can reverse analgesia as well. Doxapram does not reverse opioid induced analgesia.
- ***Ventilatory failure in patients with chronic obstructive pulmonary disease (COPD)*** (Chapter 26) : When such a patient develops hypercapnic respiratory failure and becomes drowsy or comatose and in patients in whom mechanical ventilatory support is contraindicated, doxapram may be useful to tide over the crisis; it is used by IV infusion or by slow IV injection.
- ***Primary apnoea of the newborn*** **:** Caffeine and theophylline are effective in the treatment of this condition.
- ***Pickwickian syndrome*:** See above.

Stimulants of the Spinal Cord

STRYCHNINE: Strychnine is an alkaloid obtained from the button-shaped seeds of the plant *Strychnos nux vomica*. Given, orally or parenterally in animals, it produces convulsions characterised by tonic extension of the body and opisthotonus. Death may occur as a result of asphyxia after seizures. Strychnine acts mainly on the spinal cord but it stimulates the entire neuraxis in large doses. It is believed to act as a competitive antagonist of the inhibitory transmitter glycine at the post-synaptic inhibitory sites. Excessive stimulation is followed by depression and death. Strychnine has no place in therapeutics.

The most urgent need in the treatment of strychnine poisoning is the control of convulsions with IV diazepam (10 mg. in adults, repeated as necessary). All forms of sensory stimulation must be avoided. Tracheal intubation and assisted ventilation are indicated if adequate ventilation is not restored. Only after controlling the convulsions should a gastric lavage be performed. The universal antidote if administered without delay, would adsorb the alkaloid and prevent its systemic absorption. Alternatively, oxidizing solutions like 1 : 1000 potassium permanganate or 2 per cent tannic acid (as strong tea) may be employed.

Reflex Stimulants of the Central Nervous System

Lobeline : Lobeline is an alkaloid obtained from the leaves of *Lobelia inflata*. Lobeline stimulates the CNS through the chemoreceptors of the carotid sinus. In addition to reflex stimulation of the CNS, lobeline stimulates autonomic ganglia, and the axon reflex which induces sweating. It is now rarely used as a respiratory stimulant.

Other reflex stimulants of the central nervous system such as nicotine, veratrum and apomorphine are discussed elsewhere. **Liquor ammonia** and smelling salts (ammonium carbonate) inhalation in syncope is a common household procedure which stimulates the respiratory and vasomotor centres reflexly.

Psychopharmacology 13

The term 'tranquillization' or 'ataraxia' has been defined in various ways and does not have any pharmacological basis; it is considered more or less synonymous with 'peace of mind'. Obviously, such a state can be produced by many drugs, depending upon the cause of disturbed 'peace of mind'. The term 'tranquillizer' was used originally to describe the calming effect of reserpine and chlorpromazine which have the ability to *calm without causing hypnosis*. Regardless of terminologies, *the objective of drug therapy in psychiatry is to induce an improved mental state in mentally disturbed patients. Drugs which selectively modify the behaviour pattern are known as* ***psychotropic*** *or* ***psychoactive*** *drugs.*

It is extremely difficult to define what constitutes **psyche** or **mind** which is supposed to carry out three functions :

- ***Cognition,*** the reception of environmental stimuli.
- ***Affect,*** analysing the information received and formation of a reaction pattern; and
- ***Conation,*** the actual behavioural response.

Little is known about the neurophysiological differences between normal individuals and mentally ill patients, nor is the definite biochemical basis for various psychiatric disorders known. The mind cannot be separated from the physical body. Many physical illnesses cause associated psychic problems, whereas mental illnesses can produce somatic symptoms.

The etiology of psychic illnesses ix complex, including both psychological and physiological/ biochemical factors. In some of them, psychological problems predominate, whereas in others, disturbances of endogenous neurochemicals clearly exist. When treating a mental patient, one has to assess which factor, psychological or physiological, predominates. Pure psychological problems are not likely to be helped by drugs alone, whereas drugs are most effective in treating biologically (neurochemically) based mental illnesses. However, in all patients both psychotherapy and drugs are necessary for the best results.

Evaluation of psychotropic drugs in animals : Models of psychic disturbances analogous to those seen in humans cannot be produced in animals. Further, the intellectual superiority of man over the highest primate is so great that it is difficult to predict usefulness of drugs in the treatment of human mental illnesses from the behavioural studies in animals. It is not surprising, therefore, that therapeutic application of many compounds in humans originated from accidental observations in patients getting such drugs for other purposes. Pre-clinical screening, however, gives useful information. Some of the experimental methods employed are:

- ***Natural behavioural patterns*** : Quietening property of a drug can be demonstrated by its taming effect on an aggressive monkey or on a cat in the presence of a mouse. Similarly, the modification of natural activities of various animals by drugs is helpful in evaluating their general stimulant or depressant properties.

- ***Spontaneous motor activity*:** This is usually studied in rats and mice. The animal is kept in a cage through which a beam of light passes. An electronic device records the number of times the beam is interrupted by movements of the animal. Spontaneous activity is also measured by using a jiggle cage. It is a cage suspended on springs and hence produces oscillatory movements every time the animal moves; these can be recorded.

- ***Motor co-ordination and muscle tone*:** Preliminary screening for behavioural pattern will usually reveal drug-induced ataxia. This can be quantified by rota rod test, using a horizontally mounted rod with a diameter of 2-3 cm. Normal mice maintain their position on the rod for at least five minutes while ataxic mice fall off earlier.

- ***Drug induced behavioural patterns* :** Administration of reserpine to animals induces a condition resembling retarded depression in man, where there is general reduction in activity, slowing of movements, reduced responsiveness to stimulus and neglect of activities such as feeding and sexual behaviour. Such 'model illness' has been used for testing the antidepressant properties of drugs.

Toxicity of amphetamine is considerably higher when tested on mice kept together in the same cage than on animals kept individually in separate cages. Certain drugs like phenothiazines reduce this **group toxicity**.

- ***Learning and discrimination behaviour*:** The maze has provided the psychological setting for most of these studies. Thus, drug effect on maze learning or on perfected maze habit in animals, using the time required for performance as a criterion, can give some idea about the influence of a drug on learning and discrimination behaviour.

- ***Emotional behaviour and conditioned neurosis*:** Experimental neurosis is known since the work of Pavlov. The drug effect has been studied on a variety of induced 'neurotic' reactions (phobias, compulsions etc.) in animals.

Drugs expected to inhibit selectively certain abnormal reactions or behaviour patterns such as fear and/or anxiety, without impairing the innate behaviour, are studied in 'conditioned animals'. In *conditioned avoidance* the animal first learns a response like running, pressing a bar or climbing up a pole in order to escape from an electric shock. Then it learns to avoid the shock by responding promptly to a danger signal such as a buzzer sound which precedes the shock. Antipsychotics like chlorpromazine selectively block such conditioned responses but not the non-conditioned ones, where the animal still escapes once the shock is applied. Barbiturates, on the contrary, abolish both conditioned and non-conditioned avoidance responses.

- Effects of drugs on behaviour are also studied by implanting or injecting them directly into various parts of the brain. Similarly, they can also be studied in surgically induced abnormal behaviour patterns in animals.

Clinically, the term **psychotic disorders** refers to the major mental illnesses like schizophrenia and manic depression in which (a) insight is said to be lost; and (b) the patient's experience eg. hallucinations, is outside the normal range of human experience. This is perhaps the most severe psychiatric disorder. In contrast, the term **neurotic disorders** implies the rest of recognised psychiatric conditions in which (1) insight is preserved; and (2) the patient's experience, although unpleasant and extreme, is within, the range of normal human experience. A major **affective disorder of mind** is the syndrome of mental depression.

The psychotropic drugs that reduce apomorphine-induced stereotype and amphetamine-induced hyperactivity, and inhibit conditioned avoidance responses, are likely to be useful as **antipsychotic drugs.** The animal pharmacologic test that correlates best with antipsychotic activity is the prevention of apomorphine (a dopamine agonist) induced vomiting in dogs. These effects are mediated by the mesolimbic dopamine receptors. The drugs which reduce aggressiveness but increase the exploratory activity in a maze without causing ataxia are likely to be useful as **antianxiety drugs (anxiolytics).** Drugs with possible application as **antidepressants** usually potentiate the actions of amphetamine and increase the spontaneous motor activity, but antagonize reserpine and apomorphine-induced hypothermia.

For the evaluation of psychotropic drugs in man a large number of rating scales have been designed to obtain an overall assessment of the mental state and to quantitate the drug-induced modification of parameters such as anxiety, depression and the adverse effects. Rating scales can be used to assess both objective and subjective features of the condition.

Classification: Psychoactive drugs can be classified as :

I **Antipsychotics** — used mainly in major psychoses like schizophrenia and MDP.

- ***Phenothiazines,*** e.g., Chlorpromazine, Trifluoperazine.
- ***Rauwolfia alkaloids,*** e.g., Reserpine.
- ***Butyrophenones,*** e.g., Haloperidol, Trifluperidol.
- ***Diphenylbutylpiperidines,*** e.g., Pimozide, Penfluridol and Fluspirilene.
- ***Thioxanthenes,*** e.g., Chlorprothixene and Flupentixol.
- ***Indolic derivatives,*** e.g., Molindone, Oxypertine.
- ***Dibenzodiazepines,*** e.g., Clozapine.
- ***Substituted benzamides,*** e.g., Sulpiride.
- ***Miscellaneous,*** e.g., Risperidone.

These drugs are called **neuroleptics** and also 'Major tranquillizers' because they reduce the agitation and disturbed behaviour often associated with delusions and hallucinations in schizophrenia.

II **Anti-anxiety agents (anxiolytics)** — mainly useful in anxiety states and neurosis, e.g., Benzodiazepines and Buspirone.

These drugs are also called as 'Minor tranquillizers' because they have a calming effect in anxiety states associated with neurotic personality, situational crisis or physical disease.

III **Anti-depressants** also called **mood elevators** or **psychic energizers,** such as

- ***Monoamine oxidase (MAO) inhibitors.***
- ***Tricyclic antidepressant compounds,*** e.g., Imipramine and Amitriptyline.
- ***Tetracyclic compound*** eg Maprotiline
- ***Heterocyclic compounds*** e.g. Trazodone
- ***Selective serotonin (5-HT) re-uptake inhibitors (SSRI),*** e.g., Fluoxetine.

IV **Mood stabilizers,** e.g., Lithium carbonate.

V **Psychomotor stimulants :** Methyl phenidate, Dextroamphetamine and Pemoline.

VI **Psychotogenic drugs** which induce behavioural abnormalities resembling psychosis, e.g., LSD, Cannabis and hallucinogens.

The main mechanisms of action of the psychoactive drugs are listed in Table 13.1.

Table 13.1: Mechanisms of action of psychoactive drugs

Drug class	Predominant mechanism of action
I Antipsychotics	DA receptor antagonist
II Antianxiety	GABA-A receptor agonist
III Antidepressants	(a) Inhibition of reuptake of NA or 5-HT or both (b) Inhibition of brain MAO

Antipsychotic Drugs

Introduction of antipsychotics revolutionized the treatment of schizophrenia, the most common of the serious mental illnesses.

Fig. 13.1 Phenothiazine nucleus

Phenothiazine Compounds: The first important phenothiazine compound **chlorpromazine** was synthesized in 1950 as an antihistaminic and was shown to possess an amazingly large number of actions. Phenothiazine has a three ring structure in which two benzene rings are linked by sulphur and nitrogen atoms (Fig. 13.1). According to the chemical structure, phenothiazines could be predominantly antipsychotic, anticholinergic or antihistaminic.

Mechanism of action of antipsychotics: Antipsychotic drugs produce beneficial effects probably by affecting three of the major integrating systems in the brain. viz

(i) Mesolimbic system.
(ii) Mesocortical system; and
(iii) The hypothalamus.

The drugs :

- ***Cause blockade mainly of postsynaptic dopaminergic (D2) receptors and to a smaller extent 5-HT receptors.***
- ***Modify the function of the mesolimbic system;*** and
- ***Reduce the incoming sensory stimuli by acting on the brainstem reticular formation.***

Their therapeutic efficacy is mostly related to their ability to bind and to block the dopaminergic (D_2) receptors in the mesolimbic system. At least 5 subtypes of dopamine receptors (D_1-D_5) have been described. (Chapter 17). They are distributed in the limbic region, the frontal cortex, the basal ganglia, the midbrain and the medulla. Although several of these subtypes need to be blocked simultaneously for the maximum benefit, the predominant action appears to be at the D_2. Blockade of dopamine action in the corpus striatum is responsible for the extrapyramidal reactions (EPR) often associated with these drugs.

In addition to the dopaminergic (D_2) receptor blockade, some (atypical) antipsychotics like risperidone and clozapine also block 5-HT receptors in the frontal cortex and the striatal system, which helps to lessen EPR and is related to their usefulness in improving negative symptoms. Atypical antipsychotic clozapine has wide receptor affinity and also blocks alpha 2 adrenergic receptors. Thus, the action profile of these drugs and their adverse reactions can be explained to some extent on the basis of their receptor affinity.

High dose (i.e. less potent) neuroleptics such as chlorpromazine tend to cause sedation and autonomic nervous system (ANS) adverse effects but have a lower propensity to cause EPR. **Low dose (i.e. potent) neuroleptics** such as haloperidol, fluphenazine and trifluoperazine with more specific action cause EPR more often. This is because the low dose neuroleptics are more selective in binding to the D_2 receptors.

Since chlorpromazine is the most extensively studied antipsychotic phenothiazine it is discussed as a prototype in detail. Other antipsychotic phenothiazine drugs differ from chlorpromazine mainly in potency and to a certain extent in their profile of actions. Hence, the important differences between these compounds and chlorpromazine are pointed out.

CHLORPROMAZINE (Largactil):

Introduction of chlorpromazine into psychiatric practice by Delay and Deniker in 1952 marked the beginning of modern psychopharmacology.

Pharmacological actions :

Behavioural and CNS actions : When chlorpromazine is administered to a normal monkey, the animal

- ***Loses its aggressiveness and its interest in the surroundings (quietening effect).***
- ***Shows indifference to happenings around.***
- ***Develops complete lack of initiative.***
- ***Does not attack spontaneously;*** instead, it sits motionless. There is no change in the state of wakefulness and consciousness even with high doses. Control over the muscles and withdrawal from noxious stimuli remain unaffected.

Chlorpromazine effectively blocks the conditioned avoidance responses, so that the animal forgets what it has learnt but, unlike after barbiturates, still escapes to safety as soon as a shock is felt.

In patients with major psychosis with agitation, chlorpromazine produces psychomotor slowing, emotional quietening, diminution of initiative and anxiety, without affecting wakefulness (*Neuroleptic Syndrome*). The subject sits in silence and show indifference to the events around him, responding minimally to external stimuli. Although tolerance develops rapidly to its sedative action, the antipsychotic effect resulting in amelioration of symptoms continues. Furthermore, unlike with barbiturates, there is minimal ataxia and incoordination.

Central nervous system : It causes

- ***Diminution of spontaneous motor activity.*** It produces a state of catalepsy where the body and limbs are moulded into various postures and remain immobile for prolonged periods. Catalepsy resembles but is not the same as catatonia seen in some schizophrenics; the latter is relieved by phenothiazines.
- ***Induction of sleep*** with characteristic slow wave pattern on the EEG, and normalization of sleep in schizophrenics.
- ***Improvement of cognitive and intellectual functions*** but impairment of vigilence and motor response required for a variety of tests.
- ***Antiemetic action***: Chlorpromazine depresses the chemoreceptor trigger zone (CTZ) and thus acts as a potent antiemetic. It counters the effects of apomorphine (a dopamine agonist) on the CTZ in the medulla. It, however, is not effective in vomiting due to vestibular stimulation or that caused by local GI irritation.
- ***Potentiation of the action of analgesic drugs.***
- ***Prolongation of pentobarbitone sleep in animals***.
- Phenothiazines with an aliphatic side chain (Group I, Table 13.3) increase strychnine toxicity in animals and can precipitate seizures in epileptic patients.

Autonomic nervous system: The drug acts as an autonomic suppressant. Because of its alpha adrenergic blocking action, it blocks certain actions of adrenaline and noradrenaline. It also produces moderate inhibition of actions of acetylcholine and 5-hydroxytryptamine. It has a central depressant action on the hypothalamic centre controlling sympathetic activity.

Cardiovascular system: Chlorpromazine may produce orthostatic hypotension due to inhibition of centrally mediated pressor reflexes along with peripheral adrenergic blocking action. It also dilates the blood vessels directly.

It is a myocardial depressant and may cause defects in intra-ventricular conduction. Thus, it can cause prolongation of QT interval and blunting of T waves in the ECG.

Hypothalamic-endocrine system : Chlorpromazine suppresses oestrus cycle in animals. It blocks ovulation and produces amenorrhoea and galactorrhoea due to elevation of serum prolactin levels in women. It diminishes the libido in men. These actions are due to blockade of dopamine receptors in the hypothalamus and the pituitary. It also blocks the release of growth hormone.

Miscellaneous effects: It has a potent local anaesthetic action. It prevents the shivering response to cold and thus favours the development of hypothermia.

Tolerance: In practice, patient develops tolerance to the sedative effect of phenothiazines. However, tolerance to the antipsychotic effect has not been observed.

After sudden cessation of treatment with phenothiazines, withdrawal nausea and vomiting may develop in as many as 30 per cent of individuals. Muscular discomfort, exacerbation of the psychotic state and insomnia may occur. Although some degree of dependence on phenothiazines has thus been accepted, real drug dependence has not been demonstrated. The characteristic craving is absent and the withdrawal symptoms are essentially mild.

Absorption, fate and excretion: Phenothiazines are well absorbed orally and parenterally. An active enterohepatic circulation increases the duration of action and prolongs the biological half life of chlorpromazine. Thus, chlorpromazine or its metabolites can be detected in urine even 6 to 12 months after discontinuation of therapy.

After absorption, phenothiazines are distributed in all the body tissues. Brain concentrations are lower than those in other organs, but are much higher than the plasma concentrations.

Phenothiazines are metabolized in the liver by hydroxylation and subsequent glucuronide conjugation, sulfoxidation and demethylation.

Adverse reactions: On the basis of their adverse reactions, the phenothiazines can be divided into three major groups (Table 13.2).

Table 13.2: Phenothiazines grouped according to adverse effects

	Sedation	Antimus-carinic	Extra-pyramidal
Group 1	+++	++	++
Group 2	++	+++	+
Group 3	+	+	+++

Group 1: Chlorpromazine and Triflupromazine.

Group 2: Pericyazine and Thioridazine.

Group 3: Fluphenazine, Perphenazine, Prochlorperazine and Trifluoperazine.

Neuroleptics from other chemical groups tend to resemble Group 3. They include the butyrophenones (droperidol, haloperidol and trifluperidol); diphenylbutylpiperidines (fluspirilene and pimozide); thioxanthenes (flupentixol), oxypertine; and loxapine.

Apart from common effects such as nasal stuffiness, dryness of mouth and palpitation, the adverse reactions include:

- ***Intolerance***: Skin eruptions of various types, photosensitivity and contact dermatitis are common. Rarely, yellowish brown or purple discoloration of the exposed skin may develop on prolonged therapy. The colour is due to melanin or a melanin-like substance formed by the phototoxic action of sunlight acting on the phenothiazine in the skin. The pigment also occurs in the organs like brain, liver, kidneys, retina and the cornea. Visual impairment due to pigmentary retinopathy may occur.
- ***Extrapyramidal (EP) effects***: Many patients receiving phenothiazines show EP symptoms of parkinsonism, viz, tremor, muscular rigidity, excessive salivation and akinesia. These are due to blocking of dopamine receptors in the basal ganglia and can be countered by anticholinergic drugs such as benzhexol but not by levodopa or amantidine (Chapter 14). Motor restlessness, akathisia (inability to sit still), acute dystonic reactions and dyskinesias can also occur. Tardive dyskinesia is a late-appearing neurological syndrome in patients on long term therapy.
- ***Behavioural reactions:*** These include drowsiness, impaired psychomotor function, restlessness, excitement, psychotic reactions and toxic confusional states. Fortunately, most of the patients tolerate these drugs well and such reactions are rarely serious. *However, depression, which often has an 'endogenous' character may develop after the patient has been on therapy for many weeks* and the patient may commit suicide. Such depression should be watched for and should be treated.
- ***CNS:*** The phenothiazines and other neuroleptics may occasionally produce epileptic seizures (particularly in individuals with history of seizures), disturbances in temperature regulation and respiratory irregularities, when administered in large doses. The convulsant effect is most likely to be seen with chlorpromazine, triflupromazine and the thioxanthines. The effect however, is reversible.
- ***Autonomic nervous system***: The phenothiazines, by virtue of their anticholinergic activity, may produce blurring of vision, tachycardia, constipation or even paralytic ileus, difficulty in micturition and sometimes inhibition of ejaculation. Postural hypotension can occur. Marked hypotension is uncommon but hypotensive crises on parenteral administration have been observed particularly in the elderly. Concomitant use of alcohol predisposes to this

Table 13.3: Some commonly used phenothiazine derivatives

Compound	Chemical structure of the side chain	Pharmacological properties	Daily dose (mg) *	Therapeutic uses
Group I				
Chlorpromazine (Largactil)	Propyldimethylamino	Marked sedative and autonomic effects	500 to 1000	Refer to the text
Promazine (Sparine)	Propyldimethylamino	Marked autonomic, moderate E.P. and antiemetic effects		Antipsychotic; antiemetic
Triflupromazine (Siquil)	Propyldimethylamino	Marked E.P., high antiemetic and low autonomic effects	10 to 30	Antipsychotic Antiemetic
Group II				
Thioridazine (Melleril)	Piperidine	Moderate sedative and autonomic, less E.P. and antiemetic effects.	100 to 500	Withdrawn due to cardiotoxicity
Group III				
Fluphenazine (Anatensol)	Piperazine	Moderate sedative, marked E.P. and less autonomic effects.	2.5 to 10	Antipsychotic
Trifluoperazine (Eskazine)	-do-		5 to 10	
Perphenazine (Fentazin)	-do-	Less sedative, less autonomic and marked E.P. effects	12 to 24	Antipsychotic, antiemetic
Prochlorperazine (Stemetil)	-do-	Moderate sedative, marked E.P. and less autonomic effects	10 to 30	Antipsychotic, antiemetic
Thiethylperazine maleate (Torecan)	-do-		10 to 30	Antiemetic
Group IV				
Diethazine (Diparcol)	Ethyldiethylamino	See Chapter 19		Parkinsonism
Ethopropazine (Parsidol)	Ethyldiethylamino			
Group V				
Promethazine (Phenergan)	Ethyldiethylamino	See Chapter 20		Antihistaminic

* In divided dose E.P. = extrapyramidal

effect. *Chlorpromazine should not be given IV, as fatalities due to a sudden fall in BP have been reported.*

- ***CVS*** : Thioridazine and chlorpromazine can induce ECG alterations resembling those caused by quinidine and by hypokalemia. Caution should be exercised in the use of these agents in individuals with cardiac disease.

- ***Haemopoietic system and the liver***: These drugs may rarely produce agranulocytosis, thrombocytopenia and aplastic anemia.

Intrahepatic obstructive (cholestatic) jaundice occurs in about 0.5 to 2 per cent of the patients receiving chlorpromazine. It is probably allergic in origin. Usually, it appears within first 6 weeks of therapy. Almost all the patients recover completely and spontaneously.

Administration of phenothiazines during pregnancy has been associated with increased incidence of neonatal jaundice.

- ***Endocrinal and metabolic disturbances*** : Long term therapy may occasionally produce gynaecomastia and impotence, galactorrhea and menstrual irregularities. Aggravation of diabetes mellitus and weight gain as a result of increased food intake have been reported.

- ***Neuroleptic malignant syndrome***: This is a rare but potentially fatal reaction to the neuroleptic drugs. The manifestations include hyperthermia, fluctuating level of consciousness, muscular rigidity, and autonomic dysfunction with tachycardia, sweating, urinary incontinence and labile BP. The offending drug should be discontinued as there is no proven effective treatment, although bromocriptine and dantrolene have been used. The syndrome may last for 5-15 days after the drug is discontinued.

Preparations and dosage:

(i) Chlorpromazine hydrochloride (Largactil) tablets 10, 25, 50 and 100 mg.; syrup 25 mg./(for adults) and 5 mg. (pediatric)/ml, and suppositories. Dose 25 mg. to 1000 mg.

(ii) Chlorpromazine injection 25 mg. per ml. It is usually administered IM in the dose of 25 to 50 mg. The patient should be confined to bed for 30 minutes following IM injection in order to avoid postural hypotension.

(iii) Depot phenothiazines: Esters (such as decanoate, enanthate and palmitate) of fluphenazine, perphenazine, flupentixol and oxyprothepine when given IM or SC release the active drug slowly. Satisfactory therapeutic response in schizophrenia can be obtained by injecting fluphenazine decanoate in the dose of 12.5-50 mg. every 2 to 4 weeks.

The various phenothiazines divided according to the side chain attached to the nitrogen atom are listed in Table 13.3.

Drug interactions: See Table 13.4.

Table 13.4: Interactions of phenothiazines with other drugs

- Prolongation and intensification of the CNS depressant effect of barbiturates, morphine, pethidine and alcohol.
- Precipitation of bizarre and dangerous reactions if used simultaneously with MAO inhibitors.
- Precipitation of serious hypotension if used together with such drugs as reserpine, methyldopa, and phentolamine.
- Neutralization of the hypotensive action of guanethidine and clonidine.

Therapeutic uses:

- ***Schizophrenia***: This is discussed later.

- ***Manic depressive psychosis***: Chlorpromazine and haloperidol are both effective in the treatment of mania (see later).

- ***Senile psychosis***: The phenothiazines are sometimes useful in senile psychosis for controlling delusions and hallucinations. *Care should be taken to use small doses* as these drugs can cause postural hypotension and falls.

- ***Other neuropshchiatric disorders*** e.g., Huntington's disease, where haloperidol is preferred.

- ***Drug dependence***:They are *useful* in the management of psychosis associated with chronic alcoholism (alcoholic hallucinations) but are *contraindicated* in acute withdrawl syndromes (alcohol,opiates and other sedatives) for fear of precipitating seizures.

• ***Behavioural disorders in children***: Phenothiazines are sometimes used to control the excessively aggressive and destructive behaviour in children to produce a quietening effect. In such cases, other causes of aggressiveness such as temporal lobe epilepsy, schizophrenia, hypoglycemia and drug (amphetamine) abuse should be ruled out.

• ***Antiemetic and antihiccup***: Chlorpromazine in small, nonsedating doses, is useful to control vomiting due to uraemia, radiation sickness and certain drugs. It can also be employed to treat nausea and vomiting of pregnancy; but the other phenothiazines are usually preferred. It is not effective in motion sickness (Chapter 40).

Chlorpromazine is sometimes effective in the treatment of intractable hiccup. Its mechanism, however, is not known.

• ***Miscellaneous***: Certain phenothiazines are used for preanaesthetic medication (Chapter 7).

RESERPINE: The plant *Rauwolfia serpentina* (Benth) is a climbing shrub indigenous to India. It was so named in honour of Dr. Leonard Rauwolf, a 16th century botanist, who probably was never aware of its existence. In ancient Ayurvedic medicine, the plant (*sarpagandha*) has been claimed to be useful in cases of insomnia, insanity and even snake bite. It is called serpentina because of the resemblance of its root to a snake.

From amongst the various alkaloids of this plant (reserpine, serpentine and ajmaline), **reserpine** is used in therapeutics.

Mechanism of actions: *Reserpine is of great pharmacological interest because it depletes endogenous catecholamines and 5-HT from the brain and peripheral sites by interfering with amine storage.* Such depletion can last for days or weeks. A single dose of 5 mg./kg. body weight in animals is sufficient to cause 90 per cent reduction in brain NA and 5-HT over a period of 10 days. The depletion of cerebral monoamines is believed to be responsible for its central actions.

Pharmacological actions of reserpine:

• ***Central nervous system***: It has central antipsychotic action resembling that of phenothiazines; however, it has no antihistaminic, anticholinergic or direct antiadrenergic action. Like chlopromazine, it produces a calming effect as well as EPR in man, but without clouding the consciousness.

Reserpine is less effective than phenothiazines in the treatment of schizophrenia. It may also cause mental depression precipitating suicidal tendencies; hence, it is not used as an antipsychotic.

• ***Cardiovascular system*** : Reserpine lowers BP and is useful as an antihypertensive drug (Chapter 29).

HALOPERIDOL (Serenace): This butyrophenone is a very potent antipsychotic with similar clinical effects as piperazine phenothiazines. It is more effective in highly agitated or manic patients and has less prominent sedative and autonomic effects than chlorpromazine.

It is given orally in the dose of 1.5 to 7.5 mg. bid. It can also be given IM in the dose of 2-10 mg, repeated every hour up to a total of 30 mg, in highly agitated and violent patients. Depot injectable preparations of haloperidol are also available. The incidence of EPR with this drug is high. Irreversible toxic encephalopathy has been reported in patients on lithium, given high doses of haloperidol. The other drugs of this series are **trifluperidol** (Triperidol) and **droperidol** which are used in combination with fentanyl for neuroleptanalgesia (Chapter 7).

DIPHENYL BUTYL PIPERIDINES: **Pimozide** (Orap) 2-10 mg once daily may have the advantage in that the prescribed dosage can be administered under supervision. **Penfluridol,** structurally related to haloperidol, has a long duration of action. It is given orally in the dose of 20-100 mg once a week. Orally active, long-acting neuroleptics are useful in practice to eliminate failure of patient compliance.

Other antipsychotics such as chlorprothixene, clopenthixol, centbutandol, molindone and prothipendyl mainly differ from the phenothiazines in their pharmacokinetic properties and in their sedative, autonomic and extra-pyramidal effects. Unlike other neuroleptics which react with various dopamine receptors, **sulpiride** (Dolmatil) is a more specific antagonist at post-synaptic D_2 receptors.

Atypical Antipsychotics (Second Generation)

The classic antipsychotic (neuroleptic) drugs described above have a narrow therapeutic window as these agents cause EPS even in therapeutic doses. An 'atypical' antipsychotic is an effective neuroleptic drug which:

- ***Has lower propensity to cause EPR and tardive dyskinesia.***
- ***Helps to improve negative symptoms.***
- ***Is less likely (except resperidone) to cause hyperprolactinemia;*** and
- ***Have lower affinity for D2 receptors and greater affinity for other neuro-receptors such as 5-HT, NA and muscarinic, than the standard antipsychotic drugs.***

Examples of atypical antipsychotics are **clozapine, olanzapine, quetiapine** and **risperidone.** Their receptor actions are compared in Table 13.5.

Compared to other atypical antipsychotics, quetiapine is a weaker antiphychotic but has a marked sedating effect.

Compared with placebo, a higher death rate has been reported in elderly patients with dementia receiving atypical antipsychotics for the treatment of behavioral disorders.

Table 13.5 : Actions of typical and atypical antipsychotic drugs on various CNS receptors

Drug	Receptors blocked					
	D_1	D_2	$5HT_2$	α_2	H_1	M_1
Chlorpromazine	++	+++	+	+++	++	++
Haloperidol	+	+++	+	0	+	0
Clozapine	++	++	++	+++	+++	+++
Olanzapine	+	+	+++	0	++	+++
Quetiapine	+	++	+	+	+++	++
Risperidone	—	+++	+++	++	+	0

D = Dopamine, 5-HT = 5-Hydroxytryptamine
H = Histamine, M = Muscarinic

CLOZAPINE (Clozaril): This antipsychotic drug, related to tricyclic compounds such as imipramine, was synthesized in 1960. As it was found to cause agranulocytosis, its use was abandoned. It has now staged a comeback for a specific indication viz in the treatment of schizophrenia resistant to standard therapy. It has selective effects in the limbic, dopaminergic systems. Its other actions include antiadrenergic, anti5-HT and anticholinergic actions. It differs from phenothiazines in that it causes fewer EPRs and does not cause hyperprolactinemia.

Given orally, it produces antipsychotic effects similar to the standard neuroleptics. Its major advantage is that the drug improves not only the positive symptoms but also the negative symptoms such as emotional withdrawal, blunted affect, retardation and social withdrawal. It is started in the dose of 12.5 mg once daily and gradually increased to 200-450 mg/day in divided doses.

Adverse reactions: These include nausea, vomiting, sedation, orthostatic hypotension, severe tachycardia, confusion and delirium. Its main drawback is the relatively high incidence of grand mal seizures and agranulocytosis. *Because of its toxicity, the drug should be used only in patients resistant to standard therapy (see above) and that too under supervision;* regular blood counts need to be done.

OLANZAPINE: This dibenzodiazepine is similar to clozapine in chemical structure. It causes greater 5-HT_2 than D_2 receptor blockade. Further, it does not antagonize α_2 receptor function, hence, it causes less EPR and cardiovascular toxicity. Administered orally, it is absorbed well but about 40% is metabolized during first pass through the intestinal wall. In dose of 5-25 mg per day, once daily, the drug is as effective as haloperidol in reducing psychotic symptoms. Like clozapine, it acts against negative symptoms. It has not been reported to cause agranulocytosis nor decrease the seizure threshold. The incidence of hyperprolactinemia and sexual dysfunction is also lower than with risperidone. The drug may also be useful in children with developmental CNS disorders and in patients with Tourette syndrome.

Adverse reactions: These include dry mouth, sedation, nausea, postural hypotension and constipation. It has a propensity to cause weight gain, and increase in glycosylated hemoglobin, total cholesterol and triglycerides.

It should be avoided in elderly patients, especially hypertensives, because of reported increased incidence of cerebrovascular accidents.

RISPERIDONE (Rispid, Risnia): This atypical antipsychotic has a profile similar to that of clozapine in respect of negative symptoms. The drug has action on D_2, 5-HT, alpha adrenergic and histaminergic receptors. It however, causes dyskinesias such as akathisia and has a potent hyperprolactinemic effect. Other adverse reactions include postural hypotension, dizziness, insomnia and constipation. It is as effective as haloperidol but causes lower incidence of EPR. It is less likely to precipitate epileptic seizures. The starting dose is 2 mg/day in divided doses increased gradually to 4-6 mg/day. A depot preparation is also available.

The drug also appears to be effective and well tolerated for the treatment of tantrums, aggression and self-injurious behaviour of children with autistic disorders. Risperidone and olanzapine have also been reported to be beneficial for calming agitated or aggressive patients with dementia.

Paliperidone is the primary active metabolite of risperidone. It is well absorbed orally. It is not extensively metabolized by CYP450 enzymes; hence it is less likely to have drug interactions. It is not recommend for the elderly, demented, psychic patients.

Ziprasidone and **aripiprazole** are the other, second generation antipsychotics. Ziprasidone is also claimed to possess anxiolytic and antidepressant properties because of its affinity for 5-HT receptors.

Table 13.6 summarizes the efficacy and ADR of the *second generation antipsychotics.*

Carbamazepine, an antiepileptic, is useful as an adjunct in the treatment of schizophrenic patients with aggressive or violent behaviour or agitation, who show resistance to the usual antipsychotic drugs (Chapter 9).

Management of Schizophrenia

Schizophrenia is a serious mental disorder characterised by persistent disturbance in the perception and evaluation of reality, leading to characteristic changes in the perception, thinking, affective responses and behaviour.

The word 'schizophrenia' was coined from a Greek word meaning 'split mind' to describe a mental syndrome where an individual is dominated by one set of ideas or a complex to the exclusion of others. Thus, the harmonious working of the mind is split, with one portion seizing control of the rest. The schizophrenic patient, therefore, lives in his own world, dissociated from reality. He is a victim of *illusions* (perception falsified, e.g., mistaking a rope for a snake), *hallucinations* (perception without a stimulus, e.g., hearing God talking) and *delusions* (false beliefs, not based on cultural mores, that cannot be corrected by logic and reasoning) and believes that only his behaviour and actions are rational, without realising that he

Table 13.6: Relative efficacy and toxicity of Second Generation antipsychotics

Drug	Efficacy	EPR	Serum prolactin	Prolong QTc	Blood glucose	Weight gain
Clozapine*	++++	+/-	+/-	+	+++	+++
Olanzapine	+++	+	+/-	+	+++	+++
Quetiapine	++	+/-	+/-	+	++	++
Rispirodone	+++	+++	+++	+	+	+
Paliperidone	+++	+++	+++	+	+	+
Ziprasidone	++	+	+	++	+/-	+/-

* Can cause agranulocyto myonecrosis

is ill (lack of insight). His mental functioning is sufficiently impaired to interfere grossly with his capacity to meet the ordinary demands of life. The disease is common in young people between the ages of 18 and 28, exhibits a hereditary tendency, and generally is a recurring illness. It may exist in several varieties and the paranoid form (delusional disorder), in which the individual becomes suspicious of and belligerent towards the entire society, is perhaps the most dangerous.

The etiology of schizophrenia is complex and still unknown. Although increased activity of the brain dopamine pathways is important, the role of other brain transmitters cannot be ruled out. The symptoms of schizophrenia can be both positive and negative. The *positive symptoms* include hallucinations, delusions, agitation, repetitive behaviour and thought disorder. The *negative symptoms* include psychomotor slowing, marked social withdrawal, anhedonia (inability to experience pleasure), paucity of speech, apathy, as well as lack of energy and motivation.

Phenothiazines do not cure schizophrenia but they alleviate predominantly the positive symptoms. Thus, they reduce hallucinations, aggression, agitation and anxiety and make the patient more co-operative and acceptable. Disturbed thinking, paranoid symptoms, delusions and personal neglect may improve. Although improvement with phenothiazine drugs usually commences during the first 7-21 days, it may be delayed by as much as 5-6 weeks. It is not possible to predict which cases will respond promptly, and there is a proportion of patients who do not improve with phenothiazines alone but respond well to phenothiazine and electroconvulsive therapy (ECT) combination. Patients in catatonic excitement are better controlled initially with ECT, and phenothiazine therapy started later. Unless there are physical contraindications, ECT and phenothiazines can be combined in majority of patients. Phenothiazines have made it possible for the patients, who otherwise would have needed prolonged hospitalization in mental 'asylums', to stay at home and engage in productive activity.

The drugs are started in the smallest possible dose and increased gradually as needed. The oral dose of chlorpromazine varies widely from 100 to 1000 mg. per day. The initial dose usually is 25 mg. three times a day in adults, increased gradually to 300 mg. a day. Highly agitated, rowdy and violent patients would need larger doses, sometimes given parenterally. Halopridol is administered orally in the dose of 2.5-7.5 mg bid. For most patients, high doses of neuroleptics offer little advantage over smaller doses, at least in the majority of acute psychotic episodes. Although relapse rates may be lower in patients maintained on what are regarded as **standard** doses, those maintained on lower doses may have the advantage of improved social and vocational functioning. *The present evidence indicates no significant differences in clinical efficacy between chlorpromazine and the other important phenothiazines, although in a patient with specific symptomatology, one phenothiazine may be preferred to others.* Chlorpromazine may cause more drowsiness and depression while other antipsychotics may cause more EPR. Some drugs such as thioridazine may cause less EPR but then may produce QTC prolongation and cardiac toxicity. Some authorities routinely combine phenothiazines with benzhexol for preventing EPR. Most neuroleptics, when consumed in very high doses, do not cause life-threatening coma,and the lethal dose is very high.

Patients who cannot be relied upon to take the drug properly can be treated with weekly to biweekly injections of a **depot phenothiazine**. These dosage forms are particularly useful in uncooperative patients, for maintenance therapy during relapse.

Schizophrenia is a relapsing disease; hence, after the therapeutic response is obtained, the drug should be continued without interruption in smaller maintenance doses for a long time (sometimes lifelong) even after the first episode of illness, in order to prevent it from becoming chronic. Daytime drowsiness may interfere with the patient's ability to work, but this could be reduced if he takes most of his daily dose at night. The withdrawal should be slow (6-12 months) as reappearance of symptoms following withdrawal is not uncommon. A longer maintenance period is recommended, particularly in patients with a history of relapse.

Table 13.7 gives the equipotent oral doses of various neuroleptics.

Acute schizophrenic reaction needs initiation of treatment with the equivalent of 400 mg. of chlorpromazine per day given in four divided doses. On subsequent days, the daily dose is increased by the equivalent of 200 mg. of chlorpromazine till the acute reaction is controlled. The maintenance dose for the prevention of recurrence in chronic schizophrenics is the equivalent of 75-200 mg of chlorpromazine per day.

Table 13.7 : Equipotent oral doses of neuroleptics

Drug	Oral dose (mg)
Chlorpromazine	100
Chlorproxithene	100
Thioridazine	100
Trifluoperazine	5
Haloperidol	2
Fluphenazine	2
Pimozide	2
Clozapine	50
Olanzapine	5
Risperidone	2

First generation antipsychotics (Anti-dopaminergic) such as phenothiazines and haloperidol are quite effective against positive symptoms of schizophrenia and also are cost-effective. There is no convincing evidence that **second generation drugs** such as risperidone and olanzapine are superior in this respect. Their possible advantage is that they cause fewer EPR and may show more activity against negative symptoms. However, they may cause weight gain, hyperglycemia, and disturbed lipid metabolism. They also are much more expensive. Hence, an atypical antipsychotic may be reserved for some selected patients. Clozapine is considered the most effective antipsychotic but is toxic and should be used only in patients refractory to other drugs.

The causes of non-response to treatment are listed in Table 13.8. Irrespective of the drug used large numbers of chronic schizophrenics discontinue the medication probably because of lack of efficacy, adverse reactions or lack of supervision.

The neuroleptics that stimulate the secretion

Table 13.8 Causes of non-response to neuroleptic therapy

- Inadequate doses.
- Poor patient compliance.
- Pharmacokinetic factors.
- Persistent and severe psychosocial stress.
- Substance abuse.

of prolactin are better avoided in patients with established breast cancer.

Anti-Anxiety Drugs

Anxiolytics are the drugs used for the treatment of anxiety disorders. Their CNS depressant effect is dose dependent. In smaller doses, they relieve anxiety while in larger single doses they induce sleep and can, therefore, be grouped together with sedative hypnotics. Because of their depressant effect on the motor cortex, many of them also act as anticonvulsants (Chapter 9).

BENZODIAZEPINES (BDZ) : Benzodiazepine derivatives are currently the most commonly prescribed anti-anxiety agents. All anxiolytic benzodiazepines have similar properties; however, they differ in their pharmacokinetic profiles. These drugs are described in detail in Chapter 8. **Diazepam** is the most commonly used drug.

Mechanism of action : The exact mechanism of antianxiety action is not known though they act at many levels of the neuraxis. Experimentally, they have been shown to act on the limbic system, the hypothalamus and the brain stem reticular system. They bind to BDZ receptors and facilitate the action of GABA (Chapter 8). Benzodiazepines also reduce the turnover of brain 5-HT and noradrenaline.

Pharmacological actions : In both animals and humans, BDZ produce sedation, reduce aggressiveness and thus cause a calming (taming) effect. *Unlike chlorpromazine, they block conditioned as well as unconditioned responses.* In this respect, they resemble barbiturates. Clinically, they produce beneficial effects in anxious, neurotic patients. Such therapeutic benefits are, however, difficult to assess.

BDZ, however, are capable of causing memory impairment (anterograde amnesia) and other cognitive impairment; this is their major drawback. For details, preparations and toxicity see Chapter 8.

CHLORMETHIAZOLE (Heminevrin): Chlormethiazole ethane-di-sulphonate is a thiazol derivative with sedative, hypnotic and anti-convulsant actions. Given orally, it is absorbed rapidly but undergoes extensive first pass metabolism. The drug has been used orally or by injection in delirium tremens to induce sedation. The adverse effects include tingling sensation particularly in nose and a moderate fall of BP on IV administration. Failure to produce marked respiratory depression even in excessive doses and relation of its structure to thiazol part of thiamine molecule make it a drug of pharmacological interest. It has also been used as a hypnotic in the elderly.

BUSPIRONE (Buspar) : This azaspiro decanedione (azapirone) is an anxiolytic not related to BDZ. It does not act through GABA receptors, and it lacks the sedative-hypnotic, muscle relaxant and anticonvulsant properties of BDZ.

It acts as a partial agonist of inhibitory, presynaptic 5-HT_{1A} receptors and inhibits autoreceptors; this reduces the release of 5-HT which probably explains its anxiolytic action. It also has a weak D_2 receptor antagonistic action. The drug does not potentiate the CNS depressant effect of the commonly used depressant medications and, therefore, may be particularly useful in anxious, elderly patients. The drug causes less cognitive and psychomotor impairment than diazepam.It has a short t½ (2-5 hours) and it is prescribed in the dose of 30 mg/day in divided doses. It does not cause tolerance/dependence nor interacts with alcohol. Its important drawback is that *its onset of action is slow and may take as much as two weeks. Its anxiolytic effect is weaker than that of benzodiazepines. Further, it is not useful in severe anxiety with panic disorder and in alcohol withdrawal syndrome.*

The adverse reactions include GI disturbances, nervousness, dizziness, confusion and tachycardia. Patients on MAOI can develop hypertension when given buspirone.

Gepirone, ipsapirone and trospirone are the newer analogues of buspirone.

There are many **other non-barbiturate sedatives** like hydroxyzine hydrochloride (Atarax), diphenhydramine and buclizine hydrochloride available in the market. Hydroxyzine and diphenhydramine are sedative antihistaminics and over the counter (OTC) hypnotics. More sedative tricyclic anti-depressants such as amitryptiline and doxepin are also promoted for the treatment of anxiety state. However, all these drugs also suppress the autonomic nervous system and can be called **autonomic sedatives.** They do not cause muscle relaxation and are likely to cause adverse effects such as dryness of mouth, palpitation, daytime sedation and confusion. None is superior to benzodiazepines either as anxiolytic or hypnotic; however, they are not addictive and are relatively safer.

Treatment of Anxiety Disorders

Some amount of anxiety (fear of the known or unknown) is a normal physiological response that assists the individual in solving various problems in life. *Pathological anxiety is that which has no apparent external cause, causes high intensity of symptoms, persists over time and leads to the development of harmful behavioral strategies (avoidance, compulsions etc.) that impair function.* Anxiety may be secondary to stressful situations, bodily disease or the use or withdrawal of drugs / substances of abuse. It is a cardinal symptom of many psychiatric disorders.

Primary anxiety disorders are those in which no cause is discernible. Depending on the manifestations, these disorders are given such names as : stress related adjustment disorders, phobias, panic disorders, obsessive compulsive disorder and generalised anxiety disorder (GAD).

Anxiety-associated disorder is a common condition in which anxiety is the most prominent symptom. The patient is acutely aware of his/her symptoms and complains of them. These reactions have been considered as the maladaptive results of conflict between unfulfilled desires and repressive tendencies. To some extent, they are expressions of disappointments and frustrations in life. Anxiety has two components;

- ***A psychological component*** (dread, unpleasant anticipation or a feeling of impending doom); and
- ***A physical component*** (autonomic arousal).

The reactions and emotions of a patient suffering from anxiety disorder are usually an exaggeration of those experienced by normal individuals in day to day life. Subjects generally complain of headache, tension, feeling of a tight band round the head, palpitation, tremulousness, dryness of mouth, hyperhidrosis, coldness of extremities, spasm of back muscle giving rise to vague bodyaches, and insomnia. Such patients may also suffer from bowel disturbances and phobias such as fear of dying, insanity and heart disease. Such fear complexes make them stop work. *The appetite and libido, however, are not much affected and thoughts of commiting suicide are absent unless there is associated severe mental depression or major psychosis.*

Currently, BDZ and SSRI are most commonly used to treat anxiety disorders. In general, there is little difference among the various BDZ as anti-anxiety agents. However, the high potency BDZ such as alprazolam, clonazepam and lorazepam are preferred in severe anxiety states with marked autonomic overactivity. Oxazepam in small, divided doses may be preferred in the elderly and in patients with hepatic dysfunction, because of its short duration of action.

Anxiolytic agents can reduce the somatic and autonomic disturbances, abolishing physical malaise, bodyache and anxiety. Long term studies with these drugs, however, indicate that none of the anti-anxiety agents produce permanent benefit which can come only from realization by the patient of the nature of his problems and his adjustment to them.

Drugs should be used only for short periods to lessen the patient's distress. Anti-anxiety agents are particularly useful in treating acute stress reactions. Dosage schedule should be flexible and individualized. Since insomnia is a common complaint of these patients and as most anti-anxiety drugs (not buspirone) induce sleep, the major dose should be given at bedtime. BDZ do not induce drug-metabolizing enzymes and produce remarkably little change in normal sleep patterns. Furthermore, BDZ are considered safer when suicidal tendencies are suspected since suicidal attempts usually do not succeed even with overdosage. As they are quick acting, the initial treatment always should be with BDZ.

Since anxiety is often episodic in intensity, drugs should be used to treat each episode and not be given continuously for prolonged periods. It must be emphasised that in anxious patients, placebo responses are frequent and definite. In some patients with severe anxiety, somatic symptoms such as palpitation, trembling and giddiness dominate the clinical picture. In such cases, a beta-adrenergic blocking agent like propranolol may be useful.

In practice many patients complain of 'tension' with vague symptoms without any obvious signs of illness. These are due to minor maladjustments in day to day life and do not really need drug therapy. However, in the highly technical age that we live in, one always seeks a technical solution to every problem. Unfortunately, such ideas are encouraged by drug firms and further enhanced by medical profession by publishing halfbaked confusing reports on a condition which itself is difficult to evaluate. *Drugs can temporarily modify the patient's emotional response to environmental factors. They are not expected to influence the environment or socio-economic situations.* As pointed out, "It is required that we cope actively and almost constantly with an outer environment and that we learn how to do this without disintegrating in new anxiety. To live is to be under tension, to be dissatisfied; to be anxious, sometimes unbearably so; to be angry, sometimes potently and impotently; to be everlastingly hungry; to some degree, for things that may be consciously well defined or very vague; to become depressed and discouraged; to become physically and psychosomatically ill; to worry obsessively and to become hysterically emotional. The range of normal functioning of mind is wide and flexible". Certainly, drugs should not be used every now and then to modify such normal cyclic behavioural changes without assessing the disability produced.

Indiscriminate use of anti-anxiety agents for prolonged periods may kill all the initiative in the individual and can also cause drug dependence. Effective treatment of anxiety neurosis needs the co-operation of the patient in facing his problems. The majority of patients can be helped more by a sympathetic and understanding approach of the doctor than by drugs.

Severe anxiety, however, may be extremely disabling and *often may be the presenting symptom of a more serious psychiatric disorder such as schizophrenia or depression.* In such cases appropriate treatment of the underlying disorder is important, and benzodiazepines, in general, can be added to antidepressants or anti-psychotic drugs for this purpose.

Some individuals have anxiety in specific situations (**phobic anxiety**); the intensity increases as the person approaches the feared situation such as air or ship travel and it remains as long as the exposure to that situation lasts. The person will try to avoid the situation and to terminate the exposure to it (should such exposure occur) in order to avoid / minimise anxiety. Patients with phobic anxiety may suffer from **panic attacks** if suddenly or overwhelmingly exposed to the feared situation.

The term **panic disorder** is used to describe a condition in which panic attacks appear to occur spontaneously and repeatedly. Because of marked somatic symptoms, its diagnosis is likely to be missed. Panic disorder has distinct symptoms. The patient abruptly develops a feeling of intense fear, impending disaster or death accompanied by various physical symptoms such as palpitation, sweating, trembling, feeling of choking, abdominal distress, chills or hot flushes etc. Affected individual often complains of such symptoms in an agitated state. Panic attacks are many times associated with agoraphobia, a morbid fear and avoidance of being alone or being in a public place, resulting in a marked restriction of travel. Medical conditions that are commonly noted in subjects with panic attacks include episodic high blood pressure, peptic ulcer, cardiac arrhythmias, and mitral valve prolapse. In fact, such patients may often receive treatment primarily for such secondary disorders and not the anxiety state. Hyperventilation (over-breathing) with various resulting symptoms such as carpopedal spasms is an important diagnostic feature of panic attacks.

Not all panic attacks constitute panic disorder. Often, a similar picture may be observed in *specific phobias* e.g. at heights or on seeing a snake; or in *social phobias* such as facing a stranger or an examination (where a person is likely to be scrutinized). However, patients with panic disorder may not be aware of the source of their fearfulness. Further, panic disorder is often associated with underlying major depression. Panic-like attacks may also occur in hyperthyroidism, pheochromocytoma and drug abuse.

The treatment of choice for panic disorder is:

- ***A selective serotonin reuptake inhibitor*** such as fluoxetine or paroxetine; they are all equally effective, and in addition they help to control the co-morbid depression (see later).
- ***A tricyclic (TCA) antidepressant*** such as imipramine. All TCA are as effective as the SSRI and are less expensive. Their side effects are often exaggerated. But, TCA with prominent anticholinergic effects such as amitryptiline may not be well tolerated by elderly patients.
- ***A high potency benzodiazepine,*** alprazolam, in the starting dose of 0.25 mg 2-4 times a day, works faster (in days, unlike antidepressants which take weeks), and has few other adverse effects than sedation and possible drug dependence/abuse. Other BDZ are equally effective, and the long acting ones such as clonazepam (t½ 80 hours) are easier to withdraw.

β-adrenergic blockers are useful as adjuncts for controlling tachycardia and palpitation during social phobia: By themselves, they do not counter the basic disorder.

Benzodiazepines as anxiolytics are not useful in depression, phobic or obsessional states and chronic psychosis. However, they may be used initially, concurrently with SSRI, for a speedier response. In bereavement, psychological adjustment may be inhibited by BDZ. In children, anxiolytics should only be used to relieve acute anxiety caused by fear e.g. before surgery.

Drug therapy may be combined with **cognitive-behavioral therapy** (CBT) in patients with unsatisfactory response to drugs. CBT alone may not be as helpful; but it may enhance the long term well being of the patient.

The term **general anxiety disorder** (GAD) is used when excessive anxiety and persistent worry are present on most days of the week for at least six months.The symptoms are restlessness, difficulty in concentrating, easy fatiguability, irritability, muscle tension and disturbed sleep, along with symptoms such as palpitation, dry mouth and sweating. Such symptoms are gradual in onset and do not create life threatening fears. *Major depression is the most commonly co-existing psychiatric disorder in patients with GAD*, occuring in almost 60% of the patients, whereas panic disorder occurs in 25% of the cases. The links between GAD and the personality trait in neuroticism are very strong and are controlled by genetic factors; hence, the prevention of GAD is very difficult.

The current therapy of GAD includes a combination of BDZ, SSRI and cognitive behavioral therapy. Some patients will need maintenance drug therapy almost lifelong.

The initial therapy should be with a combination of BDZ and SSRI; the dose of BDZ is tapered after 2-3 weeks when SSRI become effective. Beta blockers, though widely used for anxiety, have unproven efficacy. Severe, intractable GAD may need MAO inhibitors.

Emphasis should be on counselling, exercise, mental relaxation/meditation and behavioural therapy. Excessive intake of stimulants such as caffeine and cola in any form, and diseases such as hyperthyroidism should be excluded.

Many patients with mild anxiety symptoms are able to function well, sometimes even better than normal subjects, in daily life. Hence, the physician should step in only if symptoms interfere with normal the social functioning. Even in these, many patients are likely to respond to the minimum therapy, and one should not rush into treatment approaches that involve long term risk and expense.

Antidepressant Drugs

The syndrome of mental depression is a major affective disorder, common in the general population, and is many times underdiagnosed. Although biochemically, it is associated with depletion of brain monoamines, 5-HT and NA, its causes are complex.

Successful treatment of mental depression with drugs is one of the major advances in psychopharmacology in recent years. Several drugs are now available as 'antidepressants', sometimes also called as **'psychoanaleptics'** or **'mood elevators'.** They act by increasing the intrasynaptic availability of the monoamines in the brain.

These can be classified into:

I **Monoamine oxidase inhibitors (MAOI).**

(a) Irreversible:

- ***Hydrazine*** MAOI, e.g., Isocarboxazid, Iproniazid and Phenelzine.
- ***Nonhydrazine*** MAOI, e.g., Tranylcypromine.

(b) Reversible: e.g. Moclobemide

II **Non-selective monoamines reuptake inhibitors:**

- ***Tricyclic*:** Imipramine, Desipramine, Amitryptiline, Nortryptiline, Doxepin and Nitroxazepine and Clomipramine.
- ***Tetracyclic*:** Maproteline and Mirtazapine.
- ***Heterocyclic*:** Trazodone, Nefazodone, Venlafaxine and Bupropion.

III **Selective serotonin (5HT) reuptake inhibitors (SSRI):** Fluoxetine, Paroxetine, Fluvoxamine, Sertraline, Citalopram.

IV **Selective NA reuptake inhibitors:** Reboxetine.

V **Mood Stabilizers :** Lithium carbonate.

VI **Miscellaneous :** Carbamazepine; St. John's Wort

Monoamine Oxidase Inhibitors (MAOI)

This is a heterogeneous group of drugs which block the oxidative deamination of naturally occurring amines such as NA, 5-HT and DA.

Mechanism of action: The enzyme MAO is present intracellularly in most of the tissues, particularly the CNS, gut and liver. Relatively large amounts of 5-HT and NA are concentrated in the hypothalamus and in other subcortical regions of the brain. These amines are stored in granules in the neurons and are released following neuronal stimuli. The active amines thus liberated act on the postsynaptic receptors but do not accumulate as they are immediately metabolized by the enzyme MAO present in the brain. The two types MAO-A and MAO-B differentially affect the metabolism of neurotransmitters in humans.

- ***Inhibition of the MAO-A*** decreases the deamination of NA and 5-HT. This causes increase in local NA and 5-HT which is associated with both antidepressant action and hypertensive interactions with foods containing tyramine and with sympathomimetic drugs. In animal experiments, accumulation of these amines is associated with excitement and enhanced motor activity. Tryptophan, the precursor of 5-HT and tryptamine, taken orally, can potentiate the effect of MAOI.
- ***Selective inhibition of MAO-B***, which preferentially decreases the deamination of dopamine, is not associated with antidepressant action or hypertensive interactions, but is useful in treating parkinsonism (Chapter 14).

Given orally, these drugs exert a considerable effect on liver MAO enzymes because of their high concentration in portal circulation.

Pharmacological actions:

- ***Behavioural effects*:** These drugs elevate the mood of depressed individuals. Such subjects feel more energetic, less sleepy and more fresh. Tendency for suicidal rumination diminishes. The action is seen after a latent period of a few days to 3-4 weeks. In some cases agitation, talkativeness and restlessness may occur.
- ***Cardiovascular effects*:** There is no specific action on heart or the coronary flow. Some MAOI may, however, cause hypotension.
- ***Reserpine reversal*:** Normally, animals treated with reserpine are inert, apathetic and do not take interest in the surroundings. In animals pretreated with MAOI, administration of reserpine produces agitation and excitement due to accumulation of amines. This is known as 'reserpine reversal'.
- ***Potentiation of action of sympathomimetic amines*:** MAOI potentiate the sympathomimetic actions of other amines like amphetamine and ephedrine.
- ***Miscellaneous*:** As these drugs also inhibit MAO and other enzymes present in liver, they prevent the metabolism of many drugs and prolong their actions. This may precipitate toxicity. They are potent REM sleep inhibitors.

Absorption, fate and excretion: All compounds are well absorbed orally. Information about their metabolism in man is inadequate, but the effect of MAOI continues for 10 to 14 days after the drug is withdrawn. This is due to their irreversible action on the MAO enzyme, which may take over 2 weeks to return to normal level.

Adverse reactions:

- ***Behavioural effects*:** These include headache, excitement, agitation, hallucinations and disturbed sleep. These drugs may activate latent psychosis and their use alone in cases of schizophrenia is contraindicated.
- ***CNS effects*:** They may cause insomnia and CNS stimulation as demonstrated by tremors, twitching, ataxia, hyperreflexia, hyperthermia and even convulsions. Drugs like iproniazid and isocarboxazid sometimes cause peripheral neuritis which responds to pyridoxine.
- ***Hypertensive crisis*:** This can be precipitated by concurrent administration of *sympathomimetic pressor amines* like amphetamine and ephedrine. Sudden rise in BP may even cause subarachnoid haemorrhage. Hypertensive crisis can also occur in patients taking MAOI, if they consume *cheese* or *red wine* which contain tyramine. Normally tyramine is metabolized in the liver by MAO enzymes. MAOI, by inhibiting its metabolism, lead to tyramine accumulation which releases NA from binding sites causing a marked rise in BP. Eating of *broad beans* can also produce similar complication due to their content of DOPA. *Yeast extract* contains both tyramine and histamine. Some other foodstuffs which are incompatible with MAOI include *yoghurt, buttermilk, meat extracts, soyabeans, chocolates, ripe bananas and figs.*

A hypertensive crisis should be treated with phentolamine (Regitine) 5 mg. IV slowly or sodium nitroprusside infusion.

- ***Autonomic effects*:** Hydrazine compounds can cause antimuscarinic effects such as constipation, dry mouth, blurring of vision, impotence, difficulty in micturition and orthostatic hypotension. However, they have very little effect on cardiac conduction.

- ***Miscellaneous effects*** : Hydrazine compounds, particularly iproniazid, may cause hepatocellular jaundice. Allergic reactions are also known.

- ***Acute toxic effects*** following overdosage include agitation, hallucinations, hyperpyrexia and convulsions. Blood pressure may be low or high. The treatment is mainly symptomatic. Drugs like vasopressor agents and barbiturates should be administered cautiously.

Drug interactions: By blocking drug degradation, **MAOI** potentiate the action of several drugs (Table 13.9). Thus, the normal dose of pethidine in a patient receiving **MAOI** can cause shock, collapse, respiratory. depression and death. *The effects of adrenaline, noradrenaline and isoprenaline, however, are not enhanced as they are inactivated by catechol-o-methyl transferase, another enzyme present in the liver and blood.*

Table 13.9: Some drugs whose action is potentiated by MAOI

- Alcohol
- Sympathomimetics: Amphetamine, Ephedrine
- Anaesthetics
- Anticholinergics
- Antihistaminics
- Narcotics: Morphine, Pethidine, Barbiturates
- Antidepressants : Tricyclic, SSRI

Preparations and dosages:

(i) Isocarboxazid (Marpan) — 10 mg. tablet, usual daily dose 10-30 mg increased upto 50 mg.

(ii) Phenelzine sulfate (Nardil) — 15 mg. tablet. Usual daily dose 45-60 mg. Maximum daily dose recommended 75 mg.

(iii) Tranylcypromine (Parnate) — 10 mg. tablet, 10-20 mg. daily increased upto 30 mg.

With all these drugs, smaller doses should be used for maintenance therapy and in old people.

MOCLOBEMIDE (Manerix) : This drug acts by selective, reversible inhibition of MAO-A enzyme, and hence is termed as reversible inhibitor of MAO (RIMA). It causes less potentiation of pressor amines and lower incidence of drug interactions than irreversible MAOI. It does not need strict dietary restriction as the intestinal MAO is mainly MAO-B.

Tricyclic Antidepressants

IMIPRAMINE, a dibenzazepine derivative, is the commonly employed tricyclic antidepressant (TCA) and is discussed as a prototype.

Structurally, it differs from phenothiazines in that the sulphur is replaced by an ethylene linkage. The other cyclic antidepressants are given in Table 13.9.

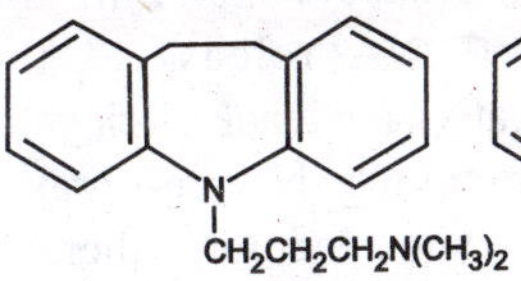

$CH_2CH_2CH_2N(CH_3)_2$

Imipramine

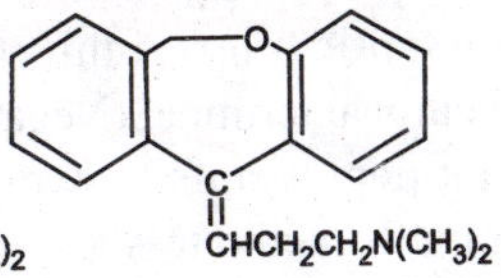

$CHCH_2CH_2N(CH_3)_2$

Doxepin

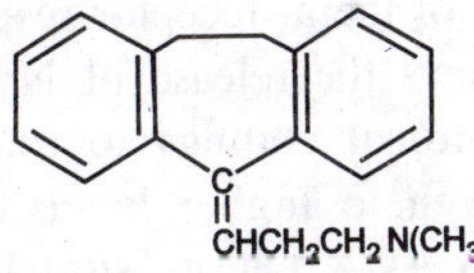

$CHCH_2CH_2N(CH_3)_2$

Amitriptyline

Fig 13.2

Mechanism of action: All drugs which modify depression or mania have distinct effects on metabolism of 5-HT, NA and DA. Normally, a large proportion of 5-HT/NA liberated at the nerve endings is inactivated by reabsorption on to its storage sites. Tricyclic antidepressants:

- ***Inhibit neuronal NA and/or 5-HT reuptake in the brain,*** causing a localized increase in NA/5-HT in the synaptic gap.

- ***Cause variable blockade of α_1 and to less extent presynaptic α_2 adreno-receptors;*** and

• ***Possess central anti-muscarinic properties.***

In general, the TCA inhibit the reuptake of NA more than that of 5-HT. Their action on 5-HT reuptake varies considerably. Imipramine and amitriptyline are potent inhibitors of 5-HT uptake whereas desipramine and protriptyline are potent reuptake inhibitors, of NA. The tricyclic and other antidepressants acting on NA uptake do not block dopamine reuptake. Nomifensine, a tetrahydroisoquinoline compound, strongly inhibits the reuptake of DA and NA, and is a weak inhibitor of 5-HT uptake; it causes less sedation. Thus, the different TCA affect several neurotransmitter systems (5-HT, NA, histamine and dopamine) to differing degrees. This may explain the differences in their action profiles.

Presynaptic α_2 adrenergic receptors play an important role in the autoregulation of neurotransmitter NA release. Activation of these receptors following release of NA in the synaptic cleft inhibits NA release at the neuronal terminal (Negative feedback). Tricyclic antidepressants, by blocking NA re-uptake, rapidly activate these auto-receptors, thereby limiting the synaptic availability of NA. Repeated drug administration, however, leads to desensitization of the a_2 receptor response. This 'adaptation' allows the release of NA from the adrenergic neuronal endings to return to the baseline or even to higher levels. Long term treatment with TCA causes similar adaptive changes and altered sensitivity of several other receptors such as muscarinic receptors and GABA-B receptors. The importance of such complex changes at the cellular and molecular levels in the therapeutic action and toxicity of the antidepressants is not clear.

Pharmacological actions:

Behavioural effects : Imipramine produces similar anti-depressant effect as MAOI, but the mechanism of action is different. The drug can reverse the depressant action of reserpine without restoring brain monoamines. It also has some anxiolytic action.

Central nervous system : A single dose of 100 mg. in normal subjects causes drowsiness and a feeling of light headedness. Clinically, it produces some degree of sedation, enhances sleep and disrupts obsessive rumination. The drug suppresses REM sleep but increases stage 4 sleep. Repeated administration of this drug in man causes sedation and may produce difficulty in concentration and thinking. The drug has no euphoriant effect and drug dependence is rare.

It lowers the seizure threshold in animals and hence, should be prescribed with caution in patients with history of seizures.

Autonomic nervous system : It has antimuscarinic effects such as dryness of mouth, constipation, blurred vision and palpitation.

Cardiovascular system: See later.

Absorption, fate and excretion: Given orally, TCA are well absorbed. They are highly lipophilic, widely distributed and get strongly bound to proteins in the various tissues. They have a large volume of distribution. Imipramine is converted in the liver to its active metabolite desmethylimipramine. It is metabolized in the liver and kidney.

The various tricyclic compounds differ in their pharmacokinetic properties. Most tricyclics are completely eliminated within 7-10 days. Their other properties vary according to their interaction with other receptor types (Table 13.9).

Adverse reactions: Some of these can be explained on the basis of *blocking of various neurotransmitter receptors* in the brain (Table 13.9). Thus, blocking of D_2 receptor is responsible for the endocrine adverse effects (eg. galactorrhoea) following clomipramine (+), amoxapine (+), trimipramine (+), amitriptyline (±), maprotiline (±) and nortriptyline (±).

• ***Allergic reactions*** like urticaria, skin rashes, pruritus and photosensitivity.

• ***Antimuscarinic effects* :** They constitute the commonest and the most troublesome adverse effects of all TCA. These include dryness of mouth, difficulty in accommodation, tachycardia, difficulty in micturition, impotence, constipation, delayed ejaculation, and rarely hyperpyrexia. The drug should be used cautiously in patients with glaucoma or enlarged prostate. Rarely, it can cause paralytic ileus.

● ***Central nervous system*** : Feeling of tiredness, lethargy, headache and sedation may be observed. Amitryptiline, trimipramine, doxepin, trazodone and mirtazepine are potent sedatives and can cause sleep. Like MAOI, these drugs can cause tremors, muscle jerking, ataxia and hyper-reflexia. They are best avoided in epileptics. Central antimuscarinic action may cause confusion, disorientation or psychosis.

● ***Cardiovascular system***: Postural hypotension, cardiomyopathy and heart failure have been reported following long term therapy. Both imipramine and amitriptyline may cause inverted or flattened T wave, prolongation of QT interval and depressed ST segment in the ECG, even in therapeutic doses. With overdosage, they can precipitate cardiac arrhythmias.

● ***Miscellaneous***: Like chlorpromazine, imipramine can cause cholestatic jaundice, agranulocytosis and edema. Unilateral or bilateral peroneal palsy has been reported following imipramine and amitriptyline. *Priapism can occur with trazodone, a heterocyclic agent.*

Tricyclic anti-depressants cross the placental barrier and can cause jitteriness, suckling problem, hyperexcitability and rarely cardiac arrhythmias in the neonate.

● ***Acute poisoning*** with tricyclics produces hyperpyrexia, hypertension or hypotension, convulsions and coma. Cardiac arrythmias may be present. It may also cause metabolic acidosis. The treatment is symptomatic. Physostigmine salicylate, given parenterally, in the dose of 1-4 mg. every 1 hour, is used to treat anticholinergic CNS manifestations.

Drug interactions: See Table 13.10.

Preparations and dosage: See Table 13.11

Therapeutic uses:

● ***Mental depression,*** discussed later.

● ***Acute panic attacks***, see earlier.

● ***Obsessive compulsive neurosis***: This disorder is characterised by obsessional pattern of thinking and ritualistic compulsive behaviour as a defence against anxiety. If such thoughts or action is prevented or interrupted, the patient becomes anxious. The treatment is either with a tricyclic antidepressant or with a selective serotonin reuptake inhibitor (SSRI, see later).

● ***Nocturnal enuresis***: Enuresis is defined as bedwetting that occurs after the age at which bladder control should have been achieved, usually between the ages 2-3 years. The disorder exists in two forms : (a) primary (persistent), and (b) secondary (acquired or regressional). Primary enuresis is the commoner of the two types. The main treatment consists of bladder training and correction of psychopathologic factors. Imipramine, in a single bedtime dose of 10 to 75 mg., has been used with variable success. The exact mechanism of action is not known. The other drugs used are amitriptyline and desmopressin (Chapter 38).

● ***Bulimia nervosa***: This is a behavioral disorder characterised by episodes of overeating, usually followed by self-induced vomiting, cathartic or diuretic abuse or fasting to undo the threat of weight gain. Antidepressants such as imipramine and SSRI are the favoured drugs treatment for this condition.

● ***Migraine,*** see Chapter 23.

● ***Deafferentiation pain,*** see Chapter 11.

● ***Attention deficit hyperactivity disorder (ADHD),*** (see later).

● ***Chronic fatigue syndrome (CFS).***

● ***Nonspecific fibromyalgias***.

Table 13.10 : Drug interactions of imipramine

● MAOI : Severe reactions like atropine poisoning (hyperpyrexia, convulsions, coma).

● Phenothiazines and thyroid preparations enhance its effects.

● Hypotensive effect of guanethidine and mecamylamine is reversed.

● Potentiation of action of phenylephrine, adrenaline and noradrenaline with potentially fatal accidents.

Table 13.11: Antidepressant compounds

Adverse reactions due to blockade of receptors

Compound	H_1 Sedative activity	M Anti-muscarinic activity	α_1 Ortho-static hypo-tension	Total daily dose mg Out patients	Total daily dose mg Hospital patients
Tricyclic Compounds					
Imipramine (Depsonil, Tofranil)	+ +	+ +	+ +	50-150	75-300
Desipramine (Norpramine)	+	+	+	50-100	75-200
Trimipramine (Surmontil)	+ + +	+ + +	+ +	50-100	75-300
Amitriptyline * (Sarotena, Tryptanol)	+ + +	+ + +	+ + +	50-100	75-200
Nortriptyline (Sensival)	+ +	+	+	25-50	50-100
Protriptyline (Vivactil)	+	+ +	+	20-40	20-60
Amoxapine (Asendir)	++	+	++	50-200	100-600
Doxepin (Sinequan)	+ + +	+ +	+ +	50-100	50-300
Dothiepin (Prothiaden)	++	+		50-100	100-200
Heterocyclic compounds					
Trazodone (Molipaxin)	+ + +	0	0	50-300	100-600
Bupropion (Welbutrin)	0	0	0	200-300	100-400
Venlafaxine (Ebflexor)	0	0	0	75-150	75-225
Selective serotonin (5-HT) reuptake inhibitors (SSRI)					
Fluoxetine (Prozac)	±	0	0	20	20-40
Fluvoxamine (Faverine)	±	0	0	50-100	100-200
Paroxetine (Seroxat)	0/+	0/+	0	20-40	20-40
Sertraline (Lustral)	0/+	+	0	100-150	100-150
Citalopram (Celexa)	±	0	0	10-40	20-40
Selective NA re-uptake inhibitor					
Reboxetine (Devadex)	0/+	+	0	8-20	8-20

* Injections 100 mg/10 ml for IM use. H_1 = Histaminic; M = Muscarinic; α_1 = Alpha$_1$ adrenergic. 0 = Negligible. + = Minimal. ++ = Moderate +++ = Marked.

Imipramine and amitryptiline are still the most cost-effective TCA for general use.

Selective Serotonin (5-HT) Reuptake Inhibitors (SSRI)

Drugs belonging to this group are listed in Table 13.10.

Mechanism of action: As the name suggests, the selective serotonin (5-HT) reuptake inhibitors (SSRI) act mainly by inhibiting the reuptake of serotonin by the tryptanergic neurons.

Pharmacological action : *They are as effective as TCA in moderate depression but may be less effective in the severely depressed patients.* Because of their selective receptor action, they cause:

- ***Less marked antimuscarinic effects.***
- ***Less sedation.***

- ***Fewer cardiovascular effects*** (bradycardia, hypotension, conduction disturbances); and they
- ***Are safer than the TCA in the elderly.***

As with TCA, repeated administration leads to gradual downregulation and desensitization of autoreceptor mechanisms over several weeks.

Absorption, fate and excretion : SSRI are well absorbed orally and have long half lives, which permits their once-a-day administration. In general, many antidepressant drugs are metabolized and eliminated slowly. Further,the metabolites of many of these compounds are also active, and some of them have half lives longer than those of the parent drugs (Table 13.12). A few drugs like trazodone, venlaflaxine and nefazodone have short half lives of 3-6 hours. Norfluoxetine, the metabolite of fluoxetine is pharmacologically active; both of them and other SSRI interfere with P450 drug metabolizing enzymes and prolong the half life of many drugs.

Table 13.12: Half-lives of anti-depressants and their metabolites

Drug	Drug t½, hours	Metabolite, t½, hours
Tricyclics		
Imipramine	12	30
Amitryptiline	16	30
Doxepin	16	30
Protryptiline	80	—
Clomipramine	32	70
SSRI		
Fluoxetine	50	240
Paroxetine	17	—
Fluvoxamine	15	—
Sertraline	24	65
Citalopram	35	—

Adverse reactions: These include nausea, anxiety, jitteriness, insomnia, headache and erectile dysfunction. They decrease sexual thoughts and desire, decrease libido, and may delay orgasm in both sexes. This side effect, however, makes them useful in the therapy of paraphilias and sexual obsession associated with increased suicidal tendencies. *Like other antidepressants, the SSRI may cause mania when used in patients with undiagnosed bipolar depression.*

If stopped suddenly, all SSRIs can produce withdrawal symptoms such as anxiety, agitation, confusion, insomnia, sweationg, tremor, vomiting and shock like syndrome. Fluoxetine with a longer t½ is less likely to cause these symptoms.

The administration of an MAOI concurrently with or immediately prior to one of these drugs can cause a **serotonergic reaction** comprising:

- ***Cognitive-behavioural symptoms:*** mainly agitation, insomnia, anxiety, hypomania and seizures.
- ***Autonomic symptoms:*** nausea, salivation, diaphoresis, diarrhoea, abdominal pain, flushed skin and hyperthermia; and
- ***Neuromuscular symptoms:*** hyperreflexia, shivering, twitching, rigidity. Rhabdomyolysis secondary to severe rigidity and hyperthermia may occur. The reaction may be fatal; fortunately, it is rare. The treatment is symptomatic and supportive.

Other drugs which increase CNS serotonin activity and may cause **serotonergic syndrome** are listed in Table 13.13.

Table 13.13: Some drugs which may induce serotonergic syndrome

- MAOI
- Pethidine
- Dextromethorphan
- Clomipramine
- Amphetamine
- Lithium
- Levodopa
- Buspirone
- Bromocriptine
- Two or more SSRI (especially fluoxetine)

Preparations and dosage :

Fluoxetine is used initially in the dose of 20 mg. once a day, in the morning, increased by 20 mg. once in several weeks, to a maximum of 80 mg. daily (less in the elderly). *Doses higher than 20 mg. should be given in divided amounts in the morning and at noon.* **Fluvoxamine** and **sertraline** are used initially in the dose of 50 mg. once a day, increased by 50 mg. once a week, to a maximum of 200 mg. daily (less in the elderly).

The other SSRI are **paroxetine, citalopram** and **zimelidine.**

Therapeutic uses : They should be given in the morning hours as they can disturb sleep. They are not the first line drugs in all depressed patients. They may be preferred in patients who:

- ***Cannot tolerate the tricyclic antidepressants.***
- ***Have a high risk of suicide.***
- ***Are accident prone,*** as the older antidepressants have sedative and autonomic adverse effects; or
- ***Have an obsessive compulsive disorder.*** A major role for serotonin system in mediation of obsessive compulsive neurosis has been suggested. However, SSRI are not only clinically effective but also have better safety and tolerability profile than tricyclics.

These drugs are also preferred in the depressed geriatric patients as the tricyclics can cause dizziness, postural hypotension, constipation and difficulty in micturition.

If used concurrently, they may increase the TCA, lithium and carbamazepine plasma levels.

SSRI should not be used:

- ***In the manic phase of bipolar depression.***
- ***Together with MAOI; and***
- ***Concurrently with ECT.***

Newer antidepressants : Newer antidepressants (**third generation**) which act more selectively on 5-HT receptor subtypes as compared to older SSRI have differing adverse effects profile while providing similar efficacy. Their properties are summarised in Table 13.14. Besides being more selective in action, in general they have low affinity for muscarinic, dopaminergic and H_1-histaminic receptors, resulting in fewer adverse reactions. Sexual dysfunction is less common with nefazodone and mirtazapine, while weight gain is not a problem with nefazodone, venlafaxine and reboxetine. Nefazodone and reboxetine relieve depression-associated sleep disturbances such as insomnia, fatigue and anergia. Further, these drugs except nefazodone cause much less cytochrome oxidase-based drug interactions. All of them are metabolized in the liver and they should not be combined with MAO-inhibitors.

Because of their more selective profile these drugs may be useful for matching individual therapeutic needs in terms of efficacy, tolerability and adverse effects in selected patients.

Choice of SSRI : All SSRIs are almost equally effective in the treatment of depression. Patient who do not respond to one drug form this class may respond to another. Because of the differences in their hepatic metabolizm, they differ in their potential for drug interactions. **Fluoxetine** is currently considered the drug of choice for routine use. **Paroxetine** may cause more weight gain as well as pose a high risk of mood changes and withdrawal syndrome. **Venlafaxine** can cause intense withdrawal syndrome. *Because of suspected effect on mood fluctuations and possible suicidal thoughts, paroxetine, mirtazapine, venlafaxine and nephazodone should be avoided in children.*

Mood Stabilizers

LITHIUM CARBONATE (Licab) : The use of lithium carbonate in mental illness was described by Cade in 1949.

Lithium is useful as a mood stabilizer in manic depressive psychosis (MDP). As compared to chlorpromazine, lithium is claimed to cause less drowsiness while controlling the marked

Table 13.14 : Newer antidepressants

Name	Mechanism of action	Adverse reactions	Drug interactions
Venlafaxine (Bi-cyclicphenyl ethylamine)	Potent 5-HT and NA reuptake inhibitor.	Nausea, dizziness, dry mouth, sexual dysfunction. May cause rise in BP.	Few
Nefazodone* (Phenylpiperazine)	$5\text{-}HT_1$ & $5\text{-}HT_2$ receptor antagonist. Weak 5HT and NA reuptake inhibition.	Nausea, dose dependent anti-muscarinic action, bradycardia, low BP, somnolence, hepatotoxicity	Inhibits hepatic metabolism of several drugs.
Mirtazapine* (Tetracyclic-piperazinoazepine)	Antagonism of $5\text{-}HT_{2A}$, $5\text{-}HT_3$ and central presynaptic alpha-2 adrenergic receptors. High affinity for H_1-receptors.	Increased appetite and weight gain, marked sedation	Few
Reboxetine (alpha-aril-oxy-benzyl derivative of morpholine)	Selective inhibitor of NA reuptake.	Tachycardia, dry mouth, constipation, sexual dysfunction	Few

* Postsynaptic 5-HT receptor blocking antidepressants

psychomotor overactivity in about 75% of the patients. The drug, however, does not exhibit positive activity in psycho-pharmacological screening in animals.

Mechanism of action: Its exact mechanism of action is not known. It could be related to one or more of the following:

(a) Inhibition of phospholipase C synthesis with resultant decrease in brain inositol triphosphate and diacyl glycerol concentration; this reduces the sensitivity of some neurons to the action of various neurotransmitters.

(b) Modification of GABA concentration in the brain.

(c) Decrease in the synthesis of DA and NA in the brain, and facilitation of their neuronal re-uptake; and

(d) Decrease in the function of brain protein kinases, leading to alterations in the release of neurotransmitters and hormones.

Absorption, fate and excretion: Given orally, it is well absorbed and gets distributed throughout the total body water. The drug is mainly excreted in the urine, the renal clearance being proportional to its plasma concentration. *Lithium decreases the sodium reabsorption by the renal tubules* leading to sodium depletion. *Patients on lithium treatment, therefore, should maintain adequate salt and water intake.*

Adverse reactions: Lithium toxicity is closely related to its serum levels and the therapeutic window is narrow. Hence, *the drug must be administered under supervision, with facilities for estimating serum lithium levels.* Blood levels exceeding 2.0 mEq/1 are associated with dangerous toxic effects. *Salt depletion from any cause including a diuretic, increases the renal tubular reabsorption of lithium and its plasma level, thus precipitating toxicity.*

- ***Mild toxicity*** includes diarrhoea, vomiting, drowsiness, muscular weakness, tremors and ataxia. Cardiac arrhythmias can occur. It can also cause allergic reactions, blurred vision, glycosuria and polyuria.

• ***Large doses*** cause sodium depletion cerebellar ataxia, epileptiform seizures, hypotension and coma.

• ***Chronic administration*** may give rise to goitre formation, hypothyroidism (rare) and abnormal ECG changes. The drug should be administered cautiously in the presence of cardiovascular, renal or brain damage. A reversible leucocytosis may occur.

• ***Embryotoxicity*** **:** Lithium is embryotoxic and increases the risk of Ebstein's anomaly in the fetus. *Because of toxicity, lithium should be prescribed only by a specialist who will also be responsible for its monitoring.*

Therapeutic uses: The principal uses are:

• ***To prevent the recurrence of mania and of depressive episodes in bipolar disorder***. Lithium salts are the first choice for long term prevention of bipolar depression.

• ***To treat acute episodes of mania***, where it is combined with an anti-psychotic like haloperidol.

• ***To treat alcohol dependence*** (Chapter 6).

The central features of the **syndrome of mania** are elevation of mood, overactivity with lack of need for sleep, and ideas of self importance. When mood is elevated, the patient appears cheerful and optimistic. *Elation is interrupted by brief episodes of depression,* characterised by low mood, poor appetite and insomnia. Manic patients are overactive; sleep is reduced; speech is often rapid and copious. Appetite and sexual desire may increase. The patient believes that his ideas are brilliant and that his work is of outstanding quality. This may be accompanied by grandiose delusions and occasionally hallucinations. However, most patients can exert some control over their symptoms, at least for a short time. The disease has a strong genetic propensity; about 50% of the patients have a positive family history. It is a highly recurrent and heterogenous illness.

Depressive and maniac symptoms sometimes occur at the same time. Patients who are overactive and talkative may be having profoundly depressive thoughts. Some manic patients may become intensely depressed for a few hours and then return quickly to manic state. The main objectives of treatment are:

(a) immediate control of acute mania or depression; and

(b) long term prevention of recurrences.

The immediate treatment is usually with anti-psychotic drugs, and haloperidol is usually preferred; chlorpromazine can also be used though it causes more sedation. They control hyperactivity and psychotic features of the severe mania. After initial large doses (IM, if necessary), the patient is maintained on smaller oral doses depending upon the degree of overactivity. Lorazepam may be used in severe cases to control over activity. Once the patient is able to cooperate, kidney and thyroid function should be tested and lithium treatment started.

Lithium salts remain the treatment of choice in acute manic state, and are generally effective as monotherapy in mania of mild to moderate severity. Lithium treatment should be used only in patients with normal sodium intake. Lithium carbonate is usually given initially in the dose of 600 mg. thrice a day. The maintenance dose recommended is 300-400 mg. twice a day. Doses are adjusted to maintain a plasma level of 0.4 to 1.0 mEq/1 12 hours after the preceding dose. As a prophylactic in MDP, the drug is used in the dose of 600-1000 mg. daily in two divided doses, 12 hours apart. *The drug may take several months to achieve its full effect.*

CARBAMAZEPINE : Carbamazepine is used as an alternative to lithium in the prophylaxis and treatment of MDP in patients who do not tolerate or do not respond to lithium. It seems particularly effective in patients who get frequent attacks (4 or more per year). It is generally used in the total daily dose of 400-600 mg., given in divided doses (Chapter 9). As a prophylactic, it is less effective than lithium.

SODIUM VALPROATE: This antiepileptic drug has also been reported to be useful as an

Table 13.15: Pharmacotherapy of bipolar depression (MDP)

	Preferred drugs	Other regimen and adjunctive drug
I **Acute mania**		
Moderate, euphoric	Lithium / carbamazepine + a benzodiazepine	Valproic acid +/– an anti-psychotic, either olanzapine or haloperidol
Severe, psychotic	Lithium / carbamazepine + an antipsychotic	Valproic acid + an antipsychotic
II **Depressive state**		
Moderate	Lithium +/- an anti-depressant such as an SSRI*	
Severe	Lithium + an SSRI*	*Levothyroxine in supraphysiological doses*
III **Long term prophylaxis**	Lithium or carbamazepine as monotherapy	Valproic acid + an atypical antipsychotic; *levothyroxine in small doses.*

SSRI = Selective serotonin (5-HT) reuptake inhibitors.
Levothyroxine is used *only* as an adjunctive drug along with other, definitive drugs

adjunct to lithium in the treatment of resistant cases of mania (Chapter 9).

Lamotrigine and **gabapentine** are also reported to be useful.

The atypical antipsychotic olanzapine and supraphysiological doses of levothyroxine have been used as add on drugs in severe and refractory bipolar depression. However, in such cases ECT is preferred because of its proven, rapid anti-depressant effect.

Pharmacotherapy of bipolar depression is summarised in Table 13.15.

St. John's Wort: This herbal product is derived from the plant *Hypericum portforetum.* Many phytoconstituents probably contribute to its action. Given orally, it is beneficial in mild to moderate depression. The ADR include G I disturbances, dry mouth, dizziness, sedation and confusion. It is a hepatic CYP 450 stimulant enzyme inducer and hence can reduce plasma levels of several drugs such as warfarin, anticonvulsants, antipsychotics and COC pills.

Treatment of Mental Depression

Mental depression is a major disorder of mood (affect) prevalent in a large percentage of the population and has a strong familial predisposition. It is a serious condition as it can disrupt the normal social life and may drive the individual to commit suicide. Hence, it is essential that it is diagnosed early as antidepressant drugs can alleviate the majority of depressive illnesses. Furthermore, such effective treatment can now be given at home by the family doctor.

Although there is no unanimity about the clinical classification of depression, it can be broadly divided into two main groups :

- ***Unipolar depressive*** disorders which involve major depression.
- ***Bipolar disorders*** (Manic Depressive Psychosis, MDP) : Patients identified as having bipolar disorders must have had mania; its management is discussed earlier.

Unipolar depression can be thought of as of two types.

(i) *Reactive, neurotic or psychological* depression, is an exaggerated reaction to adversity, manifested as gloom, unhappiness and tearfulness. It is precipitated by such factors as sudden monetary loss, failure in examinations or accidents. The individual blames the situation rather than himself. The emotional feelings are intense but there is no significant loss of self esteem. It responds favourably to moral, spiritual and social support from friends and relatives, who can share the problems and discuss the possibilities of solution. In many such **situational crises**, sedation by anxiolytics like benzodiazepines is sufficient to tide over the crisis. The patient improves with the change of situation.

Finally, the death of a close person normally results in a **grief reaction**, which resolves in course of time. Short term use of an anxiolytic can be helpful immediately after such loss; but their prolonged use may actually hinder the resolution of the grief reaction. If severe, the grief reaction may be complicated by depression, physical ill health and even suicide. The use of antidepressants in such a situation helps the depressive symptoms but does not help in the resolution of the grief reaction.

(ii) *Melancholic, earlier known as endogenous, depression* produces a varied picture. The dictionary meaning of melancholia is "a mental state characterized by dejection and misery". It usually occurs in the middle or later years of life. In its classical form, an individual suffering from this type of depression shows retardation in thoughts, movement and speech; he remains withdrawn from the usual activities. It is associated with early morning waking, occasional nightmares, feeling of guilt, anxiety and unworthiness. There is a tendency for self blaming. The subjects generally complain of various aches and pains, tiredness, loss of appetite, loss of libido, lack of concentration and loss of weight. *There is a greater tendency to commit suicide in this group*. Prompt use of antidepressants and/or ECT produces dramatic results in such cases.

Melancholic depression may have a biochemical basis in that it is probably closely related to decreased synthesis and turnover of brain 5-HT, NA and DA as well as an increased accumulation of acetylcholine; their relative importance is not clear. Patients who have attempted suicide have significantly lower CSF levels of the 5-HT metabolite, 5-Hydroxy indolacetic acid (HIAA) than those who have not. However, there appears to be no definite biological marker of depression. Hence, clinicians must rely on patient's symptom profile to assess the need for and choice of therapy.

The aims of therapy are :

(1) To reduce the symptoms and prevent suicidal tendency.

(2) To prevent relapse/recurrence of symptoms.

(3) To improve cognitive and fusnctional state; and

(4) To help in rehabilitation.

For the successful treatment of depression, doctor-patient relationship is important. One must try to create confidence in such patients. Nothing should be done to increase their guilt feeling. It is worth searching for possible external factors contributing to the depressive illness and to try to reduce their impact by modifying the environment or by psychotherapy (**Counseling**). This alone may be sufficient in mild depression.

From the various antidepressant drugs available, it is better to be familiar with a few rather than go for the unfamiliar 'latest' ones in the market. *None of the newer antidepressants appears to be consistently therapeutically superior to the TCA imipramine and amitryptiline except in a few selected subgroups of patients.* The choice from among various tricyclics should be determined by the side effects one wishes to avoid (orthostatic hypotension and anticholinergic effects) or produce (sedation). All tricyclic antidepressants are considered equally effective in uncomplicated, non-delusional depression. Considering their secondary psychotrophic effects, amitryptiline, doxepin and dothiepin are more sedative than imipramine whereas nortryptiline, desipramine and protryptiline have negligible sedating action. Patients with agitation or anxiety are best treated with a sedative antidepressant. Treatment with amitryptiline is often associated with substantial weight gain. *Imipramine/desipramine is perhaps the most suitable general purpose antidepressant,* particularly in young patients.

To begin with, imipramine is generally administered in a dose of 25 mg. bid and then increased to 50 mg. 2-3 times daily during second and third week respectively depending upon the individual response. Smaller doses are employed in elderly people. *Because of pharmacokinetic considerations, the entire daily dose of imipramine and amitryptiline may be given at bedtime.* When these drugs are given at bedtime, their sedative effect may eliminate the need for an additional hypnotic drug. However, some adverse effects may be more marked in some patients taking single large doses. No response occurs below a certain, critical drug concentration, and wide variations are known to occur in the serum concentration in different people on the same dose. *The elderly metabolize tricyclic antidepressants more slowly and may achieve therapeutic plasma concentrations with doses as low as 25-50 mg. daily.* Once the therapeutic dose has been established, the entire daily dose may be given at night. In majority of cases, improvement occurs within 4-8 weeks, but the treatment should be continued for 8-12 months. Some cases, however, may need lifelong maintenance treatment. This is because the risk of relapse after cessation of treatment is very high. Although some tolerance to the sedative and autonomic effects may develop the drugs remain clinically effective for long time.

Although the list of ADR following TCA is formidable, their incidence is not very high and they usually occur during the first few days of treatment. Anticholinergic adverse effects are the most common and are annoying, particularly in the elderly. If improvement does not occur after 3-4 weeks of therapy with recommended doses, continuation of drugs or further increase of dosage is unlikely to bring about further improvement. In such case, the use of an SSRI is indicated. The advantages of SSRI are that they are given in a single daily dose and they do not cause sedation or anticholinergic effects; hence, compliance may be better. They may be preferred in the elderly. *An antidepressant must be given for at least 4 weeks before it is judged ineffective*; in that case, a drug from a different class is prescribed.

Patients requiring long term antidepressant therapy are maintained on lower dosage schedules, determined by trial and error.

A less common adverse effect of all antidepressants is hyponatremia. It should be suspected in patients who develop drowsiness, confusion or convulsions while on antidepressants. Subjects with sexual dysfunction may benefit from trazodone or citalopram.

In general, TCA appear to be safe during pregnancy. They are, however, secreted in the breast milk.

MAOI, though faster acting, are clinically less effective and potentially more hazardous. Although it is claimed that younger patients do better with MAOI, these compounds cannot be recommended as drugs of choice. *Combination of TCA or SSRI with MAOI is hazardous and can cause agitation, convulsions, coma and death.*

A stable personality before the illness, psychomotor retardation and intermediate severity of depression with melancholia predict a good therapeutic response to antidepressants. Anti-anxiety agents like benzodiazepines (eg alprazolam) may be combined to lessen anxiety in early stages while a sedative like diazepam and flurazepam may be given at bedtime in those who complain of early waking. *Phenothiazines can be combined with tricyclic compounds in bipolar depression with accompanying agitation or psychotic symptoms.*

In severe cases with delusions, suicidal ruminations, marked retardation or severe agitation, ECT is preferred to drug therapy, as the beneficial results can be obtained more quickly. *A history of suicidal attempt or strong suicidal thoughts points to the need for immediate hospitalization.* Finally, safety of self administration of large doses with suicidal intention must be a major determinant in the choice of an antidepressant in these patients.

The relationship between depression and anxiety is complex. Depression can be precipitated as a reaction to severe anxiety. Both can coexist in a patient with neurotic illness, schizophrenia or an organic syndrome.

Although the drugs and other treatment can now achieve remarkable therapeutic results, the prophylatic effect of kindness from relatives and friends could be immense and the patient should be made to feel that he is useful to the family and community and not an unwanted, useless burden. Lastly, it must be realised that mild depressions are normal manifestations of cyclic variations in mood and they are self-limited. Antidepressant drugs, which are potentially toxic agents, should not be used indiscriminately as euphoriants in such cases. The important points to remember about depression are listed in Table 13.16.

Table 13.16: Important points to remember about depression and its therapy

- Depression is quite common in practice and limits daily functioning and well being considerably.
- It recurs in 25-30% of cases in one year.
- Upto 25% of the patients develop chronic depression, needing long term therapy.
- Many depressed patients receive no or inadequate therapy.
- Early dose reduction leads to a higher risk of relapse.
- Longer course of maintenance drug therapy is strongly recommended in patients with residual symptoms and in those with history of chronic depression or of several depressive episodes. The drug therapy should be continued for 3-5 years, even lifelong in some patients.
- Meta-analysis has revealed little evidence that any particular antidepressant or class of antidepressants is more efficacious than others, and the selection from among them is guided by their profiles of other actions.

Psychotropic drug combinations: Psychotropic agents possess varied actions and their combinations can produce dangerous drug interactions. Unfortunately, polypharmacy is widely prevalent and the number of combinations prescribed in practice is amazing. To quote Hollister "A single hospitalized psychotic patient often is given two phenothiazines (based on the unproved contention that a combination provides full therapeutic effects but only fractional side effects), a TCA (presumably because the patient may seem withdrawn or depressed), an anticholinergic antiparkinsonian drug (most often gratuitously, either in the absence of any overt Parkinson's syndrome or without awareness that the anticholinergic action of the TCA protects against EP effects), a hypnotic, such as chloral hydrate (for sleep), and a stimulant, as dextroamphetamine (to start the next day). The dangers of such combinations are:

- ***The opposing effects may attenuate the desired therapeutics effect;*** and
- ***The summation of the anticholinergic effects of phenothiazines, the tricyclics and antiparkinsonian agents may produce bladder or bowel paralysis, precipitate an attack of acute glaucoma or cause mental symptoms.***

The fact that many patients improve mentally when all such drugs are withdrawn may indicate that they were suffering from mental confusion associated with overdoses of centrally acting anticholinergic drugs."

However, the combinations should be prescribed only when they are clearly indicated and then strict vigilance maintained for possible drug interactions.

Psychomotor Stimulants

They are central stimulants with nervousness, insomnia and anorexia as the common adverse effects (Chapter 12).

CAFFEINE and AMPHETAMINE : Although these drugs stimulate the CNS and can act as "psychic energizers", they are not true antidepressants. They increase energy, alertness and confidence in some subjects. However, they do not correct the depressive state or prevent suicidal tendencies. In fact, they may aggravate them. Amphetamine evokes release of NA and dopamine and blocks reuptake of these amines. (Chapters 12 and 16).

PIPERIDYL DERIVATIVES: The drugs **pipradrol** (Meratran) and **methylphenidate** (Ritalin) have central stimulant effects intermediate between those of caffeine and amphetamine. These drugs, however, do not have peripheral sympathomimetic actions nor do they diminish appetite. Like caffeine they reduce fatigue and produce a feeling of well-being. They have no place in the treatment of depression. In large doses, they cause restlessness, insomnia, nervousness, tremors, palpitation, ataxia and even convulsions. Possibility of drug dependence is a drawback.

Therapeutic uses:

- ***Narcolepsy*** is a heritable neurologic disorder with varied manifestations which begin to appear in late teens to twenties. The manifestations are:

(a) Poor or disturbed sleep at night.

(b) Daytime Excessive Sleepiness (DES).

(c) Sudden, sleep attacks during any activity during day.

(d) Cataplexy : sudden onset of flaccid paralysis precipitated by anticipation, anger or surprise.

(e) Hypnogogic hallucinations : frightening hallucinations at the onset of sleep; and

(f) Sleep paralysis : paralysis on awakening.

The underlying biochemical abnormalities are believed to be :

(1) A widespread under-release of dopamine; and

(2) A brainstem specific hyper-response to acetylcholine.

DES and sleep attacks respond to drugs which block central, dopamine re-uptake : methyl phenidate (10 mg. 2-3 times a day) or dextroamphetamine (5-10 mg. 3-4 times a day), the last dose being given by 4 p.m. to avoid interference with night sleep. They (and cataplexy, see below) also may respond to **gamma-hydroxybutyric acid** taken at bedtime and again during the night. It is available as oral solution. The drug causes headache, nausea, dizziness, confusion and sleep walking. Its abuse has been associated with 'date-rape.'

Modafinil (Provigel) is a non-amphetamine drug which reduces DES and improves daytime performance. Its main side effects are headache, nervousness, dizziness and insomnia. It is a re-inforcing drug. It should not be used in persons with severe hepatic impairment. The dose is 200 mg (single dose) in the morning.

Cataplexy responds to TCA, imipramine or desipramine (100-200 mg./day), which suppress REM sleep, and to gamma-hydroxybutyric acid.

- ***Attention deficit hyperactivity disorder* (ADHD)** : This pediatric condition is characterized by inattentiveness and impulsiveness with or without hyperactivity, impaired learning and emotional lability. These children are easily distracted and accident prone. Psychomotor stimulants like **d-amphetamine, methylphenidate** and **pemoline** have beneficial effects when given over a period of 1-3 months. Methylphenidate is preferred. ADR include decreased appetite, weight loss, insomnia, tachycardia and abdominal pain. It is contraindicated in CV disorders, hypertension and glaucoma. **Pemoline** has lower abuse potential. It is, however, a relatively weak drug and may cause liver damage. Imipramine and nortryptiline are also used in this condition. Family counselling and psychotherapy are equally important.

Psychotogenic Drugs

These drugs, when consumed, produce psychosis— "a state characterised by maladaptive behaviour in which an individual reacts inappropriately to his environment" They produce depersonalization, changes in mood and a variety of effects on memory and learned behaviour. As some of these effects resemble those observed in psychosis such as schizophrenia, these drug are also called **psychotomimetic**; and because of their ability to produce hallucinations they are sometimes designated as **hallucinogens**.

Toxic psychosis is known following toxic doses of many pharmacological agents; but these are associated with neurological disturbances such as delirium, nystagmus and disturbances of equilibrium, speech and gait. Psychotogenic drugs, however, can produce psychotic states selectively, without delirium and neurological disturbances. The important **psychotogenic drugs** can be classified as:

- ***Indolic*** such as lysergic acid diethylamide, psilocybine, and bufotenine.
- ***Non-indolic*** such as mescaline and *Cannabis indica.*

LYSERGIC ACID DIETHYLAMIDE: LSD is an amine alkaloid, synthesized from ergot by Stoll and Hoffmann in 1938. It has some resemblance to ergometrine and possesses oxytocic action. Its central actions were recognised accidentally by Hoffmann in 1943.

Mechanism of action: The exact mechanism of the central action is not known. But, LSD is a potent agonist of central DA receptors, central 5-HT_{1A} autoreceptors and 5-HT_{2C} receptors; its hallucinogenic action is probably related to its 5-HT_2 receptor action. The drug also blocks peripheral 5-HT_2 receptors. However, there is no correlation between this peripheral blocking activity and the central psychotogenic effects.

Pharmacological actions: The drug is rapidly absorbed on oral administration and can produce its actions in doses as low as 20-25 mcg. Generally, LSD has a disintegrating effect on both inborn and learned behaviour patterns. Animal behaviour under LSD is known to be disorganized. Thus, under its influence, the garden spider produces a defective web and a fish becomes disoriented. Individuals under LSD effect exhibit marked changes in mood with emotional outbursts; they may laugh or cry on slightest provocation. It produces a blocking effect on the performance in various tests designed for evaluation and judgement. Motivation is impaired and activities such as writing and drawing become disintegrated and ultimately impossible. Many subjects experience a fear of disintegration of the self and hallucinations. The syndrome clears up after about 12 hours.

Associated with these behavioural changes, sympathomimetic actions such as dilatation of pupil, tachycardia, tremor, piloerection and hyperglycemia occur in man. These effects are probably of central origin. The drug may cause nausea and frequency of micturition.

Tolerance to behavioural effects of LSD is known, and a cross tolerance exists between LSD, mescaline and psilocybine. The drug causes psychic dependence. After a certain drug-free interval, the tolerance may disappear.

Adverse reactions: These vary markedly from species to species. In man, the margin of safety between effective dose and lethal dose appears to be wide. Sometimes, it produces suicidal tendencies. Although the psychotic changes produced by LSD are generally reversible, the drug can cause permanent psychosis and personality changes. The drug is also suspected to produce chromosomal damage.

Phenothiazines such as chlorpromazine can antagonise many acute effects of LSD while reserpine potentiates its actions.

Other agents chemically related to LSD such as psilocybine, 5-hydroxy-dimethyl tryptamine (bufotenine) and harmine produce similar psychotogenic actions.

MESCALINE: The alkaloid mescaline was isolated in 1846 from the cactus *Lophophora williamsii.* Its chemical structure was elucidated in 1918. The Red Indian tribes in Mexico and in North America were using this cactus as an intoxicant to produce ecstatic states on special religious occasions.

Given orally, the drug produces anxiety, tremors, sympatho-mimetic effects and hallucinations. The subjects get visual hallucinations of fantastic and brilliantly coloured figures, animals and people. They may get the feeling of floating in space with ever increasing feeling of dissolution. Beside such colourful hallucinations, the drug also produces delusions, depersonalization, disturbances of thought, excitement, restlessness, and intellectual and mood changes. The effects of a single dose persist for about 12 hours.

Uses: Both LSD and mescaline have been employed as an experimental tool to produce model psychosis.

CANNABIS (MARIHUANA): Cannabis is one of the oldest herbal remedies, known since 4000 BC for its therapeutic and recreational properties. It is obtained from the hemp plants, *Cannabis sativa* and *Cannabis indica.* The active ingredients are present in the resinous exudate of the tops of the female plant. The resin is known as *Hashish* or *Charas. Bhang* is prepared from the dried leaves and the flowering shoots while *ganja* is the resinous mass obtained from the small leaves and brackets of inflorescence. The term *Marihuana* is used to describe any plant part or extract containing the active principle.

The active principle of Cannabis is known as **Δ-9-tetrahydrocannabinol (THC)**, and synthetic derivatives of this have also been prepared.

Mechanism of action: Two cannabinoid receptor types (CB_1 and CB_2) have been identified. CB_1 is widely distributed in the mammalian tissues, with the highest concentration found in the brain neurons, particularly in the limbic system, cerebellum and the basal ganglia, and in the GI tract. CB_2 receptors are found in the cells of the immune system, spleen, tonsils and immune cells.

Pharmacological actions:

- ***Acute effects*** **:** These have been studied in man following the administration of synthetic THC. When smoked, THC is rapidly absorbed and effects appear within minutes and last for about 2-3 hours. Given orally, the onset of action is delayed upto 30 min–2 hours. The pulse rate increases, conjunctiva becomes red and BP may fall slightly; at higher doses, orthostatic hypotension occurs. Muscle strength is decreased; appetite may be increased, leading to increase in food intake.

CNS and behavioural effects vary according to the dose, the route of administration and the personality of the individual. There is an initial period of euphoria or "high", which is followed by drowsiness. It produces a dreamy state, feeling of well being, excitement and inner joyousness. An individual under its influence may become garrulous and hilarious, exhibiting un-controllable laughter even with minimal stimuli. Violent or aggressive behaviour, however, is rare. Time sense is altered and hearing becomes less discriminating. Vision becomes apparently sharper with many visual distortions. The drug causes depersonalization and difficulty in concentrating and thinking. Sometimes, it causes nausea, vomiting, increased urinary frequency and dryness of mouth.

- ***Chronic effects*:** The effects of chronic use are less certain. Some degree of tolerance is known to develop rapidly and a mild withdrawal reaction may occur; this is, however, not associated with craving or physical dependence. Some of the acute effects may be reversed; thus a decrease in heart rate is observed instead of tachycardia as seen following acute use. Heavy chronic cannabis users can develop an *amotivated syndrome*, with apathy and loss of academic performance in students. Such an effect is expected since cannabis is concentrated in the limbic system, the motivational centre of the brain, and also interferes with memory, cognition and psychomotor performance. Even social doses impair car driving ability because of distortions of time and space estimations, reduced vigilance and coordination; effects persist for many hours because the drug is eliminated slowly. Interestingly, the drug lowers intraocular pressure in some individuals.

Adverse reactions: Large doses of cannabis may cause an acute panic reaction, a toxic delirium, an acute paranoid state or acute mania. It seems likely that psychopathology may predispose to cannabis use rather than the other way round.

- ***Acute panic state*** is perhaps the most common psychic reaction and is characterized by anxiety, confusion and other unpleasant experiences. Occasionally it may cause a dissociative reaction, and depersonalization which may be long lasting.

Very large doses of cannabis may cause toxic delirium characterized by marked memory impairment, confusion and disorientation. Similar reactions are seen with many other drugs e.g. *Dhatura strammonium.*

A self limiting hypomania-schizophrenia-like psychosis following marihuana can occur. However, evidence for a specific type of psychosis associated with its chronic use is still elusive. Cannabis probably unmasks latent psychiatric disorders and that action probably accounts for the great variety of psychiatric reactions which can occur following its use. The drug can aggravate schizophrenia in patients controlled on neuroleptics.

Sometimes, the drug may produce "flashback" reactions in which events associated with drug use are suddenly thrust into consciousness in the non-drugged state. This phenomenon is most common with LSD and other hallucinogens, and may occur many months after the last use of such drugs. In case of cannabis, the reaction is mild.

- ***Chronic cannabis users*** may have decreased sperm production. Women may have anovulatory menstrual cycles associated with decreased LH. The drug may cause deterioration of glucose tolerance and aggravation of diabetes mellitus. 'T' cell function may be inhibited.

Chronic cannabis smokers, like tobacco smokers, can develop significant airway obstruction, bronchitis, cough and precancerous mucosal changes.

Therapeutic uses: Although cannabis possesses antiemetic, mild analgesic, muscle relaxant, anticonvulsant and sedative-hypnotic actions, it cannot be recommended for these purposes because of its adverse effects. Small doses of oral THC have been documented to be sufficient for appetite stimulation without causing serious psychotropic effects. Synthetic cannabinoid, **nabilone** (Chapter 40), is useful as an antiemetic in patients receiving cancer chemotherapy. So also is **dronabinol** which is synthetic THC (Chapter 40).

Although cannabis is illegal, marihuana is now firmly established as another social drug in the developed countries.

Rimonabant: For the uses of this selective CB_1 receptor antagonist, see below and Chapters 20, 39 and 63.

Endocannabinoids (EC): The first endogenous cannabinoid ligand was discovered in 1992 and named **Anandamide.** This name is derived from the Indian Sanskrut word *Anand* , meaning bliss, joy or tranquility. The other EC discovered was **2-arachidonoylglycerol (2-AG)**. They both are derivatives of the long chain polyunsaturated fatty acid, arachidonic acid, in the cell membrane (Chapter 24). Like "-9-THC, they bind to the G-protein coupled CB_1

and CB_2 receptors, and, as the classical cannabinoid CB agonists, exert almost identical actions.

The EC system appears to be a natural, physiological system, activation of which is believed to affect the accumulation of body fat, especially the intra-abdominal fat. The system, particularly in the brain, is believed to be relatively silent (turned off) in normal conditions, and is activated in special circumsatances. Anandamide and 2-AG are released from the cell membrane, when needed, and act immediately.

CB_1 receptors in the brain control appetite and modulate the hypothalamic neuropeptides to control the size of meals, and through the adipocytes, regulate lipid metabolism. Their stimulation by EC increases the food consumption. By acting at the hypothalamus, EC promote anabolic processes and inhibit catabolic processes. It is suggested that overweight and obesity in humans may be associated with hyperactive EC system . Apart from the CNS, the CB_1 receptors are also present in the GI tract, liver and adipocytes.

Rimonabant a selective CB_1 antagonist reduces the food intake and body weight, decreases plasma LDL-cholesterol and triglycerides, and corrects insulin resistance. Modification of the EC system by drugs may have therapeutic potential.

Drug Induced Psychiatric Syndromes

Psychiatric disturbances are often attributed to concomitantly administered drugs; yet, it is generally difficult to establish the causal relationship between the two. Such a drug-induced reaction should, however, be suspected whenever an unexpected psychiatric disturbance arises suddenly in a person of good previous personality, after a new drug has been consumed. The psychiatric reactions to drugs can be broadly categorized into:

- ***Delirium*** (acute brain syndrome, toxic confusional state): This is characterized by a fluctuating clouding of consciousness, restlessness, emotional changes usually of fear and perplexity and, in severe cases, paranoid delusions or visual hallucinations. The elderly are particularly susceptible. They may follow overdose or drug withdrawal, or may be due to intolerance to a normal therapeutic dose.

  Although many drugs can cause such states, CNS depressants (including alcohol), anticholinergics and cimetidine are the ones implicated most frequently.

- ***Psychotic states***: Hallucinogens such as LSD can induce a psychotic state with clear consciousness, paranoid delusions and visual hallucinations. States closely resembling schizophrenia with auditory hallucinations, thought disorder, aggressive behaviour and occasionally violence and suicide are seen with the CNS stimulants (cocaine and amphetamine), sympathomimetic nasal sprays, anorexiants and beta adrenergic agonists. Other drugs which cause psychotic states are beta-adrenergic blockers, anticholinergics, opioids, dopamine agonists, glucocorticoids and rarely NSAID.
- ***Manic states*** are seen with antidepressants, anticholinergics, high doses of corticosteroids, isoniazid, levodopa, dexamphetamine and clonidine.
- ***Depression*** can occur with antihypertensive drugs (reserpine, methyldopa, clonidine, propranolol and pindolol), levodopa, anti-convulsants, OC pills and cimetidine.
- ***Behaviour disorders*** that have been reported are withdrawal syndrome after cessation of benzodiazepines and akathisia during treatment with neuroleptic drugs. Pathological gambling and other compulsive behaviours such as compulsive eating and drinking have been reported in patients on non-ergoline dopamine agonists, particularly pramiprazole (Chapter 14).

Drug Therapy of Parkinsonism and Other Degenerative Disorders of the CNS

14

Parkinsonism as a clinical entity was first described by James Parkinson in 1817 (Parkinson's disease; PD; paralysis agitans). It is a syndrome of varied etiology and its important features are akinesia, muscular rigidity, postural instability, loss of associated movements and tremor. Excessive salivation, seborrhoea, depression and liver damage may occur.

Besides the idiopathic PD, arteriosclerotic and post-encephalitic forms, the syndrome is seen in hepatolenticular degeneration of Wilson's disease and can be induced by drugs like reserpine, haloperidol, triperidol, chlorpromazine and other halogenated phenothiazines. Point mutations in genes on several chromosomes have been reported in some patients.

Pathophysiology: The basal ganglia consist of the corpus striatum (the caudate nucleus and the putamen), globus pallidus, and substantia nigra. They modulate the extrapyramidal (EP) control of motor activity. The cerebral cortex and the substantia nigra pars compacta (SNpc, which is rich in dopaminergic neuronal cell bodies), both project to the corpus striatum. The latter, in turn, projects back via the globus pallidus to the thalamus and the cerebral, motor cortex, and regulates their involvement in voluntary movement. The nigro-striatal neurons make efferent connections with the striatum where they make contact with two types of striatal neurons: those bearing excitatory D_1 receptors and those bearing inhibitory D_2 receptors. The neurons which bear D_1 receptors relay impulses via a *direct (excitatory) pathway* (medial globus pallidus → thalamus) to the cerebral motor cortex to enhance stimulation by the latter of the spinal motor neurons. On the other hand, the neurons which bear D_2 receptors relay impulses via an *indirect (inhibitory) pathway* (lateral globus pallidus → subthalalmic nucleus → medial globus pallidus → thalamus) to the same cerebral motor cortical neurons to decrease stimulation by them of the same spinal motor neurons. *The excitatory segments of these relay systems are glutamatergic whereas the inhibitory segments are GABAergic.*

In health, the direct pathway predominates as the dopamine released in the neostriatum enhances the activity of the concerned neurons. In PD, dopamine deficiency, which occurs as a result of the degeneration of nigrostriatal dopaminergic neurons, leads to dominance of the indirect pathway resulting in a decrease in the stimulation by the cerebral motor cortex of the spinal motor neurons. This accounts for some of the symptoms and signs of PD. The dopamine agonist bromocriptine (see later) which is taken up by, and acts on, the striatum helps to correct this imbalance and relieves many, but not all, symptoms and signs of parkinsonism. Other defects may account for the unrelieved symptoms and signs e.g. degeneration of the noradrenergic locus caeruleus may contribute to autonomic symptoms and depression; and degeneration of the cholinergic nucleus basalis may account for the dementia which is common in these patients. Thus, the clinical features of PD can be explained by a combination of

- ***Dopamine (DA) deficiency***.
- ***Cholinergic preponderance***.
- ***NA deficiency;*** and
- ***Increased activity of GABAergic neurons.***

Initially, the dopamine deficiency is compensated for by an increased sensitivity of the denervated striatal neurons to dopamine. However, as the disease progresses more and more nigro-striatal neurons fall out. As no drug can halt the progressive loss of the nigro-striatal neurons, the disease is progressive and incurable.

In drug-induced parkinsonism, the DA receptors in the striatum are blocked; there is no deficiency of DA. Hence, the condition is reversible following omission of the offending drug.

Experimental administration of 1-methyl - 4 – phenyl, 1,2,3,6 tetrahydro pyridine (MPTP) to mice and monkeys results in selective destruction of dopaminergic neurons of the nigrostriatal pathway. This effect of MPTP is due to its conversion to a neurotoxic metabolite methyl-phenyl-pyridium (MPP) by MAO-B. The MPTP-treated primates represent the best animal model of PD. It is postulated that PD in humans may be caused by chronic exposure to MPTP-like substances in the environment, combined with effects of ageing and oxidative stress.

The aims of therapy in PD are outlined in Table 14.1.

- ***Relief of rigidity, tremors and akinesia*** : Most of the drugs reduce rigidity more than tremor and akinesia. Tremor, in fact, may be aggravated after reduction in rigidity. Levodopa ameliorates all the three. Tremor is best relieved by anticholinergic drugs. Reduction in rigidity and tremor allows the patient more free and easy movements, increases the mobility and boosts up his morale. Physiotherapy acts as a valuable adjuvant in such cases.

Table 14.1: Aims of therapy of parkinsonism

- Relief of rigidity, tremor and akinesia.
- Correction of mood changes and control of psychotic symptoms.
- Treatment of other symptoms; and
- Treatment of cause, when possible.

- ***Correction of mood changes*** : Most parkinsonian patients have a mild intellectual disability as a result of frontal lobe dysfunction. This, however, does not cause a major problem. Depression is often a marked feature of arteriosclerotic parkinsonism. If the primary drug employed fails to correct it, a tricyclic antidepressant may be helpful. A substantial minority of patients with progressive dementia are, however, difficult to treat and drug therapy itself may lead to hallucinations. Optimism is infectious and hence, the physician's attitude must be one of hope and cheerfulness.
- ***Treatment of other symptoms*** such as excessive salivation, seborrhoea and of complications like oculogyric or sweating crisis.
- ***Treatment of cause if possible***: Parkinsonism following drugs is completely reversible after stopping the drugs. Reduction in high tissue copper levels associated with Wilson's disease also results in some relief.

Successful management of parkinsonism depends on a multidisciplinary approach, and demands compassionate care of the patient. The various forms of treatment available are: (i) Drug therapy; (ii) Non-pharmacologic therapy comprising education, support, physiotherapy, nutrition; and (iii) Surgery.

Drug Therapy

The drugs used in the treatment of parkinsonism can be classified as :

I **Those that increases the dopaminergic activity:**

- ***Precursors of dopamine,*** e.g., 1-Dopa.

- ***Drugs that inhibit dopamine metabolism***
  (a) MAO-B inhibitors, e.g., Selegiline.
  (b) COMT inhibitors, e.g., Tolcapone, Entacapone.
- ***Drug sthat release dopamine,*** e.g., Amantadine.
- ***Dopamine receptor agonists,*** e.g., Bromocriptine, Lysuride, Ropinirole.

II **Those that suppress the cholinergic activity :** Atropine, and atropine substitutes such as benzhexol, procyclidine; and antihistaminics with anticholinergic properties.

Anticholinergic drugs help to diminish the cholinergic preponderance; further, some of them (eg. benztropine) inhibit active dopamine re-uptake in the striatum and increase the local dopamine concentration. In general, they are less effective but much safer than levodopa.

LEVODOPA (Larodopa, Levopa, Avodopa): Levodopa is a'universal antiparkinsonian drug'

$$(HO)_2C_6H_3-CH_2-CH(NH_2)-COOH$$

Fig 14.1: Levodopa

Mechanism of action: Levodopa, a prodrug, is a metabolic precursor of dopamine (Chapter 17). In the brain, it crosses the BB barrier by an active process mediated by a carrier of aromatic amino acids. This process may be competitively inhibited by a protein-rich diet. Levodopa is taken up by the dopaminergic neurons and is decarboxylated to dopamine. Levodopa can thus be looked upon as a 'replacement therapy' of sorts. Dopamine itself does not cross the BB barrier and hence is ineffective. In advanced PD, as there are few dopaminergic neurons remaining, levodopa becomes less and less effective. The peripheral (outside the CNS) effects of levodopa, are also mediated by dopamine to which it is converted in the peripheral tissues, such as the liver and the kidneys.

Pharmacological actions:

CNS actions: Levodopa improves all the major manifestations of PD. Akinesia responds first, followed by rigidity and tremor. Tremor may, however, be initially aggravated in some patients. Other manifestations such as seborrhoea, sialorrhoea and aphonia may also improve. The drug improves mood, memory and makes the patients more alert and interested in themselves and in their surroundings. The subjective improvement and the improvement in the general motor performance of the patient far surpass the more modest improvement in the conventional physical signs of parkinsonism. About 30% of the patients show 'impressive' improvement whereas another 30% show 'worthwhile' improvement. In general, younger patients with milder symptoms derive greater benefit than elderly, debilitated patients who may not tolerate full doses of levodopa.

Newly diagnosed patients who do not respond to 1.2 g of levodopa daily over a period of three months probably do not have PD. Improvement of parkinsonian symptoms arising from manganese poisoning has been reported. *Drug-induced Parkinsonism, however, does not respond at all to levodopa* as the dopamine receptors are blocked (see later).

Levodopa has been found to ameliorate idiopathic dystonia in children and adolescents.

Cardiovascular actions : It produces its cardiovascular effects by being converted to DA. Dopamine acts on the cardiovascular system by :

- ***Acting on specific dopaminergic receptors to cause renal and mesenteric vasodilatation*** which causes fall in BP following small doses of levodopa.
- ***Stimulating beta-adrenergic receptors in the heart (positive inotropic action)***; this effect can be blocked by beta-adrenergic blocking agents; and
- ***Stimulating alpha-adrenergic receptors in blood vessels*** to produce vasoconstriction. Thus, *large doses* of levodopa may cause rise in BP which can be countered by alpha-adrenergic blocking agents such as prazosin.

These effects do not occur following prior administration of a decarboxylase (DC) inhibitor such as carbidopa which does not cross the BBB.

Endocrine actions: Levodopa inhibits prolactin secretion and suppresses lactation by acting on the D_2 receptors on the pituitary lactotropes.

Absorption, fate and excretion : The drug is rapidly absorbed from the small intestine by active transport with peak plasma levels at 1/2-2 hours, and its plasma t½ is 1-3 hours. As more than 95% of orally taken levodopa is rapidly decarboxylated to DA in the lumen of the GI tract, liver (first pass effect) and other tissues, less than 1% is left to enter the CNS. Hence, large doses of levodopa are needed to permit enough to penetrate into the brain to raise its dopamine content. Pyridoxine accelerates its peripheral decarboxylation as the decarboxylase (DC) is pyridoxine dependent. This effect is not observed with levodopa–DC inhibitor combination.

The blood levels of levodopa can be increased by inhibiting the DC by using DC inhibitors. Since the DC inhibitors do not penetrate the BB barrier, conversion of levodopa to dopamine in the brain is not affected.

As high protein content of a meal interferes with the absorption of l-dopa, the drug is taken 1 hour before or 1 hour after a meal. Only in patients difficult to control, who need frequent doses and who have a fluctuating motor response, protein intake should be restricted. Levodopa competes with 'large neutral amino acids' for passage through the gut wall as well as into the brain. It is metabolized by both MAO and COMT. The drug is excreted in the urine partly unchanged and partly as dopamine and its principal metabolite homovanillic acid. Some of the drug is also converted to NA.

Adverse reactions : Almost every patient may show some adverse effect. GI and CVS reactions occur early in the course of therapy. Most patients develop tolerance to it. Behavioral and CNS effects occur during prolonged treatment, and as tolerance does not develop to these symptoms, they prove dose-limiting.

(A) **Early ADR :**

- ***GI*:** Nausea, vomiting and anorexia are common. They occur because of its action on CTZ and are minimized by taking levodopa with food, by increasing the dose slowly and by domperidone 10 mg. tid. Carbidopa, in addition to that present in the levodopa-carbidopa combination, in the dose of 25 mg. three times a day can help in resistant cases.
- ***Cardiovascular*:** It causes postural hypotension, generally asymptomatic, by its central action and this is not prevented by DC inhibitors. It can also cause palpitation, sinus tachycardia, increased A-V conduction and ventricular arrhythmias; these can be countered by a DC inhibitor and by beta-adrenergic blocking agents such as propranolol. Tolerance develops over weeks to postural hypotension as well as to its cardiac effects.

In view of its cardiac toxicity, the drug should be used cautiously in patients with history of MI and with ECG evidence of ectopic activity.

(B) **Late ADR :**

- ***Behavioural*:** This includes agitation, confusion, restlessness, hypomania, hallucinations, delusions and depression with attempted suicide. The drug exacerbates latent or active psychotic states, making it necessary to abandon treatment. *Patients with history of psychiatric disturbances should not be treated with levodopa.*
- ***CNS*:** On prolonged therapy, abnormal movements (choreoathetosis) involving head, neck and sometimes even the extremities may occur. They can be quite disturbing and even incapacitating. Unfortunately, they coincide with optimum therapeutic effect and correlate with the duration of therapy and the dosage. They are not prevented by a DC inhibitor.

Parkinsonian patients suffer from insomnia but do not complain of it because their daytime symptoms are more disabling. An improvement in their daytime symptoms can make them more aware of their insomnia which, in fact, neither improves nor worsens on levodopa.

A syndrome similar to the **neuroleptic malignant syndrome** (Chapter 13) can occur rarely after rapid reduction in dosage or abrupt discontinuation of levodopa.

(C) **Miscellaneous:** Some patients may show positive Coomb's test, though hemolytic anemia has not been reported. Blood urea nitrogen and serum SGOT may show a transient rise. Rise in plasma cholesterol levels and a decrease in carbohydrate tolerance can occur.

The urine is red coloured when passed and becomes dark on exposure to air or alkali. It gives a false positive test for ketone bodies with the dip-stick test.

Drug interactions : They are many and are listed in Table 14.2.

Anticholinergics, benzodiazepines, tricylic antidepressants, diuretics, oral hypoglycemic agents, antibiotics, glyceryl trinitrate, digoxin, propranolol and anti-arrhythmic agents may, however, be safely used along with levodopa.

Preparation and dosage: Levodopa is available as 100, 250 and 500 mg. tablets. The initial dose is 125 mg. bid. The total daily dose is increased progressively once in 3-4 days till satisfactory control is achieved or adverse effects appear. The majority of patients need 2-6 g. per day in four divided doses. As the drug has a short plasma t½, frequent dosage is necessary to maintain an even therapeutic effect and to minimize adverse effects. Most patients show a good response in 2-4 weeks but some may take as long as 3-4 months. *Concurrent administration of a DC inhibitor permits a 75% reduction in the daily dose of levodopa.*

Table 14.2 : Drug interactions of levodopa

- MAOI may precipitate severe hypertension. They should be stopped two weeks before starting levodopa therapy.
- Pyridoxine accelerates the peripheral decarboxylation of levodopa.
- Reserpine and phenothiazines block the effects of dopamine to which levodopa is converted and which is the active drug.
- Methyldopa intensifies the adverse effects of levodopa.
- Anticholinergics increase the stay of levodopa in the stomach and increase its degradation. They should be taken, if needed, 2 hours before levodopa.
- Sympathomimetics such as adrenaline and isoprenaline should be avoided in patients on levodopa.
- Levodopa increases the cardiac toxicity of halothane anaesthesia.

Decarboxylase inhibitors (DCI): By themselves, these drugs are inactive. They do not enter the brain. The concurrent administration of all DCI decreases the peripheral decarboxylation of levodopa. This endows certain advantages (Table 14.3).

Table 14.3 : Advantages of adding DCI to levodopa

- The dose of levodopa can be reduced by as much as 75%.
- Nausea, vomiting and cardiac effects are largely prevented.
- This permits more rapid increase in the dose of levodopa to optimum level.
- Pyridoxine does not antagonize the effects of levodopa.
- The control of symptoms is smoother and wide diurnal fluctuations are avoided; and
- The number of daily doses can be reduced without loss of control.

Postural hypotension, abnormal involuntary movements and psychiatric disturbances, all of which are central in origin, are not prevented or eliminated by concurrent use of DC inhibitors.

Carbidopa (methyl dopa hydrazine) and **benserazide** hydrochloride are the two DC inhibitors available in combination with levodopa. They are available as (a) **Sinemet** and **Syndopa** containing carbidopa and levodopa in the ratio of 1 : 10. Approximately 75-100 mg. of carbidopa is needed to totally block the effect of dopa-decarboxylase. (b) **Madopar** and **Benspar** containing benserazide and levodopa in the ratio of 1 : 4. The dose, expressed as levodopa, is initially 100-125 mg. 3-4 times a day; the maintenance dose is 0.75 to 1.5 g. per day.

The plant *Mucuna pruriens Bak* has been shown to contain levodopa and the crude seed powder has been used to treat parkinsonism.

MAO-B inhibitors :

SELEGILINE (Deprenyl, Elegin, Eldepryl): The two types of monoamine oxidases (MAO) are:

- ***Type A*** which causes oxidative deamination of noradrenaline and serotonin; and
- ***Type B*** which acts on dopamine in human platelets and brain.

Selegiline is a relatively selective, irreversible inhibitor of MAO-B. It increases the concentration and storage of dopamine within the striatum. Hence, it prolongs the duration of improvement brought about by levodopa. Further, it diminishes the diurnal fluctuations in physical strength and reduces the end-of-dose 'wearing-off' effects.

Adverse reactions : They are due to an increase in the incidence of central dopaminergic effects e.g. dyskinesia, nausea and hallucinations. As selegiline is a MAO inhibitor, the drug should be discontinued for some time before starting an antidepressant.

Its use with pethidine or an SSRI can precipiate serotonergic reaction. Selegiline is generally well tolerated in mild PD. However, in advanced disease it may accentuate the adverse motor and cognitive effects of levodopa.

Metabolites of selegiline include amphetamine and methamphetamine, which may cause anxiety and insomnia.

The daily dose is 10 mg., administered as 5 mg. at breakfast and at lunch. Administration later in the day can cause insomnia. Higher doses can cause inhibition of MAO-A as well, and should be avoided.

Rasagiline is another MAO-B inhibitor, claimed to be more potent and selective. Unlike seligiline, it does not have an active metabolite. Inhibitors of CYP1A2 such as fluoxetine and ciprpfloxacin increase the blood levels of rasagiline.

Clinical studies have indicated that the mortality due to hypertensive crises may be higher in patients treated with levodopa-carbidopa-selegiline combination than in those with levodopa-carbidopa combination. *Hence, newly diagnosed patients should not be treated with such triple drug regimens.*

COMT inhibitors :

TOLCAPONE: By inhibiting COMT, this drug reduces the central and peripheral, metabolic degradation of levodopa and prolongs its plasma t½. Given alone, it is not useful. Adverse effects reported are nausea, orthostatic hypotension, dyskinesia, diarrhoea, induction of hallucinations due to increase in the serum level of levodopa, and serious hepatotoxicity. It is used as an adjunct to l-dopa.

Entacapone, an analogue, is less hepatotoxic than tolcapone. Its action is primarily peripheral and is of shorter duration as compared to tolcapone. The main indication for this drug is to treat early 'end-of-dose' deterioration as it does not cause dyskinesia.

Dopamine releasers :

AMANTADINE (Symmetrel, Amantrel): This drug, developed originally as an antiviral agent, has been found to ameliorate akinesia, rigidity and tremor in parkinsonism. It acts by liberating dopamine from the residual intact nerve terminals. It also inhibits the activity of NMDA receptors. Its therapeutic efficacy in this respect is 15-20 per cent that of levodopa but slightly higher than that of anticholinergics. But, it produces a more rapid response (2-5 days) than levodopa and its dosage is easier to adjust. The drug is well absorbed orally and is excreted unchanged in urine.

Adverse reactions: These are similar to those of anticholinergic drugs whose adverse effects it potentiates. In general, the drug is well tolerated.

With larger doses, the adverse reactions increase disproportionately. In toxic doses, it causes convulsions and mania. (Chapter 57).

The dose is 100 mg. per day, increased to 100 mg. twice a day after 7-10 days. As restlessness is one of its major adverse effects, the second dose should not be taken late in the day.

Addition of amantadine in patients receiving near maximum benefit from levodopa causes little further improvement. The best way of using this drug may be to give it for 2-4 weeks at a time, as an adjunct to l-dopa; tolerance to it develops quickly.

Dopamine agonists:

Dopamine agonists used in the treatment of PD are summarised in Table 14.4. In general, they have substantially longer duration of action than levodopa and they are better tolerated. Their dose parkinsonism is higher than in hyperprolactinemia.

BROMOERGOCRIPTINE (Parlodel, Proctinal): This synthetic preparation (an ergoline) acts as a specific dopamine D_2 receptor agonist (Chapter 65). It crosses the BBB. Unlike levodopa, it does not have to be converted to an active metabolite. It is slower acting but less toxic than levodopa. It is used in the dose of 2.5 mg. bid to begin with, slowly increased to a maintenance dose of 20-30 mg. per day.

Table 14.4: Dopamine agonists used in parkinsonism

Drug	Dose
Ergot derived (Ergolines) :	
Bromocriptine (Proctinal)	30-40 mg/day
Non-ergot derived :	
Pramipexole (Mirapex)	Upto 4.5 mg/day
Ropinirole (Requip)	Upto 24 mg/ day
Apomorphine	Parenteral dose as needed, after priming with an antiemetic such as domperidone
Rotigotine	4-6 mg/day, transdermal patch.

All drugs except rotigotine and apomorphine are given orally.

It causes nausea by its dopaminergic action on the medullary CTZ. This can be treated by domperidone (Chapter 40), but not by phenothiazine antiemetics which worsen parkinsonism.

ROPINIROLE : This drug acts selectively at the D_2 receptors. Given orally, it is well absorbed and its actions are similar to those of bromocriptine. However, it is effective within a week or less. The adverse reactions include nausea (40%), somnolence, vomiting, dizziness and fatigue. It may cause sudden sleep attacks, postural hypotension, and rarely hallucinations. Pathological gambling and other compulsive behaviours have been reported (Chapter 13). The drug causes embryonic loss in animals.

Pramipaxole has properties similar to those of ropinirole. It has also been used to treat restless leg syndrome.

Rotigotine, an non-ergot of DA agonist, is available as transdermal patch.

All the dopamine agonists in large doses can cause severe neuro-psychiatric adverse effects. All ergolines can produce pleural as well as retroperitoneal fibrosis and digital spasms. Further, thickening and dysfunction of cardiac valves has been reported during therapy with pergolide and cabergoline; *they are not recommended in parkinsonism.* Pergolide has now been withdrawn from the market.

Anticholinergics: By their anticholinergic action, both atropine and hyoscine can relieve, to some extent, rigidity, tremor, hyperhidrosis, seborrhoea and sialorrhoea. Atropine substitutes are moderately effective and have been used for many years in the treatment of parkinsonism; they are often the only drugs patients can afford for prolonged periods. Benzhexol is discussed in detail as a prototype of the synthetic atropine substitutes.

BENZHEXOL HYDROCHLORIDE (Trihexyphenidyl, Artane, Pacitane) : Benzhexol is an effective and the most commonly used drug from this group. It has weaker peripheral anticholinergic actions and is well tolerated.

Pharmacological actions : The drug is useful in controlling muscular rigidity, tremor, sialorrhoea and seborrhoea. It improves the mood. In patients with excessive muscular rigidity; however, it may increase tremor while reducing rigidity. It does not improve bradykinesia and loss of postural reflexes significantly. Larger doses cause cerebral stimulation.

Absorption, fate and excretion: Benzhexol is well absorbed orally. It rapidly disappears from the tissues but its fate is unknown.

Adverse reactions: It is free from serious adverse reactions; however, atropine-like side effects may develop even in therapeutic doses in 10 to 20 per cent of patients. These include xerostomia, blurred vision, nausea, dizziness, restlessness and urinary retention in the presence of prostatic enlargement. Overdosage causes confusion, hallucinations and delirium, and may unmask / worsen tardive dyskinesia.

Preparations and dosage : It is available as 2 and 5 mg. tablets and 5 mg. sustained release capsules. The initial dose is 1 to 2 mg., increased gradually upto 10 to 15 mg. per day. A single dose of the sustained release capsule maintains the effect for 15 hours and may be employed after initial stabilization. The central stimulation produced by the drug can be countered by combining it with diphenhydramine.

Therapeutic use: Before the advent of levodopa, benzhexol was called a 'universal' antiparkinsonian drug as it controls, to some extent, all the signs. It can be used even in the presence of hypertension and cardiac disease. *It is effective in drug-induced parkinsonism* and is helpful in postencephalitic parkinsonism.

It is also useful in certain forms of dystonias. The other drugs used are listed in Table 14.5.

Miscellaneous: Certain antihistaminics (Table 14.5) used to treat parkinsonism also have anticholinergic action. **Diphenhydramine** (50-100 mg/day) is well tolerated, relieves rigidity but not tremor or sialorrhoea; it can cause drowsiness and giddiness. **Promethazine** (25 mg IV) is useful in rapidly controlling acute drug induced dystonic reactions, (Chapter 22).

Table 14.5: Drugs with atropine like action used in parkinsonism

Drug and Preparations	Dosage (mg/day)
Synthetic Atropine Substitutes :	
Benzhexol (Pacitane)	2-10
Cycrimine HCl (Pagitane)	5- 20
Procyclidine HCl (Kemadrine)	7.5-30
Biperiden HCl (Akineton)	2-10
Benztropine mesylate* (Cogentin)	1.5-4
Antihistaminics :	
Diphenhydramine HCl (Benadryl)	50 -100
Promethazine HCl ** (Phenergan)	25
Orphenadrine HCl (Disipal)	150-250

* A potent blocker of re-uptake of dopamine. Has a prolonged action and a sedative effect

** Useful IV, in rapidly controlling drug-induced acute dystonic reactions.

Other doses are oral.

Management of Parkinsonism

Introduction of levodopa was a landmark in the therapy of Parkinson's disease. Unlike the older drugs, it alleviates all the three cardinal features of this disease, namely rigidity, tremor and akinesia. ***Levodopa** still remains the most effective drug in the treatment of Parkinson's disease.* However, the variety and frequency of adverse effects, making continued close supervision mandatory, and the high cost put serious limitations on its routine use in all cases.

Many patients derive substantial benefit from l-dopa over the entire course of their illness. Levodopa increases life expectancy in patients with PD, and survival is significantly reduced if the administration is delayed until greater disability develops. Hence, some authorities advocate early treatment with l-dopa or dopamine agonist such as ropinirole to provide improved quality of life. However, they are expensive. Levodopa with a DC inhibitor is the only drug that promotes active life, and should be prescribed for patients who are incapacitated by restricted locomotion due to severe disease. The drug is preferred in the elderly patients (more than 70) who tolerate the anticholinergics poorly.

The major drawback of long term levodopa treatment is the occurrence of dyskinesias and rapid fluctuations in motor strength. New symptoms develop that may be resistant to levodopa. Younger patients develop fluctuations and dyskinesia to a more severe degree and sooner than the older patients. Motor complications include (a) ***Predictable* 'off' periods of immobility** or greater severity of parkinsonian signs, when the medication effect 'wears off'. This can be defined as perception of loss of mobility or dexterity usually taking place gradually over a period of minutes and having a relation to the timing of the antiparkinsonian medication; this can be helped by a COMT inhibitor (entacapone) and (b) ***Unpredictable* 'on-off' fluctuations** which are of sudden occurrence (lasting seconds) of shifts between on and off periods that are apparently not related to the timing of antiparkinsonian medication. With the passage of time, 60% of initial responders starts experiencing 'end-of-dose' wearing effect (advanced disease).

The psychiatric complications of levodopa are due to the stimulant action of levodopa on dopamine receptors in the mesolimbic and mesocortical dopamine systems. An atypical neuroleptic such as clozapine may be helpful.

Parkinsonism due to generalised degenerative brain disease and postencephalitic paskinsonism responds less well than PD to levodopa.

Bromocriptine and similar dopamine agonists though useful, have limited efficacy. About 1/3rd of the patients have a good response to these drugs and may not need l-dopa for 3-5 years. Their advantage is that these patients do not have fluctuations or dyskinesias till l-dopa is added. However, with prolonged use, their effect diminishes. Non-ergot dopamine agonists may be preferred to levodopa as they are both better tolerated and less toxic.

The synthetic atropine substitutes are still important in the treatment of parkinsonism, benzhexol being the most effective. They, in combination with physiotherapy, may be sufficient and cost effective in the relatively inactive patients with minimal disease and no functional impairment. They are particularly well tolerated by and hence preferred in the 'younger' patients (less than 50 years of age), in whom cognitive impairment is rare. However early levodopa-carbidopa therapy (see below) is indicated even in these younger patients if rapid response is essential for some reason.

Treatment with benzhexol should be started with a small dose and increased gradually. *As maximally tolerated doses do not give much more benefit than slightly smaller and better tolerated doses, no attempt should be made to push the dose to the limit of tolerance.* Some patients do not improve adequately on this drug or the initial improvement is lost due to the development of tolerance. In such cases, another synthetic atropine substitute should be tried or a drug from the other groups (antihistaminics or levodopa) may be added to benzhexol. The change over to a new drug should be gradual and overlapping. Anticholinergics may be used in combination with either amantadine or levodopa. *It is, however, best to avoid combining an anticholinergic agent and levodopa if there is history of psychosis or dementia.*

The antihistaminic diphenhydramine is particularly useful in elderly patients with mild disease, who cannot tolerate the anticholinergic drugs. Further, they help to counter the insomnia in patients on levodopa or anticholinergics.

Disease-slowing benefit observed following selegiline given initially is now thought to be due to the amelioration of symptoms. *The initial effect following selegiline was not substained and the drug did not delay the development of dyskinesias.*

Amantadine is a useful alternative to anticholinergic drugs in patients with mild PD. It can also be used as an adjunct in patients who are unable to tolerate levodopa.

The treatment strategies in PD are outlined in Table 14.6. The patient must be warned against the sudden cessation of therapy as this may prove fatal. Acute infections and surgery tend to cause rapid deterioration in the patient's health. Hence, surgery should be avoided unless it is absolutely necessary. Further, levodopa should be continued post-operatively and during an infectious illness.

Table 14.6: Treatment strategies in PD

- Therapy is initiated only when the manifestations of the disease begin to interfere with daily life.
- Selegiline with or without an anti-cholinergic may be used in mild cases.
- In patients under 70, with intact cognitive function, dopamine agonist are used. Anticholinergics can be used as an alternative.
- In younger patients with severe disease, add levodopa with or without amantadine.
- In patients over 70, start treatment with levodopa or a non-ergot dopamine agonist.
- In patients over 70 and in those with dementia, avoid anticholinergics.

Symptomatic treatment : Regular treatment with the standard drug therapy can prevent oculogyric crises which are rare except in post-encephalitic parkinsonism. Addition of dexamphetamine in the dose of 5 -10 mg. once or twice daily offers additional protection against oculogyric crises; *but, dexamphetamine must not be used along with levodopa.* Orphenadrine and trihexyphenidyl are effective in preventing and treating the rarer sweating crises.

Depression is common in PD and can occur especially in patients on levodopa. It can be treated with an antidepressant. If a patient develops an organic, confusional state or psychosis, the drug therapy should be discontinued in the following order : anticholinergics, selegiline, amantidine, and dopa agonists. Finally, the dose of levodopa should be gradually tapered. If psychosis persists, the use of antipsychotics is indicated.

Sialorrhoea is usually controlled by atropine substitutes. If dryness of the mouth is bothersome, it can be relieved by the use of hard candy. Paralysis of accommodation responds well to daily instillation of 0.5% physostigmine eye drops and seborrhoea to local therapy (Chapter 70).

Limitations of drug therapy :

- ***Drugs do not cure the disease nor retard its progression.*** All that can be expected is 20 to 70 per cent symptomatic improvement in 60-80 per cent of the patients. Tremor is not much helped by drugs except 1-dopa.
- ***Tolerance develops to most of the drugs.***
- ***Drugs with prominent anti-cholinergic actions must be used cautiously*** in patients with glaucoma and prostatic enlargement.
- ***Levodopa is not recommended during pregnancy, lactation or in children below 18 years.***
- ***Levodopa therapy is expensive***, has many adverse effects and needs regular supervision.

Education of the patient and his family is important to ensure **compliance** and **emotional and social support** to the patient. **Exercise,** especially stretching and strengthening exercises, can prevent or alleviate secondary orthopedic effects of rigidity and flexed posture such as shoulder, hip, and back pain, and may improve function in some motor tasks. The other useful exercises are brisk walking, swimming and aquatic aerobic exercises.

Nutrition : High fibre diet and adequate hydration can prevent constipation. Large, high fat meals which slow gastric emptying and interfere with drug absorption should be avoided. Dietary protein restriction becomes necessary in some patients with advanced disease and motor fluctuations in whom competition with amino acids interferes with L-dopa absorption.

Surgery : Thalamotomy, pallidotomy and deep-brain stimulation with implanted electrodes may benefit patients under 50 who suffer from severe symptoms unresponsive to drugs. Attempts are being made to transplant stem cells into the substantia nigra.

Drug Therapy of Other Extrapyramidal Syndromes

- ***Tremor*** : Propranolol in the total daily dose of 30-120 mg. is helpful in alleviating essential tremor and that due to anxiety and thyrotoxicosis; cardioselective β blockers are less effective. Primidone (in the total daily dose of 125-500 mg.) is also helpful in relieving essential tremor. It may be combined with propranolol in resistant cases.
- ***Chorea*** : Levodopa is palliative for short periods in juvenile onset Huntington's chorea; it aggravates the adult-onset disease; the latter benefits from the use of D_2 receptor blocking antipsychotic drugs such as haloperidol.
- ***Dystonias*** : A variety of drugs (trihexyphenidyl, carbamazepine, diazepam) have been tried with variable results. For the use of botulinum toxin type A, in muscle spasticity see Chapter 21.
- ***Myoclonus*** : Valproic acid, clonazepam and a combination of l-5-hydroxytryptophan with carbidopa have been reported to alleviate myoclonus.

Drug-induced Extrapyramidal Reactions (EPR)

Certain drugs used in therapeutics (phenothiazines, butyrophenones, thioxanthenes, metoclopramide, reserpine, methyldopa and levodopa) cause a variety of extra-pyramidal reactions. These reactions can be broadly grouped into four syndromes :

- ***Parkinsonism***: It is almost indistinguishable from idiopathic parkinsonism but tremor is an infrequent feature. It has been reported with all drugs mentioned above except levodopa. *Drug induced parkinsonism is treated by adding a synthetic atropine substitute and possibly withdrawing the offending agent. Levodopa is not effective.*
- ***Akathisia*** (not to sit) : In this syndrome, the patient exhibits a compulsive motor restlessness, is constantly on the move and is apprehensive. It needs to be distinguished from psychotic agitation which it resembles, because unlike the latter it is aggravated by an increase in the dose of the antipsychotic drugs. It has been reported with the antipsychotic phenothiazines and with metoclopramide. The anticholinergic benzotropine and small doses of propranolol may be helpful.
- ***Acute dystonic reactions***: These are characterized by painless, spasmodic contraction of one or more muscle groups resulting in trismus, torticollis, opisthotonus or oculogyric crisis. They are seen mainly with phenothiazines, butyrophenones, metoclopramide and prochlorperazine. Acute dystonic reactions respond well to an IV injection of an antihistaminic such as diphenylhydramine 10 mg or promethazine 25 mg., followed by 25 mg. of the same drug orally.
- ***Tardive dyskinesia***: This syndrome, reported to occur late during phenothiazine therapy, develops gradually and consists of involuntary movements such as repetitive sucking, smacking of lips, grimacing and movements of the tongue and extremities. Old age, prior brain damage, schizophrenia and cerebral hypoxia seem to predispose to it. It may persist indefinitely after stopping the drug that caused it and is assumed to be related to dopamine receptor supersensitivity. There is no satisfactory treatment but it may respond to tetrabenazine, to some extent.

In practice, episodes of EPR can be prevented by (1) prescribing the antipsychotic drugs in the minimal, effective doses; (2) concurrent administration of low doses of benzhexol with antipsychotic drugs; and (3) using less toxic drugs such as benzodiazepines for sedation or cyclizine for vomiting. Anticholinergics, however, fail to prevent the development of tardive dyskinesia. Keeping a watch for the adverse reactions during therapy is mandatory. At the first sign of EPR, the dose of the offending drug should be reduced and if possible, replaced by a less toxic drug.

Motor Neuron Disease (MND) Drug Therapy

Amyotrophic Lateral Sclerosis or Motor Neuron Disease (MND) is one of the most severe degenerative neurological disorders. Both central and peripheral neurons are affected. The course of MND is rapidly progressive and the 50% survival probability after the first signs of MND is just about 3 years. The etiology of the disease is unknown. The currently favoured hypothesis centres around glutamate.

Glutamate is the principle excitatory amino acid (EAA) neurotransmitter in the brain and the spinal cord. Excessive stimulation of glutamate receptors (excitotoxicity) may cause neuronal injury or death in various neuropathological conditions. Experimentally, selective inhibition of glutamate in the culture medium results in slowing of degeneration of motor neurons. It is suggested, therefore, that a drug that reduces the effect of glutamate may help in MND.

RILUZOLE: This 2-amino-6 trifluoro-methoxy benzothiazole, when given orally, is rapidly absorbed and easily crosses the BB barrier. It is largely metabolized in the liver. It blocks the release of glutamate from the neuronal cells as well as the postsynaptic NMDA receptors and thus protects against the excitotoxicity of glutamate. Riluzole has anticonvulsant properties in animals. Further, it protects against memory impairment and degeneration of neurons in animal models of acute cerebral ischemia.

Clincal studies indicate that riluzole retards the progression of MND and increases the duration of survival, though it does not arrest the disease. The adverse effects include nausea, diarrhoea and elevation of liver enzymes.

Baclofen, tizanidine and **dantrolene** (Chapter 21) have been tried for symptomatic treatment of spasticity in MND.

Neurotrophic factors: These naturally occurring proteins have been shown to keep the neurons alive and healthy during embryonic development and subsequently. So far, three factors are being evaluated for the treatment of MND. If the initial results with IGF-1 are confirmed, then combination therapy with riluzole-like drugs may prove more effective.

Drugs and Memory

In recent years, attempts have been made to develop drugs for improving memory in disorders of cognitive deterioration such as occurs in Alzheimer's disease and other dementias.

Alzheimer's disease is a steadily progressive, neuropsychiatric condition that is mainly characterised by cognitive deficit and debility. There is a disturbance of higher cortical functions such as memory, speech, learning, thought, orientation and judgement. Consciousness is not affected. The disease is associated with degeneration of cholinergic neurons, particularly those extending from subcortical areas such as nucleus basalis of Meynert. There is also a deficit of choline acetyltransferase, the enzyme responsible for the formation of acetylcholine. This results in decreased central cholinergic transmission. Hence, drugs that enhance central cholinergic neurotransmission are currently used to treat this condition. These are :

TACRINE (Tetrahydroaminoacridine) : This anti-ChE drug acts by preventing the degradation of ACh. The drug readily crosses the BBB and is retained in the CNS for long time. Administered in the dose of upto 160 mg/day, tacrine improves cognitive performance in 15-30% of the patients. The drug is given for 2 to 12 months. The most important and frequent adverse effect is hepatotoxicity. About 30% of the patients receiving the drug have raised values of alanine transferase. Other adverse effects are similar to those of other anti-ChEs. (Chapter 18).

Donepezil(t½ 70 hours), **galantamine** (t½ 8 hours) and **rivastigmine** (t½ 1 hour) are the selective cholinesterase inhibitors used to treat Alzheimer's disease. These drugs are less hepatotoxic, but can give rise to GI adverse reactions infrequently. They are preferred to tacrine. Rivastigmine is also available as transdermal patches.

Memantine is a non-competitive, NMDA receptor antagonist. It is believed to protect neurons from glutamate-induced excitotoxicity. Its usefulness needs confirmation.

Various vasodilators, metabolic enhancers (**Nootropics**), e.g., DHE, piracetam, estrogen, the extract of *Ginkobiloba* and antioxidants such as vitamin E have been tried in this condition with doubtful results.

The overall benefit of drug therapy is very limited.

Multiple Sclerosis (MS)

Multiple sclerosis (MS) is an autoimmune disease " in which CD_4 T cells and macrophages destroy oligodendrocytes which synthesize and maintain axonal myelin sheath in the CNS." It usually starts in early adult life. It is characterized by acute attacks which show at least a partial remission, and relapses. Pregnancy does not worsen MS; MS does not affect the course of pregnancy; but many of the drugs used in its treatment (see below) are contraindicated in pregnancy (Chapter 77). Genetic factors appear to contribute to its pathogenesis and, T cell migration to the CNS is believed to play an important role. The symptoms include impairment of vision due to optic neuritis, diplopia, sensory symptoms, a variety of motor deficits, bladder and bowel dysfunction, fatigue, depression and cognitive impairment. The diagnosis is clinical but MRI is helpful. The disease causes much disability, and shortens life expectancy. There is no cure, and the therapy includes: (a) **rest, physiotherapy and family/social support;** (b) **symptomatic treatment** e.g. carbamazepine and gabapentine to treat paroxysmal symptoms; and (c) **treatment with disease modifying drugs** e.g. glucocorticoids in pulse doses (Chapter 64) in acute attacks. They and/or the other immuno-modulators (Chapter 76) such as interferons (Chapter 24) and **glatiramer acetate/copolymer (Copaxone)** are used to reduce the frequency of relapses (Chapter 76).

Recently, two new agents have been used to treat MS with beneficial effect They are under evaluation.

(1) **Natalizumab,** a monoclonal antibody that blocks α_4-integrin-dependent adhesion of encephalitogenic cells and macrophages to micro-vessels in the CNS; and

(2) **Fingolimod,** a sphingosin1-phoshate receptor modulator which interferes with T cell migration, and thus helps to sequester circulating T lymphocytes to lymph nodes.

SECTION III
Local Anaesthetics

Cocaine, Procaine and Other Synthetic Local Anaesthetics 15

Local anaesthetics are drugs which, when applied directly to peripheral nervous tissue, block nerve conduction and abolish all sensations in the part supplied by the nerve. They are applied to somatic nerves and act on axons, cell body, dendrites and synapses.

Local anaesthetics are classified as :

I **Natural:** Cocaine.

II **Synthetic nitrogenous compounds:**

- ***Derivatives of para-aminobenzoic acid.***
  - (i) Freely soluble : Procaine, Amethocaine.
  - (ii) Poorly soluble : Benzocaine, Orthocaine.
- ***Derivatives of acetanilide,*** e.g., Lignocaine (Lidocaine).
- ***Quinoline derivatives,*** e.g., Cinchocaine (nupercaine).
- ***Acridine derivatives,*** e.g., Bucricaine

III **Synthetic non-nitrogenous compounds:** Benzyl alcohol, Propanediol.

IV **Miscellaneous drugs with local action:** e.g. Clove oil, Phenol, Chlorpromazine, certain antihistaminics e.g. Diphenhydramine. These are discussed elsewhere.

Local anaesthesia can also be produced by physical methods such as refrigeration, application of ice and ethyl chloride spray.

General properties of local anaesthetics:

Synthetic local anaesthetic drugs have many properties in common. They possess varying degrees of water and lipoidal solubility; since the nervous tissue is rich in lipid, lipoidal solubility helps the drug to move into the neuronal fibre, while water solubility helps to get the drug to the site of action from the site of injection or application. Thus, the local anaesthetic with high lipid but low water solubility will not be much useful because of difficulty in transportation through the aqueous phase surrounding the neuronal fibre. Chemically, the useful local anaesthetics consist of three parts:

(1) **A hydrophilic amino group.**

(2) **A intermediate chain;** and

(3) **A lipophilic aromatic group.**

Due to presence of amino nitrogen, these drugs are bases and form soluble salt with acids (pH 4.6). In the tissues where the pH is alkaline (pH 7.4), the free base is liberated and produces its pharmacological action on the tissues. They are thus dispensed as water soluble salts, generally as hydrochlorides (Fig. 15.1).

Majority of the clinically useful local anaesthetics are nitrogen containing compounds either in the form of esters e.g. procaine, or amides e.g. lidocaine and cinchocaines; their generic name ends with the suffix 'caine'. Non-nitrogenous compounds with local anaesthetic properties like benzyl alcohol have their generic names ending with suffix 'ol', e.g., propanediol, cyclohexanol.

Mechanism of action: Local anaesthetics block both the generation and the conduction of the nerve impulse. They bind to receptors near

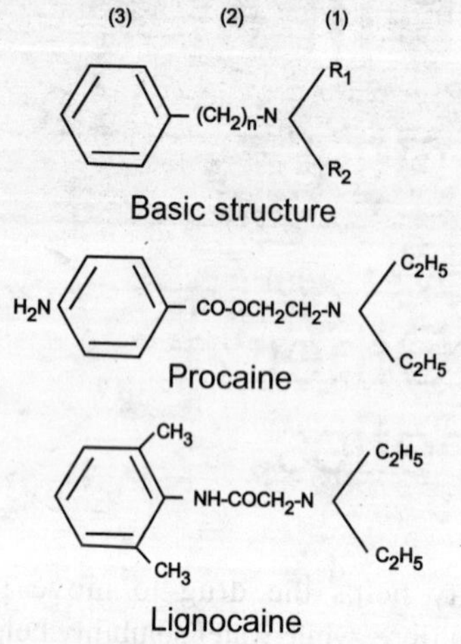

(3) (2) (1)

R_1

—$(CH_2)_n$-N

R_2

Basic structure

H_2N — $CO-OCH_2CH_2-N$ (C_2H_5)(C_2H_5)

Procaine

CH_3 — $NH-COCH_2-N$ (C_2H_5)(C_2H_5) — CH_3

Lignocaine

Fig. 15.1: Structure of local anaesthetics

the intracellular end of the voltage gated sodium channels. *This prevents the increase in permeability of the cell membrane to Na^+ ion, which is the first event in depolarization* (**Sodium Channel Block**) Thus, an action potential is not generated. This action affecting the process of depolarization, leading to failure of propagation of an impulse without affecting the resting potential, is known as '*membrane stabilizing effect*'. Increased extracellular calcium antagonizes the action of local anaesthetics on nerves and muscles, while potassium facilitates the same.

A smaller nerve fibre presents a greater surface area per unit volume for the action of an anaesthetic than a larger fibre. Smaller fibres are, therefore, blocked first. Thus, the various fibres are blocked in the following order :

- ***Autonomic fibres.***
- ***Sensory fibres conducting temperature and pain.***
- ***Sensory fibres carrying touch, pressure and vibration sensations***; and
- ***Motor fibres.***

Recovery of function occurs in the reverse order.

Local anaesthetics are less effective when injected into an inflamed area. The exact cause for this phenomenon is not known.

Pharmacological actions: Besides the local anaesthetic properties, cocaine and the other nitrogenous synthetic substitutes have important actions on other systems.

- ***Central nervous system*:** The CNS is stimulated, producing restlessness, tremors and in toxic doses, convulsions. Central stimulation is followed by depression; death is usually due to respiratory depression.

Cocaine in smaller doses acts more prominently on the higher centres causing euphoria, mental alertness and hallucinations (see later).

- ***Cardiovascular system*:** These drugs are myocardiac depressants. The heart rate and the amplitude of contraction are decreased, the excitability threshold and the refractory period are increased while conduction is slowed (membrane stabilizing effect). Higher concentrations produce change in the ECG and sometimes precipitate ventricular fibrillation or cardiac arrest. Procainamide (related to procaine) and lignocaine are used therapeutically for their cardiac depressant properties (Chapter 27).

Excepting cocaine, which is rarely used therapeutically, all the other drugs produce hypotension, by a direct action on the vessel wall; this property is related to their neuron blocking potency. Cocaine has a vasoconstrictor action.

- ***Other actions*:** Synthetic nitrogenous local anaesthetics have a direct spasmolytic action on smooth muscle and in large doses, they can produce neuromuscular blockade.

Absorption, fate and excretion: Local anaesthetics are not absorbed from unbroken skin. Applied to the mucous membrane, the absorption varies with the mucous surface. Thus, absorption is more rapid from the trachea than from the pharynx while it is poor through the urinary bladder. A considerable amount of drug can get absorbed from a raw granulating surface.

When used by infiltration, the absorption can be retarded by using vasoconstrictor agents like adrenaline along with the drug. It must be emphasized that a latent period of several minutes elapses between drug application and therapeutic effect. Failure to allow sufficient time for establishment of block may convey the erroneous impression that the dose employed is inadequate; this leads to use of unnecessarily large doses which may prove toxic and even fatal.

Many of the common local anaesthetics are esters and are metabolized by hydrolysis which occurs in both liver and plasma. The amide-like local anaesthetics such as lignocaine are degraded by liver microsomes. There is a species variation; thus, cocaine is largely detoxified in rabbits while it is excreted unchanged in human urine. Slowly and incompletely detoxified drugs would obviously produce greater systemic toxicity, if absorbed.

Local anaesthetics such as procaine, containing PABA as a component considerably decrease the clinical effectiveness of sulfonamides. Anticholinesterases increase the duration of action of procaine by inhibiting its degradation by plasma pseudocholinesterase.

Adverse reactions:

- ***Allergic reaction*:** This may manifest as a mild allergic dermatitis, a typical asthmatic attack or a severe fatal anaphylactoid reaction. It is generally seen with the local anaesthetics of the ester type and may show cross sensitivity with chemically related compounds. *Intradermal sensitivity test is recommended before using these drugs.* A negative response, however, does not rule out drug sensitivity.
- ***CVS*:** Fall of BP and cardiac arrest can occur sometimes. Hypotension should be treated with vasoconstrictor drugs such as noradrenaline and ephedrine. If the heart stops, external cardiac massage is indicated. During emergency, mouth to mouth breathing keeps the airway patent.
- ***CNS*:** This toxicity can be countered to a certain extent by preanaesthetic administration of diazepam. If convulsions occur, IV diazepam or IV thiopentone is used. Oxygen is given to prevent hypoxia; artificial ventilation is necessary in the presence of respiratory arrest.

In the presence of medullary depression, actions of local anaesthetics and barbiturates are additive and this can be dangerous.

Factors which determine the toxicity are :

- ***The rate of absorption, diffusion and inactivation of the drug.***
- ***Individual susceptibility.***
- ***Inherent toxicity of the drug.***

Prevention of toxicity: See Table 15.1.

Table 15.1: Prevention of toxicity of local anaesthetics

- Enquire about the history of allergy.
- Drugs should be given cautiously in the presence of liver and myocardial damage.
- Avoid food at least 4 hours prior to anaesthesia to prevent vomiting. Pre-anaesthetically diazepam may be given.
- Select the proper site; correct knowledge of the nerve course is needed before attempting a nerve block.
- Use minimal effective dose, well diluted, preferably with the vasoconstrictor drug, adrenaline. Avoid intravenous injection.
- Wait after injection; remember the latent period.
- Observe the face for any twitching, excitement, and pulse for tachycardia.
- Observe post-operatively for allergic reactions; warn the patient against using the drug again, if allergy is observed.

Therapeutic uses: The choice of the local anaesthetic for a particular purpose mainly depends upon the desired duration of action. Procaine is short acting, lignocaine and mepivacaine are intermediate acting, whereas tetracane and bupivacaine are long acting.

- ***Surface anaesthesia*:** Amethocaine is used as a surface anaesthetic for the eye, throat, urethra, rectum and skin. Similarly, benzocaine and lidocaine hydrochloride are used as all purpose surface anaesthetics except for the eye. Dibucaine is used for the ear, rectum and skin.

Proparacaine is used exclusively for the eye. Procaine is unsuitable as a surface anaesthetic because of its poor penetrating power.

● ***Infiltration anaesthesia*** : In this procedure the nerve endings are anaesthetised by their direct exposure to the drug. The drug is infiltrated subcutaneously. Procaine 2 per cent and lignocaine 2 per cent are most commonly used. They are mixed with adrenaline 1:200,000 to 250,000 to prolong the action. Lignocaine acts longer than procaine, but procaine is cheaper and more easily available. Adrenaline should be avoided when local anaesthetics are used to produce ring block to anaesthetize the digits or penis, in order to avoid local ischaemia and in patients with known myocardial disease.

● ***Nerve block or conduction block*** where the drug is injected very close to the nerve e.g. brachial plexus. Choice of the anaesthetic is determined by the duration of anaesthesia needed.

● ***Spinal anaesthesia*:** In this procedure the drug is injected into the subarachnoid space. Its level in the space is adjusted by using solutions with higher (hyperbaric) or lower (hypobaric) specific gravity than that of CSF, as vehicles. Usually, the injection is made 'heavy' by adding dextrose or 'light' (approximately isotonic) by adding saline. The position of the patient is also important in limiting the block to the desired level. Procaine and lignocaine are the most commonly used drugs. When the anaesthetic is injected outside the dura, the technique is known as **epidural anaesthesia.** In that case, the spread of the anaesthetic is restricted to a specific region and hence causes fewer complications.

Due to sympathetic blockade these drugs produce arteriolar dilatation, decreased venous tone, post-arteriolar pooling of blood and diminished venous return to the heart. The cardiac output is reduced and the blood pressure falls. Thus, *hypotension is one of the most important complications of spinal anaesthesia.* It is treated by:

● ***Elevation of the legs or wrapping the legs*** in elastic bandages to increase venous return.

● ***Rapid intravenous infusion of fluids*** for filling the dilated vascular bed; or

● ***Use of vasopressor drugs*** e.g. ephedrine or methoxamine to restore arteriolar and venous tone.

When used as spinal anaesthetics, lignocaine, tetracaine and other related compounds give good muscle relaxation and allow the use of cautery and electrical appliances during surgery. These drugs, however, are not suitable for surgery above the diaphragm and in apprehensive and mentally disturbed patients. Failure to block the vagus may precipitate hypotension and hiccough due to reflex stimulation during abdominal surgery. Headache, which is commonly observed following spinal anaesthesia, is probably due to leakage of cerebrospinal fluid from site of puncture and it responds to analgesic drugs.

Other complications include post-operative urinary retention and intestinal atony. Treatment of these is discussed in Chapter 18.

Systemic uses:

● ***In the treatment of cardiac arrhythmias*** (Chapter 27).

● ***As IV analgesics*** in the treatment of severe pruritus and pain due to malignancy; they are of limited use.

COCAINE is an alkaloid obtained from the leaves of the coca tree (*Erythroxylon coca*) and other species. It is the methylbenzoyl ester of ecgonine which is chemically closely related to atropine. Cocaine is not used as a local anaesthetic; but it is an important drug of abuse for its psychotropic effects.

Pharmacological actions:

● ***Local anaesthetic action*** : It acts on peripheral nerves as a membrane stabiliser (see earlier) and hence as a local anaesthetic. The concentration used to produce local anaesthesia is poisonous to many structures like leucocytes and tissue cells.

● ***Central Nervous System*** : It acts as a central stimulant. It blocks the reuptake of dopamine and causes activation of the dopaminergic system, leading to sense of euphoria (mesolimbic and mesocortical pathways), strongly reinforcing the addicting property of the drug. The euphoric effect of cocaine consumed by smoking lasts for 20 minutes whereas that following intranasal administration may last for 1-1 1/2 hours. Later, depletion of dopamine from the nerve endings gives rise to dysphoria so characteristic of cocaine withdrawal.

It impairs the homeostasis of 5-HT by blocking the uptake of tryptophan and 5-HT itself. This may account for the striking alteration of sleep-wake cycle and may enhance the central excitatory effect of dopamine.

● ***Cardiovascular system*** : It impairs the reuptake of adrenaline and noradrenaline by presynaptic nerve endings, leading to accumulation of these neurotransmitters at the synapses. This causes striking *activitation of the adrenergic system* resulting in hypertension, tachycardia and peripheral vasospasm.

Adverse reactions: These are:

● ***Acute***

(a) Allergic reactions.

(b) Activation of sympathetic nervous system produces vasoconstriction, an acute rise in BP, tachycardia and a predisposition to acute myocardial infarction, ventricular arrhythmias and convulsions. It may also result in mydriasis, hyperglycemia and hyperthermia.

(c) Sudden death after administration by any route. Since it is metabolized by plasma and liver cholinesterases, people with deficiency of these enzymes (liver disease), infants, pregnant women and old persons are at greater risk of cocaine toxicity. Most deaths are due to convulsions, respiratory failure and cardiac arrhythmias; and

● ***Chronic***

(a) Although at low dose levels cocaine delays ejaculation and orgasm and causes heightened sensory awareness, sexual dysfunction and sexual disinterest are seen in long term. Thus, cocaine is not a true aphrodisiac.

(b) Anorexia, emaciation, tremors, disturbances of sensation and emotion, hallucinations and insanity are observed in cocaine addicts.

(c) Cocaine when used by pregnant women may cause prematurity, intrauterine growth retardation and microcephaly. It has teratogenic effects on brain development. It can cause neurological symptoms including sudden death in the newborn.

Drug dependence: Persons dependent on cocaine show paranoid and suicidal tendencies. Cocaine is one of the major drugs of abuse and its withdrawal can cause severe CNS depression.

PROCAINE (Novocaine): It is the diethyl aminoethyl ester of para aminobenzoic acid. It is non-irritant and as effective as cocaine as a local anaesthetic, but is much less toxic. Its disadvantages are that it is poorly absorbed from the mucous membranes and, therefore, has no topical use. It is a vasodilator. Procaine is rapidly hydrolysed by certain enzymes in the plasma and liver and is partly excreted in the urine, conjugated with glucuronic acid and glycine.

LIGNOCAINE (Xylocaine, Lidocaine): This is the most commonly employed local anaesthetic. It is stable, can be stored for a long time at room temperature and can be autoclaved repeatedly. It has a quick onset of action and a high degree of penetration.

It is also an excellent surface anaesthetic. Its toxicity is similar to that of other local anaesthetics in equipotent doses. Following infiltration of 0.25 0.5% solution, the duration of action varies between 30 and 60 minutes. Addition of adrenaline (1 in 200,000) prolongs the action for about 2 hours. Analgesia is complete within a few minutes and recovery occurs quickly, within 2-3 hours after spinal anaesthesia. The drug is recommended for topical use, nerve blocks, infiltration and epidural injection and for dental analgesia.

It may cause drowsiness but has no vasoconstricting action. It equals procaine in toxicity in a concentration of 0.5 per cent but is probably a little more toxic in higher concentrations. It can be used in subjects allergic to procaine and other ester-type local anaesthetics. Its use in cardiac arrhythmias is discussed in Chapter 27.

Table 15.2 : Some injectable local anaesthetics

Drug	Infiltration	Nerve Block	Epidural	Subarachnoid
Procaine HCl (Novocaine)	0.25-0.5%	1.0-2.0%	--	10 %
Amethocaine HCl (Pontocaine)	--	--	--	1%
Lignocaine HCl (Xylocaine)	0.5 %	0.5-2.0%	1.0-2.0%	1.5-5.0%
Bupivacaine (Marcaine)	0.25%	0.25-0.5%	0.25-0.75%	0.5 - 0.75

(The figures in the table indicate the concentration of the solution used)

AMETHOCAINE (Tetracaine, Pontocaine) is a potent long acting local anaesthetic. It is effective when applied topically; its absorption from the vascular mucous membranes is very rapid and deaths have been reported following its use in urethra and respiratory tract. *It should never be used on inflamed, injured or very vascular surfaces.*

BUPIVACAINE (Marcaine): This local anaesthetic is about four times as potent as lignocaine and has more prolonged action (up to 8 hours). Its toxicity is similar to that of lignocaine but it is more cardiotoxic. It is used for spinal anaesthesia and epidural analgesia. It is available as 0.25% and 0.5% solutions.

Mepivacaine has N-methyl substituent in the place of the butyl group of bupivacaine.

CINCHOCAINE (Dibucaine, Nupercaine) is a potent but toxic local anaesthetic. It is not used for infiltration or nerve block anaesthesia. It can be used locally in the form of ointment and as light and heavy solutions for spinal anaesthesia.

Benzocaine is poorly water soluble and is used topically as ointment, gel or liquid spray.

BUCRICAINE (Centbucridine, Centoblock): This acridine derivative, differs from the commonly used local anaesthetics in that it has no ester, amide or tertiary amine group. The drug has been used in ophthalmic, dental and general surgical procedures in much the same way as lignocaine. Bucricaine has a longer duration of action than lignocaine. Further, the drug has some inherent vasopressor activity and, therefore, does not require the addition of a vasopressor for infiltration anaesthesia. Its CNS and cardiac toxicity appears to be less than that of lignocaine, and it can be used in patients allergic to lignocaine.

The concentrations in which various local anaesthetics are used are given in Table 15.2. An *ideal local anaesthetic* should be safe and efficient for the purpose it is used for; it should have a quick onset of action with sufficiently long duration, it should be stable, easily sterilizable and inexpensive. Associated vasoconstriction is desirable. However, there is no such ideal local anaesthetic agent.

Spinal opioid analgesia: Small amounts of morphine or a related compound fentanyl intrathecally produces analgesia without sensory loss. This technique is sometimes used for relief of chronic pain such as that of cancer. The same drugs are effective when injected epidurally (see earlier; and Chapter 10).

SECTION IV
Autonomic Nervous System

General Considerations 16

Autonomic nervous system (ANS) was so named by Langley (1898), because of the fact that unlike the somatic nervous system of the skeletal muscles, it is independent of volitional control and thus enjoys some degree of autonomy. ANS innervates the heart, the smooth muslces, the glands and the viscera and governs their functioning. Unlike the somatic structures, the structures receiving the autonomic nerve supply possess an inherent physiological activity and the nervous influences only augment or reduce the initial functional level. Interference with autonomic nerve supply, therefore, does not completely abolish the vegetative functions. This is in contrast to skeletal muscles which develop complete paralysis and atrophy following interruption of their motor supply. The presence of this inherent physiological activity appears to be a built-in protective mechanism.

The ANS comprises the **parasympathetic** (cholinergic), the **sympathetic** (adrenergic) and the **enteric nervous systems.** The parasympathetic system mainly participates in tissue building reactions while the sympathetic system enables the individual to respond to stress and prepares the body for 'flight or fight'. An animal can survive complete elimination of sympathetic but not of parasympathetic nervous system. Usually, these systems are in a state of dynamic equilibrium.

The control of autonomic functions is represented at all the levels of the CNS. The reason for this phenomenon appears to be phylogenetic. Thus, an animal or a man with the absence of entire neuraxis except the spinal cord is still capable of maintaining blood pressure and other vegetative functions except respiration. The autonomic functions are regulated through the reticular formation and its constituents, along with the cranial nerve nuclei. In the **hypothalamus**, the posterior and the lateral nuclei are regarded as being associated with sympathetic activity while the parasympathetic function is modulated by the midline nuclei. The thalamus, the centre and relay station for sensory perception, can modify the autonomic activity through its numerous connections. The limbic system is postulated to co-ordinate the autonomic reactions with emotions but the ultimate synchronization of the somatic and vegetative functions is undoubtedly achieved in the cortex.

The autonomic innervation, irrespective of whether it is parasympathetic or sympathetic nervous system, consists of a myelinated **preganglionic fibre** which forms a synapse with the cell body of a non-myelinated, second neuron, termed the **postganglionic neuron**. The postganglionic fibre in turn terminates in a synapse with the receptors of the organ supplied by it. The **synapse** may thus be defined conceptually as a structure that is formed by the close apposition of a neuron either with another neuron or with effector cell. The synapse merely transmits impulses from one neuron to another; the effect (excitation or inhibition) on the second neuron depends upon the type of neurotransmitter released and the types of receptor on which it acts. The synapse between the preganglionic and postganglionic fibres is termed as a **ganglion** while that between the postganglionic fibre and the receptors is termed the neuroeffector junction. Unlike the somatic synapses, the autonomic synapses are outside the cerebro-spinal axis. It must be emphasised that the synapse is a physiological and not an anatomical entity. Passage of an impulse across a synapse is carried out by the process of **transmission** while it is carried along the preganglionic or postganglionic fibres by the process of **conduction**.

Distribution of Parasympathetic Nervous System

The parasympathetic nervous system serves two important functions:

- It carries from the viscera the afferent impulses which reflexly modify the autonomic functions; and
- It supplies motor fibres to smooth muscle, glands, heart and viscera through its craniosacral outflow (Fig. 16.1).

Visceral afferents: The visceral afferent fibres are **non-myelinated**. They mediate visceral sensations except pain, regulate vasomotor, respiratory and viscerosomatic reflexes and co-ordinate the autonomic activity in general. The important afferents are:

- Afferents from the carotid sinus and carotid body carried through the glossopharyngeal nerves. Stimulation of these afferent fibres occurs as a result of local elevation of BP or decrease in blood pH respectively; this results in a fall in BP and bradycardia (**carotid sinus reflex**) and stimulation of respiration (*carotid body reflex*) respectively. Hypotension is attributed to a reduction of sympathetic outflow and bradycardia occurs through increased vagal tone. Respiration is stimulated by increased activity of the medullary respiratory centre.
- Afferents from the aortic arch, carried through the vagus nerve. Their stimulation also produces hypotension by reducing peripheral sympathetic outflow while the stimulation of chemoreceptors of the aortic body induces respiratory stimulation.
- Afferent fibres from the lungs, heart and the GI tract carried through the vagus. These afferents mediate visceral sensations. The reflex responses vary from hypotension (**Bezold Jarisch reflex**) to vomiting (afferents from stomach).

Craniosacral outflow: The craniosacral outflow, mainly efferent in nature, consists of

- ***Midbrain or tectal outflow*** through the Edingar Westphal nucleus of the oculomotor (IIIrd) nerve which terminates in the ciliary ganglion of the orbit. The postganglionic fibres supply the ciliary muscle and the circular fibres of sphincter pupillae (Fig. 16.1).
- ***Medullary outflow*** comprising para-sympathetic components of the facial (VIIth), glossopharyngeal (IXth) and vagus (Xth) nerves. The facial nerve supplies secretomotor and vasodilator fibres to the submaxillary and sublingual salivary glands and probably also to the lacrimal glands. The glossopharyngeal carries the para-sympathetic supply of the parotid glands via the otic ganglia, while the vagus provides secretomotor and vasodilator fibres for the thoracic and the abdominal viscera with the exception of the lower third of the GI tract.
- ***Sacral outflow*** consists of axons arising from the second, third and fourth sacral segments of the spinal cord and forms the pelvic nerves (nervi erigentis) which synapse near or within the bladder, the lower third of the GI tract including the rectum, and the sexual organs, and supplies secretomotor and vasodilator fibres to these organs.

The distribution of the parasympathetic nervous system is much more limited than that of the sympathetic nervous system. The terminal ganglia of the parasympathetic nervous system are usually located near, on or in the innervated tissue. Usually, a single preganglionic parasympathetic fibre synapses with a single postganglionic cell body of the same system. A notable exception to this rule is the vagus nerve, the preganglionic fibres of which synapse with approximately 8000 ganglion cells in the Auerbach's plexus of small intestine.

Distribution of Sympathetic Nervous System

The sympathetic division consists of the thoracolumbar outflow. The cells of the preganglionic sympathetic fibres are situated in the intermediolateral column of the spinal cord and extend from the 8th cervical to the 2nd or 3rd lumbar segments.

The sympathetic ganglia are of five types :

- ***Paravertebral.***
- ***Prevertebral.***
- ***Terminal.***
- ***Intermediate***; and
- ***The adrenal medulla.***

Paravertebral ganglia consists of 22 pairs of ganglia that form a lateral chain on either side of the vertebral column. The preganglionic sympathetic fibres emerge from the vertebral column along with the anterior spinal roots and end in the paravertebral ganglia as *white rami communicantes*. The ganglia give rise to *gray rami communicantes* which carry secretomotor fibres along the anterior spinal roots to sweat glands, pilomotor muscles, blood vessels of skeletal muscles and of the skin.

The first three pairs of the paravertebral ganglia are termed as superior, middle and inferior cervical ganglia which mainly innervate the radial muscle fibres of the sphincter pupillae, sublingual and submaxillary salivary glands and supply vasodilator and pilomotor fibres to the skin of face and neck. The sympathetic innervation of the lacrimal and parotid glands is doubtful. The fourth pair of the paravertebral ganglia is called the **stellate ganglia.**

The prevertebral ganglia lie in the abdomen and the pelvis. They are the coeliac, superior and inferior mesentric and aortico-renal ganglia. The postganglionic fibres from these supply the abdominal viscera, the urinary bladder and the external genitalia.

The terminal ganglia are few and are distributed in close proximity to the viscera such as urinary bladder and the rectum.

The intermediate ganglia are closely associated with the anterior spinal roots and lie outside the paravertebral ganglia.

A preganglionic adrenergic fibre may end in any of these ganglia. Thus, many of the preganglionic fibres arising from the 5th to the 12th thoracic segment do not synapse in the paravertebral ganglia but form the splanchnic nerves which mostly synapse into the coeliac ganglion.

The postganglionic sympathetic fibres from the upper thoracic ganglia (1st to 4th thoracic) form cardiac, oesophageal and pulmonary plexuses and thus end as arborizations in these organs.

The adrenal medulla is anatomically, embryologically and functionally a sympathetic ganglion. However, it does not have a postganglionic continuation and serves a secretory function. It secretes mainly adrenaline and small amounts of NA.

Enteric Nervous System (ENS)

The ENS, considered as the third division of the ANS, consists of collections of highly organized neurons situated in the wall of the GI tract. It includes the myenteric plexus (**Auerbach's plexus**) and the submucus plexus (**Meissner's plexus**). This network receives preganglionic fibres from the parasympathetic system and from the postganglionic sympathetic neurons.

ENS controls GI motility, secretions and the

mucosal blood flow. Stimulation of the ENS causes release of other putative transmitters, leading to relaxation or stimulation of smooth muscles. Some of the neurons have been identified as containing peptides (VIP), nucleotides (ATP), and nitric oxide (NO) which cause inhibition.On the other hand, noncholinergic, excitatory transmitters such as substance P, released locally, have also been identified in the enteric plexus. They play a modulatory role in controlling ENS functions. Some enteric neurons acts as mechanoreceptors or chemoreceptors providing local reflex pathways that can control the secretory and motor GI function without external inputs.

Although the adrenergic and cholinergic systems are traditionally believed to act antagonistically,their actions on specific tissues may be either discrete and independent or integrated and interdependent.Thus, they act as complementary in an integrated fashion on the male sexual organs to promote sexual function.

Neurohumoral Transmission

Transmission of an impulse across the synapse in the nervous system occurs mainly as a result of release of a neurohumoral transmitter substance into the synaptic cleft. Electrical transmission of impulses has, however, been demonstrated in lower organisms like crayfish and annelids; such an electrically transmitting synapse is termed **ephapse.**

Neurohumoral transmission:

Dubois Raymond in 1877 was probably the first investigator to suggest that junctional transmission could be either chemical or electrical, more probably the former, while Kuhne (1888) postulated that the motor end plate of the skeletal muscle was excited as a result of the action current of the nerve impulse. Elliott (1904), a student of Langley, suggested that sympathetic nerve impulses acted by

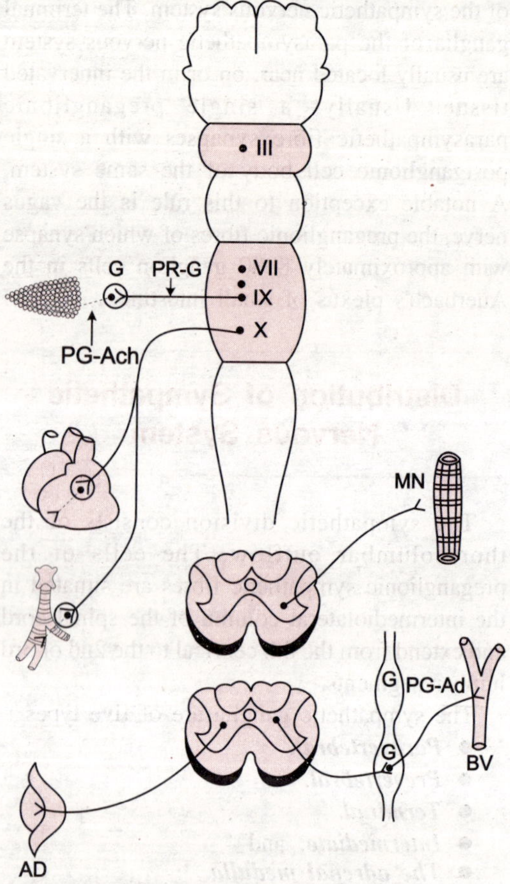

Fig. 16.1 : Schematic representation of the sites of release of neurohumoral transmitters acetylcholine (ACh) and noradrenaline. ACh is released at all the ganglia (G), postganglionic cholinergic nerve endings (PG-ACh), myoneural Junctions (Mn) And The Adrenal Medulla (Ad). Noradrenaline Is Released At Postganglionic Adrenergic Nerve Endings (Pg-Ad), Adrenaline Is Released From The Adrenal Medulla. Pr-G = Preganglionic.

liberating adrenaline at the nerve endings supplying smooth muscles. In 1905 Langley postulated the presence of excitatory and inhibitory 'receptor substances' in the effector cell and Dixon (1906) proposed that parasympathetic nerve impulses acted by liberating a muscarine-like substance.

The pioneering investigations of Otto Loewi (1921) and Loewi and Navratil (1926) showed that the vagus inhibited the heart by means of a chemical transmitter acetylcholine. Loewi allowed perfusion fluid from a frog heart (donor) to come into contact with a second frog heart (recipient). Stimulation of the vagosympathetic trunk of the donor frog produced cardiac arrest of both the donor and the recipient heart. As no anatomical communication existed between the donor and the recipient hearts, Loewi proposed that the arrest of the recipient heart was brought about by a substance released into the perfusion fluid from the donor heart on vagosympathetic stimulation. This substance was initially termed *vagusstoff*. Loewi presented evidence which established it as **acetylcholine** (ACh). He also noted that if the vagosympathetic trunk of the donor heart was stimulated after its initial atropinization, both the donor and the recipient heart accelerated. This led him to postulate another substance, released from the atropinized donor heart following vagosympathetic stimulation. He named this substance as *acceleranstoff*. Support for the release of an accelerator substance on nerve stimulation came from the work of Cannon. The accelerator neurohumoral transmitter was established as **noradrenaline** (NA) by Von Euler (1946).

The work of Dale, Gaddum, Feldberg and others led to the extension of the chemical transmitter hypothesis to the autonomic ganglia and myoneural junctions where ACh was identified as the transmitter.

Barger and Dale (1910), while describing the pharmacological actions of adrenaline and related substances, employed the term **sympathomimetic** as these actions resembled those seen following sympathetic stimulation; similarly the actions of pilocarpine, muscarine and related substances were described by them as **parasympathomimetic**. Dale in his later work (1914) used the term **Nicotinic action** to describe the ganglionic and neuromuscular actions of acetylcholine and **Muscarinic action** to describe the actions at the postganglionic parasympathetic nerve endings, because of their resemblance to those observed following the alkaloids, nicotine and muscarine respectively. Since the terms sympathetic and parasympathetic do not give any idea about the chemical transmitter at the nerve endings, Dale classified autonomic nerves as

(a) **Adrenergic**, which release NA; and

(b) **Cholinergic**, which release ACh.

A neuron can receive chemical messages at various active sites called **receptors**, three groups of which are considered important (Chapter 5):

- ***Soma-dendritic receptors*** located on the cell body and dendrites, when acted upon, primarily modify the functions of the soma-dendritic region such as generation of action potential or protein synthesis.
- ***Presynaptic receptors*** located in or near the axon terminals, when activated, primarily modify the function of the terminal region, such as facilitation or inhibition of transmitter synthesis and release (Chapter 5).

The presynaptic receptors are of two types: (1) **Autoreceptors**; and (2) **Heteroreceptors**. Autoreceptors respond to the neuron's own transmitter, and are involved in **synaptic feed back mechanism**. They are usually inhibitory to further release of the transmitter. However, somatic motor fibres of the cholinergic system have excitatory presynaptic receptors. The nerve terminals also have regulatory receptors that are activated by blood-borne agents or NT from the neighbouring cells. They are termed **heteroreceptors** e.g. AT_2 receptors on adrenergic cells.

- ***Post synaptic receptors*** are associated with the target organs/tissues (Fig. 16.3).

Neurohumoral Transmitters

ACh, NA, dopamine (DA), gamma-amino-butyric acid (GABA) and 5-hydroxytryptamine (5-HT) are considered as the classical neurotransmitters.

Steps involved in the synthesis and the storage of the **neurohumor**, its metabolism and its interaction with the receptors are potential points where a drug can act. The latter can thus mimic or antagonize the action of the corresponding neurohumor.

Table 16.1 : Sites of action of ACh

- All the preganglionic fibres of ANS i.e. at both the sympathetic and parasympathetic ganglia.
- The postganglionic parasympathetic nerve endings.
- The sympathetic postganglionic nerve endings, supplying sweat glands in humans and cats.
- The somatic motor nerve endings, supplying skeletal muscles.
- The nerve endings supplying adrenal medulla; and
- Between certain neurones within the brain and the spinal cord. Transmission from the motor neurone collateral to the Renshaw cells is cholinergic and the receptors are predominantly nicotinic. In contrast, most of the cholinergic neurones at higher levels of the CNS have predominantly muscarinic receptors.

Acetylcholine: ACh, an ester of choline, was recognised as an extremely potent pharmacological substance by Hunt in 1906. ACh acts as the neurohumoral transmitter at sites shown in Table 16.1.

ACh is synthesized inside the nerve fibre by combination of choline taken up from the ECF with an acetyl group. The acetyl group is obtained from acetylcoenzyme A, a product of the intermediary metabolism. The axon terminals contain a large number of mitochondria where acetylcoenzyme-A is synthesized.

ACh is stored in the synaptic vesicles and is released by exocytosis through the pre-junctional membrane. The coupling of choline with the acetyl group is catalyzed by the enzyme **choline acetyl transferase**. The synthesis of ACh by choline acetyl transferase is thus mainly dependent upon the continued supply of choline and glucose, the latter being essential for synthesis of acetyl coenzyme A.

It is hydrolysed into choline and acetic acid by the enzymes termed **choline esterases**. Two main types of cholinesterase have been identified:

- ***Acetylcholinesterase (AChE)* or *true cholinesterase*,** present in neurons, ganglia and at myoneural junctions, which rapidly hydrolyzes acetylcholine and another choline ester, acetyl beta methylcholine (methacholine) but not benzoylcholine.
- ***Butyrocholinesterase (BuChE)* or *pseudocholinesterase*,** present mainly in the plasma, RBCs, liver, glia and other organs, which hydrolyzes ACh slowly, but not methacholine.

The activity of the cholinesterases can be inhibited by the anticholinesterase drugs.

Noradrenaline and Dopamine: NA and DA are monoamines and act as neurohumoral transmitters at the post-ganglionic sympathetic nerve endings and certain regions within the brain. These amines are present in highest concentration in the terminal axonal processes of specific neurons, where they are synthesized and stored in the vesicles within the varicose axon terminals.

The enzymes participating in the formation of NA are synthesized in the cell bodies of the adreneregic neurons and are transported to the axon terminals.These enzymes are not completely specific as they also play a part in the synthesis of 5-HT.

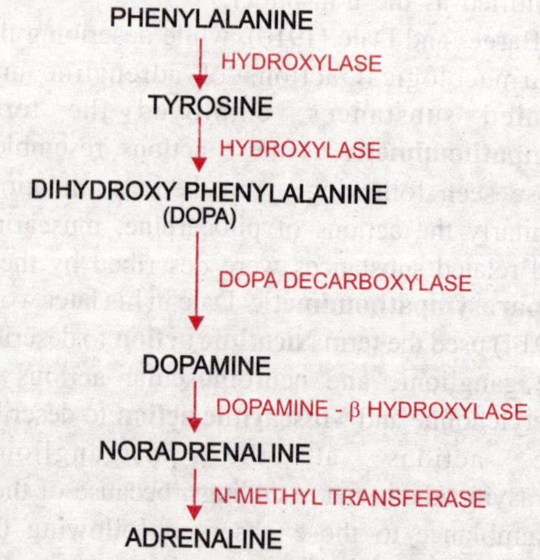

Fig 16.2 : Biosynthesis of catecholamines.

The three **catecholamines**, **dopamine, noradrenaline** and **adrenaline,** are sequentially synthesized from the amino acid phenylalanine (Figure 16.2).

The hydroxylation of tyrosine by tyrosine hydroxylase to DOPA and decarboxylation of DOPA to DA occurs in the cytoplasm. About 50% of DA is then actively transported into the vesicles containing dopamine-beta-hydroxylase enzyme, where it is converted to NA, which is stored as granules. Tyrosine hydroxylase disappears from the tissues if the sympathetic nerves degenerate. Alpha-methyl tyrosine and 3, iodotyrosine are inhibitors of this enzyme.

Unlike ACh, *NA released into the synaptic cleft is only partially degraded and a substantial part is taken up(reuptake) by the sympathetic neurons* (Fig. 16.3). The mechanism of NA metabolism is discussed in Chapter 17. The end-products of NA and adrenaline metabolism are excreted in urine in a free form and as conjugates of glucuronic and sulfuric acids.

DA is degraded predominantly by MAO-B in the brain and by MAO-A outside the CNS, and partly by COMT.

Adrenaline is formed in the adrenal medulla by methylation of NA and is stored in the chromaffin granules. The adrenline and NA forming cells in the adrenal medulla are two distinct cell types. Because of their unique blood supply, the adrenal chromaffin cells are exposed to high concentrations of glucocorticoids in the venous drainage from the adrenal cortex. Glucocorticoids cause induction of the enzyme noradrenaline-N methyl-transferase and thus control the rate of synthesis of adrenaline. It is released into the blood stream on stimulation of the adrenal medulla.

The hypothalamus plays an important role in the regulation of catecholamine secretion by adrenal medulla. Stimulation of the splanchnic nerves results in the release of ACh from the nerve endings which, by increasing the permeability of the chromaffin cells to calcium ions, increases the intracellular calcium and causes the secretion of catecholamines. Calcium is thus, important both for the release of ACh from nerve endings and for the secretion of catecholamines by chromaffin cells.

Stress stimulates the release of cortisol from the adrenal cortex (via ACTH) and of adrenaline from the adrenal medulla (via neuronal impulses). In addition, adrenaline secretion increases in response to various circulating substances such as glucagon, histamine, angiotensin II and bradykinin.

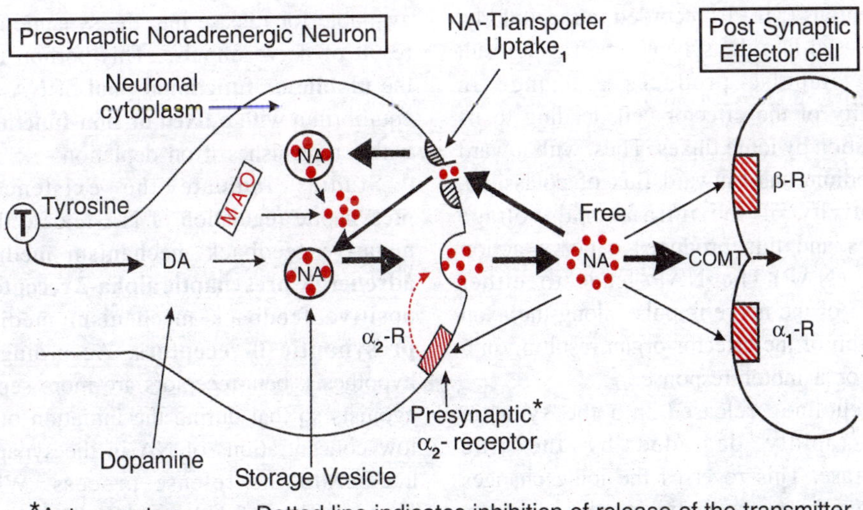

Fig. 16.3 : Synthesis and metabolism of NA at adrenergic neuronal endings

The adrenal medulla is innervated by preganglionic sympathetic neurons whose cell bodies are located in the spinal cord segments T_3 to L_3. People who have spinal cord transection at the level of T_3 or higher have reduced plasma levels of adrenaline.

Mechanisms of neurohumoral transmission: The space between the pre- and post-ganglionic fibres or that between the nerve ending and the receptor is termed the **synaptic cleft**.

The terminal portions of the pre- and post-ganglionic cholinergic axons contain spherical or oval vesicles, known as the **synaptic vesicles** in addition to mitochondria. The synaptic vesicles tend to be aggregated close to the synaptic cleft.

Acetylcholine synthesized by the choline acetyltransferase of the synaptic vesicles is termed **depot acetylcholine**. Approximately 25 per cent of this is released into the synaptic cleft from the vesicles as a result of nerve impulse. This is **releasable ACh**. Acetylcholine which is not releasable serves the function of replenishing the stores of releasable ACh.

Small quantities of Ach are released continually into the synaptic cleft and are responsible for the postjunctional miniature end plate potentials (MEPP) recorded intracellularly. ACh released into the synaptic cleft as a result of nerve impulse produces a change in permeability of the effector cell, leading to its depolarization by ionic fluxes. Thus, with inward flux of sodium and outward flux of potassium, the negativity of the intra-axonal voltage diminishes and this produces a nerve action potential (NAP).The NAP leads to either conduction of the nerve impulse along the axon or activation of the effector organ resulting in a secretory or a motor response.

Acetylcholine released into the synaptic cleft is rapidly degraded by the true cholinesterase. This reverses the ionic changes and enables the postsynaptic membrane or the receptor site to get repolarized.

Two distinctly separate but related systems exist at the level of adrenergic neuron. One is concerned with the intraneuronal amine concentrating-storage mechanism. The vesicles containing the granules have a vesicular monoamine transporter (VMAT) located in their wall; it has high affinity for NA. The other is a neuronal membrane amine pump (NET; norepinephrine transporter), responsible for the reuptake ($Uptake_1$ process) of NA following its prior release from the nerve terminals.

The maximum concentration of NA is found in the granulated vesicles at the adrenergic nerve terminals in the brain as well as the peripheral adrenergic neurons. NA in the adrenergic nerve terminals exists in several pools, the major portion, over 60 per cent, being present in protein bound form as granules. In the granules it exists with calcium and ATP. An action potential causes an influx of Ca^{++} into the axonal terminals with resultant fusion of the vesicles with the plasma membrane and exocytosis of NA. Its movement from the extracellular space back to the cytoplasm, however, involves active transport mechanisms. (**$Uptake_1$** in Fig 16.3). Thus, following a nerve impulse, NA is actively released into the synaptic cleft and binds to the receptors on the effector cells. Only a part of the stored NA is available for release into the synaptic cleft as a result of nerve impulse. This portion is termed the **mobile or functional pool** of NA and is in equilibrium with a **fixed or non-functional pool** which replenishes it on depletion.

Studies indicate the existence of a presynaptic regulation of NA release through a negative feedback mechanism mediated by **adrenergic presynaptic alpha-2 receptors** and a positive feedback mechanism mediated by **presynaptic ß-receptors**. According to this hypothesis, beta-receptors are more sensitive to agonists so that during the initiation of release, low concentrations of NA in the synaptic cleft accelerate the release process. When the concentration of NA reaches high levels, the presynaptic α_2 receptors are stimulated and the secretion is terminated by a negative feedback mechanism. Predominantly α_1 receptor antagonists such as phenoxybenzamine, on the other hand, enhance NA release. The combined effects of the positive and negative feedback mechanism may thus control the 'need oriented' release of the transmitter. It appears that a presynaptic regulating mechanism similar to that described in the periphery operates in the CNS as well. Drugs could produce actions by altering the release of these neurotransmitters centrally or peripherally, by modifying the presynaptic regulatory mechanisms (Chapter 5).

A small part of released NA is metabolized outside the cell by the enzyme catechol - O - methyl-transferase (**COMT**) but a large part (75-80%) is taken back into the cell by an active process and re-stored mostly in mobile pool. Only a small portion is metabolized intracellularly by mono-amine oxidase (**MAO**). *Rebinding of NA with the granules represents a way by which it is immobilised but can be used again. In fact, physiologically, uptake and restorage are the major routes of NA inactivation and enzymatic destruction plays only a minor role.* The enzymes MAO and COMT are widely distributed throughout the body including the brain, with the highest concentrations in the liver and the kidneys.

There are two types of MAO.

(i) 'MAO-A', which oxidizes mainly NA and 5-HT, can be selectively inhibited by very low concentration of inhibitors clorgyline and moclobemide; and

(ii) 'MAO-B', which oxidizes DA in the brain and can be selectively inhibited by the drug selegiline.

Tyramine and DA are substrates for both forms of the enzyme. The human liver contains both forms in equal amounts while the human brain MAO is predominantly type B (Chapter 14).

For details about adrenergic, DA and cholinergic receptors, see Chapters 17 and 18 respectively.

Neurotransmitter Uptake Mechanisms and Drugs

Many studies have defined the properties of the catecholamine 'uptake' mechanisms involved and their modification by drugs. The uptake processes have been designated as 'Uptake$_1$' and 'Uptake$_2$'.

(1) **Uptake$_1$** *is the picking up of catecholamines from the extracellular space by the axoplasm of the adrenergic neurons and by other extraneuronal cells.* This process demonstrates a greater affinity for NA than for adrenaline. Catecholamines taken up by 'Uptake$_1$' are then transferred to the storage vesicles in the adrenergic neurons by a separate process; both these processes are carrier-mediated transport system.

(2) **Uptake$_2$** *is the picking up of catecholamines by the effector cells in the peripheral tissues* such as the vascular smooth muscle, the heart and the exocrine glands. Such uptake is followed by rapid degradation of the catecholamines. In contrast to 'Uptake$_1$', 'Uptake$_2$' demonstrates a higher affinity for adrenaline and isoprenaline than for NA.

In the peripheral tissues, the extraneuronal sites for 'Uptake$_2$' are far more numerous than the neuronal uptake sites for 'Uptake$_1$'. *'Uptake$_1$' may be looked upon as 'uptake with retention'; by contrast, 'Uptake$_2$' is an 'uptake followed by metabolism'.* Noradrenergic Uptake$_1$ and Uptake$_2$ transport systems can be blocked selectively by a number of drugs (Table 16.2).

Table 16.2 : Inhibitors of NA Uptake$_1$ and Uptake$_2$

Inhibitors of Uptake$_1$:
Cocaine, Tricyclic Anti-depressants, Phenoxybenzamine, Amphetamine, MAOI and Chlorpromazine

Inhibitors of Uptake$_2$:
Normetanephrine, Glucocorticoids, Phenoxybenzamine.

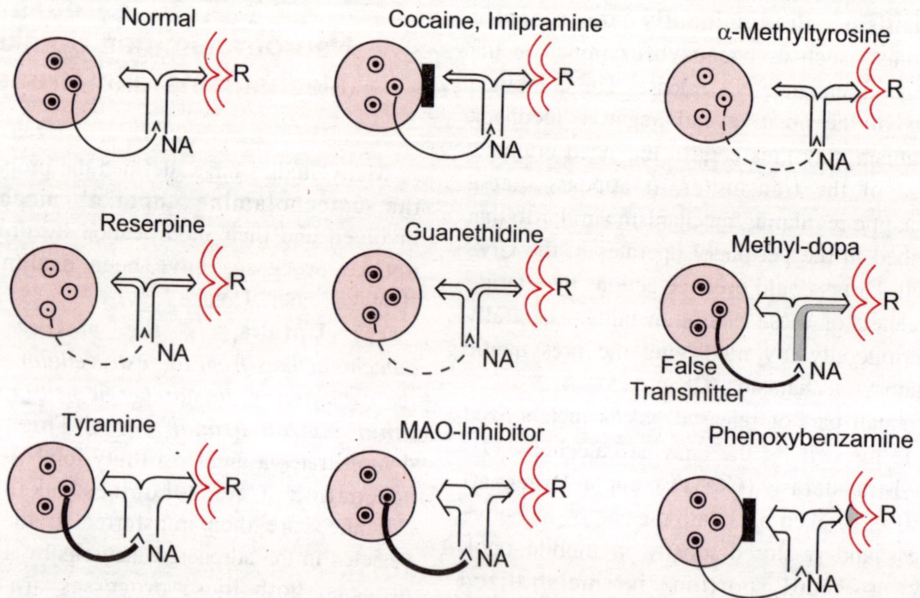

Fig. 16.4 : Schematic diagram showing the effect of some drugs on noradrenaline (NA) uptake and release mechanisms. Drugs may act by inhibiting its Uptake_1 process (impramine, cocaine), by interfering with the synthesis of transmitter, e.g., a-methyltyrosine, by depletion of NA from storage site (reserpine), by blocking the release from the storage site (guanethidine), by producing a false transmitter (methyl-dopa), by promoting the NA release (tyramine), by inhibiting the destruction of NA by MAO and by blocking both Uptake_1 and Uptake_2 mechanisms (phenoxybenzamine).

Experimentally, the actions of isoprenaline and NA on heart and aortic smooth muscle respectively are potentiated by hydrocortisone.

Many sympathomimetic amines are also taken up by "Uptake_1" process and hence, can act as competitive substrates, thus inhibiting the NA uptake. Other important drugs which are known to inhibit the "Uptake_1" mechanism are listed in Table 16.2. Some of these drugs produce their major therapeutic actions due to this blocking effect on "Uptake_1". Drugs that inhibit "Uptake_1" potentiate and prolong the responses of sympathetically innervated organs to nerve stimulation. Certain drugs like guanethidine which act as substrate for 'Uptake_1' when given in small doses, are selectively concentrated by adrenergic nerve terminals and cause a transmission block, thus reducing the effectiveness of sympathetic nerve discharge. Similarly, the drug 6-hydroxydopamine accumulates selectively through 'Uptake_1' process and produces selective destruction of adrenergic neurones (*chemical sympathectomy*) in both peripheral and central nervous system.

Various drugs known to act on the adrenergic neuron produce their effects by modifying the synthesis, storage and 'Uptake_1' mechanisms (Fig. 16.4) by:

- ***Supplying an amine precursor*** e.g. Levodopa used in Parkinson's disease is a precursor of dopamine.
- ***Blocking the Uptake1 of noradrenaline by inhibiting NET*** e.g. Tricyclic anti-depressants like imipramine used in the treatment of mental depression; cocaine.
- ***Interfering with the synthesis of NA,*** e.g., α-methyl tyrosine.
- ***Promoting the release of NA from the storage sites,*** e.g., Tyramine.
- ***Inhibiting the transport into the vesicles, thus interfere with the storage of NA, leading***

to its depletion from the sites, e.g., Antihypertensive drug Reserpine.

- ***Blocking the release of NA from the binding stores in the terminals,*** e.g., Guanethidine, a drug used in the treatment of hypertension.
- ***Promoting a synthesis of a false transmitter*** which displaces NA, e.g. Alpha methyldopa.
- ***Blocking postsynaptic receptors,*** e.g., adrenergic receptor blocking drugs.
- ***Inhibiting the intraneuronal degradation of NA,*** e.g., Monoamine oxidase (MAO) inhibitor drugs, used as antidepressants.

These mechanisms are discussed elsewhere.

Specialized uptake mechanisms, similar to that described for noradrenergic neurons, are also known to exist in dopaminergic and 5-HTergic neurons in CNS and in cholinergic neurons in the periphery and CNS. In cholinergic neurons, however, the transport mechanism is for transmitter precursor choline rather than for acetylcholine. Inhibitory action of anti-depressant drugs on 5-HT uptake at brain sites is discussed in Chapter 13.

Both ACh and NA are also termed as **local hormones** because they act at the site of their synthesis. Although ACh and NA are the main classical neurotransmitters at the autonomic nerve endings, the neurons may also possess other chemical messangers. These chemicals, when released, function as primary neurotransmitters, co-transmitters or neuro-modulators. Thus, VIP has been detected selectively in the peripheral cholinergic neurons whereas neuropeptide Y is found in the sympathetic nerve endings. Autonomic transmission may, therefore, be mediated by the release of multiple neurochemicals.

Supersensitivity: Interruption of the nerve supply of an effector organ (denervation) makes it more sensitive to the neurohumor of the system supplying it. Thus, a skeletal muscle, after sectioning the motor nerve, becomes highly sensitive to acetylcholine and the nictitating membrane becomes highly sensitive to noradrenaline after sectioning its postganglionic sympathetic supply. This phenomenon is termed **denervation supersensitivity.** The exact mechanism is not known but it coincides with the failure of uptake of NA from the extracellular fluid. It may thus be related to the elimination of the neuronal uptake mechanism. It could also partly be due to degeneration of the nerve terminals after sectioning, leading to disappearance of enzymes that normally inactivate the transmitter and are closely associated with the nerve terminals. It may also be due to an increase in receptor number (**up-regulation**) induced by the fall in the catecholamine concentration within the synaptic cleft (also Chapter 2). Supersensitivity to transmitter substances occurs also after prolonged administration of blocking agents. Increased sensitivity resulting from interruption of preganglionic autonomic supply is termed as **decentralization supersensitivity** and is of lesser magnitude.

Adrenergic and Adrenergic Blocking Drugs

17

The **sympathomimetic** or **adrenergic** drugs are agents that mimic the responses obtained as a result of stimulation of the sympathetic or adrenergic nerves. Majority of these substances contain an intact or a partially substituted amino (-NH_2) group and hence, are also called as **sympathomimetic amines**.

From the therapeutic point of view these drugs can be classified as:

I **Adrenergic drugs used for raising blood pressure,** e.g., Noradrenaline, Metaraminol and Phenylephrine.

II **Those used for their inotropic actions on the heart,** e.g., Dopamine, Dobutamine, Isoprenaline.

III **Those used as central stimulants,** e.g., Amphetamine, Dextroamphetamine and Methylphenidate.

IV **Those used as smooth muscle relaxants** e.g. (a) nonselective beta stimulants such as Adrenaline, Isoprenaline, Isoxsuprine; and (b) selective beta-$_2$ stimulants, e.g., Salbutamol and Terbutaline.

V **Those used in allergic reactions,** e.g., Adrenaline, Ephedrine.

VI **Those used for local vasoconstrictor effect,** e.g., Adrenaline, Naphazoline, Phenylephrine, Xylometazoline.

VII **Those used for suppressing the appetite** (anorectic), e.g., Fenfluramine, Phenteramine.

These drugs can also be classified as :

- ***Catecholamines,*** which are compounds containing a catechol nucleus (i.e. a benzene ring with two adjacent OH groups) and an amine-containing side-chain (Fig.17.1); and
- ***Non-catecholamines*** which lack the hydroxyl groups.

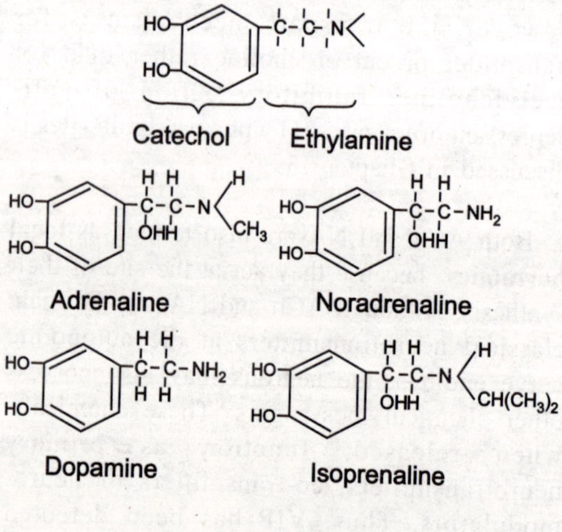

Fig. 17.1 : Catecholamines

Catecholamines

The catecholamines include the *sympathetic, neurohumoral transmitters* **noradrenaline** (NA *and* **dopamine** (DA); *the main hormone of the* *adrenal medulla* **adrenaline;** *and the synthetic compound* **isoprenaline** *(isoproterenol, isopropylarterenol).* Catecholamine content of adrenal medulla normally is 85% adrenaline and 15% NA. Dopamine not only serves as a precursor of NA but also acts as a neurohumoral sympathetic transmitter (Chapter 16). Isoprenaline is a purely synthetic compound.

The word 'nor' in noradrenaline was originally coined to indicate nitrogen (N) without (O-Ohne) a radical (R), in this case a methyl (CH_3) group.

Mechanism of action of catecholamines: The catecholamines produce their action by direct interaction with receptors located on the cell membrane. This drug receptor combination leads to either an increase (**excitation**) or a decrease (**inhibition**) in the tissue activity. In order to explain these differences in responses by different tissues, the concept of two different receptors, **alpha** and **beta**, was proposed by Ahlquist in 1948. Thus, the alpha receptor stimulation is mainly responsible for the excitatory effects of the catecholamines; the beta receptor stimulation usually produces inhibitory effects. Noradrenaline produces its pharmacological actions specifically by acting on the alpha and $beta_1$ receptors while adrenaline acts nonspecifically on both alpha and beta receptors; isoprenaline acts only on beta receptors. A given tissue may contain either alpha or beta or both types of receptors.

Even though it has been broadly stated that alpha receptors are excitatory and beta receptors inhibitory in character, there are certain exceptions to this rule. Thus, beta receptors, predominantly present in the heart, are excitatory in character; their stimulation increases the rate and force of contraction of the myocardium. Similarly, both the alpha and beta receptors of the GI tract are inhibitory in character; their stimulation produces smooth muscle relaxation.

Adrenergic receptors are classified according to their selective sensitivity to agonists and antagonists. At the molecular level,the adrenergic receptor-effector mechanism involves three interacting proteins: the receptor, the G-protein and the effector enzyme-ion channel.

Three distinct **beta receptor** subtypes have been be distinguished:

- ***$Beta_1$ receptors*** responsible for myocardial stimulation and renin release.
- ***$Beta_2$ receptors*** responsible for bronchial muscle relaxation, skeletal muscle vasodilation and uterine relaxation; and
- ***$Beta_3$ receptors*** expressed primarily in brown and white adipose tissue where they are likely to regulate NA-induced changes in energy metabolism and thermogenesis. $Beta_3$ agonists stimulate metabolic rate and induce weight loss without reducing food intake in animals. The receptor is relatively resistant to blockade by antagonists such as propranolol.

As a general rule, beta-adrenergic responses appear to result from binding of the catecholamine to beta adrenergic receptors ($beta_1$ and $beta_2$) which via the mediation of a stimulatory **G-protein** (Gs protein) stimulate a plasma membrane enzyme, **adenylyl cyclase**. This results in a rise of the intracellular cyclic AMP (see figure in Chapter 2). The cyclic AMP alters the cellular function by stimulation of a protein kinase, which then causes phosphorylation of certain enzyme proteins, resulting in activation of some and inactivation of others. This explains the stimulatory and inhibitory action of agents acting on the beta receptors.

Phosphodiesterase, another enzyme, promotes the breakdown of cyclic AMP. Drugs like caffeine, theophylline and other methyl xanthines which inhibit this enzyme potentiate the beta receptor stimulant action of adrenaline.

Presynaptic beta receptors facilitate the release of NA at the adrenergic nerve terminals. (Chapter 16).

Alpha adrenergic receptors are of two types: **$alpha_1$** and **$alpha_2$**, with three subtypes each.

Classical **α_1 adrenergic receptors** (postsynaptic) are predominantly in the vascular smooth muscles. Activation of these receptors which are excitatory in nature, increases the intracellular concentration of calcium by

Table 17.1: Distribution and responses of adrenergic receptors	
Tissue	**Response**
Predominantly alpha receptors	
(a) Medula Oblongata (α_2)	Reduction of BP and heart rate
(b) Blood vessels : (α_1)	
Skin and mucosa	Constriction
Cerebral	Constriction (slight)
(c) Skin :	
Pilomotor muscle (α_1)	Contraction
Sweat gland	Slight secretion
(d) Radial muscle of iris (α_1)	Contraction (mydriasis)
(e) Salivary glands, except parotids	Thick, viscous secretion
(f) Sex organ, male	Ejaculation
Predominantly beta receptors	
(a) Heart : (β_1, α_1)	
S-A node - β_1	Increased heart rate (positive chronotropic action)
Atria - β_1	Increased contraction (positive inotropic action)
A- V node - β_1	Faster conduction
Ventricles - β_1	Increased contractility and conductivity, increased automaticity (positive dromotropic action)
(b) Bronchial muscle - β_2	Relaxation
(c) Skeletal muscle changes - β_2	Changes in contractility
(d) Skeletal muscle blood vessels - β_2	Dilatation
Both alpha and beta receptors	
(a) G.I. tract :	
Motility and tone (α_2 β_2)	Decreased
Sphincters (α)	Contraction
Pancreas :	
Alpha$_2$	Inhibiting insulin release
Beta$_2$	Stimulation of insulin release
(b) Urinary bladder :	
Trigone - α	Contraction
Detrusor - β	Relaxation
(c) Blood vessels :	
Coronary - α, β_2	Constriction; dilatation
Pulmonary - α, β_2	Constriction; dilatation
Abdominal viscera - α, β_2	Constriction (mainly); dilatation
Renal - α, β_2	Constriction; dilatation
Skeletal muscle - α, β_2	Constriction; dilatation
(d) Adipocyte - α_2	Inhibit lipolysis
β_3	Lipolysis
Liver - α_1, β_2	Glycogenolysis, neoglucogenesis, inhibition of glycogen synthetase
(e) Leukocyte (human) - β_2	Inhibits chemotaxis and lysosomal enzyme release
Platelet (human) - α_2	Platelet aggregation
(f) Uterus :	
α_1	Stimulation
β_2	Inhibition

activation of phospholipase C in the cell membrane via stimulatory G protein (G_S). The phospholipase C then hydrolyses membrane bound phosphoinositides with the generation of two second messengers, diacylglycerol and inositol triphosphate. This results in an increase in the intracellular Ca^{++} which accounts for the vasoconstrictor effect.

Alpha$_2$ adrenergic receptors are found both in effector tissues (postsynaptic) and on the neuronal endings (presynaptic) where they are autoreceptors. Activation of the **presynaptic α_2 receptors** by agents acting through the inhibitory G protein (Gi) inhibits adenylyl cyclase and reduces the intracellular concentration of cyclic AMP. These receptors activate G-protein gated K^+ channels. The presynaptic α_2 receptor agonists produce inhibitory effects; thus, activation of the α_2 receptors in the adrenergic nerves inhibits NA release.

The activation of the **post-synaptic vascular α_2 receptors** however, causes release of 'endothelium derived relaxing factor' (EDRF, NO) which brings about vasodilatation. **Activation of venous α_2 receptors**, on the other hand, causes venoconstriction. This neuromodulatory system appears to play an important role in the control of sympathetic tone.

Activation of the **post-synaptic α_2 receptors** in the GI tract acts by inhibiting voltage sensitive calcium channels leading to inhibition.

Alpha$_2$ adrenergic receptors are also present at the post-junctional or nonjunctional sites in several tissues such as the brain. Activation of post-junctional alpha$_2$ receptors in the brain by clonidine causes the antihypertensive effect.

The presence of α receptors has been also demonstrated in human leukocytes and platelets.

The predominant receptors in various organs and the usual responses to their stimulation are given in the Table 17.1. These responses in isolated tissues may differ from those in the whole animal owing to the presence of reflex activity in the latter. Further, the initial condition of the tissue may also determine the resultant responses. Table 17.2 lists the agonists and antagonists of the adrenergic receptor subtypes and summarises their mechanism of action.

Table 17.2: Drugs acting on adrenergic receptor subtypes

	Alpha 1	Alpha 2	Beta 1	Beta 2
Agonists	Phenylephrine Methoxamine Metaraminol Mephentermine	Clonidine Apraclonidine Methyldopa Guanfacine	Dobutamine Isoproterenol	Orciprenaline Salbutamol Terbutaline Isoetharine
Antagonists	Prazosin Indoramin	Yohimbine	Propranolol Pindolol Atenolol Metoprolol	Propranolol Pindolol
Location of receptors	Postsynaptic (vessels, glands and smooth muscles)	Presynaptic Postsynaptic (vessels and brain tissue). Nonsynaptic (platelets and leukocytes)	Postsynaptic (heart and juxtaglomerular cells)	Presynaptic Postsynaptic Nonsynaptic (lymphocytes and polymorphonuclear cells)
Mechanism of action	Alteration of cellular calcium ion fluxes	Inhibition of adenylyl cyclase	Stimulation of adenylyl cyclase	Stimulation of adenylyl cyclase

Pharmacological actions of adrenaline and noradrenaline: Adrenaline acts as a nonselective α and β receptor agonist, whereas NA acts more selectively as α and β_1 agonist.

Cardiovascular system:

• ***Heart*:** Adrenaline stimulates the beta_1 receptors in the heart and increases the rate, the force of contraction and the conduction velocity. This is associated with increased metabolism of the myocardium and increased oxygen consumption. It also increases cardiac output by stimulating venoconstriction, thus increasing the venous return and increasing the force of atrial contraction which augments the ventricular diastolic volume. Very high cardiac rate, however, prevents proper diastolic filling and may produce fall in the cardiac output. Adrenaline enhances conduction across the A-V node and may produce ventricular arrhythmias.

Noradrenaline, however, usually does not increase the heart rate in an intact animal but tends to produce bradycardia due to compensatory vascular reflex activity. It should be noted, however, that NA is the physiological transmitter in the heart and its capacity to stimulate cardiac α_1 receptors is of vital importance.

The myocardial effects of adrenaline and noradrenaline can be blocked by the beta receptor blocking agents like propranolol (see later).

• ***Blood vessels and blood pressure*:** Adrenaline and NA constrict the blood vessels of the skin and mucous membranes. Adrenaline dilates the blood vessels of the skeletal muscles on account of the preponderance of β_2 receptors; and decreases the total peripheral resistance. Hence, although adrenaline raises the systolic BP mainly by its cardiac actions, it lowers the diastolic pressure by its peripheral actions; and therefore, it is not suitable for routine use in hypovolemic shock.

As the rise in systolic BP with adrenaline is only of moderate magnitude, compensatory reflexes do not antagonize the cardiac actions of adrenaline and the moderate rise in systolic BP is accompanied by tachycardia, increased cardiac output and increased stroke volume.

The rise in systolic BP produced by moderate doses of adrenaline is often followed by a fall. By stimulating the alpha receptors, it produces a rise in BP. However, the action of adrenaline on beta receptors is more persistent and hence, when the action on alpha receptors wears off, the action on beta receptors is unmasked producing a fall of BP. This blood pressure response to moderate doses of adrenaline is termed **biphasic response**. Sir Henry Dale noted that this biphasic response was converted to a depressor response by prior administration of ergot extract due to alpha receptor blocking action of ergot alkaloids, leading to stimulation

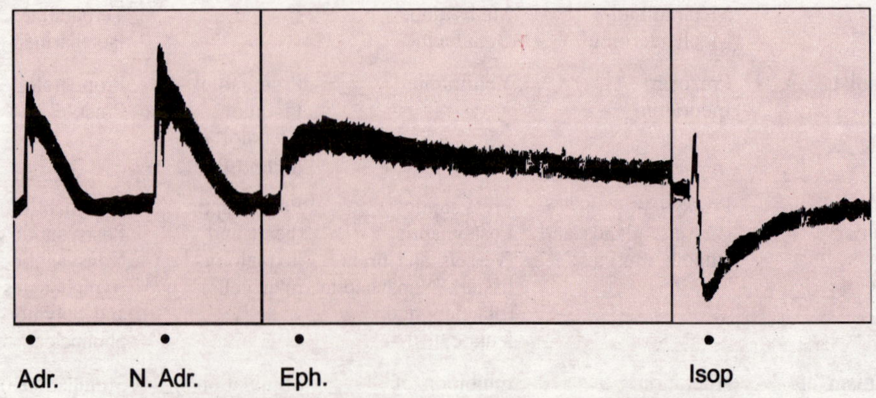

Fig. 17.2 : Effect of Adrenaline, Noradrenaline, Ephedrine, and Isoprenaline on blood pressure in anaesthetised dog.

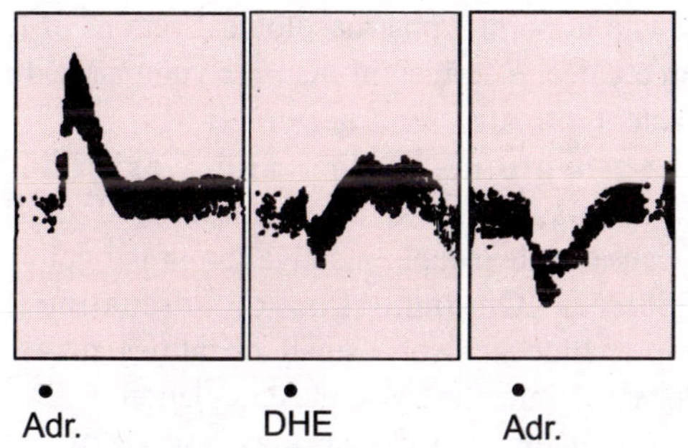

Fig. 17.3 : Dale's Vasomotor Reversal. Note the fall in BP with Adrenaline after injection of Dihydroergotamine (DHE).

of peripheral beta$_2$ receptors by adrenaline and thus causing a fall in BP. This phenomenon is termed as **Dale's vasomotor reversal** (Fig.17.3). Such reversal is not seen with NA.

Noradrenaline in an intact animal produces a rise in both systolic and diastolic BP; the pulse pressure usually remains unaltered and the mean BP increases. As compared to adrenaline, its beta$_2$ receptor actions are very feeble. Noradrenaline-induced hypertension is associated with reflex bradycardia.

Both adrenaline and NA produce a significant reduction in the renal blood flow in man even in doses that have no significant effect on BP. The urine output and urinary excretion of sodium, potassium and chloride decreases. Renin secretion is increased by direct β receptor effect, independent of vascular changes in the kidney; whereas α_2 receptors are responsible for inhibition of renin release from the kidney.

Both adrenaline and NA constrict the hepatic and mesenteric blood vessels and raise the portal venous pressure. The pulmonary arterial and venous pressures are raised by both, more by adrenaline. Constriction of the musculature of the great systemic veins tends to push the blood from the periphery into the pulmonary circulation and this may occasionally result in pulmonary edema following adrenaline administration.

Adrenaline in moderate doses increases the cerebral blood flow and oxygen consumption, probably by increasing the systemic BP. It increases the coronary blood flow by a complex mechanism.

Smooth muscle: (Table 17.1).

- ***Bronchi*:** Adrenaline by it β_2 receptor agonist activity is a potent relaxant of the bronchial smooth muscle. It antagonizes the bronchospasm produced by vagal stimulation, choline esters, histamine or an antigen-antibody reaction, bradykinin, leukotrienes or prostaglandin $F_{2\alpha}$.
- ***Uterus*:** The response of the uterus to the catecholamines varies according to species, the phase of oestrous cycle, presence or absence of gestation, period of gestation and the dose administered. The rat uterus is relaxed by these compounds irrespective of all these factors. The human non-pregnant uterine strip is stimulated to contract by adrenaline. *In the last month of pregnancy adrenaline inhibits uterine contraction and causes uterine relaxation.*
- ***Gastrointestinal tract*:** Adrenaline and NA relax the smooth muscle of the gut and reduce its motility; the sphincters are constricted.
- ***Other smooth muscles*:** Adrenaline contracts the pilomotor muscle of the hair follicle. It also produces a contraction of the vesical sphincter and the trigone (α receptor), while relaxing the detrusor muscle (β receptor). Adrenaline and NA produce contraction of the splenic capsule producing a release of erythrocytes into the peripheral circulation. This probably serves as a protective mechanism during stress such as hypoxia and haemorrhage.

Eye: Sympathetic stimulation results in mydriasis due to contraction of the radial muscle fibres of the iris, and exophthalmos due to contraction of the orbital muscles. Nictitating membrane, present in lower mammals, contracts with adrenaline. Adrenaline, on topical application, does not readily penetrate the eyeball. However, it produces a moderate reduction in intraocular tension.

Respiration : Adrenaline is a bronchodilator and weak stimulant of respiration. Given IV, both adrenaline and NA induce apnoea partly by stimulating the baroreceptors and mainly by a direct central action. Adrenaline, particularly in aerosol form, constricts the pulmonary vessels and relieves bronchial congestion; this results in an increase in the vital capacity.

Metabolic effects : Adrenaline increases:

- ***Blood sugar level*** by enhancing hepatic glycogenolysis (β_2 adrenoreceptors) and by decreasing peripheral glucose uptake.
- ***Blood lactate*** by enhancing the breakdown of glycogen to lactate in the skeletal muscles.
- ***Plasma free fatty acid concentration*** by increasing lipolysis in adipose tissue.
- ***Serum K^+ level transiently, followed by a more sustained hypokalemia.*** Both adrenaline and NA promote cellular uptake of K^+.

Activation of pancreatic α_2 adrenergic receptors by adrenaline and by severe stress (via activation of adrenergic nervous system) inhibits insulin release; β_2 adrenergic receptor agonists and vagal nerve stimulation enhance it.

Central nervous system: The catecholamines do not cross the BB barrier satisfactorily and hence, their central actions are limited. Adrenaline may produce excitement, tremor stupor, vomiting and restlessness.

Noradrenaline and dopamine are important neurotransmitters in the CNS (Chapter 5).

Skeletal muscle: Catecholamines influence skeletal muscle contractions by acting on both sides of the neuromuscular junction. The α effect on the motor nerve endings increases the amount of ACh released and is probably the main factor in the improvement of neuromuscular transmission by adrenaline. The β action on the muscle fibre itself probably contributes to the improvement of muscle contractions and tremor, sometimes observed following these drugs.

Antiallergic action : Adrenaline and similar compounds prevent the release of mediators of allergy such as histamine from the tissue mast cells (Chapter 26).

Miscellaneous : Adrenaline produces thick viscid secretion from salivary glands, leucocytosis and eosinopenia, and accelerates blood coagulation. It also stimulates platelet aggregation through alpha$_2$ receptors.

The important pharmacological actions of the three catecholamines in man are summarized in Table 17.3. Also see Chapter 31.

Absorption, fate and excretion: Catecholamines are not administered orally because of their rapid inactivation in the gut and the liver. On inhalation of adrenaline or isoprenaline aerosols, small quantities may be absorbed into the systemic circulation.

Adrenaline and NA are metabolized by :

- ***Catechol-O-methyl transferase*** (COMT) located extracellularly; and
- ***Monoamine oxidase*** (MAO), located inside the mitochondria of the adrenergic neurons.

These two enzymes act sequentially on both adrenaline and NA as shown in Fig. 17.4 and convert them into the final urinary excretory products : VMA, metanephrine (metadrenaline) and normetanephrine (normetadrenaline). A small quantity of catecholamines is excreted unchanged.

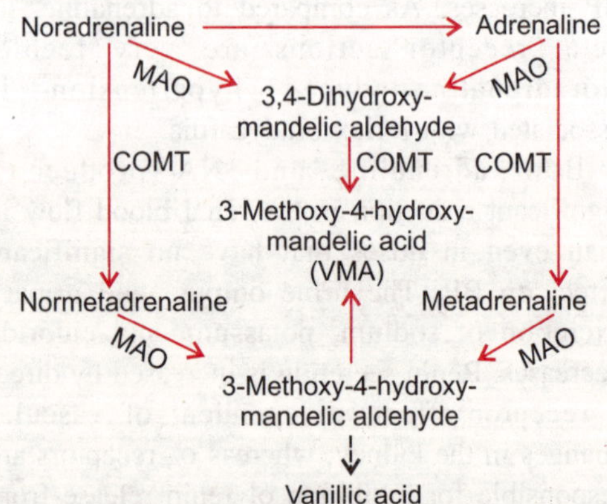

Fig. 17.4 Metabolism of Adrenaline and Noradrenaline

The normal 24 hour urinary excretion of VMA and free catecholamines is 4-8 mg. and 50-100 mcg. respectively. A significant increase in these values is considered diagnostic of pheochromocytoma, an adrenal medullary tumor, producing excessive catecholamines.

Adverse reactions: These are mostly cardiovascular and are due to extension of the pharmacological actions. Adrenaline, given SC, may produce palpitation, throbbing headache

Table 17.3: Comparison of the pharmacological actions of catecholamines in man

Effector Organ	Adrenaline	Noradrenaline	Isoprenaline
Heart			
Rate	++	-	++
Stroke volume	+++	++	+++
Cardiac output	+++	0, -	+++
Arrhythmias	+++	++	+++
Coronary blood flow	++	+	++
Blood Pressure			
Systolic	+++	+++	+, 0, -
Diastolic	+, 0, -	++	+, 0, -
Pulse	+, 0	++	0, +
Mean	+, 0	++	0
Peripheral Blood Flow			
Muscle	++	+, 0	++
Skin and mucous membrane	-	+, 0, -	+
Renal	-	-	?
Spanchnic	++	0, +	++
Cerebral	+	0, -	+
Total peripheral resistance	-	+++	-
Smooth Muscles			
Bronchi	+++	+, 0	+++
Metabolism			
Oxygen consumption	++	0, +	0
Blood sugar	+++	0, +	0
Eosinopenic response	+	0	0

+ = Increase, 0 = No change, - = Decrease.

and tremors. Noradrenaline, employed in the form of IV drip, may cause anxiety, pallor and headache.

- Both adrenaline and NA, injected rapidly, IV, may cause a sudden, marked increase in BP, precipitating subarachnoid haemorrhage and occasionally a stroke.
- They can also cause ventricular arrhythmias including fatal ventricular fibrillation. In individuals with cardiac decompensation, adrenaline may precipitate acute pulmonary edema.

Noradrenaline infusion has to be carefully titrated, and BP has to be checked at least every 15 minutes to prevent the above mentioned complications. *The infusion must never be left unattended.* Noradrenaline infusion, if stopped suddenly, may result in alarming hypotension.

- Adrenaline and NA (particularly the former) may precipitate anginal pain in persons with ischemic heart disease. Thyrotoxic or hypertensive individuals are more sensitive to the pressor effects of these agents.
- Noradrenaline infusion, if extravasated, may produce local vasospasm and sloughing.

Preparations and dosage:

(i) Adrenaline injection 0.5 or 1 ml. ampoules containing 1:1000 adrenaline in water. Dose : 0.2 to 0.5 ml. SC or IM. Rarely, the drug is administered IV, in the dose of 0.25 mg., further diluted with saline and given slowly under monitoring and supervision.

(ii) Adrenaline inhalation is a nonsterile, 1:100, aqueous solution of adrenaline tartrate.

(iii) Noradrenaline injection 0.2 per cent solution of noradrenaline bitartrate in 2 ml. ampoules. It is administered as an IV infusion. For this purpose, 2 ml. of noradrenaline bitartrate (equivalent to 4 mg. of the salt and 2 mg. of the base) is added to 500 ml. of 5 per cent *dextrose solution (which is generally acidic)* resulting in a concentration of 4 mcg of the base per ml. After judging the cardiovascular response with a test dose of 2 to 3 ml., the drug is administered at the rate of 0.5 to 1 ml. per minute. The dose is controlled according to the blood pressure response. *Noradrenaline is unstable at the neutral pH of normal saline and vitamin C (500-1000 mg) should be added to the infusion,* if noradrenaline must be infused in normal saline.

Therapeutic uses of adrenaline:

- ***Anaphylaxis and angioneurotic edema*** **:** Adrenaline is the drug of choice in the treatment of anaphylactic shock. (Chapter 22). It is life-saving in angioneurotic edema of the larynx.
- ***Bronchial asthma*** **:** Adrenaline, given SC or by inhalation is a potent bronchodilator. However, its use for this purpose has declined. (Chapter 26).
- ***Cardiopulmonary resuscitation(CPR)*:** Cardiac arrest is diagnosed if the patient collapses suddenly and becomes unconscious, is not breathing, and the carotid pulse absent. Table 17.4 summarises the guidelines for cardiopulmonary resuscitation, which comprises attention to : A (airway), B (breathing) and C (circulation).

Table 17.4: Steps of cardiopulmonary resuscitation

- Confirm unconsciousness, absent carotid pulse and apnoea.
- Shout for help.
- Clear the oropharynx.
- Blows between the shoulder blades/ Heimlich manoeuvre.
- Mouth to mouth breathing.
- Thump on the precordium.
- External cardiac massage.
- Hospitalize.
- Administer oxygen. Intubate when possible.
- ECG; IV line
- Drug(s) for cardiac asystole/ventricular fibrillation. DC shock.
- IV Sodium bicarbonate, if indicated.

Shout for help. To clear the upper airway, lay the patient supine on a hard surface such as the floor; tilt the head back, lift the chin, open the mouth and thrust the lower jaw anteriorly. With the mouth open, clear the oropharynx. If there is a foreign body (bolus) in the upper airway and the patient cannot expel it by forceful coughing, give strong blows with the flat of the hand between the shoulder blades; if the foreign body is not dislodged, apply the **Heimlich manoeuvre as a last resort**. If the carotid pulse does not return, commence **mouth-to-mouth ventilation**. If the carotid pulse is still not felt, a thump with the closed fist (from a height of 1 meter) at the junction of the middle and lower thirds of the of the sternum may initiate cardiac action. (*Remember that both Heimlich manoeuvre and the precordial thump can damage the chest wall and internal organs*).

If the carotid pulse is still not restored, begin external cardiac massage at 100 compressions/min. If two rescuers are available, continue CPR at 30 compressions followed by 2 ventilations (one CPR cycle) till help arrives or the patient reaches the hospital. If only one rescuer is available, continue chest compressions without interruption for ventilations.

In the hospital, intubate the patient, establish IV line and record ECG as soon as possible. Ventilate the patient with oxygen (room air if oxygen is not available). If the ECG shows ventricular fibrillation (VF) the patient is treated with defibrillation with DC shock, followed by IV lignocaine. In persistent VF, either bretylium tosylate is given IV, or adrenaline is injected IV in the dose of 0.5 - 1 mg (5-10 ml of 1: 10,000 solution) every 5 minutes with attempts at defibrillation between successive injections; if IV injection is not possible, 0.2 - 0.3 ml of 1: 1000 solution is injected into the trachea. *If, on the other hand, the ECG shows cardiac asystole or severe bradyarrhythmia, the patient is treated with adrenaline (used as above) and atropine (2 mg IV); defibrillation is not used in such cases.* In cases where the cardiac arrest is due to VF, post - resuscitation, lignocaine infusion is continued for 24 - 72 hours. Sodium bicarbonate infusion is used if the resuscitation has been prolonged and/or acidosis is demonstrated by arterial blood gas analysis. The underlying cause of cardiac arrest e.g. acute MI should be sought for and treated.

- ***Control of haemorrhage***: Adrenaline in the concentration of 1 : 1000 to 1 : 20,000 is sometimes used *topically* for controlling bleeding from arterioles and capillaries eg. epistaxis and bleeding after tooth extraction. It is not effective against venous oozing.
- ***Other Local Uses***: Adrenaline, because of its vasoconstrictor effect, is used in the concentration of 1 : 20,000 to 1 : 100,000 along with local anaesthetics. It reduces the systemic absorption of the local anaesthetic, thus prolonging its action and minimising its toxicity.

Adrenaline hydrochloride 0.5-2% can be used to reduce the production of aqueous humour and decrease the intra-ocular tension in patients with glaucoma. Selective $alpha_2$ agonists apraclonidine and brimonidine are preferred.

Therapeutic uses of noradrenaline:

Noradrenaline is mainly used for elevating the BP in shock (Chapter 31).

Routinely, alpha-receptor blocking drugs are used for the control of the BP before and during operative removal of a pheochromocytoma. This antagonism of alpha receptor usually does not lead to irrecoverable hypotension after removal of the tumor. However, if there is a fall in BP even after correction of hypovolemia, administration of NA may be useful.

ISOPRENALINE **(Isoproterenol, Isopropylarterenol):** Isoprenaline is the most potent, synthetic, non-selective **beta agonist.**

Pharmacological actions: Its main actions are on the heart, skeletal muscle vasculature and smooth muscles.

- ***It stimulates the heart and causes tachycardia.***
- ***It lowers the peripheral vascular resistance*** in skeletal, renal and mesenteric vascular beds and produces a fall mainly in the diastolic pressure.
- ***It relaxes the smooth muscles particularly those of bronchi and gastrointestinal tract.***
- ***Its calorigenic and FFA releasing actions are similar to those of adrenaline.***

Absorption, fate and excretion : Isoprenaline is inconsistently absorbed sublingually and orally. Absorption is quicker after IM injection and by inhalation. Given orally, it is less effective. It is rapidly inactivated by uptake into tissue and metabolized by COMT.

Adverse reactions: It can cause palpitation, tachycardia, arrhythmias, anginal pain, headache and flushing. *Combined isoprenaline-adrenaline administration in bronchial asthma may prove fatal.*

Preparations and dosage:

(i) Isoprenaline sulfate 10 mg. Dose: 5 to 10 mg. sublingually.

(ii) Isoprenaline injection (Isoprin) 2 mg/ ml. to be diluted for IV infusion.

Therapeutic uses:

- ***Stokes-Adams syndrome***: Isoprenaline, because of its lesser liability to produce cardiac arrhythmias, is preferred to adrenaline in this condition. It may be administered either IV or orally in the dose 30 to 120 mg. 6 to 8 hourly.
- ***Shock due to beta blocker overuse*** (Chapter 31).

Precautions and contraindications for catecholamines: Catecholamines should be administered cautiously in the presence of hypertension, hyperthyroidism, angina pectoris, acute left ventricular failure and hypotension during halothane anaesthesia.

DOPAMINE (DA) : (Intropin): This naturally occurring precursor of NA acts on dopaminergic and other adrenergic receptors.

Currently, two classes of **postsynaptic DA receptors** have been described: D_1-like (D_1 and D_5) and D_2-like (D_2, D_3, D_4). Table 17.5 summarises the distribution and properties of D_1 and D_2 receptors. **Presynaptic receptors** or

Table 17.5 : Distribution and properties of D_1 and D_2 receptors

Location	Type of D receptors	Functions
Limbic system	D_1 and D_2	Mood and emotional stability; stereotypy
Corpus striatum	D_1 and D_2	Motor control
Hypothalamus	Mainly D_1	Autonomic control
Pituitary	Mainly D_2	Inhibition of prolactin secretion
Blood vessels	Mainly D_1	Dilatation
Heart : muscle	Mainly D_2	Stimulation of inotropic function (Chapter 30)
Heart : sympathetic fibres	Mainly D_2	Inhibition of NA release
Mechanism of action :	D_1 Increases cAMP synthesis. D_2 Decreases cAMP synthesis.	

autoreceptors for DA are present in the brain. Dopamine is also a weak alpha and beta adrenergic receptor agonist. Like adrenaline, it is metabolized by MAO and COMT. The drug has extremely short half life. Its effects can be blocked, if necessary, by the use of alpha blocker phentolamine. Dopamine does not cross the blood brain barrier.

Table 17.6 summarises the pharmacological effects of DA at different dose levels.

Adverse reactions: These include nausea, vomiting, palpitation, ectopic beats and anginal pain. A sudden rise in BP may occur. Small doses occasionally precipitate a fall in BP. Infusion of large doses for long time may cause ischemia and gangrene of limbs.

Reduction in urine output, tachycardia and development of arrhythmias indicate toxicity.

Therapeutic uses:

- ***Shock***: See Table in Chapter 31.
- ***Threatened acute renal failure***: In low dose (less than 5 mcg /kg/min), it preferentially dilates the renal vessels and may produce diuresis. If the patient does not respond in 10-12 hours, the drug should be discontinued.

FENOLDOPAM : This D_1 receptor agonist, a peripheral vasodilator, is used in hypertensive crises (Chapter 29).

For D_2 receptor agonists, see Chapter 65.

DOBUTAMINE (Dobutrex), though structurally related to DA, has a selective β_1 receptor agonist action with predominant effect on cardiac contractility. Dopamine receptors are not involved in its action. It has negligible chronotropic and peripheral vascular actions. In patients with low-output cardiac failure, it increases the cardiac output without increasing the heart rate. Unlike DA, it does not cause renal vasodilatation. It has a short duration of action and is given by slow IV infusion in 5% dextrose, at the rate of 2.5 - 15 mcg/kg/minute. Its toxicity is similar to that of dopamine. *Like other catecholamines, dobutamine loses its effect in an alkaline medium.*

It is particularly useful in refractory, chronic, congestive heart failure, unresponsive to digoxin. It may also have beneficial hemodynamic effects in patients with bacteremic shock.

Dopexamine (Dopacard) is another inotropic agent used in heart failure associated with cardiac surgery. It stimulates cardiac DA and peripheral $beta_2$ receptors. It is administered by IV infusion via a caval catheter in the dose of 0.5-1 mcg/kg/minute, increased to a maximum of 6 mcg/kg/minute.

Noncatecholamines

The sympathomimetic amines devoid of the

Table 17.6: Pharmacological effects of dopamine

Dose (by infusion) (mcg/kg/min)	Effects
2-5 (Dopaminergic range)	Renal, mesenteric and cerebral ***vasodilation*** by action on *dopamine (D_1) receptors.*
5-10 (Dopaminergic + β_1 range)	Same as above. *Plus* ***increase in myocardial contractility*** with increase in heart rate and cardiac output, by action on dopamine and *$beta_1$ receptors.* This is of advantage in the treatment of shock. The peripheral resistance is lowered or unchanged.
11-20 (β_1 range)	***Predominantly cardiac action.***
More than 20 (α_1 range)	***Vasoconstriction***, decrease in renal blood flow and urine output, and sometimes aggravation of heart failure, by action on *$alpha_1$ adrenergic receptors.*

catechol nucleus comprise compounds like ephedrine, amphetamine and other vasopressors as well as smooth muscle relaxing compounds.

Mechanism of action: These drugs :

- ***Release NA and /or DA from the sympathetic neurons.*** Noncatecholamines are taken up in the neuron by NET and are concentrated in the vesicles by VMAT. They displace NA, which is subsequently released into the synaptic cleft by **reverse transport via NET**. Thus, this **indirect action** does not involve the usual exocytic process secondary to Ca^{++} influx, and produces mainly α effects resembling those of externally administered NA.
- ***Amphetamine and ephedrine, in particular, also inhibit the reuptake of neurotranamitters such as DA, NA and 5-HT by membrane transporters.***
- ***Act as partial agonists of NA*** and are capable of *directly stimulating* the adrenergic alpha and/or beta receptors. This explains the relaxation of the bronchial smooth muscle by ephedrine, of uterine smooth muscle by isoxsuprine, and of vascular smooth muscle by nylidrin, and stimulation of the myocardium by mephenteramine.

Compared to catecholamines, they

(1) are effective orally;

(2) are relatively resistant to the action of MAO;

(3) have longer duration of action; and

(4) cross the BBB and therefore have significant CNS effects.

EPHEDRINE is an alkaloid obtained from plants of the genus *ephedra*. The herb containing ephedrine, *ma huang*, has been employed in Chinese indigenous medicine for over 5000 years. Surprisingly, the drug has not been studied extensively in humans. Plants of this genus are commonly encountered in northern India and China.

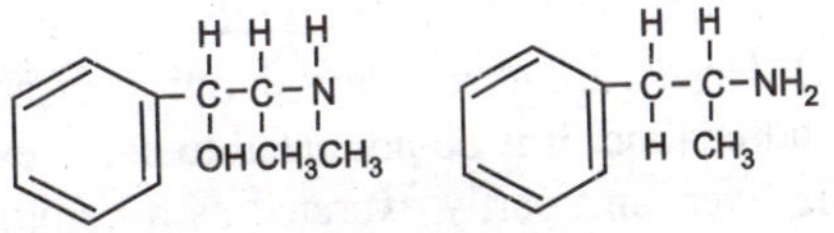

Fig. 17.5 : Ephedrine Amphetamine

Pharmacological actions: Ephedrine stimulates both the alpha and beta adrenergic receptors. It also acts indirectly by releasing NA from sympathetic nerve endings.

- ***Cardiovascular actions***: Ephedrine increases the force of myocardial contraction but its action on the heart rate is variable. The rise in BP is due to both peripheral vasoconstriction and increase in the cardiac output. Repeated administration fails to elicit the same pressor response, the phenomenon being termed **tachyphylaxis**. The pressor effect of ephedrine is antagonized by the alpha receptor blocking agents but there is no significant reversal. Qualitatively, its actions on various blood vessels are similar to those of adrenaline but it is a less potent pressor agent than adrenaline.

• ***Smooth muscles*** : Ephedrine relaxes the bronchial smooth muscle. The relaxation is less prompt than with adrenaline but persists for a longer time. Ephedrine also relaxes the uterine smooth muscle but enhances the tone of trigone and the sphincter of the bladder.

• ***CNS*** : Ephedrine stimulates the CNS probably by acting on the reticular activating system. In therapeutic doses, it often increases mental activity, restlessness, insomnia, anxiety and tremors. It enhances the monosynaptic and polysynaptic reflexes of the spinal cord and increases the depth and rate of respiration.

• ***Eye***: Ephedrine produces mydriasis on local as well as systemic administration.

• ***Metabolic effects*** : Ephedrine increases the metabolic rate and oxygen consumption. It is less effective than adrenaline in raising the blood sugar level.

Absorption, fate and excretion : Ephedrine is well absorbed orally. There is little first pass metabolism, and it is relatively resistant to MAO. Hence, it has a longer duration of action than adrenaline. It is de-aminated to some extent in the liver, and partly excreted as a conjugate. Approximately 60 to 75 per cent of the dose is eliminated unchanged in urine.

Preparations and dosage:

(i) Ephedrine hydrochloride tablet 30 mg. Dose : 15 to 30 mg. t.i.d.

(ii) Ephedrine hydrochloride elixir 15 mg. per 5 ml. Dose: 5 to 10 ml. Ephedrine pediatric syrup NF 8 mg. per 5 ml. Dose : 5 ml. per year of age to a maximum of 20 ml. per dose 4 to 6 hourly.

(iii) Ephedrine hydrochloride injection 30 mg. per ml. Dose : 15 to 45 mg. SC or IM.

(iv) Ephedrine 1% nasal drops.

Pseudoephedrine hydrochloride (Sudafed), a stereoisomer of ephedrine, 30 and 60 mg. tablets, and syrup 30 mg. in 5 ml. used as a nasal decongestant. It is less liable to produce tachycardia, increase in BP and CNS stimulation.

Adverse reactions: The adverse reactions are similar to those encountered with catecholamines. However, in therapeutic doses it is usually well tolerated. GI upset, difficulty in micturition, insomnia, tremors and rarely psychotic symptoms with paranoid hallucinations have been reported. Precautions similar to those with catecholamines should be exercised during its administration.

Therapeutic uses:

• ***Bronchial asthma***: Ephedrine is useful in treating chronic, persistent, moderate asthma and in preventing acute attacks (Chapter 26).

• ***Nasal decongestion***: Ephedrine drops are used for nasal decongestion. However, it may produce tachyphylaxis, after-congestion and palpitation.

• ***Hypotension***: Ephedrine may be employed IM to prevent or to treat hypotension during spinal anaesthesia.

• ***Stokes-Adams syndrome***: Ephedrine in the dose of 10-30 mg. 3 to 4 times daily has been used to prevent ventricular asystole. However, isoprenaline is preferred to ephedrine for this purpose.

• ***As a mydriatic***: Ephedrine eye drops 3 to 5 per cent are employed to produce mydriasis without cycloplegia.

• ***In narcolepsy*** : (Chapter 13)

• ***Miscellaneous***: Ephedrine has been used with varying success in urinary incontinence and nocturnal enuresis. It is of some value in relieving paroxysms of whooping cough and allergic brochospasm. It is sometimes used in the treatment of urticaria.

AMPHETAMINE, which is structurally related to ephedrine (Fig. 17.5), is available in racemic and dextro forms. The d-isomer is approximately 3 to 4 times as potent as the levo form in its central effects while the levo form is slightly more potent in its effects on the cardiovascular system.

Pharmacological actions:

- ***CNS actions***: It is a potent CNS stimulant and exerts its effects indirectly by releasing NA from their storage sites in the central NA neurons. Large doses also release DA. It produces a variety of psychic effects such as increased mental and physical activity, elation, euphoria and insomnia. Larger doses cause tremor, restlessness, confusion, agitation and headache. In therapeutic doses (10-30 mg. orally), amphetamine produces wakefulness, decreases and postpones fatigue and improves the physical performance. The psychic effects of amphetamine are determined by the personality of the individual and the dose. Repeated administration causes psychic dependence.

The psychic effects of amphetamine are attributed to cortical stimulation while stimulation of the reticular activating system probably accounts for its analeptic effect.

Repeated and excessive stimulation by amphetamine is followed by fatigue and depression.

- ***Cardiovascular actions***: These are similar to those of ephedrine. It increases the systolic and diastolic BP but does not elevate the cardiac output significantly. Tachyphylaxis to the hypertensive effect is known.

- ***Smooth muscles***: It contracts the sphincter of the bladder and relaxes the bronchial smooth muscle only in large doses.

- ***Appetite suppression***: See Chapter 39.

Absorption, fate and excretion: Amphetamine is well absorbed on oral and parenteral administration and readily enters CNS. Like ephedrine, it is relatively resistant to inactivation by MAO. Approximately 40 per cent of the dose is excreted unchanged in urine.

Adverse reactions:

- ***CVS and CNS toxicity***: Excessive sympathetic stimulation generally causes palpitation, restlessness, headache, tremors and agitation. CNS stimulation causes marked anxiety, confusion, erratic behaviour, paranoid psychosis, visual hallucinations and misperception. This fact and the danger of after-depression and dependence should discourage its use by students during examination season.

- ***Acute intoxication*** causes

(a) CNS effects such as restlessness, dizziness, tremors, hyperactive reflexes, irritability, and insomnia, followed by fatigue and depression.

(b) Behavioral symptoms such as delirium, confusion, acute neurotic or psychotic episodes, and suicidal/homicidal tendencies.

(c) ANS instability resulting in angina pectoris, cardiac arrhythmias, headache, chilliness, flushing, pallor, hypertension, excessive sweating and circulatory collapse.

(d) GI symptoms including anorexia, nausea, vomiting, abdominal cramps and diarrhoea; and

(e) Hyperpyrexia.

These symptoms are characteristic of serotonergic syndrome (Chapter 13), and death is usually due to convulsions and coma. Cerebral hemorrhage can also occur.

Treatment of acute poisoning is symptomatic. Sedation with diazepam is indicated to control the central stimulation. Alpha adrenergic receptor blocking agents such as phentolamine are employed to control hypertension. The urine should be acidified to promote its excretion. Peritoneal dialysis may prove useful. *Individuals on therapy with MAO inhibitors may develop an alarming rise in BP with therapeutic doses of amphetamine-like drugs.*

- ***Long term consumption*** results in irritability, aggressive and stereotyped behavior, and paranoid psychosis. Marked weight loss is observed.

- ***Dependence and withdrawal symptoms***: Amphetamine causes habituation, tolerance and drug dependence which is mainly psychic. *It is a drug of abuse.* Withdrawal symptoms are listed in Table 17.7.

Preparations and dosage: Amphetamine sulfate 5 mg. Dose : 5 to 10 mg. in the morning and at midday. Dextroamphetamine (Dexedrine) sulfate as 5 mg. tablets.

Table 17.7: Amphetamine withdrawal symptoms

- Chronic fatigue, mental depression, asthenia, tremors.
- Gastrointestinal disturbances.
- Drowsiness, prolonged sleep or lethargy.
- Intense craving

Therapeutic uses:

It is no more used for its peripheral effects; but is used for treating Attention Deficit Hyperactivity Disorder (ADHD) and narcolepsy.

- ***ADHD***: Dexamphetamine has been used with benefit in children with ADHD. The diagnosis of ADHD must be established properly as many other conditions in children which superficially resemble ADHD do not improve on dexamphetamine. Linear growth may be hampered during long term treatment, probably because of the anorectic action of the drug. (Chapter 13).
- ***Narcolepsy***: Amphetamine 30 to 40 mg. per day in divided doses ameliorates narcolepsy and prevents attacks of sleep. It should not be administered after 4 p.m. as it interferes with natural sleep (Chapter 13).

Noncatecholamines Mainly Used as Vasopressor Agents

The vasopressor agents increase the BP either by increasing the total peripheral resistance by acting on the adrenoreceptors or by augmenting cardiac output or by a combination of both. They can be classified as:

I **Nonselective,** acting on both alpha and cardiac beta receptors e.g. noradrenaline; and

II **Selective,** acting only on alpha$_1$ adrenergic receptors e.g. mephentermine, metaraminol, phenylephrine and methoxamine.

These agents are routinely administered by parenteral route :

- ***To correct hypotension due to cardiogenic shock and to prevent and treat hypotension due to neurogenic shock,*** e.g. during or after spinal anaesthesia. They are, however, of little value in treating late haemorrhagic or endotoxic shock.
- ***To correct cardiac arrhythmias associated with hypotension.***
- ***In the treatment of paroxysmal atrial tachycardia***, as some of these agents increase the vagal tone reflexly.

METARAMINOL (Aramine) : Metaraminol resembles NA in its α receptor actions except that it is less potent and has a gradual onset and longer duration of action. It raises BP mainly by peripheral vasoconstriction. However, a part of its effect is mediated through NA release. Rise in BP is usually accompanied by reflex bradycardia.

Metaraminol increases the force of ventricular contraction and the cardic output. It increases the coronary blood flow, probably as a result of increased BP, and reduces the cerebral, splanchnic, renal and limb blood flow. The pressor effect lasts for about 11/2 hour after a 5 mg. IM dose. The drug has no effect on the CNS.

It is used to treat hypotension in the dose of 2 to 10 mg IM. The IV dose is 0.5 to 10 mg. Alternatively, 15-100 mg. of the drug can be given as a slow infusion in 500 ml of 5 per cent glucose. It is also be used as a nasal decongestant and to relieve paroxymal atrial tachycardia.

MEPHENTERMINE acts directly, as well as indirectly by releasing NA. Its actions resemble those of ephedrine. It causes CNS stimulation.

PHENYLEPHRINE (Neosynephrine) : This vasopressor agent has a potent selective α$_1$ receptor stimulant action. The pressor response is accompanied by reflex bradycardia. It has minimal action on the CNS. It is used as a nasal decongestant (0.25-0.5%) and as a mydriatic (1-2 per cent).

METHOXAMINE (Vasoxine) : Methoxamine, an alpha adrenergic agonist, raises BP purely by vasoconstrictor action. Peripheral vasoconstriction is accompanied by reflex bradycardia. Its haemodynamic actions are similar to those of phenylephrine. A 0.25 per cent solution is used as a nasal decongestant.

MIDODRINE: This prodrug acts through its active metabolite, desglymidodrine, on α_1 receptors. It is used to treat postural hypotension resulting from impaired autonomic function (Chapter 43).

When using vasopressor agents, the BP should be raised only moderately above the critical level (100/70 mm. Hg.) necessary for adequate tissue perfusion. An exaggerated vasoconstriction jeopardizes tissue perfusion and defeats the very purpose of vasopressor therapy. Tachyphylaxis to certain vasopressors may develop rarely necessitating a change-over to another drug; however, *other causes of refractoriness to vasopressors like hypovolemia and metabolic acidosis should be ruled out before changing over to another agent.*

Nasal Decongestants

In addition to the vasopressor agents mentioned above, other sympathomimetic amines are available for use topically as nasal decongestants. Also, see Chapter 26.

An ideal nasal decongestant should produce a prompt, prolonged and reliable effect and should be free from tachyphylaxis, local irritation and damaging effect on nasal cilia. It should not produce after-congestion and systemic adverse effects. Only a few drugs in very dilute solution are safe; majority of them can produce temporary or even permanent damage to ciliated respiratory epithelium after repeated use, with the possibility of atrophic changes.

In many cases, simple decongestion is all that is required. **Ephedrine hydrochloride** 0.5 per cent in normal saline is satisfactory and the safest symptomatic treatment. It gives relief for several hours. **Xylometazoline hydrochloride** 0.1 per cent (Otrivin), **tuamino heptane sulfate** 1 per cent (Tuamine sulfate) and **oxymetazoline** 0.05% (Nasivion) produce similar effects, at a higher cost; only the duration of action may differ. **Propylhexedrine** by inhalation (Benzedrex) has local action similar to that of ephedrine but causes less stimulation of the CNS.

Pseudoephedrine, **phenylephrine** and **phenylpropanolamine (norephedrine)** are common constituents of various oral preparations promoted for the relief of nasal congestion. Phenylpropanolamine resembles ephedrine in its CVS actions.It can cause CNS stimulation and can suppress appetite. *The drug has been reported to increase the incidence of hemorrhagic stroke in young women.*

Selective Alpha$_2$ Receptor Stimulants

Alpha$_2$ adrenergic receptor agonists, clonidine and methyldopa, are used for treatment of hypertension where they act by stimulating central alpha$_2$ adrenergic receptors (Chapter 29). They are also used to decrease raised intraocular pressure e.g. apraclonidine (Chapter 70).

Selective β_2 Receptor Stimulants

Isoprenaline acts by stimulating both beta$_1$ and beta$_2$ receptors and, therefore when used as a bronchodilator may cause adverse cardiac effects. Drugs with predominant action on β_2 receptors are available. These are **orciprenaline (metaproterenol), salbutamol (albuterol), salmeterol, fenoterol, terbutaline, ritodrine** and **isoetharine.** Given by inhalation, they act as promptly as isoprenaline but have a longer duration of action (2-12 hours) with much less stimulant action on the heart. Adverse effects, though similar to those of isoprenaline, are less intense. (Chapter 26).

They are used as:

- ***Bronchodilators*** (Chapter 26).
- ***Uterine relaxants (tocolytics)*** (Chapter 43).

Anorectic Sympathomimetic Drugs

The use of these agents in the treatment of obesity is discussed in Chapter 39.

Miscellaneous Compounds

ISOXSUPRINE HYDROCHLORIDE (Duvadilan): This has $beta_2$ receptor actions as well as direct action on vascular and uterine smooth muscle. On this basis, the drug was being promoted in the treatment of threatened abortion, premature labour and peripheral vascular disease. There is no convincing evidence that the drug is useful clinically. It is available as 10 mg tablets and as IM/IV injection. Injections may be used to treat premature labour.

Sympathetic Blocking Drugs

The actions produced by stimulation of the sympathetic nervous system can be blocked by peripherally acting drugs :

I **Drugs that induce depletion of catecholamines from the various body tissues** e.g. Reserpine and Tetrabenazine (Chapter 29).

II **Drugs that interfere with synthesis of the adrenergic transmitter** either in the adrenergic neuron or in the adrenal medulla e.g. Alpha methyl para tyrosine (Chapter 29).

III **Drugs that interfere with transmission of impulses across the postganglionic adrenergic neurons** e.g. adrenergic neuron blocking agents like Guanethidine (Chapter 29).

IV **Drugs which block the adrenergic receptors** e.g, α and β adrenergic receptor blocking agents. They are described below.

Adrenergic Receptor Blocking Agents

Adrenergic receptor blocking agents prevent the response of effector organs to endogenous as well as exogenous adrenaline and NA. These drugs block either alpha or beta receptors.

ALPHA RECEPTOR BLOCKERS: These drugs are more effective in antagonising the alpha receptor effects of exogenously administered adrenaline and NA than those following adrenergic stimulation.They are :

I **Nonselective alpha adrenergic blockers:**

(a) Beta haloalkylamines e.g. Dibenamine and Phenoxybenzamine.

(b) Natural and hydrogenated Ergot alkaloids.

(c) Imidazoline derivatives, e.g., Tolazoline and Phentolamine.

II **Selective $alpha_1$ adrenergic blockers**: Quinazolines e.g. Prazosin, Terazosin, Doxazosin and Indoramin

III **Selective $alpha_2$ adrenergic blockers,** e.g., Yohimbine.

PHENOXYBENZAMINE (Dibenzyline) : It binds covalently to alpha receptors and causes prolonged and stable non-equilibrium (non-competitive) type of blockade, loosely termed irreversible blockade. It also blocks the $uptake_1$ mechanism.

Pharmacological actions: Phenoxybenzamine is a prodrug with an active metabolite. It is nonselective in that it blocks both postsynaptic

$alpha_1$ and presynaptic $alpha_2$ receptors. The blocking effect is established only after 1-2 hours, even on IV administration and persists for 3 to 4 days. The usual blocking doses cause only slight lowering of diastolic BP in normals but significant lowering of BP in patients with pheochromocytoma. The compound evokes Dale's vasomotor reversal. It does not antagonize the cardiac actions of catecholamines but is capable of inhibiting cardiac arrhythmias induced by adrenaline and other sympathomimetic amines. Thus, this agent *can prevent but cannot reverse* such arrhythmias.

The drug also antagonises the actions of ACh, histamine and 5-HT. In clinically effective doses, phenoxybenzamine causes orthostatic hypotension due to $alpha_1$ blockade in the blood vessels. Accumulated NA at the adrenergic neuronal endings would normally be reduced by autoreceptor action of α_2 receptors; but as they too are blocked, the released NA stimulates cardiac β receptors, causing tachycardia. Phenoxybenzamine, on slow IV infusion, often produces sedation and drowsiness, probably by its antihistaminic activity. It has no significant effect on the motility of the GI tract.

Absorption, fate and excretion : Given orally, the absorption of phenoxybenzamine is irregular. The drug may produce irritation on SC or IM administration and hence, is given orally or by IV infusion. Because of its high lipid solubility, it tends to accumulate in the body fat. Approximately 50 per cent of the IV dose of phenoxybenzamine is excreted within 12 hours and 80 per cent within 24 hours.

Adverse reactions : Besides miosis, dryness of mouth, nasal stuffiness and inhibition of ejaculation, phenoxybenzamine may cause palpitation, giddiness and postural hypotension. Large doses often produce nausea, vomiting, increased excitability and even convulsions. It can cause cumulative toxicity.

Preparations and dosage: Phenoxybenzamine (Dibenzyline) 10 mg capsules. The usual daily maintenance dose is 20-60 mg.

It is used orally to prepare a patient with a pheochromocytoma for surgery and in its long term treatment. (Chapter 29).

NATURAL AND DIHYDROGENATED ERGOT ALKALOIDS : The chemistry of the ergot alkaloids is discussed in Chapter 43. The **natural amino acid ergot alkaloids**, ergotamine, ergosine, ergocornine, ergocristine and ergocryptine (the last three collectively termed formerly as "ergotoxine") and their dihydrogenated derivatives can block the alpha adrenergic receptors. They have a direct stimulant effect on the vascular and uterine muscle. The stimulant activity on the smooth muscle decreases from the natural amino acid alkaloids to their dihydrogenated derivatives with a corresponding increase in the alpha adrenergic blockade. Thus, the natural amino acid alkaloids usually raise the BP and may constrict coronary vessels.

The **dihydrogenated alkaloids,** on the other hand, have a minimal constricting effect on coronaries and usually reduce BP, by a combination of alpha adrenergic blockade and depression of the vasomotor centre. The exception to this is **dihydroergotamine** (DHE) which retains a considerable vasoconstrictor effect in addition to adrenergic blocking activity. It has been used to treat orthostatic hypotension due to autonomic neuropathy.

Ergot alkaloids also reduce the sympathetic tone by depression of the vasomotor centre, induce bradycardia by central vagal stimulation and direct myocardial depression and may cause vomiting by stimulation of the CTZ. They are also effective antagonists of 5-HT.

The amine ergot alkaloid, **ergometrine**, is devoid of adrenergic blocking activity and is discussed in Chapter 43.

Absorption, fate and excretion : The amino acid alkaloids and their dihydrogenated derivatives are poorly absorbed on oral administration. A part of the total parenteral dose is degraded in the body.

Adverse reactions: These compounds often produce nausea, vomiting, miosis and postural hypotension. Anginal pain may occur particularly with natural amino acid alkaloids due to coronary constriction. The natural alkaloids, on prolonged administration, may also induce paraesthesiae, tingling, numbness and occasionally frank gangrene due to peripheral vasospasm. Headache, diarrhoea, confusion, depression, drowsiness and rarely hemiplegia and cerebral haemorrhage have also been reported with ergotamine. See also Chapter 43.

Preparations and dosage:

(i) Ergotamine tartrate tablet 1 mg. Dose : 1 to 2 mg. as a single dose orally, 3 to 4 mg. sublingually.

(ii) Ergotamine tartrate injection 0.5 mg. in one ml. Dose: 0.25 to 0.5 mg. SC or IM.

(iii) Dihydroergotamine injection (DHE): Dose: 1 to 1.5 mg SC or IM.

(iv) DHE tablets : Up to 20 mg/day, in divided doses, to treat orthostatic hypotension due to autonomic neuropathy.

(v) Hydergine : See Chapter 43.

IMIDAZOLINE DERIVATIVES: The compounds **tolazoline** (Priscoline) and **phentolamine** (Regitine), in addition to competitive non-selective alpha adrenergic blockade, produce an increase in the force of contraction of myocardium and tachycardia. They dilatate the peripheral blood vessels, particularly the arterioles and capillaries of the skin, and increase the gut motility and the gastric secretion. The salivary, lacrimal, respiratory and pancreatic secretions are also augmented. The compounds also exert a mild anti-5-HT activity.

Tolazoline is a partial α_1 agonist and because of its predominant cardiac effect, often evokes a mild rise in BP while phentolamine usually produces a moderate fall due to peripheral vasodilatation.

Absorption, fate and excretion : Tolazoline is well absorbed on oral and parenteral administration and eliminated mainly unchanged in urine. Phentolamine is poorly absorbed on oral administration; approximately 1/10th of its total parenteral dose is eliminated in urine while the rest is probably metabolized.

Adverse reactions: These include palpitation, flushing and apprehension. Other disturbances are a sensation of coldness, postural hypotension, piloerection, nausea, vomiting, epigastric distress and diarrhoea. Excessive doses of tolazoline may induce profuse sweating.

Preparations and dosage:

Phentolamine mesylate injection 5 mg. per ml. Dose : 1-10 mg. IV, repeated if necessary.

Quinazolines:

Fig. 17.6 : Prazosin

PRAZOSIN (Minipress) : This drug acts by blocking α_1 receptors selectively. Thus, it dilates the arteries (lowering blood pressure) and the veins (reducing the venous return and cardiac output); and it reduces the tone of the internal sphincter of the bladder (decreasing the resistance to urinary outflow in patients with benign prostatic hypertrophy). It does not cause tachycardia as it does not block presynaptic α_2 receptors. For details and advere effects, see Chapter 29.

TERAZOSIN (Hytrin) : This selective α_1 adrenergic blocker is used in the treatment of benign prostatic hypertrophy (Chapter 67). The drug is long acting and is used once a day in the dose of 1 mg (at bed time), increased at weekly intervals to 2-10 mg (single dose).

Doxazocin, alfuzosin and **tamsulosin** are the other $alpha_1$ adrenergic blockers. Tamsulosin acts more selectively on the prostatic $alpha_{1A}$ and $alpha_{1D}$ adrenergic receptors. (Chapter 67).

Miscellaneous:

INDORAMIN (Doralese): This selective $alpha_1$ blocker is used to treat benign prostatic hypertrophy in the dose of 20 mg b.i.d. (Chapter 67). The daily dose may be increased by 20 mg every 2 weeks to a maximum of 100 mg. In the elderly 20 mg once at night may be adequate. For its use in hypertension, see Chapter 29.

YOHIMBINE, an alkaloid from the West African tree *Pausinystalia chimbe,* produces a competitive blockade of $alpha_2$ receptors which persists only for a short time. Stimulation of the presynaptic $alpha_2$ receptors inhibits the release of NA from the peripheral adrenergic nerve endings. Yohimbine, by blocking these receptors, increases the sympathetic outflow and potentiates the release of NA. Given orally, the drug enjoys a reputation as an aphrodisiac and is claimed to help 50% of people with erectile dysfunction. However, prolonged therapy is needed.

Ketanserin,a 5-HT receptor antagonist, also blocks α_1 adrenergic receptors.

Alpha adrenergic blocking action of chlorpromazine and haloperidol is discussed in Chapter 13.

Therapeutic uses of alpha adrenergic blocking agents: These drugs have limited therapeutic applications, mainly owing to their adverse effects like tachycardia and postural hypotension. The important uses are:

- ***Hypertension and pheochromocytoma***: see Chapter 29.
- ***Peripheral vascular disease***: see Chapter 28. Phentolamine infiltrated in the dose of 2.5 to 5 mg. prevents cutaneous necrosis due to extravasation of NA.
- ***Benign prostatic hypertrophy:*** Prazosin is given initially in the dose of 0.5 mg b.i.d; the *first* dose is given at bedtime to avoid vascular collapse (first dose effect). After 3-7 days, the dose is adjusted to the usual maintenance dose of upto 2 mg b.i.d. The more selective α_1 blockers are now preferred (Chapter 67).
- ***Erectile dysfunction*** (Chapter 67).
- ***Scorpion sting*** (Chapter 76).

BETA ADRENERGIC BLOCKING AGENTS: These drugs block the actions of catecholamines by acting selectively and competitively on the beta-adrenoreceptors. They inhibit the activity of the cell membrane enzyme adenylyl cyclase and decrease the production of cyclic AMP. They can be classified as :

I **Cardioselective $beta_1$ blockers** e.g., Acebutolol, Atenolol, Metoprolol, Bisoprolol, Celiprolol and Esmolol. Acebutolol has intrinsic sympathomimetic activity and celiprolol has membrane stabilizing action.

II **Nonselective $beta_1$ and $beta_2$ blockers:**

(a) Beta blockers with membrane stabilizing activity e.g., Propranolol.

(b) Beta blockers with intrinsic sympathetic action e.g. Carteolol.

(c) Beta blockers with membrane stabilizing activity and intrinsic sympathomimetic activity e.g., Oxprenolol, Pindolol.

(d) Beta blockers without membrane stabilizing action e.g. Timolol, Nadolol and Sotalol. (Chapter 29).

III **Beta blockers with additional alpha blocking property** e.g., Labetalol, Bucinolol and Carvedilol.

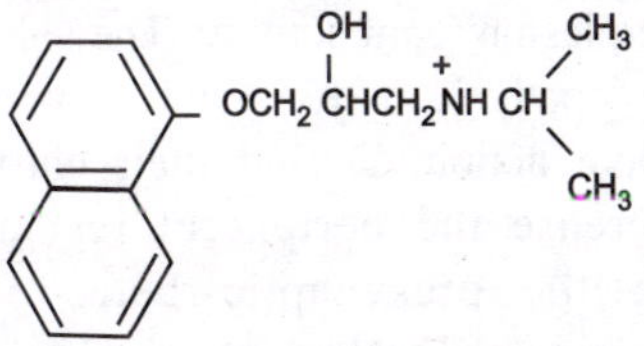

OH, CH$_3$, OCH$_2$ CHCH$_2$NH CH, CH$_3$

Fig. 17.7 : Propranolol

Pharmacological Actions:

- ***Effects of beta-blockade***: These drugs do not produce any marked effect on the normal heart in the subject at rest. In the presence of increased sympathetic tone, however, the beta-blockade in the heart

(a) Reduces the automaticity and prevents the rise in heart rate (Fig. 17.8);

(b) Reduces the myocardial contractility, cardiac output and stroke work;

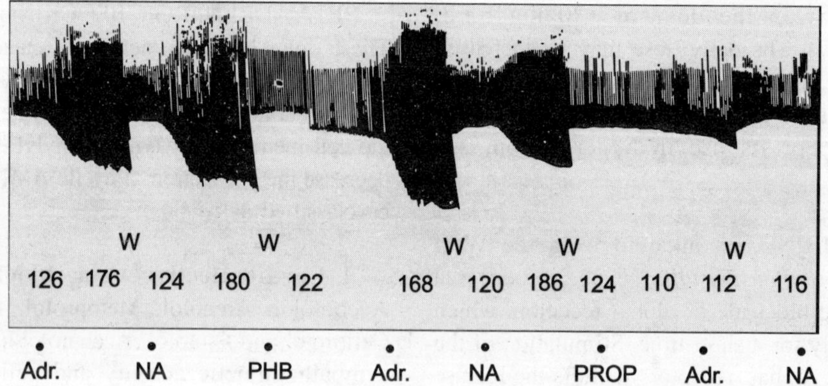

Fig. 17.8 : Effects of alpha adrenergic blocking agent phenoxybenzamine (PHB) and beta adrenergic blocking agent propranolol (PROP) on the actions of adrenaline and noradrenaline on isolated rabbit auricle. Note the reduction in the rate and the amplitude of auricular contraction with PROP in contrast to phenoxybenzamine.

(c) Slows A-V conduction; and

(d) Reduces myocardial oxygen requirement and improves exercise tolerance.

The cardiac response to exercise and to other situations in which sympathetic tone is increased, is attenuated. Certain beta-blockers are more cardioselective (beta$_1$) in action than others (Table 17.8).

Beta-blockers also reduce BP probably by their action on the heart and reduction in cardiac output. They reduce renal rennin release and lower the plasma renin activity. They also reduce central sympathetic outflow and have a central hypotensive action. During their chronic use, they decrease the peripheral resistance by blocking the presynaptic beta$_2$-receptors, resulting in reduction in the release of noradrenaline from the adrenergic nerve endings.

Some beta blockers have additional actions e.g. through NO production (celiprolol, carteolol), calcium channel blocking (carvedilol), and potassium channel opening (tilisolol). Their contribution to the therapeutic effects of BB is not clear.

The blockade of beta$_2$ receptor sites in bronchi and bronchioles causes increase in airway resistance which could be harmful in patients with asthma. Other effects include prevention of adrenaline-induced glycogenolysis in the skeletal muscle and inhibition of the release of FFA from the adipose tissue.

- ***Membrane-stabilizing action***: Propranolol and some other beta-blockers have a variable direct depressant effect on the heart similar to that of lignocaine. This membrane effect is unrelated to beta-blocking potency. It occurs only with high concentrations of the drug and is probably not relevant to the clinical use of beta blockers.

- ***Intrinsic sympathomimetic action***: Some of the beta-blockers possess beta-receptor stimulating activity (*partial agonist property*). It has been *suggested but not proved,* that beta-blocking agents with additional intrinsic sympathomimetic activity may cause less myocardiac depression and are thus less likely to precipitate congestive heart failure in the presence of damaged heart. Pindolol and oxprenolol which have partial agonistic activity may not impair A-V conduction.

It should be noted that the pharmacological actions of beta-receptor antagonism are always present at lower concentrations of the drug than either membrane stabilizing or paradoxical agonist effect. *The primary beta-blocking action of all these drugs is in fact mostly responsible for their beneficial as well as adverse effects.*

- ***Effects on the CNS***: Lipid soluble propranolol, metoprolol and labetalol can readily

Table 17.8: Properties of some beta-adrenergic blockers

Drugs	Relative lipid solubility	β_2 agonist activity	Protein binding (%)	Liver metabolism	Kidney excretion (%)	Plasma half life (hrs)
I **Nonselective :**						
Propranolol (Inderal, Ciplar)	+++	0	93	+++	0.5	3-6
Oxprenolol (Trasicor)	++	++	-	+++	5	1-2
Pindolol (Visken)	+	+++	51	++	30-40	3-4
Nadolol (Corgard)	+	0	30	+	76	20-24
Timolol (Betim)	++	0	10	+++	15	4-6
Labetolol* (Normadate)	+	+	50	+++	5	3-4
Carteolol	+	++	25-30	0	80	6
Carvedilol*	+++	0	98	+++	< 2	7-10
II **Cardioselective :**						
Atenolol (Aten, Tenormin)	+	0	6-16	+	85	6-8
Metoprolol (Lopresor)	++	0	12	++	10	3-6
Bisoprolol (Concor)	+	0	30	++	63	9-12
Acebutolol (Sectral)	+	+	26	+	30-40	2-5
Esmolol** (Brevibloc)	+	0	55	+++	2	0.15
Celiprolol	+	+	25-30	0	12-8	5-6
Nebivolol (Bistolic)	+++	0	98	+++	0.5	12-19

* Alpha receptor blocking also

** IV infusion only, in emergency management of unstable angina, threatened infarct, cardiac arrhythmias and thyrotoxic crisis + = Present. 0 = Absent.

cross the BBB. In man, propranolol alters mood and has been tried in anxiety states. Atenolol, with the lowest lipid solubility, has fewer central side effects.

● ***Metabolic effects***: Beta blockers are capable of modifying carbohydrate and lipid metabolism. Nonselective BB prevent the perception of hypoglycemia by preventing indicative symptoms such as palpitation and tremor. In addition, they prevent catecholamine-induced glycogenolysis and mobilization of glucose during hypoglycemia, and delay recovery. Further, they decrease the release of fatty acids from the adipose tissue. On long term therapy, they increase LDL cholesterol and triglycerides, and decrease HDL cholesterol. However, selective β_1 blockers such as celiprolol, carvedilol and carteolol may improve the lipid profile. The vasodilatory beta-blockers increase insulin sensitivity in patients with insulin resistance. They also increase the natriuretic peptide secretion (Chapter 36).

● ***Intraocular pressure***: β-blockers, used topically or orally, cause a reduction in intraocular pressure due to a reduction in the secretion of aqueous humour (Chapter 70). Table 17.8: list the properties of some beta-adrenergic blockers.

Absorption, fate and excretion: The effective oral dose ranges of the ß-blocking drugs are wide. Plasma concentrations vary markedly between individuals receiving the same dose. This is because although most of these compounds are completely and rapidly absorbed orally, some of them like propranolol and metoprolol are rapidly metabolized by the liver (first pass metabolism). Thus for propranolol, the relative oral bioavailability is low and variations in plasma levels are marked (almost upto 20 fold). Pindolol, acebutolol, atenolol and timolol are eliminated to variable extents by both routes. The relative oral bioavailability of pindolol and sotalol is better and variations in plasma levels are less marked.

The plasma half life of the beta-blocking drugs that are mostly metabolized by the liver is short (2-3 hours), whereas that of drugs excreted unchanged by the kidneys is longer (8-12 hours). Plasma half life is also modified by disease of the liver and of the kidney (Table 17.8) and by the metabolite(s), active or inactive e.g. the active metabolite of propranolol, 4 hydroxyproprenolol, makes twice a day administration of proprenolol possible. *The plasma half life, however, does not correlate well with the duration of the therapeutic effects of betablockers, which is relatively long lasting.* This is because the plasma level declines exponentially, thus following first order kinetics while the effect decreases linearly, following zero order kinetics. Hence, *most preparations can be given orally at much longer intervals than is suggested by their plasma half-lives.*

Adverse reactions :

- ***Cardiaovascular effects*** : These are mostly due to the *extended cardiac actions.* Thus, propranolol may cause sudden hypotension and pronounced bradycardia and cardiac arrest. The ventricular function depends on increased contractility due to sympathetic activity and beta-blockade prevents this homeostatic response leading to clinical heart failure. Congestive heart failure is thus the most important serious adverse effect of ß-blockers. Beta-blockers with additional 'quinidine like activity' may cause a direct depression of the damaged heart leading to myocardial failure.

Because of their action on A-V conduction, some of these drugs can aggravate A-V conduction defects. However, this action may be beneficial in patients with atrial fibrillation resistant to digitalis. Excessive bradycardia due to beta blockers can be countered by IV atropine 0.6 - 2.4 mg in divided doses. Hypotension refractory to atropine may require IV glucagon (Chapter 31),

If propranolol therapy is to be discontinued in angina, the dosage should be reduced gradually, as myocardial infarction may be precipitated following its abrupt withdrawal.

Cold extremities and absent pulses may sometimes be observed after beta-blockade. Raynaud's phenomenon may occasionally be troublesome and intermittent claudication may be aggravated.

- ***Metabolic effects*** : These drugs prevent the correction of hypoglycemia by adrenergic body mechanisms (**hypoglycemia unresponsiveness**) and may aggravate neurogylcopenic symptoms of hypoglycemia. However, in clinical practice beta-blockers may be used safely in most patients with T2DM (Chapter 63). If they must be used in patients on insulin, a cardioselective drug is preferred.
- ***Respiratory effects*** : Bronchospasm may occur particularly in patients with bronchial asthma. Cardioselective beta-blockers in low doses may be preferred but none is absolutely safe.
- ***CNS effects*** : Prolonged use of propranolol can cause fatigue, muscle cramps, lethargy and rarely mental depression and hallucinations.
- ***Miscellaneous*** : These include sexual dysfunction, allergic reactions, thrombocytopenia and rarely, agranulocytosis. In patient with severe renal failure, betablockers can reduce the GFR further; hence their dose needs to be adjusted appropriately. They are not teratogenic and may be used during pregnancy.

Drugs such as NSAID that cause sodium retention attenuate the antihypertensive effect of beta blockers. By reducing the hepatic blood flow by almost 30%, beta blockers can slow down the hepatic metabolism of certain drugs.

Beta blockers may increase the severity and possibly the frequency of anaphylactic

Table 17.9 : Dosage range of some beta adrenergic blocking drugs

Drug	Total daily Dose (mg)	Schedule
Propranolol	80-240	6-12 hourly
Metoprolol	100-200	12 hourly/single
Atenolol	25-100	Daily
Timolol	10-60	12 hourly
Pindolol	10-45	6 hourly
Labetalol	200-600	12 hourly

reactions to drugs, biologicals, insect stings and foods, and the reaction may prove resistant to treatment with adrenaline.

Table 17.9 shows the dosage schedules of the commonly used beta blockers.

Therapeutic uses: Clinically, in terms of beta blocking activity, no drug is demonstrably superior to others. The choice is guided by safety, pharmacological properties, ease of administration and cost. In the presence of airway obstruction or peripheral vascular disease, a cardioselective beta-blocker may be chosen, keeping in mind that cardioselectivity is not absolute. The therapeutic uses are:

I Cardiovascular :

● ***Angina pectoris***: Beta-blockers are the mainstay of the chronic, prophylactic treatment of patients with angina of effort (Chapter 28).

● ***Myocardial infarction***: Chapter 28.

● ***Cardiac arrhythmias***: Betablockers can be used successfully in the treatment of tachyarrhythmias precipitated by sympathetic overactivity as during exercise, emotion and anaesthesia. (Chapter 27).

● ***Hypertension***: Betablockers are valuable in the treatment of hypertension (Chapter 29).

● ***Congestive heart failure***: Chapter 30.

● ***Hypertrophic obstructive cardio-myopathy*** (Idiopathic hypertrophic subaortic stenosis) is characterised by a marked hypertrophy of the ventricular musculature, commonly of the left ventricle, leading to palpitation, angina, dyspnoea or syncope. Propranolol, in the dose of 60 to 400 mg. per day, causes symptomatic improvement.

● ***Pheochromocytoma***: Alpha adrenergic blocking agents are routinely used prior to surgery in patients with pheochromocytoma. In some patients, however, alpha blockade leads to a severe tachycardia particularly when atropine is used for preanaesthetic medication. Propranolol, in the dose of 1-5 mg. IV prevents this complication. It should be pointed out, however, that beta blockade without simultaneous alpha blockade may lead to severe hypertension in pheochromocytoma.

II Non-cardiovascular :

● ***Chronic open-angle glaucoma*** : Timolol maleate (Timoptal, Glucomol) 0.25-0.5% used as eye-drops is as effective as pilocarpine in lowering intraocular pressure. It has an advantage in that it does not induce spasm of accommodation nor does it affect the pupil. Further, it is convenient to administer (once or twice daily). Beta-blockers can be used in conjunction with miotics and carbonic anhydrase inhibitors in resistant cases. In general, β blockers used locally are well tolerated and reasonably safe even on long term use. Other beta blockers used in chronic open angle glaucoma are betaxolol 0.5%, metipranolol 0.1% and carteolol 1% (Chapter 70).

● ***Thyrotoxicosis***: Beta blockers are valuable adjuncts to antithyroid drugs in the treatment of thyrotoxicosis, where they produce rapid symptomatic relief (Chapter 62).

● ***Portal hypertension***: Propranolol and nadolol are used orally to prevent variceal bleeding in this condition; they act by lowering the pressure in the portal circulation.

● ***To control the withdrawal symptoms in alcohol addicts.*** (Chapter 6).

● ***Miscellaneous***: Increased adrenergic activity is prominent in **anxiety states** and propranolol can reduce the associated symptoms such as palpitation, tachycardia and sweating. Betablockers may used to decrease

Table 17.10: Contraindications to beta blockers

Absolute :

- Severe bradycardia
- Pre-existing high grade heart block
- Overt left ventricular failure (untreated)
- Cardiogenic shock
- Severe bronchospasm
- Severe depression
- Raynaud's phenomenon (active disease)

Relative : Prinzmetal's angina; concomitant use of verapamil, diltiazem or digoxin; mild asthma; insulin requiring diabetes mellitus.

cardiac symptoms prior to important meetings and public speaking engagements in susceptible individuals. Propranolol is also useful in the prevention of **migraine** and treatment of **essential tremor** as it crosses the BB barrier.

Contraindications to beta-blockers : See Table 17.10

ALPHA AND BETA-ADRENERGIC BLOCKING DRUGS:

LABETALOL (Normadate) : Labetolol is a non-selective beta blocker with selective $alpha_1$ blocking action. It is devoid of intrinsic sympthomimetic action. Given orally, it has actions similar to those of propranolol.

The drug undergoes extensive first pass metabolism.

Adverse reactions : Labetalol may cause GI disturbances, dryness of mouth and fluid retention. Cardiac effects are similar to those of other beta blockers. Postural hypotension may occur due to alpha blockade. Other reactions include nervousness, sexual dysfunction, muscle cramps and depression. Patients on long term therapy may develop antinuclear antibodies but SLE is rare. The drug accumulates in tissues with high melanin content such as the choroid, and periodic eye examination is recommended.

Therapeutic uses : It is mainly used to treat hypertension and hypertensive emergencies. (Chapter 29) as the effect comes rapidly due to concurrent α blockade.

CARVEDILOL (Cardivas) : Like labetalol, this drug is a non-selective beta adrenergic receptor antagonist, with selective $alpha_1$ adrenergic receptor blocking action. In higher concentrations, it blocks the entry of Ca^{++} into the vascular smooth muscle. It is devoid of intrinsic sympathomimetic activity but has membrane stabilizing effect. It causes vasodilatation. Carvedilol is also claimed to have antioxidant action in animal experiments. The drug is used in treatment of hypertension. Carvedilol is available as 12.5 and 25 mg tablets.

Bisoprolol (Concor): This drug is more selective than atenolol for $beta_1$ receptors and is claimed to cause adverse effects less frequently. Dose : 10 mg/day

Nebivolol is cardioselective BB with NO-mediated vasodilator properties. It is effective in hypertension as well as CHF.

Carvedilol, bisoprolol, metoprolol and nebivolol have been found to improve left ventricular function and are useful in CHF (Chapter 30).

Cholinergic Drugs

18

Cholinergic or parasympathomimetic agents are drugs which stimulate the effector cells innervated by postganglionic parasympathetic cholinergic nerves. In general, their actions are similar to those seen following the stimulation of the parasympathetic nervous system.

These drugs are classified as :

I **Esters of choline** e.g. Acetylcholine, Methacholine, Carbachol and Bethanechol.

II **Cholinomimetic alkaloids,** e.g., Pilocarpine, Muscarine and Arecholine.

III **Cholinesterase inhibitors (Anti-cholinesterases),** e.g., Physostigmine, Neostigmine, Organophosphorus compounds.

Esters of Choline

Acetylcholine (ACh) is an ester of choline with acetic acid, while carbachol and bethanechol are esters of choline and betamethylcholine respectively with carbamic acid. The base choline also possesses properties similar to acetylcholine. Esterification of choline augments the cholinergic activity markedly.

Chemically, ACh and related substances are quaternary ammonium compounds and their unique specific action is attributed to the trimethylammonium [R-N$^+$(CH3)$_3$] groupings.

ACETYLCHOLINE: Acetylcholine is available in powder form as chloride or bromide; it is extremely hygroscopic. Although it is not useful in therapeutics it is important to know its actions for understanding of cholinergic drugs used therapeutically. *There is no circulating ACh in the blood.*

$$CH_3-\overset{+}{N}(CH_3)_2-CH_2-CH_2-O-COCH_3$$

Fig. 18.1 : Acetylcholine

Mechanism of actions: ACh acts on two subtypes of cholinergic receptors :

(a) **Muscarinic**; and

(b) **Nicotinic**

• ***Muscarinic actions***: The actions produced as a result of ACh released from the postganglionic parasympathetic nerve endings or the actions resulting from exogenously administered ACh on the organs that posses M receptors are termed as *muscarinic actions,* e.g., secretory glands, smooth muscles and the heart. They are blocked by atropine. The designation muscarinic action comes from the fact that these actions are similar to those produced by the poisonous mushroom alkaloid muscarine.

Currently, five subtypes of the muscarinic receptors M_1 M_2, M_3, M_4 and M_5 have been identified.There is a great deal of homology among M_1, M_3 and M_5 receptors and between M_2 and M_4 receptors. Muscarinic receptors with M_1 sensitivity are found in the CNS and ganglia whereas M_2 sites exist in the heart and M_3 in the smooth muscle of the GI tract.

M_1 and M_3 receptors activate Gs protein that is responsible for the stimulation of phospholipase C activity. This leads to the hydrolysis of phosphatidylinositol polyphosphate (PIP) to form inositol 1-4-5 triphosphate and diacylglycerol. The former causes release of intracellular calcium from endoplasmic reticulum while the latter activates protein kinase C.

The M_2 receptors interact with a distinct group of G proteins (known as Gi) with resultant inhibition of adenylyl cyclase and activation of K^+ channels, particularly in the heart, and modulation of the activity of calcium channels in certain cell types. These effects account for both the negative chronotropic and the inotropic effects of ACh.

• ***Nicotinic actions***: The actions of ACh at the nicotinic receptors are termed nicotinic actions as they resemble those produced by the tobacco alkaloid nicotine. To demonstrate these actions, atropine has to be administered to block the muscarinic actions of ACh; in such animal preparations, injection of large doses (1-5 mg) of ACh still produces certain responses (Fig. 18.2). These actions are due to an initial stimulation and subsequent blockade of the nicotinic receptors in autonomic ganglia and the skeletal myoneural junctions.

Nicotinic receptors are ligand-gated ion channels, and their activation causes a rapid increase in the cell permeability to Na^+ and K^+ ions with resultant depolarization and excitation.

Pharmacological actions: Given orally, ACh is rapidly destroyed in the GI tract and hence, it has to be administered by IV infusion to elicit its actions. Even large IV, bolus doses of ACh have no appreciable action in man. This is because a considerable amount of ACh (bolus) given IV is destroyed in the plasma by the enzyme *pseudocholinesterase*, and at the site of action by the specific *true cholinesterase* and is thus prevented from reaching a sufficient concentration at the effector cells. The only important action seen after IV (bolus) injection of ACh is a transient fall in BP. Infusion IV can however demonstrate the other actions of ACh. Many of its actions can also be demonstrated in *in-vitro* preparations.

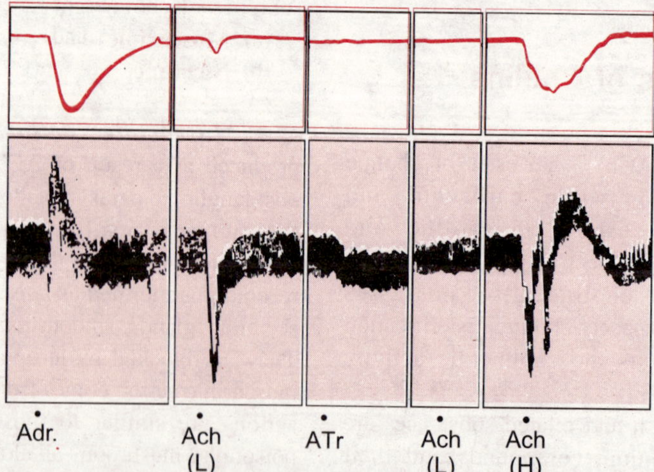

Fig. 18.2 : Blood pressure and spleen volume (upper tracing) in anaesthetised dog. Note the fall of B.P. following a low dose of acetylcholine (ACh) which is blocked by atropine (Muscarinic action). High dose of ACh in this atropinised animal produced rise in B.P. and contraction of the spleen (Nicotinic action), resembling the action of adrenaline (Adr.).

Cardiovascular system :

• ***Heart***: In mammals, the effect of ACh on the heart is similar to that obtained by stimulation of the vagus which is a cholinergic nerve. Thus, it

(1) Depresses the SA node, causes bradycardia (**negative chronotropic action**), and may cause cardiac arrest;

(2) Decreases the contractility (**negative inotropic action**);

(3) May cause A-V block; and

(4) Increases the conduction velocity in the atria. These changes are transient and can be blocked by atropine.

Acetylcholine reduces the cardiac rate in isolated heart preparation. However, in the presence of atropine, acetylcholine can stimulate the heart, causing ventricular arrhythmias.

• ***Blood vessels***: Acetylcholine dilates the blood vessels mainly of the skin and the mucous membranes by acting on the M_3 receptors located on the endothelial cells of the vessel wall. When these receptors are stimulated, the endothelial cells release nitric oxide (NO) which causes vascular relaxation. If the endothelium is damaged, ACh causes vasoconstriction. It also dilates the coronary arteries and has a doubtful vasodilator effect on the cerebral and pulmonary vessels. ACh IV in man results in flushing, a sense of warmth in the skin and throbbing headache. The BP falls owing to a decrease in the peripheral resistance and in the cardiac output (**vagal effect**) in anaesthetized animals.

Smooth muscles: Acetylcholine

• ***Increases the tone and the rhythmic activity of the smooth muscle of the GI tract and enhances peristalsis.*** The sphincters are, however, relaxed resulting in a rapid forward propulsion of the intestinal contents.

• ***Contracts the smooth muscle of the gall bladder.***

• ***Contracts the detrusor muscle of the urinary bladder while the smooth muscle of the trigonal sphincter is relaxed.***

• ***Constricts the bronchial smooth muscle and causes bronchospasm.***

• ***Usually contracts the smooth muscle of the ureter*** while that of the uterus shows inconsistent response.

Secretions: Cholinergic stimulation increases the gastric, intestinal and pancreatic secretions; the bronchial, salivary, lacrimal and nasopharyngeal secretions are also augmented. The increased bronchial secretions, accompanied by bronchospasm, may result in cough and dyspnoea. The salivary secretion is profuse and watery. *As the postganglionic sympathetic fibres supplying the sweat glands are cholinergic, ACh enhances sweating.*

Eye : Instillation of ACh in the eye is without any effect as it is not absorbed. However, intra-carotid injection after sectioning of the postganglionic fibres from superior cervical ganglion produces:

• ***Constriction of the pupil (miosis)*** by contracting the circular fibres of sphincter pupillae, resulting in reduction in intraocular tension by increasing the drainage of ocular fluid through the canal of Schlemm.

• ***Contraction of the ciliary muscle*** which results in relaxation of the suspensory ligament (zonule) of the lens. This reduces the tension on the lens and allows the lens to bulge into the anterior chamber thereby increasing its thickness and reducing the focal length. Vision is, therefore, fixed for a short distance. This is termed *spasm of accommodation.*

Autonomic ganglia: Acetylcholine-induced ganglionic stimulation results in an increased output of ACh and NA from the postganglionic parasympathetic and sympathetic nerve endings respectively. The effects of released NA can be demonstrated by using an atropinized preparation. In such a preparation the BP shows a rise due to peripheral vasoconstriction. In addition, large doses of ACh also stimulate the adrenal medulla to increase the secretion of adrenaline which further augments and sustains the rise in blood pressure (Fig. 18.2).

Myoneural junction: Acetylcholine released as a result of stimulation of the somatic nerves induces contraction of the skeletal muscle. A very high concentration of ACh at the myoneural junction can produce paralysis of the skeletal muscles by keeping the muscle in a persistently depolarized state in which it is refractory to further stimuli. Intra-arterial injection of Ach in the brachial artery of human volunteers produces fasciculations and twitching of the skeletal muscle followed by a prolonged weakness.

The action of ACh on the autonomic ganglia is blocked by ganglion blocking agents like hexamethonium whereas the action on the myoneural junction is antagonized by tubocurarine. (Chapter 21).

Miscellaneous actions: Acetylcholine is a neurohumoral transmitter at certain sites in the CNS. Both choline acetyl transferase and cholinesterase have been demonstrated in various parts of the CNS. The recurrent collaterals of the motor neurons which synapse with the Renshaw cells of the spinal cord are cholinergic and the receptors are predominantly nicotinic in nature. *In contrast, most of the cholinergic neurons at the cortical and subcortical levels of the CNS have predominately muscarinic receptors.*

Considerable experimental evidence is available indicating cholinergic involvement in behavioural responses. Patients with Huntington's disease, characterized by involuntary choreiform movements and dementia, have been found to have severe degeneration of cholinergic neurons within the basal ganglia. Patients suffering from Alzheimer's dementia have significant losses of an enzyme activity (choline acetyltransferase) in the basal ganglia, frontal cortex and hippocampus. It appears that a cholinergic system is essential to normal behaviour and cognition.

Being a quarternary ammonium compound, ACh administered IV does not cross the blood brain barrier and hence it exerts no significant central actions.

Therapeutic uses: Owing to its extremely transient action, ACh cannot be employed for any therapeutic purpose. Hence, ACh substitutes have been synthesised which are:

- ***Effective orally;***
- ***More selective in their actions;*** and
- ***Act directly as ACh receptor agonists.***

METHACHOLINE: Methacholine differs from ACh in being effective orally though its oral absorption is poor. Susceptibility of methacholine to true cholinesterase is approximately 1/3rd that of ACh. It is totally resistant to pseudocholinesterase and has a longer duration of action. It has no nicotinic actions. The drug is now rarely used.

CARBACHOL: Carbachol is resistant to both true and pseudocholinesterase. Its absorption from GI tract is incomplete. Hence, it is not useful orally.

Pharmacological actions: Unlike ACh, carbachol has a relatively selective muscarinic effect on the smooth muscle of the GI tract and the urinary bladder; it also stimulates autonomic ganglia and skeletal muscles and has a more sustained miotic effect on topical application.

Administered parenterally, it produces flushing of the face, sweating, salivation and lacrimation. *The muscarinic effects of carbachol are not adequately antagonized by atropine.*

Dose: 0.25 to 0.5 mg by injection. For ophthalmic use, 3% eye drops.

BETHANECHOL (Urecholine): Like carbachol, this choline ester is resistant to hydrolysis by both true and pseudocholinesterase. It has mainly muscarinic actions. It has negligible cardiovascular effects. However, unlike carbachol, its muscarinic effects are well antagonized by atropine.

Because of less liability to adverse drug reactions, bethanechol is preferred to carbachol in clinical practice. *Bethanechol should never be administered IV. The toxicity due to inadvertent IV injection needs immediate treatment with IV atropine.*

Preparations and dosage: Bethanechol 5 or 10 mg. tablets. Dose : 10 to 30 mg. 3-4 times daily. It is also available as injection.

Adverse reactions to choline esters: These are mostly an extension of the pharmacological actions. Besides the minor side effects like flushing, salivation, sweating and bradycardia, the serious reactions include hypotension, syncope, bronchial spasm, and occasionally cardiac arrhythmias The increased GI and urinary tract activity may produce a desire for defaecation and micturition.

Carbachol, because of its slow hydrolysis, is capable of exerting cumulative toxicity. Abdominal cramps, belching, nausea and vomiting may result. Marked hypotension, cardiac arrhythmias and death after parenteral carbachol therapy have been reported.

Therapeutic uses of choline esters:

- ***Gastrointestinal and urinary tracts*:** Bethanechol has often been employed for the treatment of post-operative paralytic ileus and abdominal distension following surgery and toxic states, for relief of gastric atony and in cases of urinary retention.

It is administered in the dose of 15 to 30 mg. 3 to 4 times a day for paralytic ileus while for gastric atony, it is given along with meals (as it increases the gastric secretion) in the dose of 10 to 20 mg. The drug is also useful in selected cases of congenital megacolon. For acute urinary retention, a dose of 5 mg is adequate. It can be repeated after 10 to 15 minutes if necessary. In chronic urinary retention 10 mg. of the drug may be given 3 to 4 times a day till voluntary or automatic voiding is established. *Presence of organic urinary obstruction (enlarged prostate) must be ruled out before using these drugs.*

Contraindication for choline esters:

(a) ***Hyperthyroidism*:** as these agents may precipitate cardiac arrhythmias.

(b) ***Bronchial asthma*:** because of the danger of aggravating or precipitating bronchospasm.

(c) ***Peptic ulcer*:** as these agents increase the gastric acid secretion.

(d) ***Myocardial infarction*:** because of the danger of hypotension and development of conduction blocks.

Cholinomimetic Alkaloids

PILOCARPINE: Pilocarpine, an alkaloid obtained from the South American shrubs *Pilocarpus microphyllus* and *Pilocarpus jaborandi,* directly stimulates cholinergic receptors and produces both muscarinic and nicotinic actions of ACh. The former are antagonized by atropine.

When applied topically to the eye, pilocarpine produces miosis, followed by a sustained fall in intraocular tension and a spasm of accommodation.

Adverse reactions: It has all the side effects of choline esters. Because of the prominent secretory response, pulmonary edema is a major hazard of systemic pilocarpine therapy.

Preparations and dosage: 1-4% Pilocarpine nitrate eye drops. (Chapter 70).

Therapeutic uses: Pilocarpine alone (0.5-4% aqueous solution) or in combination with 1 per cent physostigmine is used to reduce intraocular tension in acute congestive glaucoma. Pilocarpine-induced miosis persists for 3 to 24 hours but the spasm of accommodation disappears in about 2 hours. Pilocarpine is often used alternately with mydriatics like homatropine (2 to 5 per cent) to break adhesions between the iris and the lens (Chapter 70).

Pilocarpine ocusert is a drug delivery unit specially designed to deliver pilocarpine slowly, over a period of 7 days. However, it is far more expensive than drops.

The drug is too toxic for systemic use.

Sevimeline is an M_3 receptor agonist which increases salivary and lachrymal secretion on oral administration. It is long acting and is claimed to be less toxic than pilocarpine.

MUSCARINE AND ARECHOLINE: Muscarine is an alkaloid from the poisonous mushroom

Amanita muscaria. Acute mushroom poisoning is characterised by diarrhoea, dyspnoea, abdominal pain, lacrimation, salivation, weakness, confusion, convulsions and coma. These effects are due to muscarine and can be antagonized by large doses of atropine. *Delayed poisoning* which develops within 6 to 15 hours after ingestion of another mushroom *Amanita phalloides* is characterised by nausea, vomiting, diarrhoea, jaundice and vasomotor collapse; this is attributed to other toxins and *does not respond specifically to atropine.* Muscarine has no therapeutic application.

Arecholine, the alkaloid of betel nut *Areca catechu*, has cholinergic actions. It has no therapeutic application in humans. Betel nut is commonly used by chewing and may have mild euphoriant effect.

Cholinesterase Inhibitors

Anticholinesterase (anti ChE) drugs act by inhibiting the enzymes true and pseudocholinesterase, thus producing an accumulation of ACh at the various cholinergic sites. Their pharmacological effects resemble those of stimulation of the central, ganglionic and the peripheral cholinergic components of the nervous system. In addition, some of the anticholinesterases have independent pharmacological actions of their own. They can be classified as:

I **Reversible :** These produce reversible inhibition of cholinesterase; e.g. Physostigmine, Neostigmine etc.

II **Irreversible :** These induce almost irreversible inhibition of cholinesterase e.g. Di-isopropylflurophosphate (DFP), Octa methyl pyrophosphotetramide (OMPA) and other organophosphorus compounds.

Mechanism of action: Acetylcholine is inactivated by combination with two sites on the enzyme cholinesterase : an *anionic site* bearing a negative charge which attracts the quaternary nitrogen atom (N^+) of ACh; and an *esteratic site* which attracts the carboxylic acid group (COOH) of the ACh molecule (Fig. 18.3). As a result of the union of ACh with cholinesterase, the esteratic site of the enzyme is acetylated and this results in splitting off of choline. The acetyl group combined with the esteratic site is, however, immediately removed as a result of hydrolysis, forming acetic acid. This sets the esteratic site of the enzyme free for further inactivation of ACh.

The reversible anticholinesterases bear a structural resemblance to ACh and combine with the anionic and esteratic sites of cholinesterase as well as with ACh receptor. However, the complex which they form with the esteratic site of cholinesterase is much less readily hydrolyzed than the acetyl-esteratic site complex formed with ACh. This produces a temporary inhibition of the enzyme. In contrast to other reversible anticholinesterases, **edrophonium** forms reversible complex only with the anionic site and hence, has a shorter duration of action.

The irreversible anticholinesterases, *organophosphorus compounds,* combine only with esteratic site of cholinesterase and consequently the esteratic site is phosphorylated. The hydrolysis of the phosphorylated site, however, is slow and in certain cases does not occur at all. This produces an almost irreversible inhibition of cholinesterase. In contrast to other organophosphorus compounds, echothiophate forms complexes with both anionic and esteratic sites and hence, is much more potent than other compounds.

I **Reversible anticholinesterases** can be further subdivided into:

- ***Naturally occurring,*** e.g., Physostigmine.
- ***Synthetic*:** Neostigmine, Pyridostigmine, Ambenonium, Demecarium, Edrophonium, Tacrine and Rivastigmine.

PHYSOSTIGMINE (Eserine): This is an alkaloid obtained from the calabar bean, the dried ripe seed of an African woody climber *Physostigma venenosum.*

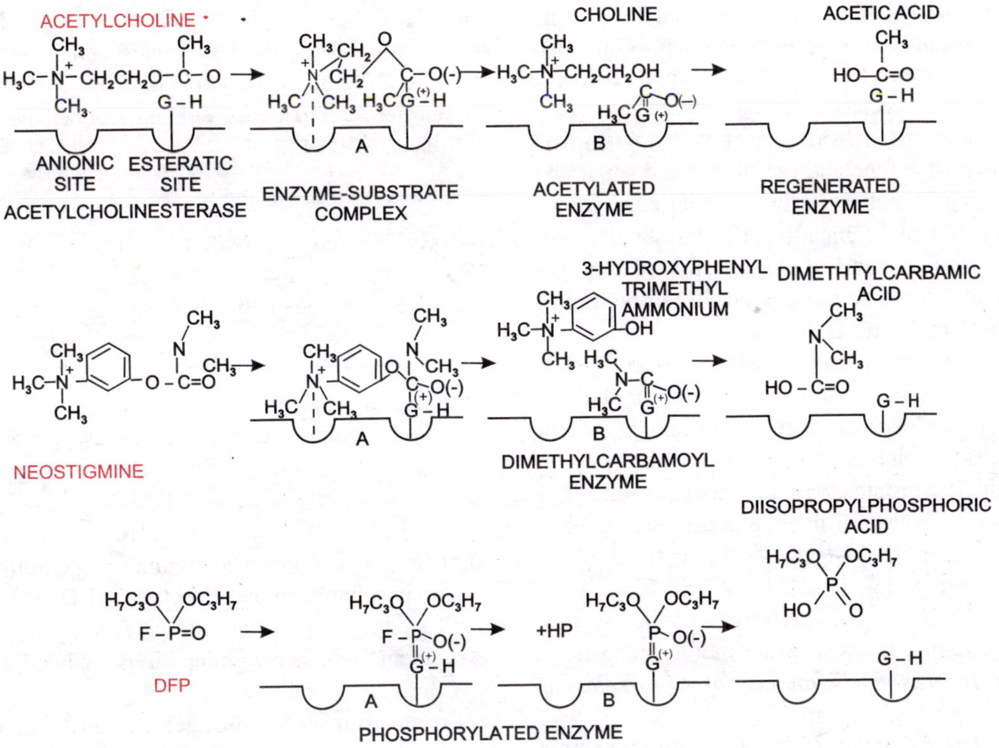

Fig. 18.3 : The inactivation of acetylcholine by cholinesterase and the mechanism of action of reversible anticholinesterase drug, Neostigmine, and irreversible anticholinesterase drug DFP G-H : a pronated acidic group of the esteratic site

Pharmacological actions: The pharmacological effects of physostigmine are similar to those of other cholinergic agents.

Topical instillation into the eye produces miosis, spasm of accommodation and a fall in intraocular tension. It has a short duration of action. It is rapidly absorbed on oral or parenteral administration, crosses the blood brain barrier and exerts central cholinergic actions.

Preparations and dosage: Physostigmine salicylate is used in eye as 0.25 - 0.50% aqueous solution or as an eye ointment. On storing, the solution becomes pink owing to the formation of decomposition products.

Physostigmine salicylate inj. 2 mg./2 ml. ampoule.

Therapeutic uses: Apart from its use in eye, physostigmine is considered relatively safe in the treatment of anticholinergic drug (atropine) intoxication, and of poisoning with phenothiazines and tricyclic antidepressants. It is particularly valuable in patients with CNS symptoms such as delirium. It is used in doses of 2 mg. SC or IV and repeated after 10-20 min. If effective, 2-4 mg. may be given every 2-4 hours.

NEOSTIGMINE (Prostigmin): It is a synthetic, quaternary ammonium compound that inhibits both true and pseudocholinesterases.

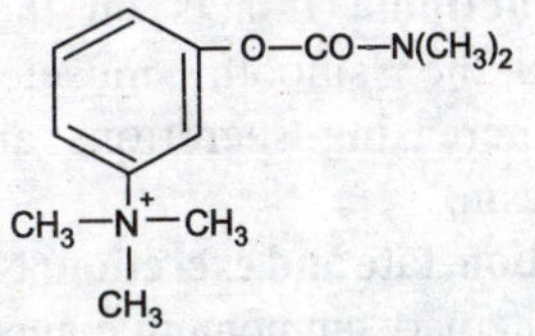

Fig. 18.4 : Neostigmine

Pharmacological actions : In addition to its anticholinesterase activity, neostigmine also directly stimulates certain organs having cholinergic receptors. Its actions are :

Gastrointestinal tract : Neostigmine increases the tone and motility of the small and large bowel, enhances the production of gastric juice; and by augmenting the intestinal motor activity, it promotes the propulsion of intestinal contents. Atropine reduces but does not abolish the intestinal effects.

Skeletal muscles : Neostigmine produces a striking increase in the strength of skeletal muscles in patients with myasthenia gravis. In contrast to physostigmine, neostigmine IV can stimulate chronically denervated muscle or a muscle in which all the cholinesterase has been inactivated. Neostigmine is postulated to improve muscle strength by:

- ***Its anti-ChE activity*** causing greater accumulation of ACh at the motor end plates.
- ***Increasing the amount of ACh released*** during each nerve impulse; and
- ***Directly stimulating the cholinoceptive receptor sites*** on the motor end plate by virtue of its structural similarity with ACh. It thus acts as a partial agonist.

Administration of neostigmine to normal subjects may cause twitchings and fasciculations of skeletal muscles but these are not encountered in myasthenic patients. It reverses the neuromuscular blockade produced by d-tubocurarine, but is not a satisfactory antagonist for benzoquinonium, and it actually enhances the paralysis of skeletal muscles causes by persistent depolarizers like succinylcholine.

Cardiovascular system: The drug reduces the heart rate and lowers BP by peripheral vasodilatation and bradycardia.

Other actions: It acts on the secretory glands and the smooth muscles of the bronchi, increasing secretions and causing bronchospasm.

Absorption, fate and excretion: Neostigmine, being a quaternary ammonium compound, is not absorbed satisfactorily orally. It is, therefore, administered SC or IM. The effect of a single IM injection starts within 10 minutes and persists for 3 to 4 hours. It is partly destroyed by the cholinesterase and partly eliminated unchanged in urine.

Preparations and dosage :

(i) Neostigmine bromide tablet 15 mg. Dose: 15 to 30 mg.

(ii) Neostigmine methyl-sulphate 0.5 mg. per 1 ml. Dose : 0.5 to 2 mg.

Distigmine (Ubretid): is a longer acting neostigmine analogue and can be used in the dose of 5-20 mg. once daily before breakfast.

PYRIDOSTIGMINE (Distinon): This compound resembles neostigmine structurally and in its pharmacological actions. The drug has a slightly longer duration of action but is less potent than neostigmine. It is claimed to have fewer visceral effects.

Preparations and dosage: Pyridostigmine bromide tablet 60 mg. Dose: 60 to 240 mg. Pyridostigmine slow release tablets have a duration of action of 4 to 10 hours with a single dose. Pyridostigmine injection 1 mg. per ml. Dose: 1 to 5 mg. SC or IM.

AMBENONIUM (Mytelase) : Ambenonium is a bisymmetrical synthetic quaternary ammonium compound which is a more potent true-cholinesterase-inhibitor than neostigmine and has a more marked direct stimulant effect on the skeletal muscle. The action is more sustained with a lower incidence of GI side effects.

It is available as 10 mg. tablets. Dose: 5-20 mg. 3-4 times a day as required.

DEMECARIUM (Humorsol): Structurally, demecarium is made up of two neostigmine molecules joined through 10 methoxy groups. The drug inhibits true cholinesterase more specifically than pseudocholinesterase. The drug is a potent miotic on topical instillation. This effect reaches a peak within 4 hours and may last for 3 to 10 days. It is accompanied by a spasm of accommodation. It is used as 0.1 to 0.25 per cent solution once or twice weekly in the treatment of glaucoma.

EDROPHONIUM (Tensilon): Edrophonium, a quaternary ammonium anticholinesterase, is structurally related to neostigmine. The drug has a weak anticholinesterase activity as compared to neostigmine but it enhances neuromuscular transmission with a dose that is too low to affect the smooth muscles, the myocardium and the glands. It has a quicker onset of action than neostigmine, and the effects of a single IV dose persists only for 10 minutes. The muscarinic side effects are mild.

Preparations and dosage: Edrophonium chloride 10 ml. vials containing 10 mg. per ml.

Adverse reactions to reversible anticholinesterases: The reversible anticholinesterases produce effects attributable mainly to their muscarinic actions. These are epigastric distress, salivation, sweating, lacrimation, paraesthesia, sense of constriction in chest, nausea, abdominal cramps, diarrhoea and fasciculations, particularly around the mouth and in the superior extremities. Hypotension and tremors have been occasionally reported.

Demecarium and physostigmine eyedrops, may pass into the nose through the nasolacrimal duct and produce muscarinic side effects. Demecarium may rarely increase intraocular tension in narrow angle glaucoma and may rarely cause retinal detachment.

When used in the treatment of myasthenia gravis, an overdose of these compounds may produce skeletal muscle paralysis by persistent depolarization. This phenomenon, termed **cholinergic crisis,** has to be differentiated from the sudden exacerbation of muscular weakness in myasthenia often associated with severe upper respiratory infection, termed **myasthenic crisis**. In myasthenic crisis, the requirement of the anti ChE agent is increased and occasionally the patient becomes resistant to anticholinesterase medication. Edrophonium 2 mg. IV brings about a prompt improvement of muscle strength in myasthenic crisis, while it exacerbates the weakness of cholinergic crisis. However, this effect is not dangerous because of the extremely short duration of action of edrophonium and its relative freedom from muscarinic side actions. If the initial dose of 2 mg. does not produce an improvement in muscle strength within 30 seconds, a dose of 8 mg. may be administered. The cholinergic crisis is treated by administration of large doses of atropine, oximes and artificial respiration.

Therapeutic uses of reversible anticholinesterases :

- ***Glaucoma:*** Chapter 70.
- ***For decurarization*** following the use of drugs like d-tubocurarine in anaesthetic procedures.
- ***Myasthenia gravis***: Myasthenia gravis is a disease characterised by easy fatiguability and progressive weakness of striated muscles and with intermittent periods of exacerbation. Pregnancy usually leads to an improvement or even temporary remission of this condition.

Myasthenia gravis is an autoimmune disease caused by a deficiency of the postsynaptic neuromuscular ACh receptor complex. Thus the receptors in myasthenic muscle are degraded and cleared much faster than normally. The number of available ACh receptors in the involved muscles is reduced by as much as 70-90%. Circulating antibodies to ACh receptors have been demonstrated in 70-90% of patients with myasthenia. Many patients with this disorder have thymic hyperplasia or a thymoma.

Another myasthenic syndrome (Lambert-Eaton syndrome) of autoimmune nature occurs in association with small cell carcinoma of the lung.

The autoantibodies are directed to the calcium channel in the nerve terminals, with resultant diminution in the release of ACh from the nerve terminals. The defect is presynaptic and does not respond to anticholiesterases but may respond to 3,4-diaminopyridine (3,4 DAP) which increases neurotransmitter release.

The diagnosis of myasthenia gravis depends upon typical clinical picture and a dramatic clinical response to either neostigmine or edrophonium. Administration of 1 to 1.5 mg. of neostigmine IM produces a marked improvement in muscle strength of myasthenic individuals, which lasts for 3 to 4 hours. Atropine sulfate 0.6 mg. is usually administered IM before or along with neostigmine to counter the muscarinic side effects of the latter.

Treatment : Neostigmine was formerly used in the treatment of myasthenia. However, because of its relatively short duration of action (< 4 hours), development of tolerance and waxing and waning of muscle strength, agents with a longer duration of action and fewer side effects, e.g. pyridostigmine (4-6 hr) and ambenonium (4-8 hr) are now preferred. These drugs may, however, be combined with neostigmine as the onset of action of neostigmine is quicker. The effect of parenteral neostigmine appears within 30 minutes while oral administration produces a response within 1 hour. The therapy is initiated with neostigmine (Prostigmine) 7.5-15 mg. or pyridostigmine 30-60 mg or ambenonium 2.5 to 5 mg. orally, at a time, and the dose is gradually increased until the maximal benefit is obtained.

The reversible antiChE are usually administered 3 to 4 hourly, orally or parenterally to ensure a smooth and sustained effect. Parenteral medication is indicated before meals so as to enable the patient to swallow his food. Most myasthenics can be improved only partially with these drugs. Thus, 80 to 90 per cent recovery occurs in 25 per cent individuals. Further increase in dosage precipitates toxic actions without appreciable increase in clinical improvement. It is, therefore, wiser to accept minor disability rather than overdose the patient and risk adverse effects which may become incapacitating. Infection increases the requirements of anticholinesterases.

Because of the probably autoimmune basis of myasthenia, prednisolone, a glucocorticoid has been used in its management in the dose of 25-100 mg. once a day. It benefits some patients who cannot be controlled adequately with antiChE, as well as older patients. Such therapy may, however, cause exacerbation of weakness in the early stages and needs supervision.

Other immunosuppresants such as azathioprine, cyclosporine as well as plasmapheresis have been used as adjunctive therapy in resistant cases.

Table 18.1 lists the drugs which aggravate the symptoms in myasthenic patients. They are best avoided in these patients.

Table 18.1: Drugs which aggravate myasthenic symptoms

- ***Antibiotics***: Aminoglycosides, Polymyxins, Norfloxacin, Ciprofloxacin, Erythromycin, Tetracyclines.
- ***Antiarrhythmics***: Procainamide, Quinidine, Lignocaine, Propranolol
- ***CNS depressants*** may depress respiration
- ***Miscellaneous***: Chlorpromazine, Lithium, Thyroid hormones, Phenytoin, Methoxyflurane, d-Tubocurarine and Penicillamine.

- ***Gastrointestinal and urinary tract*:** Neostigmine is employed parenterally in the dose of 0.5 to 1 mg. to treat postoperative paralytic ileus and urinary retention. The drug may be repeated, if necessary, at intervals of 4 to 6 hours. It is used in the treatment of achalasia and in patients with marked dilatation of the oesophagus, because of its stimulant action on the lower end of the oesophagus.

Benzpyrinium is also employed for the treatment of post-operative paralytic ileus and urinary retention.

- ***Snake venom poisoning***: An antiChE may be beneficial in the management of neurotoxicity of Asian-cobra-venom. For this purpose, atropine sulfate (0.6 mg.) is given IV, slowly, for blocking muscarinic action, and this is followed immediately by edrophonium chloride 10 mg. IV over two minutes. Edrophonium reverses oculomotor and glossopharyngeal paralysis as well as respiratory paralysis.

Following IV edrophonium, the improvement can be maintained by a longer acting antiAchE such as neostigmine methylsulfate which can be given SC or by IV or infusion.

The dose of edrophonium for children is 0.25 mg/kg; that of atropine is 50 mcg/kg.

The pathophysiologic nature of paralysis after cobra bite is very similar to that of myasthenia gravis. *Paralysis following krait bite is not likely to benefit from edrophonium therapy as the Krait beta-bungarotoxin causes pre-synaptic blockage.*

- ***Curare poisoning***: Edrophonium is preferred to neostigmine to antagonize curare induced skeletal muscle paralysis because of its short latent period of action. A single dose of 10 mg. may at times be inadequate and 2 or 3 doses may have to be administered.
- ***Alzheimer's disease*** (See Chapter 14).

II **Irreversible anticholinesterases:**

Organophosphorus compounds, the organic esters of phosphoric acid, are potent irreversible inhibitors of cholinesterase. Unlike the quaternary ammonium Anti-ChE, most of these compounds have high lipid solubility, and hence:

- ***Are absorbed by practically all the routes*** including the GI tract, the intact unbroken skin, mucous membranes and lungs; and
- ***Cross the BB barrier and affect the functions of the CNS.***

The pharmacological effects of the organophosphorus compounds are those of ACh which accumulates in the tissues on account of the prolonged inhibition of the true and pseudocholinesterases.

Table 18.2: Important organophosphorus compounds

- ***Therapeutically useful***: Diisopropyl flurophosphate (DFP), Metrifonate, Ecothiophate.
- ***Insecticides***: Fenthion (dalf), Malathion (diazone), Mipafox, Octamethylpyro-Phosphphotetramide (OMPA), Sumithion (Tik-20), Monocrotophos (Nuvaeron).
- ***Highly toxic nerve gases***: Tabun, Sarin, Soman synthesized for chemical warfare

The organophosphorus compounds are inactivated in the body almost entirely by oxidation and hydrolysis and the end products are eliminated in urine.

Table 18.2 lists the important organophosphorus compounds.

Therapeutic uses: The organophosphorus compounds have limited therapeutic uses owing to their high toxicity. They are used mainly as **Insecticides** and are, therefore, of toxicological importance.

- ***Glaucoma***: The compound currently favoured for topical use is echothiophate in the concentration of 0.06 per cent. The reduction in the intraocular tension with this drug persists for 1 to 3 weeks following a single instillation. The drug, however, produces a marked ciliary spasm, browache, headache and blurring. The major drawback of long acting anti-ChEs is the risk of development of cataract following their prolonged use (6 months or more). See Chapter 70.
- ***Worm infestation***: Dichlorovas and trichlorophos have *anthelmintic* properties (Chapter 58).

Organophosphorus Compound (OPC) Poisoning

Poisoning with organophosphorus compounds may be:

- ***Occupational*** as in persons engaged in spraying insecticides.
- ***Accidental*** e.g. by consumption of the agricultural products sprayed with these insecticides; or
- ***Suicidal*** due to intentional ingestion of any of these compounds.

Acute organophosphorus pesticide poisoning is an important cause of morbidity and mortality all over the world. Of these, 99% of the fatal poisonings occur in the developing countries, particularly among agricultural workers.

Symptomatology: The effects of acute intoxication are :

- ***Muscarinic effects***: Localized exposure of the eyes produces miosis, spasm of accommodation, headache and conjunctival hyperaemia. Inhalation results in bronchospasm, cough and augmented bronchiolar secretions and a sense of 'tightness in the chest'.

On ingestion, the GI symptoms are the earliest to appear and consist of anorexia, nausea, vomiting, abdominal cramps, tenesmus and diarrhoea. The other muscarinic effects, including those on the eye and the respiratory system, appear subsequently. Severe bronchospasm and pulmonary edema may be fatal.

- ***Nicotinic effects***: These are characterised by fasciculations, twitching, generalized weakness and a depolarization type of paralysis. There may be either tachycardia or bradycardia.
- ***Central effects***: These include giddiness, anxiety, confusion, ataxia, hypotension, respiratory depression, convulsions and coma. Death is usually due to paralysis of respiratory muscles and respiratory failure.

The duration of effect is longest with DFP and shorter with echothiophate and TEPP. It appears that even single episodes of clinically significant organophosphorus intoxication are associated with persistent decline in neuropsychological function.

- ***Neurotoxic effects*** : In addition to the acute toxic manifestations mentioned above, DFP and mipafox may produce delayed symptoms due to demyelination of the nerve tracts in the central and peripheral nervous systems e.g. the spinocerebellar tract, pyramidal tract and the sciatic nerve, producing permanent functional derangements. This is not related to ChE inhibition. This produces weakness, fatiguability, twitching and loss of tendon reflexes, leading to paralysis. Adulteration of edible olive oil with lubricating oil containing triorthocresyl phosphate (TOCP) caused thousands of deaths in a tragedy that occurred in North Africa. No treatment is available.

Treatment of acute poisoning: Table 18.3 summarises the principles of treatment of acute organophosphorus poisoning.

Table 18.3 : Principles of treatment of acute organophosphorus poisoning

- Remove soiled clothes.
- Wash soiled skin, eyes.
- Nurse in prone position.
- Clear mouth and throat.
- Insert an airway/intubate
- Gastric lavage.
- Atropine in sufficient quantities.
- Cholinesterase activator such as pralidoxime.
- Supportive measures such as oxygen, treatment of shock, prophylactic antibiotics.
- Treatment of convulsions (diazepam).
- Continued vigilance as delayed toxicity may occur as late as 2-4 weeks after apparent recovery.

As recommended by the WHO Expert Committee (Technical Report 513), "The treatment must be instituted rapidly in order to prevent a fatal outcome. In intoxication by mouth, rapid gastric lavage is imperative. For removal of secretions and maintenance of a patent airway, place the patient in a prone position with head down and to one side, the mandible elevated and the tongue pulled forward. Clear the mouth and pharynx with finger or suction. Use an oropharyngeal or nasopharyngeal airway or endotracheal intubation if airway obstruction persists. If the body is soiled with the insecticides or if vomiting or hypersalivation has occurred, clothes must be removed and the skin washed with soap and water for at least 10 minutes. Contamination of the eyes is treated by washing of the conjunctiva".

Mouth to mouth respiration is to be avoided when it is suspected that the patient has been intoxicated by mouth since vomited material may contain dangerous amounts of toxic substances.

On signs of systemic absorption, both atropine and reactivators (see below) must be given parenterally. Persons without signs of respiratory insufficiency but with manifest peripheral symptoms should be treated with 2-4 mg. of atropine sulfate and 1-2 g. of a soluble salt of pralidoxime (P-2-AM) or 250 mg. of obidoxime chloride (adult doses, see later) by slow IV injection. More atropine (with or without the reactivator) may be given depending upon the severity of the intoxication and the response to the first dose. After the administration of oximes, less atropine may be required. *Atropine is effective in antagonizing the central and peripheral muscarinic effects but does not modify the ganglionic action and the neuromuscular paralysis.* Reactivators of cholinesterase should not be used before atropine administration, as given alone they may increase muscle weakness.

Severely intoxicated, unconscious persons with respiratory difficulties and convulsions should be given atropine and a reactivator as above. *Atropine should not be given to a cyanotic patient until the cyanosis has been overcome, since this may lead to ventricular fibrillation.*

In severe intoxication, 4-6 mg. of atropine sulfate should be given initially, followed by repeated doses of 2 mg. or as much as required to maintain full atropinization. The patient's condition, including respiration, convulsions, blood pressure, pulse frequency, and salivation should be carefully observed as a guide to further administration of atropine. Initially, atropine may have to be given at 5 or 10 minute intervals. Cases are described in the literature in which several hundred mg. have been given during the first 24 hours. *Usually however, it is not necessary to exceed 50 mg.* Every 2 mg. dose gives a short-lasting improvement of respiration and reduction in cyanosis and convulsions. Tachycardia may occur and watch must be kept on salivary secretion in order to prevent over-atropinization. *The pulse rate should not be allowed to exceed 120/min.*

If possible, blood samples should be taken for cholinesterase determinations before and during the treatment. In parathion poisoning, reactivation of the enzyme activity of the red blood cells may be observed within one hour. If the patient comes late to the treatment (after 36 hours) oxime therapy is less effective.

Because most intoxications occur after exposure of the skin or after ingestion, *any deterioration in the patient's condition due to delayed absorption must be carefully watched for.* Reactivators are excreted fairly rapidly if kidney function is normal (in the case of pralidoxime 80 per cent in 2-3 hours) and repeated doses of 1 g. may be needed.

The IV injection of oximes should be made slowly, especially in small children.

Recent studies from India have shown that in "moderately severe" poisoning, pralidoxime, started within two hours of ingestion of the poison, in larger than conventional doses i.e. with a loading dose of 2g (base) by IV infusion over 30 minutes, followed by 1 g / hour by continuous IV infusion for 48 hours, is highly effective. This is followed by pralidoxime (base) 1g IV infusion every 4 hours till the patient is weaned from the ventilator. This regimen is well tolerated. The patients thus treated have lower mortality, need less intubation and ventilator support, require less atropine during the first day, and fewer develop pneumonia. As the iodide salt of pralidoxime loads the body with too large a quantity of iodide, it is preferable to use either the chloride or the methanesulfonate. The molecular weight of the compound should be taken into account while deciding the quantity injected.

After the resolution of the initial symptoms, some patients may develop the 'intermediate syndrome'. It is characterized by flaccid, proximal paralysis. Later, after a gap of 2-4 weeks, a 'delayed polyneuropathy' with sensory and motor impairment, usually of the lower limbs, may manifest. Unfortunately, there is no specific treatment.

Estimation of plasma cholinesterase may help to determine when a patient may return for work; *subjects should not be allowed to do the same work involving organophophorus until the plasma cholinesterase level exceeds 70% of normal. This usually takes several weeks.*

OXIMES (Cholinesterase reactivators): The irreversible inhibition of cholinesterase produced by the organophosphorus compounds is due to phosphorylation of the esteratic site of the enzyme (Fig. 18.3). Oximes are drugs which combine with the phosphoryl groups of these phosphorylated esteratic sites forming soluble complex. This results in setting free the esteratic site and a reactivation of the enzyme.

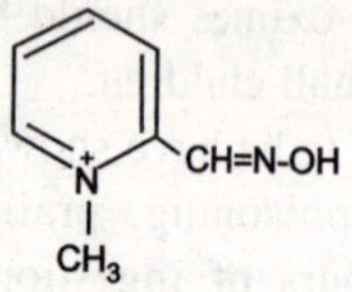

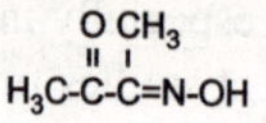

CH=N-OH, N^+, CH_3 — H_3C-C(=O)-C(=N-OH)-CH_3 (O CH_3 / H_3C-C-C=N-OH)

Fig. 18.5 : P-2-AM **DAM**

The oximes are particularly effective in reversing the neuromuscular paralysis where atropine is ineffective. Their effects on the autonomic ganglia and the CNS are not significant, except probably in the case of DAM which crosses the blood brain barrier. *These compounds are effective only when administered within a short time after poisoning.* Late administration fails to produce the expected results as by this time the phosphoryl bound with the enzyme gets more stabilized (ageing of the enzyme). Oximes are mainly metabolized in the liver and the products are eliminated in urine.

Adverse reactions: The oximes are not free from toxicity. They may produce local irritation, drowsiness, giddiness, blurred vision, diplopia, tachycardia and hypotension. Pralidoxime has weak anti-ChE activity and hence contraindicated in the treatment of overdosage with neostigmine or physostigmine. *It also does not antagonize the effects of carbamate type (Baygon / Carbaryl) of anticholinesterases.* High doses of pralidoxime and related compounds can themselves cause neuromuscular blockade.

Preparations and dosage:

(i) Pyridine-2 aldoxime chloride (2-PAM, Pralidoxime) by IV infusion (see earlier details). The dose can be repeated after 1-2 hours. It can also be given IM. It is also available for oral use.

(ii) Diacetylmonoxime (DAM) administered by IV infusion. It crosses the blood brain barrier.

(iii) Obidoxime chloride is more potent than pralidoxime. It is given IV. The dose can be repeated every 20 minutes.

Muscarinic Receptor Blocking Drugs

19

Cholinergic – muscarinic receptor blocking drugs include atropine, and related alkaloids obtained from the plants *Atropa belladonna* (the deadly nightshade), *Atropa acuminata, Hyoscyamus niger* (henbane), *Scopola carniolica* and *Datura stramonium* (Datura) and synthetic or semisynthetic atropine substitutes. They nonselectively block the muscarinic actions of ACh; the ganglionic and skeletal neuromuscular actions of ACh are not affected.

Belladonna Alkaloids

The name *Atropa belladonna* represents a paradox. For whereas Atropos is the seniormost of the Three Fates who performs the unglorious function of cutting the thread of life, the term belladonna (pretty lady) is derived from the practice by Venetian court beauties of putting the extract of these plants in the eyes, to impart them a 'lustre'. Belladonna preparations were known to ancient Hindus for many centuries.

The two important alkaloids of Belladonna are atropine (dl-hyoscyamine) and scopolamine (hyoscine). Atropine is an ester of an aromatic organic acid 'tropic acid' with a complex organic base 'tropine' while hyoscine is an ester of tropic acid with another base 'scopine' (Fig. 19.1).

Mechanism of action : The belladonna alkaloids block the muscarinic effects of ACh. The antagonism between ACh and atropine is of *competitive type* which is reversed by an increase in the concentration of ACh at the muscarinic neuroeffector site.

Atropine is more effective in blocking the effects of externally administered ACh than the effects of cholinergic nerve stimulation. The dose of the drug required to produce muscarinic blockade varies from organ to organ. Thus, salivary and bronchial secretions are extremely sensitive to atropine blockade, while the smooth muscle of the GI tract, the eye, the heart and gastric acid secretion are less affected even after relatively large doses. In the CNS, cholinergic transmission at subcortical and cortical levels is predominantly muscarinic and can be blocked by atropine.

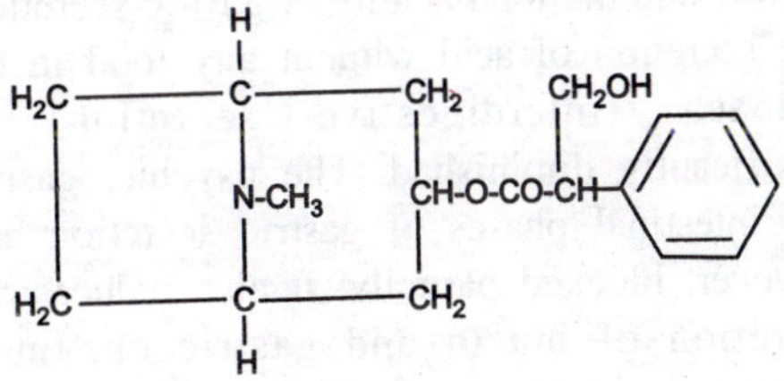

Fig. 19.1a : Atropine

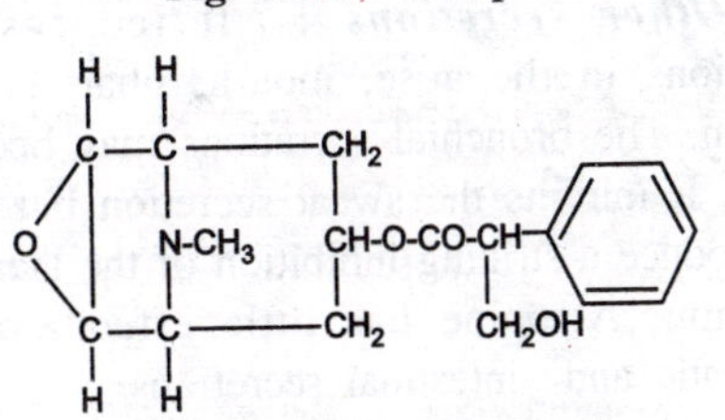

Fig. 19.1b : Scopolamine

Although atropine can completely abolish the effects of choline esters on the GI tract, it does not completely abolish the effects of vagal stimulation. This is so because it does not block noncholinergic, neurohumoral transmitters nor responses to GI peptide hormones.

In large doses, atropine blocks the nicotinic action of ACh at the autonomic ganglia; it is more marked following atropine substitutes containing the quaternary ammonium (-NH_4) ion.

Pharmacological actions: The pharmacological actions of **atropine** and **scopolamine** (hyoscine) are qualitatively similar except that *atropine is a central nervous system stimulant while scopolamine is a central depressant* and can act as a sedative. Scopolamine has more prominent effects on the iris, the ciliary body and the salivary, bronchial and sweat secretions while atropine is more active on the heart, the gut and the bronchial smooth muscle. Atropine has a longer duration of action than scopolamine.

Secretions: The belladonna alkaloids reduce the secretions of the exocrine glands except the production of milk.

- ***Salivary secretion*****:** Atropine blocks the watery salivary secretion giving rise to dryness of mouth and difficulty in swallowing.
- ***Gastric secretion*** **:** Atropine reduces the volume and the total acidity of gastric secretion. The secretion of acid without any food in the stomach (interdigestive secretion) is significantly diminished. The psychic, gastric and intestinal phases of gastric secretion are, however, blocked partially. It also reduces the secretion of mucin and gastric enzymes. (Chapter 42).
- ***Other secretions*** **:** It reduces the secretions in the nose, mouth, pharynx and bronchi. The bronchial secretions may become viscid. It inhibits the sweat secretion but does not produce a striking inhibition of the lacrimal secretion. Atropine has little effect on the pancreatic and intestinal secretions.

Smooth muscle :

- ***Gastrointestinal tract*** **:** Atropine reduces both the tone and the motility of all parts of the gut, and acts as an antispasmodic. It antagonizes the spasmogenic action of morphine on intestine and can also completely abolish the excessive motility induced by the cholinergic agents. It is, however, only partially effective in blocking the effects of vagus nerve stimulation and it does not interfere significantly with normal peristalsis.
- ***Biliary tract*** **:** Atropine exerts a weak antispasmodic (relaxant) action on the biliary tract and the gallbladder.
- ***Urinary tract*****:** Atropine produces reduction in normal as well as in drug induced ureteral peristalsis. Therapeutic doses reduce the tone of the fundus of the bladder and enhance the tone of the trigonal sphincter and can cause urinary retention.
- ***Bronchi*****:** Atropine relaxes the smooth muscles of the bronchi and bronchioles. It is par-ticularly effective in relieving bronchoconstriction produced by cholinergic agents but is much less potent than adrenaline in relieving histamine induced bronchoconstriction. Since it dries up the secretions, it is not recommended in the treatment of bronchial asthma.
- ***Uterus*****:** Atropine and scopolamine have no significant effect on the uterine smooth muscle.

Eye: On local instillation, atropine produces mydriasis by blocking the cholinergic nerves supplying the smooth muscle of the sphincter of the iris. The ciliary smooth muscle is likewise paralysed by atropine. This produces a tightening of the suspensory ligament resulting in flattening of the lens with a consequent increase in its focal length. The individual, therefore, is able to see things clearly only at a distance owing to fixing of lens for far vision. Because of sphincter paralysis, he cannot constrict the pupils for viewing near objects clearly or in response to bright light, and therefore suffers from photophobia. This phenomenon is termed as *paralysis of accommodation or cycloplegia.* Atropine is thus both a **mydriatic** and a **cycloplegic** drug. Local instillation of 1 per cent atropine drops produces maximum mydriatic response within 30 to 40 minutes and recovery occurs within 7 to 10 days. Maximum cycloplegia with atropine is seen within 1 to 3 days; it persists for 7 to 11 days. Unlike scopolamine, conventional doses of atropine administered systemically do not produce significant ocular effects.

Atropine mydriasis can be distinguished from the mydriatic effect of sympathomimetic amines as the latter do not produce cycloplegia. Atropine does not alter the intraocular tension in the normal eye but in individuals with *shallow anterior chamber* and in those with *narrow angle glaucoma,* a precipitous increase in intraocular tension may occur. It is due to relaxation of the ciliary muscle and crowding of the iris in the angle of the anterior chamber of the eye interfering with the drainage of aqueous humour.

Cardiovascular system: Atropine, in therapeutic doses, may initially decrease the heart rate owing to stimulation of the medullary vagal nuclei, followed by tachycardia, particularly in young individuals who have a high vagal tone and in whom the heart rate may increase by 30 to 40 beats per minute. Tachycardia is due to blocking of M_2 receptors in the SA nodal pacemaker. This action is sometimes not observed in old people and in infants even with large doses, probably because of the lower vagal tone. Atropine abolishes the effects of cholinergic agents on the heart rate and also the bradycardia induced by manoeuvres like carotid massage and pressure on an eyeball.

In therapeutic doses, atropine completely counters the vasodilatation and hypotension produced by cholinergic agents. However, by itself it has insignificant effect on the vasculature and does not modify the BP. Toxic doses produce dilatation of the cutaneous blood vessels resulting in 'atropine flush' and hypotension.

Central nervous system: Atropine, in therapeutic doses, causes a mild stimulation of the medullary vagal nuclei and higher cerebral centres. This occasionally produces bradycardia and an increase in the rate and depth of respiration. Respiratory depression produced by toxic doses of anticholinesterases can be antagonized appreciably by atropine administration. Atropine in moderate doses controls the tremors and rigidity in parkinsonism. In toxic doses, it produces marked excitation.

In contrast to atropine, therapeutic doses of scopolamine depress the reticular activating system, and usually produce euphoria, drowsiness, amnesia and dreamless sleep which lasts for 1 to 2 hours.

Scopolamine owes its salutary effect in motion sickness to its direct action on the vestibular function.

Absorption, fate and excretion: The belladonna alkaloids are satisfactorily absorbed from the GI tract, from parenteral sites of administration and from mucous membranes. The absorption from the eye and intact skin, however, is not significant. Atropine is partly detoxified in liver and partly excreted unchanged by kidneys. It has plasma t½ of 4 hours. Approximately 50 per cent of the parenterally administered drug appears in the urine in free form within 24 hours while 33 per cent is excreted as metabolites. Scopolamine is mostly metabolized.

Atropine crosses the placental barrier and is secreted in milk and saliva. Animals such as rabbits having atropine esterase in their plasma and liver, and rodents detoxify atropine faster than human beings and can tolerate large doses without toxicity.

Adverse reactions: Majority of these are in fact due to extension of its pharmacological actions and include dryness of mouth, difficulty in swallowing, tachycardia, fever, delirium and constipation, blurring of vision and, retention of urine in the elderly. Atropine can precipitate glaucoma especially in the elderly. Locally, atropine can give rise to allergic reactions such as dermatitis, conjunctivitis and swelling of eyelids. Infants and young children are particularly susceptible to the CNS toxicity of muscarinic receptor blocking drugs.

• ***Acute atropine poisoning***: Atropine has a wide margin of safety. The lethal dose of atropine is not known but is believed to be 10-20 mg. in children and 80-130 mg. in adults, although survival after doses over 200 mg. in adults has been reported. Scopolamine is claimed to be more toxic than atropine. Poisoning may also occur following ingestion of leaves or seeds of Datura species.

The symptoms and signs are due to:

(a) *Peripheral muscarinic blockade.* Dryness of mouth, difficulty in swallowing, intense thirst, tachycardia, palpitation, flushing, hyperpyrexia due to inhibition of sweating, dilatation of pupils, blurred vision and photophobia are the cardinal manifestations. Urinary urgency, difficulty in micturition and even retention of urine may occur due to spasm of the trigone. A rash may appear over the face, neck and upper part of the trunk, leading to desquamation of the skin; and

(b) *Central effects which* are attributed to initial stimulation and subsequent depression of the CNS. The patient shows excitement, restlessness, motor incoordination, slurring of speech, disturbance of memory, confusion, hallucinations, and occasionally mania and delirium. Nausea and vomiting are infrequent. Severe poisoning depresses the vasomotor centre, leading to vasomotor collapse. Depression following initial excitement tends to appear more quickly with scopolamine.

Belladonna poisoning may be diagnosed by adding a drop of patient's urine into a cat's eye, where it will produce pupillary dilatation. However, absence of such dilatation does not exclude belladonna poisoning. Dry mucous membranes, dilated nonreacting pupils, flushing, rash, fever and rapid feeble pulse seen in atropine poisoning may sometimes be mistaken for an exanthematous fever.

The other drugs which cause a syndrome like acute atropine intoxication include drugs possessing muscarinic blocking action such as: tricyclic antidepressants, phenothiazine antipsychotics and the anti-histaminics promethazine and diphenhydramine.

Treatment: If the poison has been ingested, prompt attempts to remove it by gastric lavage should be made. Alkaloidal inactivators like universal antidote should be administered before and after gastric lavage.

The muscarinic effects can be countered by administration of slow IV physostigmine 1-4 mg. (0.5-1 mg. in children) or neostigmine 2 to 5 mg. SC. The drugs may be repeated at intervals of 1-2 hours till satisfactory control over muscarinic blockade is established. *Physostigmine is preferred in patients with CNS symptoms as it crosses the BB barrier.* Restlessness and delirium may be treated with diazepam but this drug may augment the respiratory depression seen in later stages of atropine intoxication.

A dark room to alleviate photophobia, catheterization for urinary retention, tepid sponging for pyrexia, good nursing care, oxygen and artificial ventilation when necessary, constitute the supportive treatment.

• ***Chronic use of belladonna*** is manifested by dryness of mouth, skin eruptions, tremors and speech disturbances.

Preparations and dosage:

(i) Belladonna tincture. Dose: 0.6 to 2 ml.
(ii) Atropine sulfate 0.5 mg. tablets. Dose: 0.25 to 2 mg.
(iii) Atropine eye ointment 1 per cent.
(iv) Atropine sulfate injection 0.5 mg. in 1 ml. Dose: 0.25 mg. to 2 mg. SC or IM.
(v) Atropine methonitrate a 0.6% alcoholic solution in the dose of 0.2-0.6 mg.
(vi) Hyoscyamus tincture. Dose: 2 to 4 ml.
(vii) Hyoscine (Scopolamine) injection 0.4 mg. in 1 ml. Dose : 0.3 to 0.6 mg. by SC injection.
(viii) Hyoscine hydrobromide tablets 0.3-0.6 mg. Dose 1-2 tablets 4 times daily.
(ix) Hyoscine -N-butylbromide (Buscopan): Tablets 10 mg; Injection 20 mg./ml. Dose: 10-20 mg 3-4 times a day orally; 20 mg. IM.
(x) Hyoscine hydrobromide skin patch 1 mg (Scopoderm, TTS). Releases the drug over 72 hrs. Apply behind the ear 5-6 hours before journey. Repeat after 72 hours, if requires.

Therapeutic uses of atropine and scopolamine:

● ***Gastrointestinal colic***: Atropine is used to control hypermotility and colicky pain. Constipation due to spastic state of the bowel may be relieved after atropine. It also controls spasticity induced by lead and morphine.

● ***Other colics***: Atropine is usually administered along with morphine in the treatment of biliary colic. Morphine tends to increase the intra-biliary pressure and this effect is countered by concomitant atropine administration. Atropine morphine combination is also used for relief of renal colic.

Atropine and its substitutes are often used to allay the frequency and urgency of micturition accompanying cystitis. It acts probably by increasing the capacity of the bladder as a result of its relaxant effect on the bladder wall. Frequency of micturition associated with paraplegia is also controlled with atropine.

● ***Ocular conditions***: Atropine is used to produce **mydriasis** and **cycloplegia.** Mydriasis is necessary for a fundoscopic examination and in the treatment of acute iritis, iridocyclitis and keratitis. Atropine reduces pain in these conditions by relaxing the inflamed musculature of iris and the ciliary body. It may be instilled into the eye alternately with miotics to break the adhesions between the iris and the lens or the cornea. It also reduces the chances of adhesion formation. When maximum cycloplegia is desired e.g. in correction of accommodative esotropia, atropine is preferred.

● ***As pre-anaesthetic medication***: The details are discussed in Chapter 7. Contrary to popular belief, atropine does not abolish the laryngospasm during anaesthesia but prevents its development by reducing the respiratory secretions. It is administered at least 30 minutes before general anaesthesia. Use of atropine with non-irritant, volatile general anaesthetics may produce unpleasant sore throat postoperatively. Similarly, reduction in the bronchial secretion can lead to inspissation of the residual secretions and formation of thick bronchial plugs.

● ***Organophosphorus poisoning***: See Chapter 18. Atropine is also useful in mushroom poisoning due to muscarine.

● ***Parkinsonism*** : Chapter 14.

● ***Cardiovascular conditions*** : Atropine may be useful in abolishing A-V block due to excessive vagal activity. It is also occasionally useful in countering the syncope and bradycardia due to hypersensitive carotid sinus.

● ***Urinary incontinence***: Various synthetic substitutes like dicylomine, oxybutynin and propantheline have been used to reduce unstable detrusor contractions. (See later).

● ***Motion sickness*** : **Scopolamine hydrobromide** in the dose of 0.5 to 1 mg. by mouth is used in the treatment of motion sickness. Dryness of mouth signifies the onset of effect and the protection conferred lasts for 4 to 6 hours. The greatest advantage of the drug is that, when given orally in above doses, it has only a slight sedative effect. Hyoscine is admirably suited to control motion sickness during short journeys. In the event of prolongation of the journey, the drug may be repeated at intervals of 2 hours in the dose of 0.1 mg. Larger doses may produce excessive sedation. Atropine is much less effective than hyoscine. Hyoscine can also be given by transdermal route (Scopoderm, Chapter 40).

● ***Peptic ulcer***: Anticholinergics are now rarely used (Chapter 42).

Relative contraindications to atropine therapy: Atropine should be administered with caution in:

(a) Patients over the age of 40 as it may precipitate an attack of acute congestive glaucoma.

(b) Individuals with enlarged prostate, as retention of urine may develop.

(c) Chronic lung conditions as it may reduce the secretions and produce drying.

(d) Congestive heart failure with tachycardia and

(e) Pyloric obstruction, pylorospasm and cardiospasm which it may worsen.

Synthetic and Semisynthetic Atropine Substitutes

The need for atropine substitutes arises mainly because of the lack of its selectivity in action. Thus, the dose of atropine required to produce the therapeutic effects on GI tract invariably produces many adverse effects. Drugs have been synthesized, therefore, to produce more therapeutic selectivity. Chemically, atropine substitutes are :

I **The quaternary ammonium compounds** which are not satisfactorily orally absorbed, do not cross the blood-brain barrier,and generally exihibit a greater degree of nicotinic (ganglionic) blocking action; and

II **The tertiary amine drugs** which are better absorbed orally, cross the blood-brain barrier, and act more selectively at the muscarinic receptors.

These substitutes are employed mainly for their predominant actions :

I As mydriatics and cycloplegics in the eye.

II As antispasmodics.

III In parkinsonism; and

IV In chronic bronchitis and bronchial asthma.

I Mainly Used in Eye (Chapter 70).

II Mainly Used as Spasmolytics

These atropine substitutes are mainly used in the treatment of colics. The quaternary ammonium atropine substitutes which do not cross the blood brain barrier are relatively free from the central effects. They are more liable to produce ganglionic blockade, resulting in impotence, postural hypotension and urinary retention. They may also block neuromuscular transmission by a curarimimetic action.

ATROPINE METHONITRATE: Besides its ophthalmic use, it is administered orally in the dose of 0.2 to 0.4 mg. 4 to 6 times a day to treat congenital hypertrophic pyloric stenosis.

METHSCOPOLAMINE BROMIDE: This quaternary ammonium compound is devoid of the central effects of scopolamine and is used in the treatment of renal colic and frequency of micturition associated with cystitis. Dose : 2 to 5 mg. orally, three times a day, or parenterally in the dose of 0.25 to 1 mg. **Hyoscine-n- butyl bromide** (Buscopan) has potent smooth muscle relaxant action and similar use.

METHANTHELINE (Banthine): It is a synthetic quaternary ammonium compound with a high ratio of ganglion blocking to muscarinic blocking activity. The GI effects and the duration of action of this drug are greater than those of atropine. The drug may produce impotence, postural hypotension, urinary retention and neuromuscular blockade. Other effects like euphoria, restlessness and acute psychosis have been reported. Dose 50 to 100 mg. orally or 15 to 25 mg. IM.

PROPANTHELINE (Probanthine): It is related to methantheline and possess more potent ganglionic and muscarinic blocking actions than methantheline. It has been used as a muscle relaxant in irritable bowel syndrome and for relieving pain of diverticulitis. It is administered orally in the dose of 15 mg t.i.d.

OXYPHENONIUM (Antrenyl): This quaternary ammonium compound has a higher ratio of ganglion blocking to antimuscarinic activity than majority of other synthetic atropine substitutes. It is a potent antispasmodic. It is available as 5 mg. tablets. The usual dose is 10 mg. orally.

DICYCLOMINE (Merbentyl, Cyclopam, Colimex): A tertiary amine, also has direct relaxant properties. Dicyclomine hydrochloride is available as 10 mg. tablets and as a syrup containing 10 mg. per 5 ml. Dose : 10-20 mg. tid. Smaller doses are used in children. It is used in dysmenorrhoea and irritable bowel syndrome.

FLAVOXATE (Uripas) : This tertiary amine has local anaesthetic, analgesic and slight anticholinergic properties. It may also have a direct relaxant action on smooth muscle. It is used to treat dysuria, nocturia, suprapubic pain, and urinary urgency and frequency associated with cystitis, prostatitis and urethritis. The dose is 100-200 mg 3-4 times a day.

OXYBUTYNIN (Ditropan, Tropan) : This compound has antimuscarinic (selective M_3) direct antispasmodic and some local anaesthetic effects on the urinary bladder. It has been used in the treatment of urinary urgency, urge incontinence and urinary frequency except that following transurethral surgical procedures. The oral dose in adults in 5 mg. two to three times a day.

TROSPIUM is a nonselective antimuscarinic with efficacy and safety similar to those of oxybutynin. Dose: 20 mg. bid.

TOLTERODINE (Detrusitol, Roliten): This tertiary amine acts as a selective M_3 receptor antagonist and has been used to treat bladder detrusor instability in the treatment of urinary incontinence. It is metabolized in the liver and the metabolites possess similar actions as the parent compound. Dose : 2 mg bid.

Pirenzepine : See Chapter 42.

Some of the **other atropine substitutes** available for therapy are homatropine methylbromide, diphemanil, pipenzolate (Piptal), poldine, clidinium, procyclidine, glycopyrronium, pavatrine and drotavarine. Many of these quaternary antimuscarinic drugs in tolerated doses are claimed to be superior to atropine. None, however, can be considered as highly selective in action, and clinically effective doses will evoke some anti-cholinergic adverse effects.

III **Belladona substitutes used in the treatment of parkinsonism:** Trihexyphenidyl and Benztropine (Chapter 14).

Table 19.1: Some drugs with antimuscarinic side effects

- Antispasmodics e.g., Synthetic atropine substitutes.
- Antiparkinsonian drugs, e.g., Benzhexol.
- Antipsychotics.
- Antidepressants, e.g., Tricyclics
- Antihistaminies, e.g., Diphenhydramine.

IV **Drugs used in chronic bronchitis, COPD and bronchial asthma:** Ipratropium Bromide (Chapter 26).

Some drugs which may cause antimuscarinic side effects, when used in therapy are listed in Table 19.1.

Bladder Dysfunction – Pharmacology

Normal urinary bladder function and the act of urination (micturition) are well coordinated, involving several neurotransmitters and neuromodulators. Normal urination involves higher centres (pons), spinal cord and peripheral autonomic, somatic and afferent sensory innervation of the lower urinary tract. Disorders of any of these can contribute to the symptoms of bladder dysfunction.

Acetylcholine, by acting on the M_3 receptors, causes detrusor muscle contraction while adrenergic activity causes its relaxation through the stimulation of beta$_3$ adrenergic receptors. Stimulation of dopamine D_1 receptors suppresses bladder activity, whereas D_2 stimulation facilitates voiding. Other neurotransmitters such as GABA, encephalin, glutamate and 5-HT are also involved in the regulation of bladder function. The intern al sphincter at the bladder neck is rich in α_1 adrenoreceptors; their activation causes sphincter contraction.

Table 19.2: Drugs used in bladder dysfunction

Drugs	Mechanism of action	Use	Dose (mg)
Antimuscarinics			
Oxybutynin	Decreases bladder contraction	Urge incontinence	2.5-5.0 tid
Tolterodine	Do	Do	2 bid
Trospium	Do	Do	20 bid
Flavoxate	Do	Do	100-200 tid
Alpha$_1$ adrenergic agonist			
Pseudoephedrine	Stimulates urethral smooth muscle	Stress incontinence	30-60 tid
Alpha$_1$ adrenergic antagonists			
Terazocin	Relaxes urethra and prostate capsule smooth muscle	Urge incontinence asso. with BPH	1-10/d
Doxazocin	Do	Do	1-8/d
Tamsulocin	Do	Do	0.4 od, HS
Cholinergic agonist			
Bethanechol	Stimulates bladder contraction	Hypotonic/atonic bladder	10-30 tid
Topical estrogen *			
Cream (vaginal)	Strengthens peri-urethral tissue	Urge/stress incontinence asso. with vaginal atrophy	See foot note **
Tablets (vaginal)	Do	Do	25 mcg/day as above
Antidepressants			
Imipramine	Anticholinergic ? Central action	Nocturnal eneuresis	Chapter 13

* Long acting and transdermal estrogen preparations are available.
** 0.5-1.0 g/day for first 2 weeks; then twice weekly for 4 weeks.

The common functional abnormalities of micturition that call for treatment are :

(1) **Urinary frequency/urgency incontinence**
(2) **Hypotonic bladder** and
(3) **Nocturia/nocturnal eneuresis.**

Overactive bladder, a symptom complex, includes urinary urgency with or without urge incontinence, urinary frequency and nocturia (awakening more than once at night to void urine). It is observed in the elderly with prevalence rate of 30-40% in subjects over 75 years of age. There is no identifiable cause nor any local abnormality.

Among the types of chronic urinary incontinence, **urge incontinence** is the most common. It is characterized by sudden urgency with leakage of urine, and may be associated with increased frequency and nocturia.

Stress incontinencc; the next common type, is more common in the older females. It is associated with weakened pelvic floor muscles and consequent increased mobility of the bladder outlet and urethra. Leakage of urine occurs with increased abdominal pressure as during coughing, sneezing and laughing.

Drugs used in disturbances of bladder function are summarisee in Table 19.2.

● ***Functional urinary frequency, urgency and incontinence (overactive bladder)*** are treated with antimuscarinic drugs such as oxybutynin, flavoxate, tolterodine and trospium. They act by inhibiting the unstable detrusor contractions and thus increasing the bladder capacity. They can be used for both neurogenic and non-neurogenic overactive bladder. These drugs are also useful in detrusor muscle spasm associated with cystitis.

Solifenacin and **darifenacin** are the new drugs, claimed to be relatively 'bladder specific' in their antimuscarinic action, (M_3 antagonist) for use in overactive bladder. There is no convincing evidence of their superiority over the older drugs in either efficacy or tolerability.

Anticholinergics should be used cautiously in elderly patients with dementia. Further, obstruction due to enlarged prostate, carcinoma of the prostate and bladder stone must be ruled out.

Post-synaptic alpha$_1$ adrenergic blockers such as **terazocin** and **tamsulosin** are used to treat urinary frequency due to enlarged prostate (Chapter 67).

● ***Bladder hypotonicity*** which sometimes causes urinary retention is treated by cholinergic drugs such as **bethanechol, neostigmine** or **distigmine** (Chapter 18). Urinary retention due to benign prostatic hypertrophy, however, will be worsened by these drugs.

● ***Nocturia,*** a symptom of overactive bladder, can be due to detrusor overactivity, nocturnal polyuria or a primary sleep disorder-nocturnal eneuresis. Antidepressant **imipramine** has anticholinergic action, and possible central effect on voiding reflexes. It may be useful in some patients with stress-urge incontinence and nocturnal eneuresis (Chapter 13).

Finally, it should be remembered that the distal part of the female urethral epithelium possesses estrogen receptors. Their degeneration after menopause can cause urinary incontinence. Such patients may be helped by topical (vaginal) or oral **estrogen** therapy.

The non-pharmacological treatment of these conditions includes education about bladder function in cognitively intact, motivated patients, pelvic floor exercises and bladder training. The latter involves teaching of urge suppression and regular, scheduled voiding. Some patients can be helped by biofeedback-assisted training.

Ganglion Stimulating and Blocking Drugs

20

The ganglion stimulating agents have hardly any use in therapeutics. The important agents belonging to this group are the alkaloids nicotine and lobeline. In addition, synthetic compounds like tetramethylammonium (TMA) and dimethylphenylpiperazinium (DMPP) are mainly used as experimental tools. Although nicotine has no therapeutic utility, it is the important constituent of tobacco. Lobeline is discussed in Chapter 12.

NICOTINE : Nicotine was isolated from leaves of the tobacco plant, *Nicotiana tabacum* in 1828. It is a tertiary amine consisting of a pyridine ring and a pyrolidine ring. The actions of this compound, particularly its effects on autonomic ganglia, were studied by Langley and Dickinson in their classical experiments in 1889.

Mechanism of action: Nicotinic cholinergic receptors are present in the brain, autonomic ganglia and neuromuscular junctions, which explains the multiple effects of nicotine. Nicotinic receptors are of two types : NN form in the CNS and the autonomic ganglia; and NM form in the skeletal neuro-muscular junction. Activation of nicotine receptors facilitates the release of ACh, NA, DA, 5-HT and beta-endorphin. Nicotine also causes release of growth hormone, prolactin and ACTH.

Pharmacological actions: The amount of nicotine absorbed during smoking is sufficient to produce measurable pharmacological and psychopharmacological effects.

- ***Behavioural effects*:** These vary according to the species and the dosage used and are probably linked to DA release. In small doses, the effects are predominantly stimulant, whereas large doses cause depression. Small doses may improve attention, learning, reaction time and problem solving. Smokers often report pleasure and relaxation, and reduction in anger, tension, depression and stress.

- ***Central Nervous System*:** Nicotine stimulates the CNS and produces tremor, while large doses may produce convulsions. Small doses reflexly stimulate respiration through aortic and carotid body chemoreceptors; while large doses directly stimulate the medullary respiratory centre. The stimulation of respiration is usually followed by depression and paralysis.

Vomiting induced by nicotine is due to stimulation of the CTZ and the sensory nerve endings involved in mediation of the vomiting reflex.

Nicotine, by stimulating the supraoptic nuclei of the hypothalamus, induces the release of ADH and exerts an antidiuretic effect. In sensitive individuals, this effect may become apparent after smoking 2 or 3 cigarettes.

- ***Autonomic ganglia*:** Like ACh, nicotine initially stimulates the autonomic ganglia leading to stimulation of post-ganglionic nerves.

However, large doses of nicotine produce persistent depolarization of these ganglionic cell bodies resulting in ganglionic blockade. In still larger doses, nicotine, by competing with ACh for ganglionic receptor sites, also produces a competitive block. Nicotine in large doses, therefore, paralyses the autonomic ganglia by a dual mechanism.

• ***Adrenal medulla*** : This is anatomically and embryologically a sympathetic ganglion, is initially stimulated by nicotine, leading to discharge of adrenaline into the blood. Larger doses block the secretory response to splanchnic nerve stimulation.

The cardiovascular actions of nicotine in an intact animal usually vary according to preponderance of sympathetic or parasympathetic stimulation. The most consistent effects of smoking in humans are an increase in the heart rate and peripheral vasoconstriction. Carotid chemoreceptors are very sensitive to low levels of nicotine. Blood pressure may rise and an increase in skeletal muscle and coronary blood flow may occur. These effects result from increased release of catecholamine due to stimulation of the sympathetic ganglia and adrenal medulla. Tolerance to increase in the heart rate develops fairly rapidly.

• ***GI tract and secretions***: Nicotine increases the motility, tone and secretion of the GI tract and may cause colonic evacuation due to stimulation of the parasympathetic ganglia. Stimulation is usually followed by decrease in motility and tone, leading to constipation. Nicotine initially increases the salivary and bronchial secretions, followed by their inhibition. Salivation accompanying smoking, however, is due to irritant nature of the smoke rather than its nicotine content.

• ***Myoneural junction***: At the myoneural junction, nicotine produces a transient depolarization of the motor end plate, resulting in a stimulation of skeletal muscles and twitchings. In large doses, this stimulant effect is followed and often overshadowed by paralysis of myoneural transmission. It is usually the cause of death in nicotine poisoning. It must be pointed out, however, that nicotine has a much more prominent effect on the autonomic ganglia than on the myoneural junction.

• ***Liver enzymes***: Nicotine induces hepatic microsomal enzymes. Inhalation of cigarette smoke enhances the metabolism of several drugs including nicotine in man.

• ***Metabolic effects***: Nicotine increases the metabolic rate slightly at rest but almost doubles it during light exercise. The increase in BMR, along with appetite suppression, leads to weight loss. Nicotine, via catecholamine release, causes lipolysis and release of free fatty acids (FFA) into the circulation. Excessive release of cortisol following nicotine could affect mood and may contribute to osteoporosis.

• ***Miscellaneous***: Intradermal injection or local application of nicotine produces sweating and vasoconstriction in the area treated. This effect is attributed to cutaneous axon reflexes mediated by sympathetic nerves and serves as a basis for testing the integrity of the postganglionic sympathetic fibres. It is blocked by local anaesthetics, atropine and ganglionic blocking agents.

Tolerance and dependence: One third to one half of occasional smokers develop physical dependence. Most tobacco-dependent persons never achieve lasting abstinence and one half of all smokers die prematurely of tobacco-related diseases. A regular smoker is able to withstand large amounts of nicotine in contrast to a non-smoker. The addictive effects of tobacco smoking are largely due to nicotine.

Withdrawal syndrome, manifests as craving, depression, nervousness, restlessness, irritability, anxiety, impaired concentration, increased appetite and weight gain.

Absorption, fate and excretion: Nicotine is well absorbed from all mucous membranes and even from intact, unbroken skin. After absorption, it is concentrated in the liver, lungs and the brain. At physiologic pH, about 30% of nicotine is unionized and can cross cell membrane readily. A major portion of the alkaloid is metabolized mainly in liver to cotinine which is then glucuronidated and products are excreted by the kidney. An acidic urine enhances the excretion of ionized nicotine. Nicotine may be secreted in the milk.

Adverse reactions : Acute nicotine poisoning occurs in workers engaged in spraying nicotine as an insecticide. Nicotine poisoning may occur in children from accidental ingestion of cigarettes. Nicotine is much less toxic when swallowed in the form of tobacco than when ingested in pure form. It is, however, one of the most toxic agents and can produce death with the rapidity of cyanide. Acute nicotine poisoning is characterised by nausea, salivation, vomiting, abdominal pain and diarrhoea. Dizziness, headache, confusion and marked weakness develop. The pupils initially constrict but dilate subsequently. The initial rise in blood pressure is followed by a fall and initial bradycardia is followed by tachycardia. Cold sweat is a prominent feature. Respiration, after brief stimulation, becomes irregular. Convulsions may appear in the later stage and death occurs from respiratory paralysis.

The treatment consists of gastric lavage with 1:10,000 solution of potassium permanganate. As nicotine is rapidly metabolized in the body, attempts should be made to tide over the crisis by symptomatic therapy. Paralysis of respiration should be treated by artificial ventilation with oxygen. *The use of analeptics is dangerous.*

Chronic nicotine toxicity and tobacco smoking: Tobacco, the dried leaf of *Nicotiana tabacum,* is used in various forms as snuff, as plug for chewing and for smoking. The nicotine content of tobacco varies from 0.5 to 8 per cent. Large quantities of nicotine are absorbed from the inhaled smoke and a person who 'drags' on his cigar or cigarette absorbs larger quantities. A cigarette contains 6-11 mg. of nicotine, of which the smoker typically absorbs 1-3 mg. irrespective of the nicotine yield rating provided by the tobacco companies. The other ingredients of tobacco smoke include tar, pyridine, volatile acids, furfural, carbon monoxide and carcinogens. They also contribute to the adverse effects of tobacco smoking.

Smoking and tobacco chewing are believed to be either causative or exacerbating factors in a number of conditions including cancers. Cigarette smoking is associated with increase in morbidity and a shortening of life expectancy. The latter is related to the magnitude of cigarette consumption. It is higher in older than in younger persons, is seen especially in those who start smoking early in life and in those who inhale the smoke deeply. The increase in mortality is lower in those who give up smoking than in those who continue to smoke. Most of the increase in mortality is from cancer of various organs, chronic bronchitis, emphysema and ischemic heart disease.

- ***Carcinoma of the lung*:** The risk of carcinoma of the lung is 15-20 times higher in cigarette smokers than in non-smokers. This is especially so when cigarette smoking is combined with inhalation of asbestos dust, chromates, nickel, arsenic or radioactive material. Tobacco smoke contains several cancer initiators (carcinogens) and cancer promoters (co-carcinogens); all have not been identified but the best known is benzapyrene. Experimental cancer of the skin has been produced in animals by application of condensates of tobacco smoke and dogs who inhaled cigarette smoke through tracheostomies developed cancer of the lung.

- ***Chronic bronchitis and emphysema*:** The incidence of chronic bronchitis is higher in habitual smokers than in non-smokers. A smoker's respiratory syndrome characterised by cough, dyspnoea, wheezing, pain in chest and frequent infection of the upper respiratory tract has been described. Tobacco smoke contains a number of irritants which cause bronchoconstriction, damage to the ciliated epithelium and hypertrophy of the mucus glands. Prolonged, heavy smoking is the main cause of chronic obstructive pulmonary disease (COPD) which has two components, chronic bronchitis and emphysema. Emphysema is due to hyperinflation of the lungs coupled with destruction of the alveolar walls causing loss of elastic tissue. When younger smokers give up smoking their lung function returns to normal.

However, when older persons with established chronic bronchitis and emphysema stop smoking, the benefit is less dramatic.

● ***Ischaemic heart disease*:** Mortality from ischaemic heart disease and the frequency of angina pectoris are more in smokers than in non-smokers. Further, atherosclerotic changes are more extensive in smokers than in non-smokers. These effects are probably due to release of catecholamines from the adrenal medulla by nicotine. Catecholamines increase (a) platelet adhesiveness; (b) the concentration of blood lipids, and (c) the tendency to hypertension and cardiac arrhythmias. Further, smoking increases the concentration of carboxyhemoglobin in the blood. Thrombosis is an important mechanism of smoking-induced cardiac events.

● ***Peripheral vascular disease*:** Nicotine causes prolonged vasoconstriction in the hands and feet. Thromboangiitis obliterans (TAO) occurs far more frequently in smokers than in non-smokers and intermittent claudication is more frequent in elderly atherosclerotic smokers than in non-smokers.

● ***Tobacco amblyopia*:** Tobacco amblyopia which usually causes a gradual, but occasionally sudden, decrease in the visual acuity, particularly in the central field, is attributed to a spasm of the retinal blood vessels caused by nicotine. Fortunately, it is rare. Smoking may sometimes produce an increase in the intraocular tension in glaucomatous patients.

● ***GI disturbances*:** Nicotine causes excessive salivation, aggravation of peptic ulcer disease and constipation. Increased incidence of cancers of the mouth, larynx and esophagus has been reported in association with smoking and tobacco chewing.

● ***Miscellaneous*:** Women who smoke heavily are at risk for a premature menopause. Those who smoke during pregnancy have a higher incidence of abortions and give birth to babies with below-average birth weights. Smoking is often claimed to have a tranquillizing effect but many people feel better both physically and mentally after giving up smoking.

The polycyclic hydrocarbons present in the cigarette smoke accelerate the metabolism of many drugs by inducing hepatic microsomal enzymes (Chapter 3).

Prevention of tobacco use in any form is important. In this respect, education of children in the concept of positive health and in the harmful effect of smoking on health is of prime importance. This must be done as much by practice as by preaching since children tend to imitate the grown-ups around them and cannot be expected not to smoke as long as they see people, particularly family members, smoking or chewing tobacco all around them.

Doctors can help by inquiring about the smoking habits of all their patients, by educating them about its harmful effects, by strongly advising against smoking and by not smoking themselves!

Tobacco produces both psychological and physical dependence. Abrupt cessation of heavy smoking may cause irritability and drowsiness.

Treatment of tobacco dependence: Drugs used in treating tobacco dependence are listed in Table 20.1. Psychotic and neurotic traits are found consistently more often in smokers than in non-smokers. Attention to any underlying psychological disturbances may prove very useful.

Nicotine substitution for tobacco dependence doubles or triples the rate of success of quitting smoking. The basis of this treatment is that the re-enforcement of behavioral effects of smoking is maximum with inhalation, less

Table 20.1: Drugs used in tobacco dependence

I **Nicotine receptor agonists**
Nicotine transdermal patches
Nicotine polacrylate gum/lozenges
Nicotine nasal spray
Nicotine oral inhaler

II **Nicotine receptor partial agonist** e.g. Varenicline.

III **Dopamine/NA central re-uptake inhibitor** e.g. Bupropion.

IV **CB_1 receptor antagonist** e.g. Rimonabant.

with oral use, and least with the slow-release, transdermal nicotine patch.

The preparations used for substitution therapy are :

(i) Transdermally delivered nicotine (Nicotine patches).

(ii) Transmucosally delivered nicotine (Polacrilec); and

These preparations, in contrast to smoking, provide slower rise in, and lower and less variable plasma nicotine concentrations, thus helping the smoker to abstain from tobacco, resulting finally in cessation of smoking.

The possible mechanism by which the smoker's cessation efforts are strengthened by this medication are :

- ***Nicotine substitution decreases withdrawal symptoms.***
- ***It partially decreases the craving for cigarettes by sustaining tolerance,*** in much the same way that methadone partially decreases the craving for morphine; and
- ***It may provide some euphoria.***

VARENICLINE (Chantix) is a partial agonist of nicotinic N_N receptors. Its t½ is 14-24 hours. Oral administration of 1 mg bid, with a full glass of water, after eating, helps some patients to quit smoking. It causes nausea, headache, sleep distrubances and weight loss. Severe neutropsychiatric symptoms have been reported.

BUPROPION : Antidepressants such as **bupropion** have been claimed to help in giving up smoking in some individuals. Bupropion is used in the dose of 150-300 mg. per day, for 7 days prior to cessation of smoking and then in the dose of 300 mg per day for 6-12 weeks. It can also be used along with nicotine patches. In excessive doses, it can cause seizures in persons with a history of seizure.

Rimonabant, a CB1 receptor antagonist, has been found effective in helping patients to quit smoking. It also causes weight loss (Chapter 39).

Ganglion Blocking Agents

The ganglion blocking agents are drugs which selectively competitively block the transmission across the autonomic ganglia, both sympathetic and parasympathetic, by blocking the ACh receptors. The blockade produced by these agents, unlike that produced by nicotine, is not preceded by stimulation. They can cause adverse reactions due to parasympathetic blockade (visual disturbances, dry mouth, urinary hesitancy, constipation and sexual impotence) and sympathetic blockade (syncope from postural hypotension) (Chapter 29).

Skeletal Muscle Relaxants 21

Skeletal muscle relaxants able to reduce unwanted spasm or spasticity without interfering with consciousness and normal voluntary movements find an important application in various neurological or painful musculo-skeletal disorders. They are also valuable during operative procedures, for achieving satisfactory muscle relaxation.

Spasticity is due to increase in skeletal muscle tone associated with decrease in muscle power due to damage to the corticomotoneuronic pathways as in cerebral palsy, multiple sclerosis, CNS injury or stroke. **Spasm**, on the other hand, is an involuntary contraction of a muscle or group of muscles, usually accompanied by pain and limited function.

Skeletal muscle relaxation without the loss of consciousness can be achieved by :

I **Drugs acting centrally,** e.g., Benzodiazepines (Chapter 8), Baclofen and Tizanidine (Table 21.1).

II **Drugs acting peripherally** at neuromuscular junction. See later.

III **Drugs acting directly on muscle,** e.g., Dantrolene.

IV **Drugs effective in parkinsonism** (Chapter 14).

Centrally Acting Skeletal Muscle Relaxants

Centrally acting muscle relaxants cause muscular relaxation without loss of consciousness. Hence, they are expected to act on selective areas in the CNS. However, most of these drugs cause sedation; and sedative anxiolytic agents like diazepam also have central muscle relaxant action. The exact mechanism of muscle relaxant action is not known. However, some also have an action on the reticular neuronal mechanisms controlling the muscle tone. There is no clear evidence that any of these agents influences neuronal conduction in man. Animal experiments have shown that these drugs reduce the activity of polysynaptic reflexes in the spinal cord. But their ability to reduce decerebrate rigidity in cats does not necessarily indicate their usefulness in the cerebrate man. The commonly used agents are :

DIAZEPAM: This drug is discussed in detail in Chapter 8. It is useful alone, or in combination, for relieving spasticity especially in patients with lesions of the spinal cord, and occasionally in patients with cerebral palsy or multiple sclerosis. Painful spasms due to a spinal cord lesion are often reduced. It may be of benefit in the *stiff-man syndrome* and in localised muscle spasms due to traumatic causes. Oral dose: 2 mg. twice daily, increased gradually to maximum of 10 mg. 3-4 times daily. It is the drug of choice to control spasms in tetanus, where it can be given IM or IV. *Diazepam should not be mixed with other drugs for IV use.*

TIZANIDINE This drug reduces muscle spasm by acting centrally as an agonist of alpha2 adrenergic receptors.It is believed to enhance the presynaptic inhibition of the motor neurons.It is given in the dose of 2-4 mg at bedtime and the dose is increased gradually. Adverse reactions include dizziness, drowsiness and asthenia.

CYCLOBENZAPRINE (Flexeril) : This drug, structurally related to TCA, probably acts on descending 5-HT pathway to reduce tonic somatic motor activity. Adverse effects are dose related and include sedation, dizziness and anti cholinergic effects.

BACLOFEN (Lioresal): This compound, beta-4 (chlorophenyl)-gamma aminobutyric acid, is structurally related to GABA, an inhibitory neurotransmitter in the CNS and spinal cord. It is a potent neuronal depressant, mainly acting in the spinal cord, on presynaptic mechanisms rather than on postsynaptic GABA-B receptors. It reduces the release of excitatory transmitters, and also causes a dose-dependent 'antinociceptive' effect in the intact animal; it may thus be useful in pain syndromes.

Clinically, it produces considerable relief of painful flexor (and sometimes extensor) spasms and of increased flexor tone in patients with spinal transection. It also reduces tonic flexor dystonias of the lower extremities in patients with spinal spasticity. The drug may also improve bladder and bowel control in patients with spinal lesions. It has no action on muscle power and is not useful in other types of spasticity, such as that of cerebral origin. It has been also found to be a 'back up' drug in the treatment of trigeminal neuralgia. It is almost completely absorbed, and 80% is excreted unchanged in the urine within 72 hours.

The drug is generally well tolerated. Adverse reactions include drowsiness, lassitude, hallucinations, depression, blurred vision and GI disturbances.

It is used in the dose of 5 mg, 3-4 times a day to be increased every 3-4 days, up to a maximum of 80 mg. per day.

Centrally acting muscle relaxants are summarized in Table 21.1.

Table 21.1 : Centrally acting muscle relaxants

Name	Preparation (Tab)	Total daily dose
Benzodiazepines (Diazepam. Chap. 8)		
Carisoprodol *(Carisoma)*	0.35 g.	0.7-1.4 g.
Chlorzoxazone *(Parafon)*	0.25 g.	0.5-1.5 g.
Methocarbamol* *(Rolimax)*	0.5 g.	4-8 g.
Orphenadrine* *(Disipal)*	0.05 g.	0.1-0.2 g.
Tizanidine *(Sirdalud)*	2 mg	6-18 mg
Cyclobenzaprine *(Amrix)*	10 mg	15-30 mg

Oral doses mentioned are usually given in divided doses. * IM. and IV preparations available.

Various muscle relaxants mentioned above have been advocated as adjuvaul analgesics (Chapter 11) in such conditions as fibrositis, myalgia, myositis and spasms associated with arthritis. They are also recommended in certain spastic neurological disorders. They may be of some use in cases with localized muscle spasm but not so much in spasticity. The borderline beneficial effects observed with these agents are probably because of their central sedative and analgesic actions, and none of these compounds except benzodiazepines, dantrolene and baclofen can be recommended as effective, reliable and specific muscle relaxants.

The centrally acting skeletal muscle relaxants should be used with caution in pregnant women and in the presence of renal damage. They are contraindicated in myasthenia gravis.

Peripherally Acting Skeletal Muscle Relaxants

Physiology of skeletal muscle contraction: The steps in neuromuscular transmission leading to skeletal muscle contraction consists of:

● Release of ACh in relatively *large amounts* from the synaptic vesicles of the motor nerve into the synaptic cleft as a result of a nerve impulse which is also called nerve action potential (NAP). Even in the absence of nerve impulse, *minute quantities* of ACh are released continually in the synaptic cleft.

● Acetylcholine released into the synaptic cleft binds to the nicotinic receptors on the motor end plate, leading to the development of an end plate potential (EPP). Depolarization is due to an influx of sodium into the motor end plate (MEP).

● When the end plate potential achieves sufficient magnitude, the surrounding area of the muscle fibre membrane is excited, resulting in the development of muscle action potential (MAP) which initiates contraction as a result of release of calcium into the sarcoplasm.

● Acetylcholine is rapidly hydrolysed by acetylcholinesterase enabling the repolarization of the MEP and the muscle fibre membrane. This is achieved by reversal of the ionic fluxes. The repolarized muscle is now capable of responding to a fresh nerve impulse.

Ca^{++} ions play a crucial role in excitation—contraction (E-C) coupling in all muscle types. However, the source of these calcium ions varies in different muscle types and under different experimental conditions. Thus, in most vertebrate and invertebrate smooth muscles, calcium ions bound to the inner surface of the cell membranes are the main source of Ca^{++} for coupling. Cardiac muscles use mainly extra-cellular calcium ions while skeletal muscle uses mainly tubular membrane bound calcium for coupling. However, in both these muscles the amount of calcium that enters the myoplasm from these sources is inadequate to complete the coupling process and an amplification system consisting of Ca^{++} release from the sarcoplasmic reticulum (SR) exists. Drugs can modify this calcium-triggered calcium release from the SR in the E-C coupling process in both skeletal and cardiac muscle.

Skeletal muscle contraction can be blocked at several points as shown in Table 21.2.

Table 21.2: Ways of blocking skeletal muscle contraction in response to nerve impulse

- ***Blocking the transmission of impulse across the motor nerve,*** e.g., Local anaesthetics and certain biological toxins.
- ***Inhibiting the synthesis of acetylcholine in the motor nerve,*** e.g., Hemicholinium.
- ***Inhibiting the release of acetylcholine*** by Botulinum toxin A and Beta bungarotoxin.
- ***Modifying the MEP functional states*** so that it does not respond to ACh eg. the clinically useful skeletal muscle relaxants.
- ***Interfering with sarcoplasmic reticulum function*** e.g. Dantrolene.

In clinical practice, paralysis of skeletal muscles is usually induced by interfering with the function of motor end plate. The peripherally acting skeletal muscle relaxants can be classified according to their mode of action:

I **Agents acting by competitive blockade of ACh at the motor end plate,** e.g. d-Tubocurarine, Alcuronium, Atracurium, Vecuronium and Gallamine.

II **Agents acting by persistent depolarization of the motor end plate and the muscle fibre membrane** e.g. Succinylcholine.

III **Drugs which inhibit the release of ACh from the motor nerve terminals** e.g. Botulinum toxin Type A.

I Drugs acting by competitive blockade:

d-TUBOCURARINE (Tubarine): This is the dextrorotatory, quaternary ammonium alkaloid obtained from the plant *Chondrodendron tomentosum,* indigenous to the Western Amazon region, and plants of the Strychnos species (mainly *Strychnos lethalis*) from Eastern Amazon region of South America. Crude curare is a dark-brown to black, gummy, resinoid mass, soluble in water. The letter 'd' stands for dextro, while the prefix 'tubo' is derived from the fact that crude curare was stored and transported by the South American Indians in bamboo tubes. It was mainly used as an arrow poison. Although the mechanism of this action was studied by Claude Bernard in 1856, the alkaloid was isolated by King in 1935.

Mechanism of action : d-Tubocurarine binds to the nicotinic receptors on the MEP and thus blocks the action of ACh by **competitive blockade**. The muscle paralysed by d-tubocurarine still responds to direct electrical stimulation, showing that the drug selectively acts on the MEP. If the concentration of ACh in the synaptic cleft is increased either by augmenting its release (stronger electrical stimulation of the motor nerve) or inhibiting its degradation (by an antiChE drug), d-tubocurarine blockade is reversed (Fig. 21.1).

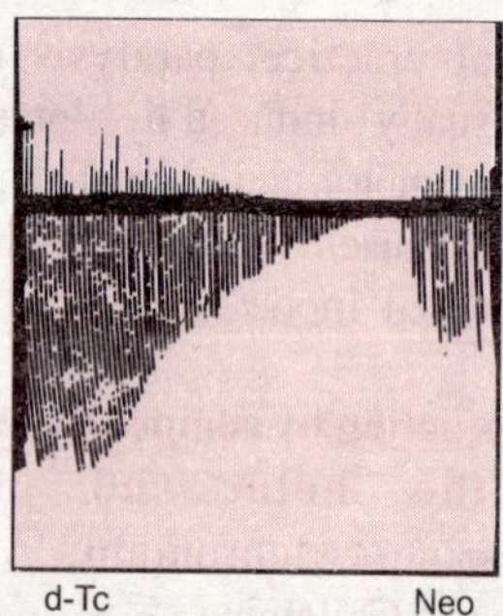

Fig. 21.1: Blocking effect of d-tubocurarine (dTc) on electrically stimulated rat phrenic nerve diaphragm preparation. Note the quick recovery following the addition of neostigmine (Neo).

Pharmacological actions:

• ***Skeletal muscle***: d-Tubocurarine, on parenteral administration, initially produces motor weakness followed by flaccid paralysis. Small, rapidly moving muscles of the fingers, toes, ears and eyes are affected first, making it impossible to perform delicate motor tasks and producing diplopia, slurred speech and difficulty in swallowing. The muscles of limbs, neck and trunk are affected later, followed by the intercostal muscles. Finally, the diaphragm is paralysed and death occurs from hypoxia. Consciousness and sensorium are unaffected. Recovery occurs in the reverse order, the diaphragm recovering first and the small muscles recovering last.

• ***Autonomic ganglia***: In the doses used clinically, d-tubocurarine can produce partial blockade of both the autonomic ganglia and adrenal medulla resulting in fall of BP, after brief initial stimulation.

• ***Histamine release***: It produces histamine release from tissues by acting directly on mast cells. This may occasionally cause bronchospasm, increased salivary, tracheo-bronchial and gastric acid secretion and contributes to production of hypotension.

Absorption, fate and excretion: d-Tubocurarine, being a quaternary ammonium compound, is not significantly absorbed from the GI tract. The drug is well absorbed on IM administration and is widely distributed in tissues. The drug owes its brief duration of action to its rapid redistribution. On IV administration, skeletal muscle paralysis becomes discernible within 1 to 1½ minutes, the peak effect is obtained within 5 to 7 minutes and the action persists for 60 to 100 minutes. About 33 per cent of the dose is eliminated unchanged in urine within 24 hours. Repeated administration can cause cumulative toxicity.

The drug does not cross the blood-brain or placental barrier. It is, therefore, devoid of CNS effects.

Adverse reactions :

• ***Hypoxia and respiratory paralysis***: Respiratory acidosis enhances neuromuscular blockate. Hypoxia should be treated with positive pressure artificial respiration with oxygen and maintenance of a patent airway till adequate recovery occurs. Neostigmine methyl sulphate, 0.5 to 2 mg., along with 0.6 to 1.2 mg. of atropine should be administered cautiously. Neostigmine, though countering skeletal muscle paralysis, enhances the bronchospasm, hypotension and hydrochloric acid secretion produced by d-tubocurarine. This can be countered by atropine. Cardiac arrest, which is liable to occur with neostigmine-atropine combination must be watched for.

• ***Hypotension***: This usually responds to IV fluids. Antihistaminics are also useful to counter bronchospasm and peripheral vasodilatation produced by release of histamine.

• ***Miscellaneous***: There may be a regurgitation of gastric juice into the oesophagus due to paralysis of the oesophageal sphincter and the diaphragm.

Drugs which synergize with d-tubocurarine are general anaesthetics (ether, halothane, isoflurane and enflurane), aminoglycosides, trimethaphan, opioids, propranolol, glucocorticoids, digitalis, chloroquine, calcium channel blockers, quinidine, diuretics and catecholamines.

Preparations and dosage:

(i) Tubocurarine injection containing 3 mg. per ml. Dose : 6 to 10 mg. IV initially repeated as per requirements.

(ii) Dimethyltubocurarine iodide (Metubine iodide) is administered IV, the initial dose being 3 mg. followed by 1 mg. after 15 minutes, if required.

Table 21.3 : Competitive neuromuscular blocking agents

Long acting (60-120 minutes)	Doxacurium, Pancuronium, Pipecuronium and Vecuronium
Intermediate acting (20-50 minutes)	Atracurium, Rocuronium
Short acting (10-20 minutes)	Mivacurium, Ropacuronium

The other synthetic competitive neuromuscular blockers are classified in Table 21.3. Chemically, they are :

(a) **Benzylisoquinolones** e.g., Atracurium, Doxacurium, Mivacurium; and

(b) **Ammoniosteroids** e.g. Pancuronium, Vecuronium, Rocuronium.

They have similar properties but differ in their relative toxicities. Broadly, they differ from tubocurarine in that they

• ***Are more selective and do not block ganglionic transmission significantly;***

• ***Have fewer cardiovascular adverse effects;*** and

• ***Are less liable to release histamine;***

GALLAMINE (Flexedil): Gallamine has d-tubocurarine-like actions, and shares its adverse effects. It is now rarely used.

Table 21.4 summarises the properties of competitive neuromuscular blocking agents.

II Drugs acting by persistent depolarization

SUCCINYLCHOLINE (Scoline, Midarine) : Succinylcholine is a quaternary ammonium compound with a structure resembling two molecules of ACh joined together. It has a short duration of action.

Mechanism of action: The drug acts like a partial agonist of acetylcholine and produces skeletal muscle depolarization, by acting on the membrane channel. This can explain the fasciculations preceding skeletal muscle paralysis with this agent. However, in contrast to ACh, the drug is destroyed much more slowly, being susceptible only to plasma and liver pseudocholinesterase. This causes a **persistent depolarization** during which the muscle is insensitive to ACh released from nerve endings and remains paralysed.

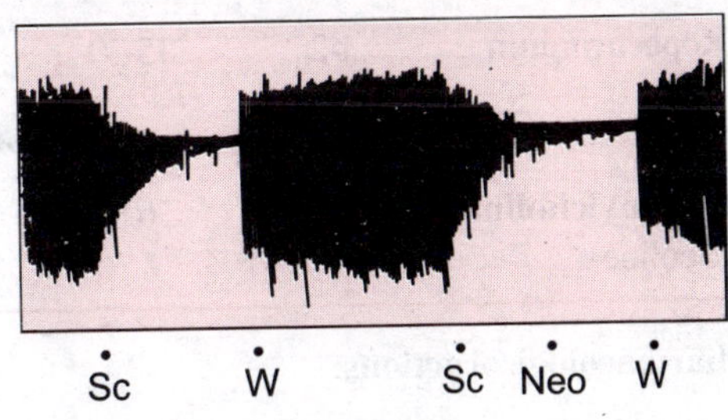

Fig 21.2: Blocking effect of succinylcholine (Sc) on electrically stimulated rat phrenic nerve diaphragm preparation. Note the worsening of the block following neostigmine (Neo) and recovery after wash (W).

Table 21.4: Neuromuscular blocking agents

Drug	Onset (min)	Duration (min)	Mode of elimination	Other actions
			Competitive	
d-Tubocurarine Tubarine	4-6	80-120	Renal and Hepatic clearance	Ganglionic blockade ++ Vagal blockade ++ Histamine release ++ (Hypotension and bronchospasm)
Pancuronium (Panconium) Zemuron	4-6	120-180	Renal	Ganglionic blockade + Vagal blockade ++ No histamine release (Slight tachycardia and increase in BP)
Vecuronium (Norcuron)	2-4	60-90	Hydrolysed in liver (to active metabolites).	No ganglionic blockade, vagal blockade or histamine release. (No tachycardia)
Rocuronium	1-2	30-40	Hepatic	Same as above
Doxacurium	4-6	90-120	Renal	No ganglionic or vagal blockade Histamine release + (Transient hypotension)
Atracurium (Tracurium)	2-4	30-40	Plasma ChE. (Spontaneous degradation).	Same as above Preferred in renal/liver impairment
Mivacurium Mivacron	2-4	12-18	Plasma ChE	Same as above.
Ropacuronium	1-2	15-30	Hepatic	
			Noncompetitive	
Succinylcholine (Scoline)	1-1.5	6-8	Plasma ChE	Ganglion stimulation Histamine release

Pharmacological actions:

● ***Skeletal muscle***: Paralysis of skeletal muscle produced by succinylcholine is preceded by transient muscular fasciculations and twitching, seen usually in the thoracic and abdominal regions. Succinylcholine relaxes the limb and neck muscles in a dose that does not significantly affect respiratory muscles. Transient apnoea is, however, usually observed with the peak effect of succinylcholine. The skeletal muscle paralysis by succinylcholine is enhanced by antiChE neostigmine which increases the local concentration of ACh.

Succinylcholine in a concentration and time dependent manner produces a dual block, initially a depolarizing block (phase 1) which later becomes non-depolarizing. The latter (phase 2), is antagonised by edrophonium. The mechanism of development of non-depolarizing blockade with large doses is not clear.

- ***Hyperkalemia:*** Prolonged depolarization may cause shift of intracellular potassium to the extracellular space. In patients with extensive soft tissue trauma or burns, as well as other condition which cause hyperkalemia, this can be life-threatening.
- ***Cardiovascular system*** : Repeated administration leads to stimulation of the vagal nuclei and sympathetic ganglia. The former produces bradycardia, cardiac arrhythmias, and hypotension. The latter causes persistent hypertension and tachycardia.
- ***Miscellaneous***: Succinylcholine is less liable to release histamine. Large doses may cause hypotension as a result of muscarinic effect and to some extent by ganglionic blockade. Because of its muscarinic action, atropine is generally given before its use.

Absorption, fate and excretion: Succinylcholine IV produces fasciculations which last for 10 to 15 seconds. Peak effect develops within 1 to 2 minutes and muscle power recovers within 5 minutes. The drug is hydrolyzed by plasma and liver pseudocholinesterase first to succinylmonocholine which has a weak competitive neuromuscular blocking effect and subsequently to succinic acid and choline. About 10 per cent of the dose is excreted unchanged in the urine. It crosses the placental barrier in insignificant amount and hence, can be used in obstetric cases.

Adverse reactions: Apart from allergic reactions, the other adverse reactions are :

- ***Cardiac arrest and arrhythmias***: High incidence of cardiac arrhythmias with the use of succinylcholine-halothane combination has been reported. The drug may occasionally produce cardiovascular collapse. Changes in K^+ distribution may cause serious arrhythmias in patients on diuretics and digitalis.
- ***Succinylcholine apnoea***: It is treated by artificial respiration and fresh blood transfusion. No antidote is available. Apnea needing respiratory support longer than 15 minutes is considered abnormal. Presence of a hereditary, abnormal plasma pseudo-cholinesterase, having a poor ability to hydrolyse succinylcholine, or acquired deficiency of normal pseudocholinesterase as in liver disease, predisposes to its development. Metabolic acidosis can also precipitate succinylcholine apnoea.
- ***Malignant hyperthermia***: The drug can rarely trigger serious malignant hyperthermic crisis in patients receiving ether or halothane.
- ***Miscellaneous***: Muscle soreness is a frequent complaint following succinylcholine. Increase in intraocular tension can also occur.
- ***Drug interactions*** : They are similar to those of d-tubocurarine. AntiChE inhibitor drugs, however, act synergistically with depolarising, blocking drugs.

Preparations and dosage: Succinylcholine chloride injection containing 50 mg. of the salt per ml. Dose : initially 1 mg. per kg. administered slowly IV, followed by 0.3 mg./kg. as needed.

Therapeutic uses of peripheral skeletal muscle relaxants:

- ***Adjuvant to anaesthesia***: The main use of skeletal muscle relaxants is to promote skeletal muscle relaxation during abdominal surgery, orthopaedic manipulations, and during various brief procedures like laryngoscopy, bronchoscopy and oesophagoscopy. When the procedure involved is of short duration, succinylcholine mivacurium or ropacuronium is obviously the drug of choice. The drug can also counter laryngeal spasm during barbiturate anaesthesia. For prolonged muscular relaxation, other newer competitive blockers are preferred.
- ***In electroconvulsive therapy***: Succinylcholine or mivacurium is often administered along with diazepam to protect the patient from injury during electroconvulsive therapy.
- ***In spastic disorders***: The curarimimetic skeletal muscle relaxants have been used to treat

the severe spasm of tetanus. This use, however, involves risk and needs expert supervision.

III BOTULINUM TOXIN TYPE A (Oculinum, Dysport) is produced by *Closrtidium botulinum.* It binds irreversibly to presynaptic, cholinergic sites and inhibits the release of ACh from the motor nerve terminals. *Local injection* of the toxin weakens the overactive muscle and decreases the hypersecretion of glands innervated by cholineregic neurons. It has been used to treat:

(1) Spastic conditions such as spasmodic torticolis, hemifacial spasm, strabismus, blepharospasm, dystonias, lower esophageal spasm and painful anal fissure; (2) Wrinkles on the face and neck; (3) Palmar hyperhidrosis. It appears to be safe and effective in these conditions. Its action lasts for 3-4 months.

Adverse reactions include ptosis, diplopia, reduced blinking leading to dry eyes, minor bruises and lid swelling; reversible muscle atrophy can occur after repeated administration.

Botulinum toxin Type B can be used in patients who have become resistant to Type A toxin.

Drugs Acting Directly on Skeletal Muscle

DANTROLENE (Dantrium): This phenytoin analogue relaxes the skeletal muscles by binding to the ryanodine (R_YR) channels on the sarcoplasmic reticulum, blocking their opening. This prevents the release of Ca^{++} from the sarcoplasmic stores. Thus, the muscle contraction is weakened without muscle paralysis. It does not alter the neuromuscular transmission. It has relatively little effect on cardiac and smooth muscle. Given orally, it is incompletely (about 1/3) absorbed and is largely metabolized in the liver. The adverse effects include generalised muscle weakness, dizziness, drowsiness, fatigue and diarrhoea. Rarely, it may cause serious hepatotoxicity. Dose: 25 mg/d, increased weekly to a maximum of 100 mg bid to qid.

Therapeutic uses:

- ***Spasticity*** : The drug is particularly useful for the treatment of spasticity (especially cerebral spasticity) in patients in whom nursing care is made difficult by muscle spasm. Patients in whom spastic, dystonic stiffness is useful as a sort of protective endogenous crutch should not be treated with dantrolene.
- ***Malignant hyperthermia***: Intravenous dantrolene (1 mg / kg, bolus, repeated if required to a maximum total dose of 100 mg) is life saving in this rare, fatal and familial disorder, triggered by any potent inhalation anaesthetic, depolarising muscle relaxant, curare-like neuromuscular blocking agent and even by stress. In susceptible individuals, these can cause excessive release of Ca^{++} from the sarcoplasmic reticulum, leading to hyperpyrexia (temperature more than 42°C), muscle rigidity, tachycardia and metabolic acidosis. It is a medical emergency.

It must be noted that management of the patient with spasticity implies more than just treatment of the spasticity. For many patients the increased tone is not harmful and may even be helpful. Active measures to reduce spasticity are only justified where the reflex hyperexcitability interferes with function, making rehabilitation, physiotherapy and nursing care difficult.

SECTION V
Other Biogenic Amines and Polypeptides

Histamine and Antihistaminic Drugs 22

HISTAMINE ('tissue amine'), a potent biogenic amine, was synthesized even before its isolation from plants and animals by Windaus and Vogt in 1907. The compound was isolated from ergot extracts by Barger and Dale in 1910 and reports regarding its pharmacological actions were published by Dale and Laidlaw in 1910-1911. The role of this extremely potent substance in the genesis of allergic and anaphylactic manifestations was forecast by the brilliant work of Lewis but even now, the exact biological functions of this compound have not been determined.

Distribution and synthesis: Histamine, an imidazole compound, is widely distributed in plant and animal tissues, and is also present in the venom of bees and wasps. In the mammals, it is formed by decarboxylation of the amino acid histidine, catalysed by an enzyme, **histidine decarboxylase**. Histamine is also synthesized by the microflora in the GI from dietary histidine. Very little, however, reaches the circulation as most of what is absorbed is rapidly metabolized in the intestinal wall and the liver. Almost all tissues in mammals synthesize histamine.

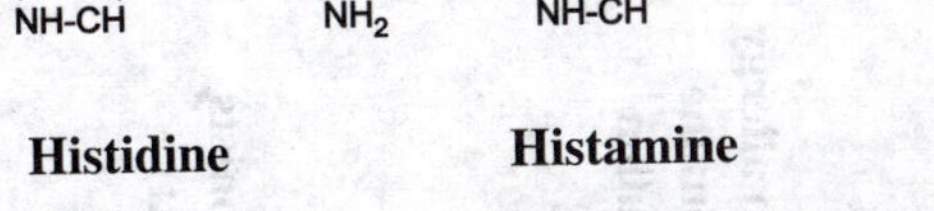

CH=N / C-CH$_2$-CH(COOH)(NH$_2$) / NH-CH → CH=N / C-CH$_2$-CH$_2$-NH$_2$ / NH-CH

Histidine **Histamine**

Fig 22.1: Biosynthesis of histamine

Histamine is present in various biological fluids, and in platelets, leucocytes, basophils and mast cells. A major portion of histamine is stored in mast cells and circulating basophils. These cells show the presence of histidine decarboxylase, and also contain specialized granules, wherein histamine is stored in a metabolically inactive form. In the mast cells of majority of animals, histamine is stored along with heparin, and in rodents, along with 5-HT. Animal lung is particularly rich in histamine, and rupture of mast cells releases free histamine into the circulation. Tissues devoid of mast cells, e.g., human epidermis, and gastric mucosa and CNS neurons also contain a significant concentration of histamine. Within the gut, the histamine concentration is highest in the stomach wall and it diminishes progressively upto the colon. In the CNS, the area postrema, the mast cells of the pituitary stalk and the hypothalamus contain significant amounts of histamine.

Mechanism of action: Four types of receptors, H_1, H_2, H_3 and H_4 have been identified and cloned. All these receptors belong to the family of GPCR (G protein coupled receptors). (Table 22.1).

- ***Activation of H_1 receptors*** causes pain, pruritus, bronchoconstriction, vasodilatation, increase in vascular permeability and in secretions. It is associated with increase in intracellular cyclic guanosine 3', 5' monophosphate (cGMP). In the tissues,

Table 22.1: Histamine receptors and their functions

Receptor	H_1	H_2	H_3	H_4
Distribution	Widespread in the neuronal system, smooth muscles endothelium and other cells	Widespread - gastric mucosa, smooth muscle heart, brain and mast cells	Mainly in the histaminergic neurons and myenteric plexus	Mainly bone marrow and eosinophils, neutrophils and CD4 T cells
General role	On stimulation : itching, pain, vasodilation, tachycardia, hypotension, increased permeability, bronchoconstriction, cough	Increased gastric acidity, vascular permeability (hypotension); and chronotropic, inotropic actions on heart; increased airway mucus production	Prevent excessive bronchoconstriction; mediate pruritus	Differentiation of myeloblasts and promyelocytes
Role in CNS	Control : sleep-awake cycle, food intake, temperature regulation, emotional behaviour, memory and learning	Neuroendocrine regulation	Presynaptic hetero-receptor; decrease histamine, NA, DA, 5-HT and ACh release	Not known
Role in allergy and immune modulation	Increased release of histamine and other mediators; promote chemotaxis of eosinophils and neutrophils; block humoral immunity and IgE production. Induction of cellular immunity	Decrease neutrophil and eosinophil chemotaxis; induce humoral immunity; suppress cellular immunity; induce IL-10 and suppress IL-12	Control neurogenic inflammation; pro-inflammatory activity	Increase eosinophil chemotaxis and IL-16 production
Antagonists (see text)	H_1 receptor blockers	H_2 receptor blockers	Under evaluation	Under evaluation

histamine serves as a chemotactic agent for neutrophils and eosinophils. *H_1 receptor effects are competitively blocked specifically by the conventional antihistaminic (H_1 receptor blockers).*

- ***Activation of H_2 receptors*** increases the gastric acid secretion and myocardial contractility. *These effects* are not blocked by the conventional antihistaminics but *are specifically blocked by H_2 receptor antagonists* such as cimetidine. **Impromidine** is a potent H_2 receptor agonist and behaves as *a competitive antagonist at the autoinhibitory receptors.*

Both H_1 and H_2 receptors appear to be involved in vascular dilatation, hypotension and edema formation.

- ***For H_3*** and ***H_4 receptors see Table 22.1.***

Pharmacological actions of histamine:

Cardiovascular system:

- ***Blood vessels*:** Although histamine may produce pulmonary and systemic vasoconstriction in certain herbivores like rabbits and guinea pigs, it causes marked vasodilatation in cats, dogs and human beings. In man, the pulmonary vessels are dilated by histamine, producing a fall in pulmonary artery pressure. The cerebral blood vessels are dilated in majority of the species. In man, it produces throbbing headache, palpable temporal pulsations, and a transient increase in the CSF pressure. The headache is attributed to stretching of sensory nerve endings around the cranial arteries. Histamine constricts large veins.

Histamine acts on the blood vessels in several ways:

(a) *Activation of H_1 receptors on the endothelial cells* causing rapid and short-lived vasodilatation.

(b) *Activation of H_2 receptors in the vascular smooth muscle* causing slower but more prolonged vasodilatation.

(c) *Direct relaxation of the smooth muscle of the capillaries and the venules* leading to their dilatation and fall in blood pressure.

In man, it causes marked flushing a sense of warmth; and marked *increase in capillary permeability after large doses* which causes edema and reduction in plasma volume.

- ***Blood pressure*:** Hypotension, induced by moderate doses of histamine is transient because of its rapid degradation and the presence of protective reflexes. Large doses, however, produce prolonged hypotension. The hypotension, if not corrected, may cause irreversible shock and death. Histamine-induced hypotension can be prevented but only partially reversed by antihistaminic agents. However, it can be reversed by adrenaline.

Triple response: When a pointed object is *drawn lightly* over the skin, the stroke line becomes blanched, i.e. white reaction, owing to contraction of the precapillary sphincters. It lasts for about 15 seconds.

When histamine (20 mcg) is injected ID or the skin is stroked firmly with the same pointed object in man, a triple response develops at the site. It comprises sequentially:

(a) **Flush** or red reaction which is a red line/spot developing within 10 seconds, owing to local dilatation of capillaries and venules; then

(b) **Wheal** which is local swelling due to edema, and mottled reddening around the injury, and lasts for about 1 ½ minute; it is due to increased permeability of capillaries and postcapillary venules, with consequent extravasation of fluid; and finally

(c) **Flare** in which the redness with irregular margins spreads out from the injury.

The triple response is a part of the normal reaction to injury. Its prevention is used to evaluate antihistaminic activity of a new drug.

- ***Heart* :** Histamine increases the sinus rate (*Positive chronotropic action*); increases the amplitude of ventricular contraction (*Positive inotropic action*); decreases A-V conduction time and increases coronary blood flow. High concentrations induce ventricular fibrillation.

Smooth muscle: Histamine stimulates the smooth muscle of various tissues directly (H_1 action). However, the individual tissue responses show a marked variation. *The bronchial and the uterine smooth muscle is* *highly sensitive to histamine.* Individuals suffering from bronchial asthma and certain other pulmonary diseases develop a sharp fall in vital capacity and considerable respiratory embarrassment in response to histamine. Histamine-induced bronchospasm is antagonised by adrenaline, isoprenaline and aminophylline but not by antihistaminics or atropine.

The GI and the ureteral smooth muscles respond moderately to histamine. Histamine, through H_1-receptors, causes gall bladder contraction while H_2-receptors mediate gall bladder relaxation.

Exocrine glands: Histamine is an important physiological mediator of gastric acid secretion. It acts by activating H_2 receptors (Chapter 42) in doses lower than those affecting the BP. It is blocked by the specific H_2 receptor antagonists.

Central nervous system: Histamine does not readily cross the BB barrier. The histamine receptors in the brain mediate the actions of locally synthesized, stored and released histamine. There are two types of histamine containing cells in the brain : histaminergic neurons and mast cells. Histamine is thought to be 'a waking amine' within the brain and is believed to act by "increasing the sensitivity of large cerebral areas to excitatory inputs". It acts through H_1 receptors which release intracellular Ca^{++}, and H_2 receptors which release intracellular cyclic AMP. Competitive blocking of H_1 receptors by the 'classical' antihistaminic drugs and of H_2 receptors by cimetidine leads to drowsiness as an adverse effect. Histamine also modulates the release of neurotransmitters via presynaptic H_3 receptors located on histaminergic and non-histaminergic neurons in the central and peripheral nervous systems.

Current evidence suggests a role of histamine as a neurotransmitter in the CNS.

Immunomodulation: All the four histamine receptors are involved in immunomodulation (Table 22.1).

Miscellaneous actions : Histamine, on intra-epidermal injection, evokes itching and pain. In large doses it produces release of adrenaline from the adrenal medulla.

Histamine has an effect on lymphocytes via H_2 receptors and it also inhibits the secretory activity of the mast cells and the basophils by a negative feedback via H_3 receptors.

Histamine facilitates pro-inflammatory activity through H_4 receptors. It also probably plays a part in embryonic development and wound healing.

Absorption, fate and excretion: Histamine is a very stable compound and is absorbed from all sites. However, only a small quantity of oral histamine reaches the circulation because of its first pass metabolism. Histamine metabolism varies according to the animal species, sex and the organ studied. In man, it is mainly converted into methylhistamine by an enzyme imidazole-n-methyltransferase and then further converted by MAO-B into l-methylimidazole acetic acid. In some species like rats, it is mainly metabolised by oxidative deamination by the enzyme diamine oxidase (histaminase) present in the liver, kidney and intestinal mucosa.

Adverse reactions: These are due to its pharmacological actions and include hypotension, flushing, headache, visual disturbances, diarrhoea and dyspnea due to bronchospasm. *Man and guinea pig are extremely sensitive to histamine while rats and mice are highly resistant.* Large quantities of histamine may be formed by bacteria in the small intestine acting on spoiled fish which may have high histidine content.Ingestion of such fish may lead to severe nausea, griping, headache and sweating. Similar reaction may be observed in susceptible subjects after consumption of red wine.

Uses : It was used to study gastric acid secretion.

BETAHISTINE HYDROCHLORIDE (Vertin): is a histamine substitute, claimed to reduce the frequency of episodes of vertigo in some patients with Meniere's syndrome. The drug causes vasodilatation and improves blood flow to the labyrinth and brainstem. The improvement is short lived. The compound may aggravate peptic ulcer and bronchial asthma.

Histamine liberators: Various agents can release tissue histamine and may thus cause histamine reactions. They are:

I Those which release histamine mainly from the mast cells with minimal tissue damage:

- ***Proteolytic enzymes*** like Trypsin, certain Venoms, Food products like crabs, lobsters and fish.
- ***Surface tension reducing substances*** like Bile salts, Anionic and Cationic surfactants.
- ***Substances with a high molecular weight*** like Dextran, and Polyvinyl pyrrollidone.
- ***Drugs***, particularly organic bases such as quaternary ammonium compounds, d-Tubocurarine, Morphine, Pethidine, Amphetamine, Hydralazine, Tolazoline, basic poly-peptides (Polymyxin B) and a few Antihistaminic drugs; and
- ***The polybasic compound 48/40 and the compound 19/35L***, the most potent histamine liberators, used in animal experiments.

II Those which release histamine accompanied by substantial tissue damage:

- ***Trauma*** due to cold and chemical, thermal or radiant energy.
- ***Antigen-antibody reactions*** (Chapter 2).

Histamine, Anaphylaxis and Allergy

The term **anaphylaxis** is used clinically to describe a medical emergency caused by allergy to a variety of agents such as drugs, foods, plants, chemicals, latex and insect/reptile bites. It is mediated by IgE (Chapter 2), and histamine is the most important of the many mediators involved in it. The clinical features in man are due to laryngeal edema, bronchospasm and hypotension (*anaphylactic shock*). An anaphylactic reaction may progress either slowly or rapidly, the latter especially after parenteral drug administration.

The term **anaphylactoid** is used for a similar condition, not IgE induced, commonly caused by hyperosmotic IV solutions of iodine containing contrast dyes. It is, however, safer to assume that all such reactions are immune mediated, and avoid future exposure to the same agent.

Treatment of anaphylactic shock:

Anaphylactic shock needs immediate treatment of : laryngeal edema, bronchospasm and hypotension.

- ***Lay the patient flat and raise his legs.***
- ***When possible, apply a tourniquet to obstruct the draining blood flow from the site of deposition of the antigen or inciting medication.***
- ***Attend to the airway.***
- ***Administer adrenaline***: Adrenaline, 1:1000 solution *IM*, produces a dramatic reversal of the hypotension, bronchospasm and laryngeal edema and is life-saving. It may be repeated cautiously after 15 to 20 minutes, if necessary. When the patient is severely ill and there is doubt about the adequacy of circulation and absorption from the IM site, adrenaline (**1:10,000, never 1:1,000, solution**) may be injected IV, slowly, in the dose of 500 mcg, at the rate of 100 mcg per minute. (Table 22.2).

Rapid IV injection of adrenaline or IV injection of the 1:1000 solution can induce lethal cardiac arrhythmias.

Table 22.2: Adrenaline doses in anaphylaxis

- ***Adults***: 0.5 ml. of a 1:1000 solution IM. or 3-5 ml. of a 1:10000 solution IM or slowly IV.
- ***Children***: 0.01 ml. of a 1:1000 solution per kg. IM or 0.1 ml. a 1.10000 solution per kg slowly IV.

In patients on a non-selective beta blocker, severe anaphylaxis may not respond to adrenaline and may need additional IV salbutamol.

• ***IV fluids***: Hypotension associated with anaphylactic shock should be corrected by immediate IV administration of large quantities of fluids (preferably colloids). If necessary, dopamine or norepinephrine can be infused IV. Cimetidine has been used in refractory cases.

• ***Glucocorticoids***: Glucocorticoids are routinely administered in the treatment of anaphylactic shock, as *they inhibit the late phase of an allergic reaction* (Chapter 26). Hydrocortisone hemisuccinate 100 mg. is given IV, followed by oral prednisolone. They do not inhibit the early phase of the anaphylactic reactions and *are not a substitute for adrenaline which is the drug of first choice.*

• ***Antihistaminic drugs***: *The antihistaminic drugs do not counter the hypotension and bronchospasm characteristic of anaphylactic shock.* This is due to involvement of mediators other than histamine in the genesis of anaphylaxis or to release of histamine in intimate contact with cells not accessible to conventional antihistaminics. However, an antihistaminic such as chlorpheniramine, 10-20 mg over one minute by slow IV injection, and repeated for upto 24-48 hours, may prevent late manifestations of allergy. *It must be given after adrenalilne.*

Injection of an H_2 receptor antagonist such as cimetidine 500 mg or ranitidine 50 mg, IV over 3-5 min may be helpful.

• ***Bronchodilators***: IV Aminophylline or nebulised salbutamol may be needed in patients with resistant bronchospasm.

• ***Supportive measures***: These include oxygen and assisted ventilation.

The methods of countering the actions of histamine in the body are listed in Table 22.3

Table 22.3: Methods of countering the actions of histamine

- Preventing antigen-antibody reaction that triggers histamine release.
- Using adrenaline which has actions opposite to those of histamine and thus acts as a *physiological antagonist.*
- Hastening the destruction of histamine by using histaminase, which is, however, clinically not effective; and
- Employing drugs that block the actions of histamine on various receptors : *H_1 receptor antagonists and H_2 receptor antagonists.*

H_1-Receptor Antagonists

In 1933, Fourneau and Bovet showed that certain phenolic ethers possessed antihistamine properties. Since then, many *specific, competitive H_1 receptor antagonists* with different chemical structures have been synthesized; *the term antihistaminics, unless qualified, refers to these agents.* In addition to their antihistaminic activity, many of them also have CNS and ANS actions.

H_1 receptor antihistaminic agents can be classified either clinically or chemically.

Clinical classification: (Table 22.4)

I **Potent and sedative**

II **Potent but less sedative**

III **Less potent and less sedative**

IV **Non-sedative** They do not cross the blood brain barrier in significant amounts.

Chemical classification: Most of the antihistaminic agents can be represented by the general formula:

$$(R_1)(R_2)X-C(H)(H)-C(H)(H)-N(R_3)(R_4)$$

Fig. 22.2 : General structure of antihistaminics

Depending upon the configuration of X, the anti-histaminic agents can be classified as :

I **Ethanolamines** where X = O, e.g. Diphenhydramine and Doxylamine.

II **Ethylenediamines** where X = N, e.g.,

Table 22.4: H_1 Receptor blocking antihistaminic agents

Drug	Adult oral dose	Remarks
	Potent and sedative $	
Diphenhydramine HC1 * (Benadryl)	25 to 50 mg. (parenteral 10 mg.)	Moderate antispasmodic, antimuscarinic.
Dimenhydrinate (Dramamine)*	25 to 100 mg.	Mainly used for motion sickness.
Promethazine HC1 * (Phenergan)	12.5 to 25 mg.	Marked antimuscarinic action.
Promethazine chloro- ** **theophyllinate** (Avomine)	25 to 75 mg.	Marked antimuscarinic action; used mainly in motion sickness. Superiority over promethazine doubtful
Pheniramine maleate (Avil) **	25 to 75 mg.	Antimuscarinic
Trimeprazine (Vallergan) **	5 to10 mg.	Mainly anti-pruritic.
	Potent and less sedative $	
Chlorpheniramine maleate * (Zeet)	4 to 20 mg. (parenteral 5 to 20 mg.)	
Triprolidine (Actidil) **	2.5 to 5.0 mg.	
Cyclizine HCl (Marzine) *	50 mg.	Used in motion sickness.
Meclizine HCl ** (Ancolan)	25 to 50 mg.	Mainly used for motion sickness.
Buclizine (Longifene)	25 to 75 mg.	Antiemetic
Methdilazine (Dilosyn)	6 to 16 mg.	Anti-pruritic
	Less potent and less sedative $	
Mepyramine maleate: * (Pyrilamine, Anthisan)	50 to 100 mg. (parenteral 25 to 50 mg.)	
Antazoline HC1 (Antistine)	50 to 100 mg.	Moderately active; antiarrhythmic
Cinnarizine (Stugeron) *	25 mg	Anti-vertigo; EP reactions
Flunarizine	5-10 mg	Anti-vertigo; EP reactions
	Non-sedative (Second generation)	
Loratadine (Alaspan) **	10 mg once daily	Less antimuscarinic and relatively free from cardiac toxicity.
Desloratadine (Deslor)	5 mg. once daily	
Fexofenadine (Allegra) **	120 mg once daily	
Acrivastine (Semprax) *	8 mg tid	
Cetirizine (Cetzine) **	5-10 mg once daily	May cause some sedation

$ First generation or classical * Short acting; ** Long acting.

Tripelennamine, Mepyramine and Antazoline. They have negligible anticholinergic and antiemetic effects.

III **Alkylamines** where X = C, e.g. Chlorpheniramine, Triprolidine, Acrivastine.

IV **Piperazines** where X = carbon in conjunction with a piperazine ring, e.g., Hydroxyzine, Buclizine, Meclizine, Cinnarizine, Cetirizine.

V **Phenothiazines** where X = nitrogen as a part of phenothiazine nucleus, e.g., Promethazine, Trimeprazine. They have potent antiemetic effect.

VI **Piperidines:** Cyproheptadine, Loratadine, Fexofenadine and Ketotifen.

VII **Dibenzoxepines :** Doxepine, an antidepressant, with potent antihistaminic properties.

Pharmacological actions of H_1 receptor antagonists:

- ***Antihistaminic actions*:** The antihistaminics competitively block histamine actions at many sites. Thus, they antagonize the stimulant action of histamine on the smooth muscle of the GI tract, the bronchi, the uterus and the blood vessels and inhibit histamine augmented salivary secretion. They also reduce histamine-induced triple response and itching, but fail to produce resorption of the edema fluid. Antihistaminics prevent the itching, edema, urticaria and increased gastric motility and to a lesser extent, the hypotension produced by the histamine releasing drugs.

Antiallergic and anti-inflammatory actions involve (a) inhibition of the release of mediators from mast cells and basophils and (b) downregulation of H_1 receptors.

Pretreatment with an oral H_1 antihistamic reduces the early response to an allergen challenge in the conjunctiva, nose, lower airways and skin. However, *as described above, the bronchospasm and hypotension during anaphylaxis are not adequately reversed by them.* This is probably because of the other mediators released during the reaction. These agents do not antagonize the cardiovascular actions of histamine.

Other actions: These actions are independent and are related to their blocking of 5-HT as well as $alpha_1$ adrenergic receptors. They are:

- ***Sedation and hypnosis* :** CNS depression is a common side effect with the classical antihistaminics. They induce varying degrees of sedation, drowsiness and sleep. Sedation is sometimes beneficial, particularly in the treatment of allergic reactions. Drugs like promethazine and diphenhydramine are potent sedative-hypnotics. Sedation is often accompanied by inability to concentrate, dizziness and disturbances of co-ordination, and thus may interfere with daily work. Sedation is negligible with fexofenadine and desloratidine.
- ***CNS stimulation*:** Stimulation is less commonly encountered than depression. Conventional doses of a few drugs such as promethazine may occasionally produce restlessness, tremors and insomnia.
- ***Autonomic nervous system*:** Majority of the **first generation** antihistaminics exhibit muscarinic blocking activity. Dryness of mouth is a common side effect. Antihistaminics, such as antazoline and phenindamine, exert an alpha adrenergic blocking effect. The **second generation** antihistaminics usually do not have these actions.
- ***Antiemetic and anti-motion sickness effects*:** Motion sickness, attributed commonly to vestibular disturbances, is benefited to a considerable extent by diphenhydramine, dimenhydrinate, promethazine and the piperazine antihistaminics. They block the histaminergic signals from the vestibular nucleus to the vomiting centre. Vomiting due to other labyrinthine disturbances, such as labyrinthitis and fenestration operation also responds to antihistaminics. These agents, except the phenothiazine antihistaminics, however, are of limited value in treating emesis due to jaundice, radiation, and alkylating agents (Chapter 40).
- ***Antiparkinsonian effect*:** Central antimuscarinic actions of some antihistaminics are useful in treating parkinsonism. (Chapter 14).

● ***Cardiovascular system***: Although therapeutic doses of antihistaminics fail to affect the cardiovascular system, rapid IV administration of diphenhydramine, antazoline, methapyrilene, and tripelennamine may produce dose related prolongation of QT interval due to their membrane stabilizing action, independently of their antihistaminic property.

● ***Local anaesthesia***: Antihistaminics such as promethazine and diphenhydramine exhibit some local anaesthetic activity.

Absorption, fate and excretion: They are absorbed well orally and parenterally; the antihistaminic effect starts within 15 to 30 minutes, peaks by 1 hour and lasts for 3 to 6 hours. *The actions of meclizine, however, persist for 12 to 24 hours.* All first generation compounds are mainly metabolized in the liver by CYP3A4, and the products are eliminated in urine. H_1 receptor antagonists can induce hepatic microsomal enzymes, facilitating their own metabolism.

Adverse reactions:They are as a rule mild and can be grouped as follows:

● ***CNS*** : The first generation antihistaminics commonly cause sedation, hypnosis and fatigue. Individuals taking antihistaminics should not drive vehicles because of drowsiness and impaired motor coordination. EP reactions (Table 22.4), excitement and delirium may occur rarely. In children less than 2 years, promethazine may cause apnoea.

● ***Antimuscarinic effects:*** The commonest effects are dry mouth, blurring of vision, bladder disturbances and rarely impotence, seen with first generation drugs.

● ***GI:*** Nausea,vomiting, and epigastric distress may occur occasionally.

● ***Miscellaneous:*** The antihistminics, in spite of their antiallergic properties,may themselves produce allergic manifestations.

Acute, first generation antihistaminic poisoning is characterised by marked central stimulation. In children the clinical picture often resembles that of atropine intoxication, while in adults, fever and flushing are uncommon, and drowsiness often precedes the development of delirium and convulsion. Blood pressure and respiration are usually well maintained. Death is due to central depression leading to cardiorespiratory collapse and coma. The treatment is symptomatic and supportive. Diazepam can control convulsions.

Preparations and dosage: The number of antihistaminic drugs available in the market far exceeds their utility. The commonly available antihistaminics are detailed in Table 22.4.

Therapeutic Uses:

● ***Allergic disorders***: The antihistaminics are beneficial in the suppression of allergic manifestations like polinosis and urticaria. They are extremely effective in the treatment of seasonal hay fever, where they reduce the sneezing, rhinorrhoea, and other manifestations associated with this condition. Their efficacy in the treatment of perennial vasomotor rhinitis, however, is much less.

Antihistaminics effectively counter the pruritus and urticaria in atopic and contact dermatitis and that induced by various drugs, chemicals and vegetables. They partially control the pruritus of eczema. Combination of a phenothiazine such as chlorpromazine with an antihistaminic may give better results in severe pruritus than the antihistaminic alone. Systemic administration also controls, to some extent, the pain and the itch due to bee or wasp stings. The antipruritic action of the antihistaminics is probably nonspecific. Their topical use is not recommended owing to the risk of sensitization and a marked tendency to cause eczema.

Adequate treatment of **pruritus** (Chapter 69) depends upon recognition of the local and/or systemic factor(s) responsible for it. For example, adequate treatment of scabies would generally relieve the itching in this condition; the itching in elderly patients, which is due to dryness of the skin, is best treated by moisturising the skin by applying a little edible oil to the affected area immediately after bath and by minimising the use of soap for washing and bathing. Itching due to inflammatory skin conditions can be relieved by a combination of a weak corticosteroid applied locally and a systemically administered antihistaminic. *Antihistaminics, however, are ineffective in itching of clinically normal skin.*

Reaginic allergy (Chapter 2) is known to be familial. A period of relative immunodeficiency may precede frank development of allergic illness in genetically predisposed children. Infants of allergic parents kept on "allergen avoidance regimen" (avoidance of exposure to cow's milk, dairy products, eggs, house dust and pets) for first six months of life may have strikingly low incidence of eczema.

Antihistaminics are of some value in controlling *mild blood transfusion reactions* but not pyrexia or hemolysis (Chapter 32). Weak atropine like activity of the classical antihistaminics and the occasional superimposition of acute cold on chronic allergic rhinitis may account for the beneficial effects of antihistaminic drugs on rhinorrhoea in a few cases of common cold (Chapter 26).

Allergic conjunctivitis is a common condition and causes itching. Local treatment with H_1 receptor antagonists (**emedastine** 0.05%, **levocabastine** (0.05%), mast cell stabilizers (**cromolyn sodium** 4%, **nedocromil sodium** 2%; Chapter 26) and drugs having both actions (**ketotifen** 0.025%; Chapter 26) can give symptomatic relief. Their use is safe. The adverse reactions are mild and include ocular irritation, burning and stinging; headache may occur. Routine long term use of local glucocorticoids (Chapter 64) is not justified for fear of causing cataract and raised intraocular pressure.

Antihistaminics are effective in the treatment of **urticaria** and **angioedema.** Urticaria may occur as acute episodes but is considered chronic when it lasts longer than six weeks. It may occur in a person with atopic history (Chapter 26) but often such history is absent. In a few cases, an *allergen* (fish, seafood, nuts, eggs; food additives such as citric acid, preservatives and colouring agents like tartrazine; drugs such as aspirin and other NSAID; vegetable gums), an *offending physical agent* (mechanical trauma, cold, heat), history of insect bites and stings, or *underlying disease* (infection, connective tissue disorder) may be identified. However, no such factor is found in majority of cases. A thorough history and a physical examination must precede laboratory tests. If a causative agent can be identified, it must be avoided if it is an external factor and treated if it is a systemic disease. But, a witch-hunt for a 'septic focus' is unrewarding.

The treatment of choice for acute urticaria (and acute angioedema) is a SC injection of adrenaline (1 : 1000 aqueous solution) in the dose of 0.3 ml, repeated if necessary. If adrenaline is contraindicated, an antihistaminics (50 mg. of diphenhydramine IM or IV) may be used.

Oral antihistaminics are the drugs of choice in chronic urticarias; they are more effective when given, prophylactically on a regular basis, than after urticarial lesions start. The newer, non-sedative antihistaminics may be preferred. Alternatives to the antihistaminics are cyproheptadine, doxepin (an antidepressant with a potent antihistaminic action) or a beta adrenergic agonist such as ephedrine. In resistant cases, an H_2 blocker such as cimetidine or ranitidine may be added to the H_1 blocker. Very few patients need corticosteroids and then, these should be used for the shortest possible period.

Topical application of calamine lotion is useful for its cooling and soothing effects and can be used alone in mild cases.

- ***Mastocytosis*:** This rare disease is characterised by an abnormal increase in mast cells in the body leading to an increase in the production of mast cell mediators mainly histamine. This gives rise to symptoms such as pruritus, diarrhoea and anaphylaxis. Partial symptomatic relief can be obtained by a combination of H_1 and H_2 receptor antagonists.
- ***Other uses:***

(i) **As hypnotics** e.g., Diphenhydramine and Promethazine.

(ii) **As antiemetics,** e.g. Dimenhydrinate and Meclizine. (Chapter 47)

(iii) **In parkinsonism** e.g. Diphenhydramine and Promethazine (Chapter 14).

(iv) **In motion sickness and vertigo** (Chapter 40).

(v) **As antitussives** e.g. Diphenhydramine.

(vi) **In drug-induced acute dystonias** Diphenhydramine, Promethazine (Chapter 14).

(vii) **As local anaesthetics** (see earlier).

Drug interactions: Sedation is enhanced when the sedative antihistaminics are used concurrently with alcohol, barbiturates, benzodiazepines or tricyclic antidepressants.

Nonsedative H_1 antihistaminics (second generation) : Most of the classical H_1 receptor blocking drugs (antihistaminics) are highly lipid soluble and have marked CNS adverse effects. They also have anticholinergic, antiserotoninergic and anti-bradykinin effects.

A **second generation** of H_1 receptor competitive blockers, which poorly cross the BBB, is now available. They are :

- ***The highly specific H_1 receptor antagonists.***
- ***Non-sedating in therapeutic doses.***
- ***Devoid of antimuscarinic, anti-serotonergic and antibradykinin action***;
- ***Relatively free from cardiac toxicity;*** and
- ***More expensive.***

Cetirizine is largely excreted as such in the urine; fexofenadine is primarily excreted in the feces. Fexofenadine is an active metabolite of terfenadine whereas cetirizine is an active metabolite of hydroxyzine.

Preparations and dosage: See Table 22.4.

Adverse reactions : Astemizole and terfenadine cause prolongation of QT interval and may cause potentially lethal ventricular arrhythmias. Their toxicity is enhanced by CYP3A4 inhibitors such as erythromycin and ketoconazole; they are no more used. Fexofenadine and desloratadine are relatively safer. Clinically relevant drug interactions are less common with these drugs.

Therapeutic uses:

- ***Allergic rhinitis but not vasomotor rhinitis*** (Chapter 26).
- ***Urticaria;*** and
- ***Dermographia.***

In practice, the choice of an antihistaminic drug depends upon efficacy, onset and duration of action, and adverse effects. These vary among different preparations, and among individuals. Sedative-hypnotic property may sometimes be beneficial. None of the preparations available is ideal for all conditions in all the patients.

H_2 Receptor Antagonists

H_2 receptors are responsible for histamine induced gastric acid secretion. (Table 22.1). They block positive chronotropic action of histamine, counter the enhanced automaticity of atria and ventricles, and prevent ventricular tachyarrhythmias induced by histamine. These agents are useful in the treatment of peptic ulcer (see Chapter 42).

H_3 and H_4 Receptors

H_3 receptors are thought to be presynaptic heteroreceptors that exert a tonic autoinhibitory control on histamine synthesis and release within the brain. **Betahistine,** a weak, partial agonist at H_1 and H_2 receptors, behaves as a weak H_3 receptor antagonist.

H_4 receptors : See Table 22.1.

5-Hydroxytryptamine (Serotonin), its Agonists and Antagonists; and Treatment of Migraine

23

5-HYDROXYTRYPTAMINE (5-HT), also termed **serotonin**, was isolated in 1948. The same compound, studied earlier independently, termed enteramine by Erspamer and co-workers, was found to have a wide tissue distribution and a variety of pharmacological actions.

Fig 23.1 : 5-Hydroxytryptamine

Distribution and synthesis : 5-HT is widely distributed in plants and in animal tissues, mast cells and platelets. In the mammalian tissues, the highest concentration (60 to 180 micrograms per g.) is present in the pineal gland, where it serves as a precursor for the synthesis of the hormone melatonin. It is also present in the venoms of wasps, bees and scorpions. Fruits like pineapples, bananas, tomatoes, plums and various nuts contain considerable amounts of 5-HT. However, it largely undergoes metabolic degradation on entering the circulation.

The compound is synthesized from the essential amino acid tryptophan (Fig. 23.2). The enzyme L-aromatic amino acid decarboxylase enzyme also decarboxylates histidine and DOPA. Within the CNS and the GI tract, 5-HT is stored in the chromaffin granules.

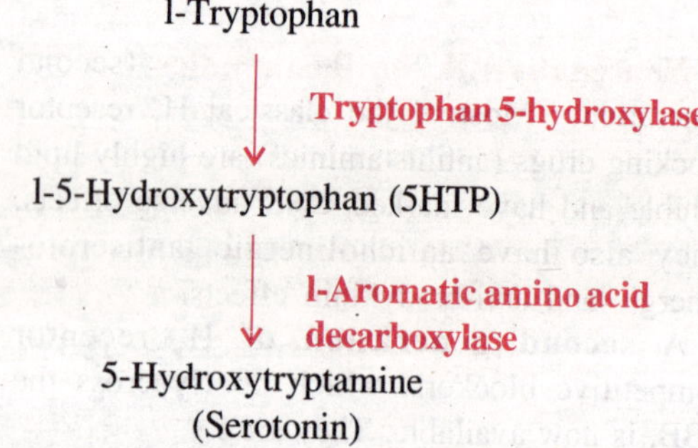

Fig 23.2: Synthesis of 5-hydroxytryptamine (5-HT)

5-HT receptors : Currently, four 5-HT receptor groups with **defined functions** have been identified: 5-HT_1, 5-HT_2, 5-HT_3 and 5-HT_4, with further subdivision into several subtypes. The 5-HT_1, 5-HT_2 and 5-HT_4 receptors belong to G-protein-coupled receptor (GPCR) families, while 5-HT_3 is a ligand-operated ion channel receptor.

The **5-HT_1 receptor** has six subtypes. Of these, 5-HT_{1A} is found in the raphe cell bodies and dendrites, and 5-HT_{1D} on the axon terminals (presynaptic). They function as autoreceptors and regulate 5-HT release. 5-HT_{1D} is also found in the substantia nigra and basal ganglia.

The **5-HT_2 receptor** has three subtypes. Of these, 5-HT_{2A} receptors are found in the frontal cortex, clustrum, GI tract and platelets.

The **5-HT_3 receptor** is a monoamine neurotransmitter receptor, located at the

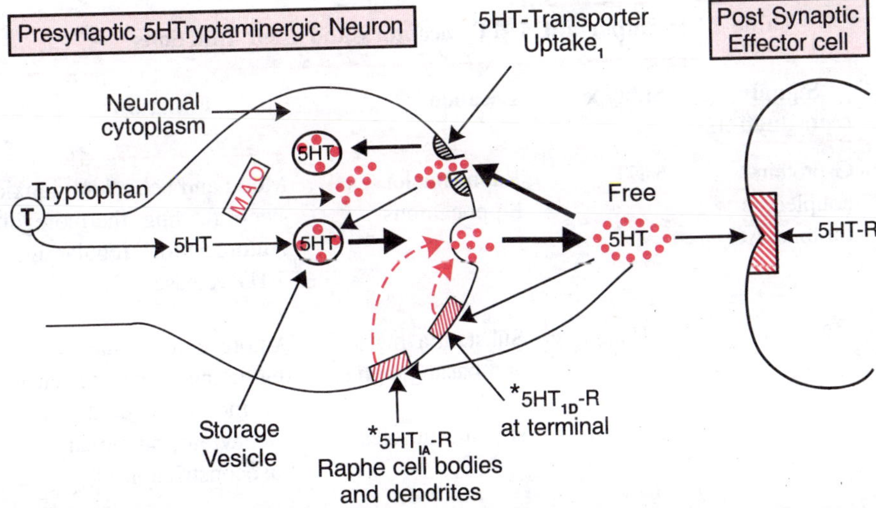

Fig. 23.3: Synthesis and metabolism of 5-HT at serotonergic neuronal endings

cholinergic terminals in the GI tract,nucleus solitarius and in the area postrema.Both the CNS and GI tract 5-HT_3 receptors participate in the process of vomiting.

The **5-HT_4 receptors** are widely distributed throughout the body, including the CNS, smooth muscles and secretory cells.Their stimulation causes increased secretion in the GI tract and facilitates the peristaltic process.

Although 5-HT_5, 5-HT_6 and 5-HT_7 receptors have been described, their exact function is not known.

The handling of 5-HT at the receptor level is similar to that of noradrenaline.Large amount of 5-HT released from the neuronal endings is retaken up (Uptake 1) and stored in the granules by the neurons (Fig. 23.3). It is metabolized by the enzyme MAO. The metabolite 5-Hydroxy-indole-acetic-acid (5-HIAA) is actively transported out of the brain by a process which can be blocked by probenecid.

Functions of various 5-HT receptors are summarised in Table 23.1.

Significance of 5-HT: The currently available information on this subject has not yet been synthesized into a unitary hypothesis. However, 5-HT does play a major role in the regulation of GI motility, acts as a central neurotransmitter and as a local hormone in the peripheral vascular system.

- ***Neurohumoral transmission*:** 5-HT is present in the nervous system of all the vertebrates and many invertebrates. Considerable evidence indicates that 5-HT is indeed a chemical transmitter released by 'tryptaminergic' neurons widely distributed in the brain. One of the important functions attributed to the tryptaminergic dorsal raphe neurons is dampening of over-reactiveness to various stimuli, and 5-HT is involved in some way in regulation of the state of consciousness. Altered tryptaminergic function may be responsible for disturbances in sleep, appetite, mood, sexual behaviour, motor activity and perception and for migraine. These neurons are also involved in other functions such as temperature regulation, endocrine control and extra-pyramidal activity. 5-HT receptors have been identified in brain areas implicated in learning and memory. Many centrally acting drugs are known to influence responses to 5-HT or alter its reuptake, synthesis, storage, release or catabolism. Prominent among these are anti-

Table 23.1: Important 5-HT receptors and their functions

Receptor	Signal transduction	Subtype	Location	Functions
5-HT_1	G-protein coupled. Inhibits AC	5-HT_{1A}	Raphe nuclei, hippocampus,	Mood and behaviour : anxiety sleep, feeding, thermoregulation. Autoreceptor regulating 5-HT release
		5-HT_{1B}	Substantia nigra and basal ganglia; vascular smooth muscles	Autoreceptors (may be regulating dopamine release); locomotor function. Behaviour; pulmonary vasoconstriction
		5-HT_{1D}	CNS; cerebral vessels	Cerebral vasoconstriction: migraine
5-HT_2	G-protein coupled. Activates PLC	5-HT_{2A}	Frontal cortex, clustrum, platelets, smooth muscles, autonomic neurons	Neural excitation; behavioral effects (of LSD); platelet aggregation; smooth muscle contraction (GI tract, bronchi, bladder)
		5-HT_{2B}	Gastric fundus	Contraction
		5-HT_{2C}	Choroid plexus	CSF secretion
5-HT_3	Ligand operated ion channels		Cholinergic terminals of GI tract; tractus solitarius; area postrema; hippocampus	Emesis Behaviour: anxiety Neuronal excitation (autonomic, nocioceptive neurons)
5-HT_4	G-protein coupled. Activates AC		Hippocampus; Myenteric neurons. smooth muscles of esophagus, secretory cells	Neuronal excitation; contraction of muscle; stimulation of secretion

AC = Adenylyl cyclase PLC = Phospholipase C

psychotic drugs like chlorpromazine, reserpine, antidepressants, hallucinogens like LSD, mescaline and even analgesics like morphine.

- ***Sleep***: 5-HT controls sleep-wakefulness cycle; depletion of 5-HT causes insomnia, which can be reversed by 5-hydroxytryptophan.

• ***Behaviour***: Disturbances in the brain 5-HT metabolism are suspected as a cause of certain psychiatric disorders such as schizophrenia and affective disorders. 5-HT_3 receptors present in brain in limbic and cortical areas are known to be involved in controlling mood, emotion, reward and memory. 5-HT_3 receptor antagonists reduce the increased psychomotor drive associated with a mesolimbic dopamine excess. Low CSF 5-HIAA is associated with impulsive,violent and suicidal behaviour, and 5-HT reuptake inhibitors are now used to treat mental depression (Chapter 13). 5-HT receptor function is altered in anorexia nervosa and bulimia, the major eating disorders.

• ***Anti-emesis and migraine***: Antiemetic activity has generally been associated with dopamine antagonist drugs such as metoclopramide but studies in animals indicate that selective 5-HT_3 receptor antagonists can prevent emesis associated with anti-cancer drugs and radiotherapy. 5-HT_3 receptors are present in high densities on afferent vagus nerves and in the area postrema and dorsal vagal complex of animals.

Role of 5-HT in migraine has been suspected for a long time. 5-HT metabolism is abnormal in patients with migraine and IV administration of 5-HT can alleviate migraine attacks. It is not clear if the relevant 5-HT receptors are vascular or neural in location. However, sumatriptan, a 5-HT_{1D} agonist, is used to treat acute attacks of migraine. (see later).

• ***Gastrointestinal tract***: Entero-chromaffin cells in the GI tract synthesize 5-HT which forms the major source of circulating 5-HT. A part of it is metabolized by the hepatic MAO during its first pass through the liver. 5-HT released by mechanical or vagal stimulation from the neuronal endings acts locally to regulate the GI motility. Because of the high concentration of 5-HT and 5-HTP in the GI, 5-HT is believed to act as a local hormone for the initiation and sustenance of intestinal peristalsis.

• ***Cardiovascular system:*** 5-HTconstricts the renal, pulmonary, splanchnic and cerebral blood vessels.It also has some positive inotropic and chronotropic action on the heart.

• ***Platelets:*** Platelets do not synthesize 5-HT but take it up from the circulation and store it. Following vascular injury, release of 5-HT occurs. It, along with other mediators of injury, activates platelets, which then promote vascular occlusion and vasoconstriction.

• ***Hormone secretion***: There is some evidence to suggest that tryptaminergic mechanisms are involved in the control of release of certain hormones. Sex hormones may affect mood and the mental state by activating the central 5-HT receptors.

• ***Carcinoid syndrome***: This clinical syndrome is associated with argentaffin cell tumours of the GI tract which secrete 5-HT. These tumours are locally invasive and may occasionally metastasize. Carcinoid syndrome is characterised by intermittent attacks of flushing, hypotension, bronchospasm, colic and diarrhoea. A picture of tricuspid incompetence and pulmonary stenosis is occasionally observed. Some of these manifestations are due to excessive production of 5-HT. The diagnosis is usually confirmed by demonstrating high plasma 5-HT and high urinary HIAA levels. It should be noted that a moderate increase in urinary HIAA levels can occur in patients with malabsorption states such as sprue and the blind loop syndrome. The drug parachlorophenylalanine (PCPA, Fenclonin) inhibits 5-HT synthesis by inhibiting tryptophan hydroxylase. PCPA in a daily dose of 2 g. results in almost complete inhibition of this enzyme leading to stoppage of diarrhoea, cramps and decrease in 5-HIAA excretion in urine. However, flushing is not much affected. The toxicity of PCPA includes allergic reactions, tinnitus, fatigue, dizziness and mental changes. Marked hypothermia following PCPA administration in man has been reported. Some benefit may also be observed by using other agents such as cyproheptadine and methysergide.

It appears that 5-HT is a mediator of acute inflammation only in rats and mice. The human skin, however, does not contain significant amounts of 5-HT and the 5-HT antagonists are not effective in controlling inflammation in human skin.

Pharmacological actions:

Cardiovascular system:

• ***Peripheral blood vessels***: 5-HT is a constrictor of majority of blood vessels including the renal, splanchnic, meningeal and pulmonary arteries. In several species, the cerebral blood vessels are constricted powerfully. It also narrows the veins and venules, but dilates the blood vessels of skeletal muscles, the coronaries and the capillaries of the skin. Administration of 5-HT in humans results in cutaneous vasodilatation, producing initially a bright red flush, that may be converted to cyanosis, probably owing to peripheral pooling of blood.

• ***Heart***: 5-HT has weak direct positive inotropic and chronotropic effects on the myocardium; these, however, are usually not demonstrable in human beings, as it also causes reflex bradycardia.

• ***Blood pressure***: A characteristic 'triphasic response' is observed after IV injection of 5-HT in majority of the species including man. It consists of:

(a) ***Initial transient depression*** attributed to increased vagal activity following stimulation of coronary and carotid chemoreceptors;

(b) ***Immediate rise in blood pressure***, due to peripheral vasoconstriction; and finally

(c) ***Sustained hypotension*** which is due to dilatation of skeletal muscle blood vessels.

Central nervous system: Considerable quantities of 5-HT are found in the midbrain, the limbic system, hypothalamus, caudate nucleus and pituitary gland. 5-HT, administered exogenously, does not readily cross the blood-brain barrier. The barrier, however, does not exist for its precursor, 5-HTP. Intraventricular administration of 5-HT in an unanaesthetized cat evokes tremors and muscular weakness, and sometimes profuse salivation. The cat becomes catatonic but not sleepy.

Smooth muscle: 5-HT stimulates smooth muscles; the most significant effect is seen on the small intestine. After stimulation of 5-HT_3 receptors in the GI tract, both the tone and the motility are initially augmented followed by an inhibition of the spontaneous activity. 5-HT also evokes bronchoconstriction.

Miscellaneous actions: It reduces the volume, acidity, and pepsin content of the gastric juice and promotes the production of mucus.

Absorption, fate and excretion: 5-HT is not significantly absorbed orally as it is degraded rapidly within the GI tract. Although platelets cannot synthesize 5-HT, they do have the capacity for its uptake and storage. It is mainly metabolized by the enzyme MAO and excreted as 5-HIAA in the urine (Fig. 23.4). The upper limit of normal urinary 5-HIAA in man is about 10 mg. per day.

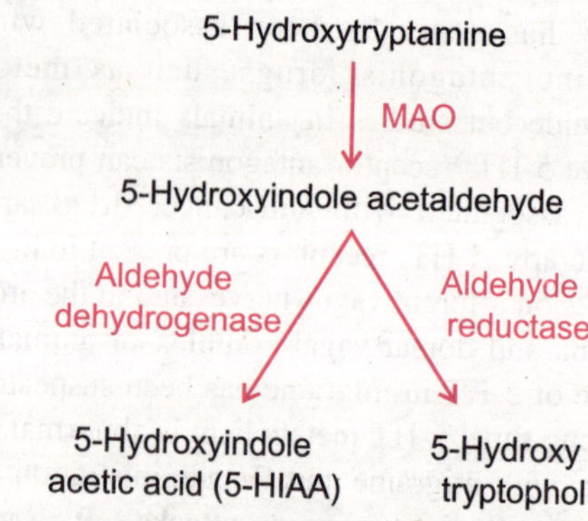

Fig. 23.4: Metabolism of 5-HT

Uses: 5-HT is not used therapeutically. However, many drugs are known to act by manipulating 5-HT at various receptor sites, centrally as well as peripherally. Drugs can also act directly on 5-HT receptors as agonists or antagonists; because of multiple types of 5-HT receptors, their actions and therapeutic uses vary. Further, some drugs in addition act on histaminergic, dopaminergic and adrenergic receptors. Some of the drugs acting through 5-HT receptors are summarized in Table 23.2.

5-HT-receptor agonists: These compounds differ in their chemical structures and actions. The important agents are:

(1) **5-HT_{1A} agonists** e.g. Buspirone used as an antianxiety agent (Chapter 13).

Table 23.2 : 5-Hydroxytryptamine and drugs

Drug	5-HT receptor	Other receptors	Uses
Agonists :			
Ergotamine	All 5- HT_1, 2_A,2_B	Dopamine; alpha-adrenergic agonist	Acute attack of migraine
LSD	2_A,2_C,1_A	—	Hallucinogen.
Triptans	1_B,1_D	—	Acute attack of migraine
Buspirone	1_A(partial agonist)	—	Anxiety states
Cisapride	5-HT_4	—	Gastroesophageal reflux disease (GERD)
		—	
Metoclopramide	5-HT_4	D_2 blocker	GERD, gastroparesis
Tcgaserod*	5-HT_4	—	Irritable bowel syndrome
Antagonists :			
Cyproheptadine	2_A,2_C	H_1-blocker Antimuscarinic	Migraine prophylaxis; carcinoid syndrome; postgastrectomy dumping syndrome
Metoclopramide	5-HT_3	D_2- blocker	Antiemetic
Methysergide	2_A, 2_C	—	Carcinoid syndrome; migraine prophylaxis
Ketanserin	2_A,2_C	H_1,Alpha-adrenergic	Migraine
Mianserin	5-HT_3,2_A, 2_C	$Alpha_2$- adrenergic	Antidepressant
Atypical antipsychotics:			
Clozapine	2_A,2_C	D_2 antagonist	Schizophrenia
Risperidone	2_A, 2_C	D_2 antagonist	Schizophrenia
Others			
Alosetron	5-HT_3	—	Irritable bowel syndrome
Ondansetron	5-HT_3	—	Antiemetic
5-HT uptake inhibitors :			
(a) Selective (SSRI) (Chapter 13)	—	H_1, antimuscarinic	Antidepressant Obsessive compulsive disorder; Panic disorder
(b) Nonselective (Chapter 13)	—	NA- reuptake inhibitor	Antidepressant Obsessive compulsive disorder
5-HT depletors :			
Reserpine	Depletion of intraneuronal stores of 5-HT and NA	—	Antihypertensive; antipsychotic

NA = Noradrenaline H = Histamine D = Dopamine * Withdrawn from market

(2) **5-HT_{1D} receptor agonists** e.g. Sumatriptan used in the treatment of migraine(see later).

(3) **5-HT_4 agonists** e.g. Cisapride used in the treatment of gastroesophageal rerflux disease.

(4) **Non-selective 5-HT agonists** e.g. LSD (Chapter 13).

SUMATRIPTAN (Imigran): This drug, an indole derivative, is a selective agonist of 5-HT_{1B} and 5-HT $_{1D}$ receptors. Activation of 5-HT_1 receptors leads to (a) blocking the release of several vasodilator neuropeptides, and (b) selective constriction of extracerebral, intracranial blood vessels. It also constricts other blood vessels such as the coronary. Triptans also reduce the increased concentration of CGRP in migraine attacks (see later). Given orally, sumatriptan is highly effective in treating acute attacks of migraine.

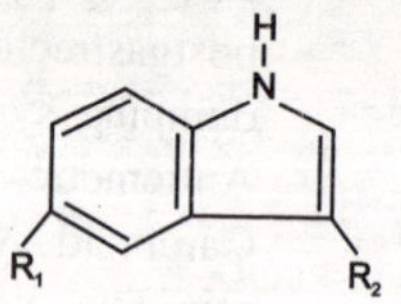

Fig. 23.5 : Triptan nucleus

The oral bioavailability is only 14%. It can also be given by nasal spray and SC. The drug is metabolized in the liver to an inactive metabolite by MAO-A enzyme. Its t½ is about 2 hours. It does not cross the BB barrier.

Adverse reactions: These are usually mild to moderate in intensity. It may cause a sensation of flushing and heat at the injection site, neck pain, dizziness, asthenia and tingling in the hands. Occasionally it may cause myocardial ischemia due to coronary vasoconstriction. It is, therefore, contraindicated in patients with symptomatic IHD, angina or hypertension. *It should not be combined with ergotamine and other vasoconstrictor drugs.*

Although analogues of sumatriptan (*triptans*) such as **Zolmitriptan**, **Rizatriptan, Almotriptan, Frovotriptan** and **Naratriptan**, have been introduced, their superiority over sumatriptan has not been established. They differ in their pharmacokinetic properties and cross the BB barrier. Naratriptan has bioavailability of 70% with a t½ of 6 hours. It is largely excreted unchanged in the urine.

Ergotamine: See Chapter 43.

Cisapride: This substituted piperidinyl benzamide compound is a prokinetic agent used previously for the treatment of gastroesophageal reflux disease and gastroparesis. It is no longer recommended because of its cardiac toxicity.

5-HT antagonists: Apart from PCPA, 5-HT synthesis can be inhibited by alpha methyldopa, some halogenated tryptophans, and phenylalanine.

A number of compounds antagonize the actions of 5-HT on the tissues. These include lysergic acid diethylamide (LSD) and its derivative 2-brom LSD or BOL (Chapter 13). By acting as agonists on the inhibitory 5-HT autoreceptors, they inhibit the release of 5-HT from the neurons in the′raphe nuclei. Other compounds like chlorpromazine, and yohimbine block the actions of 5-HT. Since there are multiple types of 5-HT receptors, a drug acting as an antagonist at one site may not act similarly at others. The 5-HT antagonists of therapeutic importance are:

METHYSERGIDE (Deseril): Methysergide, a congener of LSD, is a 5-HT_{2A} and 5-HT_{2C} antagonist. It blocks the actions of 5-HT on a variety of smooth muscles and has independent feeble vasoconstrictor and oxytocic effects.

It is an effective prophylactic agent in the management of migrainous headaches. The protective effect of the drug develops within 24 to 48 hours after initiation of therapy and persists for a similar period after its withdrawal. Rebound headaches may occur after sudden cessation of therapy. It is indicated for use in patients with resistant migraine *but is of no value in treating an acute attack and, in fact, may exacerbate it.*

Although the drug is useful in treating diarrhoea due to **carcinoid syndrome**, it is *not used* for that purpose because it has no action against the kinins released by the carcinoid tumour. The preferred treatment for malabsorption due to carcinoid tumour is the somatostatin analogue octreotide (Chapter 61) which inhibits all the mediators released by the tumour.

Adverse reactions: Significant toxicity is observed in almost 40% of the patients on chronic therapy. It includes GI irritation, nausea, drowsiness, vertigo and psychic disturbances. Postural hypotension, tachycardia, restlessness, insomnia, edema, neutropenia and paraesthesiae have been reported. A mild to severe peripheral arterial insufficiency, precipitation of angina, aggravation of peptic ulcer, retroperitoneal fibrosis with obstruction of the urinary tract pleuro-pulmonary fibrosis and cardiac valve damage are other serious, toxic effects. The drug should be avoided in pregnancy, severe hypertension, peripheral vascular disease, peptic ulcer, renal disease and coronary insufficiency.

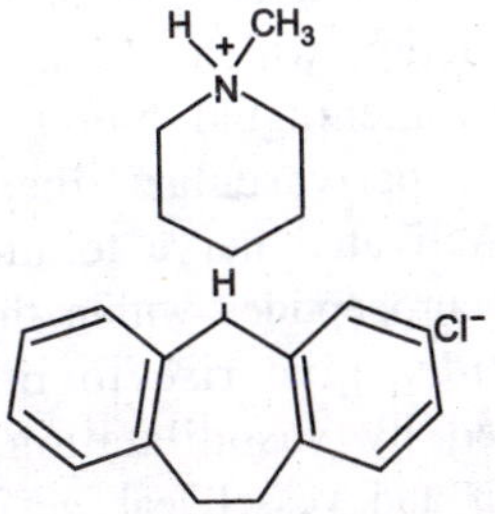

Fig. 23.6 : Cyproheptadine

CYPROHEPTADINE (Periactin): This compound, which bears some structural resemblance to phenothiazines, is a potent antagonist of 5-HT_2 receptors and to a certain extent of histamine and acetylcholine. Large doses administered to animals produce central depression. The drug also has anticonvulsant and antitremor activities. Cyproheptadine is satisfactorily absorbed from the GI tract. The metabolic fate of the compound is not known.

It stimulates appetite probably by acting directly on the hypothalamus. Weight is gained rapidly during the first few weeks of therapy and is lost again when the drug is stopped. There is evidence that 5-HT is involved in the control of ACTH secretion, possibly by stimulating corticotropin releasing factor (CRF) secretion from the hypothalamus. Administration of cyproheptadine can block the release of hydrocortisone and has, in fact, been used in the treatment of ACTH dependent Cushing's disease. It has also been shown to suppress aldosterone production in idiopathic aldosteronism.

The drug is available as 4 mg tablets. Dose : 4-20 mg/day in divided doses.

Adverse reactions: The common adverse effect is transient drowsiness which seldom necessitates withdrawal of the drug. Other adverse reactions include dryness of mouth, mental confusion, ataxia, dizziness, headache and visual hallucinations.

Therapeutic uses:

- ***Relief of pruritus*** associated with allergic dermatitis, urticaria and neurodermatosis. This action is probably due to its antihistaminic effect as the human skin does not contain significant quantities of 5-HT.
- ***Migraine prophylaxis :*** See later.
- ***Treatment of postgastrectomy dumping syndrome and carcinoid syndrome;*** its 5-HT antagonizing action is probably useful.
- ***Symptomatic relief in seasonal and perennial pollinosis*** but not bronchial asthma.
- ***As an appetite stimulant in certain conditions.*** However, its promotion as a general appetite stimulant or tonic is not justifiable and can even be dangerous.
- ***In certain cases of Cushing's disease.***

PIZOTIFEN (Sanomigran): This is an antihistaminic and 5-HT antagonist, structurally related to tricyclic antidepressants. It is effective in the prophylaxis of migraine and other vascular headaches. It may cause drowsiness, weight gain and urine retention. Dose : 0.5 to 2.0 mg. as a single dose at bedtime.

KETANSERIN: Ketanserin blocks 5-HT receptors, mainly 5-HT_{2A} and thereby antagonises vasoconstriction, platelet aggregation and bronchoconstriction. It has affinity for adrenergic $alpha_1$ and H_1 receptors which it blocks. It can cause lowering of blood pressure. The drug is used to improve digital circulation in patients with vasospastic conditions such as Raynaud's syndrome.

ONDANSETRON (Zofran, Emeset): This is a specific 5-HT_3 receptor antagonist and is useful as an antiemetic in nausea and vomiting following cytotoxic drugs and radiotherapy. Its action is partly central and partly peripheral. It is given orally in the dose of 8 mg 1 - 2 hours before treatment and in the same dose 12 hourly thereafter. The drug can also be given by slow IV infusion and as mouth dissolving tablets. It sometimes causes headache, constipation, allergic reaction and chest pain resembling MI. Unlike phenothiazine, it does not cause sedation nor EPR.

Granisetron and **Alosetron** have similar properties as ondansetron (Chapter 40).

CLOZAPINE: This atypical antipsychotic drug acts as 5-$HT_{2A/2C}$ receptor antagonist and is used in the treatment of schizophrenia.Many other antipsychotic drugs have 5-HT antagonist action (Chapter 13).

Pharmacotherapy of Migraine

Migraine is an episodic headache, unilateral or bilateral, throbbing in quality and exacerbated by physical activity. It shows a strong hereditary tendency. In practice, it is one of the most underdiagnosed and undertreated neurological disorders. According to the presence or absence of premonitory neurologic symptoms it is classified as:

- ***Migraine with aura*** (*classical migraine*); and
- ***Migraine without aura*** (*common migraine*).

Attacks of headache may be triggered by factors like food, visual stimuli, impending menstruation and relaxation after emotional tension. Classically, the headache is unilateral, may vary in duration from a few minutes to days. In 10 to 15 per cent of cases, it is preceded by visual and neurologic phenomena such as scintillating scotomata and visual field defects. These are often accompanied by nausea, vomiting, diarrhoea and prostration. *Rarely, migrainous headaches are due to structural lesions in the CNS like an aneurysm or an angioma.*

Pathophysiology : Migraine is a neurovascular disorder where there is an interaction between the intracranial nerves and blood vessels. The exact mechanism of migraine attacks is not known. According to earlier concepts, both migraine and cluster headaches result from abnormal central 5-HT transmission at diffuse sites in the CNS. According to the current concept, migraine involves a primary brain dysfunction which ultimately leads to dilatation of meningeal blood vessels and activation of perivascular trigeminal nerve terminals. Activated nerve terminals release vasoactive neuropeptides within the meninges. Those peptides give rise to inflammation characterized by vasodilatation, mast cell degranulation and vessel leakage. In addition, they are also involved in the genesis of pain and lowering of the threshold to pain response.

Evidence suggests that **calcitonin gene related peptide** (CGRP) released from the trigeminal nerve terminals plays an important role in the genesis of migraine and other vascular headaches. CGRP is a potent vasodilator of the meningeal and cerebral blood vessels, and is probably important in regulating blood flow to the brain and the pain-sensitive meninges. It is also capable of causing the release of pro-inflammatory cytokines from the meningeal mast cells. Infusion of CGRP causes migrainous headache in susceptible subjects. *Triptans which block the release of CGRP rapidly relieve the headache.*

The aims of treatment of migraine are:

- ***Amelioration of the symptoms*** during an acute attack; and
- ***Prevention of further attacks*** by behavioral or pharmacological means.

The *behavioral approach* involves education of the patient about the precipitating causes of attacks and their avoidance; a regular lifestyle with moderation in everything including regular meal hours, adequate but not excessive sleep, and minimising work-related and family stress.

Treatment of acute attacks : See Table 23.3. In all cases of migraine, aspirin (300-600 mg.) or paracetamol (500 mg.) with or without metoclopramide should be tried in the first instance. If taken at the very onset of headache and repeated every 4 hours till the headache subsides, many patients may not need any more medication. Opioids such as codeine are considered unsuitable for routine use because of their dependence liability. If nausea is prominent, an antiemetic such as chlorpromazine or prochlorperazine may be added to the above medication. An adequate dose of one of the other NSAID (ibuprofen) is as effective as aspirin in relieving an acute attack of migraine. The NSAID may be used prophylactically if headaches are predictable, as in menstrual migraine. NSAID act by inhibiting PG synthesis, thus preventing neurologically mediated inflammation in the trigemino-vascular system. *Prolonged, excessive use of any of the above medication can lead to chronic daily headache.*

Ergotamine tartrate (1 mg.) with or without caffeine (100 mg.) constitues specific therapy. It is a partial agonist of 5-HT_{1D} and 5-HT_{1B} receptors. A tablet is chewed and swallowed early during an attack, preferably during the preheadache aura phase. A repeat dose is taken 45 minutes later, if necessary. Not more than four tablets should be taken in 24 hours, nor more than 12 tablets per week. Ergotamine may make the nausea of migraine worse; this requires pretreatment with an antiemetic drug. Ergotamine tartrate is also available in sublingual form (Ergostat, 2 mg.). Dihydroergotamine (DHE) 1 mg. SC together with pretreatment with an antiemetic is effective in many cases; its main disadvantage is the need for an injection. As the tissue binding effect of ergotamine on arteries persists as long as 24 hours, repeated doses may cause a cumulative effect even after the attack subsides. *Persistent, chronic headache may be a symptom of overtreatment with ergot preparations.*

Table 23.3: Drugs used for treatment of migraine attacks

Drug	* Dose (mg)
Analgesic	
Aspirin	300-600
Paracetamol	600
Codeine**	15-60
NSAID	
Naproxen	250-500
Ibuprofen	400
Diclofenac (IM)	75
Ketorolac (IM)	30-60
5-HT_{1D} agonist	
Sumatriptan	
Oral	100
SC	6
5-HT partial agonists / antagonists	
Ergotamine	
Oral	1-4
Sublingual	1-4
DHE (SC)	1
Dopamine antagonists (IV)	
Metoclopramide	10
Haloperidol	2-10
Prochlorperazine	10

* Oral, unless specified
** For occasional use only.

Ergot preparations are contraindicated in the presence of peripheral vascular disease or coronary artery disease. They should be avoided in hypertension, during pregnancy, and in hepatic and renal disease. *Ergotamine should never be used in migraine prophylaxis.*

The **triptans** are highly effective in the treatment of an acute attack of migraine and may be preferred in a moderate to severe attack. They are given orally or by nasal spray; they can also be used SC. Sumatriptan is given orally in the dose of 25-50 mg, which may be repeated every 2 hours, if necessary, to the maximum total dose of 200 mg within 24 hours. It can also be given by nasal spray in the dose of 5-20 mg, repeated after 2 hours, if needed. It may be given SC in the dose of 4-6 mg. It is effective in 80% of patients within 2 hours. Sumatriptan and zolmitriptan nasal sprays have a faster onset of action. *A triptan should not be used until 24 hours after the last dose of ergotamine. They are not useful for prophylaxis of migraine.*

In resistant acute attacks, a 5-HT antagonist, either prochlorperazine 10 mg IV or haloperidol IM may be used.

Migraine Prophylaxis : See Table 23.4. Preventive treatment is considered when attacks occur oftener than 2-3 times a month or are severe enough to limit normal activity; and when above symptomatic therapy causes serious adverse reactions. Medications containing vasodilators should be discontinued, if possible. Therapy is started with small doses, and the lowest effective maintenance dose be used; it may take as much as 3 months to show the desired result. If the therapy is effective, the attacks become less frequent and milder in intensity, and they may respond better to analgesic drugs. Overuse of acute medication may reduce the efficacy of the preventive medication. Preventive medication may need to be maintained for long periods of time. If the response is good, the medication may be tapered gradually after 9-12 months. If headaches recur, the treatment should be restarted. *The drug should not be stopped abruptly when a cardiovascular agent such as propranolol is used.*

Table 23.4: Drugs used for prevention of migraine attacks

Drug	Dose (mg)
5-HT antagonists :	
Pizotifen	0.5-1.5 OD
Beta-adrenergic antagonists :	
Propranolol	40-240*
Atenolol	25-100 OD
Antidepressants :	
Amitriptyline	10-50 OD
Calcium channel blockers :	
Verapamil	100-200*
Anticonvulsants :	
Valproic acid	300-600*
Gabapentine	1800-2400*

* Daily-divided

The 5-HT antagonists methysergide and pizotifen (discussed earlier) and the tricyclic antidepressant amitriptyline (Chapter 13) are effective drugs for prophylaxis. *Methysergide is a toxic drug and should be used only in resistant cases.* Amitriptyline in the low dose of 5-10 mg at bedtime daily is especially useful in patients who have concomitant depression. Propranolol, a beta adrenergic blocker (Chapter 17), is considered the drug of choice in patients with attacks related to stress. Valproic acid has been reported to be useful in some patients. Menstrual migraine (attacks occurring during menses) is generally refractory and may need prophylactic treatment with amitriptyline/beta blocker, plus NSAID/ergotamine at the onset of menses. Oral diuretics are sometimes helpful in such cases by countering fluid retention.

Angiotensin, Kinins, Leukotrienes; Prostaglandins and Cytokines 24

ANGIOTENSINS are peptide hormones derived from a protein precursor angiotensinogen (a serum globulin, also called renin substrate) by the sequential actions of proteolytic enzymes in the circulation and several tissues. Angiotensinogen, synthesized by the liver, is converted by the circulating renin from the kidney into **angiotensin I, a decapeptide**; by itself,the latter is inactive. It is converted by angiotensin converting enzyme (ACE) in the plasma and the pulmonary endothelial cells into the **octapeptide angiotensin II.** Angiotensin II is further converted to either angiotensin III or angiotensin IV. The major portion of the angiotensin II in circulation is largely due to the angiotensin IV activity of membrane-bound ACE present in the endothelial cells lining the vascular walls. ACE is also found in various tissues including the brain, kidney and the adrenals. Local renin-angiotensin system in the tissues exists independently of the renal-hepatic based system. ACE is nonspecific and it acts on other natural substrates such as bradykinin, which it inactivates.

Angiotensin II is the most important, versatile and potent angiotensin. It can also be synthesized by a pathway that does not require ACE. Angiotensin II acts to raise the BP by directly constricting the blood vessels, particularly the arterioles, and perhaps more importantly indirectly by inhibiting the renal excretion of sodium and water. It acts through G protein coupled receptors, AT_1 and AT_2, to produce diverse effects.

Angiotensin III acts on the same AT_1 and AT_2 receptors, and is involved in thirst regulation and stimulation of aldosterone release.

Most of its known actions of angiotensin are mediated by the AT_1 receptors. Thus:

- ***AT_1 receptors*** mediate the potent vasoconstrictor action and the maintenance of arterial BP and renal function by it. They also bring about cell growth and hypertrophy of the arterial wall muscle, and of the ventricular wall muscle in the diseased and failing heart.
- ***AT_2 receptors*** ameliorate the above mentioned adverse effects of AT_1 receptor activation by inhibiting cell growth and hypertrophy. AT_2 receptors abound in the brain, kidneys and several other tissues in fetal life during which they may be involved in fetal tissue development and cell differentiation. AT_2 receptors are less abundant in adults.

Actions of angiotensin II : It acts at several sites in the body (Table 24.1). It increases the peripheral resistance, prevents renal sodium excretion and modulates cardiovascular morphological structure. It is a 40-50 times more potent vasoconstrictor than NA on molar basis.

- ***It causes rapid regulation of arterial BP in response to acute fall in BP,*** by constricting the arterioles, and to a smaller extent, venules.

Table 24.1: Actions of Angiotensin II via AT_1 receptors

Tissue	Action(s)
• *Artery*	Contraction and growth
• *Heart*	Contraction and ventricular hypertrophy
• *Adrenal*	Stimulates aldosterone biosynthesis
• *Kidney*	Inhibits renin release; stimulates sodium reabsorption; stimulates vasoconstriction (efferent glomerular arterioles in low concentrations, and both afferent and efferent in higher concentrations); releases PGE
• *Sympathetic nervous system*	Increased release of NA from sympathetic nerve terminals; facilitates peripheral transmission; increases adrenaline release by adrenal medulla.

• ***Long term mainenance of BP (slow response) is mediated by regulation of Na^+ excretion by the kidney.*** Angiotensin II directly promotes renal Na^+ reabsorption in the proximal tubules, and also causes Na^+ retention through the release of aldosterone.

• ***It also causes hypertrophy of the heart and thickening of the blood vessels*** (Chapter 64). Angiotensin II contributes to the pathogenesis of hypertension, cardiac hypertrophy, heart failure and diabetic renal disease which are benefited by ACE inhibitors. The direct action on some tissues by angiotensin stimulates the formation of counterregulatory substances, including vasodilating prostaglandins and nitric oxide. On the other hand, the target organs may release substances such as catecholamines, endothelin and growth factors, which may amplify the effects of angiotensin. Thus, the balance between the vasoconstrictors and the vasodilators determines the response of blood vessels to angiotensin II.

Angiotensin IV is involved in releasing plasminogen activator inhibitor-1 (PAI-1) from the endothelium and in countering the effects of angiotensin II. Angiotensin IV receptors (AT_4 receptors) have specific distribution within the hypothalamus.

Drugs are available to counter the ill effects of excess angiotensin II : inhibitors of ACE (ACEI) and AT_1 receptor blockers (ARBs). (Chapter 29).

Kinins

The kinins are vasoactive polypetides released from an $alpha_2$ globulin fraction of the plasma, termed as kininogens, by the action of enzymes termed **kallikreins**. Kininogens are present in two forms: (1) Low molecular weight kininogen (LMWK); and (2) High molecular weight kininogen (HMWK). HMWK is limited to the blood stream whereas LMWK can reach the tissues. The kallikreins (Kallikreas, the Greek name for pancreas) are highly specific proteases, and exist in two forms: (a) plasma, and (b) tissue kallikreins. Both normally exist in inactive forms called prekallikreins (PK).

Plasma prekallikrein is bound to its substrate HMWK but the protease inhibitors present in plasma prevent the proteolysis. When this system binds to a receptor complex on the endothelial cell membrane, it gets activated to kallikrein. The generated kallikrein activates clotting factor XII and cleaves HMWK to a nonapeptide, **bradykinin**.

Tissue prekallikrein is present in epithelial or secretory cells of salivary glands, pancreas, prostate, distal nephron and human neutrophils. The activation sequence of this tissue form is not well delineated but the active tissue kallikrein acts locally near the site of its origin. It converts HMWK and LMWK to a decapeptide, **kallidin** (lysyl bradykinin) (Fig. 24.1). Various factors such as tissue damage, infection, inflammation and allergic reactions can generate tissue kinins.

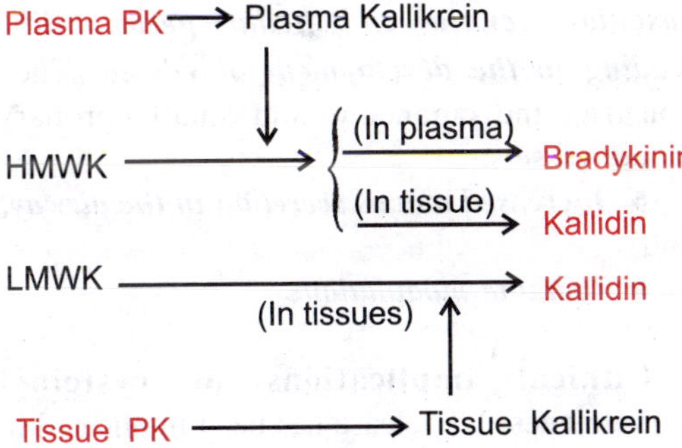

Fig. 24.1 : Kinin generation

Both **kallidin** and **bradykinin** are referred to as 'plasma kinins' and have essentially identical pharmacological properties. In addition to kallikreins, various other serine proteases like trypsin and certain snake venoms are capable of generating kinins. Preformed kinins exist in the venoms of wasps and hornets.

Physiological role: The kinins are potent vasodilators. They have been incriminated in the processes of inflammatory and allergic reactions (asthma), shock, disseminated intravascular coagulation and inflammatory bowel disease. They may also modulate migration of leucocytes and tissue cells that take part in the inflammatory process. They are also most potent activators of PG-release, including PGI_2 from vessels.

Bradykinin acts on two receptors: B_1 and B_2. B_1 are absent from the normal tissues and are induced by inflammation. In the absence of inflammation,most of the actions of the kinin are mediated through B_2 receptors which are constitutive.

Pharmacological actions :

- ***Vessels and heart*** : The kinins have about 10 times the vasodilator activity as histamine and produce mainly arteriolar dilatation in the skeletal muscle, heart, kidneys, intestines and liver, via the local release of nitric oxide and PGI_2. The kinins also have direct positive chronotropic and inotropic actions on the myocardium and in moderate doses, release adrenaline from the adrenal medulla.
- ***Smooth muscle stimulation*** : The kinins stimulate other smooth muscles including those of the uterus, the bronchi and the GI tract. The term bradykinin was coined initially to signify the slow contraction of the GI smooth muscle by the nonapeptide. They promote epithelial ion transport and fluid secretion in the airways and GI tract, leading to cough/ angioedema in the former and diarrhoea in the latter.
- ***Genesis of pain***: The kinins evoke pain (algesia) and itching on application to the base of a blister via the β_2 receptors. NSAIDs can antagonise the pain producing property of kinins.
- ***Vascular permeability***: They are more potent than histamine in increasing vascular permeability and inducing edema.
- ***Release of PGs and PAF***: Kinins can cause the release of biologically active lipids such as platelet activating factor (PAF) and prostaglandins (PGs) from a variety of cells, and some of the actions of kinins may be indirect via the release of such mediators of inflammation.

The kinins are rapidly inactivated by the plasma and erythrocyte aminopeptidases and carboxypeptidases. They have very short plasma t½ of 15 seconds. *The enzyme (ACE) that metabolises bradykinin also converts angiotensin I to angiotensin II.*

A high molecular weight polypeptide **aprotinin** (Trasylol), extracted from the parotid glands and lymph nodes of cattle, also present in mast cells, inhibits and inactivates kallikrein, trypsin and other proteolytic enzymes. It has been used in the treatment of acute pancreatitis, to prevent blood loss during open heart surgery, and in the treatment of hemorrhage due to hyperplasminemia (Chapter 32).

Leukotrienes (LTs)

Leukotrienes along with PGs, thromboxanes and lipoxins, are the major constituents of a group of biologically active, oxygenated, polyunsaturated, long chain fatty acids (**eicosanoids**). The eicosanoids are found in both animal and plants. They possess a wide range of biological activities. In the human body, they are derived *de novo* from a 20-carbon chain fatty acid arachidonic acid, which is an important constituent of the cell membrane phospholipids. The eicosanoid biosynthesis is triggered after trauma, infection and inflammation.

All the leukotrienes are derived from a common precursor, leukotriene A4 (LTA4); they are LTB4, LTC4, LTD4 and LTE4; the last three are also collectively known as *slow reacting substance* of anaphylaxis (SRS-A). The locations at which the LTs are synthesized are determined by the cellular distribution of the enzymes controlling the biosynthetic pathways. The enzymes involved are phospholipase A_2 and 5-lipooxygenase (Fig. 24.4) The distribution of 5-lipooxygenase is limited to specific number of cells types : neutrophils, eosinophils, monocytes, macrophages, mast cells, basophils and B-lymphocytes. LTs exert their biological actions through specific ligand-receptor interactions. They probably act as "local hormones". Their t/2 is very short.

Pharmacological/biological actions: LTs have several potent actions. Thus, LTB_4

(1) Is the most potent neutrophil chemotactic agent and plays an important role in the induction of neutrophil-endothelial-cell adhesion.

(2) Causes the release of substantial quantities of glucuronidase and lysozyme from the neutrophils.

(3) Stimulates myelopoiesis and proliferation of T lymphocytes; and

(4) Is probably an important mediator of inflammatory pain.

LTs — C4, D4 and E4 (SRS) are also called **sulfidopeptides** or **cysteinyl LTs.** They play an important role in the inflammatory process. They cause:

- ***Vigorous and sustained contraction of smooth muscle.*** They are the most potent vasoconstrictors known and are involved in the pathogenesis of asthma.
- ***Vasodilation and modulation of vascular (venular endothelial) permeability, leading to the development of edema.*** They constrict the cutaneous and small coronary blood vessels.
- ***Increased mucus secretion in the airway;*** and
- ***Immune modulation.***

Clinical implications of cysteinyl leukotrienes: LT release has been implicated in the pathogenesis of anaphylactic shock, asthma and various inflammatory diseases such as cystic fibrosis, glomerulonephritis, rheumatoid arthritis, psoriasis, inflammatory bowel disease and adult respiratory distress syndrome. Various LT synthesis inhibitors and antagonists are available for use in asthma (Chapter 26).

Prostaglandins (PGs)

In 1930, Kurzrok and Lieb demonstrated the activity of human semen on isolated strips of human uterine muscle. This was confirmed by von Euler (1935) who demonstrated a substance present in the extracts of human seminal fluid, which caused contraction of the isolated intestinal and uterine muscle, and vasodilatation. This substance was named as prostaglandin because of its probable origin from the prostate. Bergstrom (Nobel prize, 1982) and associates showed that the various PGs are closely related derivatives of the lipid soluble prostanoic acid (Fig. 24.2). Although human seminal fluid is the richest known source, PGs are also present in extracts of other tissues such as iris, lung, human menstrual fluid, brain, thymus, pancreas and kidneys. Prostaglandin of the human semen is a mixture of six closely related substances belonging to the groups E, F, A and B. The other human tissues contain mostly groups E and F prostaglandins, though PGD_2, PGG_2, PGH_2 and PGI_2 (Prostacyclin) have also been described. The corals, native to the Caribbean sea, contain large quantities of PGA as a natural constituent.

Fig. 24.2: Chemical structure of (a) Prostanoic acid (b) Arachidonic acid

Chemistry and biosynthesis: Fatty acids (FA) occurring in natural fats are mostly straight chain aliphatic compounds, with even number of carbon atoms connected by C-C bonds, carboxy (COOH) group at one end and methyl (CH_3) group at the other. The FA is named after the hydrocarbon with the same number and arrangement of carbon atoms, **-oic** being substituted for the final **-e** in the same hydrocarbon. The FA may be **saturated (SFA**, no double bond); or **unsaturated (UFA**, with double bonds). The UFAs may be **mono-unsaturated (MUFA** with a single double bond) or; **polyunsaturated (PUFA** with two or more double bonds). The names of the SFAs end in **–anoic** e.g. prostanoic acid (Fig. 24.2) and of the UFAs in **–enoic** e.g. eicosapentaenoic acid (see later).

Fatty acids serve many functions in the body: energy production; electrical insulation; transport of plasma lipids; maintainence of cell membrane integrity; proper development of the CNS; participation in cell communication and oxygen transport; and regulation of inflammation. Animals can synthesize SFA from carbohydrates and some amino acids. However, unlike plants, they cannot synthesize the two PUFAs, linoleic acid (LA) and alpha linolenic acid (αLNA), which are, therefore **essential** in animals. Using these two, animals synthesize all other UFAs they need e.g. arachidonic acid (AA)which is an important constituent of the cell membrane.

Eicosanoids are oxygenation products derived from 20 (eicosa) carbon UFAs: dihomo–gamma-linolenic acid (DGLA), arachidonic acid (AA) and eicosapentaenoic acid (EPA). They are ubiquitous both in animals and (together with the precursor oil) in various plants. AA is the major source of prostanoids (eicosanods) in mammals. The three respective **series** of eicosanoids viz, PG-1, PG-2 and PG-3 are defined by the number of double bonds in their side chains.

During the synthesis of eicosanoids, AA is first released from the cell membrane phospholipids by lipases. It is then oxygenated by four separate routes including by cyclo-oxygenase (COX) and lipo-oxygenase. Various factors determine the type of eicosanoid synthesized. Besides the cell type, an important factor is the nature of the precursor PUFA that is present in the respective membrane phospholipid. The PG1 and PG2 series are synthesized from LA (an $omega_6$ PUFA) and its derivative GLA via DGLA (G1 series), and from AA (G2 series), respectively. The PG3 series is derived from alpha-linolenic acid (LNA) via EPA, an $omega_{-3}$ fatty acid, and docosa-hexaeonic acid (DHA) (Fig. 24.3). Nature of the substituents in the side chain determines the **type** (A, B, C, D, E, F) of the eicosanoid. The term omega is used to denote the position of the carbon atom (3, 6 or 9 from the methyl end) after which the first double bond occurs in an FA. Prostanoids of PG2 series carry the subscript 2 e.g. PGE_2 and $PGF_{2\alpha}$.

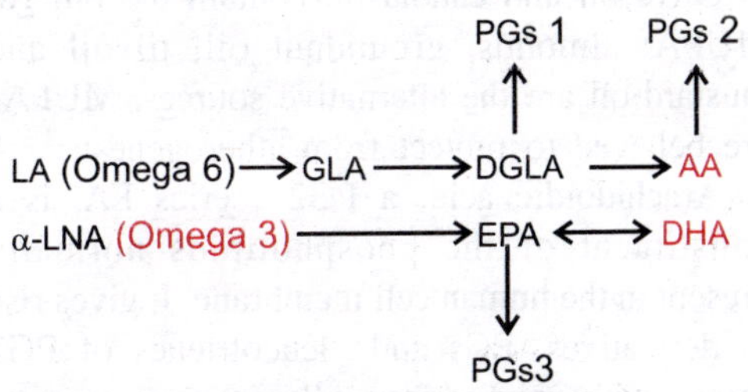

Fig. 24.3 : Biosynthesis of eicosanoids from linoleic and alpha linolenic acids. PGs = Prostaglandins, leukotrienes etc. of Series 1, 2, 3. Those of PGs 1 and 3 are less inflammatory than those of PGs2 (see text).

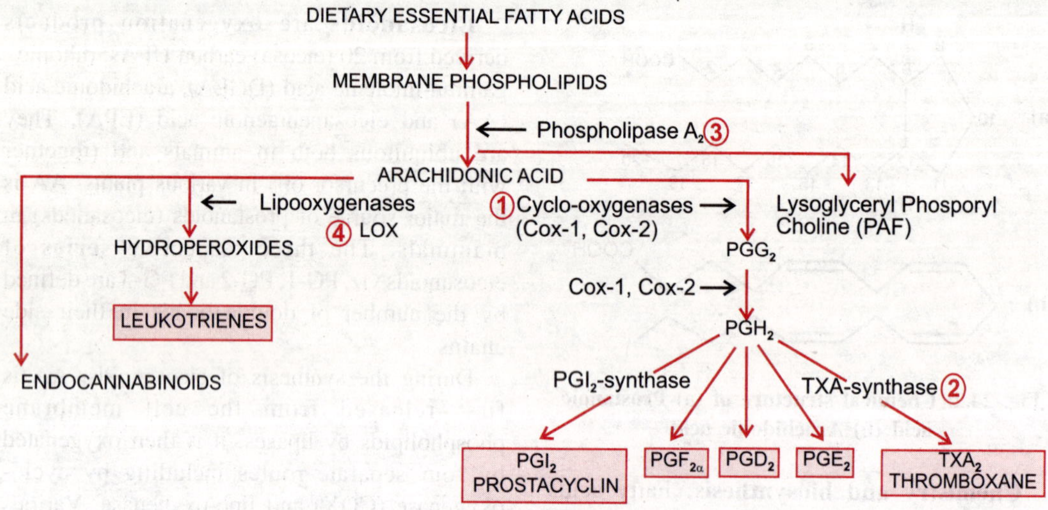

Aspirin and NSAID inhibit enzymes (1) and Dazoxiben inhibits enzyme (2) Glucocorticoids inhibit generation of arachidonic acid from cell membrane phospholipids by phospholipase A_2 (3) Zileuton inhibits 5-lipooxygenases (4).

Fig. 24.4 : Synthesis of leukotrienes and important mammalian prostaglandins

The **dietary sources** of LA are polyunsaturated vegetable oils such as safflower, sunflower and corn oils, lean meats and eggs. Hydrogenation and heating of vegetable oils for production of margarine converts the **cis** FA present in the oil into **trans FA**; *the latter behave like saturated FA metabolically and are considered atherogenic* (Chapter 39). Evening primrose oil, used for medicinal purposes, also contains GLA.

Coconut oil and animal fats contain SFAs. They are atherogenic.

Olive oil and canola oil contain the $omega_9$ MUFA; almonds, groundnut oil, til oil and mustard oil are the alternative sources. MUFAs are believed to protect from atherogenesis.

Arachidoidic acid, a PG2 series FA, is a constituent of the phospholipids normally present in the human cell membrane. It gives rise to derivatives, PGs and leucotrienes of PG2 series, with marked pro-inflammatory activity. They have been incriminated in the pathogenesis of chronic inflammatory disorders such as psoriasis and rheumatoid arthritis.

Eicosapentaenoic acid and docosahexaenoic acid (both $omega_3$ PUFA), present in fatty sea-fish, when ingested regularly, can partially replace AA (of PG2 series) with the less pro-inflammatory eicosanoids of the PG3 series (TXA3) in the tissues, and this may benefit patients with chronic, inflammatory diseases such as rheumatoid arthritis and psoriasis; it may also contribute to protection from atherosclerosis. The other dietary sources of $omega_3$ FA are flax seeds, nuts (particularly walnuts and hazelnuts), dark green leafy vegetables and soyabeans. The fatty fish contain EPA and DHA, and are a better source of $omega_3$ fatty acids than the vegetable sources which contain LNA but not EPA or DHA. It has been suggested that certain constituents of onions, apples and spices such as turmeric and red peppers (red chilly) may enhance the anti-inflammatory effect of $omega_3$ fatty acids.

Physiologically, tissue cells synthesize PGs at the site of action from the essential fatty acids LA and LNA (Fig. 24.3). The two principal mammalian PGs are PGE_2 and $PGF_{2\alpha}$.

The PGs A, B and C are artifacts that arise during extraction procedures. PGs are very active even in very low concentrations and are degraded rapidly.

Under stimulation by mechanical, thermal, chemical and bacterial insults, PGs are released in large amounts into the body Both PGE_2 and PGI_2 (Fig. 24.4) are potent vasodilators and hyperalgesic agents. PGE_2 is also a potent pyrogenic substance. In association with other mediators, PGs play an important role in the development of the inflammatory response.

Because of their instability, short duration of action and lack of tissue specificity, the natural PGs have limited clinical applications. Various synthetic derivatives available, however, overcome these limitations.

Pharmacological actions : PGs produce their effects by acting on PG receptors.

- ***Smooth muscles***: PGE_2, $PGF_{2\alpha}$ and TXA_2 stimulate the human myometrium and increase the intestinal motility. PGE inhibits the tone of tracheal and bronchial muscles and thus has a bronchodilator action.

- ***Gastrointestinal system*** : Prostaglandins are distributed throughout the gut though their concentration varies in different parts of the gut. PGE_2 and PGI_2 synthesized by COX_1 inhibit the gastric acid secretion, enhance the mucosal blood flow, and thus have a cytoprotective effect on gastric and duodenal mucosa in humans. Both PGE and PGF cause contraction of the longitudinal muscle of the gut. Further, PGs stimulate intestinal fluid secretion and cause diarrhoea when administered orally or parenterally. This suggests a possible role of PG release in certain types of diarrhoeas.

- ***Cardiovascular system***: PGE_2 and PGI_2 are potent peripheral vasodilators. The vasodilator effect is mainly localised to the arterioles, precapillary sphincters and postcapillary venules.The blood pressure falls and the blood flow to most organs increases. TXA_2 is a potent vasoconstrictor. $PGF_{2\alpha}$, however, is neutral in this respect in humans.

PGE_1 (Alprostadil) is a potent relaxant of the smooth muscle of the ductus arteriosus and preserves the ductal patency in the newborn.

- ***Kidney***: Although PGs do not maintain normal renal blood flow, their local production is important in maintaining blood flow in compromised kidneys. PGE_2 and PGI_2 cause diuresis, natriuresis and kaliuresis by direct action on the renal tubules. PGE inhibits water reabsorption induced by ADH; it also inhibits chloride reabsorption. The kidney cells that synthesize PGs contain mostly COX_1 (Chapter 11).

- ***Reproductive system***: Apart from their stimulant action on the uterine smooth muscle, PGs exert other actions on the reproductive system. In animal experiments, PGs cause regression of the corpus luteum (luteolysis) and reduction in secretion of progesterone. This can prevent the implantation of fertilized ovum. Both COX_1 and COX_2 are expressed in the uterine epithelium at different times in early pregnancy. COX_2 may play a role in the birth process and its excessive activity may be responsible for preterm or premature labour. Functions of PGs present in the semen are not clear (Chapter 43).

- ***CNS***: The role of PGs as neurotransmitters has been suggested. COX_1 is distributed in neurons throughout the brain, being most prevalent in the forebrain. COX_2 is also expressed constitutively in a few areas. PGs are probably involved in the central mechanisms that cause hyperalgesia. Further, PGE_2 is implicated in the causation of fever (Chapter 11) and the release of some anterior pituitary hormones.

- ***Platelet aggregation***: In the platelets, the only isoform detectable is COX_1. PG endoperoxide and thromboxane A_2(TXA_2), cause platelet aggregation and vasoconstriction, while PGI_2 (**Prostacyclin**) which is found in the vascular endothelium is a potent inhibitor of platelet aggregation and causes vasodilatation. When the platelets are damaged they release PG endoperoxides which cause aggregation of platelets. However, the vascular endothelial PGI_2 has anti-aggregatory effect. Damage to the endothelium reduces PGI_2 synthesis and increases the tendency to thrombosis because of the unopposed action of TXA_2. Aspirin blocks formation of both TXA_2 and PGI_2 but COX_1 in the vascular endothelial cells regenerates so that PGI_2 synthesis is reestablished. The TXA_2 synthesis is irreversibly inhibited for the lifetime (8-10 days) of the platelets in circulation (Chapter 32).

• ***Role in inflammation***: Presence of PGE and kinins in the inflammatory exudates suggests their role in the genesis of inflammation. COX_2 is clearly associated with inflammation. Selective COX_2 inhibitors may control inflammation without affecting the beneficial effects of PGE on the stomach (Chapter 11).

• ***Miscellaneous***: PGE_1 and PGE_2 block the lipolytic effect of adrenaline, ACTH and glucagon. They also produce pain when applied to an exposed blister base.

Some PGs are potent bone resorbing agents which act by stimulating osteoclasts. Experimentally, bone destruction induced by implanted metastasizing tumours in rats and rabbits, can be reduced by PG inhibition by aspirin or indomethacin.

PGE_2 also stimulates the adrenal steroid production and insulin release.

Therapeutic uses of prostaglandins:

(1) **As abortifacients and cervical ripeners** (Chapter 43).

(2) **As gastric cytoprotectives:** Misoprostol (Chapter 42).

(3) **In erectile dysfunction:** Alprostadil is injected intracavernosally (Chapter 67).

(4) **For maintenance of patency of ductus arteriosus** (Chapter 11).

(5) **In the treatment of primary pulmonary hypertension,** PGI_2 (Epoprostenol) by IV infusion, is highly effective.

Endocannabinoids, derived from AA in the brain, are the endogenous ligands for the cannabinoid receptors, and mimic some of the pharmacological actions of Δ9-tetrahydro-cannabinol, dronabinol (Chapters 13 and 40).

Cytokines

Inflammation is an integral part of the body's defence mechanisms against foreign organisms, and natural as well as acquired (specific) immunity play an important role in human defence. Several polypeptides are known to mediate some aspect or other of the inflammatory process.

The effector phases of both natural and acquired immunity are in large part mediated by protein hormones called **cytokines**, which are released from a variety of cell types in response to a number of stimuli (*induced secretion*). These cytokines activate, modulate and control various aspects of body defence and repair. In case of natural immunity, effector cytokines are mainly derived from the mononuclear phagocytes and the natural killer (NK) cells. Most cytokines in specific immunity are released from activated T lymphocytes. T cells produce several cytokines that serve primarily to regulate the growth, differentiation and activation of various lymphocyte populations (*constitutive secretion*). They activate and regulate inflammatory cells such as monocytes, neutrophils and eosinophils. Both lymphocytes and mononuclear phagocytes also produce other cytokines such as colony stimulating factors (CSF) which stimulate the growth and differentiation of immature lymphocytes in the bone marrow.

Like other polypeptide hormones, the cytokines act by binding to specific receptors on the surface of target cells. Such target cells may be (1) the same cells that secrete the cytokine (**autocrine action**); (2) nearby cells (**paracrine action**); or (3) distant cells as in the case of classical hormones (**endocrine action**).

General properties of cytokines:

• Cytokines are low molecular weight proteins secreted mainly by white blood cells and other cells, and are responsible for cell to cell communication. Many individual cytokines are produced by multiple types of cells.

Tabel 24.2: Cytokine groups according to functions

Group	Members	Major sources
Mediators of natural immunity	Interferon α and β	Macrophages, fibroblasts
	TNF α	Macrophages
	IL1	MNP, endothelial and epithelial cells
	IL6	Macrophages, endothelial cells
	IL 12	Macrophages, dendritic cells
Regulators of lymphocyte activation, growth, and differentiation	IL2	T cells
	IL4	T_H2 cells; mast cells
	IL5	T_H2 cells
	TGF β	T cells; macrophages; others
	Interferon γ	T_H1 cells, NK cells
Regulators of immune mediated inflammation and repair	Interferon γ	T cells; NK cells
	IL5	T_H2 cells
	IL10	T cells
	IL12	Macrophages and dendritic cells
	IL18	Macrophages
	Lymphotoxin	T cells
	MIF	T cells
Stimulators of immature leucocytes, growth and differentiation.	IL3	T cells
	IL7	Fibroblasts, bone marrow stromal cells
	GM CSF, M CSF, G CSF	MNP; endothelial cells; fibroblasts

TNF - Tumor Necrosis Factor; TGF - Transforming Growth Factor; MIF - Migration Inhibition Factor; CSF - Colony Stimulating Factor; GM - Granulocyte Macrophage; MNP - Mononuclear phagocytes; M - Macrophage; G - Granulocyte; IL - Interleukin

- They are produced during the effector phase of natural and specific immunity and play an important role in mediating and regulating intensity and duration of immune and inflammatory responses, including the termination of the inflammatory response, angiogenesis, healing and repair.
- They are not stored as preformed molecules. Their *constitutive* secretion is brief and self-limited. Failure of termination of their *induced* secretion can lead to chronic inflammatory disorders.
- A given cytokine has different biological effects on different cell types (pleotropism).
- Cytokines influence the synthesis of other cytokines, which may affect the other cells in turn. Thus, even if small number of cells are involved in the beginning, this cascade induction leads to amplification of the biological effects and involves a larger cellular network. It is also possible that cytokines may enhance or suppress the production of other cytokines.
- Two or more cytokines may interact with each other to produce additive, synergistic or antagonistic effects.
- For many target cells, cytokines act as regulators of cell division (growth factors).

Classification of cytokines: Based on structural studies, there exist 4 groups :

I **Hematopoietin family** (e.g. GM-CSF, erythropoietin, IL 2, IL 4);

II **Interferon family** (e.g. alpha, beta and gamma, IL10);

III **Chemokine family** (e.g. IL 8, monocyte chemotactic protein, neutrophil activating protein, platelet factor 4); and

IV **Tumor necrosis factor (TNF) family.**

Cytokines can also be classified into four groups according to their functions (Table 24.2). IL-1 and TNF have many similarities in regard to physical and biochemical properties, synthesis and release, and they possess overlapping biological properties and functions.

Functions of cytokines: The target cell responses that require cytokines fall broadly into (i) **the defence role** of alerting the body to invasion and dealing with it, and (ii) **the repair role** of cleaning up the debris and replacing lost matrix and tissue as well as controlling cellular proliferation and differentiation. IL-1 also produces metabolic responses; thereby, the necessary energy resources and rebuilding materials are mobilized, and (iii) **hematopoiesis**.

- ***Role in body defence and regulation of inflammatory responses*** : IL-1 and TNF are mediators of biological responses to endotoxins and promote inflmmation. IL-1 causes erythema, edema, chemo-attraction, and adherence as well as migration of defence cells into the sites of inflammation. Both can induce the burst in neutrophils and monocytes and the associated production of free radicals, myeloperoxide and hydrogen peroxide, that play an important role in killing the invading organisms. The cytokines activate the cells leading to release of hydrolytic enzymes and to increase in PG production. Inhibition and killing of stray tumour cells is yet another property of TNF and to a lesser extent of IL-1. These cytokines inhibit the replication of certain RNA and DNA viruses and induce viral resistance in a variety of cell types; this is not due to induction of interferons. Thus, many of the events associated with the acute inflammatory reaction and defence against infections of various kinds can be mediated by IL-1 and TNF.

TNF-α and IL-2 are potent upregulators of several cell types including fibroblasts and T cells. IL-1 is responsible for the immune component of inflammatory diseases; TNF-α by contrast has little influence on lymphocyte proliferation and immune responses.

The cytokines secreted from subpopulation of helper T cells (T_H1 and T_H2) are important determinants of the immune response generated to eliminate the pathogens. T_H1 cells secretes interferon gamma and IgG which help in defence mechanisms. Cytokines from T_H1 cells prepare body to respond to viral and intracellular pathogens. On the other hand, IL-4 and IL-5 secreted from T_H2 cells induce production of IgE. IL-5 is also responsible for eosinophil differentiation and activation. These defense mechanisms help to tackle helminth infections.

- ***Role in body repair*:** Both IL-1 and TNF appear to have considerable influence on the earlier repair events of debridement, mitogenesis and differentiation. Release of enzymes including proteoglycanase, collagenase, and gelatinase can be induced from fibroblasts, synoviocytes and chondrocytes by IL-1, and the same is true for TNF. Enzyme release is accompanied by release of PGE_2, which may also contribute to the degradation process. Local release of IL-1 and TNF could thus mediate debridement. The biological actions of TNF are related to the quantity released:

At low concentrations, TNF acts as a paracrine and autocrine regulator of leucocytes and endothelial cells. These actions are useful in generating the inflammatory responses which help to counter the microbial infections. TNF is also an endogenous pyrogen, and acts on cells in the hypothalamus to produce fever, a property which it shares with IL1.

Moderate amounts of TNF enter the blood stream and may cause systemic effects, including an increase in the acute phase proteins (APP); further. TNF may be the mediator of matrix destruction in rheumatoid arthritis.

Very high concentrations of TNF, on the other hand, cause depressed myocardial contractility, relaxation of vascular smooth muscle and intravascular thrombosis, leading to fall of BP, decreased tissue perfusion and metabolic acidosis; thus, TNF contributes in a major way to death in septic shock. It also causes depletion of hepatic and muscle glycogen. TNF and IL-1 both can induce bone resorption.

Overall, IL-1 and TNF possess the potential for mediating many of the events crucial to defence of the host, and subsequent repair; but by the same token they may also mediate much of the tissue destruction which characterizes the connective tissue diseases.

PGE_2, like cytokines, causes a rise in APP by different mechanisms. The severity and outcome of connective tissue diseases such as RA, and number of ischemic heart events during atherosclerosis correlate with APP levels.

Other cytokines like IL-10 decreses cytokine and PGE_2 formation by monocytes. TGF beta which also serves as immunosuppresant, reduces inflammation and increases extracellular matrix formation required for repair. This activity of TGF beta is kept under control by IFN gamma which inhibits collagen production and also has myelosuppressive activity.

- ***Metabolic role*: It is likely that the body wasting and cachexia seen with severe disease states is due to the catabolic properties of TNF.

Although over 200 cytokines have been detected and shown to be involved in physiological functions and mediation of certain diseases like cancer, infection, allergy etc., only a few are proven to be clinically useful.

Human recombinant IL-2 (Aldesleukin) though structurally different from native IL-2, enhances lymphocyte proliferation, cytotoxic and killer cell activity and IFN gamma activity, all of which contribute to activation of cellular immunity. It is presently used in therapy of melanoma and metastatic renal cell carcinoma. For therapeutic uses of gamma interferon, see Chapter 57; of growth factors, G CSF and GM CSF, Chapter 34; and of TNF antagonists, Chapter 71.

Platelet activating factor (PAF-acether): This ether-linked phospholipid possess a wide range of activities. It is released during mast cell degranulation and is implicated in pathophysiological states including allergic inflammation, anaphylactic shock and bronchial asthma. It is also formed by eosinophils, macrophages, neutrophils, vascular endothelium and the renal medullary cells. Like the eicosanoids, PAF is not stored in the cells but is synthesized and released in response to stimuli.

It is a potent vasodilator. It activates most inflammatory cells and is believed to be responsible for mobilisation of eosinophils, neutrophils and/or platelets in lungs after exposure to the allergen. Intradermal injection of PAF in man causes a biphasic inflammatory response in the skin, with acute and late onset components similar to the response to moderate doses of allergens in sensitized individuals. Given by aerosol inhalation, it causes dose dependent broncho-constriction and inflammation of airways. Increased microvascular permeability causes edema of the airways. Further, it also induces non-specific bronchial hyper-responsiveness in non-asthmatic human subjects. It promotes platelet aggregation and release of TXA_2, acts as a chemotactic agent and is a gastric ulcerogen.

A substance called **Ginkgolides** isolated from the extract of the tree *Ginkgo biloba* has been used in China for the treatment of asthma and other disorders. It has been reported to exert specific PAF receptor antagonistic activity. Thus, it causes inhibition of PAF induced platelet aggregation, of degranulation of isolated, human neutrophils, and of oxygen free radical production by the human neutrophils. Its possible use in the treatment of bronchial asthma and other allergic disorders is under investigation.

SECTION VI
Drugs Used in Respiratory Disorders

Pharmacotherapy of Cough 25

Cough, a protective reflex, helps to expel irritant matter from the respiratory tract. This is necessary for preventing mechanical obstruction to breathing. Stimulation of the mucosal Rapidly Adapting Receptors (RAR) and C fibre receptors/ending in the respiratory tract at sites such as pharynx, larynx, trachea or bronchi generates tussal impulses. These are carried by afferent fibres in the vagus and sympathetic nerves to the brain stem nucleus solitarius which is connected to the respiration related neurons in the central cough generator (**cough centre**). The latter initiates the act of coughing. C fibre receptors are chemoreceptors, highly sensitive to bradykinin, capsaicin and H ions (pH).

The respiratory mucosa contains cells bearing cilia which beat actively to transport the locally produced mucus towards the throat, from where it can be either coughed out or swallowed to keep the respiratory tract clean (*mucociliary clearance*). This mucociliary clearance can be defective or even absent in persons with immotile, dysfunctional or congenitally absent cilia.This leads to retention of secretions in the respiratory tract and recurrent respiratory infections including sinusitis and bronchiectasis. In turn, respiratory infection impairs the mucociliary clearance further, with worsening of the infection.Chronic cough is an important symptom in these patients.

The act of coughing involves an initial deep inspiration followed by forced expiration against a temporarily closed glottis. Closure of the glottis causes an increase in intrathoracic pressure. When the glottis opens suddenly, the pulmonary air is forced through the trachea almost at the speed of sound, throwing out the respiratory tract secretions as expectoration. The cough reflex has a tremendous reserve capacity and most coughs are greatly in excess of that required to expel particulate material. Furthermore, the strong expiration leads to a stronger succeeding inspiration and thus produces a vicious cycle in the form of a fit of coughing. Cough may be :

- ***Productive***, associated with a large amount of sputum; or
- ***Non-productive and dry.***

Environmental pollutants may cause cough by irritating the lungs, trachea or bronchi. Smoking cigarettes is a well known cause of chronic persistent cough. Cough due to the inhalation of allergens such as dust, chemicals and pollen is commonly observed in asthmatics. The commonest cause of transient cough is common cold, and is due to post-nasal drip that stimulates receptors in the upper respiratory tract. A similar mechanism probably operates in case of chronic persistent cough observed in persons with allergic rhinitis, chronic sinusitis and obstruction due to enlarged adenoids. Enlarged, infected tonsils, an abnormally elongated uvula or nasal polyps can also cause chronic persistent cough.

Other important causes of cough are :

- ***Upper respiratory tract infections***, which are self-limiting or persistent.
- ***Acute lung infections** and **pleural diseases*** where therapy of the underlying cause will relieve cough.
- ***Chronic pulmonary diseases*** like asthma, chronic bronchitis, bronchiectasis, tuberculosis and lung cancer where symptomatic treatment for cough is essential along with the specific therapy.
- ***Secondary to acute LVF***, which calls for immediate attention to the cardiac condition.
- ***Gastroesophageal reflux disease*** (GERD): (Chapter 42).
- ***Drug-induced cough*** : see Table 25.1.

Table 25.1 : Some drugs which induce cough

- ACE inhibitors such as captopril.
- Beta blockers.
- Inhaled corticosteroids and disodium chromoglycate.
- Nebulized acetylcysteine.
- Amiodarone.
- Iodides.
- Inhaled ether

Outside the respiratory tract, disorders of the external auditory canal and ear drum, pericardium and even of stomach can give rise to chronic non-productive cough. Thus, wax impacted in the ear, inflammation or eczema or even irritation of the drum by hair have all been known to cause dry cough. The entity called 'psychogenic cough' is well known; it is non-productive and not present during sleep, usually becoming worse with emotional stress.

Definitive treatment of cough depends upon its cause which should be treated. Stoppage of smoking would correct chronic cough in smokers. Mild acute cough generally does not need drugs. Only when cough serves no useful purpose and causes insomnia, or interferes with daily work, symptomatic treatment is indicated.

In case of productive cough, the patient should be encouraged to cough voluntarily in appropriate posture from time to time. In cases of bronchiectasis or lung abscess, postural drainage aided by percussion of the chest is useful. Since inflamed trachea or bronchi are irritated by cold or dry air, a warm room with humid atmosphere is beneficial, particularly during the cold season when the respiratory tract fluid is reduced in quantity. Many patients with cough feel comfortable after a cup of hot tea or even hot water; and *simple steam inhalation effectively liquifies tenacious respiratory tract secretions* (Hydroponic therapy).

Cough can be

(1) **Acute** self limiting (less than 3 weeks);

(2) **Subacute** (3-8 weeks) or

(3) **Chronic** more than 8 weeks).

Acute cough such as during and after cold is usually due to upper respiratory viral infection. Non viral causes include environmental pollution, asthma, cough –variant asthma and occupational exposure. From therapeutic point of view, chronic cough with normal chest X'ray can be either (a) **glucocorticoid responsive,** due to eosinophilic disorders as in asthma, eosinophilic bronchitis and allergic rhinitis; or (b) **inhaled glucocorticoid resistant** e.g. postnasal drip, GERD, post-respiratory infection and drug induced.

Barking cough, stridor and chest wall withdrawal are characteristic of **croup,** common in children. Cough becomes worse at night. Nebulized budesonide or oral/IM dexamethasone (0.2-0.6 mg/kg, single dose) gives dramatic relief. As dexamethasone effect lasts for 2-4 days, second dose is rarely required. Nebulized adrenaline gives immediate but short lived relief.

Drugs used in the symptomatic treatment of cough are called **antitussives** (tussis : Latin for 'cough'). They are used for immediate symptomatic relief and are not a substitutes for the specific therapy of the underlying cause.

Antitussives - classification :

I **Pharyngeal demulcents and local sialogogues,** e.g., syrups and linctuses.

II **Expectorants which increase the respiratory tract fluid,** e.g., Ammonium salt.

III **Central cough suppressants,**

- ***Opioids and related drugs*** e.g. Codeine, Hydrocodone, Dextromethorphan, Pholcodeine, Levopropoxyphene, Noscapine
- ***Non-opioids*** e.g., Caramiphene, Pipezethate.
- ***Antihistaminics*** e.g. Diphenhydramine, Chlorcyclizine.

IV **Peripherally acting compounds:**

- ***Local anaesthetics*** e.g. Benzonatate, Levodropropizine and Nebulised lignocaine.
- ***Mucolytics*** that help by liquefying thick secretions; and
- ***Anticholinergics*** e.g. Ipratropium bromide by metered dose inhalation (Chapter 26).

Pharyngeal Demulcents

Demulcents are useful in cough due to irritation of the pharyngeal mucosa above the epiglottis. They are administered in the form of lozenges, troches, cough drops or linctuses. They act by increasing the flow of saliva, the best natural demulcent which produces a protective and soothing effect. The 'syrup' part of most cough syrups serves the same function. Salivary secretion can be increased by such simple methods as using a few lemon drops, candy sugar, glycerrhiza or drops of lemon juice in a syrupy base. Costly preparations like lozenges and troches containing multiple ingredients such as menthol and antiseptics are usually unnecessary and wasteful.

Expectorants

The Latin word 'expectorare' means 'to drive from the chest'. Expectorants are the drugs which increase the production of demulcent respiratory tract fluid that covers and protects the irritated mucosa. These drugs are useful in the treatment of useless cough due to irritation of the respiratory mucosa *below the epiglottis* and respiratory conditions in which the secretion is thick and viscid, needing liquefaction.

Expectorants can stimulate the output of respiratory tract fluid either directly or reflexly; the latter group is also called as **reflex expectorants.**

Direct stimulants: Volatile oils like oil of eucalyptus, anise and lemon, administered orally or inhaled with steam, increase the respiratory secretions probably by a direct action. Alcohol and cedar wood oil (active ingredient terpene hydrochloride), added to steam inhalation, have a similar effect. Large doses of creosote and guaiacol have also been shown to possess this action in animals; and glyceryl guaiacolate forms an important ingredient of many commercial cough mixtures. However, their usefulness is limited.

Reflex expectorants: These drugs act by stimulating the gastric reflex which helps to increase the respiratory secretions. Obviously, they produce mild irritation of the gastric mucosa and may produce nausea and sometimes vomiting. Thus, emetic drugs in subemetic doses increase bronchial secretion producing a less tenacious sputum, easier to expectorate. Certain salts which produce such an action are called as **saline expectorants.**

Ipecacuanha containing an alkaloid emetine is sometimes used as an expectorant. Tincture ipecacuanha 1 ml may increase the respiratory tract fluid and lower the viscosity of the sputum. However, it often produces anorexia and nausea.

Saline expectorants:

Ammonium salts such as ammonium carbonate were used in the past as saline expectorants. They cause anorexia and nausea, and are no more used.

POTASSIUM SALTS: **Potassium iodide** is the commonly employed salt for this purpose. It probably acts both directly and reflexly. It increases the respiratory secretion, and has a reputation for liquefying the thick, viscid fluid. Potassium iodide is generally advocated in productive cough associated with chronic bronchitis, asthma and emphysema. It is administered orally in a dose of 300 mg. thrice daily in mixture form. The mixture has a slightly bitter saline taste. Watery solution decomposes on standing, liberating iodine.

Potassium iodide can cause symptoms of iodism, characterised by nasal catarrh, conjunctival swelling, edema of eyelids, lacrimation, edema of the larynx, headache and various types of skin rashes. Chronic administration occasionally gives rise to goitre and may rarely cause hypothyroidism. It should be avoided in children and pregnant women.

Potassium citrate is much less effective than potassium iodide though it is less unpleasant.

The active alkaloid, **vasicine**, and its derivative **vasicinone,** from the leaves of *Adhatoda vasaca,* possess weak bronchodilator, expectorant and mucolytic properties. The crude extract of this plant leaves in syrupy base appears to be safe and effective and has been used as a home remedy in India for ages.

Central Cough Suppressants

These drugs inhibit the cough reflex by directly acting on the cough centre in the medulla and are useful in the symptomatic relief of dry irritant cough. They are only partially successful in suppressing cough due to irritation of the carina. However, they do reduce the intensity and the frequency of cough. These drugs are invaluable in the treatment of cough due to pleural diseases. Cough suppressants are particularly useful when complications of severe cough, such as rib fracture or cough syncope, produce discomfort. They should not generally be used in patients with productive cough, especially if they are elderly, not fully alert, or neurologically impaired. However, in general, cough suppressants do not impair voluntary coughing to clear secretions. *Cough suppressants are not recommended in young children and should not be administered to those below the age of two year.* They are :

CODEINE: This alkaloid of opium resembles morphine in its actions. Like morphine, it depresses the cough centre but is less constipating. Tolerance is not common and drug dependence is rare. A commonly employed preparation is linctus codeine which contains 15 mg. of codeine phosphate in 5 ml. Dose: 5 ml. by mouth. It can also be used as an analgesic. It is a relatively safe drug and its only bothersome adverse effect is constipation. *Codeine preparations are not recommended in children.*

Codeine is unlikely to be effective in the distressful cough of terminal lung cancer. In that condition, **diamorphine** linctus (3 mg./5 ml.) in the dose of 2.5-10 ml. every 4 hours or **methadone** linctus (2 mg./5 ml.) in the dose of 2.5 - 5ml. every 4 hours is likely to be effective.

With several opioids, the dose required to suppress cough is lower than the analgesic dose. Further, the antitussive action of opioids is antagonized by naloxone to a smaller extent than their analgesic action. *This has led to the belief that distinct receptors (other than the usual opioid receptors) mediate the antitussive action of opioids.*

DEXTROMETHORPHAN HYDROBROMIDE : It is the d-isomer of codeine analogue methorphan. However, it does not act through the opioid receptors and has no analgesic or sedative property. It acts centrally to elevate the threshold for coughing. It is as effective as codeine and is much safer; hence, it is commonly used in pediatric practice. It does not depress respiration in the usual doses. It can sometimes cause excitement, irritability and confusion. Adult dose : 10-20 mg. every 6-8 hours (maximum 120 mg./day). It is a drug of abuse.

Levopropoxyphene mesylate : This levo-isomer of dextropropoxyphene, in the dose of 50-100 mg, appears to be as effective as an antitussive as 30 mg of dextropropoxyphene. It has no analgesic activity.

Pholcodeine, though related to opioids, has no opioid-like action. It is as effective as codeine as a cough suppressant, with a longer duration of action. It is non-sedative and non-addictive. It is a common constituent of OTC cough mixtures.

NOSCAPINE (Coscopin) : This opium alkaloid, belonging to benzylisoquinoline group, has a smooth muscle relaxant action like papaverine. Its antitussive action is approximately equal to that of codeine. It does not produce constipation or drowsiness. Addiction does not occur. The common side effect is occasional nausea. The antitussive dose is 15-30 mg. 3-4 times a day. *Large doses can cause bronchospasm and hypotension due to histamine release.*

The **other synthetic compounds** used include oxeladine, pipezethate and piperidone. There is no convincing evidence about their superiority over codeine. All cough suppressants are dangerous in the presence of excessive secretions as failure to expel them may produce mechanical obstruction and atelectasis of the lung. They are also contraindicated in the presence of respiratory failure.

Peripherally Acting Agents

Benzonatate (Benz), chemically related to procaine, probably acts on the stretch and cough receptors in the lungs. It also possesses some central action and can cause sedation and headache. It is not recommended below the age of 10 years. The dose is 100 mg tid.

Levodropropizine (Rapitus), another non-opioid antitussive, has mechanism of action and uses similar to those of benzonatate.

Lignocaine in nebulised form is used for suppressing cough during pharyngeal examination and bronchoscopy.

Other Antitussives

Cough may be the only symptom of bronchial hyper-responsiveness, including asthma. **Bronchodilators** are useful in these cases, as bronchospasm aggravates and may even initiate cough. The drugs commonly used are: salbutamol, orciprenaline and ephedrine.

An **inhaled glucocorticoid** (Chapter 26) may be prescribed for **a short period** (2-3 weeks) for symptomatic treatment of **persistent** cough following a viral respiratory infection.

Therapeutic usefulness of **antihistaminics** as antitussives is limited to the cases where cough is due to conditions associated with post-nasal drip. They are of little value in the treatment of allergic bronchospasm and may even have a deleterious effect because of their drying effect on the bronchial secretion. Antihistaminics with a sedative action may be useful in children who do not sleep because of cough, provided no contraindication to their use (such as bronchial pathology) exists. However, they may cause paradoxical excitement in them. Anti-infective agents such as antibiotics are useful in controlling cough due to respiratory infections.

Sympathomimetic decongestants present in some cough mixtures can cause nervousness, insomnia, hallucinations, hypertension and dystonic reactions especially in children. The use of **phenylpropanolamine** (PPA) in cough mixtures *has been banned by FDA* (USA) as it may cause hemorrhagic stroke. *Many commercially available preparations in India promoted for cough and cold contain PPA.* The safety of other oral decongestants such as pseudoephedrine and phenylephrine is unclear.

The commonest cause of cough is common cold, a viral infection which usually clears within 7 days. Most of the proprietary preparations available as "cough remedies" generally contain a central cough suppressant, an expectorant, an antihistaminic, a bronchodilator and a decongestant in pleasantly flavoured syrupy base. Multiplicity of such preparations itself indicates that there is no ideal remedy for cough. Such remedies may cause more harm than good, as they may dry up the secretions, prevent natural drainage, cause drowsiness and suppress cough, a protective reflex that helps to get rid of infective material.

Mucolytic Agents

These drugs are used to make the sputum thin and less viscid, so that it can be easily expectorated. Many patients with chest disease become dehydrated and adequate hydration along with steam inhalation or aerosolised water inhalation can help to liquify viscid sputum. Finally, oxygen should never be administered without adequate humidification as dry oxygen causes drying of the respiratory mucosa (Chapter 73).

ACETYLCYSTEINE (Airbron): This is a derivative of a naturally occurring amino acid, 1-cysteine. It reduces viscosity of sputum *in vitro*. The drug is rapidly metabolized in the body. Clinically, 2ml. of 10% solution are nebulized into a face mask every 8 hours for 5-10 days to liquefy viscous tracheobronchial secretions. It can also be administered by direct instillation into the tracheobronchial tree through a tracheostomy, a bronchoscope or a percutaneous intratracheal catheter, or as an aerosol.

Adverse reactions effects include bronchospasm, fever, nausea, vomiting, stomatitis, rhinorrhoea and haemoptysis. It reacts with most metals and with rubber.

Carbocysteine and methylcysteine (Visclair) have similar properties as acetyleysteine.

BROMHEXINE (Bisolvon) : This is a synthetic benzylamine derivative of alkaloid vasicine obtained from the plant *Adhatoda vasaca.* It is given orally, parenterally and by inhalation. Experimentally, the drug reduces the viscosity of sputum by dissolving muco-polysaccharide fibres. It is usually administered in doses of 8-16 mg. thrice daily. Adverse reactions are minor and infrequent. It can be combined with bronchodilators.

AMBROXOL (Mucolite): This is an active metabolite of bromhexine, and it is used orally in the dose of 15 mg tid as an alternative to bromhexine.

Dornase alpha : This phosphorylated, glycosylated, recombinant, human deoxyribo-nuclease, given by nebulization, can decrease the viscosity of purulent sputum by cleaving long strands of denatured DNA that are released by degenerating neutrophils. It acts extracellularly and does not affect living material. It improves lung function and is well tolerated. It is moderately effective in patients with cystic fibrosis.

It must be remembered that cough serves the useful purpose of clearing the respiratory tract. It should not be severely obtunded in patients with productive cough. Use of antitussives in sedated or debilitated patients may prove dangerous. They should be used cautiously in the acute phase of pertussis and bronchial asthma, as inspissation of mucus plugs may contribute to fatal outcome. The possible anti-tussive effect of pain relieving drugs such as morphine must be kept in mind while prescribing them in post-operative patients. *Finally, cough suppressants, especially in syrupy base, should be kept out of the reach of small children, as poisoning with them has been reported.*

Pharmacotherapy of Bronchial Asthma, COPD and Rhinitis 26

Bronchial asthma is a clinical syndrome characterized by cough/paroxysmal dyspnea and wheeze due to increased resistance to air flow through the narrowed bronchi. The narrowing of the bronchi is brought about by

- ***Bronchospasm.***
- ***Infiltration and edema of the bronchial mucosa;*** and
- ***Blockage of the bronchial lumen by inspissated mucus.***

The diagnosis of asthma is made in a patient with obstructive airway disease by objective evidence of *variability in ventilatory function over time or improvement following bronchodilator treatment.*

Pathophysiology: The etiology of bronchial asthma is multifactorial : genetic, developmental, environmental, inflammatory and immunological. Its pathogenesis is complex and involves (a) inflammation; and (b) re-modelling of the airways.

Many patients have had well defined allergen exposures which are partly or substantially responsible for the asthmatic inflammation. These patients (even the asymptomatic ones, with normal lung function and no recent acute asthmatic episode) have inflamed airways and infiltration with mast cells, basophils, eosinophils, macrophages and T lymphocytes. *Lymphocyte - directed eosinophilc bronchitis is the hallmark of asthma.* Mediators released from the eosinophils are toxic to the bronchial epithelium and cause its sloughing. Such subacute mucosal inflammation and disruption

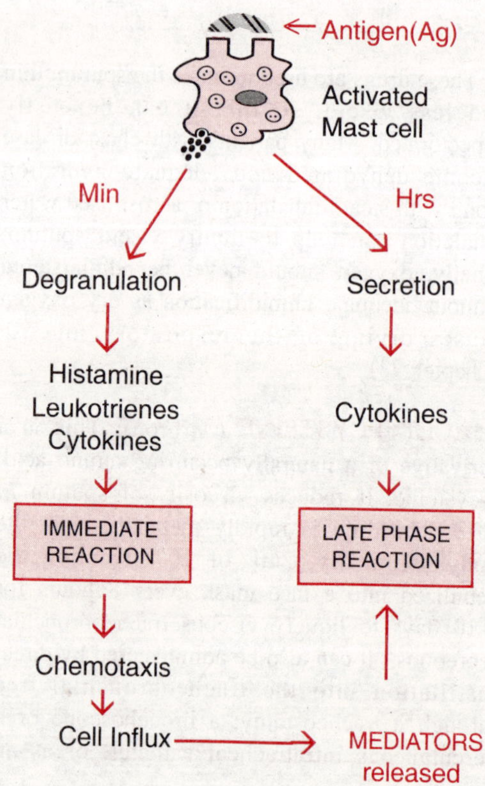

Fig. 26.1: Mast cell dependant immediate and late phase reactions

of the epithelial barrier on the mucosal surface may contribute to **bronchial hyper-responsiveness**, an exaggerated response to a variety of stimuli (*asthmatic diathesis*). This inflammation is clinically silent with no apparent bronchoconstriction during the basal state of the disease. Exposure to an antigen causes cross-linking of IgE bound to the surface of mast cells. A clinical acute attack is produced when the concerned antigen binds to the mast cell which then gets activated and degranulates, with the release of histamine and various cytokines (**Early Reaction**). This results in bronchospasm, local vasodilatation, increased capillary permeability, and chemotaxis, with consequent influx of more inflammatory cells into the walls of the bronchi. The newly arrived cells release mediators which aggravate the airway inflammation and cause further bronchoconstriction (**Late Phase Reaction**). An attack may also be triggered by factors such as viral infection, irritants like dust and other air pollutants, cold air, exercise, drugs, chemicals and histamine.Thus, the final common pathway for a clinical attack of asthma is the release of many mediators (Table 26.1) from a variety of inflammatory cells. The airway hyper-responsiveness may persist for weeks after the acute insult has abated.

Table 26.1: Some important mediators released by mast cells and leucocytes

From granules
Histamine, Heparin
Tryptase, Chymotrypsine, Proteases
From lipids
Sulfidopeptide leukotrienes
Prostaglandins, PAF
Proinflammatory cytokines
TNF α and interleukins 3, 4, 5,13.

Majority of asthmatics (80%) are **atopic**, forming IgE antibody on exposure to common environmental allergens, house-dust, mites, cockroaches, pets, pollen and so on. In such atopic subjects, challenge of the airways with allergens to which they are specifically sensitive leads to early and late phases of bronchoconstriction. Mast cells are important in the acute airway response to an allergen and may also contribute to their remodelling in chronic asthma.

The **early reaction** is rapid in onset, reaching maximum in 15-30 min. after challenge and recovering over next 24 hours. Degranulation of mast cells with mediator release is probably an important mechanism involved in early response.

Late-phase bronchoconstriction response begins 4-6 hours after challenge and lasts for up to 24 hours. During this late phase reaction, the airways become non-specifically hyper-responsive to stimuli such as histamine, which may last up to two weeks after a single allergen exposure. During this late (but not early) reaction, there occurs influx of neutrophils, eosinophils and macrophages into the airways which suggests their role in the pathogenesis of this reaction and associated increase in bronchial hyperresponsiveness. Although a large number of chemical mediators are released during allergic reaction, particular attention has been focused on the role of sulphido-peptide leukotrienes, interleukins and platelet activating factor (PAF-acether) as being candidate mediators responsible for hyperresponsiveness. The acute inflammatory response usually resolves with the repair process restoring normal structure and function.

In **chronic asthma**, the recovery is incomplete due to ineffective repair. This leads to remodelling of the airway structure. Persistent epithelial damage and the loss of its protective function expose the deeper airway structures to further insults, leading to persistent inflammation and cellular infiltration. Various mediators released cause angiogenesis, smooth muscle proliferation, fibrosis and thickening of the airways, leading to persistent obstruction to airflow. Various enzymes and growth factors are important in this remodelling process.

Asthma is considered as :

- ***Extrinsic*** when it is associated with history

of atopy in patient's childhood, a family history of allergies, illnesses like hay fever, positive skin tests, and raised serum IgE level. This type starts in childhood or at an early age and usually manifests clinically in 'episodic form;' and

- ***Intrinsic*** when it occurs in middle aged subjects with no family history of allergies, and clinically assumes a 'chronic form'; there is a lack of identifiable allergen; plasma IgE is not raised.

This classification would appear to imply that there is an allergic factor in extrinsic asthma but none in intrinsic asthma. This is not strictly true and an allergic factor may be involved in many cases of intrinsic asthma as well.

Bronchial narrowing causes hyperinflation of the alveoli and disruption of alveolar walls with loss of elastic tissue (emphysema-like picture). It promotes infection distal to the obstruction and leads to hypoxemia (reduction in arterial oxygen tension) and hypercapnia (increase in arterial CO_2 tension). Prolonged hypoxemia may cause pulmonary hypertension and right ventricular failure. Hypercapnia causes cerebral vasodilatation, rise in intracranial tension, mental confusion, twitching, drowsiness and finally coma. In severely ill patients, unregulated treatment with oxygen aggravates hypercapnia and the respiratory failure.

Prolonged asthmatic attacks produce dehydration as the patient cannot eat or drink during the illness.

Clinically, bronchial asthma presents as :

I **Mild intermittent asthma :** The patient gets discrete, infrequent, acute attacks, which are relieved by bronchodilator drugs with no disability between the attacks. In these cases, there is often a recognisable precipitating factor such as allergy, an upper respiratory tract infection or psychological trauma.

II **Chronic persistent asthma:** This is generally due to the presence of inflammation and thickening of mucosa of the bronchioles with resultant excessive secretion of mucus, decreased elastic recoil of the lung tissue because of destructive changes in the alveolar walls and finally hyperreactivity of the bronchi with bronchospasm. In such patients, symptoms are persistent and relief of bronchospasm with drugs is incomplete.

Chronic form can be subdivided into **mild, moderate** and **severe** grades, depending on the interference with daily activities and with sleep, and the degree of incapacity. Clinically, there is more or less persistent dyspnoea and wheeze, with superadded **acute attacks**. In some patients, chronic asthma co-exists with COPD.

III **Severe acute asthma (Status asthmaticus):** This is a condition where an acute attack is severe, persistent and does not respond to standard treatment with beta adrenergic stimulants; it is accompanied by evidence of respiratory insufficiency or failure.

IV **Exercise-induced asthma** in which the attack is precipitated by exercise or following inhalation of cold air.

Principles of therapy: Treatment is directed toward (1) relieving bronchospasm; and (2) reducing the inflammation. The important aims of therapy are prevention of repeated attacks and enabling the subject to live as normal a life as possible, including normal exercise tolerance, without causing severe adverse reactions.

The focus of treatment has now shifted from bronchodilator therapy to anti-inflammatory therapy. The available therapeutic measures are:

- ***Elimination of the trigger factors,*** e.g., allergens, upper respiratory infection and environmental pollution.
- ***Avoiding respiratory irritants,*** eg., smoking and environmental — occupational pollutants.
- ***Drug therapy***, which forms the most important part of the management, includes the use of bronchodilators and anti-inflammatory drugs.
- ***Correction of dehydration and acidosis in severe acute attack.***
- ***Controlled administration of oxygen, when needed.***
- ***Physical exercise*: A programme of graded exercise training to improve the sense of well

being and exercise tolerance. As physical exercise tends to precipitate acute attacks in some patients, an exercise which does not precipitate such attacks (e.g., swimming) is preferred in these patients; and

- ***Psychological treatment*** which by itself is rarely of much help, except in functional cases. A sympathetic discussion of the patient's problems and patient education about his disease are, however, very helpful.

Antiasthmatics - classification :

I **Bronchodilators:**

- ***Selective beta$_2$ adrenergic receptor agonists***:

(a) *Short acting* e.g. Salbutamol, Isoetharine, Bitolterol, (a prodrug), Fenoterol and Rimeterol; and (b) *Long acting* such as Salmeterol and Formoterol.

- ***Non-selective beta adrenergic agonists*** e.g. Orciprenaline, Adrenaline and Ephedrine.
- ***Phosphodiesterase inhibitors*** : theophylline derivatives such as Aminophylline.
- ***Anticholinergics*** such as Ipratropium bromide.

II **Anti-inflammatory drugs:**

- ***Glucocorticoids***.
- ***Leukotriene (LT) modifiers***:

(a) LT receptor antagonists: Montelukast; Zafirlukast.

(b) LT synthesis inhibitors: Zileuton;

- ***Mast cell stabilizers*** : Sodium cromoglycate; Nedocromil.
- ***PAF antagonists***: Ketotifen.

III **Anti IgE antibody :** Omalizumab.

Whenever possible, the drug therapy should be given by inhalation. This route is convenient, promptly effective and reduces the systemic toxicity. It is carried out by using:

(1) **Pressurised, metered dose (aerosol) inhalers** (PMDI) which deliver small doses of the drugs.

(2) **Nebulisers** which deliver much larger doses; and

(3) **Dry powder inhalers:** The disadvantages of this method are the irritation of the airways; less stability during storage; and the difficulty that the children, the old and the very ill may have in generating the high inspiratory air flow needed to operate the system.

Faulty inhalation technique is an important cause of treatment failure. Patients who find the inhalation route inconvenient or difficult to follow are given oral drug therapy which invariably causes more systemic adverse effects.

Drug Therapy During an Acute Attack

Drugs used to treat an acute attack are called **rescue drugs**. *Beta$_2$ adrenergic receptor agonists are the rescue drugs par excellence as both airway smooth muscle and mast cells have beta$_2$-adrenergic receptors.* These drugs

- ***Relax the smooth muscle of all airways*** from trachea to the terminal bronchi, irrespective of the spasmogen involved. Therefore, they serve as **physiological antagonists**.
- ***Enhance mucociliary clearance from the respiratory tract.***
- ***Suppress microvascular leakage in the airway.***
- ***Inhibit mediator release from the mast cells and the basophils, and cytokine release from the inflammatory cells in the airway;*** and
- ***May inhibit release of acetylcholine*** from the postganglionic cholinergic nerves in the respiratory tract.

These drugs, however, do not inhibit either the late response to allergens or the subsequent bronchial hyper-responsiveness.

The short acting selective beta$_2$ adrenergic stimulants are the preferred rescue drugs. As the pathophysiology of asthma is restricted to the airways, their direct, local delivery to the airways is the preferred method of administration. With all the methods of local administration, only about 10-30% of the administered drug reaches the desired site, the distal bronchial tree. The rest is swallowed but undergoes extensive first pass metabolism, thus minimizing the systemic adverse effects. There is no evidence that any drug from this class or any method of administration is superior to others, except with regard to the duration of action. The choice depends upon the convenience and the cost. Salbutamol is described as the prototype of this class.

SALBUTAMOL (Albuterol, Ventolin, Asthalin): This selective β_2-adrenergic agonist is chemically related to isoprenaline. (Chapter 17)

- ***It has a prominent bronchodilator action of rapid onset*** (1-5 minutes after inhalation).
- ***It has poor cardiac (beta$_1$ receptor) action.*** Hence, it causes less palpitation or a rise of blood pressure; and
- ***It is resistant to inactivation by COMT and, therefore, has a longer duration of action.*** The action of a single inhalation or a single oral dose lasts for about 4-6 hours.

Methods of Administration: It is more rapidly effective ***by pressurised metered dose inhalation (MDI)*** (dose 100 micrograms / puff) than orally (dose 2-4 mg.). Each inhalation may improve the effectiveness of subsequent inhalations. The dose must be prescribed clearly as "so many puffs at a time and the maximum number of puffs per day." It may also be given SC or IM in the dose of 0.5 mg. every 4 hours and IV slowly, in the dose of 0.25 mg. at the rate of 5-10 mcg. per minute. Tremor, particularly of the hands, is an adverse effect.

When a patient is prescribed an inhaler, he must be taught to synchronise the actuation of the inhaler with inspiration, in order to maximise the delivery of the drug to the lungs (Table 26.2).

Table 26.2: Technique of using a pressurised inhaler when a spacer is not available

- Shake the container thoroughly.
- Hold the mouthpiece of the inhaler 4 cm. away from the open mouth or use the spacer.
- Breathe out slowly and completely.
- Discharge the inhaler while taking a slow, deep breath (5-6 seconds).
- Hold the breath in full inspiration for 10 seconds.

Children, old people and those who are breathless find such synchronisation difficult. Further, the velocity of the aerosol causes the latter to impinge on the oropharynx, leading to the decreased delivery of the drug to airways. *Spacers* are available (Fig. 26.2) which reduce the velocity of the aerosol and allow more of the drug to reach the airways. The coordination between actuation of the aerosol and inspiration is less critical when a spacer is used.

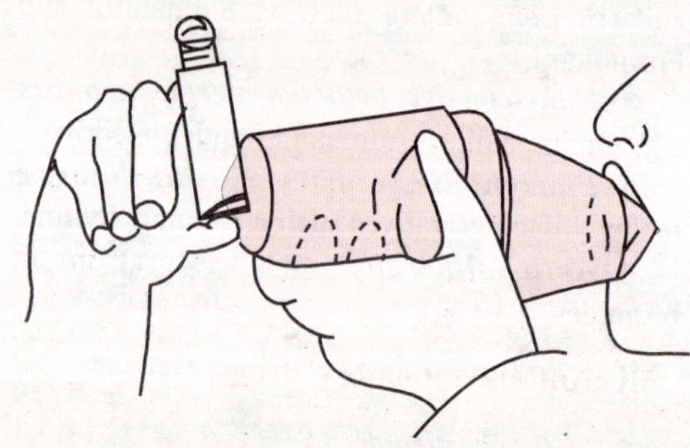

Fig. 26.2 : Spacer

Salbutamol may also be administered **by a nebuliser.** The dose administered (2-5 mg.) is much larger than that by a puff of the inhaler (100 mcg.). The drug can also be administered **by a dry-powder inhaler.**

Salbutamol is used in mild intermittent asthma on 'as needed' basis. In an acute attack, it must be administered in adequate doses such as 10-12 puffs in one hour. Inadequate dosage is the cause of apparent 'resistance'.

Levosalbutamol (Levolin): Salbutamol is a racemate. The active compound levosalbutamol is available in 50 mcg/puff MDI. It is claimed to be superior to salbutamol.

Isoetharine, terbutaline, fenoterol, bitolterol and rimiterol are other selective short acting β_2

agonists with similar properties as salbutamol.

Short acting beta$_2$ adrenergic agonists are very effective for:

(1) Treating acute attacks of asthma; and

(2) Prevention of exercise-induced asthma.

They are less useful when taken regularly, and hence should be used only as needed.

They are safe during pregnancy.

Beta$_2$ agonists are also useful in treating wheezing following upper respiratory tract viral infection in infants and children under 5 years and are used orally in **syrup** form or by a nebuliser.

They are likely to be ineffective in the occasional patient who uses a beta blocker. In such a patient, aminophylline is preferred.

All beta$_2$ agonists can cause muscle tremor. The use of fenoterol, a more potent beta$_2$ agonist than salbutamol, has been associated with greater cardiac toxicity in patients with acute asthma. *Excessive use of beta$_2$ agonists has been associated with asthma deaths.*

It must be kept in mind that all beta-adrenergic agonists may cause hypokalemia; the latter can be aggravated by concurrent use of theophylline and its derivatives, diuretics and glucocorticoids, and by hypoxemia.

ORCIPRENALINE (Metaproterenol, Alupent): This derivative of isoprenaline is effective orally, parenterally and by inhalation. *It stimulates both β_1 and β_2 receptors.* Thus it is less selective than salbutamol. It is given orally (20 mg qid); or IM/SC 0.5-1 mg.

Adrenaline hydrochloride: This is a potent bronchodilator. It also relieves pulmonary congestion by constricting the pulmonary arterioles.

It is administered SC in the dose of 0.2 to 0.5 ml. of a 1 in 1000 aqueous solution. It is effective within a few minutes. The drug is injected slowly and no further injection is given if the attack subsides. The relief of an acute attack by adrenaline is generally dramatic but may be accompanied by unpleasant palpitation and tremulousness. To be maximally effective, it has to be injected early in an attack and hence, it is an advantage for the patient to be able to inject it himself. *This, however, carries the risk of overtreatment by the patient. Further, before injecting the drug, one must be certain that the tip of the needle is not in a vein.*

The use of adrenaline in the presence of cardiac damage and/or hypoxia can cause sudden death. It can cause serious toxicity in patients receiving tricyclic antidepressants like imipramine (Chapter 13). Because of the inconvenience of the parenteral administration and its toxicity, *it is no more recommended for routine use. Adrenaline solution that is even slightly coloured must not be used.*

Ephedrine (15-30 mg), if taken early, orally may abort an acute attack. It is a cheap, easily available and relatively safe medication for treating mild acute attacks of asthma, but lacks selectivity (Chapter 17). It was used extensively in the past.

AMINOPHYLLINE: This is a stable mixture of theophylline and ethylene diamine; the latter makes theophylline more water soluble (Chapter 12). Given IV slowly, it:

- ***Causes bronchodilatation by its weak and non-selective inhibition of pulmonary enzyme PDE4.***
- ***Inhibits adenosine receptors in the airways.***
- ***Inhibits the late response to allergens*** but does not inhibit the release of mediators.
- ***Acts synergistically with beta adrenergic agonists.***

It is less effective orally. Given rapidly IV, it may cause nausea, vomiting, cardiac arrhythmias and collapse. *Deaths have been reported following rapid IV aminophylline, particularly in the presence of cardiac damage.* Rapid IV administration can also cause twitching of the facial muscles, severe hyperventilation and seizures. This can be controlled by diazepam or phenytoin. The repeated use of theophylline in children may cause learning difficulties and sleep disturbances. It is safer than adrenaline in hypoxic subjects in status asthmaticus, and in patients with concomitant cardiac disease. *It is especially helpful when one cannot decide whether a given attack is one of bronchial or cardiac asthma.*

Therapeutic uses:

- ***Acute attack of asthma*:** If treatment with inhaled selective beta$_2$ agonists in adequate doses fails to relieve an acute attack in about half to one hour, **aminophylline** is administered by IV infusion in a dose of 5 mg./kg. over 15-30 minutes, followed by 0.5-1 mg./kg. per hour for several hours. The infusion rate should be reduced in patients with cirrhosis, pneumonia, acute viral infection and congestive heart failure and in patients receiving cimetidine and erythromycin which interfere with metabolic degradation of drugs by the hepatic microsomal CYP450. Smokers may need a larger dose.
- ***Chronic persistent asthma*:** Slow release preparations may be useful in patients with persistent bronchospasm between acute attacks and in preventing nocturnal attacks. However, these preparations may also prolong the toxic effects as peak plasma level is reached 12-24 hours after the ingestion.

If an acute asthmatic attack is not terminated within 2 hours by above measures, the patient should be treated as a case of severe acute asthma (status asthmaticus).

Selective and potent PDE-4 inhibitors with anti-inflammatory action, **cilomilast** and **roflumilast** are being evaluated in asthma and COPD.

Anticholinergics: As the airways have parasympathetic innervation, atropine-like drugs can induce bronchodilatation and have been used as a remedy for bronchial asthma :

IPRATROPIUM BROMIDE is a congener of methylatropine. Administered by inhalation (Atrovent) in the dose of 1-2 puffs (40 - 80 mcg) tid, it is as effective as 200 mcg of salbutamol by inhalation in relieving bronchospasm in patients with chronic bronchitis, and in prolonged bronchial hyperresponsiveness following viral respiratory infections. It is the preferred drug in patients with COPD. It is used in nebulized form for treating acute attacks and appears to have fewer systemic adverse effects than beta adrenergic agonists as it is not much absorbed.

It has a slow onset of action (30 min.) and lower efficacy than β_2 agonists in the management of acute attacks of asthma. It is particularly useful in patients with concomitant heart disease. A combination of ipratropium and a beta adrenergic agonist by inhalation produces additive effects because ipratropium acts on large and medium sized bronchi whereas β_2 agonist act on the smaller bronchi.

Oxitropium bromide and **tiotropium bromide** are other analogues with similar properties; tiotropium has a longer duration of action.

Prevention of Acute Attacks

Avoidance of the causal factors, such as an allergen, may eliminate acute attacks. This is not easy, and if the allergen is not easily detected, extensive skin testing and desensitisation are unlikely to yield much success. Patients in whom acute attacks are precipitated by a psychologically unpleasant situation are likely to benefit from some readjustment in their family and social life; in case of children, a discussion with the parents is helpful.

The drugs used in the prevention of acute attacks *(***maintenance therapy***)* are: salmeterol, formoterol, ephedrine hydrochloride, theophylline, glucocorticoids and leukotriene modifiers. *As the beta-adrenergic agonists and theophylline act by different mechanisms, their concurrent use has an additive effect.*

GLUCOCORTICOIDS: When attacks are frequent, are not easily relieved by the inhaled bronchodilators and interfere with daily activities and with sleep, the current practice is to start prophylactic inhaled glucocorticoids, on a regular basis. The glucocorticoids **beclomethasone**, **budesonide** and **fluticasone** have the advantages that they are potent, lipid soluble and effective promptly in small doses. Further, because of their low bioavailability due to high first pass metabolism, their systemic toxicity is low, although almost 80% of the drug is swallowed during inhalation.

SALMETEROL (Serobid) is a **long acting** β_2 adrenergic agonist, weaker than salbutamol. It is used as the drug of choice in the prevention of nocturnal asthmatic attacks and those induced by exercise. Its onset of action is slow (10-15 min.) and the duration of action long (12 hours). *It is not useful in relieving acute attacks.* It is available in pressurised MDI delivering 25 mcg per puff. The dose is 1-2 puffs every 12 hours. It should not be used more than twice a day.

Formoterol, an analogue, has quicker onset (3-5 min.) than and similar duration of action as salmeterol.

Tolerance develops to these two drugs during long term therapy. *They are always used in combination with an inhaled glucocorticoid.*

Cromolyn sodium: See later.

EPHEDRINE HYDROCHLORIDE: This sympathomimetic drug, given orally in the dose of 30 mg. at bed time, was considered useful in preventing nocturnal asthmatic attacks. Patients who get daytime attacks need 60 mg. on waking and 30 mg. at mid-day. Taken later in the day, it may cause insomnia. Sometimes, it causes palpitation and difficulty in passing urine, particularly in the elderly. It also raises the BP in hypertensive patients. Tolerance to ephedrine develops after several weeks of continuous therapy but it is reversible (Chapter 17).

THEOPHYLLINE and aminophylline may not be tolerated orally in therapeutically effective doses (1 g. daily in divided doses) because of nausea. However, given in the form of tablets, they are cost effective for general use. Their major drawback is the variability in bioavailability. Slow release preparations of theophylline given in the evening may be useful as adjuncts in preventing nocturnal attacks.

Leukotriene Modifiers

Leukotrienes liberated during inflammation are more potent and longer acting than histamine as bronchoconstrictors (Chapter 24). They increase bronchial mucus secretion, decrease mucociliary clearance, and increase vascular permeability. Drugs can modify the leukotriene system by :

(1) **Acting as competitive antagonist** eg. Montelukast; or

(2) **Blocking the leukotriene synthesis** e.g. Zileuton.

Leukotriene modifiers have no bronchodilator action and cannot be used as rescue drugs. For prevention of acute attacks, they are less potent than low dose inhaled glucocorticoids. Combined use of glucocorticoids and leukotriene modifiers may permit a reduction in steroid dose. They can be used as an alternative to low dose inhaled glucocorticoid therapy in mild asthma, and in children. *Their use mandates periodic monitoring of hepatic function.* Their superiority over the older drugs is not established. They are expensive.

MONTELUKAST: This is a competitive and selective LT_1 receptor antagonist. Its oral bioavailability is 60-70% and t½ 3-6 hours. It is highly protein bound and metabolized by the liver. It is effective in asthma with once to twice daily administration.

Adverse reactions: These are mild, self-limited and include dyspepsia, headache, eosinophilia and raised liver enzymes. The drug may rarely cause sytemic vasculitis.

Therapeutic uses :

- ***Aspirin-induced bronchospasm.***
- ***Cold-air-induced airway obstruction.***

- *Exercise-induced bronchospasm;* and
- ***Mild to moderate chronic persistent asthma.***
- ***Allergic rhinitis.***

Pranlukast and **Zafirlukast** are the analogues of montelucast. The latter can cause severe hepatitis, and can interact with warfarin to enhance its effect.

Zileuton, a leukotriene synthesis inhibitor, is as effective as montelukast but has been withdrawn from the market in the USA because of safety concerns.

Treatment of Chronic Persistent Asthma

Over and above the treatment during acute attack, patients with persistent asthma need some form of maintenance therapy.

Bronchodilator drugs: Salmeterol and formoterol are the beta$_2$ agonists of choice for this purpose. However, their use is generally less effective in such cases because they lack anti-inflammatory action. Further, their efficacy diminishes with continued use owing to development of tolerance. *They are best used concurrently with an inhaled glucocorticoid.*

Salbutamol should be used additionally (preferably by inhalation) to treat acute attacks when they occur. However, *inappropriate administration of repeated doses of potent sympathomimetics can induce lethal cardiac arrhythmias.*

Antiinflammatory drugs: A glucocorticoid by inhalation is the **first-line therapy** for chronic persistent asthma since chronic inflammation is important in its pathogenesis. Glucocorticoids block the inflammatory response and improve lung function at multiple levels. They:

- ***Inhibit phospholipase A$_2$*** and thereby reduce the cellular histamine and SRS-A content.
- ***Stabilize the cellular lysosomal membranes.***
- ***Inhibit the influx of inflammatory cells*** into the lungs after exposure to an allergen.
- ***Prevent and reverse the downregulation of the beta adrenergic receptors,*** and thus maintain/restore the responsiveness of the airway smooth muscle to beta$_2$ agonists.
- ***Inhibit the release of mediators from the macrophages*** and the eosinophils but not from the mast cells, in the lungs. *Therefore, they are useful in blocking the late response and the consequent bronchial hyper-responsiveness.*
- ***Long term administration also reduces the immediate response to allergens, and prevents exercise-induced asthma.***

Clinically, they reduce the frequency of acute attacks as well as interval symptoms; and thus improve the quality of life. During long term steroid therapy, the reduction in bronchial hyper-responsiveness is gradual, and may take several months. Effective, long term suppression of airway inflammation reduces the need for bronchodilators, and may reduce the morbidity and perhaps mortality in bronchial asthma. Concurrent use of glucocorticods and a long acting beta$_2$ agonist is beneficial.

The important limitations of inhaled glucocorticoids are :

(1) Whereas small doses are highly effective, higher doses produce limited additional benefits; and

(2) Long term use of high doses may cause systemic adverse effects such as osteoporosis, cataract, glaucoma and growth retardation.

The macrolide antibiotics (erythromycin, trioleandomycin, clarithromycin) increase the half life of glucocorticoids and theophylline in the body. Hence, the dose of the latter drugs needs to be adjusted if concurrent administration of a macrolide becomes necessary.

BECLOMETHASONE DIPROPIONATE (Becotide/Beclate Inhaler): This halogenated glucocorticoid ester is used in an MDI which delivers 50 micrograms of the drug per puff.

It suppresses asthma by a topical anti-inflammatory action without causing systemic toxicity. The usual dose recommended is 2 puffs (200 mcg) 3-4 times a day. Modest but significant decrease in

Table 26.3: Doses of inhaled steroids

Drug	mcg/puff	Low dose, mcg	High dose, mcg/day, in divided doses
Beclomethasone	100, 200, 250	100 - 400 bid	800 - 2000
Budesonide	100, 200, 400	100 - 400 bid	800 - 2000
Fluticasone	50, 125, 250	50 - 200 bid	400 - 1000
Ciclesonide	80, 160	80- 320 bid	-
Mometasone furoate	30, 60, 120	200- 400 bid	800 OD

bone mineral density (BMD) occurs in women receiving doses as low as 500 mcg/day. Doses up to 1.5 mg. daily *in adults* do not cause significant suppression of the hypothalamopituitary axis, and this is its major advantage. However, localized infection with *Candida albicans* in the mouth or the throat can occur. This can be prevented by rinsing the mouth after every administration of the drug. It may interfere with the growth of lung and other organs in young children; and hence should be avoided in them in mild asthma. A flare up of allergic rhinitis and nasal polyps has been reported on stopping treatment. *Steroid inhalation is of no value in treating acute attacks.*

BUDESONIDE (Pulmicort): This drug has a higher ratio of topical to systemic activity and is more potent than beclomethasone. Its uses and limitations are similar to those of beclomethasone. The total daily dose is upto 2000 mcg. Its major advantage is that it is effective in the dose of 1-2 puffs bid; this improves patient compliance.

Fluticasone has properties similar to those of beclomethasone and budesonide. The total daily dose is upto 1000 mcg. It is expensive.

The adverse reactions to budesonide and fluticasone are similar to those to beclomethasone.

Mometasone furoate is another glucocorticoid used as a powder for inhalation.

Table 26.3 lists the doses of inhaled steroids.

DISODIUM CHROMOGLYCATE (Cromolyn, Ifiral, Intal): This is the sodium salt of 1,3-bis-(2-carboxychromon-5-yloxy)-2 hydroxy propane. It is useful in preventing attacks of bronchial asthma in selected cases.

Fig 26.3: Disodium chromoglycate

Pharmacological actions: The drug acts by altering the function of the delayed chloride channels in the cell membrane, thereby preventing mast cell and eosinophil activation. It stabilizes the mast cell membrane and inhibits release of spasmogenic autocoids after combination of the antigen and antibody. In this respect, like glucocorticoids, it acts as an anti-inflammatory agent. It also prevents the early response to allergens and exercise, and the subsequent bronchial hyper-responsiveness, by acting on inflammatory cells such as eosinophils. The drug relieves coughing due to asthma. It has few other significant pharmacological actions. Tolerance to cromolyn during long term use has not been reported so far.

Absorption, fate and excretion: It is absorbed poorly after oral administration (0.5%) and after inhalation (5%). The absorbed portion is rapidly eliminated unchanged in urine and bile.

Adverse reactions: Except some local irritation, no serious toxicity has been observed with this drug.

Preparation and dosage: Disodium chromoglycate is administered in 20 mg. capsules, given by inhalation, 3-4 times daily. It is inhaled by using a **spinhaler** in which the capsule is punctured and spun by the patient's own inspiratory effort in order to release the drug. Its effect is enhanced when the patient's ventilation is improved by *prior* (but not simultaneous) inhalation of a beta stimulant. It is also available as powder for nasal insufflation and as 2% aqueous eye drops and ointment.

Therapeutic uses:

- ***Allergic bronchial asthma*:** When inhaled during a symptom-free interval, it protects against an attack for several hours in most patients with extrinsic asthma. It is, however, ineffective when used after the beginning of an attack. The results in patients with intrinsic asthma are less satisfactory. However, it is worth trying this drug in all cases of asthma not responding to conventional therapy. It is more likely to work in patients with clear evidence of allergic factors and in those with **exercise-induced bronchospasm.** A single dose taken 15-30 minutes before exercise may prevent an acute attack for 1-2 hours. When effective, it reduces the number of attacks, cough and sputum, and the requirements of glucocorticoids and bronchodilator drugs. Some patients have to take the drug for 3-4 weeks before they notice its beneficial effects. Cromolyn is probably the anti-inflammatory drug of first choice in children because it has few side effects.
- ***Other respiratory allergies*:** It has been used in allergic alveolitis and in allergic rhinitis.
- ***Miscellaneous*:** The drug has also been used in the treatment of aphthous stomatitis, ulcerative colitis, food allergy and systemic mastocytosis with variable results.

Nedocromil sodium has properties similar to those of cromolyn but is effective orally. It also inhibits PAF. *Nedocromil and its analogues have now been largely superceded by low dose inhaled glucocorticoids.*

KETOTIFEN, a cromolyn analogue, is an antihistaminic which is claimed to be useful in asthma. It is believed to inhibit airway inflammation induced by platelet activating factor (PAF) in primates. It can cause drowsiness. Its usefulness in asthma is equivocal.

OMALIZUMAB (Xolair): This is a recombinant, humanized anti-IgE monoclonal antibody. It binds to IgE and prevents it from binding to IgE receptors on mast cells and basophils. It thus prevents the allergic reaction at a very early step. Plasma level of IgE diminishes markedly. It is administered as a single SC injection once in 2-4 weeks. The IgE-Ab complex is degraded by the RE system in the

Table 26.4: Stepwise management of asthma

Mild, intermittent asthma: Inhaled, short acting $beta_2$ agonist as needed

Mild chronic persistent asthma: as above *plus daily use of*

- Inhaled low dose glucocorticoids; or
- Chromoglycate sodium; or
- Inhaled long acting $beta_2$ agonist

Moderate chronic persistent asthma :

- Inhaled high dose glucocorticoids plus
- Inhaled long acting $beta_2$ agonist or
- Inhaled ipratropium or
- Leukotriene modifier/oral aminophylline

Severe chronic persistent asthma: As above *plus* oral glucocorticoids (prednisolone 30 mg/day for 5-7 days)

Acute attack (in any of the above categories) : Additional treatment : Inhaled $beta_2$ agonists in adequate doses (see earlier) nebulised beta agonists; aminophylline IV

Status asthmaticus: See later.

liver; the elimination t½ is 26 days. The drug is not a bronchodilator. In adults with allergic, moderate-to-severe persistent asthma, it reduces the dependance on glucocorticoids and decreases the frequency of asthma exacerbations. It may also be useful in seasonal allergic rhinitis and food allergy. It is generally well tolerated, but may cause local reactions and, rarely, anaphylaxis. Its use is not recommended in children below the age of 12 years. It is very expensive.

Other concurrent medications: Most chronic asthmatic patients have associated chronic bronchitis and lung damage. Such cases should receive **antimicrobial therapy** whenever the sputum turns yellow or other signs of infection develop. Those who are prone to get repeated infections, may need continuous prophylactic antimicrobial therapy during winter or monsoon seasons.

Antihistaminic drugs are not so useful in the treatment of asthma except in the presence of definite allergy, where they may prevent the onset of an attack. They may, however, produce drowsiness and dry the respiratory secretions. They are not recommended routinely.

Although most of the cases of asthma can now be controlled by a stepwise approach (Table 26.4) using a β-adrenergic agonist, glucocorticoids and theophylline, a few cases may still be difficult to manage. These may be benefited by oral glucocorticoid therapy in larger doses. In such cases, careful monitoring for adverse effects is necessary (Chapter 64).

Table 26.5 lists the drugs which cause bronchospasm and may precipitate asthma.

Table 26.5: Some drugs known to cause bronchospasm

- Aspirin and other NSAID.
- Beta adrenergic blockers.
- Cholinergic drugs.
- Quinine.
- Morphine.

Table 26.6: Points to remember in asthma

- Inhaled glucocorticoids or cromolyn is the treatment of first choice for maintenance therapy of persistent chronic asthma.
- Where symptoms of asthma persist in spite of low dose inhaled glucocorticoids, add inhaled long acting beta agonists instead of increasing the dose of inhaled glucocorticoids.
- High dose inhaled glucocorticoids (more than 1500 mcg/ day) increase the risk of skin bruising, cataract, low bone density and suppression of hypothalamo-pituitary-adrenal axis.
- Long acting $beta_2$ agonists are highly effective as prophylactics in exercise-induced and nocturnal asthma.
- Inhaled long acting beta agonists should not be used as monotherapy but combined with inhaled glucocorticoids for long term treatment of asthma.
- Oral aminophylline is much less effective than inhaled glucocorticoids.

Table 26.6 enumerates the important points to remember in the management of asthma.

Treatment of Severe Acute Asthma (Status Asthmaticus)

Severe acute asthma (Status asthmaticus) is a serious medical emergency, requiring urgent hospitalization and vigorous therapy. It is often precipitated by:

- ***An acute respiratory infection.***
- ***Abrupt cessation of glucocorticoid therapy.***
- ***Drugs*** (aspirin or NSAID) or ***inhaled allergens;*** or
- ***Acute emotional stress.***

A patient in status is markedly dyspnoeic, exhausted, cyanosed and dehydrated. He has tachycardia, may have pulsus paradoxus and may become drowsy if respiratory failure supervenes. Signs of right ventricular failure including a gallop may occur as a further complication. *Pulsus paradoxus, prominence of the sternomastoid muscles and high pitched wheezing with absent breath sounds are indicative of the severity of status asthmaticus.* Silent chest, feeble respiratory efforts, cyanosis, bradycardia, hypotension, exhaustion, confusion and coma are **life-threatening** features in status asthmaticus.

Relief of tachycardia and dyspnoea and evidence of better oxygenation, including a clearer mental state, are evidence of favourable response to therapy if repeated measurements of FEV_1 are not available or are not possible because the patient is too ill to cooperate. The intensity of wheezing can be misleading; it may decrease with worsening obstruction.

Table 26.7 outlines the principles of management of a severe acute asthma.

Glucocorticoids in large doses are the mainstay of therapy. Hydrocortisone is administered IV in the dose of 200-300 mg. every 4-6 hours. Equivalent doses of another glucocorticoid, e.g., methylprednisolone 30-40 mg. by slow IV infusion may be used. Prednisolone 30-60 mg. orally every 6-8 hours is equally effective. *The bronchodilator therapy should be continued in full dose*, using nebulised salbutamol ± ipratropium, as glucocorticoids need at least 6 hours to produce a beneficial effect. If such bronchodilator administration is not effective, either aminophylline or salbutamol may be administered by slow IV infusion.

Table 26.7: Management of severe acute asthma

Initial treatment

- Correct dehydration
- Oxygen administered carefully.
- Nebulised salbutamol and ipratropium.
- Oral glucocorticoids.

If poor response to above in 1 hour

- Hospitalize.
- Correct dehydration and acidosis.
- Repeat nebulised salbutamol every 30 minutes.
- Repeat nebulised ipratropium.
- IV glucocorticoids.
- IV infusion of aminophylline or salbutamol.
- Monitor serum K^+.
- Antibiotics for chest infection.
- Exclude pneumothorax (X'ray chest).

If still poor response after 1 hour

- Shift to intensive care unit.

Once the patient shows improvement, he should be switched to oral glucocorticoids; 50-60 mg. of prednisolone should be given as a single morning dose. If the patient continues to improve, the dose should be reduced by 5 mg. every 3-4 days. If it is not possible to discontinue the glucocorticoid altogether, it should be continued in the minimum effective dose. An attempt should be made to change the treatment to a glucocorticoid by MDI. *Alternate day glucocorticoid therapy has not been successful in the management of asthma, as the patient deteriorates on the 'steroid-off' day.*

Rehydration of the patient either by mouth (using liquids to which glucose and salt have been added) or by parenteral administration of 5 per cent glucose-saline (with appropriate quantities of potassium) is essential. It not only corrects dehydration but also makes the bronchial secretions less tenacious. Correction of acidosis by means of IV sodium bicarbonate is likely to restore the patient's sensitivity to the bronchodilators. Some cases would need treatment for acute respiratory failure.

Sedatives, tranquillizers and antihistaminics should be avoided in status asthmaticus. They make the patient drowsy, diminish the voluntary ventilatory drive and thus aggravate the hypoxemia. Morphine is contraindicated as it constricts the bronchi and depresses the respiratory centre.

Steroid resistant asthma: Rarely, inspite of adequate doses, glucocorticoids may not be effective. Glucocorticoids act by binding to nuclear receptors and attach to DNA sites that code for cytokine production. Glucocorticoid resistance has been related to defective DNA binding, a decrease in number of glucocorticoid receptors and decreased ligand receptor affinity. Interestingly, glucocorticoid resistance in these cases is confined to T-cells. In such cases increase in dosage will cause toxicity without any relief from asthma.

COPD – Management

Chronic Obstructive Pulmonary Disease (COPD) is a syndrome of progressive air inflow limitation caused by chronic inflammation of small airways and lung parenchymatous tissue.It is a major cause of mortality and morbidity all over the world. It is characterized by slow, progressive loss of lung function that is irreversible (emphysema).

COPD is a heterogeneous disorder, and responds differently according to its phenotype. The main physiological abnormality in COPD is an accelerated rate of decrease in the **Forced Expiratory Volume** (FEV_1) compared to that in normals. There is hyperinflation which is present at rest and worsens on exercise, increasing the work of breahing. The CO_2 diffusing capacity decreases with resultant hypoxemia.

The current therapy of COPD includes:

- ***Inhaled bronchodilators.***
- ***Inhaled glucocorticoids.***
- ***Oxygen inhalation;*** and
- ***Physiotherapy, pulmonary rehabiltation and education..***

Inhaled bronchodilators are the mainstay of therapy, and any one of the regimens given in Table 26.8 may be used. However, combination therapy with an **inhaled glucocorticoid** and a long acting beta agonist gives better benefits with acceptable side effects. Inhaled glucocorticoids probably help to reduce the number of exacerbations; but they alone do not substantially modify airway obstruction in COPD. They are better avoided in older patients because of possible ADR. Addition of **theophylline** may be beneficial in some subjects.

Intermittently inhaled oxygen improves long term survival in COPD and home oxygen therapy should be used along with pulmonary

Table 26.8 : Bronchodilator regimens in COPD

Drug	Duration of action (hr)	Dose
	Short acting	
Salbutamol sulfate	4-6	2 puffs every 4 hours (MDI 100 mcg/puff)
Ipratropium bromide	4-6	2 puffs every 4 hours (MDI 20 mcg/puff)
	Long acting	
Formoterol fumarate	8-12	One inhalation twice a day (DPI 12 mcg/inhalation)
Salmeterol xinafoate	8-12	One inhalation twice a day (DPI 50 mcg/inhalation)
Triotropium bromide	>24	One inhalation once a day (DPI 18 mcg/inhalation)
Arformoterol	8-12	One nebulization, 15 mcg twice a day

MDI = Metered dose inhaler. DPI= Dry powder inhaler

rehabilitation. Some severe cases may need **oral glucocorticoid therepy**.

An exacerbation of COPD can be defined as " an event in the natural course of the chronic disease, characterized by change in the baseline dyspnea, cough and sputum beyond the normal variation ".It is usually triggered by bacteria, viruses and pollutants. The most common viruses are rhinovirus, coronavirus and influenza virus. The common bacteria involved are *H. influenzae, Moraxella catarrhalis, S. pneumoniae* and *Ps. pyogenes.* Purulent sputum is a reliable marker for bacterial infection, and should be treated promptly with **antibiotics**. **Mucolytic agents**, by and large, are not useful for reducing the frequency of exacerbations.

Treatment of Acute Respiratory Failure

Respiratory insufficiency indicates impaired ability of the lungs to eliminate carbon dioxide or to take up oxygen. It may become apparent at rest or only on exercise. Respiratory failure is said to exist when a serious abnormality of blood gases (arterial CO_2 tension of over 50 mm. Hg. or arterial O_2 tension of 60 mm Hg or less) is present at rest. Respiratory failure may be either:

- *Ventilatory failure;* or
- *Oxygenation failure.*

In the commoner variety of **acute ventilatory failure** in patients with COPD, prolonged bronchial narrowing and their obstruction by secretions are responsible for the failure in patients with already badly damaged lungs. This leads to an inadequate uptake of oxygen and inefficient elimination of carbon dioxide. Hence, the immediate need is to correct the reduced oxygen tension of the blood. Since oxygen lack stimulates the respiration reflexly, its correction leads to a reduction of ventilatory drive, with the result that carbon dioxide accumulates further; the patient may thus become drowsy or even comatose. To avoid this, oxygen is given continuously, preferably in a concentration of 25-30 per cent. (Chapter 73).

The patient should be made to cough vigorously while his chest wall is being percussed. Coughing out mucus plugs may result in significant improvement and this is further helped by humidification.

Respiratory stimulants (*analeptics*) may be used to increase ventilation in patients in whom oxygen therapy is followed by a reduction in ventilation. They may also help by stimulating coughing and thus helping the patient to expel secretions. They are usually given IV and have to be repeated frequently. Satisfactory response is characterised by a return of deeper breathing and consciousness, and a reduction in carbon dioxide tension in the blood. Later, this may be maintained by oral administration of these drugs. *There is no drug which could selectively, safely and in a controlled manner stimulate the respiratory centre.* The drug which is generally used is **doxapram**, given as an IV infusion of 1.5-4.0 mg/min., adjusted according to the patient's response. It may be useful as a short term measure in conjunction with assisted ventilation, but is not useful in the long term management of respiratory insufficiency.

Other supportive measures in acute ventilatory failure in COPD include bronchodilators, antibiotics, large doses of glucocorticoids, a diuretic (furosemide) to treat cardiac failure and correction of acid-base and electrolyte imbalance. If these conservative measures do not help the patient sufficiently, aspiration of secretions from the respiratory passages through a bronchoscope or a cuffed endotracheal tube may be needed.

In acute ventilatory failure due to disorders of the CNS (narcotic poisoning, stroke, head injuries), peripheral nervous system and respiratory muscles, intensive nursing care, assisted mechanical ventilation, and other life supporting measures are the mainstay of treatment. In some cases e.g. morphine poisoning, specific antidote therapy is helpful.

In the syndrome of **oxygenation failure,** which occurs in patients with diffuse interstitial fibrosis, there is no tendency to retention of carbon dioxide, and oxygen can be administered without any reservation and safely. The response is, however, disappointing.

Surfactants and the Respiratory Distress Syndrome

Surfactant is a complex mixture of phospholipids, proteins and carbohydrates secreted by the type II pneumocytes within the alveolar epithelium of the lungs, into the alveolar lumen. By its local action, it:

- ***Reduces surface tension within the alveoli*** and facilitates their aeration at lower ventilatory pressures; this increases the lung compliance and reduces the work of breathing.
- ***Aids in keeping the alveoli dry (antiedema action).***
- ***Enhances oxygenation of blood at lower intra-alveolar, partial oxygen pressure;*** and
- ***May play a role in the immune defence system of the lungs.***

The secretion of the surfactant is stimulated by cortisol, adrenergic agonists, cholinergic agonists and prostaglandins.

Deficiency of surfactant action may be due to:

- ***Diminished production*** as in full term infants delivered by caeserian section (where stimulation of the adrenocortical production of cortisol occurring during vaginal delivery is absent); and in prematurely born infants with immature secretory mechanisms. This is the cause of widespread atelectasis and Neonatal Respiratory Distress Syndrome (Neonatal RDS).
- ***More rapid degradation*** of the surfactant by the macrophages; and
- ***Abnormal composition of*** the surfactant.

The last two factors probably are at work in Adult Respiratory Distress Syndrome (ARDS).

The surfactants available for therapy are bovine-lung derived **Calfactant** and **Beractant;** porcine-lung derived **poractant alpha;** and the rDNA synthetic **calfasceril.**

Adverse reactions include bradycardia, hypotension and endotracheal tube blockage. Allergic reactions are rare.

Therapeutic uses : Instillation of surfactant into the trachea of the newborns at risk of developing or already having RDS reduces the morbidity and mortality. The results in adult ARDS are less encouraging. *Neonates born by caeserian section can be protected from RDS by administration of dexamethasone to the mother 24 hours prior to the surgery.*

Drug Therapy of Rhinitis

Rhinitis is inflammation of the nasal mucosa and can be:

- ***Noninfectious*** e.g., allergic and nonallergic rhinitis; or
- ***Infectious*** e.g., viral common cold and bacterial infection.

Noninfectious rhinitis is frequently caused by seasonal allergy (e.g., hay fever, pollinosis) and leads to sneezing, nasal stuffiness, ocular pruritus, lacrimation and a postnasal drip.

Chronic or nonseasonal rhinitis, often referred to as perennial rhinitis, results in daily episodes of rhinorrhoea, nasal congestion and sneezing that are present for several weeks during most months of the year. It is caused by various allergic and nonallergic nasal disorders. It includes (1) **vasomotor rhinitis (VMR),** a nonallergic, noninfectious rhinitis in which eosinophils are generally absent on nasal smear; and (2) **nonallergic, non-infectious rhinitis with eosinophilia (NARES).**

Chronic rhinitis can also be produced by drugs such as adrenergic blockers, cholinesterase inhibitors, estrogen preparations (including oral contraceptives), and by the presence of a foreign body, nasal polyps, tumours and nasociliary disorders.

Non-Drug therapy for all types of rhinitis is

similar. Exposure to cigarette smoke, pollutants, allergens and other irritants should be avoided. In patients with pharyngitis, saline gargles, steam inhalation and warm mist therapy may be helpful. Local instillation of hyperheated, humidified air directly into the nasal passages significantly relieves symptoms of allergic rhinitis. When nasal congestion is severe, nasal irrigation with warm saline solution, prepared by dissolving one tablespoonful each of table salt and baking soda in a pint of warm (37°C) tap water, may relieve the congestion. The patient should drink plenty of fluids.

Drug Therapy: No drug is likely to abolish the symptoms completely. In general, drugs are more effective in allergic rhinitis than in nonallergic forms of rhinitis. Acute rhinitis usually responds more favourably than the chronic form. *The treatment is directed at preventing the release of inflammatory mediators such as histamine and leucotrienes, or blocking their effects after they are released.*

The drugs used to treat rhinitis are:

- ***Antihistaminics.***
- ***Nasal decongestants.***
- ***Antiallergic drugs.***
- ***Anticholinergic drugs***; and
- ***Local corticosteroids.***

The selection of drugs in individual patients requires that the noninfectious, allergic forms be distinguished from the infectious forms (common cold) because the agents useful in the former, antihistaminics, cromolyn sodium and intranasal corticosteroids, have little value in the latter. Nasal decongestants, however, are beneficial in both. Antibiotics should be reserved only for patients with bacterial infections.

Antihistaminics: These are the most widely used drugs for allergic rhinitis and are often chosen for initial therapy. They help to relieve rhinorrhoea, sneezing, nasal pruritus and conjunctivitis but do not affect nasal congestion. They are usually effective in seasonal allergic rhinitis when sneezing and rhinorrhoea predominate and edema and congestion are minimal. They are more effective if taken before the symptoms occur, and should be taken regularly by susceptible patients during the allergen exposure period even when symptoms are absent. A single daily dose of an antihistaminic with a long half life, taken at bedtime, may relieve symptoms the following day. The non-sedating antihistaminics such as cetirizine and loratadine, are preferred (Chapter 22) when sedation needs to be avoided: They are not useful in controlling cough.

Nasal decongestants: Nasal decongestants shrink the swollen turbinates, and are the most effective agents for nasal congestion. These drugs are synthetic alpha-adrenergic agonists (Chapter 17). When used locally by spray or as drops, they constrict the dilated blood vessels in the mucosa and help to reduce edema. The drugs commonly used are:

- Ephedrine 0.5%.
- Phenylephrine 0.25%.
- Naphazoline 0.05%; and
- Oxymetazoline 0.05%.

They increase the nasal patency, lower nasal resistance and provide subjective relief of nasal symptoms. They provide temporary symptomatic relief in common cold, and acute rhinitis associated with other respiratory infections, as well as in allergic rhinitis, NARES, sinusitis, and in acute otitis media with eustachian tube blockage. Oral decongestants such as pseudophedrine may be preferred when sinuses are involved. They are not useful in VMR.

The most common adverse effects of the orally administered nasal decongestants (phenylephrine, pseudoephedrine) are insomnia and irritability. Topical decongestants sometimes cause local discomfort, stinging, burning, dryness of the mucosa, rebound congestion and *rhinitis medicamentosa.*

Nasal decongestants are only palliative. Only a few drugs in very dilute solution are safe. Simple ephedrine in isotonic saline, used as nasal drops, is as effective as any other drug, and cost effective. In infants and children, imidazole drugs such as naphazoline and tetrahydrozoline are known to cause disturbance of body temperature, CNS depression and even coma. *Hence, decongestants should be stored beyond the reach of children.*

Antiallergic drugs: These drugs prevent the release of inflammatory mediators (e.g. glucocorticoids and cromolyn sodium), and inhibit their action on the target cells (e.g. H_1 blockers). The nasal spray of cromolyn sodium is as effective as an oral antihistaminic in preventing the symptoms of allergic rhinitis. Patients with seasonal allergic rhinitis are more responsive than those with the chronic form. They are reasonably safe.

Anticholinergic drugs: Rhinorrhoea, a common symptom in patients with rhinitis, is primarily the result of glandular hypersecretion, mediated by the cholinergic innervation of the nasal mucosa. Some patients with severe rhinorrhoea and congestion obtain more relief from antimuscarinics than from nasal decongestants. Intranasal administration of **ipratropium bromide,** an atropine substitute significantly reduces the nasal hypersecretion.

Topical glucocorticoids exert a marked anti-inflammatory effect on the nasal mucosa by inhibiting the release of inflammatory mediators from the mast cells and basophils, and by blocking the inflammatory effect of leucocytes in the nose. Intranasal glucocorticoids are safe, and are the most effective agents available for the prophylaxis and treatment of seasonal and non-seasonal allergic rhinitis and for weaning the patients with rhinitis medicamentosa from topical decongestants. NARES also responds to local glucocorticoids, but their effectiveness in VMR is limited. Topical glucocorticoids occasionally shrink nasal polyps and reduce nasal obstruction significantly. Small polyps may even disappear.

The efficacy of nasal spray preparation of beclomethasone dipropionate, flunisolide, budesonide, fluocortil butyl and fluticasone is similar. However, *local use of dexamethasone formulations is contraindicated as the drug is rapidly absorbed and can cause systemic adverse effects.* After the initial application of the nasal steroid, stinging and burning may occur, but they usually abate with continued use. Sneezing, headache, drying and nasal bleeding can occur after the use of these drugs. Topical steroids, if required, should be used along with appropriate systemic antibacterial therapy in patients with infection. *They should be used with caution in patients with ocular herpes zoster.*

Injudicious use of commercially promoted combinations of decongestants with antihistaminics, glucocorticoids and antibiotics may be hazardous and is not recommended.

Hyposensitization: This comprises carrying out skin tests with several antigens individually, followed by serial injections of desensitizing vaccines prepared from the 'offending' allergens. The use of such vaccines may benefit (a) patients with allergy to pollens (causing seasonal hay fever); and (b) those with allergy to wasp and bee venom. It is currently felt that:

(a) Most atopic (allergic) patients are allergic to multiple allergens and are not likely to benefit from vaccines prepared from single allergens.

(b) Diagnostic tests are unreliable, if used by themselves.

(c) The allergen extract desensitizing vaccines can precipitate either severe asthma or anaphylaxis.

(d) Vaccines prepared from house dust, house dust mite, animal danders and foods have not been shown to be effective.

All such vaccines should be avoided in asthmatics, pregnant women, children under 5 years and those taking beta-blockers.

SECTION VII
Cardiovascular Drugs

Pharmacotherapy of Cardiac Arrhythmias 27

Cardiac arrythmia occurs when there is a disturbance of initiation or condution of cardiac impulse. The mortality rate in acute myocardiac infarction (MI) can be reduced by early recognition and prompt treatment of various arrhythmias. **Anti-arrhythmic drugs** are the compounds used to prevent or correct cardiac arrhythmias. The *antifibrillatory* drugs are compounds which prevent the development of atrial and/or ventricular fibrillation. The antifibrillatory drugs must be differentiated from the **defibrillatory drugs** i.e. drugs capable of restoring normal sinus rhythm of the heart under atrial and/or ventricular fibrillation. Although many drugs are able to arrest rapid atrial and ventricular arrhythmias, no drug is available that can consistently restore normal rhythm to a fibrillating ventricle.

Electrophysiology of cardiac tissue: The cardiac cell is bounded by a lipoprotein membrane which has *receptor channels* crossing it. These are ion-selective membrane-spanning proteins which permit passive movement of ions (Na^+, K^+, Ca^{++} and Cl^-) down their electrochemical gradients during the open but not during the closed state of the channels. The Na^+ channels are known as 'fast' channels and are present in the myocytes of the atria, ventricles and the His-Purkinje tissue; they are absent from the SA node and the AV node. The other ion channels are present in all the cardiac tissues. The rapid depolarisation (Phase 0) is due to the influx of Na^+ into the cell, with the late addition of Ca^{++}, through the 'fast' channels. However, the SA and AV nodes depend upon the inward movement of Ca^{++} through the 'slow' Ca^{++} channels. The outward movement of K^+ is responsible for the repolarisation (Phases 1 to 3) of all cardiac tissues (Fig. 27.1).

In addition to the above mentioned 'channels', there are two, energy requiring *exchange pumps* in the cardiac myocyte cell membrane : (1) the adenosine triphosphatase (ATP ase) energized Na^+ - K^+ exchange pump which pumps Na^+ out of the cell and K^+ into the interior of the cell (see below); and (2) the Na^+- Ca^{++} exchange pump, which mainly extrudes Ca^{++} from the cell to the exterior. Such extrusion is dependent on the activity of the Na^+- K^+ pump, and diminishes when the latter is made inoperative by digoxin (Chapter 30).

Normally, Na^+ ions are concentrated extracellularly and K^+ ions intracellularly. Ordinarily, this would lead to diffusion of these ions across the cell membrane along their concentration gradients and to equalization of concentrations on its two sides. Such diffusion is, however, opposed by the membrane Na^+ - K^+ pump which actively pushes Na^+ ions out of the cell and K^+ ions into the cell. For every three Na^+ ions pushed out of the cell, the pump pushes two K^+ ions into the cell, and the pump is thus electrogenic. *The Na^+- K^+ pump operates continuously and does not switch on and off* *during the action potential of the cardiac cells.* Further, during the diastole more K^+ ions leave the cell than the Na^+ ions that enter it, because of the differences in the membrane permeability. As these cations carry positive electrical charges, there is a net loss of positive charges from the cell during the diastole. Further, the anions Cl^- and proteins do not leave the cell along with K^+ because the cell membrane is impermeable to them, contributing to the intracellular negativity. Thus, the inside of the resting myocardial cell remains (about 90 millivolts) negative to its outside; the cell membrane is said to be *polarized.*

During the excitation of the cell, larger quantities of Na^+ and K^+ ions cross the cell membrane. These ion fluxes are too small to be measured directly but show themselves by and are, in fact, responsible for the more easily measurable phenomenon of the continuously varying potential difference *(transmembrane electrical potential)* across the cell membrane. These variations can be recorded as an **action potential** by inserting a microelectrode into the myocardial cells. Figure 27.1 shows the action potentials as recorded from the Ca^{++} driven tissues (SA and AV nodes wherein the resting potential is 30 to 40 mv.) (Fig 27.1 A) and Na^+ driven tissues (others) of the heart (Fig 27.1 B).

In the normal heart, only the SA node and the AV node are capable of *spontaneous depolarisation* i.e. generating an action potential without external stimulation; as the frequency of spontaneous discharge at the SA node (70/min) is faster than at the AV node (45/min), the former acts as the pace-maker. The other cardiac tissues merely respond by depolarisation to an action potential generated by the SA node. *The diseased heart,* may contain other sites capable of spontaneous depolarisation, giving rise to arrhythmias.

When an atrial or a ventricular cell receives an action potential, it starts depolarising in response to it, and Na^+ starts entering it; the intracellular negativity starts diminishing. When such depolarisation reaches a **threshold potential** (T P in Fig. 27.1), the sodium channels open abruptly and Na^+ enters the cell in large quantities. ***Phase '0'*** of the action potential (Fig. 27.1) indicates rapid depolarisation of the cardiac cell membrane associated with fast selective inflow of Na^+ions. During the latter part of Phase 0, Ca^{++} also enters the cell via the Na^+ channels. The entry of Ca^{++} continues through Phases 1 and 2 via the slow Ca^{++} channels. The Ca^{++} which enters the cell in this manner causes release of Ca^{++} stored in the sarcoplasmic reticulum of the cardiac myocytes, raising the concentration of Ca^{++} within these cells. This intracellular free calcium interacts with the troponin-actin-myosin system and causes

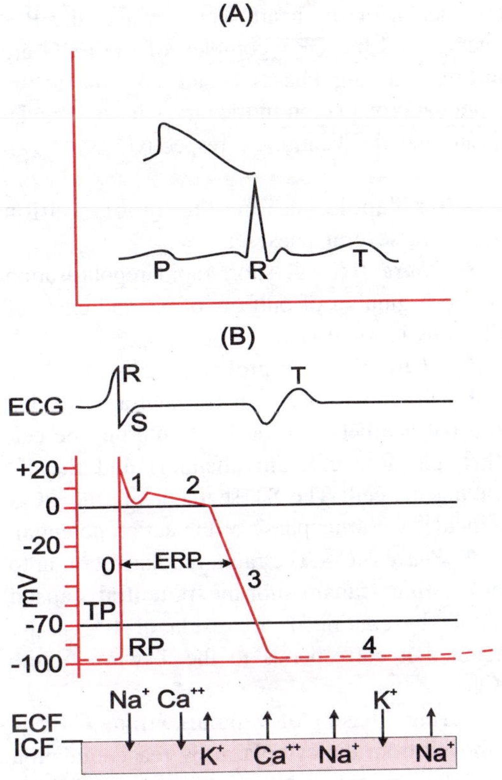

Fig. 27.1 : Relationship between transmembrane cationic fluxes, ECG recording and transmembrane action potential recorded from mammalian (A) sinus node and (B) His-Purkinje fibre

RP = Resting potential. TP = Threshold potential

(O) = Phase of depolarization

(1,2,3,) = Phases of repolarization

(4) = Resting period

contraction of the heart. The P wave, the P-R interval and the QRS complex of the ECG are inscribed during Phases 0 and 1 of the action potential propagation in the atria, the A V nodal tissue and the ventricles, respectively.

After depolarisation, the repolarisation occurs in several phases :

- ***Phase '1'*** – A short rapid repolarisation due to beginning of outflow of K^+ and entry of Cl^- ions into the cells.
- ***Phase '2'*** – A prolonged plateau phase (delay in repolarisation) at the neutral level due to a balance between the Ca^{++} entering the cell (through slow calcium channel) and the K^+ leaving the cell. The ST segment of the ECG coincides with this phase of the action potential.
- ***Phase '3'*** – The rapid repolarisation upto the resting transmembrane potential caused mainly by continued extrusion of K^+ via K^+ channel; it corresponds to the T wave of the ECG.

During Phase3 of repolarisation, Ca^{++} is removed from the cytoplasm by reaccumulation into the sarcoplasmic reticulum sacs and by extrusion from the cell. The lowering of Ca^{++} concentration in the cytoplasm allows the cardiac muscle fibre to relax; and

- ***Phase '4'***– In this resting phase, the final ionic reconstitution of the cell is achieved by the Na^+- K^+ exchange pump which actively pushes Na^+ out of the cell and K^+ into the cell. The cycle is then repeated. In the atria and the ventricles, the membrane potential is steady throughout the diastole; in contrast, the SA node, the AV node and the His-Purkinje tissue depolarize spontaneously because the cell membrane is leaky to Na^+.

During the greater part of the action potential, the cardiac muscle is resistant to further stimulation (refractoriness, Fig. 27.2). The earliest transient depolarization that can be produced (without propagation) marks the end of the **absolute refractory period** (ARP, Phases 1and 2). The part of the action potential during which a stimulus can evoke only a local, non-propated response is called **effective refractory period** (ERP). The ERP is slightly longer than and includes the ARP. **Relative refractory period** extends from the end of ERP to the time that the cardiac tissue has recovered fully; during this period, a stimulus of greater than threshold strength is needed to evoke response that is propagated, though slowly.

The above concepts are important for understanding the mechanisms of action of various antiarrhythmic drugs in terms of sodium-channel blocking, calcium-channel blocking and potassium-channel blocking.

Certain terms appear repeatedly during a discussion of cardioactive drugs; they are

- ***Automaticity*** is the capacity of a cell to undergo spontaneous diastolic depolarization. In the normal heart, it is maximum in the SA node (pacemaker). In the diseased heart, other areas of the myocardium may develop automaticity and act as ectopic foci.
- ***Excitability*** is the ability of a cell to respond to an external stimulus by depolarization. It can be conceived in terms of the minimum intensity of a stimulus required to depolarize the cell membrane. It depends upon the level of the resting (diastolic) intracellular negativity; if the negativity decreases (say from -90 to -70 mv), the excitability of the cell increases.
- ***Threshold potential*** (TP) is the level of intracellular negativity at which abrupt and complete depolarization occurs. If the TP is raised (i.e. changed from -70 to -60 mv), the automaticity of the tissue is suppressed.
- ***The conduction velocity of an impulse*** is determined primarily by the slope of action potential and amplitude of Phase 0 (Fig. 27.1) in that tissue; any reduction in the slope leads to depression of conduction.

Propagation of an impulse in the cardiac tissue depends upon (a) the ERP of the tissue and (b) its conduction velocity.

- ***Inotropic action*** is the action of a drug on the contractility of the mycoardium.
- ***Chronotropic action*** is the action of a drug on the heart rate.

• ***Lusitropic action*** is the action on relaxation (diastolic function) of the heart.

The autonomic nervous system modulates the inotropic state of the myocardium by regulating the transmembrane ion movements, e.g., beta adrenergic stimulation allows entry of larger amounts of Ca^+ through the *slow channels* and exerts a positive inotropic effect. Beta adrenergic blockers counter this adrenergic influence on the heart and thus exert a negative inotropic effect. Digoxin (Chapter 30) exerts its positive inotropic effect by inhibiting the Na^+ - K^+ pump in the cardiac cell membrane. Ca^+ channel blockers (Chapter 28) act by blocking the entry of Ca^+ through the *slow channels.*

Cardiac arrhythmias, mechanisms: Cardiac arrhythmias arise as the result either of (a) disorders of impulse formation and/or (b) disorders of impulse conduction.

• ***Tachyarrhythmias due to disturbed impulse formation*** are associated with spontaneous, irregular and rhythmic discharge from ectopic pacemaker activity from areas other than the SA node. Production of such ectopic impulse involves an abnormality of the spontaneous diastolic depolarization (Phases 3 and 4), leading to *ectopic areas of automaticity.*

The differences among various atrial arrhythmias could be explained on the basis of the rate of discharge of the ectopic focus. Thus, an ectopic pacemaker with a rate 160-180/min. would cause **atrial tachycardia.** If the ectopic rate becomes more rapid, 220-300/min., it would produce **atrial flutter**, while very rapid rates over 350/min. would result in **atrial fubrillatin** (AF).

• ***Disorders of impulse conduction,*** commonly referred to as *re-entry disturbances,* are probably the commoner of the two mechanisms of arrhythmias. According to this theory, the affected myocardium has areas of depressed function with prolonged refractory period. Due to that, an impulse approaching such an area would be diverted to adjacent excitable tissue. It is possible that the same impulse, after taking a circuitous route through normal tissue, will again reach the depressed area which by then becomes excitable. Upon traversing it, the excitatory process is free to re-enter normal regions and restimulate the chamber or entire heart. Repetition of this cycle would produce an ectopic tachycardia. The presence of a single re-entry mechanism within the ventricle may account for ventricular premature systoles, ventricular tachycardia and ventricular flutter. The presence of a similar mechanism within the atria, usually termed the *circus phenomenon,* could cause atrial flutter. It is postulated that atrial and ventricular fibrillation are caused by the fragmentation of single re-entrant path into multiple smaller cycles. In *arrhythmias of the re-entrant type,* conduction velocity and duration of refractory period are the two most critical electrophysiological properties which could be altered by drugs.

Clinically, it is usually not possible to determine whether an arrhythmia represents a disorder of impulse formation or impulse conduction. Identical arrhythmias on the ECG may result from disparate mechanisms in different patients, or even in the same individual at different times. Hence, except in a few cases, an antiarrhythmic drug cannot be selected simply on the basis of its effect on electrophysiological properties relative to a clinical tachyarrhythmia.

Not all arrhythmias need the same aggressive drug therapy. If an arrhythmia is precipitated by hypotension, restitution of BP by vasopressor agents like DA or NA may re-establish normal sinus rhythm. Further, sinus tachycardia and sinus bradycardia generally need no treatment other than that of the underlying cause. Only those which are lethal (VF), herald more dangerous rhythm (ventricular premature beats in acute MI) or seriously compromise cardiac output (AF with fast ventricular rate) require rapid and effective therapy.

Every patient with an arrhythmia should be evaluated for : a primary cardiovascular disorder (myocardial disease or shock); pulmonary disease; autonomic disorders (hypersensitive

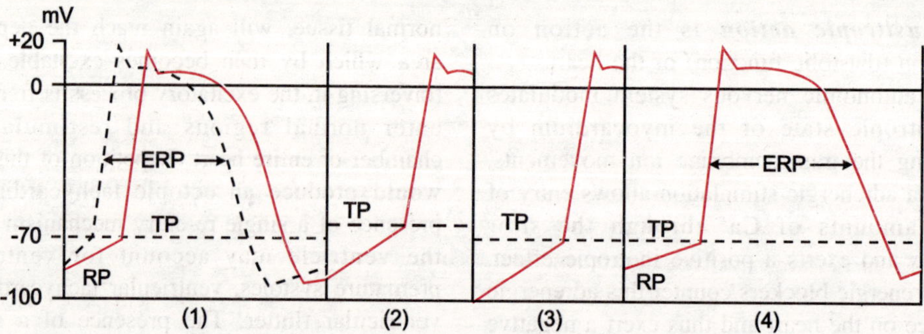

Fig. 27.2: The normal pattern (dotted line) of transmembrane action potential of a pacemaker cardiac cell and mechanisms of action of antiarrhythmic drugs: (1) Delaying the spontaneous diastolic depolarization from the resting potential (RP), thus decreasing the rate (all drugs); (2) Increasing excitation threshold potential (TP) e.g. quinidine, procainamide, propranolol; (3) Prolonging the resting period in part by increasing maximum diastolic intracellular negativity e.g. phenytoin and (4) Increasing the effective refractory period (ERP) e.g. quinidine, procainamide.

carotid sinus syndrome); electrolyte disturbances (acidosis, hypercalemia, hypokalemia); systemic disease; and drug induced toxicity. Correction of an identifiable factor should precede the administration of an anti-arrhythmic drug. *In many situations, arrhythmias tend to be benign. Their treatment should be expectant, and potentially toxic drugs should be avoided.*

The basic electrophysiological actions of antiarrhythmic drugs (Fig. 27.2) are as follows:

- ***Decreasing the slope of Phase 4*** (diastolic depolarization) of the action potential in the excitable cardiac tissues. This action is possessed by all antiarrhythmic drugs and suppresses the enhanced automaticity of ectopic foci.
- ***Shifting the threshold potential towards zero*** (i.e., making it less negative). This again suppresses the automaticity of ectopic foci. Quinidine, Procainamide, Propranolol and Potassium possess this action.
- ***Shifting the resting potential away from zero*** (i.e. making it more negative), which also slows the rate of diastolic depolarization and suppressing automaticity. Lignocaine and Phenytoin possess this action.
- ***Increase in the duration of the action potential***, thus increasing the effective refractory period (ERP) and blocking re-entrant impulses. Quinidine, Procainamide, Propranolol and Potassium possess this action.
- ***Shortening of the duration of action potential*** by Lignocaine and Phenytoin,on the other hand, reduces the refractoriness of the AV junctional tissue.
- ***Decreasing the slope of Phase 0 of the action potential and slowing the conduction velocity of a propagated impulse***. This blocks the re-entrant impulses responsible for an arrhythmia. Quinidine, Procainamide, Disopyramide, Lignocaine (in large doses) and Verapamil possess this action.

Antiarrhythmic drugs, classification: They are generally classified according to their mechanism of action as:

Class I : **Sodium channel blockers:** Although the drugs belonging to group I act predominantly by blocking the sodium channels, in higher concentrations, they also block nerve conduction due to their local anaesthetic action. With the usual doses, most drugs, other than group IC, have little discernible action on the normal conduction system. They act on the initial rapid depolarization and slow the phase 0 depolarization rate,without altering the resting potential and are sometimes called *membrane stabilizers* (Chapter 15). Class I drugs are subdivided into 3 subgroups according to their effect on action potential duration which determines the refractoriness of the cardiac tissue:

(IA) ***Those which prolong repolarization*** (refractoriness, *phase 3)* and hence, moderately suppress conduction and prolong the action potential duration, in addition to suppression of automaticity e.g. Quinidine, Procainamide, Disopyramide;

(IB) ***Those which shorten repolariation*** (refractoriness, *phase 3)* and action potential duration. They suppress automaticity; have little influence on conduction velocity; and shorten the refractory period e.g. Lignocaine, Phenytoin, Mexiletine, Tocainide, and

(IC) ***Those which have no effect on action potential duration and repolarization but mainly slow phase 0 depolarization rate,*** e.g., Flecainide, Propafenone; they markedly slow conduction.

Class II : **Beta adrenergic blockers** which block the beta$_1$ cardiac receptors and mainly suppress phase 4 depolarization (diastolic depolarization). They do not prolong repolarization (phase 3).

Class III : **Potassium channel blockers:** They act by **markedly prolonging Action Potential duration** (prolong repolarization — phase 3) without affecting the conduction velocity, e.g., Amiodarone, Sotalol, Ibutilide. Sotalol is a non-cardioselective beta blocker with additional class II activity.

Class IV : **Calcium channel blockers** (Verapamil but not Nifedipine) which shorten the action potential duration and depress the slow inward Ca^{++} current (phase 2). Their action is mostly limited to SA and AV node where the electrical activities are more calcium dependent. They slow conduction and increase ERP.

Class V : **Miscellaneous:**

(a) Those which do not cause prolongation of repolarization, e.g. Adenosine.

(b) **Digitalis** (Chapter 30); Potassium; Magnesium.

Although such a classification may help the clinician in understanding the mechanism of action of specific drugs, most of the antiarrhythmic drugs have multiple actions. Further, the metabolites of these drugs contribute to or even are primarily responsible for the antiarrhythmic action of some drugs. Thus, the procainamide metabolite, n-acetylprocainamide, has class III action (prolongation of repolarization).

The antiarrhythmic drugs can also be classified clinically as:

I **Those used for supraventricular arrhythmias,** viz. Adenosine, Verapamil and Diltiazem.

II **Those used for both supraventricular and ventricular arrhythmias,** viz. Amiodarone, Beta blockers, Disopyramide, Quinidine and Procainamide; and

III **Those used for ventricular arrhythmias,** viz Lignocaine, Mexiletine and Bretylium tosylate.

The choice of anti-arrhythmic agent in a given arrhythmia depends on :

- ***Correct diagnosis.***
- ***Urgency for treatment.***
- ***Route of administration.***
- ***Extent of cardiac damage***; and
- ***The risk-benefit ratio of the drug concerned.***

All the anti-arrhythmic drugs have both cardiac and non-cardiac adverse effects which vary in severity. Although the drug may be indicated for a particular arrhythmia it may not be effective in every patient; this is particularly true for recurrent ventricular arrhythmias.

Table 27.1 lists the major risks with Group I antiarrhythmics. All drugs that block the sodium channels have the capacity to reduce ventricular function. This propensity is highest with flecainide (IC). Class III agents are also pro-arrhythmic but to a smaller extent. Further, flecainide is known to cause (a) incessant, sustained ventricular tachycardia; (b) ventricular fibrillation; this is particularly likely to occur in

Table 27.1: Cardiovascular risks with Group I antiarrhythmic agents

- Bradycardia, heart block.
- Heart failure.
- New or worsened arrhythmias
  Torsade de pointes
  Increased frequency of ventricular tachycardia.
- Increased mortality during long term treatment.

patients with poor ventricular function and in those on diuretics or digitalis, and (c) unexplained, sudden deaths.

Therefore, although ventricular premature beats and non-sustained ventricular tachycardia increase the risk in patients with recent MI, asymptomatic and mildly symptomatic patients with such arrhythmias may not benefit from antiarrhythmic drugs other than beta adrenergic blocking agents.

QUINIDINE: Quinidine is discussed here as the prototype of Group IA. It is an isomer of the antimalarial drug quinine, one of the alkaloids occurring in the cinchona bark. The beneficial effect of quinine on AF was first noted by a Dutch colonial with atrial fibrillation, who took quinine for malaria. Later, Wenckebach, an Austrian cardiologist confirmed this observation and introduced quinine as an antiarrhythmic drug.

Pharmacological actions: These can be conveniently considered as,

I Cardiac actions and
II Extracardiac actions.

The cardiac actions are mainly due to its vagolytic and myocardiac depressant properties.

Quinidine gets bound to the cardiac cell membrane and blocks the sodium channels, thereby modifying the various electrophysiological properties of cardiac tissue. It also inhibits potassium channels in the cardiac cells.

- ***Automaticity*** **:** Quinidine depresses diastolic depolarization and hence, automaticity in all tissues, especially the ectopic pacemaker. This action helps to suppress the arrhythmias due to enhanced impulse formation. Quinidine does not suppress the automaticity of the normal SA node although it can do so in the case of a diseased SA node (sick sinus syndrome).
- ***Excitability*****:** Quinidine depresses the excitability of the cardiac tissue and hence a weak ectopic impulse becomes ineffective.
- ***Conduction velocity*****:** Quinidine slows the conduction velocity in all the cardiac tissues. This property, along with the increased RP and decreased excitability, contributes to a decreased cardiac rate in arrhythmias due to the presence of an ectopic focus.
- ***Refractory period*****:** Quinidine blocks delayed rectifier potassium current, thus depressing the potassium efflux during repolarization. Thus, it prolongs (by a direct action) repolarization and hence, the RP of cardiac tissues. However, its vagolytic action increases the atrial RP, shortens that of the A-V node while leaving that of the ventricles unaltered. The overall action of quinidine in the intact animal is (a) to prolong the RP markedly in the atria, (b) to increase it in the ventricles to a smaller extent and (c) to decrease it in the A-V node.

Simple prolongation of RP prevents the heart from responding to premature or rapid stimulation. Re-entry movement is intercepted, since the re-entrant impulse may find the originally depolarized tissue still inexcitable. Quinidine thus abolishes the arrhythmias due to re-entrant circuits.

- ***A-V conduction*****:** Quinidine depresses conduction predominantly within the atria and the His-Purkinje system. However, its vagolytic (antimuscarinic) effect appears to permit or even enhance conduction in the A-V node, causing tachycardia. Thus, the occurrence of sudden ventricular acceleration in patients with atrial flutter treated with quinidine is most likely to be due to both slowing of the flutter rate and improved conduction across the A-V node.

Quinidine is contraindicated in the presence of intraventricular conduction disturbances.

- ***Contractility*** **:** Quinidine exerts a negative inotropic action on the heart. This obviously is a disadvantage. Elevation of the serum potassium enhances the depressant effects of quinidine, while its action is reduced in hypokalemia.

- ***Effects on ECG*** **:** Early changes comprise increase in Q-T interval. Decrease in amplitude or inversion of T wave and depression of S-T segment may also occur. Later changes include widening and frequent notching of the P wave, and prolonged P-R interval.

Widening of the QRS complex signifies reduction of conduction velocity, and if accompanied by a considerable increase in the RP of the ventricle, might lead to the development of ventricular tachycardia and eventually to ventricular fibrillation (VF). If ventricular extrasystoles fail to respond to quinidine in spite of widening of the QRS complex, further increase in quinidine dosage may precipitate VF. When, the QRS complex is widened by 25 to 50 per cent or above 0.12 to 0.14 second, quinidine should be withheld.

Quinidine is known to cause unpredictable abnormalities of rhythm in digitalized heart and as it is usually employed after initial digitalization in the treatment of AF, a careful surveillance of the patient is necessary.

Extracardiac actions :

- ***Blood pressure*****:** Quinidine causes a significant lowering of the BP in most patients. The subsequent circulatory adjustments, however, depend on the physiological status of the subject. Thus, if the cardiac output is normal, quinidine does not produce any significant change; but if the cardiac output is low, quinidine may shift it towards normal. This is accomplished by a reduction in BP which reduces the left ventricular load, permitting a more complete emptying of the ventricle.

- ***Miscellaneous actions*** **:** Quinidine depresses the skeletal muscle and like quinine, shows antimalarial, antipyretic and oxytocic activities.

Absorption, fate and excretion : Quinidine is almost completely absorbed from the gut. Following a single oral dose, the peak effects are reached within 2 to 3 hours and persist for 6 to 8 hours. Quinidine given IV could be very toxic.

Quinidine is bound to plasma albumin (80 per cent). It is primarily metabolized (75%) in the liver with half life of 4-8 hours. One metabolite 3-hydroxyquinidine is as potent as quinidine. About 25 per cent of the drug is excreted in an unchanged form.

With the same quinidine regimen, there are wide differences in the serum quinidine levels in different persons. Electrophysiological and toxic effects correlate better with serum levels than with dosage of quinidine. Hence, frequent clinical and ECG monitoring of the patient is mandatory.

Adverse reactions :

Cardiac toxicity : The drug causes bradycardia, conduction defects and heart failure. The risk of heart failure is maximum in patients with marked cardiac damage. Further, there may be increased frequency of ventricular premature beats. In addition, two distinct, drug-induced ventricular arrhythmias may occur :

- ***Torsade de pointes;*** and
- ***Incessant ventricular tachycardia.***

All antiarrhythmic drugs that prolong QT interval markedly can precipitate a polymorphic ventricular tachycardia known as *torsade de pointes*, which may result in syncope and sudden death. Other drugs which can produce a similar effect are : amiodarone, amitryptiline, cisapride, chlorpromazine, sotalol and quinine.

When used in conjunction with digitalis, quinidine may precipitate VF or cardiac arrest.

These are caused by extreme depression of the S-A node and the A-V conduction.

Hypotension: Hypotension has been observed more commonly in older patients, even with relatively small doses.

Embolic phenomena: Sudden restoration of sinus rhythm by quinidine in a patient with chronic AF may dislodge the mural thrombi attached to auricular appendages. This might precipitate embolic occlusion of the vessels of the vital organs and may even cause sudden death. Fortunately, this occurs rarely. Prophylactic anticoagulant therapy is used before conversion in patients with AF.

Miscellaneous toxicity:

- ***Allergic Reactions*:** The manifestations of intolerance include skin rashes, fever and thrombocytopenic purpura.
- ***Gastrointestinal*:** Nausea, vomiting and diarrhoea are common.
- ***Cerebral*:** Headache, dizziness and convulsions may result from a direct effect of quinidine on the CNS.
- ***Cinchonism*:** It results from cumulative overdosage and includes impairment of hearing, ringing in ears, vertigo, blurred vision, light headedness, giddiness and tremor.

Drug interactions: Quinidine is metabolized by hepatic cytochrome P450 enzymes and hence, induction or inhibition of these enzymes affects plasma concentration of quinidine. These enzymes are inhibited by erythromycin and ketoconazole, which can result in higher plasma concentration while induction of these enzymes by rifampicin and other drug causes increased clearance of quinidine. Quinidine also increases the plasma digoxin level.

Preparations and dosage: Quinidine sulfate, 200 mg. Dose 200-400 mg. every 6 hours.

Therapeutic uses:

- ***Atrial fibrillation (AF) and atrial flutter*:** Asymptomatic patients with these conditions need no treatment; in some of these patients, anticoagulant therapy may be commenced. Patients in whom *symptoms persist* in spite of control of the ventricular rate with drugs such as diltiazem, propranolol or digoxin may benefit from conversion to sinus rhythm with quinidine-like drugs. Such patients need careful monitoring of cardiac rhythm. *Quinidine-like drugs are not recommended in the long term treatment of AF as this increases the mortality.*

Quinidine, when used for the conversion of AF to normal sinus rhythm, restores normal rhythm in 70 to 80 per cent of patients. *However, it is a potentially dangerous drug and inconvenient to use in view of the long period of observation required for its safe use.* DC conversion is considered the preferred method of restoring sinus rhythm.

The main use of quinidine is to reduce the risk of recurrent AF after conversion to sinus rhythm. When normal sinus rhythm is established, prophylactic maintenance dose, 0.2 to 0.4 g. 3 to 4 times a day is continued for a few days. *Patients with AF are digitalized prior to quinidine therapy.* This is because, digitalis corrects the cardiac failure often present in association with fibrillation. Further, quinidine therapy alone may result in a rapid ventricular rate during conversion of fibrillation to sinus rhythm. *It should be remembered, however, that both digitalis and quinidine can cause conduction blocks.*

Table 27.2 summarizes the principles of treatment of (AF).

AF is often an incidental finding in a patient with some cardiovascular disease and it needs to be treated. In subjects with short history (a few days) and with normal sized atrium cardioversion may be attempted. Pharmacological correction can be achieved by amiodarone; ibutilide and amiodarone are also useful in patients with recurrent AF after earlier DC conversion.

- ***Paroxysmal atrial and nodal tachycardia and ventricular tachycardia*:** Although quinidine can be used in these conditions, other measures such as carotid massage, propranolol, digitalis, IV verapamil, vasopressor agents and parasympathomimetic drugs should be tried first.
- ***Atrial, nodal and ventricular premature beats*:** Most premature beats, particularly if the frequency is below 100 per 24 hours, without definite pathology, cause no complaints and require no therapy except the occasional use of sedatives. The development of ventricular

Table 27.2: Principles of treatment of atrial fibrillation (AF)

- ***Control of ventricular rate***

(a) Urgent DC cardioversion in patients hemodynamically unstable because of rapid ventricular rate; needed more often in flutter than in fibrillation.

(b) Antiarrhythmic drugs in patients with stable hemodynamics: IV diltiazem, verapamil, metoprolol (which act within 5-10 min), ibutilide, amiodarone or digoxin (which starts acting in 3 hours). The same drugs may be used orally in less acute situations.

(c) Long-term rate control: Digoxin controls the resting rate; beta blockers control the exercising rate; CCB (diltiazem and verapamil) control both resting and exercise rates.

(d) Surgical or catheter ablation (see later) of the A-V junction in resistant cases.

- ***Restoration of sinus rhythm*** (Cardioversion): Either drugs (amiodarone, procainamide or disopyramide) or DC cardioversion. Treatment of an underlying or precipitating factor that is reversible may cause the rhythm to revert to sinus rhythm.
- ***Maintenance of sinus rhythm***: This improves the hemodynamic status and may obviate the need for anticoagulation. Infrequent (fewer than once a year) episodes of atrial fibrillation may be treated as they arise. If the episodes are more frequent, long term antiarrhythmic drug therapy should be considered.
- ***Anticoagulation and antiplatelet therapy***: Anticoagulation with warfarin and to a smaller extent aspirin reduce the risk of thromboembolism. Anticoagulation is carried out before cardioversion if AF is more than 48 hours in duration or of uncertain duration. It is also recommended in patients with chronic AF.

premature beats during acute MI may herald the onset of ventricular tachycardia and in such cases, quinidine therapy may be instituted; however, *other drugs are preferred.*

Drugs are of no use in the treatment of VF and flutter; and electroversion is the treatment of choice. Quinidine can, however, be used to prevent their recurrence after electroversion.

Contraindications to quinidine therapy:

- ***QT prolongation***
- ***Chronic heart failure***
- ***History of quinidine intolerance.***
- ***Ventricular tachycardia associated with complete A-V block.***
- ***Hypotension.***
- ***Stokes-Adams syndrome.***
- ***Myasthenia gravis***

Quinidine should be given with caution in bundle branch block and in extensive myocardial damage as suggested by gross cardiomegaly. *Quinidine must not be used to treat digitalis-induced arrhythmias.*

Although quinidine is useful in patients with symptomatic ventricular arrhythmias and impaired ventricular function, other drugs are now preferred.

PROCAINAMIDE (Pronestyl): Procaine, a local anaesthetic, suppresses the excitability of the ventricular muscle. It is, however, not effective orally. It can cause stimulation of the CNS resulting in convulsions. Further, the action is of short duration as it is degraded by an esterase in the plasma (Chapter 15). Procainamide, a derivative of procaine, is effective orally, IM and IV; it is not destroyed by esterase, and is almost free from CNS toxicity. The local anaesthetic properties of procainamide are comparable to those of procaine but it does not produce nerve block.

Pharmacological actions: The cardiac and hemodynamic effects of procainamide are similar to those of quinidine.

Absorption, fate and excretion: Procainamide is rapidly and almost completely absorbed from the gut. Given orally, peak plasma level is reached within 1 hour and declines by 4 hours. Intramuscular administration produces peak level within 5 to 30 minutes and the level gradually declines by 6 hours. Peak level with IV route is reached within 4 minutes. It is minimally bound to plasma proteins and is largely (60%) excreted unchanged in urine. A small part is hydrolysed by plasma esterases. Impairment of renal function can produce cumulative toxicity.

Adverse reactions:

- ***Allergic reactions*** which include chills, fever, itching, skin rash and angioedema.
- ***Cardiotoxicity*** is similar to that of quinidine. Hypotension (or a shock-like state) occurs most often with the IV use.
- ***Mental symptoms*** simulating psychosis develop occasionally.
- ***Gastrointestinal effects*** such as anorexia, nausea and vomiting.
- ***Blood***: Agranulocytosis and SLE are rare but serious manifestations.

Preparations and dosage:

(i) Procainamide hydrochloride (Pronestyl) tablet 250 mg.

(ii) Procainamide hydrochloride injection, 100 mg. per ml.

It is administered orally in the dose of 0.25 to 0.5 g. every 4 to 6 hours. In serious cases, 0.5 to 1 g. may be given every 2 to 4 hours. The maintenance dose is 0.25 to 0.5 g. 6 hourly.

It may be administered IM in the dose of 0.25 to 0.5 g. every 4 to 6 hours. For IV use, after initial dose of 100 mg., 100 mg. may be injected every 5 minutes, the total dose not exceeding 1 gm. This route is indicated when conversion to normal sinus rhythm is urgent, as in shock-like states and during surgery. A constant watch on the ECG and BP is essential.

Therapeutic uses: Procainamide, being safer than quinidine, is used as a substitute for quinidine. It is not recommended for more than 6 months' treatment because of the risk of SLE.

DISOPYRAMIDE PHOSPHATE (Norpace, Regubeat): This drug has membrane depressant (quinidine like) and anticholinergic properties. Its therapeutic effects and toxicity are similar to those of quinidine but it is better tolerated. Given orally, it is completely absorbed and has a plasma half life of 6 hours. About 70% of the drug is excreted in urine and the rest in the bile. It can also be given IV.

Common adverse effects include prominent anticholinergic effects such as dryness of mouth, retention of urine, and constipation; less common are mental depression, erectile dysfunction and hypotension.

It was the most favoured drug in its class for treating the ventricular arrhythmias and to a smaller extent in the supraventricular arrhythmias. It is contraindicated in the presence of acute pulmonary edema, untreated cardiac failure and shock. It is now rarely used.

LIGNOCAINE (Lidocaine, Xylocard): This drug is a local anaesthetic (Chapter 15). Given IV, it:

- ***Selectively acts on diseased or ischemic myocardium.***
- ***Has a rapid onset and short duration of action.***
- ***Depresses diastolic depolarization and automaticity in ventricular tissue.***
- ***Shortens the ventricular action potential.***
- ***Has little influence on conduction velocity in normal tissues.***
- ***Does not significantly affect the electrophysiological function of the atria, SA node and AV node, and causes hardly any change in the surface ECG; and***
- ***Has no hemodynamic adverse effects.***
- ***Toxicity, if it occurs, is of short duration.***

Since the electrophysiological effects of lignocaine are primarily limited to ventricular myocardium, it is most useful in abolishing ventricular arrhythmias. Its lack of action on A-V nodal conduction velocity, makes it a suitable drug in the treatment of digitalis induced ventricular arrhythmia.

The drug is usually given IV, although it can also be used IM. *The IV preparation must not contain a preservative nor a sympathomimetic or other vasoconstrictor. The common local anaesthetic preparation should not be used intravenously.* It is not effective orally because of extensive hepatic first pass metabolism. Its plasma-protein-binding is 60-80%. The plasma half-life after a single injection is from 15 to 30 minutes.

Adverse reactions : In recommended dosage, lignocaine is a relatively safe drug. Adverse reactions include drowsiness, disorientation, muscle twitchings and rarely convulsions. It diminishes the cardiac output and may rarely cause hypotension, bradycardia and apnea. *An IV preparation of a barbiturate or diazepam should be at hand while using IV lignocaine.* It should not be used in the presence of liver damage.

Therapeutic uses: It is the drug of choice for :

(1) Treating severe ventricular arrhythmias of many etiologies in an acute setting.

(2) Emergency termination of ventricular tachycardia following recent MI and that occurring during cardiac surgery and cardiac catheterization; and

(3) Treating digitalis-induced ventricular arrythmias.

Because of its immediate effect and short duration of action (10 min.), lignocaine is given as a single large initial IV bolus, 1-2 mg./kg. in 30 sec., followed by a continuous IV infusion at the rate of 1-4 mg/min. to maintain the effect. Smaller doses (50%) are used in patients with congestive heart failure, shock, hepatic dysfunction and in those over 70 years.

PHENYTOIN SODIUM (Diphenylhydantoin): The hypothesis that the excitatory processes or substances initiating the discharge of impulses in cardiac arrhythmias may be similar to those responsible for epilepsy, led to the use of phenytoin in the treatment of cardiac arrhythmias (Chapter 9).

Phenytoin depresses the ventricular automaticity; but like lignocaine it does not decrease the conduction velocity between the ventricular fibres. It also accelerates the A-V conduction. Similar to lignocaine, it reduces the duration of the action potential. Phenytoin has little effect on the surface electrocardiogram although it may shorten the QT interval.

It is administered orally in the dosage of 100-200 mg. 4 times daily for the suppression of ectopic beats and for prophylaxis against recurrent paroxysmal tachycardia. Because of its long half life, the therapeutic effect can be maintained by oral administration of 1.0 g. on the first day, 0.6 g. on the second and third days and 0.4 g. per day thereafter.

Therapeutic uses: The main use of IV phenytoin is to terminate digitalis induced cardiac arrhythmias where it was preferred as it does not aggravate the A-V block. Further, it does not cause any adverse effect on intraventricular conduction or myocardial contractility. The reversibility of the adverse effects and freedom from hypotension after therapeutic doses are important advantages. However, as lignocaine is more effective for this purpose, the use of IV phenytoin has declined.

It is given by slow IV injection. A constant IV infusion is more liable to cause phlebitis because of the high pH, and should be avoided.

In digitalis-induced ventricular tachycardia, when procainamide has to be discontinued because of QRS widening, phenytoin can still be used since it can reverse the conduction block while accentuating the depression of automaticity. Its use in controlling other arrhythmias is disappointing.

MEXILETINE (Maxitil): This drug resembles lignocaine, chemically as well as in its pharmacological actions. It is, however, effective orally and can be used to treat ventricular arrhythmias. Adverse reactions are common and are dose related. They include vomitting, tremor, ataxia, blurred vision and hypotension. The dose is 400 mg. followed by 200 mg. tid.

TOCAINIDE: This is an amine analogue of lignocaine and can be given orally in the dose of 400-800 mg. every 8 hours. It can cause serious dose related neurological adverse effects.

Table 27.3: Principal effects of some antiarrhythmic drugs on the heart

	Group IA (Quinidine, Procainamide, Disopyramide)	Group IB (Lignocaine, Phenytoin)	Group II (Propranolol)	Group IV (Verapamil)
Electrophysiological				
Automaticity	Decrease	Decrease	Decrease	Decrease
Excitability	Decrease	No change	Decrease	Decrease
Conduction velocity	Decrease	No change or increase	Decrease	Decrease
ERP	Increase	Decrease	Increase	Increase
Electrocardiogram				
PR duration	No change or increase	No change or decrease	No change or increase	No change or increase
QRS duration	Increase	No change	No change	No change
Q-T duration	Increase	No change or decrease	No change or decrease	No change
Hemodynamic				
Blood pressure	No change or decrease	No change or decrease	No change or decrease	No change or decrease
Cardiac output	Decrease	No change or decrease	Decrease	Decrease
Contractility	Decrease	No change or decrease	Decrease	Decrease
Left ventricular end diastolic pressure	May increase	No change or increase	May increase	May increase
Adverse effects	Proarrhythmic Negative inotropic effect Conduction block	Negative inotropic effect	Sinus bradycardia Conduction block Negative inotropic effect	Conduction block Negative inotropic effect

FLECAINIDE (Tambocor): This fluorinated analogue of procainamide is well absorbed on oral administration. It is highly effective but causes marked prolongation of PR and QRS intervals and minimal changes in the QT interval, and is liable to cause arrythmias and sudden death. It also has negative inotropic effect. It can also be given IV slowly. It is a specialist's drug.

ENCAINIDE (Enkaid): It has properties similar to flecainide and is effective orally. It has mild negative inotropic action. Both flecainide and encainide are used as substitutes for quinidine. *Although encainide and flecainide readily suppress ventricular premature beats, they can promote incessant ventricular tachycardia which is difficult to terminate.*

PROPAFENONE : This class 1C antiarrythmic drug also has mild beta blocker and calcium channel blocker activities. It is relatively safe for suppression of supraventricular arrythmia including WPW syndrome and recurrent AF. It is also used for treating life threatening ventricular arrythmia provided there is no associated structural heart disease. At the onset of paroxysm, 600 mg is administered orally, followed by 300 mg 8 hourly.

The adverse effects are dose related and include prolongation of PR and QRS complex, conduction blocks, inhibition of sinus node and precipitation of cardiac heart failure.

Moricizine: This phenothiazine derivative belongs to class IC and is used to treat supraventricular arrhythmias. It is given orally in the dose of 200-300 mg tid. Its active metabolites contribute to its long t½. Dizziness and nausea are the common adverse effects.

Adrenergic Blocking Agents: Alpha-adrenergic blocking drugs like phenoxybenzamine, administered prophylactically, can prevent the cardiac arrhythmias occurring during surgery of pheochromocytoma (Chapter 17).

Myocardiac sympathetic ß-receptor stimulation increases automaticity, enhances A-V conduction velocity and shortens the refractory period especially in supraventricular tissues. **Beta-adrenergic blocking agents** are useful because they :

- ***Antagonise the effects of beta-adrenoreceptor activation on SA node*** and some ectopic foci.
- ***Prolong the refractoriness of AV node*** and slow down the ventricular rate.
- ***Have a membrane stabilising properties*** (propranolol and oxprenolol).
- ***Reduce myocardial oxygen demand,*** particularly in the presence of IHD; and
- ***Are generally well tolerated and are much safer than class I group of drugs.***

The detailed pharmacology of ß-adrenergic receptor blocking drugs is discussed in Chapter 17.

PROPRANOLOL antagonises the tachyarrhythmias precipitated by sympathetic discharge during exercise, emotion or anaesthesia and in patients with thyrotoxicosis. It is a useful adjunct in patients with AF refractory to digitalis.

The plasma half life of propranolol is 2 to 3 hours following IV administration and 4 to 6 hours after oral use. The drug is given slowly IV at the rate of 1 mg. over 1 minute, repeated at 2 minutes interval upto a total dose of 0.1 mg./kg. Orally it is used in the dose of 10-40 mg. every 6 to 8 hours. Other beta blockers may also be used. Severe propranolol toxicity may result in progressive bradycardia and cardiac asystole.

Long term therapy with beta adrenergic antagonists reduces the frequency of sudden death after MI despite the patients having a relative contraindication (Chapter 30). They exhibit synergistic effect when combined with other antiarrhythmic drugs from class I and III. Broad spectrum of antiarrhythmic activity and established safety record make them agents of choice for general use as antiarrhythmic agents. (Chapter 31).

Beta blockers may potentiate the negative inotropic action of antiarrhythmic drugs, particularly verapamil, which can result in marked bradycardia and even asystole.

Esmolol (Breviblock, Miniblock) is a rapidly acting cardioselective beta blocker with a short duration of action (t½ 9 minutes). It is given IV in the dose of 500 g/kg over one minute, followed by a 4 min. infusion of 50 g/kg/min. It may be preferred to propranolol.

SOTALOL (Betacardone): This drug is a non-cardioselective beta adrenergic blocking agent with beta blocking potency similar to that of propranolol. However, unlike propranolol it has no membrane stabilizing action.

(a) It prolongs the duration of action potentials in the atria and the ventricles in a concentration-dependent fashion.

(b) It prolongs the ERP of all cardiac tissues, including the A-V node and His-Purkinje system.

These actions are unrelated to its beta blocking action.

(c) It has no negative inotropic effect in isolated cardiac tissue, and clinically it does not reduce the left ventricular ejection fraction in the majority of cases.

(d) Experimentally, IV sotalol increases the ventricular fibrillation threshold in normal and ischemic myocardium.

The surface ECG shows prolongation of QT interval.

Absorption, fate and excretion: Given orally, it is absorbed completely and does not undergo first pass metabolism in the liver. It is excreted unchanged (90%) in the urine. Its apparent plasma t½ is 7 to 18 hours.

Adverse reactions : These are due to its beta blocking properties viz. sinus bradycardia, conduction blocks and hypotension; and due to its property of prolonging the QT interval viz. *torsade de pointes* (similar to quinidine).

Preparations and dosage : Sotalol hydrochloride tablets (40, 80 and 200 mg.) and a solution (10 mg./ml.) for IV injection. The oral dose is 80-160 mg. per day in divided doses (maximum oral dose 640 mg./day). It is important to avoid hypokalemia during its use.

Therapeutic uses: Although sotalol is relatively safe in patients who have arrhythmias after MI, it is not recommended routinely as a substitute for other beta blockers. It has been found to be specifically useful in :

- ***Unsustained ventricular arrhythmias such as ventricular ectopic beats,*** even in patients with reduced left ventricular function.
- ***Sustained ventricular tachycardia.***
- ***W-P-W syndrome or recurrent atrioventricular nodal tachycardia;*** and
- ***Prevention of inducible ventricular tachycardia and fibrillation.***

The main advantage of sotalol is that its use is associated with low incidence of adverse effects as compared to the sodium channel blocking antiarrhythmic (class I) agents. It can also be used in the treatment of hypertension and angina. It is very expensive.

IBUTILIDE: This class III agent is used for chemical cardioversion of atrial flutter and fibrillation. It prolongs the atrial and ventricular RP with minimal effect on conduction, probably through its K^+ channel inhibiting action. It also activates the inward Na^+ current. Given IV, it acts within 1 to 2 hours.

Dofetilide has similar properties as ibutilide but can be given orally. It blocks the delayed rectifier current in dose-dependent manner; the effects are more in hypokalemia. Given orally, 80% undergoes renal excretion unchanged.

AMIODARONE (Cordarone): This drug, structurally related to thyroxine, possesses antiadrenergic properties. It:

- ***Depresses sinus, atrial and A-V nodal function.***
- ***Prolongs the effective refractory period of A-V node and ventricles;*** and
- ***Slows the conduction in A-V node and specialized conducting tissues.***

Its hemodynamic effects include bradycardia, increase in cardiac output and a fall in peripheral and coronary vascular resistance. It can be used orally as well as IV. It has a large apparent volume of distribution and is stored in fat and tissues. *Its half ife is 18-60 days* and it is metabolized in the liver. In an emergency, it must be given by IV infusion. Oral therapy is helpful in chronic prophylactic use.

Adverse reactions : *It has a wide spectrum of adverse effects* which are mainly dose-dependent. These include anorexia, nausea, abdominal pain, tremor, hallucinations, peripheral neuropathy, elevation of SGPT, hypotension, A-V block, hypersensitivity pneumonitis pulmonary fibrosis and asymptomatic corneal microdeposits. It enhances the bradycardia caused by beta blockers. It contains iodine and can cause disorders of thyroid function (Chapter 62). *The drug is embryotoxic.*

Therapeutic uses: Amiodarone is a potent but toxic drug useful in preventing and treating both supraventricular and ventricular tachyarrhythmias. It is particularly useful in patients with sustained ventricular tachycardia. Its beneficial effects are seen after 5 to 10 days and full improvement may not occur for 4 to 6 weeks of therapy. However, it should be considered only if other alternatives are not suitable. It is a difficult drug to handle. Even its short term use can precipitate serious toxicity.

Aprinidine, like amiodarone, is useful in controlling refractory ventricular (and, to a smaller extent, supraventricular) tachyarrhythmias. Its electrophysiological effects resemble those of quinidine.

VERAPAMIL (Isoptin, Cordilox): This calcium channel blocker (Chapter 28) is the drug of choice for rapid conversion to sinus rhythm in cases of paroxysmal supraventricular tachycardia. It is given IV in the dose of 5-10 mg. injected over a period 2 to 3 minutes; and can be repeated, if necessary, after 30 minutes. It can also be given orally in the dose of 40-120 mg. three times a day. Verapamil can also be used to reduce the ventricular rate in patients with AF and atrial flutter. *Verapamil IV is absolutely contraindicated in patients on beta blockers, quinidine or disopyramide* (Chapter 28).

DILTIAZEM has similar uses as verapamil in supra-ventricular arrythmias. In fact, it may be the preferred drug because of its less marked negative inotropic effect. Like verapamil, it may be used orally or IV. The IV dose is 0.25-0.35 mg/kg over 10 minutes, followed by 5-15 mg/hour.

Calcium channel blockers are not likely tobe useful in the prevention or suppression of most clinically important ventricular arrhythmias.

ADENOSINE (Adenocarg): This is a naturally occurring purine nucleoside which is released during myocardial ischemia. It has antiarrhythmic and potent vasodilator properties. Its exact mechanism of action is not known. It probably acts as a K^+ channel opener, thereby controlling supraventricular tachycardia. It also blocks inward calcium current in the myocytes. It is rapidly metabolized by circulating adenosine deaminase and has a very short plasma t½ (4 to 8 seconds). Given IV, as a rapid bolus, it suppresses SA node automaticity and depresses A-V nodal conduction. The drug can rapidly terminate paroxysmal, supraventricular tachycardia and is safer than verapamil. It is not effective in converting AF or ventricular tachycardia into sinus rhythm. Unlike verapamil, adenosine may be used after a beta blocker. It is contraindicated in the presence of asthma, sick sinus syndrome or A-V block. Adverse effects include nausea, dyspnoe a, headache, flushing, ventricular ectopy and severe bradycardia.

Digoxin, because of its positive inotropric action, is an important antiarrhythmic agent useful in slowing A-V conduction in AF with increased ventricular rate. (Chapter 30).

POTASSIUM: The basic cardiac effects of potassium administration without causing hyperkalemia are :

- ***Reduction in conduction velocity.***
- ***Prolongation of the refractory period***; and
- ***Diminution in the automaticity.***

These effects differ in degree in different cardiac tissues and are most marked in the Purkinje fibres. In toxic doses, it is more likely to cause intraventricular conduction defects than A-V block. Hypokalemia predisposes to digitalis toxicity (Chapter 30). Slight, induced hyper-kalemia can protect against arrhythmias arising after cardiac surgery (Chapter 36). Correction of hypokalemia, hypoxia and acid base distur-bances often restores sinus rhythm without the use of antiarrhythmic drugs.

The administration of antiarrhythmic agents in the presence of high serum potassium levels may be disastrous.

Magnesium, as magnesium sulfate 2-4 g by slow IV injection over 10-15 minutes, repeated once if necessary, is useful in the emergency treatment of ventricular tachycardia, including digoxin-induced and polymorphic ventricular tachycardia (especially torsades de points). It is especially indicated in the presence of hypokalemia where hypomagnesemia may also be present.

Table 27.4: Drug treatment of cardiac arrhythmias

Arrhythmia	Emergency Treatment*		Chronic treatment and prophylaxis
	Preferred treatment	Other treatment	
SA Node:			
Sinus arrhythmia	Needs no treatment	-	-
Sinus tachycardia	Sedative, Propranolol	Treat the cause	-
Sinus bradycardia	Atropine	Treat the cause	-
Atria:			
Premature beats	Sedative, Propranolol	Quinidine, Procainamide, Disopyramide	Quinidine, Procainamide, Disopyramide, Digitalis*
Paroxysmal atrial tachycardia (PAT)	Vagal manoevres, IV Verapamil Diltiazem	IV Propranolol IV Adenosine	Quinidine, Disopyramide, Procainamide, Propranolol, Digitalis*
PAT with hemodynamic compromise	DC cardioversion		Quinidine
Atrial fibrillation and Atrial Flutter	To control ventricular rate : IV Verapamil, Diltiazem Beta blockers	To terminate fibrillation: a) Amiodarone/Ibutilide b) DC cardioversion c) Digitalis + Quinidine	Digitalis or Propranolol
Ventricles:			
Premature beats	IV Lignocaine, Beta blockers, Amiodarone	Quinidine, Procainamide, Disopyramide.	Procainamide, Disopyramide, Digoxin**, Propranolol***
Paroxysmal ventricular tachycardia (PVT)	Same as above	Same as above	Same as above
PVT with hemodynamic compromise	DC cardioversion		Quinidine
Ventricular fibrillation	Defibrillation	Lignocaine, IV Bretylium	Quinidine, Procainamide, Disopyramide.
Digitalis induced tachyarrhythmias	Lignocaine	IV Phenytoin	
Complete A-V Block	Atropine	Isoprenaline	Pacemaker

* = When using digoxin, verapamil or a beta blocker IV, drugs such as atropine and isoprenaline and cardiac pacemaker equipment should be at hand in the event of complete A-V block; in case of verapamil, calcium gluconate 1 g IV is also effective for this purpose.
** = If related to congestive cardiac failure, *** = Useful when ventricular tachyarrhythmias are associated with increased sympathetic tone or circulating catecholamines.

Cholinergic and anticholinergic drugs: Similar to vagal action, acetylcholine decreases the automaticity and slows conduction through the A-V node, increases its refractory period and may cause A-V block. **Edrophonium,** a short acting cholinesterase inhibitor, is sometimes useful in the treatment of supraventricular arrhythmia (Chapter 19).

Atropine, an anticholinergic drug, blocks the effects of vagal stimulation. It is of some value for the diagnosis of sinus bradycardia, where it increases the heart rate, and in the treatment of heart block, if the latter is due to vagal influences. Its indiscriminate use, however, to treat sinus bradycardia after MI may precipitate ventricular arrhythmias because the sympathetic activity is no longer moderated by vagal influences.

Table 27.4 summarises the drug therapy of cardiac arrhythmias.

Drugs Used in the Treatment of Heart-Block

ISOPRENALINE (Isoproterenol): The effects of isoprenaline in enhancing the rhythmicity of sinus as well as subsidiary nodal and ventricular pacemakers have proved invaluable in the treatment of advanced second degree and high grade A-V block. In emergency, the drug is administered IV in the dose of 2 mg. in 500 ml. of 5 per cent dextrose under ECG control. In less urgent situations, it is generally given sublingually in the dose of 10-15 mg. every 4 to 6 hours. Isoprenaline is also effective in abolishing ventricular tachycardia in the presence of advanced AV block. It acts by:

- ***Accelerating the basic sinoauricular pacemaker*** resulting in the suppression of ectopic ventricular activity,
- ***Enhancing A-V conduction,*** and
- ***Increasing the cardiac output*** as a result of increased heart rate. This tends to augment the coronary flow.

Other sympathomimetic drugs like adrenaline and ephedrine are less effective than isoprenaline.

A-V conduction can also be improved during an emergency by **atropine** 0.6 mg. IV.

Glucocorticoids are helpful when the heart block is due to an inflammatory disorder such as rheumatic fever.

Electrical depolarization of the heart: Electroversion has been used successfully in supraventricular tachycardias (AF, flutter and paroxysmal atrial tachycardia). *It is a life-saving procedure in case of ventricular tachycardia and fibrillation.* However, electrical cardioversion does not obviate the need for antiarrhythmic drugs which must be used frequently to prevent the recurrence of the arrhythmias.

It is contraindicated in digitalis-induced arrhythmias. When it is used for treating other types of arrhythmias, digitalis is generally omitted for 24 hours before electroversion. It may induce VF if employed in patients with advanced A-V block.

DC shock is used under IV diazepam cover.

Surgical or radiofrequency (RF) ablation of the focus of arrhythmias is now available and has been reported to result in 'cure' of the arrhythmias in selected cases.

Vasodilator Drugs and Pharmacotherapy of Angina Pectoris

28

Angina pectoris is not a disease but a symptom of myocardial ischemia produced in a variety of ways. It develops as a result of an imbalance between the oxygen supply and the oxygen demand of the myocardium. Its onset and clinical modalities, therefore, are related to :

- ***The physiology of the coronary circulation.***
- ***The factors governing myocardial metabolism; and***
- **The mechanism regulating the genesis and appreciation of pain.**

The design of the coronary circulation has three bad features:

- ***The coronary arteries are functionally end arteries.*** In health, there is little communication between the larger branches of coronary arteries although collateral circulation does develop in patients who have had MI.
- ***Unlike the skeletal muscle, the cardiac muscle shows almost maximum oxygen extraction at rest***, as shown by the comparative values of oxygen saturation of coronary sinus blood (30 per cent) and skeletal muscle venous blood (60-70 per cent). Hence, during exercise the tissue demand for increased oxygen supply is met, at least partly, by increased oxygen extraction in the case of skeletal muscle, but in the case of cardiac muscle it can only be met by increasing the coronary blood flow. Such increase can be severely limited by coronary artery disease. Moreover, unlike the skeletal muscle the cardiac muscle has extremely limited capacity for anaerobic metabolism and, therefore, cannot incur 'oxygen debt'.
- ***The coronary blood flow is influenced by the inflow (aortic) pressure and the resistance of the coronary vascular bed.*** The latter depends on: (a) the state of dilatation of the coronary arterioles, determined largely by local metabolites, and (b) the pressure exerted upon the coronary vessels from the exterior by the contracting myocardium of the left ventricle during systole. Thus, in contrast to other areas where the arterial blood flow is continuous, coronary arterial blood flow to the left ventricle is intermittent and mainly diastolic; whereas in the absence of pulmonary hypertension it is both systolic and diastolic in case of the right ventricle.

In spite of these limiting features, the coronary circulation has a very large reserve and the coronary flow can increase upto 500 per cent of the resting value in exercising healthy dogs.

Physiologically, vascular endothelial cells control the vascular tone by producing (a) vasodilators such as prostacyclin (Chapter 24) and NO/EDRF; and (b) vasoconstrictors such as endothelin and thromboxane A_2.

NITRIC OXIDE (Endothelium derived

relaxing factor EDRF) : Robert Furchgott (1980) first demonstrated that the endothelial cells release a labile factor that causes vascular relaxation. He designated it as EDRF, which later was identified as NO. Nitric oxide (NO), a simple diatomic molecule, is biosynthesized through the action of a class of enzymes **nitric oxide synthases** (NOS). These enzymes utilise the amino acid l-arginine as the endogenous substrate for NO generation. The organic **nitrates**, after conversion to **nitrites** in the body, act as the pharmacological substrate for NO synthesis. Three NOS isoforms have been identified :

(1) nNOS (NOS-1), is found in high concentrations in central and peripheral neurons and some non-neural tissues such as endometrium and skeletal muscle.

(2) aNOS (NOS-2), is found in macrophages, Kupffer cells, fibroblasts, vascular smooth muscle cells, neutrophils and endothelial cells; and

(3) eNOS (NOS-3), first identified as the enzyme that produces EDRF and found in the vascular endothelium, brain and heart.

Both types, 1 and 3, often grouped as *constitutive NOS*, are expressed constitutively, and their activities are regulated by intracellular calcium. These isoenzymes produce on demand short bursts of NO in small amounts. Type 2, on the other hand, is not expressed in resting cells and is the *inducible NOS*.When macrophages and other cells are activated,this enzyme triggers the production of large amounts of NO.

NO causes both (a) **Direct effects**, partly mediated by NO molecule itself and mainly by the interaction of NO with soluble guanylyl cyclase (which acts as the receptor for NO), resulting in the production of 3'5'-cyclic guanosine monophosphate (cGMP); and (b) **Indirect effects** mediated by the interaction of reactive nitrogen species (intermediates in NO synthesis) with oxygen and superoxide radicals, to yeild cytotoxic peroxynitrite anion.

NO is a highly diffusible second messenger that can produce effects far from its site of production. The source of NO and its concentration are the major factors which determine its biological effects. At low concentrations, the direct (physiological) effects of NO predominate. When NO production is induced, high concentrations are produced which cause indirect and often toxic effects.

Functions of NO :

- ***NO and the vascular system*:** NO causes vascular smooth muscle relaxation and vasodilatation that helps to regulate blood flow and BP. NO release from the endothelial cells is primarily the result of an influx of Ca^{++} into the endothelial cells. Thus, any agent or stimulus capable of eliciting an influx of Ca^{++} into these cells such as acetylcholine, bradykinin or shear force, can activate NO biosynthesis. The NO then acts through cyclic GMP and causes vascular muscle relaxation by lowering Ca^{++} influx.(Fig. 28.1)

Endothelial dysfunction (impaired NO production), is implicated in hypertension, cerebral and coronary vasospasm, atherosclerosis and ischemic reperfusion injury.

- ***NO and RBCs:*** NO appears to be a critical factor in the prevention of sickling of RBCs. Its precursor l-arginine is used to treat pulmonary hypertension in sickle cell disease.

- ***NO and the platelets:*** NO causes inhibition of platelet aggregation and adhesion. The NO that diffuses from the vascular endothelial cells may function primarily to inhibit the adhesion of platelets to the vascular endothelial cells. The anti-aggregatory and anti-adhesive effects of NO are a result of increased cyclic GMP within the platelets.

- ***NO and the CNS* :** Neurons which are neither adrenergic nor cholinergic innervate a variety of smooth muscles, such as those of the GI tract, the corpus cavernosus and the esophagus. These are called non-adrenergic, non-cholinergic (NANC) neurons. These neurons contain the NO-cyclic-GMP pathway, and the exclusive neurotransmitter in the NANC is NO. NO is the physiological mediator of penile erection (Chapter 67) and gastric emptying.

- ***NO and immune system* :** When the macrophages are exposed to infective agents, there is a dramatic local increase in NO production. NO synthesis by activated macrophages represents an immune response to infection. NO appears to be utilized by the immune system as a cytotoxic agent.

Adverse effects of NO : It is an important mediator of inflammation and neurodegenerative disorders. Exposure to bacterial endotoxins can lead to overproduction of NO, which can cause severe hypotension and/or endotoxic shock. NO production by the macrophages can be toxic to the pancreatic islet cells.

ENDOTHELIN (ET) : This 21 residue polypeptide, originally isolated from cultured vascular endothelium, is now known to be present in several other tissues (brain, kidney, intestine, adrenal glands) in the body. It is a potent endogenous vasoconstrictor that also has proliferative, pro-fibrotic and pro-inflammatory effects. It also stimulates secretion of many hormones. Three types of ETs have been identified so far : ET-1, ET-2 and ET-3. Of these ET-1 is the most potent, long acting vasoconstrictor which is continuously formed in the cells of resistance vessels and contributes to peripheral vascular resistance. It controls the utero-placental blood flow and is involved in the development of cardiorespiratory system. Patients with pulmonary arterial hypertension (PAH) have raised plasma and lung levels of ET-1. It is also present in thyroid follicles and is involved in thyroglobulin synthesis.

There are **two types of ET receptors :** ET_A and ET_B. ET_A is expressed on vascular smooth muscles, heart, lung and kidney. ET-1 preferentially activates ET_A which, results in vasoconstriction, bronchoconstriction, aldosterone release and smooth muscle proliferation. ET_B is mainly expressed in brain, but moderate expression is observed in vessels, heart, lungs, kidney and adrenals. In contrast to ET_A, ET_B is highly expressed on the endothelial cells (ET_{B1}) and causes vasodilatation by stimulating NO and PGI_2 synthesis in response to ETs. ET_B found on smooth muscles (ET_{B2}) is responsible for vasoconstrictor effects.

BOSENTAN (Tracleer) : This substituted pyrimidine derivative acts as a **nonselective competitive antagonist of ET_1**. It binds to both ET_A receptors in vascular smooth muscles and ET_B receptors in the brain, smooth muscles, and endothelium. Given orally in patients with PAH, it reduces the pulmonary vascular resistance and lowers the pulmonary arterial pressure.

The drug is well absorbed orally, and food does not interfere with its absorption.It is highly (98%) protein bound and has a t½ of 3 hours. It is metabolized in the liver, and the metabolites excreted in the bile. Inhibition of hepatic microsomal enzymes by ketoconazole and fluvastatin can increase its plasma levels. Bosentan can cause decrease in the serum levels of drugs such as warfarin and oral contraceptives. Cyclosporin-A increases its plasma concentration.

Adverse reactions: These include nausea, anemia and liver damage. It is teratogenic and carcinogenic in mice and rats, and is contraindicated during pregnancy.

Therapeutic uses: It has been used to treat severe pulmonary arterial hypertension (PAH), in the dose of 62.5-125 mg bid.

Sitasextan and Ambrisextan, selective, newer, analogues of bosentan are used for similar purpose as bosentan.

The other drugs used in PAH are CCB, nifedipine and diltiazen, orally; prostacyclin by IV infusion; sildenafil orally; and warfarin to counter the tendency to thrombosis.

Methods of Assessing Coronary Circulation

Experimentally, the coronary blood flow can be studied either in animals or isolated hearts. The data obtained from such studies, however, are many times inapplicable to humans. Even in human studies, it has been observed that the responses of atherosclerosed and normal coronary vessels to a given drug differ. Important methods used clinically are :

● ***Methods using a radionuclide (^{201}Thallium) or a radiopharmaceutical (^{99}m Technetium pyrophosphate) to study myocardial ischemia*** : The former localizes in the healthy, well perfused myocardium but not in the ischemic one; the latter localizes in the necrosed myocardium. These methods, with or without the use of exercise, permit detection, localization and quantification of myocardial ischemia; they also permit assessment of LV function in the form of ejection fraction and localized wall motion abnormalities. In patients who are unable to exercise, pharmacological stress testing can be carried out by infusing IV adenosine, dipyridamole or dobutamine.

● ***Coronary angiography:*** This is the definitive method of diagnosing coronary artery disease and has shown important differences between the response of normal and atherosclerotic arteries to drugs. Coronary angiography can be combined with pharmacological or exercise stress testing to assess the physiological significance of the observed coronary artery stenotic lesions. However, angina can occur even in the presence of normal coronary arteriograms.

● ***Coronary CT/MR angiography*** : They give information about calcification and patency of coronary arteries but not about condition of the mycocardium.

● ***Computerised stress test*:** This test is used for evaluating anti-anginal drugs. Patients with angina pectoris are subjected to exercise, and the amount of exercise which they can tolerate without the development of pain with concomitant ECG changes is noted. The procedure is then repeated after the drug. An increase in the exercise tolerance, as shown by a delay in the development of precordial pain and ECG changes, is a measure of anti-anginal activity of the drug.

Manifestations of ischemic heart disease (IHD): They are

(1) Silent (asymptomatic) ischemia.
(2) Angina pectoris.
(3) Acute coronary syndrome (ACS)
  (a) Unstable angina (UA)
  (b) Acute myocardial infarction (AMI)
  Non-ST-Segment Elevation MI (NSTEMI)
  ST-Segment Elevation MI (STEMI)
(4) Congestive heart failure (CHF) and
(5) Sudden cardiac death (SCD)

Angina Pectoris

Angina pectoris is a symptom which arises when there is an imbalance between the demand for oxygen by, and its supply to, the myocardium. Its occurrence depends upon two factors (a) Coronary blood flow; and (b) Oxygen consumption by the myocardium. The former may be compromised by either obstructive (athersclerotic) or vasospastic disease of the coronary arteries.

Cardiac O_2 consumption increases with increase in:

● ***Heart size.***
● ***Heart rate.***
● ***Systemic blood pressure;*** *and*
● ***Myocardial contractility,*** which is the rate at which the cardiac muscle fibre shortens.

The last three are increased by heightened sympathetic activity. The myocardial oxygen consumption increases significantly during exercise and other states (emotional excitement, exposure to cold) with increased sympathetic activity. If, for any reason, the increase in coronary blood flow is unable to match this increased oxygen demand, angina develops. It is generally described by the patient as retrosternal pain, heaviness or discomfort which may radiate to the neck, shoulder, back or the arm. It occurs **during** exercise, severe cold or stress. In each patient, there exists at a given time a threshold (**angina index = heart rate x systolic BP**) at which angina occurs. The angina index is a measure of the myocardial oxygen consumption. Spasm of the coronary arteries is also important in the production of angina.

The common clinical types of angina are:

● ***Stable exertional angina*** : This

commonest form is usually provoked by unusual physical exertion or emotional stress and is relieved by rest and nitrates. It is diagnosed when the chest pain has remained unchanged in severity, frequency and duration over several weeks. The main pathophysiological factor appears to be increased myocardial oxygen demand, induced by tachycardia and rise of BP, in a person with fixed, atherosclerotic narrowing of epicardial, coronary arteries. The ECG shows depression of ST segment during the attack.

• ***Cardiac metabolic syndrome X :*** More common in women, this condition comprises angina or angina-like chest pain on exercise; ST segment depression on treadmill exercise testing; and normal coronary angiography, with no spontaneous or inducible epicardial coronary artery spasm on ergonovine provocation. "Sensitive heart " is believed to be mechanism of the pain. Response to physical training and to beta blockers, and less satisfactory response to nitrates and CCB, aid in its diagnosis.

• ***Variant angina of Prinzmetal*** (Vasospastic angina): It is characterised by chest pain at rest rather than during exertion or stress, and ST elevation rather than depression in the ECG. Spasm of large epicardial coronary arteries is responsible for this entity. It is relatively uncommon.

Unstable angina (UA) which includes a variety of clinical pictures such as new onset angina, angina occurring at rest or with minimal exertion, progressive angina with prolonged or more frequent attacks superimposed on chronic stable angina (Cresendo angina); it can progress to MI and sudden death (pre-infarction angina). The diagnosis is made on the basis of the ECG showing ST depression, and a negative troponin test.

Drugs Used in Angina Pectoris

The drugs effective in the treatment of angina pectoris act by (a) dilating the coronary arteries and /or (b) reducing the cardiac workload by reducing pre- and after load (Fig. 28.1). The agents currently used are:

I **Organic nitrates.**
II **Beta-adrenergic blocking agents.**
III **Calcium channel blockers (CCB);** and
IV **Potassium channel activators.**

Additional beneficial effects can be obtained by using adjuncts such as :

- ***Antiplatelet drugs.***
- ***Treatment of hyperlipidemia;*** and
- ***Cytoprotectives.***

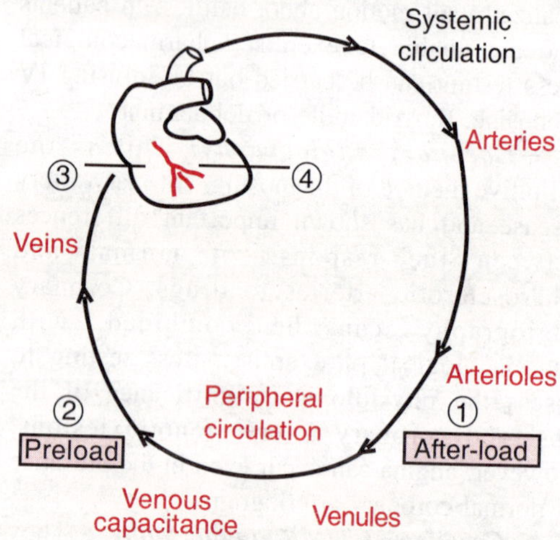

Fig. 28.1 : Antianginal drugs - sites of action

(1) **Reduce after-load** - Calcium blockers, b-blockers, nitrates.
(2) **Reduce pre-load** – Nitrates.
(3) **Negative inotropic action**-Beta-blockers, Calcium channel blockers (verapamil, diltiazem).
(4) **Coronary dilators** – Nitrates, calcium channel blockers.

ORGANIC NITRATES: Organic nitrates which are polyol esters of nitric acid are potent vasodilators and have been used successfully in the therapy of angina for over a hundred years. Usefulness of nitroglycerine was discovered by William Murrell, a physician, in 1879.

Mechanism of action: All the effects of nitrates, except those produced by toxic doses, are mediated through the direct relaxant action on smooth muscles. Organic nitrates are reduced to organic nitrites, which are then converted to

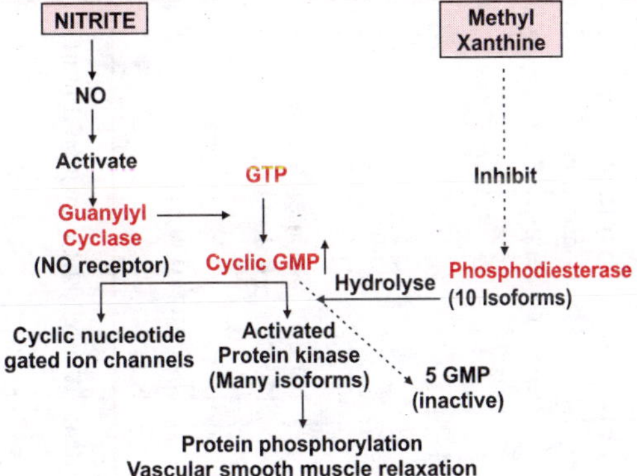

GTP:Guanosine triphosphate. Cyclic GMP:Cyclic guanosine monophosphate.

Fig. 28.2 : NO-Cyclic-AMP pathway and mechanism of action of nitrites and meythylexanthine as vasodilators

NO which acts as a direct vasodilator. (Fig. 28.2) Thus, they serve as exogenous sources of NO without involving endothelial cells (NO donors).

Pharmacological actions

I Cardiovascular system :

• ***Hemodynamic actions*:** Nitrates cause a relaxation of the systemic venous and arteriolar bed. Venodilatation causes peripheral pooling of blood and a reduction in venous return and in cardiac output. On the arterial side, relaxation is maximum in the large arteries (resulting in bounding pulse), followed by the arterioles (resulting in lowered impedence). The BP falls, the systolic more than the diastolic, and reflex tachycardia occurs due to compensatory sympathetic overactivity. Syncope may occur if the patient is standing.

These actions on the systemic venous (capacitance) and arteriolar (impedence) vascular beds reduce respectively the **preload** (end-diastolic left ventricular pressure) and the **afterload** (resistance to left ventricular ejection) on the heart. The left ventricular work load and energy expenditure thus decrease. *The improvement in the left ventricular function as a result of this generally outlasts the measured pharmacological actions of individual doses of nitrates;* this is of great importance in the therapy of angina pectoris.

Sublingual nitroglycerine (NTG) in clinically used doses is predominantly a venodilator causing reduction of ventricular preload. By contrast, inhalation of amyl nitrite, which acts very rapidly, has preferential systemic arteriolar dilator action which primarily reduces the afterload. Rapid arteriolar dilatation causes distinct fall in BP. Compensatory rise in sympathetic activity causes tachycardia and increased myocardial oxygen requirement. This is a disadvantage.

• ***Coronary circulation*:** A decrease in the coronary resistance and an increase in the total coronary flow occur in normal man; but these effects are transient. In patients with angina nitrates bring about :

(a) **Dilatation of the large epicardial coronary arteries** without affecting the resistance of the arterioles.

(b) **Dilatation of collateral vessels,** and

(c) **A redistribution of the coronary blood flow** along collaterals and from epicardial to endocardial region with improved perfusion of ischemic subendocardial areas.

Chronic administration of nitrates also promotes the development of inter-arterial anastomoses within the myocardium.

• ***Effects in angina pectoris*:** Nitrates help most patients with angina by increasing their exercise tolerance but without increasing their 'angina index'. They probably achieve this by reducing the oxygen consumption of the heart at submaximal exercise levels and thus extending the duration of such exercise. In such patients, they prevent the appearance of ECG changes of cardiac ischemia during exercise. They, however, do not increase the maximum aerobic capacity of the heart.

• ***Other vascular beds*:** Nitrates cause dilatation of other vascular beds as well, viz. (a) the skin, giving rise to flushing, (b) the meningeal vessels, resulting in throbbing headache, (c) pulmonary vessels, with fall in pulmonary arterial pressure, and (d) kidneys, with a reduction in renal flow.

II **Other smooth muscles:** Nitrates relax the

Table 28.1 : Nitrate and nitrite preparations for clinical use

Drug Preparations	Dose	Onset	Duration	Schedule	Remarks
Glyceryl trinitrate (Nitroglycerine, Angised) Tab 0.3, 0.4 and 0.6 mg.	0.3-0.6 mg. SL.*	1-2 min.	15-40 min.	SOS	Volatile. Unstable in plastic containers. Store tablets in tightly closed amber, glass bottles, without cotton plugs, preferably in a fridge. Once a bottle is opened, it should be discarded after 8 weeks and fresh supply obtained. Sublingual tablets give immediate relief. Capsules, oral tablets and ointment for prophylaxis.
Sustained release caps. (Nitromack) (2.5 mg.)	2.5 - 5.0 mg. P O	60 min.	8 - 12 hrs.	8-12 hrly.	
Sublingual spray (Nitrolingual)	0.4 mg./metered dose	1-2 min	15-40 min	every 5 minutes for 3 doses	
2% skin ointment (15 mg. per inch) (Nitrobid)	½ - 2 inch applied without rubbing	20-60 min.	4-6 hrs.	4-6 hrly	
Transdermal patches	5-15 mg.	30-60 min.	12 hrs.	once daily	
Isosorbide dinitrate (Sorbitrate, Isordil) Tab. sublingual 2.5-10 mg.	2.5-10 mg. SL.	10-30 min.	1-2 hrs.	3-4 hrly.	Hepatic metabolism to isosorbide mononitrate. Useful in immediate relief and in prophylaxis.
Buccal spray (Dinospray)	1.25 mg / actuation	2-5 min	-	-	
Tab Oral 10, 20, 40 mg.	10-40 mg. P O	30-60 min.	4 hrs.	6 hrly.	
Tab sustained release	40-80 mg. P O	60 min.	6-12 hrs	8-12 hrly.	
Isosorbide mononitrate (Ismo) Tab. 10, 20 mg.	10-20 mg. P O	30-60 min.	6-8 hrs	8-12 hrly	No first pass metabolism Used in prophylaxis.
Pentaerythritol tetranitrate (Peritrate) Tab. 30 mg.	30 mg. P O	15-30 min.	4-6 hrs.	8-12 hrly	Used in prophylaxis.

* When the tablet, placed under the tongue, fails to produce local burning, flushing of the face and pounding in the head, it should be considered inert. Tab. = tablets. Cap. = capsules; SL. = sublingually; P O = orally.

smooth muscles of the gall bladder, the biliary ducts, the sphincter of Oddi, the bronchi and the GI tract. The ureteral and uterine smooth muscle are also relaxed.

Absorption, fate and excretion: Organic nitrates are readily absorbed from the *sublingual* mucosa, and their effects are more rapid and more predictable by this route. This is because after sublingual administration, they bypass the liver where normally they are rapidly metabolized by denitration. With *relatively small sublingual doses*, the various organic nitrates have similar duration of action, 10-45 minutes.

Small oral doses (0.6 mg. of NTG or 5 mg. of isosorbide dinitrate) are of doubtful value as antianginal agents. **Large oral doses** (6.5 mg. of NTG, 30 mg. of isosorbide dinitrate or 40-80 mg. of pentaerythritol tetranitrate, every 4-6 hours) which exceed the metabolizing capacity of the liver, however, produce beneficial hemodynamic effects and are useful in prophylaxis. NTG skin ointment and transdermal patches have similar prolonged effect and are useful in prophylaxis. NTG lingual aerosol has onset and duration of action similar to those of the sublingual tablet.

Preparations and dosage: See Table 28.1. For IV use, NTG is diluted in 5% dextrose or 0.9% saline. It is administered in the dose of 5 mcg/min, increasing the rate every 3-5 minutes upto 80-100 mcg/min. It is useful in the treatment of refractory chest pain of myocardial ischemia or MI, and in patients with refractory, variant angina.

Adverse reactions :

- ***Headache* :** Although this is common, it usually decreases gradually on repeated administration and can be controlled by aspirin.
- ***Hypotension and syncope*:** Transient episodes of giddiness, weakness and other signs of cerebral ischemia associated with postural hypotension may develop. These are seen especially when the patient stands immobile. Hypoxemia may stimulate the central vagal nuclei and cold sweats, nausea, vomiting, involuntary passage of urine and faeces may accompany postural hypotension. Head-low position to augment the venous return quickly corrects the nitrite syncope. *Marked hypotension may occur when nitrates are used along with potent anti-hypertensive drugs especially vasodilators; it is also seen following the ingestion of alcoholic beverages or sildenafil* (Chapter 67).
- ***Tolerance*** to various actions of nitrates and to headache develops after repeated administration. Cross tolerance is common. *Tolerance to the anti-anginal action develops commonly when the patient is exposed to nitrate for all the 24 hours of the day.* Hence, it is more common with long acting nitrate preparations such as SR tablets and transdermal preparations; this can be avoided by omitting the night-time dose of long acting preparations. However, during such nitrate-free periods, the patient needs to be covered by another anti-anginal drug, especially if he has severe angina. *Tolerance is rare with sublingual nitrate because of the intermittent exposure.*
- ***Withdrawal symptoms*** : Sudden stoppage of nitrates during chronic administration may precipitate severe angina due to coronary spasm; such abrupt cessation should be avoided.
- ***Miscellaneous*** : Drug rash may occasionally be observed, most commonly with pentaerythritol tetranitrate.

Therapeutic uses of nitrates :

- ***All varieties of angina pectoris*:** Discussed later.
- ***At the onset of pain of acute MI*** (Chapter 31) except in those with inferior wall infarct (with right ventricular involvement).
- ***Later in the course of acute MI***, as a prelude to or a substitute for IV NTG.
- ***Paroxysmal nocturnal dyspnoea*:** NTG may give dramatic relief in paroxysmal nocturnal dyspnoea due to LVF.
- ***Acute LVF* :** Nitroglycerine by IV infusion is useful in this condition.
- ***Congestive heart failure*:** Organic nitrates are sometimes used in the long term

management of chronic heart failure due to ischemic heart disease (Chapter 30).

- ***Acute anal fissure*** : Chapter 41.
- ***Cyanide poisoning***: Amyl nitrite inhalation and IV sodium nitrite are used to treat cyanide poisoning. Nitrites convert hemoglobin to methemoglobin and methemoglobin competes with cytochrome oxidase for the cyanide ion. Combination of methemoglobin with cyanide forms cyanmethemoglobin, a relatively non-toxic product.

BETA-ADRENERGIC BLOCKING AGENTS:

These drugs are a cornerstone of the therapy of all stages of ischemic heart disease, except Prinzmetal's, vasospastic, variant angina. Only their actions relevant to angina are discussed below (also see Chapter 17).

Pharmacological actions: Exercise and emotional excitement induce angina in susceptible subjects by the increase in heart rate, BP, myocardial contractility and oxidative metabolism, which they cause through increased sympathetic activity. Beta blockers prevent angina by blocking all these effects. Moreover, they help to control BP in hypertensive patients. Like the nitrates, beta-blockers increase the exercise tolerance without increasing the angina index; they prevent both subjective and ECG manifestations of cardiac ischemia. They also prevent arrhythmias precipitated by exercise, emotion and other conditions involving excessive sympathetic activity. They reduce the frequency of anginal attacks and decrease the NTG requirement. In most patients, the net effect is a beneficial reduction in cardiac work load and myocardial oxygen consumption. However, they are not useful in acute attacks.

Long term studies have demonstrated definite prophylactic value of beta blockers in angina pectoris. They also decrease the incidence of MI in these patients. For chronic prophylaxis, they are usually combined with nitrates. *If there is evidence of cardiac decompensation, the patient should be digitalized before starting a beta-blocker.*

For use of beta blockers immediately after acute MI, see Chapter 31. They are used IV within the first 12-24 hours of onset of MI.

Long term use of beta blockers after MI has been shown to reduce the rate of re-infarction and sudden death. In experimental animals, their use reduces the size of the infarct.

Clinically, all beta blockers are probably equally effective in angina of effort. Generally, the more selective beta-blockers, atenolol, metoprolol and bisoprolol are preferred.

Beta blockers are not useful in the therapy of Prinzmetal's, vasospastic, variant angina.

Absorption, fate and excretion: Chapter 17.

Adverse reactions: The adverse reactions of relevance to antianginal therapy are:

(a) Precipitation or aggravation of congestive heart failure. Patients receiving both digoxin and a beta-blocker should be watched for the development of heart block.

(b) Development of severe syncope on using NTG or amyl nitrite in patients on a beta-blocker.

Abrupt withdrawal of beta-blockers especially when large doses are being used, can cause aggravation of angina and even precipitation of MI (Chapter 17).

CALCIUM CHANNEL BLOCKERS (CCB):

Calcium is necessary for the excitation-contraction coupling in the skeletal, cardiac and smooth muscle. However, in contrast to the contractile activity of the skeletal muscle, the contractility of the cardiac and vascular muscle is highly dependent on the extracellular calcium.

Calcium transport in myocardial and vascular smooth muscle involves :

- ***Voltage dependent channel*** which is controlled by a gate that opens and closes in response to a voltage gradient. There are 2 types of calcium channels: the L and T. Of these, the L-channels make the calcium ions available in the cytoplasm, that are required for initiation of contraction. These ions in turn induce calcium release from the sarcoplasmic reticulum. T-channels open at more negative potentials than the L-channels and play a role in the initial depolarization of sinus and AV nodal tissue.

• ***Receptor operated channel***, normally activated by an alpha adrenergic agonist, such as NA, or angiotensin interacting with the alpha adrenergic receptors. They increase degree of contraction of arterioles. Similarly, $beta_1$ agonists increase calcium influx in cardiac muscles and enhance contraction, frequency and conduction velocity of heart.

• ***Sodium-calcium exchange*** which is an electrogenic mechanism. It operates bidirectionally to mediate the movement of calcium ions across the sarcolemma.

• ***Calcium ATPase*** which extrudes calcium from the cell in an energy dependent way.

Sarcoplasmic calcium is also regulated by uptake and release of calcium by sarcoplasmic reticulum, mitochondria and by buffering of calcium by various intracellular proteins such as calmodulin and troponin C.

Mechanism of action: CCB bind to alpha-1 subunit of L-channel, and act by inhibiting the entry of calcium into the myocardial and vascular smooth muscles, thus decreasing availability of the intra-cellular calcium.

CCBs belong to 3 chemically distinct classes:

I **Phenylalkylamines** e.g. Verapamil

II **Dihydropyridines** (DHP) e.g. Nifedipine and Amlodipine.

III **Benzothiazepines** e.g. Diltiazem.

Cardiovascular actions:

• ***Negative inotropic effect*:** CCBs depress myocardial contractility, and decrease the cardiac workload and oxygen consumption. This effect is beneficial in the treatment of angina of effort. *Verapamil and diltiazem have negative inotropic actions and hence should not be combined with beta-blockers in the treatment of angina of effort*; however, nifedipine can be used together with beta-blockers (but see later).

• ***Antiarrhythmic effect*:** Calcium channel blockers decrease the rate of discharge of the SA node, suppress ectopic pacemaker activity, increase the refractoriness of the AV node and slow the conduction (Chapter 27). The slowing of the conduction prevents re-entrant excitation. This effect plus the improvement of cardiac ischemia (by decreasing myocardial oxygen consumption) account for the potent (though selective) antiarrhythmic action. Verapamil and diltiazem are particularly potent in this respect. Verapamil and diltiazem (but not nifedipine), however, can aggravate AV block.

• ***Coronary artery dilatation*** : These drugs are more potent than NTG as coronary artery dilators. Nitroglycerine dilates the large epicardial branches of coronary arteries but not the smaller intramyocardial coronary arterioles; CCBs dilate both, even in the presence of coronary artery spasm. Further, they can prevent the spasm even in diseased, atherosclerotic coronary arteries. This effect accounts for their efficacy in Prinzmetal angina; it contributes to their effectiveness in angina of effort.

• ***Effect on peripheral blood vessels*:** Calcium channel blockers relax the vascular smooth muscle in systemic as well as pulmonary arterial circulations. They thus decrease the vascular resistance and the BP in both territories, and are useful in the treatment of systemic and pulmonary hypertension. Further, reduction in the afterload contributes to their efficacy in angina of effort. Nifedipine is a more potent vasodilator than verapamil. The reduction in BP is accompanied by reflex tachycardia in the case of nifedipine but not in the case of verapamil which depresses the SA node. They have little effect on the venous (capacitance) bed and do not alter the cardiac preload.

• ***Antianginal action*** of these drugs is probably due to (1) improvement in the coronary blood flow; and (2) decrease in the oxygen demand of the heart due to reduction in systemic vascular resistance (vasodilatation) and BP (afterload). Verapamil, in addition, reduces the heart rate. *As a group, these drugs can be used in anginal patients with COPD in whom beta-blockers are contraindicated.*

VERAPAMIL (Isoptin, Calaptin): This drug is a synthetic papaverine derivative. It causes:

- Suppression of SA and AV nodes which are Ca^{++} dependent.
- ***Coronary and peripheral vasodilatation.***
- ***Potent antiarrhythmic effect;*** and
- ***Potent negative inotropic effect.***
- ***AV block.***

It does not cause reflex sympathetic overactivity and tachycardia.

Given orally, it is absorbed completely but is substantially metabolized by first pass hepatic metabolism. In the circulation, it is highly protein bound. Adverse effects include constipation, vertigo, bradycardia, heart block, CHF, hypotension and rarely cardiac asystole.

It is available as 40 mg. tablets and as sustained release tablets. It is used in the treatment of angina in the dose of 40-80 mg. 3-4 times a day.

Its use in paroxysmal supraventricular tachycardia is described in Chapter 27.

DILTIAZEM (Dilzem): This drug has pharmacological properties intermediate between those of verapamil and nifedipine (see Table 28.2). It has less negative inotropic effect than verapamil and less vasodilating effect than nifedipine and verapamil. It should be avoided in patients in CHF, and in the presence of heart block or concurrent therapy with digitalis / beta blockers. It can be combined with nitrates.

Fig. 28.3 : Nifedipine

NIFEDIPINE (Depin, Calcigard, Adalat): The pharmacological properties of this dihydropyridine derivative are shown in Table 28.3. In contrast to verapamil, it has negligible negative inotropic effect, is a more potent coronary and peripheral vasodilator, and causes tachycardia. It is a potent inhibitor of platelet aggregation. It also relaxes bronchial, ureteric and uterine smooth muscle. It is available as tablets and capsules, and can be used either orally or (for a rapid effect) sublingually. However, for long term use a sustained release formulation in the dose of 30-90 mg. OD is preferred.

Adverse reactions: These include headache, tachycardia, dizziness, fatigue, orthostatic hypotension, leg cramps, skin rashes and gingival hyperplasia. Occasionally, CHF may be precipitated. Coronary artery spasm has been reported following rapid withdrawal during chronic therapy.

Therapeutic uses: Its main use is in the treatment of variant angina refractory to nitrate therapy. It is also used to treat hypertension and Raynaud's syndrome (Chapter 29).

Nicardipine (Cardene) and **isradipine** (Trescal) are other dihydropyridine compounds with pharmacological properties and uses similar to those of nifedipine.

Amlodipine and **felodipine**, with long t½ are the second generation dihydropyridine CCBs. They are potent coronary and peripheral vasodilators; bradycardia and AV block are less liable to occur with their use.

Nimodipine (Vasotop) is related to nifedipine but is claimed to have a preferential vasodilating action on the cerebral arteries in animal studies. Its use is confined to the prevention of vascular spasm following subarachnoid hemorrhage; its usefulness for this purpose is uncertain. It is given in the dose of 60 mg. every four hours for the first few days.

Other uses of CCBs : See Chapters 23, 38 and 43 for their use in migraine, mountain sickness and as tocolytics, respectively.

Table 28.2 lists the important differences among different calcium channel blockers.

Contraindications to CCBs are:

- ***Tight aortic stenosis.***
- ***Severe myocardial depression and heart block.***

Table 28.2: Properties of some calcium channel blockers

	Verapamil	Diltiazem	Nifedipine	Amlodipine
Chemical class	Diphenylalkylamine	Benzothiazepine	Dihydropyridine	Dihydropyridine
Bioavailability	20-35%	40%	40-70%	40-70%
Plasma half-life	6-12 hr	3-5 hr	2-5 hr	35 hr
Blocks A-V conduction	+++	++	0	0
Antiarrthymic effect	+	+	0	0
Negative inotropic effect	++	+	±	±
Vasodilatation	++	+	+++	+++
Heart rate	↓	N or ↓	↑	N
Blocks reflex sympathetic effects	+	++	0	0
Dose (mg/day) in hypertension	120-240	60-120	30-60	2.5-10
Dose (mg/day) in angina	240-480	120-360	15-60	2.5-10
Dosage schedule	8 hourly	8 hourly	6-8 hourly	O.D.
Adverse effects	A-V. block, constipation, nausea, possibly LVF	A-V block, hypotension, Rarely LVF	Palpitation, hypotension, nausea, edema	Palpitation, hypotension, nausea, edema

+ = Mild effect; ++ = Moderate effect; +++ = Potent effect.

- ***Clinical heart failure.***
- ***Unstable angina;*** and
- ***Preexisting hypotension***

They should be used in pregnancy only if absolutely necessary. It is unwise to use them in patients on digoxin or a beta blocker, as they may exacerbate A-V block or heart failure.

Potassium Channel Activators

These are discussed in Chapter 29.

NICORANDIL (Zynicor): In addition to acting as a potassium channel activator, nicorandil produces vasodilatation by acting as a NO donor. Though it preferentially acts on the venous side and reduces the preload, it also acts on the arteriolar side and reduces the afterload. Given orally in the dose of 10-20 mg bid, it is equivalent to standard dose of a beta-blocker or a CCB in angina of effort. Adverse effects are mostly due to vasodilator action and include headache, dizziness and dose dependent hypotension. Nicorandil is perhaps useful but expensive background therapy for patients with angina pectoris. It is particularly useful as an alternative to nitrates when tolerance is a problem. It can be used in the presence of asthma or cardiac failure.

Pinacidil is similar to nicorandil in its properties, adverse reactions and uses. Its duration of action is about 6 hours; the controlled release preparation (37.5 mg capsule) acts for about 12 hours.

Antiplatelet Drugs

ASPIRIN: Prophylactic aspirin reduces the incidence of MI in patients with chronic stable and unstable angina (Chapter 32).

DIPYRIDAMOLE (Persantin): This drug is a coronary dilator; but unlike nitrates which dilate conductance vessels it is claimed to dilate coronary resistance vessels. It is a weak platelet inhibitor. It is used as an antithrombotic drug (Chapter 32).

Cytoprotectives

Trimetazidine (Flavedon, Travedon):This drug is a **P**artial inhibitor of **F**atty acid **Ox**idation (PFOX) pathway, in the myocardium, thereby improving its metabolism in the presence of ischemia. It is claimed to maintain normal left ventricular function without exerting any hemodynamic effect. It has been used to treat stable angina of effort. Its superiority over standard treatment, however, needs further studies.

Ranolazine: This drug is chemically related to trimetazidine. Its mechanism of action is not known. Clinically, it produces modest improvement in exercise tolerance. It's side effects are dizziness, nausea, asthenia and constipation. Prolongation of QT interval can occur. It may be used as an add-on drug when the standard treatment fails. The drug is under evaluation.

Ivabradine: It is a selective sodium channel blocker, which is claimed to be as effective as a CCB in reducing anginal attacks.

Treatment of Angina Pectoris

Exertional angina (angina of effort) : Table 28.3 outlines the principles of treatment of angina of effort.

Relief and prevention of individual attacks: Nitroglycerine (NTG) is the drug of choice *in all types of angina.* The patient is advised to carry the tablets, and to put one sublingually as soon as premonitory symptoms develop. He should be advised to use NTG while sitting, to avoid possible syncope. If symptoms are not relieved immediately, additional tablets may be used at 5 minute intervals, but not more than three tablets should be used in a 15 minute interval. The remnant of the tablet should be discarded soon

Table 28.3: Principles of treatment of angina of effort

I **General**

- ***Reassurance***
- ***Measures to prevent progression***

(a) Treatment of IHD risk factors e.g., hypertension, hyperlipidaemia, diabetes, obesity.

(b) Use of anti-atherogenic agents, e.g. statins (Chapter 39).

(c) Advise about life style modification (control of emotional excitement, alcohol and smoking and weight control).

(d) Supervised, graded, physical exercises.

- Treatment of associated conditions which increase oxygen demand, e.g. hyperthyroidism, anaemia, valvular disease, heart failure.
- Avoidance of preparations containing sympathomimetic amines (cold remedies, anti-asthmatic and anorectic agents), atropine, aminophylline and antidepressants

II **Specific**

- Drugs for relief from acute attack e.g. a nitrate (See Table 26.1).
- Chronic prophylaxis (prevention of MI and improved survival) (See text).

(a) Aspirin

(b) Use of nitrates, beta blockers, calcium channel blockers

III **Surgical revascularization**

after pain relief as excessive absorption of the drug would lead to hypotension. One may use as many tablets per day as needed.

NTG or isosorbide dinitrate, used sublingually 10-15 minutes before a period of increased activity such as walking, climbing or sexual intercourse, can frequently prevent the attack. This is the preferred method of using these drugs for prophylaxis. The acute prophylactic effect of sublingual NTG and isosorbide dinitrate persists for about 30 minutes and 2 hours respectively. Longer prophylactic effect (upto 4 hours) is obtained with NTG cutaneous ointment as NTG is absorbed slowly and bypasses the liver. Generally, isosorbide dinitrate causes less headache than NTG.

Chronic prophylaxis: This comprises

- ***Nitrates*:** Large oral doses of organic nitrates decrease the frequency of anginal attacks and increase the exercise tolerance. They are useful in chronic prophylaxis of angina. They, however, increase the risk of hypotension, tachycardia and tolerance. Small oral doses are of doubtful value for this purpose. Nitrates may be combined with beta-blockers or diltiazem but not with nifedipine or verapamil. (Table 28.4).
- ***Beta-blockers*:** All beta-blockers seem to be equally effective as anti-anginal drugs and are the drugs of choice for chronic prophylaxis of angina of effort. They can be combined, if necessary, with nitrates for this purpose. Beta adrenergic blockers are particularly preferred for the treatment of asymptomatic (silent) myocardial ischemia. Generally, propranolol is started in the dose of 10 mg. 3-4 times a day. The daily dose is gradually increased by 20-30 mg. once in 3-4 days until the resting pulse rate is lowered to about 60/minute and the symptoms are relieved without the development of CHF. Weight gain is a useful early indicator of the latter. The average, effective, daily dose of propranolol is about 100-200 mg. But some patients may require larger doses. Alternatively, a selective beta-blocker such as metoprolol (50-100 mg. twice a day) or atenolol (50 - 100 mg. once a day) can be used. Beta-blockers are the drugs of choice in cardiac syndrome X but are not particularly effective against angina at rest or on minimal exercise since their beneficial effect in the absence of sympathetic overactivity is small. Long term treatment with beta blockers is relatively safe.
- ***Calcium channel blockers*:** Variant angina is generally relieved rapidly by NTG. CCB are valuable in its prophylaxis. Long acting nifedipine and verapamil are equally effective in this respect, and the choice between them rests on other considerations. In patients with angina of effort, these drugs appear to be as effective as beta-blockers as prophylactics but they are less well tolerated. Their advantage is that they can be used in patients with COPD who do not tolerate the beta-blockers. Verapamil can be used instead of a beta blocker to control tachycardia in thyrotoxic patients with asthma.

In patients with stable angina, the dose of nifedipine needs to be titrated very finely. If a patient benefits from 10 mg. tid, he is likely to deteriorate on a higher dose. Calcium channel blockers have no beneficial effect, and may even be detrimental, in acute MI.

- ***Combination of a beta blocker and a CCB*** is additive but not synergistic. *Verapamil should not be combined with betablockers.* Diltiazem may be combined with betablockers only in patients with normal cardiac function and without conduction defects. Nifedipine or amlodipine and betablockers have complimentary actions on the coronary blood supply and myocardial oxygen demand.The former dilate the coronaries and decrease the BP whereas the latter slow the heart rate and reduce the myocardial contractility. The second generation dihydropyridines (e.g. amlodipine) are particularly useful in patients with angina associated with hypertension.

Table 28.4 outlines a step-wise approach to the drug treatment of angina.

- ***Advice about the life style*:** Excitement and emotional upset can precipitate anginal attacks. A patient who suspects that he has 'heart pain' is worried, and reassurance can give

Table 28.4: Stepwise approach to drug therapy of angina

All patients are prescribed aspirin 75-150 mg/day orally and glyceryl trinitrate sublingually, by lingual aerosol or transdermally.	
Control risk factors	• Obesity, hyperlipidemia, hypertension, diabetes, smoking. Consider using a statin.
Treat concomitant diseases	• Anemia, thyrotoxicosis, valvular disease, heart failure.
Mild to moderate symptoms	• Betablockers; if contraindicated, calcium channel blockers. • If both are not tolerated, use prophylactic isosorbide dinitrate/mononitrate, or nicorandil.
If symptoms persist	• Combine betablockers with a calcium channel blocker nifedipine/amlodipine; or A calcium channel blocker plus (nitrate/nicorandil); or Nitrates plus (betablocker or calcium channel blocker)
If severe and not responding	• Refer for revascularization.

much relief. Rest, choice of occupation not involving heavy manual work and mental relaxation are important. In fact, the value of such an approach is more than that of any known drug. A placebo can diminish the severity of the symptoms in many patients; hence, one should be wary of accepting a cleverly advertised antianginal drug or manoeuvre which has helped "many" patients.

The patient should be advised to avoid overeating, exercise after eating, and extremes of heat, cold and humidity. He should avoid any type, amount or pace of activity known to precipitate angina in him; if it is unavoidable the prophylactic use of NTG or isosorbide dinitrate sublingually 10-15 minutes before commencing the activity is recommended. Sexual activity can be permitted in most patients.

Alcohol should be avoided by patients with angina. It is not a coronary vasodilator. By removing the higher inhibitory controls in the CNS, it may induce an individual to ignore the anginal pain, leading to more exertion and an aggravation of the cardiac ischemia. A further disadvantage is the liberation of catecholamines by acetaldehyde, a metabolite of alcohol. Alcohol has a negative inotropic action on the heart damaged by coronary artery disease. However, in alcohol addicts, its abrupt withdrawal may precipitate undesirable effects, and small amounts of alcohol may be permitted.

• ***Cessation of smoking***: Patients with angina must be advised to give up smoking which increases the heart rate and oxygen consumption of the myocardium. Further, absorption of carbon monoxide from the inhaled smoke increases the concentration of carboxyhemoglobin; this reduces the oxygen carrying capacity of blood.

• ***Treatment of associated diseases***: Weight reduction in obese patients and treatment of associated hyperlipidemia, anemia, hypertension or thyrotoxicosis help in prophylaxis of angina. Vasodilator anti-hypertensive drugs can aggravate angina by causing tachycardia; but this can be countered by using a beta-blocker.

• ***Supervised, graded, exercise training*** improves exercise tolerance in anginal patients probably by increasing oxygen extraction in the peripheral circulation. This allows more physical activity with less increase in heart rate and in cardiac output. The cardiac work load is thus kept below the angina index. Isometric physical activity of any type may, however, be harmful and should be avoided.

Variant angina of Prinzmetal: The treatment of this condition comprises (a) NTG sublingually or nifedipine first chewed and then swallowed, for rapid onset of action in acute attacks; and (b) long acting nitrates or CCBs for prevention of attacks. *Beta-blockers are contraindicated.*

Unstable angina: It requires aggressive treatment in an ICCU to prevent MI or sudden death. The patient is treated with aspirin (150-300 mg); sublingual NTG or IV isosorbide dinitrate/NTG, continued till the patient remains pain-free for 24 hours. A beta blocker is administered to lower the heart rate to 50-60/ minute. The combined use of aspirin and clopidogrel is synergistic. Routine anticoagulation with heparin is helpful. A CCB such as diltiazem is substituted in patients in whom beta blockers are contraindicated; but, it does not reduce the risk of MI. *Thrombolytic therapy (Chapter 32) is not indicated in these patients as it may worsen the condition.*

Drugs Used in the Treatment of Peripheral Vascular Disorders

Peripheral vascular disease may be:

I **Obstructive :** Atherosclerosis or thromboangiitis obliterans (TAO) with large vessel involvement, or diabetes with small vessel involvement); or

II **Vasospastic :** Raynaud's syndrome.

I **Obstructive peripheral vascular disease:** In these patients vasodilator drugs are of little avail as they fail to increase the blood flow to ischemic areas with blocked arteries/arterioles. Further, the associated generalised vasodilatation can produce severe adverse reactions. Such patients may benefit from

- ***Correction of remediable underlying factors*** such as CHF, anemia or diabetes mellitus.
- ***Cessation of smoking.***
- ***Daily physical exercise*** (such as walking) which can increase the walking distance.
- ***Foot care*** (cleanliness, avoidance of any injury and prompt treatment of infection).
- ***Drugs:*** Aspirin (antiplatelet action), statins (cholesteral lowering action) and pentoxyphylline (hemorheologic action) have been used with variable success, (Chapter 32).

Naftidofuryl oxalate (Praxilene) 100 mg orally 2-3 times a day alleviates symptoms and increases pain-free walking distance in moderate peripheral obstructive vascular disease. It is not a direct vasodilator but may increase the supply of ATP and reduce lactate level in muscles.

Cilostazol (Pletal) 100 mg bid (30 minutes before or 2 hrs after food) may be useful in patients without rest pain and no peripheral tissue necrosis.

- ***Endarterectomy*** or peripheral arterial bypass surgery in selected cases.

II **Vasospastic diseases :** Drugs useful in these conditions are:

- ***Calcium channel antagonists,*** e.g., Nifedipine and Diltiazem are preferred.
- ***Beta adrenergic stimulants*:** Nylidrin and Isoxsuprine (Chapter 17).
- ***Alpha adrenergic blocking agents*:** Tolazoline and Prazosin (Chapter 17).
- ***Anticoagulants*:** Heparin and Warfarin, discussed in Chapter 32.

In Raynaud's syndrome, prazosin is used in the dose of 0.5 mg. bid (first dose at bed time); the maintenance dose is 1-2 mg. bid. Nifedipine is used in the dose of 5-20 mg. tid.

Other drugs claimed to be useful are nicotinic acid derivatives, cyclandelate (Cyclospasmol), pentoxyphylline (Chapter 32), ketanserin (Chapter 23) and prostacycline.

The drug therapy must always be combined with non-pharmacological measures such as exercise, avoidance of exposure to cold and cessation of smoking.

Pharmacotherapy of Hypertension 29

Hypertension, as a clinical entity, can be divided into two major divisions :

I **Primary or essential hypertension,** where definite cause for the rise in blood pressure (BP) is not known; and

II **Secondary hypertension,** secondary to renal (chronic diffuse glomerulonephritis, pyelonephritis, polycystic kidneys), endocrine (Cushing's snydrome, pheochromocytoma, primary hyperaldosteronism) and vascular (renal artery disease, coarctation of aorta) lesions.

The syndrome of **essential hypertension** is characterised by elevation of the diastolic BP, a normal cardiac output (in most cases) and increased peripheral vascular resistance, with documented natural history and with characteristic pathologic changes in the arterioles.

The Joint National Committee for Detection, Evaluation and Treatment of High BP has defined 'Normal' BP **in adults** as that *below* 120/80 mm Hg; and 'High Normal' BP (prehypertension) as 130 to 139 mm Hg systolic *and* 80 to 85 mm Hg diastolic. *BP above 139 mm Hg systolic or above 85 mm Hg diastolic on several occasions qualifies as hypertension,* **at all ages**. Systolic BP above 140 mm Hg *plus* diastolic BP of below 90 mm Hg in the elderly is termed *isolated systolic hypertension.* Individuals with prehypertension are more likely to progress to hypertension.

Hypertension, if left untreated, leads to a variety of disabling cardiac, cerebrovascular, and renal complications, with shortened life expectancy, regardless of the etiology of hypertension.

Further, *the risk of morbidity and mortality rises with BP and there is no clearly defined cut-off point for increased risk.*

The etiology of primary hypertension is not clear but certain factors are implicated in its genesis:

- In adult populations, the BP rises with age. However, the rise in BP with age in a population as a whole is not uniform, but is due to the development of hypertension in a discrete group of individuals with advancement of age. These individuals, therefore, are presumed to differ qualitatively from the remainder of the population in their BP regulation.
- There is a strong familial clustering of essential hypertension and the inheritance seems to be polygenic.
- The arterial pressure is a function of the cardiac output and the peripheral resistance. Both can be readily affected by various factors. Resistance to the blood flow resides chiefly in the arterioles. The resistance offered by the arteries, veins and capillaries is much smaller. Changes in the calibre of the arterioles, therefore, produce enormous changes in the peripheral resistance.

Arteriolar walls have very reactive smooth muscle. Factors which tend to diminish their radius augment the total peripheral resistance

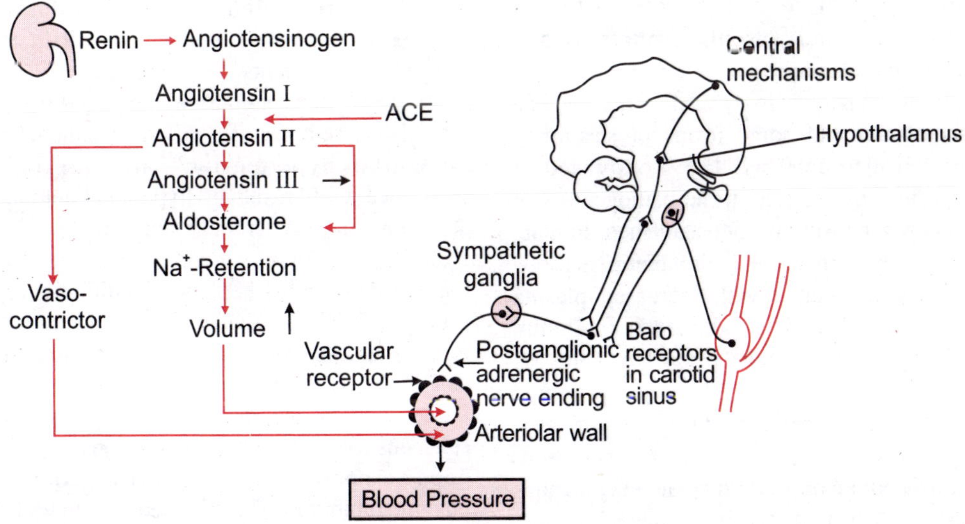

Fig. 29.1 : Physiology of BP control

and consequently, the BP.

- Normally, the BP is controlled by two main types of systems (Fig. 29.1).

(a) **The adrenergic nervous system** which operates through the baroreceptors and is mainly responsible for the counteracting acute changes in the BP. Baroreceptor reflexes protect the circulation against stresses that alter arterial pressure acutely. When one stands up from the lying down position, the cardiac output tends to fall due to reduced venous return to the heart. This may lead to a fall in BP and fainting. Normally, it is prevented by a reflex increase in heart rate and in peripheral resistance through the baroreceptor mechanism.

(b) **The humoral renin-angiotensin-aldesteronal system,** which has a slow response and is important in long term regulation of BP. It operates through the kidneys and involves various humoral agents. It is increasingly incriminated particularly in the genesis of rapidly progressing hypertension (Fig. 29.1).

Renin, a proteolytic enzyme, is produced and stored in the kidneys. It is released in response to (a) reduction in renal perfusion pressure, (b) reduction in sodium delivery to the macula densa, (c) increase in the sympathetic activity, and (d) certain humoral factors. The reaction between renin and the serum globulin **angiotensinogen** results in the generation of an inactive decapeptide, 'angiotension I.' The latter, during its passage through the lungs, is converted into an octapeptide, 'angiotension II' by the action of enzyme **Angiotensin Converting Enzyme** (ACE). **Angiotensin II** is the most potent direct vasoconstrictor agent, effective in as small a dose as 0.1 mcg per kg. body weight. Angiotensin II also stimulates the synthesis and release of aldosterone from the adrenal cortex and thus regulates the ECF volume. In the circulation, angiotensin II is converted into a heptapeptide Angiotensin III which is as potent as angiotensin II in its action on the adrenal cortex but is weaker in its other actions. *"The kidney thus plays an important role in determining the BP level, doing so via renin-angiotensin -aldosterone system activity, which presides over both vasoconstriction and volume, the two major determinants of BP and of tissue flow."*

Renin and angiotensin are also produced locally in many tissues including blood vessels, brain, kidney, heart and adrenal glands. It is likely that these tissue angiotensin-generating systems are involved in the local control of cardiac, renal and vascular function, and cardiovascular damage.

The renin-angiotensin system is involved in the pathogenesis of some forms of secondary hypertension such as the renovascular hypertension; but its role in the pathogenesis of essential hypertension is not established. In man, procedures that increase sympathetic nervous activity are associated with increased plasma renin activity (PRA). It is claimed that morbidity in the hypertensives is related to PRA. Whereas the adrenergic blockers, methyldopa, reserpine and propranolol reduce PRA, vasodilator antihypertensives such as hydralazine, diazoxide, sodium nitroprusside and the thiazides increase PRA in hypertensive patients.

- There is deficient vascular synthesis and release of nitric oxide (NO) in hypertensives.
- Some patients with labile hypertension and mild essential hypertension have tachycardia and increased cardiac output but normal peripheral resistance, indicative of a hyperkinetic circulatory state due to increased beta adrenergic activity. These patients also have elevated PRA (HREH, High Renin Essential Hypertension). Some other patients with essential hypertension have either normal or even low PRA (LREH, Low Renin Essential Hypertension). By contrast, majority of patients with essential hypertension have normal PRA.
- There is a positive correlation between total body sodium and BP, and a negative one between total body potassium and BP, in hypertensive patients. Primary (essential) hypertension and age-related increase in BP are virtually absent in populations where less than 50 mmol of Na^+ (< 3.00 g of salt) is consumed daily. It appears that both excess of body sodium and deficit of body potassium contribute to the development of hypertension. Increase in intracellular Na^+ stimulates Na^+-Ca^{++} exchange pump, driving Ca^{++} into the cell. Increased cytosolic Ca^{++} triggers vascular smooth muscle contraction. Further, sodium retention in the cell decreases NO synthesis by endothelial cells whereas high potassium diet causes endothelium-dependent vasodilatation. Clinically, salt restriction reduces BP in many hypertensive patients.
- The other endocrine abnormalities that have been demonstrated in some patients with "essential hypertension" are: (a) insulin resistance with resultant hyperinsulinemia; (b) secretion of a structurally abnormal steroid (a hybrid between cortisol and aldosterone) by the adrenal cortex; this heritable condition is called glucocorticoid-remediable aldosteronism (GRA) and (c) an inherited defect in the modulation by salt of the local renin-angiotensin system in the kidney and the adrenals; these subjects have a salt sensitive form of hypertension that shows good response to the angiotensin converting enzyme inhibitors. This is called "nonmodulating hypertension".

Experimental evaluation of anti-hypertensive drugs: Although many techniques exist for causing a sustained rise in the BP in various species, none has duplicated, in every detail, the picture of human essential hypertension. The important experimental models for evaluating antihypertensive drugs are:

- ***Nephrogenic hypertension***: (a) Dogs can be made hypertensive by partial constriction of one renal artery, accompanied by removal of the other kidney (Goldblatt). (b) Similar hypertension can be produced in the rat without removing the other kidney.
- ***Neurogenic hypertension***: (a) Sectioning of the carotid sinus and the aortic arch nerves produces hypertension in dogs. (b) Other methods include subjecting rats to intermittent loud noise and injection of kaolin into the cisterna magna of dogs.
- ***Hormonal hypertension***: The methods used include (a) Prolonged administration of deoxycorticosterone acetate (DOCA) or aldosterone together with sodium chloride in chicks and rats; (b) Severe hypertension can be produced in uninephrectomized and uniadrenalectomized, salt treated rats during regeneration of the enucleated adrenal cortex.
- ***Spontaneously hypertensive rats*** (SHR)

are available. They would seem to come closest to human essential hypertension.

Ingestion of salt is necessary for the development of hypertension in many animal models. Drugs like methyldopa and beta blockers have little hypotensive effect in animals; but they are highly effective in hypertensive patients. Hence, the final evaluation has to be done in hypertensive human subjects.

Antihypertensives, classification : *The drugs used in the treatment of hypertension act by reducing the cardiac output and/or the total peripheral resistance, without correcting the cause.* They can be classified according to site of action : (Fig. 29.1).

I **Drugs acting centrally:**

(a) $Alpha_2$ adrenergic receptor stimulants, e.g., Clonidine and Methyldopa.

(b) Selective imidazole receptor (I-receptor) stimulants, e.g., Moxonidine.

II **Drugs acting on the autonomic ganglia:** Ganglion blocking agents, eg., Trimethaphan.

III **Drugs acting on the postganglionic sympathetic nerve endings:**

(a) Adrenergic neuron blockers : Guanethidine, Bethanidine, Debrisoquine, Bretylium.

(b) Catecholamine depletors : Reserpine.

IV **Drugs acting on adrenergic receptors:**

(a) Alpha-adrenergic blocking agents: Phentolamine, Phenoxybenzamine, Prazosin, Indoramin.

(b) Beta-adrenergic blocking agents: Propranolol, Atenolol, Metoprolol.

(c) Both alpha and beta adrenergic blocking drugs: Labetalol.

V **Drugs acting directly on the vascular smooth muscle (Vasodilators):**

(a) Arteriolar vasodilators: CCB, Hydralazine, Diazoxide, Minoxidil.

(b) Arteriolar-venular vasodilators: Sodium nitroprusside.

VI **Potassium channel activators:** Diazoxide, Minoxidil, Pinacidil, Nicorandil.

VII **Drugs which block renin-angiotensin-aldosterone axis:**

(a) Those which block renin release : Beta-adrenergic blockers.

(b) Those that inhibit PRA action e.g. Aliskiren.

(c) Those which block the conversion of angiotensin I to angiotensin II by inhibiting the ACE: Captopril, Enalapril.

(d) Those which competitively block angiotensin II vascular receptors (ARB): Losartan.

(e) Those which counterer the action of aldosterone (Aldosterone antagonist) : Spironolactone.

VIII **Oral diuretics:** Thiazides.

IX **Miscellaneous:** Metyrosine.

Various *antihypertensive drugs may ultimately reduce BP by more than one mechanism.* Further, the hemodynamic alterations produced by a single parenteral dose of a given drug may differ from those resulting from its prolonged oral use. Moreover, the degree of hypotensive effect produced also differs in hypertensive and normotensive subjects.

Drugs Acting Centrally

CLONIDINE (Catapres, Arkamin): This imidazoline derivative is a potent antihypertensive drug.

Fig. 29.2: Clonidine

Mechanism of action: Clonidine mainly acts centrally as agonist at postsynaptic adrenergic $alpha_2$ receptors in the vasomotor centre and the hypothalamus. Activation of these receptors suppresses the sympathetic outflow and decreases the release of NA from the neuronal terminals, leading to lowering of BP. Almost all the central effects of clonidine can be blocked by the $alpha_2$ receptor blocker yohimbine.

With higher doses, clonidine stimulates the peripheral inhibitory presynaptic $alpha_2$ adrenoreceptors (autoreceptors). This reduces the peripheral NA release.

Clonidine reduces the PRA. It also produces sedation and many symptoms of behavioral depression in laboratory animals.

Since alpha adrenoreceptors are widely distributed, their interaction with clonidine can produce other effects such as increase in the level of plasma growth hormone. It potentiates the analgesic action of opioids.

Clonidine binds to CNS nonadrenoreceptor sites (imidazoline receptor), which may also contribute to its antihypertensive effect.

Pharmacological actions: *Given IV* in normal and hypertensive man, it produces a transient hypertensive response followed by a prolonged fall in both systolic and diastolic BP accompanied by bradycardia. Such initial hypertensive effect is not seen after its *oral administration*. The rise in BP is blocked by alpha-adrenergic receptor blocking drug phentolamine. Acute oral administration of clonidine promptly reduces the plasma noradrenaline levels in normals but not in patients with pheochromocytoma.

Chronic administration of 0.3 to 1.5 mg./day reduces both supine and standing BP in hypertensive patients. Baroreceptor reflex activity is relatively normal and circulatory reflexes are intact; postural hypotension is not much of a problem during clonidine therapy. Addition of a diuretic potentiates its effect.

Clonidine causes a decrease in the cardiac output due to both a decrease in stroke volume and bradycardia. It also causes significant reduction in the total peripheral resistance in the standing position. The renal and muscle blood flow is not much affected; this is an advantage. Tolerance to antihypertensive effect develops on prolonged use.

Absorption, fate and excretion: It is a lipid soluble drug and is well absorbed from the gut. It has a high volume of distribution. Its t½ is about 12 hours and hence, two doses per day would be sufficient in therapy. About half of the drug is excreted unchanged in the urine.

Preparations: Clonidine hydrochloride 0.1 mg. tablets. A transdermal preparation is also available; its effect lasts for 7 days.

Adverse reactions: It commonly causes drowsiness (**central sedative action**) and oral dryness due to central inhibition of salivation. Vertigo, constipation, parotid pain, impotence, GI disturbances, allergic reactions and hallucinations may also occur. Orthostatic symptoms, however, are uncommon. Toxic doses cause marked bradycardia, miosis and hypotension.

Abrupt cessation of clonidine therapy can cause hyperirritability and a dangerous and sometimes lethal *rebound rise of BP*. The treatment of such rebound hypertension is either reinstitution of clonidine or use of a combined α and β adrenergic blocking agent e.g. labetalol. Therefore, when clonidine must be withdrawn, gradual tapering is recommended.

Clonidine produces sodium and fluid retention and rapid development of tolerance to its antihypertensive effect unless it is combined with a diuretic. Combination of clonidine and a beta-blocker can cause severe drowsiness.

Tricyclic anti-depressants like desipramine may impair the hypotensive action of clonidine.

Therapeutic Uses:

- ***Hypertension***: Discussed later.
- ***Menopausal hot flushes*** (Chapter 65).
- ***Opiate, alcohol and nicotine withdrawal, to control adrenergic symptoms.***
- ***Miscellaneous***: Diagnosis of growth hormone deficiency (Chapter 61).

Guanfacine is related to clonidine and has actions similar to clonidine. Duration of action, however, is prolonged.

ALPHA METHYLDOPA (Aldomet, Emdopa): This isomer of methyldopa which bears a close similarity to dihydroxy-phenylalanine (DOPA) was introduced in the treatment of hypertension in 1960 by Sjoerdesma. It is a prodrug that acts

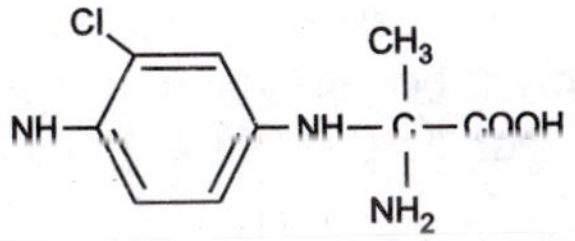

Fig. 29.3 : Alpha Methyldopa

via active metabolite alphamethyl-noradrenaline.

Mechanism of action: It is metabolized in the adrenergic neurons to alphamethyl-noradrenaline which acts, like clonidine, centrally by activating the alpha$_2$-adrenergic receptors in the vasomotor centre. Methyldopa also inhibits renin release by the kidneys, and has some direct action on blood vessels.

Pharmacological actions: After oral or IV administration, the hypotensive effect appears after a latent period of 3-6 hours and 1-2 hours, respectively.

- The heart rate diminishes.
- The cardiovascular reflexes remain intact.
- Postural hypotension is not a problem.
- The hypotensive effect is associated with a reduction in cardiac output, total peripheral resistance, or both. With time, this reduction in cardiac output becomes less apparent.
- The renal blood flow and the GFR are not affected; hence, the drug is valuable in patients with compromised renal function.
- Its hypotensive effect is enhanced by simultaneous use of a thiazide diuretic.

Absorption, fate and excretion: Given orally, 50 per cent of the drug is absorbed and is carried into the brain via aromatic amino acid transporters. Peak effects are produced after 2 to 4 hours. As the drug metabolite gets stored in the neuronal endings the effect lasts longer (24 hours) even after its disappearance from the circulation. The drug is almost completely excreted in urine in 12 hours. In patients with severely impaired renal function, the drug may accumulate during chronic administration.

Adverse reactions: Commonly, it produces sedation, headache and fatigue. These usually disappear with continuation of therapy. Other effects referable to the CNS are diminished intellectual drive, drowsiness, forgetfulness, nightmares, hyperprolactinemia, gynecomastia mental depression and parkinsonism. The drug may also cause retention of sodium and water. GI upset, constipation, failure of ejaculation, arthralgia and skin rashes can occur. Tolerance to the antihypertensive effect may occur.

Alpha methyldopa produces fever accompanied by abnormal liver function tests, and parenchymal/cholestatic jaundice in a few cases. Rarely it causes thrombocytopenia. Methyldopa produces positive direct antibody (Coomb's) test in upto 25% of patients.

Preparations: Alpha methyldopa hydrocloride 250 mg. tablets; injection 50 mg. per ml.

MOXONIDINE: This is claimed to be a *selective imidazole receptor (I_1 receptor) agonist*. Discharge at central sympathetic neurons in the rostroventral medulla maintains arteriolar smooth muscle tone, and hence peripheral vascular resistance. Moxonidine activates I_1 receptor in the medulla, thereby reducing central sympathetic drive and peripheral vascular resistance. Plasma concentrations of catecholamines and renin are reduced. Moxonidine has similar hypotensive action as clonidine and methyldopa. However, it causes less adverse effects related to co-stimulation of medullary α_2 adrenoceptors. The drug is claimed to have beneficial effects on lipid and carbohydrate metabolism. However, its clinical superiority over clonidine needs confirmation.

Ganglionic Blocking Agents

These drugs competitively block the nicotinic receptors in both sympthetic and parasympathetic ganglia.

Pharmacological actions: Hexamethonium blocks the cholinergic receptors on the postganglionic neurons in the sympathetic and parasympathetic ganglia . This blockade reduces the amount of NA released from the postganglionic sympathetic nerve endings leading, to a reduction in the peripheral sympathetic tone and a fall in BP. The normal protective vasomotor reflexes mediated through the baroreceptors and the sympathetic nervous system are blocked, which causes marked postural hypotension.

The ganglion blocking drugs, once used to treat hypertension, are now obsolete because of the high incidence of adverse effects (Chapter 20).

Trimethaphan camphor sulfonate (Arfonad): Because of its extremely transient action, it is used by IV infusion to produce controlled hypotension for short periods, during surgery and is the drug of choice in the treatment of dissection of the aorta.

Adrenergic Neuron Blockers

Adrenergic neuron blocking agents are the drugs that block release of NA from the postganglionic adrenergic neurons in response to impulses or nerve stimulation. The ganglionic transmission is unaffected and the effector organs are fully responsive to injected NA. Guanethidine, the prototype of this group of drugs, is described below.

GUANETHIDINE (Ismelin) was synthesized in 1961 by Maxwell, Mull and Plummer. Given alone or in conjunction with other hypotensive agents, it was employed in the treatment of severe hypertension resistant to other drugs.

Mechanism of action: The drug is selectively taken up by adrenergic neuron, the uptake mechanism being similar to uptake of NA (uptake$_1$). It causes adrenergic neuron blockade resulting in:

- ***Inhibition of the release of NA at the adrenergic nerve terminals.*** This is its main action.
- ***Blockade of re-uptake of NA*** by the adrenergic nerve endings, observed following higher doses (Fig. 26.6). This effect may account for the transient sympathomimetic overactivity following IV guanethidine.
- ***Depletion of NA stores*** at the adrenergic nerve endings and tissues such as the heart and the aorta. This is because the drug replaces NA stores in the adrenergic neuronal endings.

Pharmacological actions:

Following oral administration: The antihypertensive action of guanethidine is usually delayed for 48-72 hours.

- The ensuing fall of BP is prolonged.
- It abolishes the protective cardiovascular reflexes mediated by the sympathetic nervous system and the carotid baroreceptors, and thus produces severe postural hypotension.
- Cardiovascular responses to exercise and the cold pressor response are impared.
- The renal blood flow diminishes markedly.
- It augments the pressor response to exogenous adrenaline and NA.
- The heart rate usually diminishes and so does the pulse pressure.

On IV administration in animals, guanethidine exerts a triphasic response: an initial, transient fall in BP due to membrane stabilising action on the heart; followed by a transient rise in BP (sympathomimetic action); and finally a marked and prolonged fall in BP. This is accompanied by an increased heart rate.

Adverse reaction: These are due to marked sympathetic blockade (postural hypotension, failure to ejaculate) and consequent predominance of cholinergic system (diarrhoea, parotid pain). It reduces renal blood flow markedly and cause fluid retention. Tricyclic antidepressants inhibit the entry of guanethidine into the adrenergic neuron and can antagonize its antihypertensive action.

Bethanidine and **Debrisoquine** have properties and uses almost similar to those of guanethidine. These drugs are now obsolete.

Catecholamine Depletors

RESERPINE: The root of the plant *Rauwolfia serpentina* has been in medicinal use in India since ancient times. It was considered useful for such diverse conditions as insomnia, snake bite and insanity. The root contains alkaloids reserpine, rescinnamine, deserpidine and ajmaline. Reserpine is by far the most potent of all hypotensive alkaloids whereas ajmaline has quinidine-like properties (Chapter 13).

Mechanism of action: *Reserpine depletes the catecholamines, adrenaline, NA and dopamine, from the various storage sites in the body.* This is accompanied by depletion of 5-HT as well, particularly from the CNS. The depletion of NA stores in the peripheral sympathetic nerve endings, including those of heart, explains the antihypertensive action of reserpine.

Normally, the NA released at the sympathetic nerve endings is metabolized partly by specific enzyme catechol-O-methyl transferase (COMT), but is largely taken up by the adrenergic neuronal endings (Chapter 16).

A part of NA in adrenergic nerve endings is taken up by intracellular 'granules' or 'vesicles' and is subsequently stored.

Reserpine binds to storage vesicles in adrenergic neurons.This binding persists for a long time, leading to inhibition of both granular uptake and storage of catecholamines and 5-HT. Thus, *the reserpine action leads to depletion of the transmitter and consequently to peripheral sympathetic blockade*. The transmitter which 'leaks out' from the storage granules is inactivated by the mitochondrial MAO. It is for this reason that reserpine does not exhibit any sympathomimetic activity; however, if the enzyme MAO is inhibited by an MAO inhibitor, the subsequent reserpine administration produces a rise in BP (**reserpine reversal**).

The drug also inhibits the release of renin.

Pharmacological actions:

Cardiovascular system:

- The hypotensive effect appears 30 minutes after IV administration of a single dose, whereas, the maximum effect develops after 2 to 4 weeks of repeated oral medication. Hypotension is usually accompanied by bradycardia. Although there is a decrease in the peripheral resistance, reduction in the cardiac output as a cause of hypotension cannot be ruled out completely.
- In therapeutic doses, reserpine has less action on the homeostatic reflexes in man and postural hypotension is not a problem.
- It acts synergistically with other hypotensive agents, particularly the diuretics.

Reserpine pretreatment enhances the pressor response to sympathomimetic amines like adrenaline and NA, and this must be kept in mind when the sympathomimetic amines have to be employed in individuals on reserpine therapy.

CNS: Reserpine has sedative and antipsychotic actions due to depletion of biogenic amines, e.g. 5-HT from the CNS (Chapter 13).

GI system: It causes increased gastric acid secretion and augmentation of peristalsis. The drug has been used to induce experimental peptic ulceration in animals.

Absorption, fate and excretion: Reserpine is readily absorbed from the gut and from the parenteral sites of injection. The drug appears to be rapidly taken up by lipid rich tissues and is distributed fairly uniformly in the various parts of the CNS. The metabolic pathway of reserpine is not known. The central and the peripheral effects of reserpine are established slowly and maintained for a long time even after complete elimination of the drug.

Adverse reactions: These usually develop as an extension of its pharmacological actions.

- ***Parasympathetic predominance*** due to peripheral sympathetic blockade causes excessive salivation, cutaneous vasodilatation, nasal congestion, increased motility of the gut and increased gastric acidity. *Reserpine should be avoided in individuals with history of hyperacidity and/or peptic ulcer.* It can prolong A-V conduction time, particularly if administered along with digitalis.
- ***Orthostatic hypotension*** as a result of sympathetic blockade may occur infrequently.
- ***Mental depression*** is by far the most serious but uncommon, **dose-related** adverse effect. It may assume serious proportions

resulting in nightmares, insomnia and suicidal tendencies in some cases. Hence, *it is contraindicated in the presence of depression.* Further, *reserpine-induced depression* lasts for a long time after stopping the drug and *is resistant to treatment with tricyclic anti-depressants.* Reserpine may also exacerbate epilepsy.

• ***Weight gain*** is due to an increased appetite and retention of sodium and water. Release of ADH by the central action of reserpine probably plays some part in water retention. The use of diuretics with reserpine reduces the danger of salt and water retention.

• ***Parkinsonism*** can occur due to depletion of DA following large doses of reserpine. This is reversible and can be controlled by antiparkinsonian drugs.

• ***Endocrine disturbances*** such as gynecomastia and impotence in males and reduction in fertility in females can occur with relatively large doses of reserpine.

• ***Allergic manifestations*** are rare. These include thrombocytopenia and purpura.

• ***Hypotension and death during induction of anaesthesia*** have been reported in patients receiving reserpine. *Surgery should, therefore, be done in such patients with full access to resuscitative procedures.*

Notwithstanding the above listed ADR, they are uncommon with therapeutic doses (less than 0.25 mg/day). In general, reserpine is well tolerated, was used extensively in the past, and is cost-effective. However, its use has declined. It has been suggested that *"reserpine is a tragic victim of myth, marketing and fashionable prescribing."*

Preparations and dosage:

(i) Rauwolfia tablet (Serpina) containing powdered root-bark standardised to contain 4 mg. of total alkaloids. The daily dose is 2-4 mg.

(ii) Reserpine tablet (Serpasil) 0.25 mg. It is used once daily the dose 0.25 mg or less. As little as 0.05 mg per day may be effective when used in combination with a diuretic.

(iii) Reserpine injection (Serpasil), 2 and 10 ml. ampoules containing 2.5 mg. per ml.

Adrenergic Receptor Blockers

I **Alpha adrenergic blocking agents:** Peripheral vascular alpha-receptors are of two types:

• ***Postsynaptic alpha$_1$ receptors*** which are stimulatory in nature; and

• ***Presynaptic alpha$_2$-receptors*** (autoreceptors), which are inhibitory in nature.

Blockade of alpha$_1$ causes fall in BP. However, simultaneous blocking of alpha$_2$ results in enhanced output of noradrenaline leading to tachycardia. The alpha adrenergic blocking agents like phentolamine are of relatively little value in the treatment of essential hypertension because their use leads to preponderance of the beta adrenergic activity, palpitation and tachycardia (Chapter 17).

PHENTOLAMINE (Regitine): Phentolamine, an alpha adrenergic blocking agent with a short duration of action, is used in the diagnosis of pheochromocytoma, the tumour of adrenal medulla which secretes adrenaline and NA. Phentolamine mesylate 5 mg IV produces a fall of BP, 35 mm. systolic and 25 mm. diastolic, or greater, within 2 minutes in an individual with pheochromocytoma. A similar degree of fall of BP may occur in patients with essential hypertension who are on a sedative or an antihypertensive drug or who have concomitant renal failure. Phentolamine may also be administered IV in the dose of 2.5 to 10 mg. to prevent or treat severe hypertension due to release of catecholamines during removal of pheochromocytoma. It may also be used to treat the severe hypertension induced by abrupt clonidine withdrawal (Chapter 17).

PHENOXYBENZAMINE: This long acting alpha adrenergic blocking drug is used in the preoperative preparation of patients with pheochromocytoma. Its use controls hypertension and causes an expansion of plasma volume; intraoperative hypertensive episodes are prevented. It is also used for long term management of inoperable cases of pheochromocytoma, where it is combined with a beta-adrenergic blocker.

PRAZOSIN (Minipress): This quinazoline derivative is a peripheral vasodilator (Chapter 17). It acts by selective alpha$_1$ adrenergic receptor blockade. The drug is relatively ineffective in blocking presynaptic alpha$_2$-receptors which are inhibitory. Prazosin, is thus less likely to cause reflex tachycardia. In contrast to the direct peripheral vasodilators (hydralazine, diazoxide and minoxidil), prazosin produces little or no tachycardia at rest. Though it has a short plasma half life (2.5-4 hours), its effect lasts much longer (10 hours). It controls both supine and standing BP with minimum of postural hypotension. Prazosin does not seem to affect renal function, cardiac output or the renin-angiotensin axis. It is effective in all grades of severity of hypertension but its main use is for the treatment of moderate to severe hypertension as an adjunct to other drugs such as diuretics and beta-blockers.Selective α_1 antagonists may decrease total cholesterol and thyroxine levels and increase HDL cholesterol levels.

Adverse reactions: These are giddiness, drowsiness, tiredness, weakness, nausea, diarrhoea, fluid retention, palpitation and nervousness. The **first dose** should be 0.5 mg. or less and should be taken on retiring to bed at night, as some patients have adverse reactions such as palpitation, dizziness and even collapse and loss of consciousness following the first dose.

The therapy is started with 1-3 mg./ day in divided doses. The maintenance dose is 3 to 7.5 mg/day. A sustained release prepartion (Minipres XL) is also available. Prazosin is also used to treat CHF (Chapter 30) and benign prostatic hypertrophy with obstructive symptoms (Chapter 67).

Terazosin, doxazosin and **alfuzosin** are the other analogues of prazosin. Doxazosin has t½ of eight hours. The initial dose is 1 mg daily, doubled at 1-2 weeks intervals, according to response, upto a maximum of 8 mg daily: the usual maintenance dose is 2-4 mg daily. All these drugs are extensively metabolized in the liver.

INDORAMIN (Doralese): This selective alpha$_1$ adrenergic blocker lowers the BP in a manner similar to that of prazosin.

For other uses of alpha blockers, see Chapter 17.

Dihydrogenated ergot alkaloids (Hydergine): These are discussed in Chapters 17 and 43. Hydergine is a mixture of the dihydro derivatives of the three alkaloids of the ergotoxine group, namely ergocornine, ergocristine and ergocryptine. It is now rarely used in antihypertensive therapy.

II **Beta-adrenergic blocking agents:** Their detailed pharmacology is discussed in Chapter 17. Only their antihypertensive effects are discussed below.

Mechanism of action: Their antihypertensive effect seems to correlate best with their β_1 blocking action. Peripheral resistance is lowered during chronic administration. Reduction in cardiac output and lowering of plasma renin are variable. They also increase the natriuretic peptide secretion 2-3 fold. The lipid soluble agents (e.g. propranolol) have some central effect on catecholaminergic neurons.

Beta blockers also reduce the tyrosine hydroxylase and dopamine-β hydroxylase activities in the peripheral sympathetic nervous system.The relative role of these actions in producing the therapeutic effect is not clear.

Pharmacological actions:

- Beta-adrenergic blocking drugs reduce elevated BP in hypertensive patients. All of them seem to be equal in their ability to control hypertension and if one drug fails to control the BP in the maximally tolerated doses, a change to another one generally does not help.

- Both systolic and diastolic BP are lowered, both in the supine and standing positions.
- There is no accompanying tachycardia and in fact tachycardia caused by a drug such as hydralazine is prevented by a beta-blocker.
- They protect against stress-induced hypertension.
- They do not block baroreceptor mechanisms and postural hypotension is not a problem. Protective, alpha receptor constrictor mechanisms remain intact.
- They are cardioprotective and are especially valuable in patients with concurrent ischemic heart disease (Chapter 28).
- They do not impair the kidney function.
- They are generally safe, and many of them are economical.

Absorption, fate and excretion: See Chapter 17 for details. The clinical hypotensive effect of a single dose lasts longer than the t/2 (2-5 hours) would suggest and hence, most of these drugs can be used on a twice a day basis. Longer acting drugs such as atenolol can be used on a once a day basis. The onset of antihypertensive effect is dose-related but generally takes 5-7 days to become manifest. Highly lipid soluble agents such as propranolol, metoprolol and oxprenolol are metabolized in the liver while highly water soluble atenolol, nadolol are excreted by the kidney.

Adverse reactions: In general, these drugs are well tolerated and cause minimal ADR. Because beta receptor density increases during chronic administration, abrupt withdrawal of beta blocker therapy can result in potentially dangerous tachycardia, rebound rise of BP and angina pectoris. Cardiac enlargement is a relative contraindication to their use. Concurrent use of clonidine and propranolol results in excessive drowsiness. In a patient with pheochromocytoma, the use of a beta blocker can cause a dangerous rise of BP unless it is combined with an alpha-blocker. Deterioration of renal function in some patients with established renal disease may occur.

Most NSAIDs reduce the antihypertensive effect of beta blockers, and cause sodium retention probably because of inhibition of formation of renal prostacyclin. Highly lipid soluble beta blockers such as propranolol are likely to cause CNS adverse effects (Chapter 17).

Preparations and Dose: See Chapter 17.

Therapeutic uses : Beta blockers are used to treat all grades of hypertension (see later).

III Alpha and beta adrenergic blockers:

LABETALOL (Normadate): For details see Chapter 17. It is given orally in the dose of 100 mg. twice daily and increased gradually upto 400 - 800 mg daily. The evidence that labetalol has an important advantage over other beta blockers is lacking. However, it can be given IV to treat hypertensive emergencies (see later).

Carvedilol (6.25 mg.bid.) has similar actions as labetalol. It is also used in CHF (Chapter 30).

Vasodilator Drugs

HYDRALAZINE (Apresoline): Hydralazine was first synthesized and tested for antihistaminic activity. However, subsequent investigations demonstrated its hypotensive action instead of antihistaminic activity.

N
N
NH–NH_2

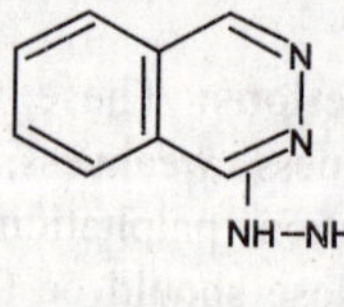

Fig. 29.4: Hydralazine

Pharmacological actions:

- Hydralazine lowers the BP by causing a direct relaxation of the arteriolar wall.
- The effect is slow in onset but prolonged. Even on its IV administration, the BP falls only after 15-20 minutes.
- The fall in BP is accompanied by a decrease in the total peripheral resistance, and by a compensatory tachycardia, increase in stroke volume and in cardiac output. Orthostatic hypotension is rare.

- It can cause increase in plasma renin activity and fluid retention.
- The splanchnic, coronary, cerebral and renal blood flow may increase.

Absorption, fate and excretion: It is well absorbed after oral and parenteral administration. Maximal blood levels are reached within 3 to 4 hours after oral administration. The drug is acetylated and there may be 'fast acetylators' and 'slow acetylators'. Elimination of the drug is almost complete within 24 hours. Less than 5 per cent of an oral dose is excreted unchanged in urine. Hence, it can be used even in the presence of renal damage.

Although the plasma half life (t½ - one hour) is short, its action is much longer.

Adverse reactions: The high incidence of ADR is the main drawback of hydralazine therapy. The manifestations are:

- ***Gastrointestinal irritation*** producing nausea, vomiting, gastric hypersecretion, anorexia and diarrhoea.
- ***Cardiac effects***: These include palpitation, tachycardia and anginal attacks.
- ***Others like*** headache, nasal congestion, flushing, tremors and dizziness. It causes renin release and secondary salt and water retention.
- ***Intolerance***: The manifestations are fever, skin rash and polyneuritis. GI haemorrhage and pancytopenia are serious manifestations.
- A syndrome like acute rheumatoid arthritis or disseminated systemic lupus erythematosus (SLE) may develop with large doses (over 600 mg./day) for prolonged periods (over 6 months).

Preparations and dosage:

(i) Hydralazine hydrochloride tablets 10, 25, and 50 mg. Maximum dose 100 mg.daily s.

(ii) Dihydralazine sulphate 25 mg. tablet (Nepresol).

(iii) Injection: Available as 1 ml. ampoule containing 20 mg. for IM/IV use.

SODIUM NITROPRUSSIDE (Nipride, Sonide): This drug, known since 1850, has been used as a colour indicator for acetone and aldehydes. It was regarded as a poison because of its cyanide group. Given IV in small doses, it has a specific, vascular smooth-muscle relaxant action. It is metabolized to active compound NO which causes relaxation of arterioles and veins. This results in the reduction in peripheral resistance and venous tone, lowering the after load (impedence to LV ejection) and the preload (LV filling pressure) respectively. This results in reduced myocardial oxygen consumption and improved myocardial function in low output states. Heart rate and the regional blood flow are little affected. It increases plasma renin activity.

The action is of rapid onset but of very short duration. Hence, it is administered by IV drip. It is rapidly metabolized to thiocyanate.

Sodium nitroprusside is supplied as 50 mg. powder to be dissolved in 500 ml of 5% dextrose in water, just prior to administration. When it is exposed to light, it is converted to cyanide; hence a brown or black paper bag over the IV fluid container is necessary. Translucent plastic tubing may need taping. *Only freshly prepared solution should be used.*

Adverse reactions: High doses or renal insufficiency tends to precipitate thiocyanate toxicity whereas hepatic dysfunction may result due to toxic cyanide ion. The drug may cause fatigue, anorexia, nausea, vomiting, sweating, disorientation, psychotic behaviour and muscle twitchings. Larger doses may cause ataxia, rigidity, convulsions and metabolic acidosis.

Therapeutic Uses: Apart from its use in the emergency treatment of hypertension, nitroprusside has also been used to produce controlled hypotension during surgery and to improve left ventricular function in acute MI and other low output states. It is infused IV slowly in the dose of 0.5-5 mcg/kg/min. In the treatment of severe hypertension, if the BP is not adequately controlled after 10 minutes of infusion at the maximal rate, the drug should be stopped immediately for fear of drug toxicity. On the other hand, nitroprusside must not be stopped abruptly during treatment of heart failure because of the danger of rebound hypertension.

CALCIUM CHANNEL BLOCKERS: Their properties and uses are discussed in detail in Chapter 28. They are used in the long term treatment of hypertension. Nifedipine has also been used in the management of hypertensive emergencies. It is particularly useful in patients with impaired renal function or asthma, and during pregnancy. Further, it may be used as a single drug in hypertensive patients with diabetes mellitus as it does not affect the secretion of glucoregulatory hormones. CCB have no significant CNS effects.

There is some concern about the long term safety of the short acting dihydropyridines. Hence, the standard formulations (used for immediate relief) of nifedipine and other short half-life dihydropyridines are not recommended for long term treatment of hypertrension. Diltiazem and amlodipine are as effective as diuretics, beta-blockers or their combination, in the long term treatment of essential hypertension.

Nitrates have a synergistic vasodilator effect with the vasodilator drugs and, therefore, the use of nitroglycerine by a patient receiving a peripheral vasodilator drug e.g. a CCB can lead to sudden fall of BP and collapse.

Potassium Channel Activators

The group includes: **diazoxide** and **minoxidil** used in hypertension; and **nicorandil** and **pinacidil** used in angina (Chapter 28).

Mechanism of actions: Potassium channels play an important role in the regulation of membrane potential and excitability of cells. Potassium channel activators combine with ATP modulated potassium channels; opening these channels causes potassium ions to leak out from the cell. This action hyperpolarizes and stabilises the cell membrane of the vascular smooth muscle, and prevents its contraction, leading to its relaxation. Thus, they act as arterial vasodilators.

In the heart, the drugs reduce the excitability of the myocytes. They may have a role in the management of myocardial ischemia because the ATP modulated potassium channels are believed to be crucial in myocardial adaptation to ischemic injury via 'preconditioning'.

DIAZOXIDE (Eudemine) is a compound structurally related to the diuretic chlorothiazide. It is a potent, direct arteriolar vasodilator with t½ of 36 hour. As with hydralazine, compensatory reactions include tachycardia, increased cardiac contractility and sodium retention. It is highly protein bound and must be injected by IV bolus. It has no diuretic activity (Chapter 63).

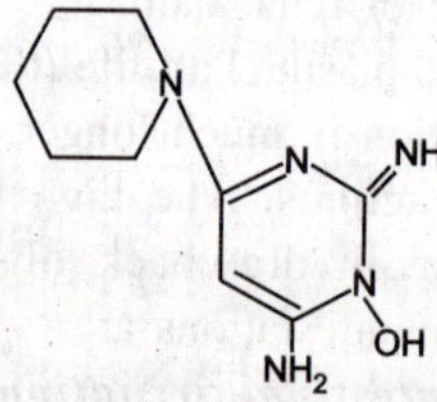

Fig. 29.5: Minoxidil

MINOXIDIL (Loniten) used orally is a peripheral vasodilator. Its actions are similar to those of hydralazine, but it is more potent and more toxic. It causes compensatory tachycardia, increased cardiac contractility, palpitation, angina and sodium retention. It can also cause pulmonary hypertension, hypertrichosis and headache. Pericardial effusion and cardiac tamponade have been reported. Its effective dose range is wide, 5-40 mg./ day. Because of its toxicity, the drug is reserved for resistant cases.

See Chapter 69 for its use in alopecia.

All arteriolar vasodilators cause reflex tachycardia.

Renin Inhibitors

Aliskiren: Renin cleaves angoitensinogen from the liver to form angiotensin I, which is then converted to angiotensin II (Fig.29.1). Oral, nonpeptide, renin inhibitor, aliskiren, causes dose-dependent, direct inhibition of the plasma renin activity (PRA i.e. angiotensin I generation) and thereby reduces both angiotensin I and II levels, and produces fall in BP. Angiotensin II functions within the RAAS as a negative inhibitory feedback mechanism. Reduced levels of angiotensin II due to aliskiren lead to increase in plasma renin levels; yet renin activity remains blocked. Thus in contrast to ACEI and ARB, which increase both plasma renin levels and PRA, aliskiren increases only renin levels. It is under evaluation.

Angiotensin Converting Enzyme Inhibitors (ACEI)

CAPTOPRIL (Capoten, Aceten): This orally effective inhibitor of angiotensin converting enzyme (ACE) is chemically D-3- mercapto-2-methyl propanoyl-L-proline.

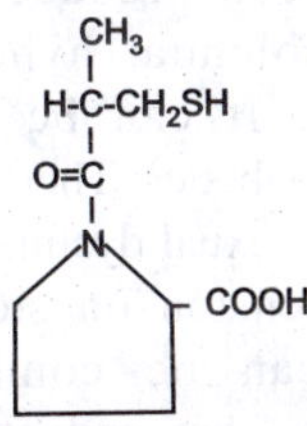

Fig. 29.6: Captopril

Mechanism of actions: ACE inhibitors competitively inhibit the conversion of angiotensin I to angiotensin II. They thus prevent (a) the pressor effect (angiotensin II); and (b) stimulation of aldosterone synthesis and secretion. As a consequence, the plasma levels of renin and angiotensin I show a marked compensatory rise.

ACE also metabolizes bradykinin (Chapter 24). Inhibition of ACE raises the levels of bradykinin, a potent vasodilator, which may also contribute to the antihypertensive and cardioprotective effects of ACEI. It has been suggested that blockade of generation of angiotensin II in the tissues (vascular, cardiac and renal) by ACEI may be responsible for their beneficial effect.

Pharmacological actions:

In healthy, sodium replete humans, a single oral dose of captopril lowers the systemic BP only slightly; the effect is more marked on repeated administration. By contrast, a single dose of captopril causes substantial lowering of BP in salt depleted subjects.

In hypertensive subjects:

- Captopril lowers systemic arterial resistance, as well as both systolic and diastolic BP. The drug acts even in the presence of low plasma renin activity.
- Captopril increases the compliance of large arteries and thus contributes to the reduction in systolic BP.
- The antihypertensive effect is seen in all varieties of hypertension except that due to primary aldosteronism; it is most marked in patients with renovascular hypertension. It is potentiated by the concurrent use of a diuretic.
- It causes vascular dilatation and increases the renal, cerebral and coronary blood flow.
- Baroreceptor function is reset, cardiovascular reflexes are not compromised and responses to posture and exercise are not impaired. Postural hypotension is not a problem.
- Secretion of aldosterone is reduced but adequate levels are maintained by other secretogogues, ACTH and potassium. As these secretogogues need a permissive level of angiotensin II for their action, the inhibition of ACE is not complete.

In patients with chronic CHF: captopril produces several beneficial effects.

- As a result of decreased peripheral arterial resistance, it reduces the afterload without causing a reflex activation of the adrenergic system. The cardiac output increases and the heart rate diminishes. Systemic BP falls initially but tends to return to pre-treatment levels.
- It causes natriuresis following hemodynamic changes and reduction in

aldosterone secretion. The venous return to the heart diminishes, decreasing the preload.

- Pulmonary arterial pressure, pulmonary capillary wedge pressure and of left atrial and left ventricular filling pressure (preload) are reduced.
- Exercise tolerance increases. In this respect, the drug is more specific and superior to hydralazine and prazosin.
- It prolongs survival in these patients.

In diabetic patients, captopril and other ACEI improve kidney function and reduce microalbuminuria. (renoprotection).

In patients with acute MI (Chapter 31).

Absorption, fate and excretion: Captopril is rapidly absorbed from the gut with a bioavailability of about 65%. Its absorption is reduced by food and so it is given 1 hour before a meal. It is cleared rapidly from the body by renal excretion (95%); about ½ is excreted as captopril and the other half as metabolites.

Adverse reactions: Captopril is generally well tolerated. Most adverse effects are the result of the specific inhibition of ACE. A steep fall in BP may occur after the first dose in subjects with severe hypertension who are on multidrug regimes including a diuretic, and generally in all salt depleted patients. *In such patients, captopril should be started in very small doses, preferably after stopping the diuretic.* Serious hyperkalemia is uncommon. However, potassium retention can, occur in patients with renal insufficiency and in those taking a potassium sparing diuretic. It should be used with caution in patients taking an NSAID or a betablocker.

In patients with severe bilateral renal artery stenosis or severe stenosis of the artery supplying a single functioning kidney, ACE inhibitors reduce glomerular filtration, and are likely to cause progressive renal failure.

Relatively common adverse effect is persistent dry cough (10-15%). It is believed to be due to raised bradykinin. The other adverse effects are skin rashes, disturbances of the sense of taste, vitiligo, headache, GI disturbances and muscle cramps. Proteinuria (>1 g/day) has been described. Rarely it causes serious angioedema. *The drug causes foetal toxicity in animals and should be avoided in pregnancy.*

Preparation and dosage: Captopril 25, 50 or 100 mg. tablets. It should be taken 1 hour before a meal. The starting dose in adults is 12.5 mg. bid. It is increased once in 1-2 weeks to a maximum of 50 mg. bid; a dose larger than 150 mg. per day is rarely required. In patients taking diuretics, the initial dose should be 6.25 mg. or less. Because of reduced clearance, smaller doses are indicated in patients with impaired renal function.

Therapeutic uses:

- ***Hypertension*****:** Captopril is useful in hypertension of all grades, including malignant hypertension. Used alone, it is roughly comparable to a thiazide diuretic or a beta adrenergic blocker. When combined with a thiazide, it can reduce hypokalemia, hypercholesterolemia, hyperglycemia and hyperuricemia. It can be used safely in asthmatics and diabetics. There is little tendency to weakness and sexual dysfunction. There is no rebound hypertension on stopping the drug abruptly. It can be combined with an antihypertensive from any other class and is generally well tolerated by the elderly.
- ***Chronic congestive heart failure*****:** ACEI are indicated in all clinical manifestations of heart failure and in individuals with asymptomatic LV dysfunction (Chapter 30).
- ***Diabetic nephropathy :*** Captopril and enalapril protect kidneys and decrease microalbuminuria in patients with insulin dependent diabetes mellitus and nephropathy.
- ***Acute MI*** (Chapter 31).

ENALAPRIL (Nuril): This congener of captopril, without an SH group, has actions similar to those of captopril and the same precautions apply to its use.

It differs from captopril in that:

- It is a prodrug and is converted in the body to the active metabolite enalaprilat.

- Food does not interfere with its absorption.
- It is more potent than captopril.
- Its action is slower but lasts longer.
- Hypotension and renal insufficiency are far commoner with enalapril than with captopril.
- It is less liable to cause taste disturbances leucopenia and glomerulopathy.

Urticaria, cough and angioedema have also been reported with enalapril.

In patients with congestive heart failure, the starting dose should be 2.5 mg./day in subjects over 60 years of age and 5 mg./day in subjects younger than 60. It is available as 5, 10 and 20 mg. tablets. It is given once daily. Usual maintenance dose is 10-20 mg. per day. As with captopril, the addition of enalapril to con-ventional treatment in patients with severe CHF can reduce mortality and improve symptoms.

Table 29.1 lists currently used ACEI .

Table 29.1: ACE inhibitors in current use

Drug	t ½ * (hrs)	Usual dosage (mg) $ in hypertension	
Captopril	1.9	12.5-50	bid
Lisinopril	11-12	5-40	od
Enalapril	11 12	5 20	od
Ramipril	13-17	2.5-20	od
Benazepril	10-11	10-40	od
Fosinopril	12	10-40	od
Quinapril	3	10-80	od

Drugs other than captopril and lisinopril are prodrugs.

* Of active drug/metabolite

$ Smaller doses in patients on diuretics, in CHF and with renal insufficiency.

Contraindication for ACEI:

(1) Severe renal artery stenosis.
(2) Aortic stenosis
(3) Coarctation of the aorta
(4) Pregnancy.

Angiotensin Receptor Blockers (ARB)

SARALASIN: This synthetic analogue of angiotensin II is a competitive inhibitor of angiotensin II; however, it has significant partial agonist properties. Infused IV, it lowers the BP in patients with angiotensin dependent hypertension (renovascular hypertension and malignant hypertension). It is used as a diagnostic agent.

LOSARTAN (Losacar, Cozac): This phenyl tetrazole substituted imidazole compound acts as a *selective, competitive antagonist of angiotensin II receptor type 1 (AT_1) (ARB)* and decreases peripheral vascular resistance. Conventional ACE inhibitors such as captopril inhibit ACE which is not a specific enzyme, and has other substrates (bradykinin, substance P and neurokinins); inhibition of these may be responsible for ADR such as cough and angioedema. Even ARBs can increase bradykinin due to AT_2 activation. Its action is potentiated by thiazides and it has some uricosuric action.

Given orally, it is well absorbed and undergoes hepatic first pass metabolism, being partly converted to a more active metabolite. Its effect on the CV hemodynamics are similar to those of captopril.

Adverse reactions: Like the ACEI it can cause fetotoxicity and should not be used during pregnancy. It can precipitate renal failure in patients with bilateral renal artery stenosis and in those with low, fixed renal blood flow. It can cause skin rashes and neuropsychiatric distur-bances such as insomnia, confusion, nightmares, agitation and depression. Even cough and angioedema can occur.

The drug is used to treat essential hypertension.

Valsartan, Irbesartan, Eprosartan and **Candesartan** are the other analogues of losartan. They are expensive.

ACEI and ARB are equally effective for treatment of hypertension. The choice between them depands upon familiarity and cost. Whether ARBs offer the same degree of cardioprotection as ACEI is not known. ARB have similar contraindications as ACEI.

Aldosterone Antagonist

SPIRONOLACTONE (Aldactone): This aldosterone antagonist is discussed in Chapter 38. As an add-on drug, it may be particularly useful in hypertensive patients with significant hyperuricemia, hypokalemia, or glucose intolerance. It is the *drug* of choice in primary hyperaldosteronism. It is now also recommended in small doses as an *add-on* drug in congestive heart failure (Chapter 30).

Eprenolol : See Chapter 38.

Diuretics as Antihypertensives

The **thiazide** group and related compound chlorthalidone have proved extremely valuable in the treatment of mild to moderate hypertension. In addition, they enhance the effect of other antihypertensive agents. They are described in detail in Chapter 38.

Mechanism of action: The thiazides probably reduce the BP by several mechanisms. The sodium depletion and consequent reduction in plasma volume and cardiac output produced by them are important in the initial days of treatment of essential hypertension. The same is probably true of the sodium- and water-dependent form of hypertension in chronic renal failure. Severe dietary restriction of sodium can produce a similar fall in BP.

After a few weeks of thiazide therapy, the plasma volume and the cardiac output, however, return to the pre-treatment level. From then on, decreased systemic vascular resistance, probably due to changes in the ionic composition of the vascular wall, is important in maintaining the antihypertensive effect. Diuretics may produce cellular sodium loss and increased entry of potassium into the cells. Activation of the K^+ channels may also contribute to thiazide-induced vasodilatation.

When GFR is reduced by 50% or more, thiazides lose most of their diuretic and antihypertensive effects. Thiazides also increase the PRA which may contribute to the development of tolerance.

Pharmacological actions : The antihypertensive effect of thiazides develops slowly. There is a reduction in the systolic and the diastolic BP. The hypotensive action is moderate, the maximum effect being obtained with 50 mg of **hydrochlorothiazide** or an equivalent amount of any of its congeners. *Increase in the dose does not enhance the hypotensive effect and there appears little difference in their antihypertensive action in equivalent doses.* Differences do exist, however, in their duration of action. (Chapter 38). The very potent diuretic furosemide is not recommended for the long term management of hypertension because of its short duration of action and the serious electrolyte disturbances. However, it can be valuable in patients with chronic kidney disease who do not respond to thiazides. In recommended doses, (25-50 mg) hydrochlorothiazide usually does not cause orthostatic hypotension or tachycardia, nor does it decrease renal blood flow. However, tolerance may develop after prolonged use. Thiazides are not useful in patients with markedly decreased GFR. Further, they are less effective than ACEI in reducing left ventricular hypertrophy.

Adverse reactions: These include hypokalemia, hyperuricemia and hyperglycemia (Chapter 38). With the recommended doses, hypokalemia is generally not a problem. Data indicate that (a) in the absence of digitalis and possibly overt heart disease, hypokalemia is not associated with increased occurrence of ventricular arrhythmias; and (b) although serum LDL cholesterol levels do rise modestly after thiazide diuretic dosing, the levels usually revert to the pre-treatment levels during long term use. Routine potassium supplementation during thiazides use is not necessary. Those at high risk of developing complications of hypokalemia (patients with IHD, arrhythmias, diabetes, severe hepatic disease as well as those on digitalis or glucocorticoids) should receive prophylactic potassium supplements or potassium sparing diuretics .

In general, *the oral thiazides still remain the most valuable, safe and highly cost-effective antihypertensive drugs.*

INDAPAMIDE (Natrilix, Lorvas): This compound, an indole derivative of chlorosulphonamide, is chemically related to chlorthalidone. Like the latter drug, it has a long duration of action with a plasma t½ of about 18 hours. Given orally in the dose of 2.5 mg. once daily, it reduces the BP in mild and moderate hypertension. Larger doses cause diuresis. It has similar therapeutic activity as chlorthalidone and is available as 2.5 mg. tablets and as 1.5 mg sustained release (SR) tablets.

XIPAMIDE (Xipamid): This is 4-chloro-5-sulfamoyl-2'- 6' salicyloxlidide. The drug has diuretic and hypotensive effects as well as adverse effects similar to thiazides. It also resembles furosemide in that it is an effective diuretic in patients with renal failure. It is generally administered in a single daily dose of 20-40 mg. It is available as 20 mg. tablets. It can also be used as a diuretic.

Miscellaneous Drugs

METYROSINE (Alpha methyl tyrosine, Demser): This drug blocks the synthesis of catecholamines by inhibiting tyrosine hydroxylase. It is useful in the preoperative treatment of patients with pheochromocytoma, and in the long term management of those in whom surgery is not feasible. The ADR include sedation, GI symptoms, extrapyramidal effects, crystalluria, nasal congestion, gynecomastia, galactorrhoea and peripheral edema. It is available as 250 mg capsules. Therapy is commenced with 250 mg qid, gradually increased to a maximum of 3 g daily. *It is not indicated in essential hypertension.*

Hypertension – Therapy

Effective treatment of hypertension is an important part of any programme to reduce the toll of cardiovascular disease, viz end-organ damage and mortality, in the society. This is so because any elevation of BP significantly increases morbidity and mortality which are directly related to the level of the BP.

The drug treatment of essential hypertension is still ‘empiric’, as these drugs reduce the BP without correcting the cause. However, it is now accepted that the reduction of BP (even suboptimally) prevents or postpones renal, cardiac and cerebral complications and prolongs life. The control of hypertension in diabetics also helps to delay the onset of retinal and renal damage. Complications arising from associated atherosclerosis are now the chief cause of death. Therefore, control of the other modifiable cardiovascular risk factors is an essential part of the treatment of hypertension.

Pretreatment evaluation should include:

- ***Multiple BP readings*** in supine and standing positions after sufficient rest, especially in elderly individuals.
- ***Assessment for target organ damage***

(a) Detailed history and physical examination: Dyspnoea; polyuria; nocturia; edema; cardiomegaly.

(b) Kidneys : Urine examination; serum creatinine; serum electrolytes.

(c) Heart : ECG, X'ray chest

(d) Fundoscopy: The condition of the retinal vessels reflects that of the cerebral vessels.

- ***Assessment for other cardiovascular risk factors :*** Salt intake; alcohol consumption; smoking; obesity; diabetes; hyperlipidemia; premature CV death in close relatives.
- ***Special investigations to identify the cause of hypertensions :*** USG of the urinary tract/renal blood vessels; renal angiography; tests for pheochromocytoma, aldosteronoma, etc. These are done if indications exist; or if the hypertension is drug-resistant.

It should be noted that:

(a) Every patient who knows that his/her BP is elevated requires treatment, though not necessarily with antihypertensive drugs.

(b) Systolic hypertension is as damaging as diastolic hypertension.

(c) Treatment with antihypertensives, once started, will *generally* have to be continued for life.

(d) Success of the treatment depends upon the care and the time spent by the doctor upon educating and counseling the patient; and the patient's compliance.

Reassurance by a physician and lifestyle modifications (Table 29.2) are necessary in all patients, including the prehypertensives. They may suffice in those with uncomplicated, mild hypertension and should be tried in them for 2-3 months.

Table 29.2: Lifestyle modification in hypertensives

- Weight reduction in obese persons.
- Restriction of salt consumption to 4-6 g. (about 2-3 g. of sodium) a day*
- Increase in *dietary* potassium (fruits and vegetables) consumption.*
- Restriction of fat consumption (Chapter 39).
- Physical exercise such as brisk walking; and mental relaxation.
- Reduction in alcohol and caffeine consumption.
- Cessation of smoking.
- Better adjustment at work and in family life.

* Increased salt intake is a necessary but not sufficient cause for hypertension. Reduction in salt intake reduces BP in hypertensives as well as those with high normal BP. It may also prevent a recurrence in those who were previously normotensives on drugs. Salt restriction needs to be at least moderate (a reduction of salt intake to 4g or less/day), sustained, and may take several weeks to be effective. Salt restriction also minimizes the age-related rise in BP. Chloride is as important as sodium in elevating BP, and their effect is additive; other salts such as sodium citrate are less liable to elevate the BP. Liability for BP to be elevated by salt (*salt sensitivity)* is partly genetic. It is also seen in insulin resistance, hyperlipidemia and microalbuminuria. It is alleviated by increased postassium intake. *Extreme salt restriction has been reported to be harmful.*

Clinically, hypertension can be divided into **mild, moderate**, **severe** and **very severe** grades (Table 29.3).

- ***Patients with very severe hypertension*** are at grave risk of developing one of the typically a 'hypertensive complications' such as cerebral hemorrhage, hypertensive encephalopathy, acute left ventricular failure, renal failure or dissection of the aorta. These patients and those with papilloedema (**malignant hypertension**) need urgent and aggressive treatment.
- ***Patients with severe hypertension*** are also at risk of developing the same 'hypertensive complications', especially if they are old or have long-standing hypertention.

Although the risk of a fatal complication is less in young patients, they are more liable to suddenly develop malignant hypertension. Prompt treatment of these patients can ward off a 'hypertensive complication' but unfortunately does not slow down the accelerated rate of atherosclerosis.

- ***Patients with moderate hypertension*** are also at risk if they have a bad family history " (a near relative has had a 'hypertensive complication'), or if they have cardiomegaly,

Table 29.3: Classification of hypertension

Category	Systolic BP (mm.Hg.)		Diastolic BP (mm.Hg.)	Recommendation
Normal	<120	**and**	<80	Recheck in 2 years.
High Normal (prehypertension)	120-139	or	80-89	Recheck in 6 months.
Hypertension				
Mild*	140-159	or	90-99	Confirm and treat within 2 months.
Moderate**	160-179	or	100-109	Treat within 1 month.
Severe**	180-209	or	110-119	Treat within 1 week.
Very severe**	>210	or	>120	Treat immediately.

* = Stage 1. ** = Stage 2.

fundus changes or ECG abnormalities. They too require energetic treatment.

- ***If the hypertension is mild***, the need for drug treatment is determined by the patient's age. Studies by the Veterans' Administration have shown that young patients in this group definitely benefit from aggressive treatment of their hypertension. *Aggressive reduction of BP is, however, likely to prove dangerous in elderly, arteriosclerotic individuals with elevated systolic but normal diastolic BP.*

In mild hypertension nonpharmacological treatment should be given a trial for 2-3 months. If it does not lower the diastolic BP to less than 90 mm Hg, treatment with drug is indicated, especially if additional cardiovascular risk factors such as diabetes mellitus or hyperlipidemia are present. If diastolic BP is below 90 mm Hg but other cardiovascular risk factors are present, non-pharmacological treatment should be initiated.

- ***In patients with hypertension and renal failure,*** there may be an initial deterioration of renal function after starting aggressive antihypertensive drug treatment. In the long run, however, effective control of hypertension halts the downhill progress of renal failure and prolongs life.

- ***In patients with diabetes mellitus***, low dose thiazides, betablockers, ACE inhibitors and dihydropyridine CCB are used for long term therapy (see later).

Antihypertensive drugs should be used cautiously in patients who have had a recent MI or a stroke, as a rapid lowering of BP can worsen their condition.

The duration of drug treatment is lifelong in most patients. An occasional patient may be able to give up his treatment and remain normotensive thereafter. How often this happens is not known.

Principles of Drug Therapy

The aims of treatment of hypertension are:

(a) Maintaining the BP, including the early morning BP, as near normal as possible (less than 140/89 mm Hg) without undue side effects.

(b) Maintaining/improving the quality of life, including the intellectual and sexual functions.

(c) Reduction in left ventricular mass.

(d) Prevention of cardiac arrhythmias, heart failure and other complications.

(e) Control of other CHD risk factors; and

(f) Doing all this in a cost-effective manner.

Principles of treatment :

- In the long run, one aims at keeping the BP in the erect posture as near normal as possible. This generally means a systolic BP (SBP) of less than 140 mm. Hg and a diastolic blood pressure (DBP) of less than 90 mm Hg. (less than 130/80 in diabetes mellitus and chronic renal failure). However, a higher level of BP may have to be accepted in elderly patients, in patients with impaired renal function and in those with ischemic heart disease or cerebrovascular disease. This is done in order to avoid the unpleasant symptoms and the possible complications (including myocardial and cerebral ischemia) of postural hypotension.

- Antihypertensive drugs are started in small doses, increased gradually and only infrequently (every 3-4 weeks) as the maximum effect of a drug or drug combination at a given dose level may take some days or weeks.

However, in severe and very severe hypertension, one generally initiates the treatment with full doses of drugs, often using more than one drug from the start.

- Having found a regimen that controls BP in the best possible manner, it is wrong to change the schedule unless there is a good reason to do so. However, in hot weather the patient may be asked to reduce the doses of antihypertensive drugs slightly in order to avoid postural hypotension. The fall in standing pressure may be exaggerated by exercise or sudden change of position and the patient should be warned of the possibility of fainting.
- With drugs such as ACEI, beta-blockers and methyldopa, which do not cause significant postural hypotension, it is possible to maintain both standing and supine BP normal or near normal in some patients. If this can be done safely and continuously, then this is almost ideal antihypertensive therapy.
- In patients with severe and very severe hypertension (see Table 29.3), the diastolic BP should be lowered to 100-110 mm Hg in the first 24 hours; further lowering to target levels should be carried out over the next 2-3 days.
- During chronic therapy, adjustments occur in homeostatic mechanisms including the reflex cardiovascular responses and in the end organ receptor concentration; for example, the number of beta adrenergic receptors increases during chronic beta-blocker therapy. The reaction of the patient to the abrupt cessation of drug therapy depends upon the dose and duration of action of the drug, and the readjustment time for the homeostatic mechanisms activated during drug therapy. If the former is much shorter than the latter (as is the case with propranolol and clonidine) rebound cardiovascular changes are likely to occur, with occasional lethal consequences such as cerebral hemorrhage. If, on the other hand, the former is prolonged compared to the latter (as is the case of reserpine) no such rebound occurs.
- In practice, it is difficult to be familiar with more than a few preparations and hence, it is wise to continue using the one or two preparations which one knows best, and change them only if they are ineffective or adverse effects are troublesome.
- Patients should be educated about the drugs they are receiving and their adverse effects. Watch for possible drug interaction when the patient is on more than one drug.
- The patient must be given a card bearing the names and doses of the drugs he is receiving.
- Impress upon the patient the hazards of uncontrolled or intermittently controlled hypertension and the rewards of keeping the BP under check continuously and lifelong.

Choice of Drug Therapy

Although many antihypertensive drugs are useful in controlling high BP, the initial choice is still debated.

Long term studies indicate that there are no important differences as regards efficacy, adverse effects or quality of life among patients who receive thiazides, beta blockers, calcium channel antagonists, ACEI, ARB or alpha blockers, except in certain selected group of patients. Further, thiazides, ACEI and calcium channel blockers do not increase the frequency of development of diabetes when they are used in non-diabetic hypertensive subjects.

Analysis of many clinical trials reconfirms that the low-dose thiazide/thiazide-type diuretics alone or in combination (depending upon the severity) remain the first line therapy in majority of the patients with hypertension. The 'diabetogenic' and 'hyperlipidemic' effects of the thiazides and beta-blockers are often overstressed. Similarly, unless specifically contraindicated, reserpine is a useful and cost effective drug. An ACEI or CCB is considered a reasonable, but more expensive, alternative first choice. Patients with special problems (Table 29.4) benefit from a non-diuretic as a first line drug eg. ACEI in patients with LV dysfunction or diabetes mellitus; or a beta-blocker/CCB in patient with stable angina pectoris. *Half the patients, however, in long term, would need a minimum of two drugs for controlling their BP.*

Use of Drug Combinations

An appropriate combination of anti-hypertensive drugs can produce beneficial effects on:

- ***Blood pressure.***
- ***Adverse reactions;*** and
- ***Hemodynamic effects.***

In practice, except perhaps those with mild hypertension, many patients would need combination drug therapy. Drug combinations not only help to achieve better BP control but also reduce the incidence of ADR from individual drugs because of reduction in their doses. These combinations also reduce the ADR by pharmacological means. Fixed-dose combinations ensure better compliance. They however, should be chosen by the physician with the full knowledge of the clinical pharmacology of the drugs.

It is rational to combine antihypertensive drugs with different pharmacodynamic actions or with different anatomical sites of action, e.g., a diuretic can be combined with a beta-blocker, a vasodilator, methyldopa or ACEI. Drugs with similar adverse effects should generally not be combined. e.g. methyldope and clomidine. Extra care should be taken in patients who are at risk for postural hypotension.

The drugs which interfere with the adrenergic system tend to produce fluid retention with consequent diminution in the drug's therapeutic effect (*pseudotolerance*). Addition of a thiazide effectively counteracts fluid retention, enhances the therapeutic effect and permits the use of smaller doses of other drugs.

Management with Drugs

The major factors in human hypertension are:

- ***Peripheral vasoconstriction.***
- ***Expansion of plasma volume;*** and
- ***Hyperdynamic heart action, particularly in the young.***

Since *the majority of hypertensive subjects will have BP reduction no matter what drug is used,* the initial choice of the drug should depend upon such factors as safety, cost, likely patient compliance and associated medical problems which may either benefit from a given drug or increase the liability to adverse effects. Such *symptom drug profiling* (Table 29.4) is very useful in practice.

Generally, a *stepped-care approach* is recommended in drug treatment of hypertension. Initially, treatment is started with a small dose of a single drug (monotherapy). The dose is gradually increased till the desired BP level is achieved without undue ADR or the maximum recommended dose is reached. At that point, a another drug is substituted or added, if needed. This requires the application of a flexible, individualized approach to drug prescription.

The therapeutic guidelines that can be derived from the various outcome studies are:

(1) Start the therapy with low dose of an agent, appropriate for a given patient, depending upon the co-morbid conditions such nas diabetes mellitus, angina, pregnancy and so on (Table 29.4). If the BP is not controlled, the dose should be increased in small increments (**start low, go slow**).

(2) If the BP is still not controlled, another drug from a different class may be added which

is likely to be well tolerated, as the compliance and the long term efficacy of drugs depend upon their long term tolerability.

(3) When two agents are used, one of them should be a diuretic, preferably a low dose of a thiazide e.g. hydrochlorthiazide 25 mg or less/ day,or its equivalent,in nearly all cases.

(4) Use low dose combination therapy, if indicated, as initial therapy :

(a) A diuretic + (a beta blocker or an ACEI or an ARB); or

(b) A long acting CCB + an ACEI.

(5) A two drug combination will control BP in almost 90 % of patients. If this is not achieved,the primary agent should be increased to the full dose e.g. enalapril 20 mg,atenolol 50 mg or diltiazem 360 mg. This may be combined with reduction in salt intake to less than 4 gm/ day and increased intake of potassium in the form of fresh vegetables and fruits, (the latter not in combination with ACEI or ARB).

(6) In resistant cases, the primary agent **other than thiazide** should be replaced by a drug from another class. Triple drug therapy with a diuretic + an ACEI/ARB + hydralazine may also be effective. *In still resistant cases, the patient should be investigated in detail for a possible cause of secondary hypertension.*

(7) Once the BP is controlled and maintained consistently, an attempt should be made to reduce the dose step-wise and possibly omit one of the drugs, to determine the minimal therapeutic regimen that will maintain the BP less than 140/90 mm Hg or less, without any inconvenient, adverse effects.This will ensure long term compliance.

Mild hypertension: The basic drug is a thiazide such as hydrochlorothiazide or chlorthalidone unless a specific contraindication exists. Hydrochlorothiazide is administered in the dose of 25 mg. od; any of its congeners can be employed in equivalent dosage. *Increasing the dose of hydrochlorothiazide beyond 50 mg. daily usually does not produce any further therapeutic benefit.* The antihypertensive effect is usually established within 2 to 3 weeks. Subsequently, smaller doses (12.5 mg OD) can be administered for maintenance therapy. If the BP is not adequately controlled by thiazides, the therapy can be intensified with the addition of a beta-blocker or a CCB.

If the patient is younger than 50 years of age and has evidence of tachycardia and hyperdynamic cardiac action, a beta-blocker may be initial drug of choice, especially if there is no evidence of peripheral vascular disease. Beta-blockers are also preferred in hypertensive patients with IHD. Atenolol 12.5-50 mg. per day is usually preferred. In patients with diabetes mellitus, ACEI would be the first drug of choice.

Alpha blockers should not be first line therapy.

In patients with repeated BP readings of more than 160/100 mm Hg. it is justifiable to start the therapy with two drugs, one of which preferably should be a thiazide diuretic.

Moderate hypertension: In moderate hypertension, hydrochlorothiazide or chlorthalidone in combination with a beta-blocker may not be able to control the BP effectively. In such patients, a CCB or an ACEI may be substituted for (mono therapy) or added to the above mentioned drugs.

Calcium channel blockers such as diltiazem, amlodipine or felodipine or a sustained release preparation of nifedipine are effective anti-hypertensive agents. *Diltiazem is contraindicated if congestive heart failure or AV block is present and in patients on digitalis or a beta blocker. Short acting nifedipine formulations are not suitable for long term use.*

An ACEI such as captopril/enalapril may be a good drug to add to thiazide, especially if the patient is also in congestive heart failure. ACEI is the preferred drug in hypertensive patients with *diabetic nephropathy* for several reasons:

- ***It does not alter or may even improve glucose tolerance.***
- ***It does not mask the symptoms and signs of, nor interfere with recovery from hypoglycemia.***
- ***ACE inhibitors protect the kidney in the long term.***

Table 29.4: Symptom profiling of antihypertensive drugs

Associated Problem	Recommended	Not Recommended	Associated Problem	Recommended	Not Recommended
Migraine	BB		**Hyper-lipidemia**	Low dose thiazides, alpha-blockers, ACEI	High dose thiazides, BB
Depression	Diuretics ACE inhibitors CCB Vasodilators Alpha blockers	Reserpine Clonidine Methyldopa BB	**Essential tremor**	Propranolol	
Bronchospasm	CCB Vasodilators	BB esp. propranolol	**Open angle glaucoma**	BB	
Palpitation	BB Diltiazem	Vasodilators	**Diabetes mellitus**	ACEI, ARB CCB	Potassium sparing diuretics
Angina pectoris	BB CCB	Vasodilators	**Azotemia**	Loop diuretics Direct acting vasodilators BB Alpha methyl-dopa Alpha$_1$ blockers	ACEI Potassium sparing diuretics Guanethidine
Old MI	BB ACEI				
Congestive heart failure	Diuretics ACE inhibitors Vasodilators	BB CCB			
Bradycardia		BB, Verapamil Diltiazem	**History of sexual dysfunction**	Gradual reduction of blood pressure (CCB, ACEI, and Alpha$_1$ blockers are preferred)	Rapid reduction of blood pressure
Mitral valve prolapse syndrome	BB	Drugs causing tachycardia or orthostatic hypotension			
Left ventricular hypertrophy	ACE inhibitors	Direct acting vasodilators			
Raynaud's phenomenon	CCB Alpha blockers	BB	**Benign prostatic hypertrophy**	Alpha$_1$ blockers relieve prostatism	
Fluid retention	Diuretics	Vasodilators Clonidine BB	**Osteoporosis**	Thiazides	Loop diuretics
Thyrotoxi-cosis	BB	Drugs causing tachycardia	**Renal calculi**	Thiazides	Loop diuretics

BB - Beta blockers. CCB - Calcium channel blockers.

Severe and very severe hypertension: These patients usually have damaged kidneys and heart. A sudden reduction in BP may produce azotemia or coronary insufficiency. If, however, the diastolic BP is above 120 mm Hg and there is no evidence of target organ damage, vigorous therapy is advocated.

Treatment of severe hypertension may need combination with additional drugs such as an alpha adrenergic blocker (prazosin), a centrally acting drug (alpha methyl dopa), a direct acting peripheral vasodilator (hydralazine, or in resistant cases minoxidil). Minoxidil is a difficult drug to use because of its ADR.

An alpha blocker e.g. prazosin is especially useful in patients having concurrent symptomatic benign prostatic hypertrophy.

Alpha methyldopa may be used along with a thiazide. Intial dose is 250 mg. 2-4 times a day and it is increased by 250 mg. at intervals of 2 to 7 days to a maintenance level. *Doses of methyldopa larger than 1.5 g. daily should be avoided* as it can cause mental apathy.

Hydralazine is usually started in a small dose, 10 mg bid, which is then gradually increased to 50 - 100 mg bid. The upper limit of 400 mg should not be exceeded for fear of appearance of rheumatoid arthritis-like syndrome. Hydralazine is particularly useful in the presence of kidney damage as it dilates the renal vessels. It is contraindicated in patients with arteriosclerotic hypertension, angina, MI or peptic ulcer.

Hypertension in the Elderly

Both diastolic and isolated systolic high BP are cardiovascular risk factors in the elderly. The beta adrenergic responses of vascular smooth muscle and plasma renin levels decline with age. The most consistent cardiovascular physiologic change in elderly patients is increased peripheral resistance.

Not all hypertension in all old people needs drug treatment; this is especially so in patients over 70 years of age. Treatment should be considered for those elderly patients whose BP exceeds 140/85 mm Hg. Rapid lowering of BP and postural hypotension can be dangerous. Sometimes, unpleasant hypotension can occur on exertion. The low dose thiazides or atenolol would appear to be relatively safe in these patients. Doses of diuretic larger than the equivalent of 25 mg. of hydrochlorothiazide per day should probably be avoided and even mild hypokalemia treated with potassium supplement or potassium sparing diuretic, provided kidney function is normal. Calcium channel blockers and ACE inhibitors are also well tolerated. Reserpine may cause serious depression. Clonidine and prazosin are also better avoided because of their possible adverse effects.

Swedish studies with chlorthalidone 12.5 - 25 mg. daily, with atenolol 25-50 mg., added if necessary, showed that this therapy is effective in old (70-84 years) hypertensives and that it significantly reduces the incidence of stroke and coronary events. Further, as per ALLHAT trial in elderly high risk patients over 55 years, chlorthalidone 12.5-25 mg./day alone or in combination was found as effective as ACEI or CCB in preventing the cardiovascular events. Chlorthalidone is twice as potent as hydrochlorothiazide and has a longer duration of action. Hence, *low dose thiazides including chlorthalidone ± atenolol (12.5-25 mg.)* appears to be suitable first line therapy in the vast majority of elderly hypertensive subjects. Such regimens are effective, simple, inexpensive and well tolerated.

Complex, multiple-drug regimes are best avoided in the elderly as they may be confusing. Hypertension which persists after cardiac failure is corrected needs treatment with an antihypertensive drug whereas a patient with an established stroke in old age does not benefit from such therapy. In fact, some patients of the latter group may show an intellectual deterioration on lowering of the BP.

The aim of therapy in the elderly should be to lower the BP as much below 180/100 mm Hg as the patient can tolerate comfortably, preferably to 160/85 mm. Hg. or less. No attempt should be made to make the BP 'normal'.

Further, **isolated systolic hypertension** (defined as systolic BP over 140 mm Hg and diastolic BP less than 90 mm Hg) is often resistant to treatment; attempts to treat it aggressively lowers the diastolic BP to such an extent as to compromise blood flow to vital organs. It may be treated with a diuretic or a beta blocker, (or both), or with amlodipine alone.

Hypertension in Pregnancy

Hypertension in pregnant women may be diagnosed when the systolic BP is 135 mm. Hg. or more or when the diastolic BP is 85 mm. Hg. or more. Hypertension during pregnancy may be:

- ***Chronic hypertension***, either essential or secondary, dating from before the pregnancy.
- ***Transient hypertension*** developing after midpregnancy; this is usually mild and the BP returns to normal postpartum. Such women are liable to develop hypertension subsequently; or
- ***Pre-eclampsia*** with moderate to severe hypertension, edema, proteinuria and disturbances of liver function and coagulation. It can lead to eclampsia with generalized convulsions and fetal death.

Chronic hypertension dating from before pregnancy, especially *when secondary, long standing* and associated with organ damage, predisposes to pre-eclampsia. However, *more than 85% of women with mild pre-exisitng chronic, essential hypertension have uncomplicated pregnancies.* Hypertension during pregnancy needs treatment in order to possibly prevent pre-eclampsia; however, no treatment guaranteedly prevents pre-eclampsia.

Women with secondary hypertension and those with diastolic BP of 95 mm. Hg. or higher need aggressive treatment. Women with risk factors such as renal disease or end organ damage should be treated even at lower levels of diastolic BP. **Methyldopa** is effective, and is safe for the mother and the baby; it is the preferred antihypertensive drug in pregnant women. The alternative to methyldopa is beta-blockers; they are safe in the third tremester of pregnancy but may cause intrauterine growth retardation when prescribed earlier. However, by causing fetal bradycardia beta blockers remove an important index of fetal distress, viz. fetal bradycardia. In acute episodes of hypertension during pregnancy, nifedipine can be used safely.

Labetalol may be hepatotoxic whereas the use of ACE inhibitors is associated with oligohydramnios and neonatal renal failure. *ACE inhibitors and ARBs are absolutely contraindicated during pregnancy.* Diuretics should not be used as first-line agents to treat hypertension in pregnancy as they can deplete maternal intravascular volume, and may rarely cause neonatal thrombocytopenia. However, they are useful in patients with edema. Clonidine is better avoided in pregnant women unless hypertension fails to be controlled by methyldopa. Hydralazine is not considered desirable in pregnant women.

Severe hypertension may develop near term or during labour. When such is the case or when preeclampsia is suspected at any time during the pregnancy, the patient should be hospitalized and put to complete bed rest. The urgent need is to lower the diastolic BP to between 90 and 100 mm Hg. For this purpose, IV labetalol or sublingual/oral nifedipine (see later) given every 30 min as needed is the treatment of choice. **Magnesium sulfate IV** is the drug of choice for prevention and treatment of eclamptic convulsions. However, its anti-hypertensive action is slight and unpredictable. It should be continued upto 24 hours postpartum. Sodium nitroprusside is likely to have adverse effects on the fetus. If the patient's condition deteriorates or if eclampsia supervenes, the pregnancy is terminated regardless of its duration.

Supportive Treatment of Hypertension

General treatment: Adequate rest, relaxation

and sleep are desirable. Ambitions may have to be curbed or sacrificed for reasons of health. Reassurance and a benzodiazepine could benefit the patient. The patient should be explained in detail what 'moderation in all things' actually means. Yoga, meditation and relaxation techniques may be helpful. Very strict restrictions are, however, often unnecessary, as Page has aptly remarked, "I firmly believe that those who follow directions minutely do better than the careless. But there are important areas of living in which we physicians know no more than others. Often when we don't know what to do, we proscribe instead of prescribing — we forbid this or that of the things people often most enjoy. I suppose this characteristic is a hangover from the days when anything that was pleasurable was sinful. Whether we forbid smoking, alcohol and such, may make a good deal of difference as to whether people will think life worth living. I should therefore remind you that smoke and alcohol were the oldest known preservatives and that Winston Churchill was 100 proof of this observation."

Weight reduction by diet control in obese patients is beneficial. Centrally acting anti-obesity drugs should be avoided as they tend to increase the BP. Although sodium restriction is known to help the reduction in BP, with the present day diuretic drug treatment rigid restriction of salt intake is rarely necessary. (Also see Table 29.2).

Prevention of cardiovascular disease: Aspirin in daily dose of 75-150 mg can reduce major cardiovascular events in hypertensive patients. Hence, for primary prevention it is recommended in patients aged 50 years or over, only after BP is controlled.

In patients under the age of 70 years, who have total serum cholesterol of more than 180 mg/d1, a statin may be used on long term basis (Chapter 39).

Resistant hypertension may be defined as BP persistently higher than 140/90 mm Hg in most hypertensive patients, and 130/80 mm Hg or more in diabetics and subjects with renal disease, despite prescription of three drugs including a diuretic. The common causes of inadequate response to antihypertensive treatment (**resistant hypertension**) are listed in Table 29.5. The commonest cause is non-compliance, probably present in 50-70% of patients. Apparent resistance is commonly due to faulty BP apparatus and/or faulty technique employed for measurement.

Table 29.5: Common causes of inadequate response to antihypertensive treatment

- Visceral obesity.
- Poor patient compliance.
- Continued stress.
- Inadequate drug therapy .
- Concomitant use of certain drugs (Table 29.9).
- Excesive sodium intake (including that in medications).
- Smoking, too much of alcohol; and
- Secondary hypertension.

Treatment of Hypertensive Crises

Extremely high BP (130 mm Hg or higher DBP) may sometimes be found in completely asymptomatic patients. Long term treatment with *gradual reduction of BP* is sufficient in them to prevent severe organ damage.

On the other hand, in many situations *BP must be reduced in several hours or even within one hour* to prevent death or severe damage to vital organ functions; they constitute **hypertensive crises** (Table 29.6). They usually occur in patients with known hypertension,but may occur in previously normotensive persons. They are characterized by *some or all* of the following:

- ***Sudden or sustained rise of DBP to 120 mm Hg or higher.***
- ***Papilledema*** (not always present).
- ***Decrease in renal function.***

Table 29.6: Hypertensive crises

(A) **Hypertensive urgencies:**These may be defined as sudden or severe elevation of BP, usually with DBP of 120 mm Hg or higher ***with an impending complication***. Such patients need immediate treatment, preferably in an ICU. The diastolic blood pressure needs to be reduced to 100-110 mm Hg *within 24-48 hours* without the use a loading dose. The BP may then be reduced further, gradually, over the next several days.
Severe epistaxis
Severe perioperative hypertension
Unstable angina pectoris
Diabetic retinopathy
Pre-eclampsia
Tyramine ingestion during MAOI therapy
Amphetamine or cocaine intoxication
Hypertension with papilledema
Rapidly progressing renal failure with vitreous hemorrage

(B) **Hypertensive emergencies**:These may be defined as severe elevation of BP to 210/120-130 mm Hg, ***with evidence of target organ damage or dysfunction***. Such patients also require admission into an ICU and rapid, but not too rapid, lowering of BP to 150-160/100-110 *within 1hour;* the BP should be maintained at that level for a few days, before lowering it, slowly, still further.
Hypertensive encephalopathy
Intracranial hemorrhage
Acute myocardial infarction
Acute LVF with pulmonary edema
Acute aortic dissection
Eclampsia
Hypertensive crisis in pheochromocytoma
Most hypertensive emergencies are characterized by vasoconstriction and normal or reduced plasma volume. Therefore, drugs which do not cause reduction in renal blood flow (CCBs, fenoldopam and sodium nitroprusside) are preferred.

- ***Neurological dysfunction;*** and
- ***Acute LVF.***

The severity of a hypertensive crisis depends not only upon the absolute BP but also on the rapidity of its rise to the present level.

Hypertensive crises should be treated in a hospital ICU with facilities for invasive BP monitoring. *In their absence, IV antihypertensives should be avoided.* Drugs which reduce the perfusion of vital organs minimally are preferred. *Patients should be treated in a strictly supine position to avoid orthostatic complications.* If renal function is greatly impaired, even a small reduction in GFR may worsen it. Drastic lowering of BP in a few minutes is hazardous and may cause cerebral ischemia leaving permanent neurological deficit, angina, MI, blindness or stroke.

BP can be reduced rapidly by using:

Sodium nitroprusside: This agent has almost instantaneous onset of action and is most consistently effective. Since it can cause a precipitous fall in BP, the infusion should be titrated very carefully. This is its main disadvantage. However, it is the drug of choice in the presence of MI or pulmonary edema. It is also helpful in a hypertensive crisis due to pheochromocytoma, the use of sympathonimetic drugs, and drug interactions of MAO (Chapter 13).

Nitroglycerine (NTG) : Nitroglycerine is useful in lowering the BP in a few minutes. It is the preferred agent in severe CAD or advanced renal or hepatic insufficiency where nitroprusside is contraindicated. Since it reduces the preload more than the afterload, it should be avoided in patients with inferior wall MI with RV involvement. NTG may also be administered sublingually.

Labetalol, IV, reduces the BP in a dose-dependent manner, even in severe cases, including patients in the early phase of acute MI, and it affects the heart rate and cardiac output minimally. Since its t/2 is 5-8 hours, the IV infusion should be discontinued before starting oral therapy with 200 mg., and continuing with 200-400 mg. 6-12 hourly.

Table 29.7 : Some parenteral/oral drugs in hypertensive emergencies

Drug	Dose	Onset	Duration	Remarks
Arteriolar and venous dilator				
Sodium nitropruside	0.25-10 mcg/kg/min, IV infusion	Immediate	2-3 min.	Thiocyanate toxicity
Nitroglycerine	5-100 mcg/min, IV infusion	2-5 min	5-10 min.	Preferred in pts.with IHD
Arteriolar dilator				
Hydralazine	5-10 mg IV bolus every 30 min. or 10-50 mg IM	10-20 min	2-4 hrs	May ppt. angina, MI, Used in pregnancy
D_1 receptor agonist				
Fenoldopam	0.1-0.6 mcg/kg/min IV infusion	3-5 min	10-30 min	Maintains renal perfusion
Alpha and beta adrenergic blocker				
Labetalol	20-80 mg IV bolus every 10 min. to max. total dose of 300 mg or 2mg/min IV infusion	5-10 min.	3-6 hrs	Avoid in pts.with cardiogenic shock or marked bradycardia
Nonseletive alpha blocker				
Phentolamine	5-15 mg IV	1-2 min.	3-10 min	For pheochromocytoma and MAO interactions
Beta adrenergic blocker				
Esmolol	250-500 mcg/kg/min for 1 min; then 50-300 mcg for 1 min; then 50-300 mcg/kg/min for 4-5 min	3-5 min	10-20 min.	For post-op.hyertension
CCB				
Nifedipine	SL 10 mg, then 10 mg PO 6 hrly.	2-3 min	2-3 hrs	May cause fluctuation in BP
Nicardipine	5 mg IV bolus, repeated every 10-15 min., max. 15 mg/hr	1-5 min	3-6 hrs	Can cause reflex tachycardia
Clevidipine	1-2 mg /hr.IV, increased slowly to 4-6 mg/hr	2-4 min.	5-15 min.	Do.
ACE blockers				
Enalapritalat	1.25-5 mg IV bolus 6 hrly	15-30min	6 hrs	—

Labetalol IV (infusion or bolus doses) is the drug of choice in hypertensive crisis in pregnancy.

Fenoldopam: This drug is a peripheral, dopamine (D_1) receptor agonist with a short action. It causes peripheral and renal vasodilatation, and natriuresis. It is as effective as sodium nitroprusside in the treatment of hypertensive emergencies. It can cause headache, flushing and raised intra-ocular pressure.

The other drugs used and the regimens are outlined in Table 29.7.

Nifedipine: Sublingual nifedipine is effective in lowering the BP rapidly. It is given in the dose of 10 mg, acts within 2-3 minutes and the action lasts for 2-3 hours. In less urgent cases, it is given orally in the dose of 10 mg 6 hourly. If a sublingual preparation is not available, the patient can *chew* a 10 mg. tablet for immediate local absorption and should *swallow* a second 10 mg tablet at the same time. Nifedipine is the drug least liable to aggravate regional blood flow imbalances and to cause ischemia of the brain, eyes or kidney; but it can cause undesirable fluctuations in BP. *Although not an ideal drug, given under supervision, it is the preferred drug when intensive care facilities are not available.* Nifedipine should be avoided in patients with CAD or with ECG evidence of LVH.

Captopril, 12.5-25 mg sublingually, may be used as an alternative to nifedipine.

Diuretics should be used only to treat salt retention or acute LVF with pulmonary edema.

An immediate fall of BP to below the autoregulatory range of cerebral blood flow (which in hypertensives can be as high as 120-160 mm Hg systolic) can cause severe brain damage. The initial reduction in DBP should be about 20%; further reduction of 10% every two to four hours till the diastolic pressure reaches 90-100 mm Hg is desirable. Drugs with long plasma t/2 may cause extended hypotension with its attendant risk of acute neurological damage. *Close monitoring by frequent BP measurements is, therefore, mandatory.*

Drugs like reserpine, methyldopa and hydralazine have unpredictable onset and duration of action in hypertensive emergencies. Sodium nitroprusside allows precise titration; but it needs monitoring.

Although parenteral drugs are administered with precaution and care, an occasional patient may develop excessive hypotension. Hence, noradrenaline should be kept ready to treat drug induced hypotension. Similarly, if diuretics are used, attention must be given for maintaining adequate hydration to avoid oligemia.

Drug Induced Hypertension

Some drugs used in therapeutics may cause a rise in BP as their adverse effect (Table 29.8). Further, some dietary supplements such as *bitter orange* have been reported to increase BP.

It is imperative, therefore, to enquire whether the patient is taking any such drug while evaluating a hypertensive subject.

Table 29.8 : Some drugs causing hypertension

- ***Hormones***: Glucocorticoids, fludrocortisone, testosterone, ethinyl estradiol.
- ***Vasoconstrictors***: Adrenergic agents, ergot alkaloids, anorexiants, decongestants.
- ***MAO inhibitors.***
- ***Salt retaining drugs:*** NSAID, liquorice.
- ***Miscellaneous***: Bromocriptine, Alcohol, Caffeine in excess, Epoeitin alpha, Cyclosporine.

Many proprietary 'cold cures' and 'cough mixtures' contain adrenergic drugs e.g. ephedrine, phenylephrine, phenylpropanolamine or phenteramine. Hence, it is best to warn the patients on antihypertensives to avoid such preparations as they may cause a sudden rise of BP, particularly in those receiving adrenergic neuron blockers.

Pharmacotherapy of Heart Failure 30

Heart failure is a common and serious condition with high morbidity and mortality. Since the introduction of digitalis in its treatment in 1776, the pharmacotherapy of heart failure has made spectacular advances, resulting in better prognosis.

The normal heart is capable of increasing the cardiac output upto 3-4 times the resting value during exercise and in other states of increased need. **Heart failure** may be defined as the inability of the heart to maintain the cardiac output adequate to meet the metabolic demands of the body at all times. It manifests as :

(1) **Acute heart failure as after MI;** or

(2) **Chronic heart failure.**

The aims of therapy in acute heart failure differ from those in chronic heart failure. For rational therapy of heart failure, it is necessary to understand the physiology of cardiac contraction and the pathophysiology of failure of the heart as a pump.

Physiology of cardiac contraction: The structural and functional unit of the cardiac muscle (myocyte) is a sarcomere. It is made up of two interdigitating myofilaments: the thicker filament made of the protein **myosin** and the thinner one made of the protein **actin**. Myosin has intrinsic enzymatic (ATPase) activity sites. Actin possesses the ability to combine reversibly with myosin in the presence of ATPase and Ca^{++}. Calcium ions activate myosin ATPase, which in turn breaks down ATP, the energy source for excitation-contraction coupling in cardiac muscle.

The principal mediator for the inotropic state of the heart is increased intracytoplasmic Ca^{++}. Cardiac contraction and relaxation result from the changing concentration of Ca^{++} in the myocyte cytosol. During depolarization (Chapter 27), calcium ions enter the myocyte via the calcium channels and trigger the release of more Ca^{++} from the sarcoplasmic reticulum, and thereby initiate the cardiac contraction-relaxation cycle. According to Starling's law of the heart, "the force of contraction of the cardiac muscle is a function of the end-diastolic length of the muscle fibre", which in turn closely relates to the ventricular end-diastolic volume. Upto a limit, increase in the muscle fibre length increases the force of contraction, resulting in increase in cardiac output.

Among the neurohumoral influences that affect the cardiac contractility, the most important is the adrenergic system which acts via the neurotransmitter noradrenaline that stimulates the cardiac $beta_1$ receptors.

The cardiac output is determined by:

(1) **Preload**, the length of the ventricular muscle fibre at the onset of contraction, which reflects the ventricular end-diastolic pressure.

(2) **Myocardial contractility**; and

(3) **Afterload,** defined as the tension or stress developed in the ventricular wall during

ejection.It is dependent on aortic pressure as well as the volume of the ventricular cavity and the thickness of the ventrticular wall.The aortic pressure in turn is regulated by the peripheral resistance and the condition of the arterial wall. When myocardial contractility is impaired and the ventricle dilates, afterload rises and the cardiac output dimishes. The resultant neural and humoral stimuli following decrease in cardiac output in turn contribute to increase in the afterload. This reduces the cardiac output further while increasing the myocardiac oxygen requirement, thus establishing a viscious cycle.

Among the techniques used to assess the global cardiac function, the most clinically convenient is the evaluation of **left ventricular ejection fraction** (LVEF), the ratio of the stroke volume to the end-diastolic volume of the left ventricle (normal value about 65%). LVEF may be depressed to less than 45% in **systolic heart failure**, even when the stroke volume itself is normal. Alternatively, in a patient in clinical heart failure, a normal or almost normal LVEF indicates **diastolic heart failure**.

Pathophysiology of congestive heart failure (CHF) : A failing heart is characterized by inability to provide a cardiac output sufficient for the body's metabolic needs, initially during exercise, but later even at rest. Basically, heart failure is failure of the heart as a pump, the left ventricle more often than and earlier than the right ventricle. This can arise in several ways:

(a) ***Pressure overload*** as in hypertension and stenosis of cardiac valves (mitral or aortic).

(b) ***Volume overload*** as in congenital heart disease and in regurgitant lesions of the mitral and aortic valves.

(c) ***Loss of cardiac muscle*** due to infarction or chronic ischemic damage.

(d) ***Impaired cardiac contractility*** due to causes such as myocarditis; and

(e) ***Restriction of cardiac filling*** as in constrictive pericarditis **(diastolic heart failure)**.

The syndrome of heart failure is worsened by (a) factors which increase the need for a higher cardiac output such as, e.g., fever, anemia or thyrotoxicosis; and (b) hypoxia, acidosis and cardiac arrhythmias which impair contractility.

In a failing heart, the diminished cardiac output causes fatigue, diminution in exercise tolerance and a variety of compensatory circulatory changes. LVEF may be as low as 20% in patients with severe cardiac failure. The increased venous pressure behind the failing ventricle is responsible for (a) **pulmonary venous congestion**, pulmonary edema and dyspnoea of left ventricular failure, and (b) **systemic venous congestion**, liver enlargement and peripheral edema of right ventricular failure.

The important event in heart failure is the loss of functioning cardiac tissue following cardiac injury. To compensate for this loss, both hemodynamic and neurohumoral adaptive mechanisms are activated to improve the force of ventricular contraction and so preserve the cardiac function. (Fig 30.1). The compensatory mechanisms involved are:

- ***Increase in diastolic tension (preload)*** which in early stages enhances the force of contraction according to Frank-Starling principle.
- ***Activation of adrenergic nervous system,*** leading to increase in the circulating NA; chronic stimulation of the adrenergic system, however, causes increased afterload.
- ***Activation of renin-angiotensin-aldosterone system;***
- ***Atrial stretch, stimulating secretion of atrial natriuretic peptide – ANP*** (Chapter 36); and
- ***Release of endothelin.***

In response to these mechanisms, ventricular remodeling occurs : the ventricle hypertrophies, and in severe cases there is loss of myocytes with interstitial fibrosis. The atrial stretch stimulates the baroreceptors to produce bradycardia which counteracts the effects of sympathetic outflow. The atrial distention stimulates the release of ANP, which causes vasodilatation, and natriuresis, thus opposing the actions of angiotensin II and aldosterone (Chapter 36). Thus, the cardiac output is maintained and the cardiac tissue is protected to a certain extent from the adverse effects of

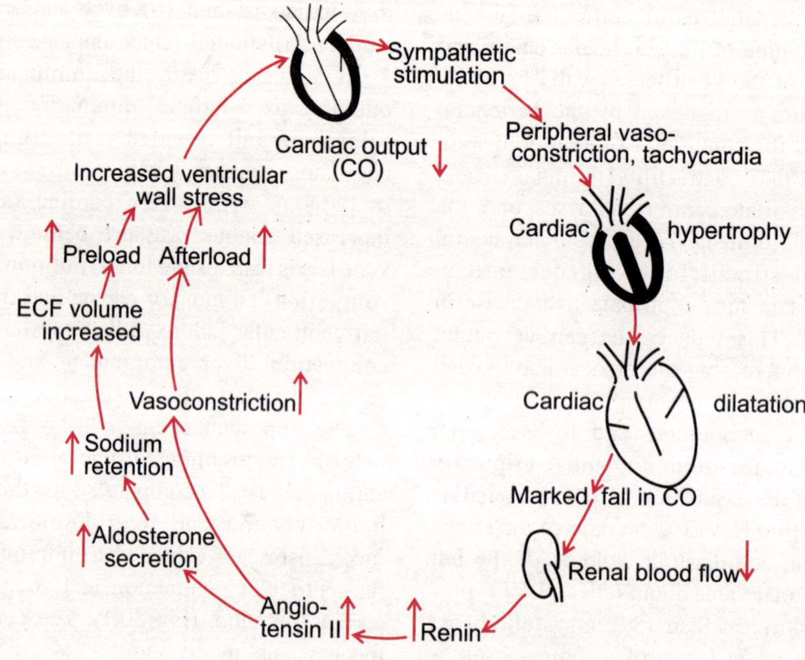

Fig. 30.1 : Pathophysiology of CHF

Key events are:
- Reduced myocardial contractility
- Peripheral vasoconstriction due to activated adrenergic and renin-angiotensin-aldosterone systems
- Increased ECF volume due to aldosterone secretion and sodium retention

ventricular dilatation and sympathetic activation. However, prolonged ventricular distension leads to progressive dilatation of the ventricles and to a gradual loss of inhibitory control over the adrenergic stimulation, which becomes progressively activated; decompensated heart failure begins. The failing heart is not able to maintain the cardiac output. Further, increased responsiveness to alpha-adrenergic stimuli in the peripheral vessels causes vasoconstriction, leading to further increase in the load on the ventricles (afterload).

When the cardiac output falls, systemic perfusion pressure is maintained by two mechanisms: (1) peripheral vasoconstriction and (2) sodium retention. The adrenergic system is activated early in the disease process during ventricular dilatation. By the time the patient is symptomatic, the *renin-angiotensin system* is triggered leading to increase in circulating angiotensin II and aldosterone. In the terminal phases of cardiac disease, vasopressin is also released (**decompensated heart failure**). *Thus, the heart failure is not only a disease of the heart (a systolic dysfunction of the left ventricle), but is also a* ***disorder of the circulation****, involving both hemodynamic and neurohumoral factors.*

Three important pathophysiological factors that contribute to the ventricular wall stress are:

- ***Reduced cardiac contractility.***
- ***Peripheral vasoconstriction due to activation of sympathetic and renin-angiotensin aldosterone systems;*** and
- ***Sodium and water retention.***

In **acute heart failure** such as acute LVF, load reduction and maintenance of cardiac

Table 30.1: Rational therapy of chronic heart failure

Reduction in ventricular wall stress by
- Bed rest.
- Vasodilators.

Reduction in neurohumoral activation by
- ACE inhibitors.
- Beta blockers

Countering sodium and fluid retention by
- Restriction of sodium intake (< 2 g/day).
- Restriction of fluid to < 1.5 L/ day.
- Promotion of sodium excretion by using a diuretic, furosemide 20-40 mg.

Treatment of the cause e.g. hypertension, arrhythmias, anemia, thyrotoxicosis.

Use of aldosterone antagonist: Spironolactone

Use of an inotropic drug, e.g., Digoxin.

function as well as optimal blood pressure are the *immediate aims* of therapy. In **chronic heart failure,** the *long term aims* include:

- ***Relief of symptoms and signs;***
- ***Stabilization of hemodynamics;*** and
- ***Improvement in quality of life and reduction in mortality.***

The principles of rational therapy of chronic heart failure are outlined in Table 30.1. The current therapy targets more than one pathophysiological mechanisms.

ACEI and Vasodilators in Heart Failure

Reduced cardiac output in CHF activates the neurohumoral mechanisms leading to increase in the systemic vascular resistance and venous return. Thus, the body tries to maintain an adequate pressure – head to perfuse the vital organs. Unfortunately, such vasoconstriction of arterioles causes increased impedence (afterload) to left ventricular ejection and further increases the work load of the heart. Increase in venous return increases the end diastolic ventricular filling pressure (preload), which also increases the cardiac work. A reduction in either the afterload or in the preload increases the cardiac output. *Vasodilators, particularly ACEI, are now considered the cornerstone of the therapy of patients with heart failure.*

Vasodilator drugs are of three types (Table 30.2):

- ***Arterial*** e.g. Hydralazine. It reduces the afterload on the heart.
- ***Venous*** e.g. Nitrates. They reduce the preload on the heart.
- ***Combined, balanced arteriolar plus venous*** e.g. Prazosin; ACEI, Angiotensin receptor antagonists ARB, Nitroprusside. They reduce both preload and afterload.

The vasodilator drugs currently used in *chronic congestive heart failure* (CHF) are shown in Table 30.3. Parenteral vasodilators such as sodium nitroprusside, nitroglycerine and enalaprilat should be reserved for patients with severe heart failure.

Many clinicians treat heart failure with sinus rhythm, at least initially, with bed rest

Table 30.2: Beneficial effects of vasodilators in cardiac failure

Vasodilator type	Preload	Afterload	VEDV	Stroke volume
Arterial	No change	Reduced	No change	Increased
Venous	Reduced	No change	Reduced	No change
Combined	Reduced	Reduced	Reduced	Increased

VEDV = Ventricular end diastolic volume.

Table 30.3: Vasodilators used in chronic congestive heart failure

- Captopril (6.25-50 mg. tid), enalapril (10 mg. bid), lisinopril 5 mg od.
- Isosorbide dinitrate (20-40 mg. orally or 2.5-10 mg. sublingually, 6 hourly) or nitroglycerine ointment.
- Hydrallazine (50-75 mg. 6 hourly).
- Prazosin (5 mg. 8 hourly).

and ACEI (Chapter 29) which are now recommended for all patients with LV systolic dysfunction; ACEI has several advantages:

- ***They are beneficial clinically and hemodynamically even in resistant heart failure.***
- ***They control hypertension which is an important risk factor.***
- ***They prolong survival in chronic heart failure.***
- ***Tolerance is rare.***
- ***By blocking the local generation of angiotensin II, they reduce its direct toxic effects on the myocardium (cardiac remodeling) and also reduce the risk of coronary ischemic events.***

Table 30.4: Use of ACEI in heart failure

- Start with small doses (captopril 6.25 mg., enalapril 2.5 mg, lisinopril 2.5 mg or ramipril 2.5 mg. a day)
- Maximum doses are captopril 50 mg tid, enalapril 10 mg bid, lisinopril 30 mg. od, or ramipril 5 mg bid.
- Stop potassium supplements and potassium sparing diuretics before starting ACEI.
- Stop other diuretics 24 hours before the first dose of ACEI. They may be restarted the next day.
- Patient should be sitting or lying down for 2-4 hours, depending on the drug used, after the first dose of ACEI.

- ***They reduce the mortality rate and the risk of hemodynamic and clinical progression in asymptomatic patient with left ventricular dysfunction following acute MI.***

All patients with asymptomatic or symptomatic LV dysfunction or LV enlargement should be treated with ACE inhibitors. Patients who do not tolerate ACEI or remain symptomatic while on them may be treated with **hydralazine + isosorbide dinitrate combination** as it is the only other vasodilator regimen documented to improve exercise tolerance and increase life expectancy in CHF. It is, however, less effective than ACEI.

In the management of **acute congestive heart failure** due to MI, the therapy of choice is an infusion of sodium nitroprusside or nitroglycerine (Chapter 29). The use of such infusions requires the facilities of an intensive cardiac care unit. In their absence nitroglycerine ointment may be used.

The other indications for vasodilator therapy are:

- ***Hypertensive crisis*** especially malignant hypertension and dissecting aortic aneurysm; and
- ***Acute or chronic mitral or aortic regurgitaion,*** and ventricular septal defect, in patients awaiting surgery.

Vasopeptidase inhibitors : These new drugs inhibit both ACE and neutral endopeptidase (NEP). NEP is found mainly in the renal tubules but is also present in other tissues such as lungs, intestines, brain, heart and blood vessels. It catalyses the breakdown of atrial natriuretic peptide (ANP) and some other peptide hormones including bradykinin. Its inhibition by vasopeptidase inhibitors causes vasodilation and sodium excretion by preventing the breakdown of ANP. They also inhibit the production of angiotensin II. Thus, they may be useful in the treatment of CHF and hypertension.

OMAPATRILAT : This vasopeptidase inhibitor drug, given orally, is rapidly absorbed with plasma half life of 14-19 hrs. It causes both arterial and venous dilatation and natriuresis. It inhibits the serum ACE activity and increases the renal excretion of natriuretic peptide in a dose dependant manner. Toxicity reported includes dizziness, cough and angioedema.

NESIRITIDE (Natrecor) : This is a recombinant human B type natriuretic peptide (BNP). Given IV, it binds to surface receptors on the vascular smooth muscle and endothelial cells and activates cGMP. It causes both arterial and venous vasodilatation and natriuresis. It also supresses the renin-angiotensin-aldosterone system. Because of its short t ½ (18 mins), it is given by IV bolus followed by IV infusion. It causes dose-dependant hypotension, nausea, vomiting, nervousness and renal damage. It has been used to treat severely decompensated heart failure resistant to nitroprusside.

Beta-adrenergic Blocking Agents in Heart failure

Although the beta-adrenergic blockers can block the adverse cardiac effects of catecholamines, their use *in large doses* to begin the therapy with can worsen the heart failure owing to their negative inotropic action. However, the use of gradually increasing doses (*start low, go slow*) of drugs such as **metoprolol/carvedilol/ bisoprolol** over weeks improves the symptoms of and reduces the all-cause mortality in heart failure.

They attentuate the adverse effects of the sympathetic drive (including apoptosis) on the heart, upregulate the beta receptors and reduce the remodeling. They are recommended in all patients in a stable condition, in whom LVEF is less than 35%, without substantial salt and water retention and without recent exacerbation of heart failure requiring inotropic therapy. Their long term effects are uniformly beneficial. Combination of an ACEI and a beta blocker is currently the cornerstone of the treatment of patients with left ventricular systolic dysfunction. Metoprolol is a selective beta locker whereas carvedilol is nonselective. Once started, beta blockers should not be stopped abruptly.

Beta blockers are not indicated in heart failure after acute MI nor in those with heart failure and normal LVEF (i.e. diastolic heart failure). They are also not indicated in patients with heart rate less than 60/min, AV block, asthma or COPD. They are not indicated when the heart failure is severe or unstable.

Diuretics in Heart Failure

Diuretics are used in heart failure to relieve sodium and water accumulation **(volume overload)** and thus reduce peripheral edema, and dyspnoea due to pulmonary congestion. This gives quick symptomatic relief. But, their use *alone* has limitations: they do not increase cardiac output nor do they improve ventricular function (which ACEI and digoxin do). Further, with the excessive use of diuretics, cardiac output and renal perfusion may diminish, with resultant fatigue, hypotension and impairment of renal function. Therefore, diuretics alone are not recommended. They should be combined with either ACEI or digoxin, both of which improve the LV function. *Diuretics have no place in the absence of overt heart failure.* Table 30.5 outlines the principles of safe diuretic therapy of

Table 30.5: Diuretic therapy of heart failure

- Use diuretics in moderation 2-3 times a week; avoid excessive doses.
- Exploit synergism between diuretics from different groups (Chapter 38), especially in resistant cases.
- Monitor blood chemistry, especially Na^+, K^+ and creatinine; serum K^+ should be at least 4 mEq/L
- Use diuretics in combination with an ACEI or digoxin.

heart failure. For pharmacology of diuretics, see Chapter 38.

Aldosterone Antagonists in Heart Failure

It is known that ACEI in therapeutic doses do not completely abolish the secretion of aldosterone. In addition to its classic mineralocorticoid properties, excess aldosterone causes coronary and renovascular remodeling, endothelial cell and baroreceptor dysfunction, potassium excretion and inhibition of myocardial noradrenaline uptake (Chapter 62). Morphological studies indicate that chronic excess of aldosterone and salt loading cause fibrosis in the atria, ventricles, kidney and other organs. The **aldosterone antagonist spironolactone** (Chapter 38) in the dose of 12.5-25 mg OD has been shown to decrease the hospitalisation and mortality rates in patients with severe CHF who are already on the drugs discussed earlier. Further, the risk of hyperkalemia is very low when such small doses of spironolactone are used in combination with ACEI. For **eplerenone**, see Chapter 38.

Digitalis and Other Inotropic Agents in Heart Failure

In 1776, William Withering, the master physician and botanist from Birmingham, identified digitalis as the active ingredient from a mixture of twenty different herbs used by an old woman in Shropshire for the treatment of dropsy. The old woman's medicine, according to Withering, had worked 'miracle' in a few 'hopeless' cases of dropsy. In 1785, Withering published his treatise entitled 'An Account of the Foxglove and Some of its Medical Uses : with Practical Remarks on Dropsy and other Diseases', which remains a classic even today. He, however, thought it to be a diuretic. Later a

Table 30.6: Important cardiac glycosides

Source	Glycoside	Aglycone or Genin
Digitalis purpurea	Digitoxin Gitoxin Gitalin	Digitoxigenin Gitoxigenin Gitaligenin
Digitalis lanata	Digitoxin Gitoxin Digoxin	Digitoxigenin Gitoxigenin Digoxigenin

number of active glycosides were identified and shown to have specific and potent actions on the heart (**cardiac glycosides**).

Chemistry of the cardiac glycosides: Besides the plant *Digitalis purpurea* or foxglove, many other plants also serve as a source of cardiac glycosides. The glycoside strophanthin is obtained from the seeds of *Strophanthus kombe* or *hispidus* and another glycoside ouabain is derived from the seeds of *Strophanthus gratus.* Other less important and less prevalent sources include squill, the dried fleshy bulb of the 'sea onion' and the plants *Convallaria majalis* and *Thevetia neriifolia* (yellow oleander).

The cardiac glycosides exist in plants as precursors, called *'native'*, *'natural'* or *'genuine'* glycosides. These have to be hydrolysed for the release of the active glycosides. The seeds of *Strophanthus gratus,* however, yield the glycosides directly. Each glycoside represents the combination of an *aglycone* or *genin,* with a sugar (Table 30.6). If the sugar is glucose, the glycoside is called as

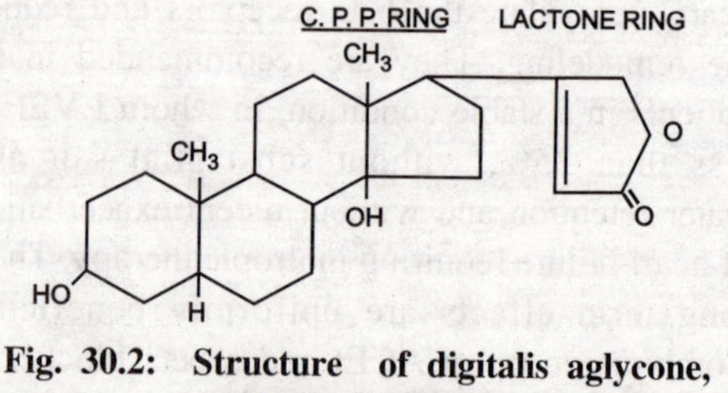

C. P. P. RING   LACTONE RING
CH_3 CH_3 OH HO H O O

Fig. 30.2: Structure of digitalis aglycone, digitoxigenin.

a glucoside, e.g., strophanthin. Structurally, the aglycone has a steroid nucleus with an attached lactone ring (Fig. 30.2). Acid hydrolysis of the glycoside results in separation of the aglycone and the sugar.

The pharmacological activity is contained in the aglycone, which has however, a less potent and shorter action than the parent glycoside. The sugars ensure increased water solubility, cell penetrability and potency of the aglycones.

Mechanism of action: Sarcolemmal membrane structures that regulate calcium entry into the cell include the slow (L type) calcium channel, the sodium-calcium exchanger, calcium ATPase, and (indirectly) the sodium – potassium-activated ATPase, and the sodium-hydrogen exchanger. *Digitalis acts as a potent positive inotropic agent by directly inhibiting the membrane bound sodium potassium ATPase which acts as a digitalis receptor* (**direct action**). This prevents extrusion of sodium and hastens the entry of sodium into the cell during the resting phase (diastolic depolarization). Along with sodium, some calcium also moves in and remains intracellularly because of the depressed function of the Na^+- Ca^{++} exchange pump. The accumulated intracellular sodium exchanges for the extracellular calcium thus increasing the cytoplasmic calcium concentration. The increased calcium is stored within the sarcoplasmic reticulum sacs. This permits faster release and dispersal of calcium from these sacs into the cytoplasm. Increase in intracellular calcium activates the light chain of myosin; the latter combines with actin to form actomyosin, and the muscle contracts. This enhances the contractility, automaticity and ectopic pacemaker activity in the heart.

Decrease in the resting intracellular negativity increases the excitability of the atrial and ventricular automatic tissues. Alterations of transmembrane fluxes of sodium and potassium are responsible for the electrophysiological effects including changes in the surface ECG. Digitalis depresses the conduction of the A-V junctional tissue by a complex mechanism.

The inhibition of the sodium pump prevents reentry of potassium into the cell after repolarization is complete, leading to depletion of intracellular potassium. This potassium depleting action of digitalis is not confined to the cardiac muscle but also involves the skeletal muscle and the liver.

Digitalis also exerts **indirect action** on the heart, mainly by enhancing the vagal activity and thus influencing the activity of the SA node, the atria and the AV node (see below).

Pharmacological actions of digitalis: These can be divided into

I Cardiovascular actions; and

II Extracardiac actions.

Cardiovascular system: The CV actions are explained by an *indirect* and a *direct* actions of digitalis on the heart.

In a normal individual cardiac glycosides augment the strength and speed of myocardial contraction and raise the cardiac output. However, they constrict the smooth muscle of the peripheral arterial and venous beds. This action counters the effects of increased force of contraction and hence, in the normal individual, digitalis in small doses fails to produce any significant alteration in the cardiac output even though the stroke volume and the mean arterial pressure may be increased.

In the presence of CHF, digitalis has the following actions :

- ***Contractility*** : By direct action, it increases the force of contraction of the heart muscle. This results in more complete ventricular emptying with a rise in stroke output, as well as an enhanced capacity to propel blood against increased peripheral resistance. At the same time, duration of the systole is shortened, allowing greater time for both ventricular filling. and cardiac rest. The diastolic size of the heart is reduced. Since the oxygen consumption is a function of the initial diastolic fibre length, such a reduction in size diminishes the oxygen consumption for a given work output. *The digitalized heart, thus, can do the same work with less energy expenditure (oxygen* *utilization) or more work for the same energy expenditure, than before digitalization.* Digitalis, therefore, is called a 'cardiotonic'. Such increase in the cardiac output also occurs in cases wth 'latent' heart failure, that is, in subjects with heart disease but not in clinical failure.

• ***Heart rate* (HR):** In normals, digitalis produces no significant alteration in the heart rate, while in an individual with CHF the heart rate diminishes. However, digitalis is not effective in tachycardia without cardiac decompensation as in sinus tachycardia due to fever or thyrotoxicosis.

Small doses of digitalis reduce the HR predominantly by stimulation of the vagus **(the vagal effect)**. This vagal effect can be abolished by atropine and exercise.

Full digitalising dose reduces the HR by **direct cardiac action**; this effect cannot be abolished by exercise or atropine. In an individual with CHF, the sympathetic activity is increased as a compensatory phenomenon. This leads to tachycardia and increased venous pressure. Digitalis, by improving the circulation, decreases the sympathetic tone thus helping in reducing the heart rate and venous pressure.

• ***Refractory period* (RP):** Digitalis exerts varying effects on the RP of different cardiac tissues.

It shortens the *atrial* RP with small doses **(vagal action)** and prolongs it with larger doses **(direct action)**.

It prolongs the effective RP of *A-V node* through the vagus and directly. This leads to a decrease in the transmission of the number of stimuli arising from the supraventricular pacemakers to the ventricle. *This action is of major importance in slowing the rapid ventricular rate in a patient with AF.*

In contrast, digitalis shortens the *ventricular* RP by direct action, as observed in ECG as a shortening in the Q-T interval.

• ***Conduction velocity*:** The resultant effects of the *'vagal'* and the *direct cardiac* actions on conduction are:

(i) The conduction velocity is slightly increased in the atria and the ventricles by small doses of digitalis (vagal action) while larger doses depress the conduction velocity (direct action).

(ii) *Conduction through the A-V node is depressed by both vagal and direct actions, this effect being therapeutically useful.* The action of digitalis on A-V conduction and refractory period is mainly due to increased vagal tone and only to a minimal extent due to its direct effect.

(iii) Conduction through the Purkinje fibre system of the ventricles is depressed by the direct action.

• ***Automaticity*:** Digitalis increases the ability of the Purkinje cells and the ventricular muscle to initiate impulses. This leads to the development of ventricular extrasystoles, bigeminy, and if accompanied by depression of the conduction velocity, even to ventricular fibrillation.

• ***Blood pressure*:** IV injection of a digitalis glycoside in normal humans increases the mean arterial pressure while persons with CHF show no such increase. The effects of oral digitalis upon arterial pressure in patients with failure are secondary to improvement in the circulation.

• ***Coronary circulation*:** Improvement in coronary flow is secondary to the improvement in cardiac output and slowing of the heart.

• ***Venous system*:** The decrease in venous pressure in individuals with CHF is secondary to the improvement of circulation.

• ***Digitalis and potassium*:** Discussed later.

• ***Digitalis and calcium*:** Calcium ions increase the force of cardiac contraction. Digitalis acts synergistically with calcium; and digitalis toxicity is enhanced by excess of calcium ions. *IV calcium should be avoided in individuals on digoxin.*

• ***Effect of digitalis on the electrocardiogram*** (ECG): Digitalis produces characteristic ECG changes.

(a) *Changes in the T wave and ST segments* are the earliest to appear, sometimes as early as within 2 to 4 hours of an oral dose. These include depression or 'scooping out' of ST segment, and inversion of the first portion of T wave. These changes may occur simultaneously or independently and may confuse the diagnosis of cardiac pathology. The changes, however, are no guide to adequacy or toxicity of digitalis dosage and severe digitalis poisoning can occur even in the absence of such changes.

(b) *Changes in the P wave and P R interval* appear later. The PR interval may be prolonged, usually to not more than 0.25 seconds.

(c) The *Q-T interval* is shortened by digitalis, an indication that the drug shortens ventricular systole. Large doses may produce extrasystoles, various degrees of A-V block and ventricular fibrillation as the terminal event.

Almost every type of ECG abnormality associated with cardiac disease has been seen in patients on digitalis. However, *QRS widening in the presence of sinus rhythm is not caused by digitalis; it is due to the concurrent heart disease.*

Extracardiac actions:

- ***Kidney*:** Diuresis is often one of the first manifestations of digitalis action in edematous patients with CHF. The increased urinary output observed in edematous patients is due to:

(a) Decrease in the venous pressure bringing about shifting of the edema fluid into the circulation.

(b) Improvement in renal circulation resulting in an increased excretion of sodium; and

(c) Inhibition of renin release from the kidney because of the decreased activity of the renal sodium pump.

- ***Gastrointestinal tract*:** Digitalis, can produce anorexia, nausea, vomiting and diarrhoea. The nausea and vomiting are of central origin due to stimulation of the CTZ.

Absorption, fate and excretion: No fundamental differences have been found among the digitalis glycosides in their effects on heart; the dissimilarities encountered are quantitative and related to the differences in pharmacokinetics. These drugs are usually administered orally or IV. Absorption is mostly from the small intestine. *Absorption after SC or IM administration is unreliable* and they may cause local irritation.

The pharmacokinetics of the two digitalis glycosides (digoxin used more commonly than digitoxin) is summarised in Table 30.7. Digitoxin, a non polar compound, is absorbed almost completely and rapidly from the gut whereas the more polar digoxin is absorbed to the extent of 70-80%. Further, absorption of digoxin is slowed by the presence of food in the GI tract and by malabsorption syndrome.

As about 50-75% of digoxin is excreted by the kidneys, its excretion is prolonged in renal insufficiency and hence its dose needs to be reduced in renal failure.

Table 30.7: Pharmacokinetics of oral digoxin and digitoxin

	Digoxin	Digitoxin
Absorption	70-80%*	90-100%
Plasma Protein binding	25%	90% or more
Disposal	Renal excretion of unchanged drug 50-75%	Metabolized in liver**
Enterophepatic recycling	6-8%	Extensive
Plasma half-life	24-48 hours	5 - 7 days
Therapeutic plasma concentration	0.5-2ng/ml	10-35 ng/ml
Time for max. effect of a single dose***	4-6 hours	6-12 hours
Persistence of effect after stopping drug	3-6 days	18 days
Time for digitalization without loading dose	5-7 days	25-30 days

* Liquid filled capsules of digoxin (Lanoxicaps) have higher bioavailability.

** One of the metabolites is digoxin.

***Corresponding figures after IV dose are 1.5-3 hours (digoxin) and 4-8 hours (digitoxin).

The body eliminates per day not a fixed quantity of digoxin and digitoxin but a fixed proportion of that present in the body at the beginning of the day (**exponential elimination**). The figure is 30 per cent in the case of digoxin and 10 per cent in the case of digitoxin. Therefore, on repeated daily administration, these compounds accumulate in the body until the daily dose equals the amount eliminated by the body per day. After this, a steady state is reached. It is reached much faster if initial loading dose is employed but is eventually reached even with the use of a daily maintenance dose right from the first day without any initial loading dose; only it takes longer. Thus, *it is possible to digitalize a patient without using any loading dose.*

Adverse reactions: Digoxin can cause cardiac and extracardiac adverse effects :

(1) **Cardiac toxicity:** Digoxin produces cardiac arrhythmias either due to :

- ***Disturbed impulse formation.***
- ***Disturbed impulse conduction;*** or
- ***Both.***

The disorders of impulse formation are due to ectopic pacemaker activity. The commonest are multifocal extrasystoles and bigeminy, followed by partial or complete AV block. Less common are AV dissociation, sinoatrial block, paroxysmal atrial tachycardia with block, sinoatrial arrest, ventricular tachycardia and VF. *In fact, any arrhythmia occurring in a patient receiving digoxin should be assumed to be due to drug toxicity until proved otherwise.*

Occasionally, in chronic AF, digoxin toxicity is manifested by an increase in the ventricular rate, and this is mostly due to the developement of paroxysmal atrial tachycardia with block (PATB). In such cases continuation of digoxin therapy, unwittingly, to reduce the ventricular rate may lead to death. Pre-existing extra-systoles in themselves, however, do not constitute a contraindication to digoxin therapy.

Factors which can modify the cardiac toxicity of digitalis are :

- ***Age:*** An elderly patient needs a smaller dose than a young adult.

Table 30.8: Causes of hypokalemia leading to digoxin toxicity

- Secondary hyperaldosteronism of congestive heart failure.
- Diuretic therapy, which may precipitate acute digoxin toxicity.
- Nausea, vomiting or diarrhea, with resultant inadequate intake.
- Hypoxia, metabolic acidosis and prolonged exercise which increase urinary potassium loss.
- Administration of large quantities of glucose, bicarbonate or insulin which shift potassium from extracellular space into the cells.
- Chronic metabolic alkalosis

- ***Hypokalemia*:** Hypokalemia from any cause (Table 30.8) enhances digoxin toxicity. The serum potassium level, however, is not a reliable guide to the severity of depletion of myocardial potassium. Digoxin cardiotoxicity in fact can occur even in the presence of a normal or elevated serum potassium level.
- ***Hypercalcemia*** : See earlier.
- ***Impaired renal function***
- ***Cor pulmonale*** : Vigorous therapy of cor pulmonale with digoxin without correction of the other abnormalities with measures such as diuretics, bronchodilators, oxygen and antibiotics can precipitate cardiac toxicity. Cor pulmonale produces hypoxia which results in tachycardia and an increased blood volume due to compensatory polycythemia. Hypoxia also produces pulmonary vasoconstriction resulting in pulmonary hypertension. The right ventricle has to force an increased volume of blood against an increased vascular resistance (because of pulmonary hypertension) into a grossly reduced pulmonary vascular bed (due to emphysema). Inability of the right ventricle to achieve this results in right ventricular failure. Such patients might become worse following the administration of digoxin, as increase in the right ventricular stroke volume may further increase

the load on the already compromised pulmonary circulation. This leads to the development of pulmonary hypertension.

• *Cardiac status*: Recent myocardial infarction, hypoxemia and acidosis increase the liability to digoxin induced arrhythmias.

In patients with AF and CHF, slowing down of the ventricular rate provides a good guide to digoxin therapy. But, this is not so in patients with sinus rhythm, in whom improvement in the cardiac status can occur without much reduction in the heart rate; increasing the dose of digoxin in order to slow down the heart rate to an arbitrary level in such patients can lead to digoxin toxicity. Persistence of tachycardia and cardiac failure can be due to such factors as myocarditis, pulmonary infarcts or emboli, hypoxia or a mechanical problem such as very tight mitral stenosis. Increasing the dose of digoxin in such cases may lead to digoxin toxicity.

• ***Hormones***: Adrenergic drugs enhance the digoxin cardiotoxicity. Digoxin toxicity is more easily provoked in hypothyroidism because of diminished digoxin disposal but is rare in hyperthyroidism.

• ***Inappropriate use of digoxin***: A common cause of digoxin toxicity is the use of increasing doses of digoxin for non-cardiac dyspnoea. Unless CHF is present, digoxin is ineffective.

(2) **Gastrointestinal toxicity:** Although anorexia, nausea and vomiting are generally the earliest toxic effects, cardiotoxicity may sometimes occur without them. Diarrhoea is less common. It is necessary to distinguish vomiting due to digoxin from that due to CHF.

(3) **Neurological toxicity:** About 25 per cent of patients with digoxin toxicity experience a true vertigo. Visual disturbances include blurring, photophobia and disturbances of colour vision. Headache is fairly common. Lassitude, confusion, disorientation, delirium, neuralgic pains, and psychotic behaviour may appear.

(4) **Miscellaneous toxicity:** These include skin rashes, eosinophilia and gynecomastia; cardiac glycosides have a structural resemblance to estrogens.

Digoxin crosses the placental barrier, producing foetal concentration higher than the maternal concentration. Large doses to the mother, therefore, may lead to premature delivery, and the newborn may present with ECG abnormalities.

Table 30.9: Drug interactions of digoxin

(a) **Drugs which increase serum digoxin levels:** Quinidine; Verapamil; Methyldopa; Indomethacin. Antibiotics (see text); Amiodarone.

(b) **Drugs which reduce serum digoxin levels:**

- ***By induction of hepatic microsomal enzymes***: Rifampicin.
- ***By reducing the bioavailability***: Antacids; Kaolin-pectin preparations; Neomycin; Cholestyramine
- Drugs acting indirectly by interfering with serum K^+ and Ca^{++} levels, e.g., diuretics and IV calcium.

Drug interactions: See Table 30.9. About 10% of patients convert large amounts of digoxin to inactive metabolites in the gut; in such patients oral antibiotics can cause a sudden increase in serum digoxin level.

Recognition of overdigitalization: Overdigitalization is to be suspected when any of the aforementioned symptoms or signs arise in a patient on digitalis therapy. A detailed analysis of the clinical situation, with special reference to past digitalization, the amount and the speed of digoxin administration during the present illness, the nature of the disease process, and the patient's electrolyte and renal status, is necessary because the ECG may not be of help in diagnosing digoxin toxicity.

Determination of *plasma digoxin level* by radioimmunoassay is valuable

(a) In pharmacokinetic studies;

(b) In adjusting the maintenance dose of digoxin; and

(c) In detecting such unsuspected factors as poor patient compliance or poor bioavailability.

Higher than expected levels suggest renal

failure which may otherwise go undetected unless creatinine clearance is determined. *Its value in diagnosing digoxin toxicity is not established.* Therapeutic serum levels of digoxin generally range from 0.5 to 2.0 ng/ml. Although levels are higher in patients showing toxicity than in those without it, one cannot rely on plasma level alone for the diagnosis of digoxin toxicity. *A thorough clinical* assessment of the patient is more important in making this diagnosis than plasma *digoxin level.*

Table 30.10: Principles of treatment of digoxin toxicity

- Stop digoxin.
- Stop diuretics.
- Estimate serum potassium.
- Bradycardia: atropine.
- *Mild toxicity* : oral potassium.
- *Supraventricular tachyarrhythmias* : oral/IV propranolol. Verapamil is contraindicated as it elevates serum digoxin concentration.
- *Ventricular tachycardia*: lignocaine or phenytoin, IV.
- *Severe toxicity* : antidigoxin antibodies.
- Potassium is contraindicated in the presence of A-V block, hyperkalemia or severe renal insufficiency.

Treatment of digitalis toxicity: See Table 30.10.

Mild toxicity (stable, ventricular premature beats especially bigemini) can be treated by administration of **potassium salts**, 5 to 7.5 g. of potassium chloride orally, daily, in divided doses. In *more serious arrhythmias* a solution containing 40 mEq of potassium chloride in 500 ml. of 5 per cent glucose can be administered IV over 2-4 hours with ECG as a guide.

Tachyarrhythmias and ectopic impulse generation caused by digoxin are associated with intracellular loss of potassium and can be corrected by potassium administration; however, potassium loss does not appear to be related to the other cardiac toxic actions of digoxin.

Potassium has little effect on the myocardial binding of digoxin that has already occurred; it can only reduce further uptake of the glycoside by the heart. Although it is probably the drug of choice in treating tachyarrhythmias induced by digoxin, the cation itself prolongs the refractory period of the A-V node and hence, is contraindicated in the presence of A-V block. It is usually preferred, even in the presence of normal serum potassium level, when there is an evidence of ventricular irritability. However, it should be avoided in the presence of hyperkalemia and / or severe renal impairment. The administration of a potassium salt for treating digoxin toxicity does not counteract the positive inotropic properties of the glycoside.

The supraventricular tachyarrhythmias complicating digoxin therapy are best treated with a **beta-adrenergic blocking drug**. Propranolol is used orally in the dose of 10-40 mg. every 6 hours or IV in the dose of 0.5 to 1 mg.

Ventricular tachycardia is best treated with either **lignocaine hydrochloride** or **phenytoin sodium** IV. In the case of lignocaine, an initial dose of 1-2 mg./kg. is followed either by similar doses at 20-30 minute intervals or by drip at the rate of 1-2 mg. per minute. Phenytoin sodium is injected IV in the dose of 250 mg. well diluted, over 3-5 minutes. Phenytoin sodium has the added advantage of countering the depression of A-V conduction by digitalis.

In severe digoxin toxicity (which usually involves suicidal overdose), hyperkalemia is commonly present and administration of an antiarrhythmic agent may lead to cardiac arrest. Such patients are best treated with **antidigoxin specific antibodies** (Digibind).

Preparations:

(i) Digoxin tablet (Lanoxin) 0.125 or 0.25 mg.
(ii) Digoxin injection 0.25 mg per ml of 70% ethanol.
(iii) Digitoxin tablet 0.1 mg. Digitoxin injection 0.2 mg. per ml. of 40 to 50 per cent alcohol.
(iv) Liquid-filled capsules of digoxin (Lanoxicaps) 100 mcg and 200 mcg (Table 30.7).

(v) Elixir Digoxin 1 ml equivalent to 0.05 mg. of digoxin.

Therapeutic uses:

- ***Heart failure*** : For its positive inotropic action; (see below); and
- ***Cardiac arrythmias*** for its action on the conducting system of the heart.

Larger doses of digoxin are required to control arrhythmias than CHF.

Table 30.11 summarises the therapeutic usefulness of digoxin in various cardiac conditions.

(1) **Congestive heart failure (CHF) :** Digoxin, by increasing the cardiac output, brings about more complete emptying of the ventricles during systole. This reduces pulmonary congestion and edema (relief from orthopnea, disappearance of basal rales) and reduces systemic venous pressure (disappearance of hepatojugular reflux). As a result of improved cardiac output, the compensatory circulation changes abate, providing further clinical relief. Thus, tachycardia improves and diuresis is established as a result of diminution in the augmented sympathetic drive and reduction in various hormonal levels in the blood.

Table 30.11: Therapeutic usefulness of digoxin

- ***Very useful*** in heart failure associated with atrial fibrillation and rapid ventricular rate.
- ***Useful*** in low output failure in valvular, hypertensive, ischemic and congenital heart disease.
- ***Of limited value*** in high output failure in anemia, thyrotoxicosis, beriberi and arterio-venous fistula; and in heart failure due to myocarditis and cor pulmonale.
- ***Not effective*** in mitral stenosis, constrictive pericarditis and restrictive cardiomyopathy.
- ***Contraindicated*** in patients with A-V block and in those with dynamic outflow block such as hypertrophic cardiomyopathy. (Refer text for details).

In **acute heart failure** associated with such catastrophies as acute myocardial infarction, acute onset mitral regurgitation and papillary muscle dysfunction, digoxin has *no place in treatment*. These conditions are best treated by reduction of afterload.

Studies have re-confirmed the usefulness of digoxin in improving the clinical status and LV function in patients with CHF. The consensus is that:

- ***Digoxin (in maintensance doses 0.125-0.25 mg/day) is an effective, generally safe and inexpensive drug for the relief of symptoms of CHF.*** It prevents worsening of heart failure, improves exercise tolerance and reduces the repeated hospitalization.
- ***It does not alter the natural history of the disease;***
- ***It does not substantially increase survival,*** in contrast to ACEI; and
- ***Maintenance of lower serum digoxin level (0.5-1.0 mg/ml) as effective as and much safer than higher levels.***

Digoxin may be prescribed particularly in patients with persistent symptoms after the administration of ACEI.

(2) **Left ventricular failure (LVF) :** Digoxin is helpful in the treatment of *chronic, pure, left ventricular failure* in patients with hypertensive or ischemic heart disease and aortic valve disease. It relieves orthopnoea in these patients. If significant hypertension is present, it should be treated with an antihypertensive drug.

Acute left ventricular failure with pulmonary edema is a medical emergency and is treated with IV furosemide, nitrate and ACEI (Table 30.12).

The patient is made to lie in **a semi-upright position** either by raising the head end of the bed or by using a back-rest, preferably with the legs hanging over the edge of the bed. Application of **tourniquets** to three limbs at a time, with rotation of the free limb every 15-20 minutes, helps to pool the blood in the limbs and to reduce the preload. **Oxygen** is administered at

Table 30.12: Management of acute LVF with pulmonary edema

- Semi-upright posture.
- Tourniquets to three limbs in rotation.
- Oxygen.
- Furosemide 40-80 mg. IV.
- Morphine IV.
- Aminophylline IV slowly.
- Sublingual nitroglycerine/IV sodium nitroprusside or nitroglycerine.
- Digoxin IV in patients with atrial fibrillation/supraventricular tachycardia and heart failure.
- Continued management of heart disease/ heart failure, after resolution of acute heart failure.

the rate of 6-8 litres a minute. **Furosemide** is injected IV in the dose of 40-60 mg, repeated every 30 minutes until diuresis sets in. It acts by causing venodilatation, in addition to diuresis. **IV morphine** 2 to 5 mg. every 15 minutes to a total of 15 mg. is effective in this condition. In addition to allaying anxiety and improving patient comfort, morphine also brings about peripheral pooling of blood by central reduction in sympathetic activity (Chapter 10). If the patient has associated bronchospasm, **aminophylline** is given IV in the dose of 250-500 mg over 15 minutes, followed by an infusion. In resistant cases, careful use of **sodium nitroprusside infusion** (as a balanced preload and afterload reducer) may be helpful; it requires the facilities of an intensive care unit. If such facilities are not available, **sublingual nitroglycerine** (0.4 mg) may temporarily reduce the pulmonary capillary pressure by producing venodilatation; it may be repeated every 10-15 minutes. Blood pressure should be monitored carefully in patients receiving nitroglycerine, as it may cause severe hypotension in some patients. If inotropic effect is desired, drugs such as **dopamine** or **dobutamine** may be preferred to **digoxin.** However, IV digoxin, 0.5 mg. injected over 15 minutes, can be valuable in patients with atrial fibrillation or supraventricular tachycardia. After resolution of acute heart failure, the patient should be investigated for the possible cause of heart failure, and treated accordingly.

Table 30.13 lists important points to remember in the management of systolic LV dysfunction.

Table 30.13: Points to remember in management of left ventricular systolic dysfunction

- Diuretics are needed for relief of pulmonary congestion and peripheral edema.
- ACEI are recommended in all patients.
- Beta blockers in low doses substantially reduce morbidity and mortality, and can be combined with ACEI.
- Aldosterone antagonists are recommended for patients remaining symptomaic despite treatment with ACEI and beta blockers.
- Digoxin has a limited role in patients with sinus rhythm. It improves symptoms and quality of life but does not reduce mortality.
- Patients with persistent angina may receive additional nitrate or a CCB such as amlodipine.

(3) **Atrial fibrillation (AF) :** Digoxin is indicated in (a) *patients of AF with rapid ventricular rate;* and (b) *those with AF and cardiac failure, even if the heart rate is not rapid.*

The aim of **digoxin** therapy in patients with AF is to reduce the ventricular rate, and thus improve the circulation. If failure is present, digoxin relieves it. In the absence of failure, digoxin can protect the ventricles from too rapid atrial impulses by depressing conduction across the A-V node and the A-V bundle, mainly by its vagal action. The dosage should be adjusted to maintain a ventricular rate of 60-80/minute at rest and less than 100/minute during physical activity. Unlike quinidine digoxin does not restore sinus rhythm in AF. Verapamil or diltizem is now preferred to digoxin in the absence of heart failure (Chapter 27),

Electrical cardioversion *is dangerous in patients with overt digoxin toxicity, who can develop fatal ventricular arrhythmias.*

Digoxin is not indicated in patients with AF

with normal or slow ventricular rate. In such patients, **warfarin** is recommended to prevent stroke if any clinical or echocardiographic risk factor is present; the risk factors are a history of transient ischemic attacks, clinical heart failure, enlarged left atrium or impaired left ventricular function. In the absence of such risk factors, these patients should receive aspirin in the daily dose of 150 mg, (Chapter 27).

(4) **Atrial flutter: Digoxin** corrects any associated cardiac failure. Ventricular rate is slowed by augmentation of A-V block. **Propranolol** can be added in patients resistant to digoxin. Atrial flutter is often converted into atrial fibrillation by digoxin, and its **withdrawal** at this stage may restore sinus rhythm.

(5) **Paroxysmal atrial tachycardia (PAT) :** Digoxin is the drug of choice in the treatment of *PAT - associated with heart failure.* In patients without heart failure, other drugs such as verapamil or diltiazem are preferred (Chapter 27). Physical measures such as pressure on the carotid sinus may occasionally be helpful. Digoxin terminates PAT probably by its indirect (i.e. vagal) action. It should be noted that digoxin therapy itself sometimes converts atrial fibrillation into PAT with A-V block (PATB) and hence, it is imperative to enquire about previous digitalization before the institution of therapy. *Spontaneous PAT without obvious cause could be benign but PATB induced by digoxin is a serious complication.*

Digitalization: The patient should be digitalized, avoiding even the mildest digoxin toxicity. This, however, may not always be possible. The important determinant of daily digoxin dose is the renal function. *The therapeutic benefit, though proportionately smaller, comes even from partial digitalization, because there is a linear dose-response relationship in the case of digoxin* and there is no threshold for the positive inotropic effect of digoxin. *Hence, except in special circumstances, the use of initial, large loading dose of digoxin should be avoided.*

The recommended schedules for digoxin therapy are summarized in Table 30.14.

Table 30.14: Digoxin dosage (mg) in adults in heart failure

For routine, oral digitalization: 0.25 mg once in 24 hours (maintenance dose);smaller doses in the the elderly and in those in renal failure; digitalization occurs in 5-7 days.

For rapid, oral digitalization : Loading dose of 0.75 mg in 24 hours, followed by maintenance dose.

For IV digitalization : 0.5 –1.0 mg.

In a patient with mild cardiac failure, especially when he is treated on an out-patient or domiciliary basis, digoxin should be administered in *maintenance dose* from the first day. Estimation of serum level may be useful for dose adjustment in renal failure.

A *loading dose* should be used only when it is necessary to digitalize a patient rapidly (in 24-36 hours) as in:

- ***Severe LVF***; or
- ***Acute heart failure due to paroxysmal atrial fibrillation with rapid ventricular rate.***

The loading dose, if used, should be three times the expected maintenance dose and should be given in divided doses in the first 24 hours. History of digoxin therapy should be enquired into before using the loading dose. A baseline ECG should be recorded.

IV digitalization is a potentially dangerous procedure, to be employed only in emergency. The preparation to be administered should be diluted with isotonic sodium chloride solution and injected slowly over 10-15 min.

Once started, digoxin therapy is generally required for life in most patients. During long term therapy with digoxin, the patient's condition should be reviewed periodically to ascertain that the maintenance dose is optimum and to look for digoxin toxicity.

Bioavailability of digoxin varies among different brands of tablets because of differences in the dissolution rates of tablets. Change to a different brand may suddenly increase the plasma level of digoxin and precipitate toxicity.

Contraindications to digoxin therapy: The only absolute contraindication to digoxin therapy is digoxin toxicity. Except for partial and complete heart block and perhaps paroxysmal ventricular tachycardia, no other cardiac arrhythmia, unless digoxin induced, is a contraindication to digoxin therapy, and even in these cases, it may be used if CHF is present.

Table 30.15 describes one of the proposed protocols for the management of CHF.

As there is no single measurement that appears to be a sensitive indicator of the effectiveness of therapy, progress can be monitored by observing the following:

Symptoms and signs of improvement:

(a) Increased urinary output.

(b) Relief from fatigue, insomnia, orthopnoea and disappearance of basal rales.

(c) Improved exercise tolerance.

(d) Diminution in jugular venous pressure, hepatojugular reflux and in liver size.

(e) Disappearance of tachycardia and ventricular gallop; and

(f) Change of dry and paper like skin to normal, moist and elastic type.

Symptoms and signs of digoxin toxicity:

(a) Anorexia, nausea and vomiting.

(b) Decrease in the pulse rate below 60 per minute, presence of extrasystoles, especially bigeminy or any other arrhythmia.

Ouabain (Strophanthin – G) : Ouabain is a pure crystalline glycoside derived from the plant *Strophanthus gratus.* It is rarely used now.

Other inotropic agents: These agents stimulate the myocardium either by stimulating

Table 30.15: Protocol for management of heart failure

Stage $	Risk factors for heart failure*	Symptoms of heart failure**	Structural abnormalities in the heart ***	Treatment recommended
A: High risk only	Present	Never	None	Treat risk factors Patient education. ACEI or ARB in some patients
B: Asymptomatic LV dysfunction		Never	Detectable	ACEI/ARB + beta blockers for all.
C: Symptomatic heart failure		Currently present or H/O such symptoms	Detectable	ACEI + beta blockers in all +/- Diuretics +/- Digoxin, +/- ARB +/- Aldosterone antagonist +/- Vasodilator
D: End stage heart failure		Refractory heart failure with marked symptoms at rest, resistant to maximal therapy	Obvious	Difficult to treat No beta blockers May use inotropes Ventricular assist device/ Surgery

$ = Stages as per the guidelines of the American College of Cardiology and The American Heart Association.
* = Hypertension; Diabetes mellitus; Ischemic heart disease; Chronic lung disease; Heavy smoking/alcohol consumption; H/O rheumatic fever. ** = Symptoms (current or past) of either left or right sided heart failure.
*** = Cardiac chamber enlargement; Valvular heart disease; H/O myocardial infarction; signs of left or right ventricular hypertrophy/failure.

Table 30.16: Drugs to be avoided in CHF

Antiarrhythmics except beta blockers and amiodarone
Calcium channel blockers
NSAID
Glucocorticoids
Thiazolinediones
Metformin
Cilostazol
Sildenafil
Amrinone

the β_1 receptors or inhibiting the breakdown of cAMP by phosphodiesterase (aminophylline). Their usefulness is limited.

Beta-adrenergic agonists, **dopamine** and **dobutamine** increase myocardial contractility, particularly in selected patients with severe heart failure.They are administered by IV infusion in an ICU.

AMRINONE (Inocor): This bipyridine derivative is a non-adrenergic, positive inotropic agent. It increases the force of contraction and rate of shortening of the cardiac muscle. It acts by inhibiting cardiac phosphodiesterase activity and its inotropic effect is additive to that of digitalis. It is a vasodilator and, reduces peripheral resistance. It has been used with beneficial effects in patients resistant to digoxin. A common adverse effect is dose related thrombocytopenia. The drug has no clear benefits over digoxin and may infact, increase the mortality.

Milrinone has similar action as amrinone but has a prominent vasodilator component.

Table 30.16 lists drugs to be avoided/used cautiously in CHF.

Diastolic heart failure : Diastolic cardiac dysfunction involves an abnormality of diastolic distensibility, filling or relaxation of the left ventricle, irrespective of the ejection fraction which is normal. The patient may be symptomatic or asymptomatic. Doppler echocardiography plays a critical diagnostic role in such patients, partly because the physical examination, chest X'ray and ECG do not provide definite information that differentiates diastolic from systolic failure. It occurs in some patients with hypertension, diabetes mellitus and IHD. The management primarily comprises the treatment of the specific underlying cause. Digitalis, diuretics and vasodilators are less effective than in systolic heart failure and must be used with great caution.

Nonpharmacological Treatment of Heart Failure

This is outlined in Table 30.17.

Table 30.17 : Nonpharmacological treatment of heart failure

- Salt and water restriction : advise sodium intake less than 2-3 g/day.
- Weight reduction in the obese.
- Cessation of smoking and alcohol consumption.
- Limit physical activity in the acute phase of illness.
- ***Stop any drug contributing to heart failure,*** (Table 30.16).
- Influenza and pneumococcal vaccination has been recommended.
- Supervised rehabilitation therapy including regular graded physical exercise which improves peak exercise capacity and the quality of life.
- Surgical treatment, when appropriate.

Chronic heart failure in many cases is preventable by :

- ***Controlling risk factors such as hypertension, DM and correcting the structural anomalies like valve damage/stenosis.***
- ***Controlling body weight and the sodium intake.***
- ***Use of ACEI after MI and in patients with asymptomatic LV dysfunction.***
- ***Avoidance of certain drug*** (Table 30.16).

Pharmacotherapy of Shock 31

Shock may be defined as a state of acute systemic circulatory failure associated with hypoperfusion of tissues, which is incompatible with life if untreated and persisting for more than a short time. It may be initiated by trauma, acute blood loss, depletion of body fluids, severe infection or acute myocardiac dysfunction. In these conditions, it may be mediated by one or more of the following mechanisms; of these, hypovolemia is the most important.

Mechanisms of shock:

- ***Hypovolemic***: This may be defined as a reduction in the circulating blood volume, and can arise in many different ways. When present, it evokes, through the baroreceptors, a generalized, compensatory sympatho-adrenal discharge and peripheral vasoconstriction. The latter is responsible for many of the clinical manifestations of shock. Though it helps to maintain the cardiac output and is important in short-term survival, it aggravates the hypovolemia by making the microcirculation very sluggish, pooling the blood in the periphery and thus reducing the effective intravascular volume.

The excessive sympatho-adrenal discharge causes a redistribution of the cardiac output with reduction in the blood flow to the skin, the intestines and the kidneys. The BP is stabilized but the tissue perfusion is impaired. Excessive vasoconstriction results in slowing of the blood flow, local hemoconcentration from loss of fluid from the capillaries into the tissues and in local formation of thrombi in the microcirculation. This causes tissue hypoxia leading to acidosis and to liberation of substances such as histamine, kinins, prostaglandins and cardiodepressant peptides into the circulation. Tissue hypoxia damages intracellular structures. The coronary filling is mainly diastolic and excessive fall in diastolic BP (together with cardiodepressant peptides) adds a cardiogenic element to any other variety of shock. Inadequate cerebral blood flow leads to mental changes. Microcirculatory changes in the lungs lead to pulmonary odema (shock lung); this is abetted by neurogenic and mechanical factors which lead to ventilatory failure, and by multiorgan dysfunction. Oligemic acute renal shut down completes the devastating picture.

- ***Cardiogenic*** : Failure of the heart as a pump as in acute myocardial infarction (MI). Rarely, in some cases, there is complete failure of the compensatory sympathoadrenal discharge.
- ***Obstructive*** : Extracardial obstructive diseases impair cardiac filling.
- ***Distributive*** : In shock due to sepsis and burns, the peripheral resistance is initially low (warm shock); the cardiac output is elevated but is maldistributed exactly as in shock with low cardiac output, with all the disastrous consequences detailed above. In the later stages,

the cardiac output falls and the peripheral resistance rises markedly.

The events leading to septic shock are initiated by the toxins released by the micro-organisms: exotoxins (as in the case of Toxic Shock Syndrome (TSS) due to staphylococci or streptococci); or endotoxins (as with gram-negative bacilli). In the circulation, these substances cause the release of tumour necrosis factor alpha (TNF alpha) and a variety of interleukins especially IL-1ß, and the platelet activating factor (PAF) from the mononuclear phagocytes and the endothelial cells. These cytokines cause a further cascade of synthesis and release of substances such as leukotrienes, PGs and thromboxane A2. They injure the vascular endothelium, increase its permeability, and cause fluid loss from the circulation leading to hypovolemia. They also depress the myocardium. There is a diffuse cell injury resulting in multiple organ failure. Distributive shock may also occur following anaphylaxis and spinal cord or neurologic injury. Many patients with septic shock have partial adrenocortical insufficiency.

The **clinical picture** of shock is variable but generally consists of pallor, sweating, cold extremities, rapid and thready pulse and air hunger, all due to the sympatho-adrenal discharge. Cyanosis of the extremities may or may not be seen. Rarely, the extremities may be warm (even in the absence of fever) whereas the circulation to the vital organs may be critically compromised. Oliguria (urine output less than 25 ml per hour for 4 hours or less than 500 ml/24 hours in adults), mental changes (somnolence, confusion, restlessness), acidosis and a marked difference in the temperature between the rectum and the skin are all indicators of reduced cardiac output and reduced tissue perfusion. Central venous pressure (CVP) is the best guide to hypovolemia. If it is low to begin with and fails to rise during intravenous infusion of fluid at the rate of 10-20 ml per minute for 10-15 minutes, hypovolemia can be diagnosed. If during such infusion, the CVP exceeds 15 cm of water or rises more than 5 cm of water over the basal level, pump failure is a major component of the shock. In patients with chronic lung disease and after acute MI, CVP does not truthfully reflect left ventricular filling pressure. In such patients monitoring of pulmonary artery occlusive pressure (PAOP) is a better index of left ventricular filling pressure.

By the time the BP falls, there is already a 25% deficit in the effective intravascular volume and hence *an attempt should be made to diagnose and treat shock before the BP falls significantly.* The femoral pulses are the best guide to the level of arterial pressure, since they are weak in hypotension but bounding in the presence of peripheral vasoconstriction with adequate arterial pressure. On the other hand, thready or absent radial or brachial pulses may be due to either severe hypotension or to reduction in extremity blood flow due to peripheral vasoconstriction. A low BP recorded by means of a blood pressure cuff has the same significance as weak brachial or radial pulses.

Arterial hypoxemia (reduced PaO_2), lactic acidosis and acidemia are the biochemical reflections of severe tissue hypoxia. It is customary to talk about 'irreversible' shock when the latter does not respond easily to treatment. It may be better to give up this term which admits defeat and call it 'refractory'.

Successful management of circulatory failure aims at:

- ***Early recognition of the shock state.***
- ***Correction of the initiating insult*** (defibrillation, antibiotics, hemostasis, IV fluids, surgical removal of necrotic tissue).
- ***Correction of secondary consequences of shock*** (e.g., acidosis, hypoxemia).
- ***Maintenance of function of vital organs*** (e.g., cardiac output, B.P., urine output); and
- ***Identification and correction of aggravating factors.***

All the five factors must be handled concurrently.

Hemodynamic and biochemical monitoring of the patient's response to treatment is critical to success of the treatment. Heart rate, respiratory rate, systemic BP, CVP, mental state, urine output, ECG, serum electrolytes and arterial blood gases — all need repeated monitoring. After successful treatment the metabolic parameters (mental state, urine output and blood gases) are likely to return to normal earlier than the hemodynamic parameters.

Restoration of blood volume: *Since increased blood flow to vital organs increases the likelihood of survival, therapy should augment cardiac output.* This is best achieved by restoring the intravascular blood volume as quickly as possible and may be the only treatment necessary, except in shock due to MI where the function of the heart itself is impaired. Fluid administration should be monitored by measurement of CVP and mean arterial BP. Rise in CVP without a corresponding rise in arterial blood pressure during IV fluid therapy denotes an overloading of the circulation. To avoid such overloading, CVP should be maintained below 15 cm of water.

Various types of fluids used for volume replacement are:

I **Whole blood and plasma.**

II **Colloidal plasma substitutes :** Dextran, hydroxyethyl starches, polyvinylpyrrolidone and oxypolygelatin.

III **Crystalloid plasma substitutes :** Normal sodium chloride solution and 5% dextrose solution.

Whole Blood, Plasma and Plasma Fractions

BLOOD, obtained from human donors by aseptic technique, is preserved with either CPD (citrate-phosphate-dextrose) or CPDA (citrate-phosphate-dextrose-adenine) solution. Blood is stored at a constant temperature between 2°C and 6°C; storage below 2°C damages the red blood cells. It is vital to maintain the temperature constantly below 6°C. This prevents the multiplication of bacterial contaminants. "However, some bacilli can multiply at a temperature below 6pC if they have previously been stimulated by exposure to a higher temperature. As the degree of hemolysis produced by such organisms is too insignificant for detection, *a bottle once taken out from the refrigerator and exposed to room temperature for a period of 30 minutes or more should be discarded.*

The supernatant straw colour of the plasma serves as a convenient indicator to judge the suitability of blood sample for use. Pink or red stained plasma indicates hemolysis.

The expiry date for blood preserved in CPD solution is 21 days and that for blood stored in CPDA solution is 35 days; however, the local FDA regulations must be followed in this matter. Blood should not be used after the stipulated period as the fragility of the erythrocytes increases after that period. Supernatant plasma, however, is stable and can be used.

In the absence of an unusual hemolytic state or factor, the transfused erythrocytes have an average life of 4 months.

While transfusing **whole blood**, care must be taken to use only blood belonging to the *same* ABO blood group but preferably not from a genetically related donor (see GVH below). While using *packed red blood cells*, it is permissible to transfuse cells from an O group person (universal donor) into a person with any ABO group; similarly a person with AB group may receive packed RBCs from a donor of any ABO group. Rh positive blood should not be given to Rh negative individual if it can be avoided; at least, it should not be repeated in a Rh negative individual who has received Rh positive blood transfusion previously.

Autologous blood transfusion: Blood collected from a patient awaiting elective surgery which is likely to require a blood transfusion, can be infused back into the donor, when the need arises. The main advantages of this procedure are avoidance of immunological mismatch and/or disease transmission; and conservation of the available blood resources. The disadvantages are reinfusion of contaminants, dilutional coagulopathy and undesired infusion of anticoagulants; further, hemolyzed red cells in the blood may cause renal insufficiency.

Indications for blood transfusion:

(1) **Acute hemorrhage:** Assesment of blood loss is relatively easy in case of external injuries or gynaecological emergencies. Many times, however, one has to rely mainly on clinical signs such as pallor, tachycardia and hypotension to gauge the degree of blood loss.

While treating acute blood loss, an attempt should be made to maintain (1) blood volume at 90% or more of normal; (2) hemoglobin level of at least 10 g/dl; (3) total serum proteins level of at least 60% of normal; (4) platelets above 50,000/cu mm; and (6) plasma coagulation factors above 35% of normal. When the blood loss is mild (25% or less of the total blood volume) a crystalloid solution (see later) should be infused in amounts 3-4 times the estimated blood loss. With moderate blood loss (26-50% of the total blood volume), colloid plasma expanders are indicated. With larger estimated blood losses, either packed blood cells or whole blood are needed to achieve adequate tissue oxygenation; *this may be in addition to crystalloid and colloid solutions.*

Adequacy of transfusion can be judged clinically from the reappearance ot colour and warmth in the patient, filling of veins and the improvement in pulse and BP.

(2) **Anemia:** Blood transfusion is indicated in:

- ***Symptomatic anemia with hemoglobin below 20 per cent (8 g.%).***
- ***Aplastic and refractory anemias.***
- ***Thalassemia and other haemolytic anemias.***
- ***Cases of dyshaemopoiesis.***
- ***As a pre-operative measure.***

Ten ml. of whole blood per kg raise the hemoglobin level by 1 gm per cent in adults. Children with weight less than 25 kg. should be given 20 ml./kg. of blood and premature infants 10 ml./kg.

In chronic severe anemia and in sepsis, the myocardium is on the verge of ischemia, and the rate of transfusion should not exceed 10-15 drops per minute. Failure to observe this precaution may result in heart failure.

(3) **Other hematological disorders:** In this case blood transfusion is given :

- ***To provide clotting factors and platelets*** and
- ***To provide leucocytes in cases of agranulocytosis. Fresh blood is preferred as the leucocytes deteriorate on storage.***

(4) **Miscellaneous:**

- ***Supply of antibodies in severe infections.***
- ***Exsanguination transfusion with withdrawal of the patient's blood*** and simultaneous replacement with donor's blood. This can be life-saving in kernicterus in the newborn. It has also been used with success in hepatic coma due to acute infective hepatitis.
- ***Intrauterine transfusion:*** Transfusion of fresh blood in the Rh positive foetus of a Rh negative mother has been achieved in utero. It has given encouraging results in reducing the mortality due to erythroblastosis foetalis.

Complications of blood transfusion:

- ***Nonhemolytic pyrexial reaction*:** Rigor, a common manifestation, is mainly due to imperfect sterilization of the apparatus. In the event of a rigor, the transfusion should be stopped. The patient is covered with blankets. In severe cases aspirin, anti-histaminics and glucocorticoids are employed. Usually, it is due to pyrogens but occasionally it can be caused by antibodies against antigens on donor leucocytes or platelets, stimulated by a previous transfusion or pregnancy.
- ***Allergy*:** Antihistaminics and adrenaline are used to treat this manifestation. It is mandatory to enquire about previous history of urticaria in the donor to prevent this complication.
- ***Air embolism.***
- ***Myocardial failure*** due to hypervolemia and circulatory overload.

• ***Transmission of disease***: (i) **Acute viral hepatitis B** or **C** is one of the most serious adverse reactions. Type C virus is the infective agent most frequently transmitted by blood. (ii) **Acquired immuno-deficiency syndrome** (AIDS) due to HIV. (iii) **Syphilis. Treponema pallidum** does not survive refrigeration for more than three days. In an emergency, prophylactic use of penicillin can prevent this complication. (iv) **Malaria.**

There is also the possibility of the recepient coming to harm if the donor has received certain medications in recent or remote past. Blood for homologous transfusion should not be collected if the prospective donor has been given:

(a) A blood transfusion or a blood product or any hormone derived from the human pituitary, ever in the past;

(b) Isotretinoin or etretinate (Chapter 69) in the past 3 years;

(c) Rabies vaccine in the past one year;

(d) Any other vaccine in the past 4 weeks;

(e) An antiplatelet agent such as aspirin or another NSAID (Chapter 11), clopidogrel or ticlopidine (Chapter 32), in the past 7 days, especially if the recepient requires platelets;

(f) An androgen or a antiandrogen, especially one with long half life (danazol or cyproterone acetate); or

(g) Is currently taking any drug.

• ***Hemolytic reaction*** due to mismatched transfusion is characterised by rigor, pain in loins, jaundice, hemoglobinuria, oliguria, bleeding and coma. The treatment of an acute hemolytic reaction is aimed at prevention of acute renal shut down. Mannitol 20 g. (20%) should be administered rapidly, to initiate diuresis. If diuresis occurs, it should be maintained at 100 ml./hour by giving normal saline, and IV furosemide, and by maintaining BP above 100 mm systolic. Alkalinizing the urine with 40-50 mEq of sodium bicarbonate, given IV, helps to hasten the excretion of free hemoglobin. If diuresis fails to occur, patient is treated for acute renal failure.

• ***Hyperkalemia***: Storing of blood at a temperature below 6^{0}C causes an efflux of potassium from erythrocytes into the plasma. When the blood is brought back to room temperature, potassium re-enters the erythrocytes. *Failure to re-warm the blood to room temperature may lead to hyperkalemia.*

• ***Graft-versus-host disease (GVHD)*** in which the donor lymphocytes attack and damage the host immune system. The mortality rate is high. It may be prevented either by avoiding transfusing blood from a genetically related donor or by irradiating such blood before transfusing it.

• ***Iron overload*** can occur in an adult after he/she has received 60-210 (mean 120) units of blood. It is successfully treated by iron chelation (Chapter 32).

• ***Citrate intoxication*** leading to cardiac irregularities and metabolic alkalosis due to metabolic conversion of citrate to bicarbonate, is a rare complication seen only after massive blood transfusions (generally more than 5 units of blood).

Other complications after massive blood transfusion are : hypocalcemia; hyperkalemia; pulmonary insufficiency with adult respiratory distress syndrome (due to debris comprising of platelets, leucocytes and fibrin, in the stored blood); hypothermia (if blood is transfused without warming it to body temperature); and hemorrhagic diathesis (due to dilution of platelets and clotting factors in patient's own blood or due to disseminated intravascular coagulation).

Packed red cells can be transfused when it is desired to increase the oxygen carrying capacity of blood without increasing its volume. A packed red cell preparation is made by removal of 40 per cent of the supernatant plasma. The red cell content of the remaining packed cells should be at least 5.5 million per cubic millimeter. Concentrated red cells have to be infused within twelve hours of preparation. Fifteen ml./kg. of red cells increase the hemoglobin level by 2 g. per cent. The amount of packed cells administered should not exceed 500 ml. at a time.

The amount administered in children under 25 kg. is usually 15 ml./kg. of body weight while 10 ml./kg. are administered in premature infants.

PLASMA: **Fresh plasma** is prepared by separating a single unit of blood immediately after collection, for immediate infusion; and **fresh-frozen plasma** is prepared by separating a single unit of blood within 8 hours of collection and then storing the plasma at -18°C or lower. Fresh plasma and fresh frozen plasma contain all the stable proteins (albumin, globulin) and the coagulation factors; their main use is to treat/ prevent bleeding due to deficiencies of coagulation factors.

Plasma can also be prepared by separating stored blood within five days after its expiry date; it may be prepared by separating single units of blood individually; or by first mixing together blood of many donors (preferably small in number, say 10-12), and then separating that mixture. Such plasma may then be freeze dried and stored. Plasma prepared in this last manner lacks the labile coagulation factors but has the advantage of easy and prolonged storage upto 5 years. *The use of pooled plasma is, however, discouraged* because of the statutory requirement of sterilizing it free of viruses. The use of plasma merely to maintain blood volume is not recommended.

NORMAL HUMAN SERUM ALBUMIN: This sterile preparation is obtained from human whole blood. It is used to raise the serum protein and reduce edema level in hypoproteinemia, in hypovolemic shock, and as a vehicle for transfusing packed red cells. It is usually non-toxic and does not interfere with normal coagulation mechanisms. It is given as 5% or 25% solution. The 5% solution is given undiluted usually at a rate of 2 to 4 ml./min. The 25% solution can be administered undiluted or diluted with sterile saline or 5% dextrose. Undiluted solution is used to treat the presence of edema. In patients with low cardiac reserve, the rate of administration should be slow, (1 ml./min).

Plasma fractions: Plasma may also be used, by fractionating it, to prepare:

- ***Individual coagulation factor concentrates, such as Factor VIII concentrate, to treat deficiencies of specific factors;***
- ***Human gamma globulin;***
- ***Fibrinogen;***
- ***Human and bovine thrombin,*** and
- ***Human fibrin foam.***

These are discussed elsewhere.

Colloidal Plasma Expanders

Colloidal plasma expanders are substances of relatively high molecular weight, which, when infused, augment the blood volume by increasing its oncotic pressure.

Requirements of an ideal plasma expander:

(a) It should have an oncotic pressure comparable to that of plasma.

(b) It should remain in the circulation for an adequate period to perform its function and yet be eventually disposed of either by metabolic degradation or by excretion.

(c) It should not affect any visceral function adversely and should not have antigenic, allergenic or pyrogenic effects.

(d) It should not interfere with blood grouping or cross-matching.

(e) It should remain stable over a long period and at usual variations in environmental temperature. It should be easily sterilized and have a viscosity suitable for infusion.

(f) It should be easily available.

The plasma expanders are used to treat oligemic shock when blood and plasma are not available immediately. The artificial, colloidal, plasma expanders are:

DEXTRAN: Dextran is isolated from beet root, where it is formed by the action of a contaminating bacterium *Leuconstoc mesenteroides*. Native dextran has a very high molecular weight (40 million) and from it can be prepared low molecular weight dextrans. Those used in therapeutics are **Dextran 70** (Macrodex, M.W. 70,000) and **Dextran 40** (Lomodex, M.W. 40,000). Dextran 70 is available as a 6% solution and Dextran 40 as a 10% solution, in either isotonic saline or 5 percent dextrose. They are infused in the dose of 10 ml per kg. body weight.

The oncotic pressure of dextrans is similar to that of plasma proteins and they persist in the plasma with an effective half life of about 24 hours. The dextrans also inhibit rouleaux formation by RBCs and have an antisludging effect on blood; they are claimed to improve the microcirculation independently of volume expansion. They may not interfere with typing, crossmatching or Rh determination. However, they coat the platelets and coagulation factors, and interfere with their function. In large doses, dextrans can cause widespread hemorrhages.

Dextran 70 tends to be retained in the body especially in the liver and the reticuloendothelial system. Dextran 40 is rapidly excreted by the kidneys; as much as 50 per cent is excreted in 24 hours and the remainder in 4-7 days. Dextran molecules not excreted are slowly degraded enzymatically to glucose over a period of weeks.

Dextrans are potent antigens especially when administered in small doses by the subcutaneous route. However, administration of massive doses IV does not induce antibody formation, probably because of immunological paralysis. Allergic reactions including fatal shock are seen in about 10 per cent of persons, including those who have never received it in the past.

During its excretion through the renal tubules, dextran 40 can clog them and is known to precipitate acute oliguric renal failure which is gradual in onset (3-6 days) and hence may be missed initially. The following precautions should be taken to guard against this possibility; dextran should not be used:

(a) In quantities larger than 1 litre (20 ml/kg) on day one and 10 ml/kg/day on subsequent days.

(b) If the urine output is less than 1500 ml per day or the blood urea is 60 mg/dl or higher.

(c) If the urine output drops further or the specific gravity of the urine rises above 1045 during its administration; in such cases an attempt may be made to keep the urine output high with the use of diuretics and a high fluid intake; and

(d) For more than 5 days.

Dextrans can be easily sterilized by either filtration or autoclaving. They can be stored without any special precautions for upto 10 years and thus can be stockpiled for emergency use.

They are **contraindicated** in those who are known to be allergic to them; in patients in heart failure; in existing or threatened acute oliguric renal failure; and in patients with hypofibrinogenemia or marked thrombocytopenia.

HYDROXYETHYL STARCHES: Addition of hydroxyethyl groups to starch molecules makes them resistant to hydrolysis by amylase and prolongs their intravascular half-life. One preparation (Hetastarch, Expan, MW 450,000) of hydroxyethyl starch has been extensively tried in treating shock. Compared to dextrans, hetastarch

- ***Maintains blood volume longer.***
- ***Is non-allergenic***; and
- ***Does not cause acute renal failure or coagulation disturbances.***

POLYVINYLPYRROLIDONE (PVP): This is a synthetic, water soluble, hydrophilic polymer of heterogenous molecular sizes with an average molecular weight between 35,000 and 40,000.

It is given IV, as a clear, amber coloured, 40 per cent solution in buffered normal saline.

Much of the PVP is rapidly excreted; 50 to 75 per cent of the administered dose is recovered from the urine within 48 to 72 hours. About 10 per cent is excreted in bile. The remainder (fraction of molecular weight above 120,000) is not metabolised and is apparently stored indefinitely in the skin, skeletal muscle and the reticuloendothelial system. It may interfere with antibody formation.

PVP can bind drugs like penicillin and insulin

and has a tendency to produce agglutination of erythrocytes. Hence, it interferes with blood grouping. The compound remains in the Kupffer cells of the liver many months after its administration.

GELATIN POLYMERS: Various gelatin polymers have been investigated as plasma substitutes. One such polymer of degraded gelatin available commercially (**Haemaccel**) is a polypeptide with molecular weight of about 30,000-35,000. It is dissolved in an electrolyte solution with the final pH of the infusion 7.2-7.3. In this state, it can remain stable for 3 years at room temperature. Given IV, its mean serum half life is 4 to 5 hours. Approximately 60-80 per cent of the gelatin is excreted unchanged by the kidneys. The preparation exerts osmotic activity similar to that of albumin. It does not interfere with coagulation, blood grouping and cross matching and is non-antigenic. Occasionally, it may cause flushing, urticaria and rigors. Bronchospasm and fall in blood pressure can also occur. It is available as 3.5 per cent gelatin polymer in 500 ml. infusion solution.

Crystalloid Plasma Expanders

NORMAL SALINE, 0.9 per cent, is the most widely used IV preparation. As its osmolality (308 m Osm/Kg) matches that of serum, it is an excellent fluid for volume replacement. It distributes itself in the extracellular space, and infusion of 1 litre of normal saline raises the blood volume by about 300 ml. It is mainly useful to replace lost sodium, chloride and water, particularly in cases of dehydration where it is used to correct the hypovolemia immediately. It is also used as a vehicle for giving IV drugs by drip. Though normal saline is adequate to raise the effective blood volume and BP in emergencies, it leaves the blood rapidly and hence, has a very limited duration of effect. Too rapid an administration of large quantities of normal saline can produce pulmonary edema. The febrile reaction that sometimes occurs is usually due to the presence of pyrogens.

It is important to note that *noradrenaline is unstable at the neutral pH of normal saline but is stable at the acidic pH of dextrose solution.*

DEXTROSE 5 per cent in water: When the glucose metabolism is normal, this solution is equivalent to administration of water alone. As its osmolality is lower than that of serum, it is not optimum for volume replacement. Water distributes itself in the total body water, and infusion of 1 litre of dextrose in water raises the blood volume by about 100 ml only. It is particularly useful when the kidney function is impaired. It supplies nutrition. It can be used as a vehicle for drugs, especially noradrenaline. However, *phenytoin should not be infused in glucose-containing fluids.*

In general, colloids are superior to crystalloids in maintaining blood volume. But they are expensive and they may not always be available. Hence 0.9% sodium chloride or Ringer-lactate is used commonly.

Cardiovascular Drugs in Shock

The major cardiovascular drugs used in shock are summarized in Tables 31.1 and 31.2. **Dopamine** is indicated for reversing hemodynamically significant hypotension following MI, trauma, sepsis, kidney failure, overt heart failure and chronic CHF, when volume resuscitation is unsuccessful. For **dobutamine**, see Chapter 17. **Noradrenaline** may be required for severe hypotension. The other drugs used are mephentermine, metaraminol and methoxamine. **Mephentermine** acts chiefly by increasing the cardiac output. **Metaraminol** acts like noradrenaline but is less potent. As it acts by releasing NA from the nerve endings, prior treatment with reserpine (which depletes catecholamine stores) makes the patient unresponsive to this drug. **Methoxamine**, being

Table 31.1: Actions of drugs used in shock

Drug	Receptors			
	Dopamine	$Beta_1$	$Beta_2$	Alpha
Adrenaline $	-	+++	+++	++
Noradrenaline $$	-	++ (small doses)	-	++ (large doses)
Dopamine*	++	+	-	+
Dobutamine	-	+++⊗⊗	±	±
Phenylephrine	-	-	-	++
Isoprenaline	-	+++	+++	-

Glucagon: Positive inotropic and chronotropic action independent of beta-adrenergic receptors.

$ Low doses elevate systolic and decrease diastolic pressure; higher doses elevate both.
$$ Both systolic and diastolic pressures elevated.
* The action of dopamine varies with the dose. See Table in Chapter 15.
⊗⊗ Dobutamine is a more potent ionotropic agent than isoprenaline.

a pure alpha adrenergic stimulant, is useful only in neurogenic shock (Chapter 17). Correction of acidosis restores sensitivity to the sympathetic amine drugs. The main problem with sympathomimetics is the loss of responsiveness to them, apparently due to downregulation of adrenergic receptors, which may become evident within 8 hours of continuous infusion. Therefore, some workers recommend intermittent use of sympathomimetics in shock.

Except as a desperate resuscitative measure, the use of vasopressors should be preceded by expansion of intravascular volume. The systolic blood pressure should be maintained around 90-100 mm. Hg. (or in previously hypertensive patients, 30 mm. Hg. below their usual pressure) during vasopressor infusion, as at infusion rates needed to raise the pressure higher, peripheral resistance rises disproportionately and compromises tissue perfusion. Use of isoprenaline should be monitored by PAOP measurement and measurement of arterial BP; heart rate over 120/ minute may cause cardiac arrhythmias and should be avoided.

Treatment of Shock

Clinically, shock can be classified as:

I **Hypovolemic or oligemic shock** due to acute loss of plasma or blood as in burns and hemorrhage; or due to dehydration and sodium depletion as in excessive vomiting, diarrhoea, diabetic ketoacidosis and Addison's disease.

II **Bacteremic endotoxic or septic shock** produced as a result of severe infection usually with gram negative bacteria like *E. coli.* Gram positive organisms, particularly resistant staphylococci, are also capable of producing shock by releasing an exotoxin called toxic shock syndrome toxin-1 (TSST-1) into the circulation. Deficiency of adrenal gland function and vasopressin production occurs in about half and one-third patients respectively. The mortality is still 40-60%.

III **Cardiogenic shock** due to acute heart failure e.g., myocardial infarction, acute myocarditis or severe paroxysmal tachycardia.

IV **Anaphylactic shock** which is due to

Table 31.2 : Principles of management of shock

Treatment	Hypovolemic shock	Endotoxic shock	Cardiogenic shock	Anaphylactic shock
Volume replacement	Yes	Yes	Usually no	Possibly
Dopamine	Yes	Yes	Yes	Possibly
Dobutamine*	Possibly	Yes	Yes	No
Noradrenaline (only if severely hypotensive)	Yes	Yes	Yes	Yes
Adrenaline	No	No	No	Drug of choice
Vasodilators (Sodium nitroprusside, nitroglycerine)	Possibly	No	Possibly	No
Phenylephrine**	No	Sometimes	No	Sometimes
Isoprenaline***	No	No	No	No
Glucocorticoids	In Addison's disease	Yes	No	Yes
Antihistaminics	No	No	No	Yes

* May also be used along with dopamine.

** Also useful in spinal shock.

*** Useful in toxicity due to betablockers if bradycardia is the main problem (atropine may also be used for the same purpose); glucagon, dopamine and dobutamine are useful if hypotension is the main problem.

release of histamine and various other mediators (Chapters 2 and 22).

V **Neurogenic shock** due to pooling of blood in post-capillary capacitance blood vessels, e.g. shock encountered with spinal anaesthesia, spinal cord injury, abdominal and testicular trauma and perforation of a hollow viscus. In fact, it is a form of distributive shock.

VI **Haemo-obstructive shock** produced as a result of obstruction of a main vascular channel, e.g. shock due to massive pulmonary embolism.

I **Hypovolemic shock:**

- Immediate treatment is directed towards restoration of effective blood volume by suitable fluids given IV. Hypovolemic shock is usually associated with metabolic acidosis as tissue hypoxia increases the production of lactic acid. This can be corrected by administration of sodium bicarbonate. Associated diseases such as diabetes or Addison's disease must be treated.
- Abnormalities of electrolyte balance should be corrected.
- As soon as the clinical state of the patient permits, the causative factor should be corrected, if possible.
- Morphine is administered IV to relieve pain if shock is not associated with head injury or suspected acute abdomen.
- Vasopressor agents (DA or NA see Table 30.2) may be employed to correct hypotension. However, *fluid deficit must be corrected before using vasopressors.* Without such correction, the use of vasopressor agents may worsen the

patient's condition by reducing renal and cerebral blood flow and by increasing the oxygen consumption of the myocardium.

- Oxygen administration to correct arterial hypoxemia. Central venous O_2 saturation should be maintained at more than 70%.

II **Bacteremic shock** (Endotoxic shock): This is caused by severe infection and tissue hypoperfusion, leading to organ dysfunction. Emergency treatment comprises the use of broad spectrum antibiotic, surgical intervention (if necessary), correction of acidosis, blood volume expansion, and therapy for hypotension. As active lung injury often complicates severe sepsis, lung-protective ventilation, meaning the use of relatively low tidal volumes (6ml/kg of ideal body weight), is reported to be beneficial in reducing mortality. Excessive tidal volume, however, causes lung injury. Anti-endotoxin and monoclonal antibodies to TNF-α for the treatment of endotoxic shock are under evaluation.

Drotrecogin alpha (Xigris) is the first, activated, DNA recombinant human protein C, which can be used for treatment, in combination with standard therapy, of critically ill adults with severe sepsis and high risk of death. Severe sepsis results from an excessive inflammatory response to infection,combined with inapppropriate coagulation and impaired fibrinolysis. Protein C inhibits coagulation, increases fibrinolysis,and *in vitro* inhibits synthesis of TNF-α which also has been implicated in the sepsis syndrome.The drug is given by IV infusion in the dose of 24 mcg/kg/hour for 96 hours. Its main adverse effect is bleeding, including intracranial bleeding. It is reserved for the ''sickest patients''.

III **Shock due to myocardial infarction (MI):** Table 31.3 summarises the treatment of acute myocardial infarction.

Relief of pain: In mild cases, *sublingual nitroglycerine* may suffice. Transdermal or IV nitrate therapy is helpful in relieving persistent pain. In patients with severe pain, the slow IV administration of 10 mg. of *morphine* hydrochloride over 10 minutes ensures rapid relief from pain and thereby minimises the shock. Morphine SC is less useful in such cases because of peripheral circulatory collapse which delays its absorption. **Morphine** may be repeated, if necessary, after 30 minutes. Alternatively, **pethidine hydrochloride** 25 to 50 mg. may be given IV, particularly in the presence of bradycardia. Both morphine and pethidine produce release of histamine and can produce

Table 31.3: Principles of treatment of acute myocardial infarction

Before hospitalization

- For prompt relief of pain

(a) Sublingual nitroglycerine 0.4 mg. every 5 minutes till pain is relieved (max. 3 doses) in mild cases and in the absence of hypotension (systolic BP 90 mm.).

(b) IV morphine, 1 mg per minute, titrated to a maximum total dose of 10 mg, together with IV metoclopramide 10 mg. (antiemetic).

(c) Oxygen.

- Aspirin 75 to 150 mg. (antiplatelet action).

After hospitalization

- Bed rest.
- Treatment of hypotension.
- IV betablocker.
- ACE inhibitor
- Thrombolytic therapy; anticoagulants.
- Treatment of complications.
- General measures (sedation, diet, bowel care, activity).

Discharge and rehabilitation

- Graded increase in physical activity, including exercise therapy.
- Aspirin.
- ACE inhibitors.
- Betablockers.
- Modification of cardiac risk factors : smoking (including nicotine substitution), alcohol, hypertension, diabetes mellitus, hyperlipidemia, obesity.

hypotension. This can be corrected by elevating the lower limbs. Morphine may cause sinus bradycardia and respiratory depression.

• ***Oxygen and rest***: The patient should be confined to bed and made to breathe 100 per cent oxygen by means of a face mask. Even a slight increase in activity could worsen the condition.

• ***Antiplatelet therapy***: Aspirin, administered as soon as the diagnosis of MI is made, and continued throughout convalescence and after recovery, significantly reduces the mortality.

• ***Thrombolytic therapy*** (Chapter 32). This is most useful in patients with ST elevation MI (STEMI)

• ***Maintenance of effective blood volume***: The effective circulating volume is reduced in cardiogenic shock. This should be corrected by:

(i) Elevating the lower limbs and thus increasing the venous return to the heart and,

(ii) Infusing 5 per cent dextrose. Excessive infusion, however, may cause pulmonary edema. This can be averted by a careful monitoring of CVP or PAOP and arterial blood pressure.

• ***Vasopressors and inotropic drugs***: Dopamine and dobutamine are the drugs of choice in this condition. Dobutamine is less likely to cause arrhythmias and sinus tachycardia. If they are not available, NA may be used. *Isoprenaline is contraindicated in shock due to myocardial infarction.*

• ***Vasodilators***: see later.

• ***Prevention and treatment of arrhythmias***: *Prophylactic therapy with Class I antiarrhythmic drugs is not recommended in patients without an arrhythmia.* It is best not to give drug empiricals for a paroxysmal tachyarrhythmia or rapid irregularity of the pulse until an ECG is recorded. Ventricular ectopic beats at a frequency of 5/min. herald the possibility of serious ventricular arrhythmia and should be treated with (a) IV infusion of lignocaine, given at a rate of 1 to 2 mg./min., or (b) procainamide, 100 mg. IV every 5 minutes, to a total dose of not more than 1 gm. Alternatively, lignocaine may be given IM in the dose of 400 mg. and repeated if necessary. Ventricular tachycardia is a serious complication needing immediate therapy with IV infusion of lignocaine or D.C. shock. Atrial fibrillation and flutter may need digitalization or DC shock. Sinus or nodal bradycardia is treated with IV atropine sulfate 0.3 to 2 mg., or isoprenaline 0.05 mg., respectively Digoxin may be given if CHF develops.

• ***Beta blockers***: Given IV within 4-6 hours of the onset of symptoms, propranolol, atenolol and metoprolol may limit the infarct size and reduce early mortality. They are of maximum benefit in patients with continued pain, evidence of sympathetic overactivity and absence of heart failure. The contraindications to the use of these drugs are: bronchospasm, resting bradycardia (less than 55/min), low systolic BP (less than 95 mm. Hg.) and heart block. **Propranolol** IV has been used in the dose of 0.1 mg./kg. divided into three doses at 5-10 minutes, followed by 20-40 mg. orally every 6-8 hours. **Atenolol** has been used in the IV dose of 5-10 mg., followed by 100 mg. orally once daily. **Metoprolol** has been used in the IV dose of 5 mg. over 2 minutes, repeated every 5 minutes (total 3 doses), followed by 50-100 mg. orally every 12 hours. Currently, it is recommended that a betablocker should be given to all patients who do not have a contraindication (Chapter 17). Intravenous therapy should be commenced as soon as possible after hospitalization, at least within 24 hours of onset of symptoms; oral therapy should be given in patients who are admitted late. Long term use of beta-blockers has been shown to be beneficial following MI. If tolerated, the therapy may be continued for 2-3 years, and perhaps longer.

• ***ACE inhibitors (ACEI):*** They should be administered to all patients within 24 hours of the onset of symptoms, if important contra-indications (hypotension, bilateral renal artery stenosis, renal failure or history of intolerance to these drugs) are absent. ACEI reduce LV dysfunction and slow the progression of CHF. They should be used, in the first instance, for 5-6 weeks; if signs of LV dysfunction are present, with or without symptoms, they should be continued indefinitely.

• ***Anticoagulants***: Anticoagulants should be given to all patients with ST-Elevated MI (STEMI), except those who are given a non-selective fibrinolytic; and in all patients with Non-ST-Elevated MI (Non-STEMI). They prevent venous thrombosis, pulmobary embolism, and stroke in patients with severe LV dysfunction after MI. Heparin, especially LMWH, is the preferred drug for this purpose (Chapter 32).

• ***General measures***: Sedation with a benzodiazepine is useful in the initial days of illness to allay anxiety. The diet should be liquid on the first day; subsequently, it should be soft, with no added salt and low in calories. Caffeinated beverages and very hot or very cold liquids should be avoided. A stool softener is administered routinely as straining at stool (a Valsalva manoeuvre) can precipitate cardiac arrhythmias.

• ***Rehabilitation and long term drug treatment***: Modification of cardiac risk factors (see Table 29.3) is a must. Every effort must be made to persuade and help the patient to give up smoking (Chapter 20). Lifelong continuation of **aspirin** in the dose of 75-100 mg. once daily is valuable to reduce the re-infarction rate. However, patients with large infarcts and severe left ventricular dysfunction should be considered for long term anticoagulant therapy to reduce the risk of systemic embolization. **Beta-adrenergic blockers** (propranolol 20-80 mg. qid or metoprolol 100 mg. bid) have been shown to reduce mortality, sudden deaths and reinfarction after MI; this therapy should be used for at least 2 years after acute infarction. **ACE inhibitors** reduce mortality, incidence of heart failure and re-infarction. They can be stopped after 1-2 years in many patients but must be continued lifelong in patients with severe left ventricular dysfunction.

Calcium channel blockers have no place in the treatment of acute MI. Antioxidant and /or vitamin therapy after MI has not been shown to be useful in reducing mortality.

IV **Anaphylactic shock :** See Chapters 2 and 22.

V **Neurogenic shock :** This should be treated like hypovolemic shock. Use of a vasopressor IV (Tables 31.1 and 31.2) is indicated. Alternatively, ephedrine 0.5 to 1 ml of 45 mg/ml solution may be injected IM prophylactically.

VI **Hemo-obstructive shock :** This should be treated like cardiogenic shock.

Vasodilators in shock: Their use is restricted to the treatment of continued ischemic pain or cardiogenic shock in acute MI. Nitroglycerin IV infusion, along with dobutamine infusion is the preferred regimen.

Glucocorticoids in shock: Glucocorticoids are of definite value in shock due to adrenocortical insufficiency and anaphylaxis. As many patients in septic shock may have partial, adrenocortical insufficiency, early administration of low doses of a glucocorticoid (200 mg hydrocortisone per 24 hours by continuous IV infusion, or equivalent doses IM of methylprednisolone, betamethasone, or dexamethasone) for 5-7 days may be helpful. The first dose should be administered as soon as septic shock is suspected. In resistant cases, the addition of fludrocortisone, 50 mcg/day, orally, is recommended. *Treatment of septic shock with corticosteroids is, however, not accepted by all experts.* It is of no value in cardiogenic, hypovolemic and traumatic shock.

Section VIII
Drugs Acting on Blood and Blood Forming Organs

Drugs and Blood Coagulation 32

Drugs are often used in therapeutics to prevent blood coagulation and to arrest blood loss. They do that by acting on various stages of coagulation:

- ***Platelet aggregation.***
- ***Clot or fibrin formation;*** or
- ***Fibrinolysis.***

Hemostasis is the spontaneous arrest of bleeding from damaged blood vessels. When cut, the precapillary vessels constrict. Platelets adhere to the exposed collagen fibrils in the subendothelium of the injured vessel via a specific, platelet-collagen receptor, **glycoprotein Ia/IIa** (*platelet adhesion*). This causes platelet activation leading to release of preformed platelet granule constituents and *de novo* generation of mediators of coagulation including adenosine diphosphate (ADP). This promotes platelet aggregation (more platelets sticking to each other), thus forming a primary hemostatic plug. Activated platelets lose their individual membranes, form a viscous mass and promote the assembly of clotting factors, thereby amplifying thrombin formation. Activated platelets generate thromboxane A_2, a potent platelet agonist that also stimulates additional platelets. The other platelet agonists include shear stress, collagen, ADP, adrenaline and thrombin.

Circulating fibrinogen binds to an activated platelet receptor **glycoprotein IIb/IIIa** (Integrin). Fibrinogen is then converted to fibrin. *The process of deposition of fibrin is called coagulation.*

Coagulation of blood comprises the formation of fibrin by a series of interactions among various protein factors and other substances (Kallekrein, calcium, platelet factor) present in the plasma. *The clotting factors* (listed in Table 32.1) are synthesized by the liver. Some of the factors (II or prothrombin; VII, IX and X) are *vitamin K dependent* for the final stage of their synthesis in the liver. In the process of clotting, each factor undergoes partial proteolysis to form an enzyme (activated factor labelled by the subscript 'a' after the Roman number indicating the factor e.g. Xa). The activated factor then brings about similar proteolysis of the next factor in the cascade of coagulation, leading ultimately to conversion of fibrinogen into soluble fibrin (friable clot) and finally, conversion of soluble fibrin into insoluble fibrin (firm clot). Figure 32.1 depicts the current concept of the sequence in which the various clotting factors are 'activated' leading to the formation of a clot.

The coagulation is *initiated in vitro by the* **intrinsic pathway** *whereas it is initiated in vivo by* **extrinsic pathway** (Fig. 32.1). The two pathways merge with the generation of factor Xa. All the reactants necessary for the intrinsic pathway are already present in the blood in inactive form. The initial event in the intrinsic

Table 32.1: Blood clotting factors

Factor No.	Common name
I	Fibrinogen
II	Prothrombin
III	Thromboplastin
IV	Ionic calcium
V	Hereditary labile factor, Activator (AC) globulin, Proaccelerin.
VI	Accelerin, supposed to be active form of Factor V
VII	Proconvertin; Serum prothrombin conversion accelerator (SPCA)
VIII	Antihemophilic factor (AHF)
IX	Plasma thromboplastin component (PTC; Christmas factor)
X	Stuart-Prower factor
XI	Plasma thromboplastin antecedent (PTA)
XII	Hageman factor
XIII	Fibrin stabilizing factor, Fibrinase
XIV	Prekallekrein
XV	Kallekrein
XVI	Platelet factor

pathway appears to be the activation of factor XII to factor XIIa by an undefined mechanism following a contact with a foreign surface such as glass. The initiators of the extrinsic pathway are not normally present in the blood; they are added following tissue injury; in their presence, factor VII converts factors IX and X to active factors IXa and Xa respectively. The two pathways have the common objective of generating factor Xa from factor X. The intrinsic pathway is a slow pathway and minutes are required for the formation of activated factor X (factor Xa); the extrinsic pathway takes only seconds for the same.

Normally, the blood is kept fluid by :

- ***The rapid flow of blood,*** which keeps the local concentration of clotting factors low.
- ***Antithrombin III*** which inactivates all the clotting factors in the blood as well as any thrombin formed in the circulation; and
- ***Removal by fibrinolysis of traces of fibrin formed in the circulation.***

Disturbances in hemostasis include hypercoagulability and excessive bleeding. The latter may be due to deficiency of platelets or clotting factors. Hypercoagulability is due to:

- ***Stasis within the venous system.***

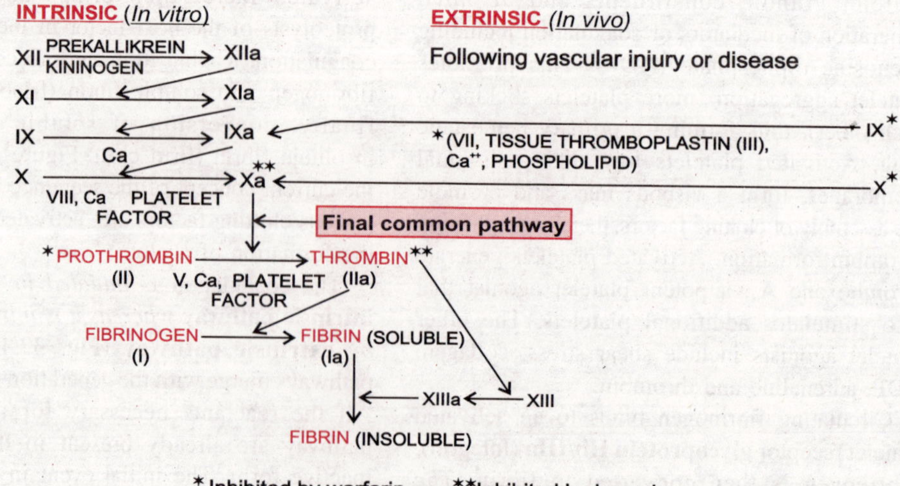

Fig. 32.1: Clotting factors and blood clotting

- ***Injury to or disease of the vessel wall;*** and
- ***A hypercoagulable state of blood.***

Thrombogenesis is a pathological process, leading to an intravascular thrombus formation. It is normally prevented by several regulatory mechanisms such as normal vascular endothelium, PGI_2, antithrombin, protein C and heparan sulfate proteoglycans synthesized by the vascular endothelium.

There are two types of thrombi: (1) arterial (white thrombus); and (2) venous (red thrombus). The process of formation of an **arterial thrombus** is an extension of the processes of platelet adhesion, granule release and platelet aggregation. The arterial thromus is predominantly made up of aggregated platelets and contains little thrombin. The arterial thrombus via platelet receptor glycoprotein IIb/IIIa (Gp II b /III a) may occlude the artery or, by disintegrating, embolize the distal arterial tree. It may lead to ischemic necrosis of the tissue such as heart. By contrast, a **venous thrombus** forms in an area of venous stasis (slow blood flow). It is largely a mass of fibrin with RBCs entangled in its mesh and resembles a clot formed in a test tube. It has few platelets.

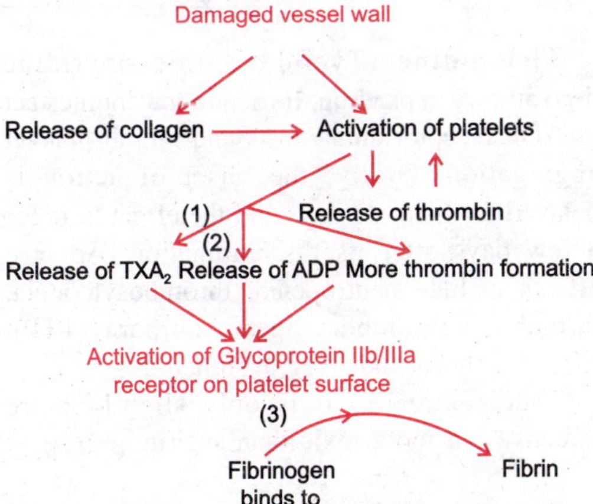

Fig. 32.2: Mechanism of thrombosis and its inhibition by drugs (1) Aspirin; (2) Ticlopidine; and (3) Glycoprotein IIb/IIIa antagonists. Prostacyclin is a physiological inhibitor (see text).

Figure 32.2 depicts the steps in thrombosis and their inhibitors. Drugs used in the prevention and treatment of thrombosis are:

- ***Antiplatelet agents.***
- ***Hemorrheological agents.***
- ***Anticoagulants;*** and
- ***Thrombolytic agents.***

Antiplatelet Agents

Platelets play an important role in hemostasis. It is generally accepted that intravascular thrombosis is initiated by platelet adhesion and aggregation and is completed by the formation of fibrin.

Prostacyclin (PGI_2) and thromboxane (TXA_2) are both derived from arachidonic acid. Unlike PGI_2 which is formed by the vascular endothelium, TXA_2, mostly generated by the platelets, is a potent vasoconstrictor, and promotes platelet aggregation. PGI_2 is an important circulating hormone that plays a major role in the natural resistance to intra-arterial thrombosis. A balance between platelet TXA_2 and vascular PGI_2 regulates the platelet aggregability. Circulating platelets normally do not adhere to the healthy endothelium, mainly because of the adequate PGI_2 formed locally.

Exposed collagen from the subendothelial matrix of damaged vessel wall initiates platelet attachment and simultaneously the release of TXA_2 and ADP from the platelets. Additional platelets are then recruited.

Platelet cyclic AMP plays an important role in platelet adhesion/aggregation. Endothelial PGI_2 stimulates adenylate cyclase and the formation of cAMP. TXA_2 within the platelets, on the other hand, inhibits adenylyl cyclase and lowers cAMP concen-tration. High concentration of intraplatelet cAMP inhibits, whereas low concentration accelerates, platelet aggregation. Platelet adhesion and thrombosis seen in atheromatous plaques are due to failure of local generation of PGI_2 by the vascular endothelial cells (**Endothelial dysfunction**). Apart from PGI_2, the endothelial cells also produce NO which increases the platelet cAMP resulting in inhibition of platelet aggregation. Prevention of platelet aggregation can prevent thrombosis.

Antiplatelet agents can be classified as:

I **Prostacyclin PGI2.**

II **Inhibitors of TXA2 formation** e.g., Aspirin.

III **ADP receptor antagonists** e.g., Ticlopidine, Clopidogrel.

IV **Phosphodiesterase inhibitors** e.g., Dipyridamole; and

V **Glycoprotein IIb/IIIa antagonists.**

PROSTACYCLIN (PGI_2) *is naturally* produced by the endothelial cells lining the blood vessels. It is also present in other tissues such as the brain, the gut and the kidney. It is formed from PG-endoperoxide (Chapter 24).

In man, prostacyclin infusion, in addition to inhibiting platelets, causes vasodilatation, resulting in hypotension, tachycardia, headache and intense facial flushing. It causes renin release. The compound is very unstable and has a short half life of 3 minutes.

Prostacyclin (Epoprostanol) is avaiable for preventing platelet aggregation during hemodialysis and to treat primary pulmonary hypertension (Chapter 24).

ASPIRIN: Aspirin is highly active against platelet cyclo-oxygenase which it acetylates irreversibly (Chapter 11). However, the enzyme of vessel walls is less sensitive to aspirin than is that of platelets. *Hence, small doses of aspirin inhibit the synthesis of TXA_2 by platelets whereas higher doses inhibit prostacyclin formation in the vessel wall as well.* The present evidence indicates that in the oral dose of 75-150 mg. daily, it is useful in:

- Decreasing the incidence of CHD in adults with high risk factors (Primary prevention).
- Preventing MI in patients with angina.
- Acute coronary syndromes (ACS) such as unstable angina. As immediate platelet inhibition is desirable, the dose of aspirin should be 150-300 mg.
- Patients undergoing coronary bypass surgery or angioplasty, or other revascularization procedures.
- Preventing stroke in patients with cerebrovascular disease and history of transient ischemic attacks (TIA).
- Preventing ischemic limb complications in patients with atherosclerotic peripheral vascular disease.
- Preventing re-infarction in patients with MI and ischemic heart disease.
- Preventing the development of pre-eclampsia in pregnant women at high risk of developing that condition; for this purpose, it is started between the 12th and 16th weeks of pregnancy. *Its routine use in all pregnant women to prevent pre-eclampsia is, however, not recommended.* It does not prevent the development of eclampsia if started after the onset of pre-eclampsia.

In hypertensive patients, aspirin therapy should not be initiated until the BP is controlled.

The low dose aspirin therapy can cause adverse effects including G.I. bleeding, and rarely, intracranial hemorrhage.

Dazoxiben is a substituted imidazole which selectively blocks production of TXA_2 without affecting the production of PGI_2. However, aspirin is safer and far superior.

Ticlopidine (Tyclid), a thienopyridine derivative, is a prodrug. Its active metabolites act as ADP receptor antagonists and inhibit platelet aggregation. Orally, the onset of action is delayed for hours to days and the effect lasts for a few days after its discontinuation. Adverse effects include neutropenia, thrombosytopenia, thrombotic thrombocytopenic purpura (TTP), rash, diarrhoea and liver dysfunction.

Therapeutically, it is only slightly more effective but more toxic than aspirin.

CLOPIDOGREL (Clopid) : It is related chemically to ticlopidine, has similar properties but is less toxic. It is a prodrug with slow onset of action. The usual dose is 75 mg/day. Given alone, it is equivalent to aspirin but is much more expensive. Its superiority over aspirin remains to be established. Substitution of clopidogrel for aspirin may provide marginal benefit at higher cost for the secondary prevention of serious vascular events. Combination of aspirin and clopidogrel is synergistic. Such combination offers no advantage over aspirin for primary prevention of CV disease. However, it may be beneficial in acute coronary syndromes, and in patients undergoing percutaneous, coronary intervention and other vascularization procedures. Excess bleeding is a clear hazard during long term use of the combination.

Low dose aspirin still remains the relatively safe, efficacious and cost-effective antiplatelet regimen for routine use.

DIPYRIDAMOLE (Persantin): This vasodilator inhibits the platelet phosphodiesterase enzyme leading to increase in the intraplatelet cyclic AMP, resulting in potentiation of platelet inhibition caused by the vessel wall prostacyclin. It has a weak therapeutic effect. Its main use is as an adjunct to warfarin in patients with artificial heart valves. It is used orally in the dose of 100 mg. qid. By itself, it is hardly of any benefit.

Glycoprotein (GP) II b / IIIa antagonists:
These are:

(1) **A monoclonal antibody against the platelet receptor,** e.g., Abciximab.

(2) **Synthetic inhibitors of glycoprotein IIb/IIIa** e.g., Tirofiban - *a non-peptide*; Eptifibatide - *a cyclic peptide*.

These agents compete with fibrinogen to occupy the glycoprotein IIb/IIIa receptors. They inhibit the final common pathway of platelet aggregation and thus, are effective against any platelet aggregating agent.

ABCIXIMAB (Reo-Pro) : This monoclonal antibody causes platelet receptor blockade and inhibits platelet aggregation. Given as IV bolus, followed by infusion for 12 hours, it produces an immediate effect which lasts for 48 hours after stopping the infusion. Small amounts of the drug can be detected on circulating platelets for 7-14 days. It is an effective antithrombotic agent in ACS that requires percutaneous coronary intervention. It acts synergistically with aspirin and heparin. The beneficial effect is reported to last for at least 6 months. The drug is effective in refractory unstable angina and has also been used in ischemic stroke. The major adverse effect is thrombocytopenia, which is reversed by platelet transfusion.

Tirofiban and **Eptifibatide** are competitive inhibitors of the GP IIb/IIIa complex, with a plasma t½ of 2-2.5 hrs. Their effect disappears within 4-6 hours after stopping the infusion. Their action cannot be reversed.

The use of antiplatelet drugs may unmask an underlying defect in hemostasis.

Hemorrheological agent :

PENTOXIFYLLINE (Trental): This analogue of xanthines is claimed to increase the deformability of the RBCs in circulation and thus improve the microcirculation (hemorrheological action). It has been claimed to be useful in patients with cerebrovascular disease, especially those getting transient ischemic attacks; in those with intermittent claudication and in those with ischemic ulcers on legs. The clinical results have been variable and difficult to predict. The drug may reduce plasma fibrinogen level and inhibit platelet aggregation. It causes mild gastrointestinal upset and CNS adverse effects. It is available as 400 mg. sustained release tablets. The dose is one tablet 2-3 times a day after food.

Anticoagulants - classification :

I **Those used for preventing clotting of blood inside the intact vasculature.**

- ***Fast acting,*** e.g., Heparin, Bivalirudin, Dabigatran.
- ***Slow acting,*** *e.g.,* (i) Coumarin derivatives e.g. Bishydroxycoumarin, Ethyl biscoumacetate and Warfarin sodium. (ii) Indandione derivatives e.g. Phenindione.

II **Those used to prevent clotting of blood in *vitro*.**

The division is necessarily arbitrary as certain drugs can be used both *in vivo* as well as *in vitro.*

Fast Acting Anticoagulants

HEPARIN: Heparin was discovered in 1916 by McLean, a medical student, who was looking for a coagulant in the liver. It is a naturally occurring substance of marked molecular heterogeneity, found in the metachromatically staining granules of mast cells. These cells are abundant in the liver (hence the name heparin), and in the lung. When released, it is rapidly degraded by macrophages and hence heparin cannot be detected in normal plasma. Commercial heparin is obtained from the lung and the intestinal mucosa of pigs and cattle. It is generally believed that heparin is the naturally occurring anticoagulant responsible for fluidity of the blood.

Purified, *unfractionated (native)* heparin preparations from different animals have different activities. The bioassay of heparin depends upon the capacity of heparin to prevent clotting of sheep or cattle plasma under standardized conditions. This activity is compared with that of the standard heparin powder; 1 mg. of dry material obtained from the cattle lung equals 150 USP units.

Heparin is a mucopolysaccharide composed of a number of sulfated D-glucosamine and D-glucuronic acid units linked through an oxygen bridge (glucosaminoglycans). The content of esterified sulfuric acid is very high, which makes heparin a strongly electronegative compound. It is thus the strongest organic acid occurring in the body. *The anticoagulant activity is attributed to its strong electronegative charge.* It is used as the sodium salt.

Pharmacological actions of heparin:

- ***Blood coagulation*:** Heparin prevents the clotting of blood both *in vivo* and *in vitro.* It probably acts on all the three stages of coagulation.

Heparin binds to and activates antithrombin, (antithrombin III), which then inactivates factor IXa, Xa, and thrombin. It increases the formation of thrombin-antithrombin complex several fold. The formation of fibrin monomer and its polymerization are prevented. *Even small doses of heparin that have much less antithrombin activity inhibit factor Xa which is a critical moiety in both intrinsic and extrinsic coagulation system. It has no action on thrombin bound to fibrin.*

The therapeutic doses prolongs the clotting time (2 to 2½ times the control) and activated partial thromboplastin time (APTT) to 1.5 to 2 times the control. Clinically, the dose-response relation is not linear; instead, the anticoagulant response increases disproportionately in intensity and duration with increasing doses.

- ***Heparin and lipoprotein lipase*:** Heparin abolishes the cloudiness of the hyperlipemic plasma (Tyndall effect) within minutes after its administration. This action occurs only *in vivo* in doses too small to exert an anticoagulant effect. It is attributed to an enzyme called lipoprotein lipase activated by heparin.

- ***Miscellaneous actions*:** Heparin inhibits aldosterone secretion and causes hyperkalemia. Heparin inhibits the growth of many cells such as vascular muscle and endothelium in culture. It also has some antiinflammatory action.

Absorption, fate and excretion: Heparin is not effective orally. It is well absorbed after SC injection. Usually, it is given IV. It circulates bound to several plasma proteins. The mast cells take up heparin in their metachromatic granules and may act as a storage depot for exogenously administered heparin. It is also taken up by the endothelial cells.

The onset of anticoagulant action with an IV dose is almost immediate and reaches peak within 5 to 10 minutes; whereas after SC administration, it is delayed upto 1 hour. The clotting time returns to normal within 2 to 4 hours with a t½ of about 60 minutes. The aqueous preparation is, therefore, administered at 2 to 4 hourly interval. In general, the duration of anticoagulant activity increases with the size of the dose.

Heparin is metabolized mainly by a liver enzyme termed heparinase. Following IV administration, 25 to 50 per cent of a single dose may appear in the urine in active form. *Heparin does not cross the placental barrier and is not secreted in the milk.*

Adverse reactions :

- ***Allergic and anaphylactoid reactions*** are rare and include asthma, urticaria, rhinitis, and fever. It is advisable to give a trial dose of 1000 units of heparin.
- ***Bleeding***: Excessive or injudicious use of heparin may produce hemorrhage from various sites such as peptic ulcer, kidneys and hemorrhoids, and may cause hemarthrosis or wound hematoma. Patients can bleed with even normal aPTT value. It is advisable to avoid aspirin and other drugs which interfere with platelet function during heparin therapy.
- ***Thrombocytopenia***: Heparin causes transient, mild thrombocytopenia in 25% of patients and severe thrombocytopenia in a few. The mild reaction results from heparin induced platelet aggregation. The severe form, which occurs on 8th to 12th day of treatment, is due to the formation of heparin dependent antiplatelet antibodies; this can result in tolerance to the anti-coagulant action of heparin and recurrent thromboembolic disease. The thrombocytopenia improves after discontinuation of heparin. It has been reported even during 'low dose' heparin therapy. Low molecular weight (LMW) heparins reportedly interact less readily with platelets than unfractionated heparin. It is recommended that a platelet count should be obtained before starting heparin therapy and frequently during therapy, and that heparin should be discontinued if platelet count falls below 1,00,000/cu mm.
- ***Alopecia***: Transient alopecia may occur after prolonged heparin therapy.
- ***Osteoporosis***: Use of heparin in the dose of 15,000 units daily for a period of 6 months or more has been reported to cause osteoporosis and spontaneous fractures of ribs and vertebrae.
- ***Miscellaneous***: SGOT and SGPT levels may rise during therapy with heparin.

Preparations and dosage: Heparin is available as sodium or calcium heparin. Since the commercial preparations of heparin vary in their potency (as units/mg), the dosage of heparin must be prescribed in units.

Small fixed doses of heparin are given deep SC to prevent venous thromboembolism. Larger doses are used either SC or IV to prevent the propagation of an established thrombus; still larger doses may be necessary in acute pulmonary embolism. When large doses are used, they must be adjusted according to the results of clotting time and activated partial thromboplastin time (aPTT) (see below).

Heparin should not be injected IM as it can cause a hematoma.

(i) *Low fixed dose, SC regimen* (Prophylactic): 5,000 u given every 8 - 12 hours, starting 1-2 hours before the operation and continuing till the patient is discharged. Injection is given with a small needle and the smallest possible volume is employed, to prevent local hematoma. Determination of aPTT is not needed.

(ii) *Dose adjusted SC regimen* (Therapeutic): This regimen employs either 8000-10,000 u hourly or 15,000-20,000 u 12 hourly, the actual dose being adjusted in either instance according to the results of aPTT.

(iii) *IV Intermittent regimen* (Therapeutic) : 10,000 u initially (in a 70 kg man) followed by 5000 to 10,000 u every 4-6 hours. In children, the dose is 50-100 u/kg initially, followed by a similar dose every 4 hours.

(iv) *IV infusion* (Therapeutic): Initially, 5000u into the tubing of infusion, followed by 20,000 to 30,000 u daily at the rate of 0.5 u/kg/min (1000 u/hour in a 70 kg man) in isotonic saline. Not more than 25,000 units of heparin should be added to one bag for IV infusion.

Table 32.2: Doses of commonly used LMWH

Preparation	For prophylaxis of deep vein thrombosis (DVT)	For treatment of DVT and pulmonary embolism
Enoxaparin	2000 units s c 2 hrs before surgery; then 2000 units every 24 hrs for 7-10 days	100 units/kg s c every 12 hrs for 5 days
Dalteparin	2500 units s c 1-2 hrs before surgery; then 2500 units every 24 hrs for 5-7 days	100 units/kg s c twice daily for 5 days
Tinzaparin	3500 units s c 2 hrs before surgery; then 3500 units every 24 hrs for 7-10 days	175 units/kg s c once daily for 6 days
Fondaparinux	2.5 mg, s c once daily	—

Low molecular weight heparins (LMWH): are commercially prepared by fractionation of native heparin; they are more homogeneous molecularly and have molecular weight between 4000 and 6500. When given SC once or twice daily, these compounds have at least as much antithrombotic activity as native heparin given SC or by continuous IV infusion. Further, they:

- ***Are absorbed more uniformly*** than the native heparins after SC administration.
- ***Have a longer duration of action.***
- ***Inactivate factor Xa selectively;*** their action against thrombin is minimal.
- ***Have a predictable anticoagulant effect because they bind less avidly to cells and to heparin binding proteins.***
- ***Interact relatively less with platelets*** and lead to fewer bleeding episodes; and
- ***Are less antigenic*** and cause thrombocytopenia and osteoporosis less frequently.

Table 32.3: Monitoring heparin therapy

- ***Whole blood clotting time*** (Lee-White), which should be kept at 2-3 times the normal; and
- ***Activated partial thromboplastin time (aPTT)*** which should be kept at 1½-2 times the normal.

These properties would make their use attractive for outpatient and domiciliary use. However, they are expensive. Examples of LMW heparins are **enoxaparin** (Clexane), **dalteparin** sodium (Fragmin), **tinzaparin** (Logiparin), **parnaparin** (Fluxum) and **reviparin** (Clivarine). Their uses are similar to those of native heparin. (Table 32.2). *However, native heparin still remains the parenteral anticogualant of choice in ICU, operation theatre and in patients with renal impairment.*

Table 32.3 lists the methods of monitoring heparin therapy. Small doses of heparin given SC, for prophylaxis, and LMWH do not generally require monitoring of blood samples.

Heparin antagonists: The anticoagulant effects of heparin can be promptly arrested by the administration of strongly basic compounds which react with the strongly acidic groups of heparin, thereby abolishing the anticoagulant activity e.g. protamine sulfate.

PROTAMINE SULFATE: Protamine is a mixture of simple, low molecular weight polypeptides, found in the sperms of certain fish. It binds firmly to heparin and inactivates it. Protamine sulfate as 1 per cent solution, is administered slowly, IV, not more than 50 mg. over a 10 minute period. One mg. of protamine sulfate neutralizes the anti-coagulant effect of 100 units of heparin activity. If more than 30 minutes have elapsed after heparin administration half of this dosage is required. A patient given protamine should be observed for recurrence of bleeding as protamine sulfate itself has anticoagulant activity and the action of heparin lasts longer than that of protamine.

It is considered unsafe to exceed the dose of 50-100 mg. over a short period. Protamine IV injection may cause a sudden fall in BP, bradycardia, dyspnoea and transitory flushing.

HIRUDIN: This is a potent antithrombin polypeptide obtained from the leech *Hirudo medicinalis.* It has now been synthesized by recombinant DNA technique (**lepirudin**). Unlike heparin, hirudin binds tightly to thrombin. It inactivates free as well as fibrin–bound thrombin. *The effect of hirudin does not require antithrombin or other co-factors.* It not only prevents conversion of fibrinogen to fibrin, but also blocks thrombin-catalyzed platelet aggregation, and activation of other clotting factors. It inhibits disseminated intravascular coagulation, and venous and arterial thrombosis more effectively than heparin in animal experiments. Its activity is monitored by the same tests as that of heparin. Its action is very short and it has to be given by IV infusion. *There is no antidote to lepirudin.*

Biviluridin is an analogue of hirudin, with rapid onset and offset of action. It is claimed to be safer than the latter.

Dabigatran: Dabigatran etexilate is a prodrug. Given orally, it is converted to the active agent dabigatran which is a direct inhibitor of thrombin. Given once daily, it is claimed to be as effective as enoxaparin for the prevention of venous thomboembolism. The drug appears to have an ADR profile similar to that of enoxaparin. The major advantage of this drug is that it is effective orally without the need for coagulation monitoring unlike heparin. It is under evaluation.

Argabatrine is also a direct thrombin inhibitor, given as IV infusion. It is used an alternative to lepuridin.

Rivaroxaban: It is an orally acting, **direct, selective Factor Xa inhibitor** for prevention and treatment of arterial and venous thromboemlism. It does not require monitoring.

Danaparoid: This heparinoid, obtained from porcine intestinal mucosa, is a mixture of glucosaminoglycans and inhibits Xa. It is given SC twice a day, for prophylaxis. It does not cause thrombocytopenia and *has no antidote.* It is used as a heparin substitute to prevent postoperative DVT.

HUMAN ANTITHROMBIN CONCENTRATE : This is prepared from pooled human plasma. It is heat treated in solution at 60°C for at least 10 hours in order to inactivate the pathogenic viruses. It is used either alone or along with heparin to treat patients with a rare heriditary disorder, antithrombin III deficiency.

Slow Acting Anticoagulants

These drugs are known as **oral anticoagulants** because, in contrast to heparin, they are effective orally. They have a slow onset of action.

Fig. 32.3: Coumarin ring

COUMARIN DERIVATIVES: Bis-hydroxycoumarin or dicoumaral, the first coumarin compound, was isolated from spoilt sweet clover in 1943-1944 and was proved to be the causative factor in a cattle disease termed 'Sweet Clover Disease', characterised by a severe haemorrhagic tendency. Many chemically related compounds have since been studied but only a few are clinically useful. The most commonly used drug is warfarin sodium.

Pharmacological actions: The various coumarin drugs exert qualitatively similar pharmacological actions.

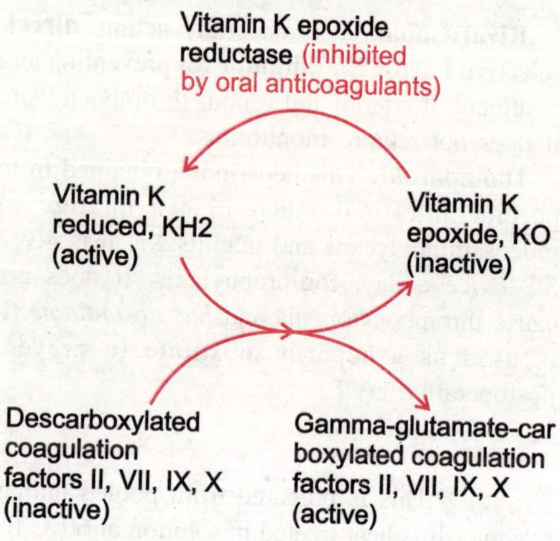

Fig. 32.4: Vitamin K cycle and site of action of Coumarin anticoagulants

- ***Anticoagulant action***: Unlike heparin, coumarins have no anticoagulant action *in vitro*. Coagulation factors II, VII, IX and X are synthesized in the liver but are biologically inactive until the amino terminal glutamic acid residues are carboxylated. Carboxylation is directly coupled to the oxidation of vitamin K to its epoxide.To sustain the carboxylation,the epoxide is converted back to the reduced form of vitamin K by the enzyme vitamin K epoxide reductase (Fig. 32.4). This enzyme complex is inhibited by coumarins, leading to prevention of regeneration of reduced form of vitamin K and therefore to inhibition of carboxylation. Because of the long half lives of the already circulating coagulation factors, it takes several days to achieve the desired therapeutic effect. Unlike heparin, oral anticoagulants have no direct effect on the circulating coagulation factors. Coumarin therapy is controlled by estimating prothrombin time of the blood which is expressed as *International Normalised Ratio (INR)*. Bleeding time is unaltered.

- ***Miscellaneous actions***: Coumarin therapy is found to increase the plasma antithrombin levels. Both coumarin and indandione derivatives produce a uricosuric effect, by interfering with the renal urate reabsorption.

Absorption, fate and excretion: The absorption of coumarin from the intestine is slow and incomplete. The drugs are extensively bound to plasma proteins. They cross the placental barrier and are also secreted in milk. They are mainly metabolized in the liver. There is a considerable individual variation (as much as 14 fold) in the rate of detoxification.

In contrast to heparin, there is a considerable lag (usually 24 to 48 hours) between the time of peak plasma level of coumarins and the therapeutic response. This is because they prevent the formation of active essential clotting factors by the liver but do not destroy the already circulating ones. It takes 3-7 days for prothrombin time to return to normal after cessation of therapy.

Adverse reactions:

- ***Bleeding*** : The incidence of hemorrhage is 5-6 per cent. There is no correlation between the onset of hemorrhage and the dose, nor between the occurrence of hemorrhage and the prothrombin, coagulation or bleeding time. In fact, controlled studies indicate that similar degree of hypoprothrombinemia may be found in patients who bleed and those who do not.

Bleeding from an unsuspected peptic ulcer or neoplasm can often be fatal and sometimes the patient may come with symptoms of acute intestinal obstruction. Such patients are poor surgical risks.

The hemorrhage induced by coumarin compounds can be treated by large doses of vitamin K_1 oxide which enables the liver to synthesize active clotting factors. However, even the IV administration of vitamin K is associated with a latent period of several hours. Therefore, *in the immediate treatment of severe hemorrhage, prompt administration of fresh whole blood is necessary. Menadione (synthetic Vitamin K, Vitamin K_3) is ineffective in countering the bleeding caused by oral anticoagulants.*

- ***Fetal toxicity***: *Coumarin anticoagulants may cause fatal hemorrhage in the fetus; further they are teratogenic* (Chapter 77).

- ***Cutaneous gangrene***: Petechiae that

coalesce to painful ecchymoses, hemorrhagic bullae and finally to necrosis/gangrene occur occasionally within 3-8 days after starting treatment with large doses of warfarin. The lesions affect women more often than men and involve the adipose tissue of breasts, buttocks, thighs and the distal lower extremities. Debridement and even amputation of the affected tissue, limb or breast have been necessary in severe cases.

- ***Miscellaneous***: Rarely, coumarins may cause urticaria, anorexia, vomiting and diarrhoea.

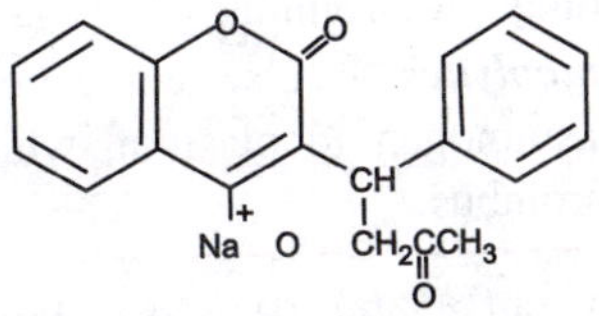

Fig. 32.5 : Warfarin

WARFARIN SODIUM (Uniwarfin): This compound, originally employed as a rodent poison, is the most widely used coumarin anticoagulant and is considered to be the drug of choice. It is a racemic mixture of two isomers, S (t ½ 35 hours) and R (t ½ 50 hours), in almost equal proportions. After initiating therapy with the maintenance dose 5-10mg/day (*no loading dose is used*), therapeutic INR level is usually achieved in 36 hours. The drug's duration of action is 2-5 days. Approximately 97 per cent of the drug is bound to plasma albumin. Its advantages are:

- ***It is almost 99% absorbed*** and gives more steady plasma levels;
- ***It has rapid onset and predictable duration of action;*** therefore,the therapy is easier to regulate; and
- ***It is water soluble and can be given parenterally.*** Parenteral administration, however, does not accelerate the speed of anticoagulation.

If warfarin is employed for long-term anticoagulant therapy, it takes about 3 days for the prothrombin time to return to normal after drug discontinuation. Warfarin has the unique property of being water soluble, among the 'antiprothrombin' drugs.

Adverse reactions : Comparatively few toxic effects other than haemorrhage have been reported. These include alopecia, urticaria and dermatitis. It can cross the placenta but is *not secreted in the milk.* It is contraindicated during pregnancy. *Women on long term warfarin therapy should avoid pregnancy. The major drawback of this drug is the possibility of multiple drug interactions* (see below).

The action of warfarin can be antagonised by vitamin K (see later).

Preparation and dosage : Warfarin sodium 5 mg. tablets. It is used once a day in the dose of 2.5–10 mg. The drug has a cumulative action and the maintenance dose may have to be gradually decreased after the first week or so. *No loading dose is used to initiate therapy; maintenance doses are used from the beginning.*

Depending upon the reason for anticoagulation and risks involved, the dose of warfarin is adjusted by measuring INR, which is generally maintained between 2.0 and 4.0.

The other bishydroxycoumarin drugs such as acenocoumarin are now rarely used.

Table 32.4: Drug interactions of coumarin anticoagulants

- **Drugs which prolong prothrombin time and may cause bleeding:** Aspirin, phenylbutazone, other NSAID, heparin, clofibrate, thyroxine, amiodarone, anabolic steroids, cimetidine, omeprazole, metronidazole, co-trimoxazole, high doses of penicillins, erythromycin, some cephalosporins, moxalactam.
- **Drugs which shorten prothrombin time:** Barbiturates, chloral hydrate, meprobamate, rifampicin, griseofulvin, cholestyramine, carbamazepine (see above). When these drugs are stopped, bleeding may occur in a patient on oral anticoagulants.

INDANDIONE DERIVATIVES: These include the compounds **phenindione**, *and* **anisindione.** The anticoagulant activity of these compounds is essentially similar to the coumarin compounds. Because of their toxicity, they are now almost obsolete.

Drug interactions: See Table 32.4. Coumarins can cause drug interactions by :

Inhibiting the platelet function (aspirin, NSAID).

- ***Stimulating hepatic microsomal catabolism of warfarin*** (barbiturates, rifampicin, griseofulvin, carbamazepine).
- ***Displacing warfarin from protein binding*** (sulfonamides, phenylbutazone, chlorpropamide); or
- ***Inhibiting the metabolic clearance of warfarin*** (cimetidine, omeprazole, amiodarone).

Drugs like tolbutamide and phenytoin may accumulate in the body following coumarins and hence, doses of these drugs must be reduced.

Other factors affecting the dosage and activity of the oral anticoagulants are listed in Table 32.5.

Table 32.6 summarises the main actions of antithrombotic drugs.

Therapeutic uses of anticoagulants : Arterial and venous thrombosis differ in their causes, pathologic effects and management. To understand the usefulness and limitations of anticoagulants it is essential to realize the difference between a **thrombus** (White thrombus) and a **clot** (Red thrombus). In the case of an artery, because of the rapid blood flow, the thrombotic mass does not have red cells, is pale, friable and non-homogeneous. This, then, is a thrombus. *Platelet aggregation is the more important event in the initiation of arterial thrombus.* In contrast to this is a typical clot, which is soft, dark red, and homogeneous. It is made up of red cells, platelets, white cells and fibrin. The slow blood flow in a vein encourages the formation of 'clot' which has a much smaller platelet-leucocyte element and a considerable clot-like tail. In venous 'thrombosis' and pulmonary embolism the structure responsible for the clinical state is usually a clot, and not a 'thrombus' as occurs in artery. *The drugs which interfere with the clotting mechanism may not necessarily modify the arterial thrombus formation unless they affect the platelet behaviour.* Although such drugs may satisfy the conventional definition of an 'anticoagulant' they are not 'antithrombotic' agents.

Conventional anticoagulant therapy can prevent the extension of an existing venous thrombus and the development of additional thrombi in the vascular bed. *It does not influence the established thrombus, nor can it reverse ischemic tissue damage.*

Table 32.5: Factors affecting the dosage of oral anticoagulants

- Genetic differences in the rate of drug metabolism.
- Age and sex.
- Vitamin K deficiency caused by poor diet, bowel disease or biliary disease enhances the response to oral anticoagulants.
- Chronic alcoholism, liver disease, kidney disease and vitamin C deficiency enhance the response.
- Hypermetabolic states.

Table 32.6 : Main actions of antithrombotic drugs

- ***Heparin*** accelerates inactivation of thrombin by antithrombin III.
- ***LMWHs***, in addition, inactivate factor Xa (activated factor X).
- ***Hirudin*** inactivates thrombin.
- ***Gp IIb/IIIa (a platelet receptor) antagonists*** block the receptor and thus inhibit activation/aggregation of platelets.
- ***Warfarin*** inhibits the synthesis of several active coagulation factors, including prothrombin.
- ***Thrombolytics*** accelarate the conversion of plasminogen to plasmin, which lyses the thrombus.

Heparin is the drug of choice when rapid induction of anticoagulation is desired. It can be used safely during late pregnancy. The disadvantages of heparin are its narrow therapeutic window, high cost, the need for parenteral administration, and the frequency of local reactions at the site of injection. The oral anticoagulants have the disadvantages of delayed onset of action, variable therapeutic effect and need for an elaborate laboratory control. The maximum therapeutic response to oral warfarin is achieved 3-5 days after the initial dose. Hence, in order to obtain immediate therapeutic response, heparin is given IV, intermittently at 4-8 hour interval. Institution of combined IV heparin and oral warfarin gives the patients the advantage of immediate and prolonged anticoagulation with minimal discomfort and maximum economy.

Invasive procedures and intramuscular injections should be minimized and antiplatelet drugs (aspirin and NSAID) should be avoided in patients on anticoagulants. Further, if a patient on anticoagulant therapy bleeds it should not automatically be attributed to the anticoagulant therapy, but an effort should be made to rule out an underlying lesion such as a malignancy.

Indications for anticoagulant therapy :

- ***Prevention and treatment of deep venous thrombosis and pulmonary embolism:*** Anticoagulants are most useful in the prevention and treatment of venous thrombosis and pulmonary embolism.

Low fixed dose heparin considerably reduces the incidence of pulmonary embolism, if used **prophylactically** in post-operative therapy and in patients with acute MI. For this purpose, heparin is given SC in doses of 5000 units every 8-12 hours, the first dose being given 2 hours before surgery. *Laboratory monitoring is not necessary.* A highly concentrated solution of heparin should be used. Pressure over the injection site minimizes local bleeding into the tissues. The risk of hemorrhage following low doses is minimal.

Such prophylactic use of heparin **in low doses** is also justified for prevention of deep vein thrombosis particularly in patients confined to prolonged bed rest for some reason.

Patients with recurrent venous thromboembolism should receive long term, perhaps indefinite, anticoagulant therapy to minimize the risk of pulmonary embolism. Similarly, patients with chronic atrial fibrillation should receive long term anticoagulant therapy to prevent arterial thromboembolism. Adequate anticoagulation for three weeks is indicated prior to conversion to sinus rhythm in such patients.

For patients who have *confirmed acute proximal DVT or pulmonary embolism, immediate anticoagulation with full dose IV heparin and oral warfarin is recommended.* Subcutaneous heparin takes 12 hours to exert full anticoagulant effect and is not as useful in such patients. Oral anticoagulants should be continued for 3-6 months in these patients. Patients with calf vein thrombosis without proximal extension are less liable to develop pulmonary embolism and may not require such intensive anticoagulation.

Table 32.7: Contraindications to anticoagulant therapy

- Haemorrhagic tendency and blood dyscrasias.
- Benign or malignant ulcers, such as in the gut, colitis, diverticulitis, recent operation upon the CNS, eye or prostate gland.
- In subacute bacterial endocarditis, anticoagulants may cause detachment of the bacterial vegetations from the damaged valves into general circulation.
- Threatened abortion, injury to the brain the spinal cord and stroke.
- Regional and lumbar block anaesthesia.
- Prothrombin deficiency, severe hepatic, renal impairment and severe uncontrolled hypertension.
- An uncooperative patient, inadequate laboratory facility and uninformed or casual medical supervision.
- Pregnancy

• ***Myocardiac infarction***: Refer to Chapter 31.

• ***Rheumatic heart disease***: The occurrence of emboli associated with rheumatic valve disease with AF is an indication for long term anticoagulant treatment.

• ***Cerebrovascular disease***: As a rule, anticoagulants are not indicated in cerebrovascular disease for fear of causing cerebral hemorrhage. Their therapeutic usefulness is doubtful, except perhaps in the intermittent insufficiency syndromes, and stroke due to emboli from the heart; the possibility of hemorrhage should be rued out.

• ***Miscellaneous***: They are also used in case of artificial heart valves in order to prevent emboli and during cardiac bypass surgery.

Contraindications to anticoagulants: See Table 32.7.

Long acting oral anticoagulants such as diphenindione, pindone and broadifacum are used as rodenticides.

In Vitro Anticoagulants

Physical methods: Clotting can be delayed by cooling the blood or by collecting it in coated vessels so that platelets are not broken up. The coating used is paraffin, collodion or silicone.

Oxalates and **citrates:** These act by removal of calcium ions. Potassium oxalate 0.1 per cent precipitates serum calcium as calcium oxalate. Sodium citrate combines with calcium and forms calcium sodium citrate. The anticoagulant solution (B.P.) contains 2.5 per cent of sodium citrate in 0.9 per cent saline. Citrate is usually employed as an anticoagulant for blood to be transfused. The final strength of citrate is 3.8 per cent. Potassium oxalate produces convulsions and hence is not employed *in vivo.*

EDTA (Ethylenediamine tetraacetic acid) a chelating agent, has a great affinity for calcium and its sodium salt has been used as an anticoagulant (see also Chapter 72).

Heparin: discussed earlier.

Thrombolytic Agents

The process of fibrinolysis or dissolution of blood clot is schematically represented in Fig. 32.6. Normally, the euglobulin fraction of the plasma contains the inactive precursor plasminogen. Plasminogen is converted to the **fibrinolytic enzyme plasmin** by an activator substances (tPA, Urokinase) present in tissues. The active proteolytic enzyme plasmin is capable of breaking down fibrin clots. Plasmin is relatively nonspecific in action and it can also act on proteins and clotting factors.

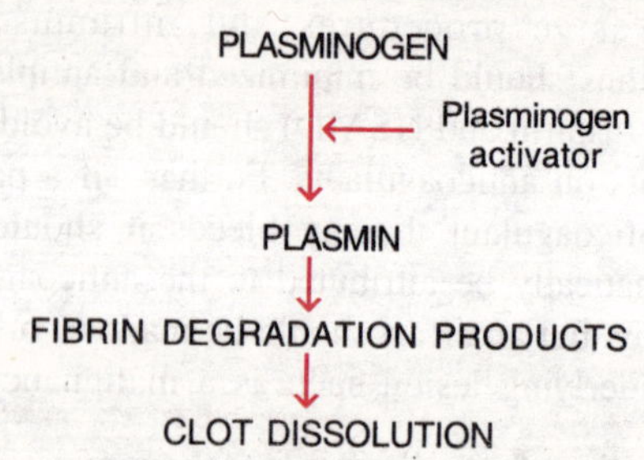

Fig. 32.6: Mechanism of fibrinolysis

Plasminogen is the inactive proteolytic enzyme of plasma and binds to fibrin during the formation of a thrombus. This binding endows specific fibrinolytic properties on the plasminogen-plasmin enzyme system, since fibrin-bound plasminogen is more susceptible to the activation than is plasma plasminogen.

All thrombolytic agents in use act directly or indirectly as plasminogen activators. These are:

• ***Streptokinase*** (Streptase).

• ***Recombinant tissue-type plasminogen activators*** Alteplase (rt-PA, Actilyse), Reteplase (Retavase), Tenecteplase (TNKase).

• ***Urokinase*** (Ukidan).

• ***Acylated plasminogen-streptokinase activator (APSAC) complex*** (Anistreplase).

Table 32.8: Properties of thrombolytic agents

Characteristic	Streptokinase	Urokinase	Alteplase*
Plasma half life (t½ min.)	15-25	15-20	4-8
Fibrin specificity	Minimal	Moderate	Maximum
Plasminogen binding	Indirect	Direct	Direct
Potential for allergic reaction/hypotension	Yes	No	No
Total dose	1.5 million units	3-4 million units	100 mg
Administration for MI	1.5 MU IV	3 lacs IV in 10 min, then 3 lacs/hr for 12 hrs.	15 mg IV bolus, then 50 mg over 30 min, then 35 mg over 1hr

* Appears to result in a higher rate of early coronary reperfusion compared to streptokinase.
(MU = million units)

These agents differ in their propensity to activate plasma plasminogen; the rt-PA and single-chain urokinase plasminogen activator are termed **fibrin specific** because of their high ratio of activity for fibrin-bound plasminogen to that for plasma plasminogen. *Streptokinase, anistreplase and urokinase are* **fibrin-nonspecific**, and are not well absorbed by fibrin thrombi. They are direct activators of plasminogen in circulation. With the doses used in the treatment of acute MI, the lytic activity is greatest with streptokinase, intermediate with urokinase and least with rt-PA. Given IV, the plasma t½ of these agents differs (Table 32.8). Thus, differences in pharmacokinetics and patient's tolerance and the disease state dictate the duration of administration necessary to achieve an appropriate thrombolytic effect. *Alteplase, reteplase* and *tenecteplase* more **fibrin-specific**. They bind strongly to fibrin and are capable of dissolving resistant thrombi better than fibrin-nonspecific agents.

Therapeutically, when treatment is begun within the first 6 hours of the onset of chest pain in MI, a similar incidence of reperfusion is provided by all the agents, but there are considerable differences in the ease with which they can be adminstered (see later). Re-thrombosis, after re-perfusion, occurs in roughly inverse proportion to the length of the plasma half life of the drug used, with the lowest incidence with urokinase and streptokinase, and the highest with rt-PA. Hence, heparin is administered simultaneously with rt-PA, primarily to enhance re-perfusion and decrease the rate of re-thrombosis. Since streptokinase and urokinase produce more prolonged and extensive coagulation defect, simultaneous administration of heparin is not required.

Adverse reactions:

- ***Bleeding*** is the commonest adverse effect with all these agents. Thrombolytic therapy induces a marked hemostatic defect by combined action on blood components, the vessel wall and the hemostatic plug. It is probably much less with selective agents such as rt-PA.
- ***Mutiple microemboli*** can occur following disintegration of existing thrombus in the vascular system.
- ***Allergic reactions***: Streptokinase, being a

bacterial protein, is antigenic. Hence, it may cause allergic response and rarely (0.1%) anaphylactoid reaction; therapy with urokinase does not provoke allergic reaction.

- ***Hypotension*** may occur more often with rapid administration of streptokinase.
- ***Hemorrhagic stroke*** is a dreaded complication of thrombolytic therapy.

The therapeutic goal is to re-establish the blood flow through the occluded vessel within a short time, so as to prevent organ damage. The optimal dose that would produce the highest rate of reperfusion and the lowest incidence of bleeding complications and rethrombosis is difficult to decide precisely. Because thrombolytic agents do not distinguish between the fibrin of a thrombus and the fibrin of a hemostatic plug, they are double edged weapons. From the experience with heparin, it appears that a hypocoagulable state is itself well tolerated and an unlikely initiator of bleeding in patients with an intact vascular system and in the absence of such risk factors as recent surgery, DU, thrombocytopenia or administration of other antithrombotic medication. *Vascular injury, rather than changes in blood coagulation is the main cause of bleeding.* The important contraindications to thrombolytic therapy are listed in Table 32.9.

Table 32.9: Contraindications to thrombolytic therapy

- Active bleeding, bleeding tendency.
- Recent major trauma.
- Invasive or surgical procedure in the past 10 days.
- GI or genitourinary bleeding in the past 10 days.
- Recent prolonged cardiopulmonary resuscitation.
- Neurosurgical procedure in the past 2 months.
- Stroke or transient cerebral ischemic attack in the past 12 months.
- History of cerebral tumour, aneurysm or arteriovenous malformation.
- Active peptic ulcer disease.
- Hypertension (severe, uncontrolled).
- Diabetes mellitus with proliferative retinopathy.
- Pregnancy.

Probably 10-20% of reperfused arteries undergo re-thrombosis. The ideal antithrombotic regimen to sustain reperfusion has not been definitively established; but heparin in the dose of 5000 units (IV bolus) followed by 1000 units hourly (by IV infusion) for 3-5 days and aspirin (150 mg/day) have been recommended. The most popular approach to preventing rethrombosis in arteries is a combination of anticoagulation and angioplasty. Rethrombosis of veins is probably most often related to incomplete lysis of the original thrombus, and the present management emphasizes adequate anti-coagulation with heparin as the best approach to preventing rethrombosis.

Therapeutic uses: The use of a fibrinolytic agent accelerates the rate of vascular reperfusion, and improves rapidly the physiologic and laboratory manifestations of vessel occlusion.

- ***Myocardial infarction (MI)*:** Thrombolytic therapy is most useful in patients with STEMI (Chapter 28). Patients without ST elevation or those with unstable angina are only marginally benefited.

As progression of ischemia and infarction from the subendocardium to the epicardium occurs in about 6 hours, thrombolytic therapy, begun soon after an acute MI (within 6 hours of the onset) reduces mortality and preserves LV function.

Among various thrombolytic agents available, streptokinase (SK) and recombinant tissue plasminogen activator (rt-PA) are commonly used. The classical *indications* for thrombolytic therapy in acute MI are chest pain characteristic of infarction, lasting for at least 30 minutes but not more than 6 hours, with 0.1 mV (1 mm.) or more ST-segment elevation in at least two contiguous leads in the ECG, in a patient younger than 75 years. However, survival may improve even when patients are treated within upto 24 hours after the onset of pain. Although such therapy is useful, it rarely prevents the subsequent ECG and enzymatic changes indicating infarction, even when used within the first hour after MI.

Streptokinase is given IV in the dose of 1.5 million units over 60 min.; rt-PA (Alteplase) is given IV in the dose of 100 mg over 1½ hours. This is followed by 75-150 mg of aspirin by mouth, daily, for 4 weeks. *Heparin is also given concurrently if alteplase is used.* There appears to be little difference in left ventricular function or predischarge patency rates whether SK or alteplase is used. SK sometimes aggravates hypotension and this should be watched for. *Patients are not routinely treated with thrombolytics later than six hours after infarction unless they are at high risk; they can, however, be given aspirin.*

- ***Ischemic stroke*:** Because of the risk of conversion of a non-hemorrhagic stroke into a hemorrhagic one, such therapy is highly controversial in ischemic strokes. IV rt-PA has been used within 3 hours (0.9 mg/kg to maximum of 90 mg) to treat acute ischemic stroke, with reported success of 50% near complete recovery at 3 months. *However, in such cases occlusion by clot must be demonstrated by MRI.*
- ***Pulmonary embolism*:** Heparin is the mainstay of treatment of pulmonary embolism. "A thrombolytic agent may be a useful adjunct in patients with severe pulmonary embolism and right ventricular dysfunction.
- ***Acute peripheral arterial occlusion*:** It is used especially for dissolving occlusion of small arteries that cannot be surgically treated. Further, it may serve as a prelude to vascular surgery. Thrombolytic therapy for arterial thrombi in locations other than the limbs or the coronary arteries has been reported for virtually all organs. For this, the drug may be administered systemically or by regional infusion.
- ***Deep venous thrombosis (DVT)*:** Anticoagulation is the treatment of choice in this condition (see earlier). Thrombolytic therapy has been used with some benefit to treat axillary vein thrombosis, a condition that may not respond to conventional anticoagulant therapy.

All the plasminogen activators are effective thrombolytic agents when given in correct dosage for proper duration, at an appropriate time. The biochemical properties of all agents dictate the treatment regimen. Because of their longer half-life, SK and urokinase can be administered by bolus injection, or short infusion without *simultaneous* administration of heparin, which can be given later, when recovery from the plasma coagulation defect begins. In contrast, rt-PA must be infused for 3 or more hours concurrently with heparin, in order to provide a continuous supply of fresh agent to the thrombus to prevent rethrombosis. SK and anistreplase also induce the formation of antibodies, which may limit the response to future administration of these agents.

Aspirin is administered as soon as the thrombolytic therapy is begun and continued as described earlier.

Clinically, no large differences are seen between SK and rtPA, though theoretically and experimentally rtPA, being selective, appears to be superior. But, it needs heparin supplementation to prevent early re-closure of the vessels, whereas the incidence of stroke is higher than with SK. SK is more cost-effective than rtPA and is preferred for routine use. *If, however, the patient has received SK even 4 days earlier, rtPA is preferred.*

***Unstable angina*:** *Administration of heparin and aspirin remains the mainstay of treatment in this condition. Thrombolytic therapy is not useful and is not recommended.*

STREPTOKINASE (Streptase, Kabikinase): It is used in the treatment of DVT in the dose of 250,000 units IV in 30 minutes, followed by 100,000 units every hour for 24-72 hours. (Chapter 74). A loading dose is given to neutralize the antibodies following any previous dose.

ALTEPLASE, rtPA (Recombinant tissue-type plasminogen activator, Actilyse), natural protein in man, is now prepared by recombinant DNA technology. It preferentially activates plasminogen bound to fibrin clot and thus avoids systemic activation of plasminogen; fibrinogen depletion and bleeding are thus minimized. It is as effective as streptokinase but may be safer. It has a short t½ of 8 min. It is metabolized by the liver. For doses see Table 32.8. Patients weighing less than 67 kg. should receive a total dose of 1.5 mg./kg. Heparin 5000 u is given IV bolus prior to administration of rt-PA.

Reteplase and **tenecteplase** are the other recombinant analogues of human rt-PA available for therapy. They have long plasma half lives and can be given as bolus injection.

UROKINASE (Abokinase): This enzyme, originally isolated from human urine, is now obtained from cultured human renal cells. It is a potent direct plasminogen activator. Unlike streptokinase, it is *non-antigenic, non-pyrogenic and does not cause allergic reactions.* However, it lacks fibrin specificity. and is very expensive. For doses, see Table 32.8. Its use is followed by administration of heparin and still later by oral anticoagulants. It is also used to lyse fibrin or blood deposits in the anterior chamber of the eye. For this purpose, 5000 units of the enzyme in 2 ml of sterile physiological saline at pH 7.2 to 7.6 are usually instilled into the anterior chamber.

ARVIN (Ancord): Arvin is a purified enzyme obtained from the venom of the Malayan Pit Viper, *Agkistroden rhodostoma.* The enzyme :

- ***Converts fibrinogen to an imperfect fibrin polymer that breaks up easily in the circulation and is lysed.***
- ***Produces fibrinogen depletion independently of the coagulation and fibrinolytic enzyme systems.***
- ***Does not affect platelet function.***

The therapy is controlled by measuring plasma fibrinogen.

The enzyme has been used with encouraging results in the treatment of venous thrombosis. It is administered IV in the dose of 2-3 units per kg. over a period of 6-8 hours, followed by slow IV injection of 2 units/kg every 12 hours. It reduces the fibrinogen levels, the peak anticoagulant activity occurring 8 to 12 hours after its administration, and fibrinogen levels return to normal within 3 weeks after cessation of therapy. It can also be used IM/SC.

The major advantage of the enzyme appears to be that unlike the conventional anticoagulants, it does not cause a hemorrhagic tendency. However, bleeding may occur from a silent peptic ulcer or a surgical wound. Hemolytic anemia, urticaria and unilateral impairment of vision have been reported. Specific antivenom antidote is available to treat the toxicity. Resistance to the enzyme may occur due to antibody formation.

Hemostatic Agents

Bleeding can be controlled by physical methods such as application of direct pressure, tourniquet, cold and use of cautery. Drugs like desmopressin and adrenaline can be used to produce vasoconstriction. Thus, pitressin (synthetic, 8-L-Arginine vasopressin) 20 units is used by infusion to reduce the portal venous pressure, thereby reducing the bleeding from oesophageal varices in cirrhosis. Adrenaline is used in the form of nasal pack to control epistaxis.

When bleeding is the consequence of a specific defect in hemostasis such as hemophilia, the ideal treatment is to correct the defect. Such specific treatment, however, may not be possible because the bleeding may be due to multiple defects or no specific cause can be identified. Major blood loss commonly occurs during surgery, trauma and some medical conditions. In such cases nonspecific hemostatic therapy has to be employed.

Drugs used for hemostatic therapy can be classified as:

I **Agents acting locally**

II **Transfusional agents** such as specific coagulation factors

III **Nontransfusional agents,** e.g., Vitamin K and Epsilon amino-caproic acid.

I **Agents acting locally:** These agents control oozing of blood from minute vessels but are not effective in controlling bleeding from large vessels. They are:

THROMBIN: Thrombin is obtained from bovine/human plasma. It is stable as a dry powder stored between 2 to 8pC. It is, however, inactive below pH 5. Thrombin therapy is restricted to local application in oozing of blood. It has also been used, mixed with plasma, to anchor skin grafts.

THROMBOPLASTIN: Thromboplastin is a powder prepared from the acetone extracts of brain and/or lung tissue of freshly killed rabbits. It is used for determination of prothrombin time and as a local haemostatic in surgery.

FIBRIN: Fibrin obtained from human plasma is used in the dehydrated form as sheets to cover bleeding surfaces. When used in combination with a thrombin solution, it also acts as a mechanical barrier and holds thrombin in position over the bleeding area.

GEL FOAM: Gel foam is a porous, pressed form of gelatin sponge used in conjunction with thrombin to control oozing of blood from surface wounds. Gel foam is moistened with isotonic saline before use. It is completely absorbed within 4 to 6 weeks and hence, may be left in place after suturing of a wound. It is available as cones, packs, sponges and powder.

OXIDIZED CELLULOSE (Oxycel): Oxycel is surgical gauze treated with nitrogen dioxide. It promotes clotting by a reaction between hemoglobin and cellulosic acid. Oxycel, when wet with tissue juice, becomes sticky and gummy and exerts its haemostatic effect by mechanical blockage. Oxycel is usually absorbed completely within 2 to 10 days. It interferes with bone regeneration.

MICROFIBRILLAR COLLAGEN (Avitene): This hemostatic material is prepared from purified, bovine corium collagen. When applied to a bleeding surface, it attracts platelets to initiate formation of a platelet plug followed by a natural clot. Used along with manual pressure, it is effective in controlling capillary bleeding, even in patients on heparin or oral anticoagulants, and in hemophiliacs. It is non-allergenic but can promote local infection, abscess formation, and rupture of cutaneous incisions. It may conceal deep hemorrhage/hematoma in a penetrating wound. The residual unused material should be discarded. It is inactivated by autoclaving and hence should not be sterilised. Care should be taken to avoid spillage over nonbleeding surfaces, especially abdominal or thoracic viscera.

II **Transfusional agents:**

HUMAN FIBRINOGEN: Fibrinogen, a sterile fraction from human plasma, is used for restoring normal fibrinogen levels in haemorrhagic complications caused by acute afibrinogenemia. Fibrinogen and thrombin may be employed together for local haemostasis.

ANTIHAEMOPHILIC GLOBULIN (AHG): Haemophilia A and Christmas disease (haemophilia B) are the two commonest hereditary haemorrhagic states, due to deficiency of specific clotting factors VIII and IX respectively. Antihaemophilic globulin or concentrate of factor VIII (AHG) is highly effective in the treatment of classical haemophilia-A. High potency human AHG is prepared from pooled, normal, human plasma; it is now prepared by recombinant DNA technique. It is given in the dose of 15-60 units/kg. daily. Simultaneous use of fibrinolytic inhibitors like EACA can reduce the dose of AHG required. In case of non-availability of AHG, fresh plasma or blood transfusion is used. The half-life of injected factor VIII in a haemophiliac, is about 12 hours. Desmopressin (Chapter 38), which causes release of AHG from its stores, transiently increases its blood level and is helpful mild-moderate hemophilic bleeding.

Pure recombinant factor VIII, factor IX and activated factor VII (rFVII$_\alpha$) are available. They are very expensive and may be associated with a greater risk of inducing IgG antibodies to factor VIII, thus reducing the efficacy of specific therapy. rFVLL$_\alpha$ has also been used in major bleeding from surgery, trauma and other medical causes. It probably acts locally at the site of tissue injury and vascular disruption. Finally, treatment should be guided by the physician experienced in the case of hemophilia.

In patients with Christmas disease, fresh or stored plasma infusion is indicated to replenish the factor IX which is stable on storage.

PLASMA or BLOOD: Fresh frozen plasma is suitable for the treatment of most coagulation disorders, since it provides all the clotting factors. Concentrate of factor VIII (purified) and a partially purified preparation containing factors II, VII, IX and X are also available for specific deficiencies. Whole blood for replacement of coagulation factors may not be ideal as large volumes required carry the risk of transfusion reactions.

III Non-transfusional agents:

VITAMIN K: Vitamin K comprises three distinct fat soluble, naphthoquinone compounds which participate in the biosynthesis of several clotting factors. Vitamin K_1 (phytonadione) is found in several foods and is also prepared synthetically. Vitamin K_2 is produced by the bacteria in the GI tract and supplies almost 50% of the human requirements. Vitamin K_3 (menadione) is a synthetic compound used for therapeutic purposes. The diphosphate salt of menadione is water soluble.

Pharmacological actions: Vitamin K is essential for the biosynthesis of 'active' coagulation related proteins (coagulation factors). It participates in the carboxylation of the glutamic acid residues of prothrombin and factors VII, IX and X in the final stage of their synthesis (see earlier). Vitamin K is also shown to be involved in electron transport (coenzyme) and oxidative phosphorylation.

Absorption, fate and excretion: Vitamin K is produced by the flora of the human intestine. The fat soluble vitamin K_1 and K_2 are absorbed in the presence of bile salts, while the water soluble menadione salts can be absorbed even in their absence. The exact daily requirement of vitamin K is not known. Both the lipid and water soluble preparations are satisfactorily absorbed on parenteral administration.

Adverse reactions: These are rare after oral administration. However, serious anaphylactoid reactions can occur after IV use. Large doses of synthetic menadione have produced haemolytic anaemia, hyper-bilirubinemia and kernicterus in newborn, especially in premature infants. Menadione competes with bile salts for glucuronide detoxification mechanism causing the accumulation of bile salts in the blood and this results in jaundice. Haemolysis with menadione is usually seen in infants, whose erythrocytes lack the enzyme G6PD. Patients with liver disease should not be given repeated, large doses of vitamin K if the response to the initial dose is unsatisfactory.

Therapeutic uses:

- ***Adult vitamin K deficiency*** which may be produced by (a) Malabsorption syndrome or obstructive jaundice. (b) Long term intravenous feeding (prophylactic use). (c) Prolonged periods of malnutrition. Menadione may be used.
- ***Vitamin K deficiency in infants*** during acute diarrhea. Menadione may be used.
- ***Neonatal vitamin K deficiency,*** for prevention and treatment.
- ***Bleeding state during oral anticoagulant therapy.***

Vitamin K can generally be given orally but requires the presence of bile salts for its absorption, except in the case of the water soluble menadione preparation. It can also be given SC, IM or IV.

Menadione preparations are ***not*** *useful in treating oral anticoagulant induced bleeding, and may cause adverse reactions in neonates with vitamin K deficiency. They should not be used in the last weeks of pregnancy to avoid neonatal hemorrhagic disease.*

Preparations:

(i) Vitamin K_1 (Kapilin) tablets and injection for IV use. Dose: 25 mg. orally; 0.5 to 25 mg IV (not faster than 1 mg. per minute; IV route to be used only when other routes are not feasible).

(ii) Menadione (Synkavite) 5 mg. tablets. Dose 5-10 mg. daily.

(iii) Menadione sodium diphosphate (Synkavite) injection, 5 and 10 mg. per ml. Dose 5-15 mg. once or twice daily, SC, IM or IV.

EPSILON AMINO-CAPROIC ACID: (EACA, Amicar, Hemocid): This is a water soluble analogue of the amino acid lysine.

Mechanism of action: Lysine analogues reversibly occupy the lysine binding sites on plasminogen. This results in inhibition of fibrin binding to plasminogen. Activation of plasminogen to plasmin is thus inhibited. This impairs fibrinolysis with consequent stabilisation of clot.

$$H_2NCH_2(CH_2)_3CH_2\overset{O}{\overset{\|}{C}}OH$$

Fig. 32.7: Aminocaproic acid

Orally, it is rapidly absorbed; the peak level after a single dose is achieved in about 2 hours. About 60-90% of the dose is excreted in the urine within 24 hours. A blood level of 13 mg. per 100 ml. is required for plasminogen inhibition, whereas 130 mg. per 100 ml. inhibits plasmin activity.

Adverse reactions: The drug has been reported to produce minor side effects such as nasal stuffiness, abdominal discomfort, dyspepsia, hypotension, conjunctival erythema, nausea, vomiting, diarrhoea and skin rash. A rare, lethal complication is disseminated intravascular thrombosis.

Preparation and dosage: See below.

Therapeutic uses: The drug has been found to be useful in preventing the hyperplasminaemic bleeding state following the damage to tissues rich in plasmihogen activator, e.g.

- ***Primary menorrhagia*** (Chapter 65).
- ***During prostatic surgery.***
- ***Upper GI bleeding.***
- ***Bleeding following dental extraction in patients with coagulation disorders;*** and
- ***Bleeding associated with thrombocytopenia and postpartum hemmorrage.***

It is given in the dose of 100 mg/kg loading dose (upto 10 g), and 50 mg/kg (upto 5 g) 6 hourly for 2-3 days.No more than 30 g should be given in 24 hours. It is also given IV during surgery. Although the drug has been employed to control bleeding during prostetactomy, it is contraindicated in the event of hematuria because of the risk of ureteral occlusion by unlysed clot.

TRANEXAMIC ACID (TA), also a derivative of lysine, is about 10 times more potent than EACA and has a longer duration of action. It is used in the dose of 1–1.5 g 3–4 times daily. Indications are similar to those for EACA. Mouthwashes containing TA are claimed to be effective for the prevention of oral bleeding in patients with hemophilia. Adverse reactions are mild and include nausea, diarrhoea and hypotension.

Both EACA and TA are contraindicated in patients with subarachnoid bleeding because they may induce vasospasm and ischemic stroke.

ETHAMSYLATE (Ethamsyl, Dicynene) is used for similar indications as EACA and TA. It probably acts by correcting abnormal platelet adhesion. It does not stabilize fibrin. The oral dose is 500 mg four times a day.

Aprotinin : It is a polypeptide obtained from bovine lung. It inhibits the action of several proteases such as plasmin, trypsin, chymotrypsin and kallikrein by formation of reversible enzyme-inhibitor complex. Hence, aprotinin inhibits the initiation of both coagulation and fibrinolysis. The drug was used mainly during cardiac surgery to reduce blood loss. But, *because of cardiovascular toxicity it is now withdrawn.*

DESMOPRESSIN: This analogue of arginine vasopressin (Chapter 38), given IV or SC, increases for a short time the plasma concentration of factor VIII in hemophiliacs, and of von Willebrand factor, the adhesive protein that is deficient or defective, in patients with von Willebrand disease. Demopressin is considered a treatment of choice for patients with mild hemophillia-A or type I von Willebrand disease. It shortens or normalises the bleeding time in patients with congenital defects of platelet function. It has also been found of some use in acquired bleeding disorders such as during uremia, and following drugs like aspirin. It has no role in the treatment of Hemophillia B, which is caused by factor IX deficiency. Adverse effects are mild and include headache, water retention and hyponatremia.

The major risk involved in using agents that potentiate hemostasis is thrombotic complications.

CONJUGATED ESTROGENS (Chapter 65): Given IV in the dose of 0.6 mg/kg, daily, they improve platelet function, shorten the prolonged bleeding time, and reduce or stop bleeding in uremic patients. Compared to desmopressin, they have a delayed onset but much longer duration of action on bleeding time. They can be combined with desmopressin for synergistic effect. They have been used daily for 5-7 days with hardly any adverse reaction.

VITAMIN C : Vitamin C (50-100 mg tid) specifically controls bleeding due to scurvy.

SNAKE VENOMS: Snake venoms, especially Russel Viper and Copper Head snake venoms, enhance coagulation by stimulating thrombokinase.

Sclerosing Agents

Sclerosing agents are irritating substances employed to obliterate varicose veins. They have also been employed for sclerosing esophageal varices and uncomplicated piles.

The important preparations are:

- ***Sodium tetradecyl sulfate*** is an anionic detergent, marketed as 0.5-3.0% solution: given IV as 0.5-1.0 ml at upto 4 sites.
- ***Ethoxy skleral*** (3%) in 5% aqueous ethanol (Polidocanol), a nonionic detergent.
- ***Phenol***, 5% in vegetable oil, in the dose of 2 - 3 ml, given into the submucosal layer at the base of each pile; maximum total dose 10 ml at any one time.
- ***Sodium linoleate.*** The dose varies from 0.5 to 5 ml. by intravenous route, locally.
- ***Ethanolamine oleate*** 5%. Dose: 2-5 ml. divided between 3-4 sites.
- ***Sodium morrhuate*** 1-2 ml of 5% solution per site. Total 15-25 ml at one sitting.

Drugs Effective in Iron Deficiency and Other Related Anemias 33

Anemia is one of the most common disorder in clinical practice. It is characterized by a decrease in the oxygen carrying capacity of the blood. The oxygen carrying capacity is determined by the haemoglobin content of the erythrocytes. Hence, a reduction in the blood haemoglobin level and in the number of circulating erythrocytes are the hallmarks of anemia.

Erythropoiesis: The erythrocytes are produced in the bone marrow and are destroyed by the reticuloendothelial system. The maturation of erythrocytes occurs through several stages. The precursor cell in the bone marrow is the proerythroblast or haemocytoblast, which is subsequently converted to early, intermediate and late normoblast. The nucleus of the late normoblast becomes pyknotic along with the appearance of a reticulum in the cytoplasm, resulting in the formation of a reticulocyte. It takes the reticulocyte approximately 4 days to mature into a normal erythrocyte. The normal life span of a human erythrocyte is roughly 110 to 120 days.

Various factors such as oxygen lack, vitamin C, growth hormone and thyroxine stimulate erythropoiesis. The red cell mass is continually adjusted to the optimum quantity for its function as an oxygen carrier by messages transmitted to the bone marrow from an oxygen sensor in the kidneys. These messages are mediated by a glycoprotein hormone, **erythropoietin (EP)**, produced by the kidneys. Deficiency of dietary factors such as iron, folic acid and vitamin B_{12}, and of EP disturbs the normal erythropoiesis resulting in anemia.

Anemias may, thus, be classified according to their etiology:

I **Anemias due to dietary deficiency or malabsorption of factors essential for normal blood formation,** e.g., Iron, Folic acid, Vitamin B_{12}, Vitamin C, and Pyridoxine.

II **Anemias due to blood loss** such as menorrhagia, GI loss and hookworm infestation.

III **Anemias due to excessive blood destruction,** e.g., thalassemia, sickle cell anemia and autoimmune haemolytic anemia.

IV **Anemias due to aplasia or hypoplasia of the bone marrow,** such as idiopathic or following certain drugs such as anticancer drugs and chloramphenicol.

V **Anemia due to deficiencies of erythropoietin** as in chronic renal disease.

VI **Anemias of uncertain origin,** e.g., due to chronic infections, rheumatoid arthritis, liver disease and cancer.

Iron Metabolism

Iron deficiency anemia is caused by deficient synthesis of hemoglobin of which iron is an essential constituent. Iron is present in every cell in the body. The total iron content of the body varies between 2 and 3 gm. depending upon the body weight and hemoglobin level. There is a difference between men and women. In adult males the iron content is estimated to be about 50 mg. per kg. body weight as compared to only 35 mg. per kg. body weight in adult females. The body iron is distributed as:

- ***Heme***, in hemoglobin, myoglobin, and in cytochrome oxidase and other enzymes.
- ***Iron bound to protein,*** without heme formation, as the storage compounds, water soluble ferritin and insoluble hemosiderin; and
- ***Transport iron*** bound to transferrin.

Hemoglobin has an iron-containing moiety, metalloporphyrin or heme, combined with the protein globin. The molecular weight of hemoglobin is 64,500. Porphyrin consisting of 4 pyrrole rings and the protein globin are both synthesized in the body. About 2/3rds of the total body iron is in the form of hemoglobin.

Myoglobin is the heme protein of skeletal and cardiac muscle with molecular weight 16,800.

Parenchymal iron exists as a component of various cellular enzymes. Many iron compounds in the body are not related to erythropoiesis. Some are concerned with tissue respiration while others are linked to metabolic enzymes.

Iron absorption: The amount of iron available from food depends upon its iron content as well as absorbability which differs with different foods. Iron from animal foods is better absorbed than that from vegetable foods. Heme iron is by far the most available (20-40%) and its absorption is independent of the food composition. However, non-heme fraction represents by far the largest amount in a vegetarian diet. Green vegetables, peas and beans, bananas, spinach, some cereals, egg yolk, meat and liver are rich in iron.

The mean absorption of iron from vegetable foods ranges from 1% for rice, 5% for wheat to 6% for soyabeans, while for animal foods it ranges from 11% for fish, 12% for hemoglobin to 13% for liver. *Milk and milk products are a poor source of iron.* Use of iron cooking utensils increases the iron content of food. Absorption of inorganic iron salts can occur from any part of the GI tract; however, there exists an absorption gradient, decreasing from the duodenum to colon. Maximum iron absorption occurs in the duodenum.

Mechanism of iron absorption: The iron is absorbed via the brush borders of the intestinal lining cells. The absorption depends as much on its form as on its absolute amount. Two mechanisms for iron absorption have been postulated. These are:

- ***An active transport process*** which actively transports iron from intestinal lumen to mucosal cells with the help of a carrier protein. The absorption of iron is probably controlled by the availability of apoferritin, a protein present in the mucosal cells. The absorbed iron combines with apoferritin to form ferritin and is stored and released into blood as Fe^{+++} as per body needs. When apoferritin gets fully saturated to ferritin, no more iron is absorbed. Thus, in normal individuals the body is protected from possible excessive absorption of the metal. This regulation by the mucosa, however, is relative and partial.

Iron deficiency, decreased iron stores and accelerated erythropoiesis due to any cause increase iron absorption. It is less influenced by plasma iron level.

Within the mucosal cells, iron exists as:

(1) Mobile iron - Fe^{+++} and

(2) Storage iron - ferritin.

In iron replete subjects, most of the iron fails to pass through the mucosal cells but becomes bound to apoferritin to form ferritin. This intracellular ferritin is eventually excreted during desquamation of the epithelial cells, as a part of the regular shedding of the intestinal mucosa. In iron deficiency, however, the amount of apoferritin synthesized is reduced and iron passes through the cells into the blood.

- ***A passive transport process,*** by which iron diffuses across the intestinal villi, perhaps in combination with amino acids such as glycine and serine, has been described. This mechanism probably operates primarily at doses of iron exceeding the amounts in a normal diet.

Factors affecting iron absorption:

- ***Type of iron*:** In man, food iron must be reduced from ferric to ferrous form before it is absorbed. This reduction begins in the stomach and continues in the small intestine. Ionisation of food iron takes place in the stomach under the influence of gastric acid, pH lower than 5 being essential for adequate ionization. Hypochlorhydria may thus reduce the amount of iron absorbed from the food. However, iron deficiency is not common in pernicious anemia, where achlorhydria is characteristic. Heme iron present in animal foods is absorbed better than non-heme iron. Ferric hydroxide iron complexes present in the vegetarian foods are absorbed poorly.
- ***Reducing agents present in the diet,*** such as ascorbate, succinate, and the SH groups of amino acids like cysteine, and proteins convert ferric iron to ferrous form and help the iron absorption.
- ***A diet poor in phosphorus*** enhances iron absorption, while phytates and organic phosphates (as in vegetarian foods) interfere with iron absorption by forming insoluble and unabsorbable complexes. Wheat is rich in phytates and consequently only about 5 per cent of wheat iron is absorbed, which increases to only about 7 per cent during iron deficiency. Egg iron is strongly complexed to the phosphate of yolk phosphoproteins and is poorly absorbed.
- ***Antacids*** such as calcium carbonate, aluminium hydroxide and magnesium hydroxide reduce iron absorption.
- ***Other drugs*** like tetracycline, levodopa, fluroquinolones, captopril, biphosphonate and thyroxine interfere with iron absorption.
- ***Administration of iron along with or after food reduces its absorption.*** However, in practice, ferrous salts are usually administered after food to minimize gastric irritation.
- ***Pancreatic secretion has an inhibitory effect on iron*** absorption and prevents iron overload. In severe chronic pancreatitis and liver cirrhosis, iron absorption is greatly increased. Pyridoxine deficiency also enhances iron absorption despite elevated plasma iron levels.
- ***Iron deficiency accelerates iron absorption.*** Individuals with iron deficiency absorb 20 to 30 per cent of the food iron (compared to 5-10% in normals), while the absorption of iron in organic form (vegetables and meat) is approximately doubled, and that of inorganic iron is increased 5 to 6 fold.
- ***Pica*** **:** Iron deficiency can promote appetite for bizarre foods (pica). If clay is consumed (geophagia), there occurs chelation of iron in the gut, worsening the iron deficiency.
- ***GI Disorders:*** Partial gastrectomy and extensive bowel surgery reduce absorption of food iron. Absorption of inorganic iron salts, however, is less impaired. Cachexia, infectious diseases and malabsorption syndrome reduce iron absorption.

Hepcidine, an iron-regulatory peptide, plays an important negative role in iron absorption. It is 'an acute phase protein', and in acute and chronic inflammatory diseases and cancer, hepcidine synthesis by the liver increases. It inhibits iron transport accross the cell membranes, and reduces the GI absorption of dietary iron as well as iron storage. Anemia of chronic inflammation is usually associated with hypoferrimia and low transferrin saturation. Such patients respond poorly to oral iron.

Iron transport and utilisation: After absorption, iron circulates in the blood bound to a beta globulin fraction, siderophilin or **transferrin.** Transferrin present in the plasma and the extravascular space serves to transport iron from the sites of absorption and storage to the sites of its intracellular utilization. In iron deficiency, increased number of transferrin receptors increase the cellular iron uptake. The liver parenchymal cells are the major site of transferrin synthesis.

Transferrin is normally one-third saturated with iron. Plasma iron is normally in equilibrium with iron stores. The normal plasma iron level varies between 66-146 mcg./100 ml. The plasma iron level and plasma unsaturated binding capacity are modified by:

(a) Iron deficiency which is associated with a reduction in serum iron levels and an increase in iron binding capacity.

(b) Haemochromatosis which is associated with high serum iron levels and reduced binding capacity. A similar picture is seen in pernicious and aplastic anemias; and

(c) Acute and chronic infections which are generally associated with reduced serum iron and decreased binding capacity (see later).

The **labile iron pool** is that part of body iron which is readily available for utilization for haemoglobin synthesis. Iron quickly enters this pool after absorption from the intestine, after release from the RBC breakdown and following an injection. If the amount entering this labile pool is in excess of needs, then it is transferred into **storage pool.**

The daily iron turnover has been estimated to be approximately 35 mg. The major contribution to this, 21 mg., comes from the normal red cell destruction; iron thus released is reutilised. About 11 mg. of iron is contributed by that fraction which is not used for hemoglobin production during its stay in the marrow while the remaining 2-3 mg. comes from the storage sites, intestinal absorption and the ECF.

From these 35 mg. of iron, about 32 mg. enter the 'erythropoietic labile pool', a poorly defined compartment, primarily in the bone, for erythropoiesis. Approximately 1 mg. of iron goes for storage and into the ECF each, and about 1 mg. is excreted, mainly in urine and sweat.

Iron transfer to maturing erythrocytes (erythron) occurs mainly by release from transferrin to specific receptor sites on the membrane of the erythrocyte precursors. The insertion of iron into the porphyrin ring to form heme is now considered to be controlled by enzymes situated in the cell mitochondria. Failure of this process causes 'sideroachrestic anemias'. The anemias of lead poisoning and of thalassemia are of this type. In such cases iron granules are seen in the cytoplasm of erythroblasts.

Iron storage: About 30 per cent of the total body iron is in the form of storage iron. This amount is vital, since iron deficiency anemia does not appear until the stores are largely depleted. Iron is stored predominantly in the form of ferritin and hemosiderin in bone marrow, liver, spleen and other areas with prominent reticuloendothelial components. Hemosiderin is probably a polymer of ferritin but unlike ferritin, it is not soluble in water. Conversion of iron to ferritin in the body is rapid, the normal stores being 0.5 to 1.5g. Both ferritin and hemosiderin are available for heme synthesis.

The concentration of ferritin is normally directly related to body iron stores. *Serum ferritin measurement, therefore, can be used to evaluate body iron stores.* Usually 1 mcg/1. of serum ferritin corresponds to 8 mg. of storage iron.

Iron excretion: Iron is tenaciously conserved. The body iron is regulated mostly by regulation of iron absorption by the gut. The total iron excreted daily is 0.5 to 1 mg. via :

- ***Intestine***: Iron is excreted in the faeces with the exfoliation of the villous cells. Iron is also lost by desquamation of the skin and hair.
- ***Bile and sweat***: Traces of iron are lost in bile and sweat. However, in tropical climate like in India, sweat may be a major channel of iron loss and amounts as high as 2 to 3 mg. may be excreted daily in sweat.
- ***Urine*** : Urinary iron excretion is 0.1 mg. daily but may increase with proteinuria or iron overload.
- ***Menstrual blood*** : One ml of blood contains 0.5mg of iron and the iron loss due to menstruation, spread evenly over the 28 days of the cycle, is 0.3 to 0.6 mg. per day.
- ***Milk:*** Upto 1.5 mg. appears in milk daily during lactation.

Iron requirements and sources: Table 33.1 gives the daily iron requirements. Vegetable foods rich in iron (containing 10 mg of iron per 100 g.) include cereals like bajra, rice bran, whole wheat flour, pulses like Bengal gram, many leafy vegetables, condiments like turmeric

Table 33.1: Daily dietary iron requirements*

- ***Children*** 8-18 mg.
- ***Adult men*** 10-15 mg.
- ***Menstruating women*** 15-20 mg.**
- ***Pregnant and lactating women*** 20-25 mg.***

*	Based on 5-10% absorption of food iron.
**	Based on the monthly loss of 50 ml. of blood (= 25 mg. of iron).
***	Based on the fetal accumulation of 200-400 mg. of iron and loss during child birth.

and tamarind pulp and jaggery. The iron content of milk is so poor (0.2 mg.%) that an infant fed on cow's milk alone would need 10 litres of milk daily to get its daily requirement of iron! Among the non-vegetarian foods, egg yolk, crab muscle, meat, liver and heart are rich in iron.

Preparations and dosage: Table 33.2 lists the commonly used iron salts for oral use.

(i) Dried ferrous sulfate tablet 200 mg.

(ii) Ferrous sulfate syrup. 60 mg. of ferrous sulfate (12 mg. of iron) in 5 millilitres.

(iii) Ferrous sulfate paediatric drops for infants contain 125 mg. of ferrous sulfate (25 mg. of iron) in each millilitre.

(iv) Ferrous gluconate 300 mg. tablets. Elixir of ferrous gluconate 36 mg. of iron per 5 ml.

(v) Ferrous fumarate: 200 mg. tablets.

(vi) Iron and ammonium citrate is a scaly ferric preparation soluble in water and is administered in the form of a mixture in the dose of 2 g. three times a day.

(vii) Ferric hydroxide polymaltose complex (100mg of elemental iron per tablet). This is an expensive preparation which offers hardly any advantage. Therapeutic failures have been reported with this preparation.

Therapeutic uses: Iron should generally be administered orally. Many iron preparations are marketed but there is little to recommend them over the cost effective ferrous sulfate. Sustained release and enteric coated iron preparations are generally poorly dissolved in the gastric and intestinal secretions, and may be lost in the feces.

Indications for iron therapy are summarised in Table 33.3.

As iron deficiency develops, iron stores diminish, as reflected by reduced and later absent stainable iron, hemosiderin. The most sensitive diagnostic test for detection of early or mild iron deficiency is the iron staining of the bone marrow. In fact, prelatent iron deficiency is characterized by the absence of stainable iron in the bone marrow, increased iron absorption but no decrease in either serum iron or hemoglobin concentration.

The iron deficiency anemia is characterised by the presence of small erythrocytes (microcytosis) poorly filled with hemoglobin

Table 33.2: Iron preparations for oral therapy

Preparation	Therapeutic * dose mg./day	Total iron content mg.	Per cent utilisation of iron
Exsiccated ferrous sulfate	600	180	15
Ferrous gluconate	900	108	11
Ferrous fumarate	600	198	15
Iron and ammonium citrate	6000	1200	1.5 to 3
Ferrous succinate	300	105	-

1 to 3 and 5 given either as tablets or in liquid form; 4 given only in liquid form.
* Prophylactic dose 1/3rd or less.

Table 33.3 : Indications for iron therapy

Prophylactic: Pregnancy; infancy; rapidly growing children; menstruating women; professional blood donors; following partial gastrectomy.

Therapeutic: i. e. to treat existing iron deficiency anemia.

- ***Nutritional deficiency*** due to deficient intake or decreased absorption.
- ***Anemia of pregnancy, infancy, prematurity and prolonged breast feeding.***
- ***Anemia due to acute or chronic blood loss*** as in menorrhagia, peptic ulcer and hook-worm infestation. (Blood loss of 100 ml. corresponds to a loss of 50 mg. of iron)

(hypochromia) and many cells of bizarre shapes (poikilocytosis) and variable sizes (anisocytosis). All hypochromic anemias, however, are not due to iron deficiency. There is now considerable evidence available that the metabolic importance of iron extends far beyond the red cell. *Even in the absence of anemia, iron deficiency can produce adverse effects on brain function and abnormalities in behaviour; mental performance in children with iron deficiency improves after iron therapy. Rule out thalassemia trait before starting long term iron therapy unless the cause of iron deficiency (e.g. bleeding) is obvious.*

The aims of treatment of iron deficiency anemia are:

- ***Correction of hemoglobin.***
- ***Correction of the underlying cause; and***
- ***Building up body iron stores.***

Evidence to show that any one of the oral iron preparations is superior to others in raising the hemoglobin level or in reducing the ADR is lacking. Ferrous sulphate is the cheapest iron preparation, and is to be preferred. Tablets are more convenient than fluid preparations; further, they do not blacken the teeth and the tongue. The fluid preparations, however, are preferred in children and in the presence of dysphagia and peptic ulcer.

The great majority of patients do not experience any significant adverse effects with 200 mg. of dry ferrous sulfate three times daily after food. Absorption of ferrous sulfate in the usual therapeutic dose varies from 20 to 50 per cent in iron deficient patients. Dose should be increased at weekly intervals to reduce G.I. disturbances. If it is not tolerated, the dose should be reduced or other preparations such as ferrous gluconate or ferrous fumarate may be tried.

During pregnancy, women should receive oral iron supplements (equivalent to 100 mg. of elemental iron daily) prophylactically from the fourth month onwards and this should be continued during the lactation period.

Prophylactic iron therapy is also advocated for infants and children, more so in those with low birth weights, the average daily dose of ferrous sulfate varies from 100 to 200 mg.

Professional blood donors should receive routinely 300 mg. of ferrous sulfate daily for 1 month after each donation of 500 ml.

Following oral iron, normal hemoglobin level is usually attained within 1 to 3 months, depending mainly on the initial hemoglobin level. It is important, however, to continue with the therapy for 12-20 weeks after the hemoglobin level has returned to normal, in order to replenish the depleted iron stores.

The response to iron therapy is quite predictable. The **reticulocyte count** in the peripheral blood begins to rise within a week, reaches a peak at 10 to 14 days and returns to normal after about 3 weeks. Reticulocyte response is more striking in children than in adults; however, in children with hemoglobin more than 7.5 g. per cent and in adults, the rise in hemoglobin level may be the only indication of response to iron therapy.

The response to oral iron is considered satisfactory when the hemoglobin level increases by about 1.5 g./100 ml. of blood) within three weeks. Most patients respond to oral therapy satisfactorily if iron is taken regularly and it is absorbed. Table 33.4 lists the causes of failure of oral iron therapy.

Table 33.4 : Causes of failure of oral iron therapy

- Incorrect diagnosis.
- Non-compliance.
- Continued loss of blood .
- Defective iron absorption.
- Superimposed infection or inflammation; and
- Underlying uremia or malignancy.

Adverse reactions to oral iron: All iron preparations are probably equally toxic per unit mass of soluble iron. They produce mild GI disturbances characterised by colicky pain, nausea, vomiting, diarrhoea or constipation, and gastric distress in about 6 to 12 per cent of individuals. These disturbances can be minimised by giving iron with food and by a gradual increase in the dosage. The daily dose should not exceed six 200 mg. tablets of exsiccated ferrous sulfate (180 mg of elementary iron). Iron administered in liquid form may combine with sulfide ions in the mouth forming black iron sulfide which causes blackening of teeth; this can be avoided by using a straw for drinking. Oral iron invariably makes the faeces black due to iron sulfide; this may interfere with detection of occult blood in the stools with old tests, but not by newer tests.

Acute iron poisoning is rare in adults but is not uncommon in children and infants. Doses of 1 g. or more of ferrous sulfate are considered toxic in children. Ingestion of large doses of iron is associated with severe GI irritation resulting in hematemesis, vomiting, diarrhoea, cardiovascular collapse and shock. Death may occur within 12 to 48 hours. Some may develop jaundice, hypoglycemia and convulsions. Even if recovery occurs, sequelae such as GI obstruction may prove troublesome. *Every patient should be warned to keep the tablets away from children who may mistake them for sweets.*

Indications for parenteral iron: It must be emphasized that *response to oral or parenteral iron preparations is essentially similar, with average daily hemoglobin rise of about 0.2 g%.* Hence, parenteral therapy is used only under special circumstances (Table 33.5).

Table 33.5: Indications for parenteral iron therapy

- Failure to absorb adequate amounts of oral iron e.g. malabsorption or extensive bowel resection.
- Inability to tolerate oral iron
- Ulcerative colitis, colostomy and intestinal shunts.
- Depleted iron stores as in patients with chronic bleeding, in whom the average daily iron loss equals or exceeds absorption of iron from oral iron preparations.
- When the patient cannot be relied upon to take oral iron medication.

Parenteral iron preparations used are :

For IM use:

(i) Iron-dextran (Imferon) : 15 ml vial, 50 mg of *elemental* iron/ml.

(ii) Iron-Sorbitol-Citric acid complex (Jectocos) : 1.5 ml vial, 50 mg of iron/ml.

For IV use:

(i) High molecular weight iron dextran (Imferon), 1-2 ml vial, 50 mg iron/ml

(ii) Low molecular iron dextran (Cosmofer) 2ml vial, 50 mg of iron /ml

(iii) Iron saccharate (Ferric hydroxide complexed with sucrose), 5ml vial, 20 mg of iron/ml

(iv) Ferric gluconate, 5 ml vial, 12.5 mg iron/ml

The dose is calculated on the basis that 25 mg. of elemental iron are needed to correct 1% deficit of hemoglobin by Sahli's method. To this dose is added half of the calculated amount for replenishing body iron stores.

Iron dextran and iron sorbitol citric acid complex are the two commonly used preparations. They are injected deep into the upper and outer quadrant of the buttock. The injection is made by 'Z' technique, pulling the skin and subcutaneous tissue to one side before entering the muscle to avoid leakage and skin staining. After an initial test dose of 25 mg., 100 mg. are given daily or every few days till the total calculated dose is administered. A single dose should not exceed 25 mg. for infants, 50 mg. for children and 100 mg. for adults.

Iron sorbisol is rapidly absorbed into the blood, and saturates transferrin. It is mostly stored in the liver and bone marrow. Excess, unbound fraction is excreted in the urine.

Mobilization of iron dextran from IM injection site varies from 50-90 per cent. Iron dextran, unlike iron sorbitol citric acid, does not saturate transferrin rapidly. It is absorbed from the muscle via the lymphatics and is converted by hepatic parenchymal cells into ferritin which in turn releases iron for hemoglobin synthesis.

Utilization of IV iron is 70 to 100 per cent. The initial dose of IV iron preparations is usually 20 to 30 mg. of iron (1-1.5 ml.). It is gradually increased to 100 to 200 mg. (5-10 ml.) and repeated daily, till the total dose is given. Excess unbound iron is excreted in urine.

Intravenous infusion of total dose of iron dextran in 500 ml 5 per cent glucose or normal saline, given over 3-4 hours has been reported; the drug concentration in the infusion must not exceed 5 per cent. The initial rate of the infusion is 10 drops per minute. If no ill effects are seen over 30 minutes, the rate may be increased to 30-40 drops. The IV administration of prednisolone before and after the infusion decreases the incidence of myalgias and arthralgias. Although a satisfactory response is obtained, there is no evidence to indicate that the response is more rapid than that obtained by other conventional methods. The incidence of severe adverse reactions varies from 1 to 6 per cent and hospitalization is essential. The incidence is claimed to be much less with low molecular weight dextran-iron preparations. The merit of IV therapy is that the patient gets the required iron in one dose and the iron stores may be rapidly restored, which would take months to achieve by the oral route.

As there are reports of abnormalities in the offspring of animals given large single doses of iron dextran parenterally, *the preparation is contraindicated in early pregnancy.* However, IV iron dextran seems to be safe during late pregnancy.

Alternatively, ferric gluconate or iron saccharose is used in repeated IV boluses in the dose of 100-200 mg of elemental iron. Doses larger than 100 mg may be diluted in normal saline and infused over 30 minutes. Lower doses can be injected slowly over 2 minutes. Prior test dose or medication is not needed. These preparations are not preferred for total dose infusion because they may cause dose-dependent GI or vasoactive reactions at doses above 200 mg.

Parenteral and oral iron preparations should not be administered concomitantly.

Adverse reactions to parenteral iron:

- ***IM preparations*** cause local pain, permanent skin discoloration and local inflammation and regional lymphadenopathy. The systemic toxicity which may develop within 10 minutes of injection includes headache, fever, myalgia, arthralgia, backache, tachycardia, flushing, haemolysis and circulatory collapse. These effects are probably due to excessive amounts of free iron in the plasma. Iron sorbitol, in addition, may cause disorientation and temporary loss of taste.

- ***With IV therapy***, the systemic reactions are similar to those observed following IM iron. Anaphylactoid reactions can occur within the first few minutes of administration. Severe chest pain, respiratory distress and circulatory collapse have been reported. In general, local inflammatory reactions are much less frequent with IV than with IM iron. Extravasation into the subcutaneous tissue can cause abscess formation.

- The urine of a person on iron sorbitol therapy turns black on standing, probably due to conversion of excreted iron into iron sulfide and the patient should be warned about this effect.

Treatment of Iron Poisoning

Acute Oral Iron Poisoning:

(a) Milk and egg yolk mixture is administered to bind the iron.

(b) Desferrioxamine 1-2 g IM is administered.

(c) Gastric lavage with water containing desferrioxamine is given initially, followed by 5-10 g of the same in 100 ml of water being left in the stomach to adsorb any more iron. If desferrioxamine is not available, calcium disodium edetatae 35-40 mg/kg may be used.

(d) An IV infusion of desferrioxamine (see below).

(e) Early replacement of body fluids and electrolytes using isotonic saline, correction of metabolic acidosis and hypotension by using ringer lactate and vasopressor agents, respectively, are indicated.

(f) Diazepam may be necessary to control convulsions.

DESFERRIOXAMINE MESYLATE (Desferal): This compound, obtained from *Streptomyces pilosus*, is a potent and specific chelator of iron. It readily binds ferric iron to form ferrioxamine, a stable and water soluble chelate. Ferrioxamine is excreted 2/3 in the urine and 1/3 in the bile. It colours the urine reddish brown. Desferrioxamine also removes iron from hemosiderin except that in the bone marrow; desferrioxamine 100 mg. binds 8.5 mg. of iron.

The drug is generally well tolerated. Rapid IV injection can produce hypotension, tachycardia and anaphylactoid reactions and urticaria. Allergic reactions and cataract formation are known to occur during its chronic administration for iron storage diseases. It is contraindicated in patients with severe renal disease or anuria, and in pregnant women. It is available as lyophilized powder (500 mg.) and is administered by IV infusion or IM.

Therapeutic uses:

- ***Acute iron intoxication***: In severe cases (in shock), the drug is administered by IV infusion: 10-15 mg./kg./hour to a maximum of 80 mg./kg. in 24 hours. In less severe cases (without shock), it is given in the dose of 1-2 g. every 3-12 hours; maximum dose 6 g. in 24 hours. In less severe cases (without shock), it is given IM in the dose of 40 mg./kg. every 4-2 hours.
- ***Hemochromatosis***: Desferrioxamine is useful in the *prevention and treatment* of iron overload in patients with chronic anemia such as in thalassemia major treated with multiple transfusions. In these patients, it is administered by continuous IV infusion in the dose of 2 g. over a period of 12 hours once daily. Concomitant oral administration of ascorbic acid (0.5 to 1 g. twice a day) improves its action.

The drug is less effective than phlebotomy in primary (genetic) hemochromatosis, but may be used when phlebotomy is contraindicated.

Deferiprone: This is an orally effective iron chelator which, though less effective than desferrioxamine, is an alternative to it in patients who refuse to use the latter because of its complex administration or cannot afford its high cost. It can cause blood dyscrasias, especially neutropenia. It is under evaluation.

Deferasirox (Exjade, Desirox): This oral, selective iron chelator is given once daily. The drug-iron complex is excreted in the feces. Its uses are similar to those of desferrioxime. It is under evaluation.

Adjuvants to Iron Therapy

Various substances claimed to enhance the efficacy of iron are vitamin C, cobalt, copper, zinc and manganese. Vitamin C may increase the iron absorption but it is not necessary to use costly iron preparations incorporating vitamin C to achieve this effect. Copper is said to mobilize iron from storage, while cobalt is claimed to stimulate erythropoietin production. Cobalt is potentially toxic. Angina, goitre and CHF are some of the adverse effects reported with the use of cobaltous chloride. The therapeutic value of these supplements in the treatment of iron deficiency anemia is doubtful. However, nutritional iron defficiency is commonly associated with folate defficiency and folic acid is combined with iron with beneficial effects.

In the treatment of pure iron-deficiency anemia, *the use of expensive pills containing several minerals and vitamins along with iron is unnecessary and wasteful.*

Anemia of Chronic Disease (ACD)

ACD occurs in patients with chronic infections (tuberculosis), inflammatory diseases (rheumatoid arthritis), cancer and trauma. It is usually moderate in degree. Hypoferremia in the presence of bone marrow iron overload is a constant feature. The presence of hypoferrimia and microcytosis may confuse it with iron deficiency anemia. In ACD, there is deficient delivery of iron to the developing RBCs. *This anemia does not respond to iron therapy.* ACD may respond to erythropoietin.

Erythropoietin (EP) and Anemia

Anemia is an almost invariable feature of chronic renal failure. The critical defect is probably inadequate secretion of erythropoietin, the major hormonal regulator of red cell production, produced by the kidney. Recombinant human erythropoietin is now available.

ERYTHROPOIETIN (Epoetin a and b) has molecular weight about 36,000. It is a glycoprotein hormone mainly synthesized by the kidney in response to hypoxemia. Some amount of erythropoietin is also produced by the liver, which is its important source to maintain erythropoiesis in patients who are anephric or have degenerated kidneys.

Thyroxine, growth hormone, prolactin, testosterone, $beta_2$ adrenergic agonists, PG's and angiotensin II stimulate erythropoietin production, while alkylating agents, estrogens and beta-adrenergic blocking drugs inhibit it.

Commercial recombinant DNA-EP has the same amino acid sequence as the natural human erythropoietin. Given IV, it has a plasma t/2 of 6-8 hours. The target cell for erythropoietin is the early erythroid colony forming unit. It is metabolised primarily in the liver.

Adverse reactions are aggravation of hypertension, associated with a too-rapid rise in hematocrit, increased viscocity, stroke and an increased tendency to blocking of vascular access in dialysis patients. The drug appears to be non-immunogenic and causes no significant allergic reaction.

Therapeutic uses:

- ***Anaemia of end stage renal failure***: It is a normochromic, normocytic, hypoproliferative anaemia. The IV or SC administration of erythropoietin causes in a dose dependent rise in the hematocrit and eliminates the need for transfusions. Most patients respond to a dose of 35-80 i.u./kg. three times a week, which is needed to maintain the lowest hemoglobin level required to avoid blood transfusion. Correction of co-existing iron deficiency should be done before erythropoietin therapy.
- ***Anemia in premature babies.***
- ***To permit the autologous blood transfusion*** : Injection of 600 IU/kg of erythropoietin thrice a week makes it possible both to donate more blood and to maintain higher hematocrit at the time of elective surgery in an individual.

Patients with aplastic anemia, hematologic cancers and severe hemolytic anemia usually have high erythropoietin levels and are unlikely to be benefited by exogenous erythropoietin.

Darbepoietin is a long acting, r-DNA synthetic analogue of epoietin. Its properties and uses are similar to those of epoietin. It can be injected once a week.

Drugs Effective in Megaloblastic Anemias and Neutropenia

34

The story of megaloblastic anemias really began in the middle of the nineteenth century when Thomson Addison, a physician from Guy's Hospital, London, described pernicious (deadly) anemia, so designated because of its fatal outcome. The brilliant discovery by Minot and Murphy in 1926, demonstrating the dramatic effectiveness of liver preparations in pernicious anemia, forms one of the landmarks in the history of therapeutics. This was followed by the work of Castle (1932) who postulated the hypothesis that 'an intrinsic factor' from the normal human gastric juice reacts with 'an extrinsic factor' in the food to produce 'antipernicious anemia principle'. Crystalline vitamin B_{12} was isolated from the liver in 1948 and soon after, the 'extrinsic' factor and 'antipernicious anemia principle' in Castle's hypothesis were shown to be vitamin B_{12}. Another anti-anemic factor from the liver, useful in macrocytic anemia of pregnancy, was isolated in 1943 and identified as pteroyl-monoglutamic acid, which turned out to be the same as 'folic acid' described by Mitchel and co-workers in 1941 and so named because of its isolation from the leafy vegetable, spinach.

Megaloblastic anemia : Megaloblastic anemias are characterised by the presence of abnormally large, nucleated, red cell precursors, known as megaloblasts, in the bone marrow. A megaloblast is viewed as an example of the unbalanced growth between the cytoplasm and the nucleus due to defective synthesis of nucleoproteins. In almost 95 per cent of the cases with megaloblastic bone marrow, vitamin B_{12} and/or folic acid deficiency is present.

Although folic acid and vitamin B_{12} influence different metabolic pathways in the synthesis of nucleoproteins, the final result of deficiency of either of these is defective DNA (deoxyribonucleic acid) synthesis. Since DNA is present in every cell, the basic abnormality affects all proliferating cells such as those in buccal cavity, tongue and GI tract leading to glossitis, stomatitis and intestinal malabsorption. Other organs affected include the cervical and vaginal squamous epithelium, the ovary and testes. The precursors of white cells (giant metamyelocytes) and those of platelets show abnormal mitotic activity. These abnormally large cells give rise to abnormally large offsprings that appear in the peripheral blood, which shows fully hemoglobinized (hyperchromic), large, red cells called macrocytes, polymorphonuclear leucocytes with hypersegmented nuclei and giant platelets. The anemia is thus described as 'macrocytic hyperchromic'. Such abnormal cells have a shortened life span and may undergo early hemolysis, which sometimes gives rise to associated jaundice. The anemia is also associated with pancytopenia (leucopenia, neutropenia and thrombocytopenia). Vitamin B_{12} deficiency causes damage to myelin in peripheral nerves, spinal cord and brain. With folate deficiency, the loss of body weight is much more marked and nervous instability may be present; but, the damage to the myelin is doubtful.

Although the megaloblastic anemia due to vitamin B_{12} and/or folic acid deficiency produces peripheral macrocytosis, not all the macrocytic anemias are megaloblastic. Thus, the macrocytic anemias due to liver disease, myxedema, following certain hemolytic states, and leukemias usually have normoblastic bone marrow; these obviously do not respond to vitamin B_{12} and/or folic acid.

Physiological role of Vitamin B_{12} and folic acid: Physiologically, both these vitamins are closely related and play an important role in the synthesis of DNA and RNA. The deficiency picture produced by both is clinically indistinguishable except that the neurological disturbances are commoner with vitamin B_{12} deficiency than with folic acid deficiency; the peripheral blood picture and bone marrow changes are also similar and only certain special tests and blood levels of these vitamins give the correct clue about the precise diagnosis.

Small 'physiological' doses of either folic acid or vitamin B_{12} will selectively improve the blood picture only in those persons suffering from a deficiency of the particular vitamin being administered; large 'pharmacologic' doses of either vitamin, however, will cause a hematological response irrespective of the type of deficiency, vitamin B_{12} or folic acid or both.

Although it is believed that folate deficiency may lead *directly* to megaloblastic anemia, such a direct effect is doubted in case of vitamin B_{12}. Since the deficiency of one vitamin is known to affect the metabolism and utilisation of the other, it is believed that vitamin B_{12} produces its actions *indirectly* by influencing folate metabolism and megaloblastic anemia produced by vitamin B_{12} deficiency is partly due to deranged folate metabolism (see below).

COBALAMINS: Chemically, vitamin B_{12} belongs to the family of cobalamins which are cobalt containing carrinoid compounds. Cobalamins are dark red crystalline hygroscopic powders, readily soluble in water. The solution is stable at room temperature. These compounds differ from each other in the groups attached to the cobalt atom. In case of **cyanocobalamin**, a cyanide group is attached to the cobalt atom. A cobalamin with hydroxy (OH) group is known as **hydroxocobalamin**. Cyanocobalamin, on exposure to light, is converted to hydroxocobalamin, while hydroxocobalamin in the presence of cyanide gets changed into cyanocobalamin. Other cobalamins of physiological importance are aquocobalamin, nitrocobalamin, methyl-cobalamin and 5'-deoxyadenosine coenzyme.

Cyanocobalamin and hydroxo-cobalamin are commonly used therapeutically. They are discussed below under the general heading 'Vitamin B_{12}'.

VITAMIN B_{12}: Vitamin B_{12} is synthesized solely by micro-organisms in soil, water and animal intestine or rumen. It is almost absent in plant products. In man, as in animals, it is synthesized in the colon by micro-organisms; however, it is hardly absorbed from this site and hence, is excreted (about 3-5 mcg. daily) in feces. Some of the animals like rabbits and rats eat their own feces (coprophagy) and hence, they have very high serum B_{12} levels. Nonvegetarian foods like muscle, liver, kidney, oysters, fish and egg yolk are rich in B_{12}. Dairy food contains smaller amounts of B_{12}. The vitamin B_{12} content of cow's milk is considerably more than that of human milk.

The daily dietary intake of B_{12} varies considerably and is high in non-vegetarians and likely to be very low in vegetarians, some of whom may not even consume sufficient amount of milk or milk products; however, vegetarians may obtain enough vitamin B_{12} from contaminated water and in the form of co-enzyme B_{12} by ingesting legumes and nodules of root vegetable in which vitamin B_{12} is synthesized by micro-organisms.

The minimum daily requirement of B_{12} in adults is not exactly known but is believed to be extremely small, about 1 mcg per day. Taking into consideration the incomplete absorption of the food B_{12}, the recommended daily dietary intake is 2 mcg for adults, 3 mcg in pregnancy and lactation and 0.3 mcg for infants.

Absorption of vitamin B_{12}: The cobalamins in food exist in a bound form and are metabolically inactive until they are released by heat (cooking) and by proteolysis in the stomach or intestines.

Vitamin B_{12}, given in microgram doses, such as are present in the diet, is absorbed only in the presence of intrinsic factor, produced by the parietal cells of the gastric mucosa. Thus, very little or none is absorbed in cases with pernicious anemia and after gastrectomy as the intrinsic factor is absent.

The **intrinsic factor** (IF) is a glycoprotein. It is produced by the fundus and the body of the stomach. It binds to vitamin B_{12} and acts as a carrier. The presence of hydrochloric acid facilitates this binding. Many naturally occurring substances can also bind B_{12} but they are not intrinsic factors. Intrinsic factor thus escorts B_{12} to the site of absorption, which is ileum in man and facilitates its absorption. It is antigenic and antibodies against intrinsic factor are known.

The gastric juice contains another cobalamin binding protein from saliva, called R-type protein. This protein binds cobalamine with higher affinity than does IF. Thus, at acidic pH the dietary cobalamine enters the duodenum bound to R-type protein.

Pancreatic proteases degrade this complex in the jejunum, whereafter it is presented to the IF. High affinity, specific receptors for the absorption of cobalamine are located on the ileal mucosal cells.

Ionic calcium is necessary for the initial binding of the intrinsic factor - B_{12} complex to the ileal receptor site. Low ionic calcium concentration and a low pH as observed in chronic pancreatitis may cause vitamin B_{12} malabsorption.

The maximum absorption of vitamin B_{12} occurs within 8-12 hours following a physiological dose (1-5 mcg), uninfluenced by the concentration of vitamin B_{12} in the blood.

Given SC or IM, cyanocobalamin is rapidly absorbed and the plasma level reaches the peak in 1 hour. Cyanocobalamin can also get absorbed without the help of intrinsic factor, but the dose needed is much higher (*500-1000 mcg*). This type of absorption occurs by simple diffusion, probably by mass action, although such absorption is inefficient.

Vitamin B_{12} transport and storage: Absorbed vitamin B_{12} is transported in the plasma, bound to $beta_2$ globulin called **transcobalamin II.** Only 1-10 per cent circulates as a free fraction. The transcobalamin II is taken up by cells by endocytosis. During the process, the transcobalamin is degraded and the released cobalamin is converted to two coenzymes, viz., methylcobalamin and adenosyl cobalamin. The major form of vitamin B_{12} in the serum is methylcobalamin attached to a globulin; this may be a circulating storage form of vitamin B_{12}. The total body stores of cobalamin in normal adult are estimated at about 3-5 mg., of which about 50-90% is present in the liver. Not all of this, however, is available for hemopoesis.

Turnover of vitamin B_{12} is very slow and in long-term studies only 0.2-0.3 per cent of the total B_{12} contained in the body is excreted per day. Vitamin B_{12} is excreted in the bile but most of it is reabsorbed, so that there is a closed enterohepatic circulation. This is how the body conserves B_{12} and this would explain partly why even strict vegans with a very low intake of this vitamin do not commonly develop clinical vitamin B_{12} deficiency syndrome. The lack of intrinsic factor or defective absorption due to intestinal pathology in such cases, however, will lead to a rapid depletion of B_{12} stores.

Excretion: The daily urinary loss of vitamin B_{12} is very small, ranging between 0 and 0.25 mcg. Only the cobalamin not bound to proteins is capable of being excreted by glomerular filtration. Conservation of the vitamin by enterohepatic circulation and its very slow excretion explain why it takes a long time, perhaps 10 years, for deficiency to develop in the presence of deficient intake or absorption. The half life of a tracer dose of radioactive vitamin B_{12} in the liver is about 12 months.

If vitamin B_{12} is injected, only the amount necessary for the saturation of the binding sites is retained; the remaining excess is excreted in the urine. It is calculated that 80-95 per cent of a 50 mcg dose of injected vitamin B_{12} is retained. As the dose exceeds 100 mcg, large proportions (50-98%) of the injected dose may appear in the urine within 48 hours in healthy individuals.

Vitamin B_{12} crosses the placental barrier and the cord blood level of vitamin B_{12} is significantly higher than the maternal blood levels.

Metabolic actions of vitamin B_{12}: Cyanocobalamin itself has no metabolic activity in man. After absorption it is converted by cellular enzymes in tissues to the coenzyme forms which are active. Cobalamin functions as an essential cofactor for two enzymes in the human cells : (1) methionine synthetase (methyl transferase); and (2) l-methyl-malonyl coenzyme-A transmutase (Fig. 34.1).

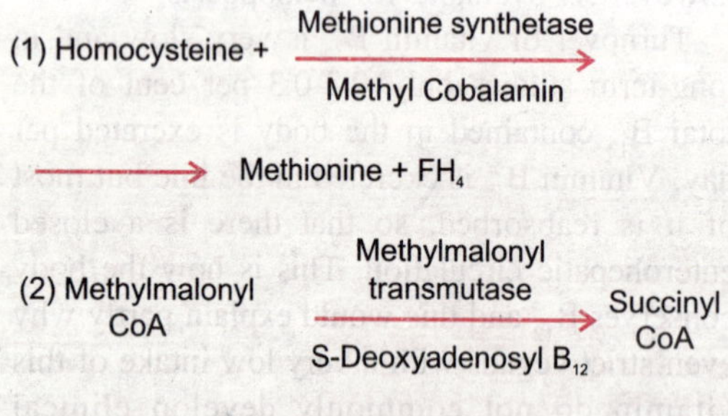

Fig. 34.1: Important metabolic actions of vitamin B_{12}

(1) Vitamin B_{12} exists intracellularly as an active enzyme, methyl cobalamin; on entry into the cell, methyl group from Nu-methyl tetrahydrofolic acid ($MeFH_4$) is transferred to cobalamin to form methyl cobalamin. The methyl group from methyl cobalamin is transferred to homocysteine to form methyl-homocysteine also called methionine (Fig. 34.1). In the absence of B_{12}, the conversion of dietary and stored folate ($MeFH_4$) to FH_4 is blocked (Fig. 34.2), resulting in deficiency of essential folate co-factors and accumulation of $MeFH_4$, 'methyltetrahydrofolate trap'. This may explain the similarity of GI lesions and peripheral blood picture seen in megaloblastic anemia due to deficiency of either vitamin B_{12} or folic acid.

(2) Because the neurons do not divide, impaired DNA synthesis cannot explain the demyelination that occurs in vitamin B_{12} deficiency. Various hypotheses have been proposed to explain the neurological damage. The most favoured hypothesis suggests that tissue deficiency of S-AM and failure of transmethylation reactions are important in causing deficiency of myelin synthesis. The major pathway of propionic acid utilisation in animal tissues involves the conversion of propionyl co-enzyme (CoA) to succinyl CoA. Thus, propionyl CoA is first converted to methyl malonyl CoA. Vitamin B_{12} CoA is necessary for the conversion of methyl malonyl CoA to succinyl CoA. (Fig. 34.1). Deficiency of this enzyme interferes with the production of lipoprotein in myelin tissue and may explain the neurological complications such as peripheral neuritis, optic atrophy and subacute combined degeneration of the spinal cord.

(3) Purine biosynthesis is reduced in cobalamin deficiency and this abnormality may also contribute to defective DNA synthesis. Both methyl tetrahydrofolate trapping and lack of S-adenosyl methionine (S-AM) contribute to impairment of purine synthesis.

Methylmalonyl coenzyme – A accumulates in cobalamin deficiency due to lack of adenosyl cobalamin.

Human red blood cells show low folate stores in the presence of vitamin B_{12} deficiency. The red cell folate rises after B_{12} therapy, suggesting that B_{12} plays some role in folate uptake and storage.

It has been demonstrated in animals that supplementing the diet with vitamin B_{12} has a growth promoting effect. It is used in poultry farming for increasing the bird weight and for fattening the pigs. No such growth acceleration effect, however, has been observed in normal or premature human infants.

Vitamin B_{12} does not seem to have any other significant pharmacological actions, even in large doses.

Assay of vitamin B_{12} and blood levels: Vitamin B_{12} in biological samples is assayed microbiologically using *Euglena gracilis* or *Lactobacillus leichmanii* as the test organism. The serum level in normals consuming non-vegetarian food varies between 140 and 750 pg./ml. The levels in healthy subjects consuming vegetarian food are considerably lower, some of them even below 100 pg./ml.; they may not, however, show any clinical or hematological evidence of deficiency. The factors controlling the levels of serum B_{12} and folic acid are unknown. Although B_{12} deficiency anemia is accompanied by low serum levels, it is doubtful whether a low serum level of B_{12} by itself signifies tissue deficiency in otherwise healthy vegetarians. Plasma B_{12} can also be assayed by using a radioisotopic competitive protein binding assay.

Preparations and dosage:

(i) Cyanocobalamin, pink coloured injection, contains 100 mcg per ml. *It should be administered either IM or SC.*

(ii) Hydroxycobalamin injection, 100,500 or 1000 mcg per ml.

(iii) Vitamin B_{12} for oral administration is available as a part of multivitamin formulations. Such preparations may be helpful in treating *dietary* deficiency of vitamin B_{12} but are ineffective in B_{12} deficiency from other causes and in patients with severe B_{12} deficiency. *Oral formulations of vitamin B_{12} are not recommended to treat established B_{12} deficiency.*

Adverse reactions: Vitamin B_{12} given orally is very safe. Cyanocobalamin IV has been reported to cause transient exanthema and even anaphylactoid reactions very rarely. Hence, *cyanocobalamin should never be injected IV. The use of hydroxycobalamin can lead to the development of antibodies to the transcobalamin-vitamin B_{12} complex* and consequent refractoriness to treatment. Hence, cyanocobalamin, IM or SC is the treatment of choice in vitamin B_{12} deficiency.

Therapeutic uses:

(1) **Megaloblastic anemia due to vitamin B_{12} deficiency due to:**

- ***Deficient intake*** in nutritional megaloblastic anemia as seen in strict vegans. As the daily B_{12} requirement is extremely small, nutritional deficiency due to pure B_{12} is uncommon even among the vegetarians in India. Majority of the nutritional megaloblastic anemias observed in India are mainly due to folic acid deficiency. The nutritional B_{12} deficiency can be corrected by parenteral administration of B_{12}.
- ***Impaired absorption*** of Vitamin B_{12} as observed in pernicious anemia (due to lack of intrinsic factor), after gastrectomy or resection of small bowel, in malabsorption syndromes and in gastrointestinal diseases involving stomach and intestine such as malignancy, and chronic pancreatitis. In all these conditions, absorption of orally administered radioactive B_{12} is markedly diminished. Correction of this absorption defect by simultaneous administration of intrinsic factor suggests its absence as observed in patients with pernicious anemia. This forms the basis for *Schilling's test.* In all these cases, B_{12} should be given *parenterally.*

Cyanocobalamin is the drug of choice. Initially, it is given in the dose of 200-1000 mcg. IM daily for 1-2 weeks to replenish the body stores. Then, a similar dose may be given IM once a month. The reticulocyte response occurs on 3rd to 4th day and reaches the peak by 5 to 8 days. In patients with pernicious anemia and in cases with incurable gastrointestinal lesions, the treatment has to be continued lifelong.

- ***Infestation with the fish tapeworm*** also causes megaloblastic anemia due to preferential uptake of dietary B_{12} by the worm. This is not common in India but heavy infestation with other worms may possibly contribute to such a deficiency.
- ***Inadequate utilisation*** of B_{12} which may occur in infants who inherit the deficiency of certain enzymes necessary for conversion of vitamin B_{12} to its co-enzyme forms.

(2) **Vitamin B_{12} deficiency neuropathies** such as tropical neuropathy, subacute combined degeneration, tobacco and tropical amblyopia, which sometimes occur without clearcut megaloblastic anemia, respond to parenteral B_{12} therapy. The sensory component inproves much less than the motor component. The exact mechanism of action is not known. There is some evidence to suggest that certain well defined neurological and ophthalmic syndrome (tobacco amblyopia) may represent the chronic neurotoxic effects of cyanide, and that hydroxocobalamin may help in the detoxication of cyanide by binding it.

Vitamin B_{12}, given in massive doses, has been claimed to be effective in such varied conditions as infective hepatitis, sterility, psoriasis, multiple sclerosis, herpes zoster, toxic amblyopia and trigeminal neuralgia; there is no clear evidence to suggest that this vitamin is of any value in such conditions. Nor there is any conclusive evidence to suggest its usefulness in patients with mental disorders.

HYDROXOCOBALAMIN: Hydroxocobalamin, when injected, is absorbed slowly from the injection site and is more protein bound than cyanocobalamin. It is excreted slowly and hence, higher blood levels are maintained over a longer period than with cyanocobalamin. In pernicious anemia, it is given initially in the dose of 1mg. IM every 2-3 days for five doses. Maintenance dose is 1 mg. every three months. Similar doses may be used to treat nutritional B_{12} deficiency.

Methylcobalamin : There is no evidence for superiority of this analogue over cyanocobalamin and hydroxycobalamin. It is very expensive.

FOLIC ACID (PTEROYLMONO-GLUTAMIC ACID) : Folic acid occurs as yellow, spear shaped crystals. Its disodium salt is soluble in water in the concentration of 1.5 mcg. per cent. Chemically, folic acid molecule contains pteridine, para-aminobenzoic acid and glutamic acid. It is named folic acid because it is commonly present in green leaves. The term 'folate' is used in the generic sense and includes other chemical forms.

Folate is present in abundance in green vegetables, liver and yeast. Moderate amounts are present in eggs, meat, fish and dairy foods. Most of the folic acid in vegetables is in conjugated form, where one or more glutamic acid molecules are incorporated in the structure. These are usually triglutamic and heptaglutamic acid conjugates. Prolonged boiling of food during cooking destroys most of the folate in the food. As in the case of vitamin B_{12} many microorganisms including those in the colon synthesize folic acid. It is doubtful, however, whether the folic acid synthesized in the colon is available for utilisation in man.

Absorption: Folic acid conjugates are hydrolysed to pteroylmonoglutamic acid by enzymes, conjugases, present in vegetable and mammalian tissues. A conjugase is found throughout the gastrointestinal mucosa and in pancreas, the highest level being in the duodenum and jejunum. Pteroylmonoglutamic acid is absorbed almost completely in the small intestine, particularly in the jejunum. As in the case of vitamin B_{12} physiological doses (1 mg.) are absorbed by an active process while large doses can get absorbed by diffusion. Absorption of food folate as such, however, is incomplete. Further, inhibition of conjugase by certain drugs or its decreased concentration due to intestinal pathology may cause malabsorption of polyglutamates in the diet.

Transport, storage and fate: Given orally, folic acid appears in the blood within 30 minutes. It circulates in the plasma mainly as N-methyl tetrahydrofolate. The majority is loosely bound to albumin, from which it is readily taken up by the cells. Inside the cells, it is converted to tetrahydrofolate (FH_4) by the cobalamine dependent enzyme, methionine synthetase.

The amount of folic acid excreted in the urine is dependent on the dose. Only a small amount appears in the urine following ingestion of

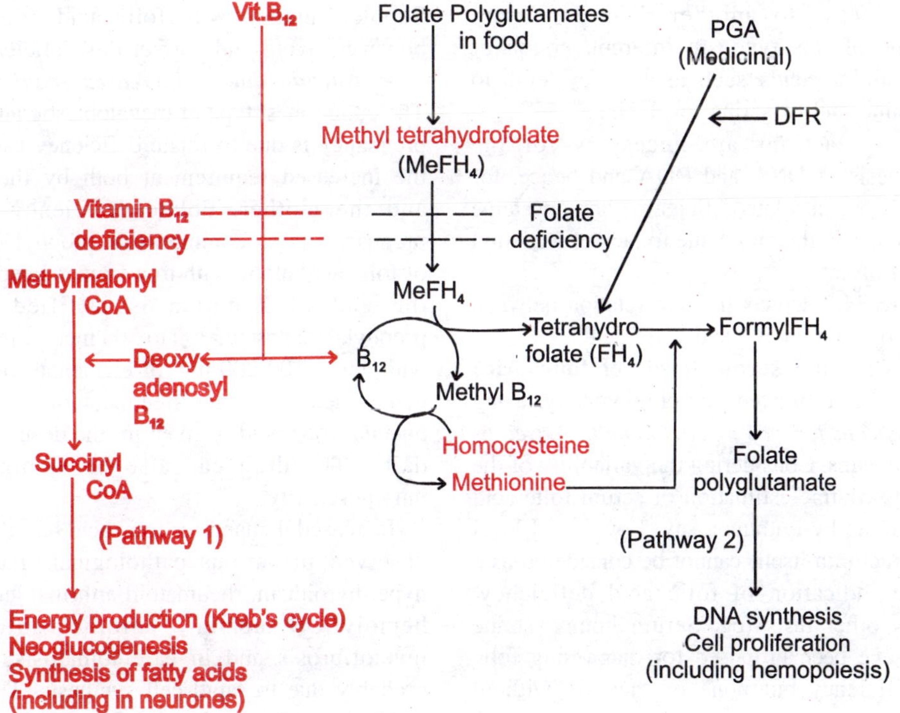

Fig. 34.2 : Interrelation between B12 and folate actions.

0.1 mg. of folic acid, while almost 90 per cent is excreted after 15 mg. dose. Folate appears in the urine within 6 hours after ingestion, and excretion is complete within 24 hours.

Vitamin C protects the reduced product, tetrahydrofolic acid, from oxidative destruction. It also protects the folate in the food. Hence, food poor in vitamin C content is generally low in folate content as well. There is no evidence, however, that vitamin C in any way potentiates the therapeutic effects of folic acid in man.

The total body folate is estimated to be in the range of 5-10 mg. of which almost one-third is present in the liver mostly as methylfolate. Unlike vitamin B_{12}, folate gets selectively concentrated in the spinal fluid.

Folate is incorporated in red cells during erythropoiesis and the amount decreases only slightly during their life span. Red cell folate is, therefore a useful indicator of body folate status.

The exact daily requirement of folate in humans is not known; but it appears to be about 200 mcg in adults, 100 mcg for children and 300-400 mcg in pregnancy and lactation. Since the net folate losses from the body appear to be about 50% of the amount ingested, the recommended daily intake is 400 mcg for adults, 200 mcg for children and 600-800 mcg in pregnancy.

Metabolic actions of folate: Like vitamin B_{12}, folic acid by itself is inactive. Folate functions to transfer one carbon units such as methyl and formyl groups to various substrates in enzymatic reactions. Folate co-enzymes are involved in various metabolic reactions.

- Biosynthesis of purine and pyrimidine nucleotides; and
- FH_4 is able to accept one carbon fragment such as methyl, formyl and methylene groups; the folate co-enzymes participate in reactions in which one carbon fragment is transferred from

one molecule to another. The important reactions of this type are interconversion of certain amino acids such as homocysteine to methionine and of serine to glycine.

These reactions are necessary for the biosynthesis of DNA and RNA and hence, for cell division. In folate deficiency, homocysteine accumulates in the blood due to lack of 5-methyl tetrahydrofolate.

Figure 34.2 depicts the interrelation between actions of vitamin B_{12} and folic acid.

Bioassay and serum levels of folic acid: Folic acid is estimated microbiologically, using *Streptococcus faecalis or Lactobacillus casei* as test organisms. Considering the variability of the bioassay, routine estimation of serum folic acid is now done by immunoassay. Low blood level of folic acid, in itself, cannot be considered as a definite indication of folic acid deficiency. Various other tests (eg. Serum homocysteine level) have been proposed for diagnosing folic acid deficiency but none of these is without fallacies.

Adverse reactions: Folic acid is almost non-toxic in man and no adverse effects have been reported except a rare and doubtful allergic reaction to parenteral preparations.

Preparations and dosage: Folic acid tablet contains 5 mg. of the drug. Dose 1-5 mg. It can also be given parenterally.

Therapeutic uses: Folic acid is used in the treatment of megaloblastic anemias due to folate deficiency. These are:

- ***Dietary deficiency:*** Nutritional megaloblastic anemia is the commonest type of megaloblastic anemia in India and other tropical countries, and is mainly due to dietary deficiency because of undernutrition. Megaloblastic anemia of protein caloric undernutrition of infancy and childhood is mostly due to folic acid deficiency. Cooking habits involving prolonged boiling of food with spices, which destroys folic acid, and possibly loss of folate in sweat contribute further to the development of its deficiency. It must be realised that wherever there is deficiency of folate there is also a lack of other nutrients and the ideal treatment lies in correcting the diet. Supplementation with folic acid orally can, however, avoid and correct this deficiency.

- ***Anemia due to increased requirements*:** The commonest type of megaloblastic anemia in pregnancy is due to folate deficiency caused by the increased requirement both by the foetus and the mother. Folate deficiency during pregnancy is so common that prophylactic use of folic acid along with iron from conception till the end of lactation is justified. Daily prophylactic dose of 300 to 500 mcg of folic acid with about 100-200 mg. of elemental iron is all that is needed. In the treatment of *established anemia*, folic acid is given in the dose of 5 mg. daily. The drug can also be administered intramuscularly.

Increased demand for folic acid has also been observed in various pathological states like hyperthyroidism, rheumatoid arthritis, leukemia, hemolytic anemia, chronic infections myelofibrosis and in carcinomatosis; this is probably due to rapid cell synthesis. This may add to or aggravate the already existing anemia.

- ***Anemia due to impaired absorption*:** This is observed in malabsorption syndrome associated with tropical sprue, extensive organic disease of the jejunum and in blind loop syndrome.

In other types of malabsorptive states such as idiopathic steatorrhoea, adult celiac disease and nontropical sprue, sensitivity to the gluten fraction of wheat protein is often the offending cause. In such cases and in gluten enteropathy in children, administration of gluten-free diet gives dramatic results; many patients in this group, however, also suffer from folic acid deficiency. In such conditions folic acid is given IM in a dose of 5 mg. daily, followed by oral therapy as soon as the diarrhoea ceases.

- ***Anemia due to impaired utilisation*:** Certain anti-epileptic drugs like phenobarbitone, phenytoin and primidone may cause folic acid deficiency anemia probably by impairing its absorption and/or its utilisation. Drugs like methotrexate, the anti-malarial pyrimethamine and the antibacterial drug trimethoprim can also cause folate deficiency by blocking the conversion of folic acid to tetrahydrofolate. A supplement of folic acid, 1 mg. daily, orally, can correct this deficiency. The antiepileptic treatment, if required, need not be stopped.

- ***Certain other megaloblastic anemias as*** in liver disease, chronic alcoholism and scurvy are usually associated with folate deficiency.
- ***Prevention of neural tube defects (NTD)***: Any woman who can become pregnant should be prescribed 400 mcg of folic acid daily, as otherwise the conceptus might develop NTD which are liable to occur during the first week of gestation, even before the subject knows that she is pregnant. Further, if the woman is at high risk for NTD (has past/family history of NTD, or is taking carbamazepine or valproate), she should be prescribed 4-5 mg of a folic acid daily around a planned conception.
- ***Folate deficiency of ageing*** may be associated with elevated serum homocysteine levels and degenerating vascular disease in the elderly and that folate supplementation (400-1000 mcg/day), particularly in the elderly, may be a useful prophylactic health manoeuvre.

Folate deficiency as a cause of neuropathy is not universally accepted, although cases of encephalopathy giving rise to a confusional state, usually diagnosed as senile dementia and/ or myelopathy, responding to folic acid have been reported. Hence, folic acid may be tried empirically in obscure chronic neurological disorder not responding to B_{12} therapy.

Administration of folic acid alone is contra-indicated in pernicious anemia as, although it may correct the hematological abnormality, it can precipitate or worsen the neurological complications. The precise reason for this phenomenon is not known. It has been suggested that folic acid accelerates the utilisation of the meagre vitamin B_{12} stores (Pathway 2 in Fig. 34.2) in an already deficient subject and may thus aggravate deficiency of B_{12} which is essential for maintaining the integrity of the nervous system (Pathway 1 in Fig. 34.2). In a few cases of pernicious anemia, however, the folate stores are so low that there is only little response to vitamin B_{12} therapy until folic acid is also administered.

Following initiation of treatment with folic acid, subjective improvement such as feeling of well being and decrease in the soreness in the mouth occur early. Objective responses including disappearance of megaloblasts from the peripheral blood occur within 48 hours, with reticulocyte peak within 7 days.Rise in hemoglobin is observed in 10-15 days.

FOLINIC ACID (Citrovorum factor): This is the term used for N5 formyl tetrahydrofolinic acid. It was originally found in the liver and was demonstrated to have a growth promoting effect on the organism *Leuconostoc citrovorum*. It is available in 1 ml. ampoules containing 3 mg. of the vitamin. Its only use is in the treatment of toxicity due to folic acid antagonists like methotrexate.

Drugs Used in Neutropenia

Recombinant preparations of human granulocyte colony stimulating factor (G-CSF) and granulocyte/macrophage colony stimulating factor (GM-CSF) are available for the treatment of nutropenia.

FILGRASTIM (Neupogen) is a glycoprotein which is not glycosylated unlike the natural GCSF. It stimulates neutrophil progenitors to produce mature neutrophils, stimulates their release from bone marrow storage pool and also increases their functional activity.

MOLGRASTIM (Sargrastim, Leucomax, Leukine) stimulates proliferation and differentiation of partially committed hemopoietic progenitor cells to produce end cells of granulocyte and monocyte/macrophage lineages. It also activates some of the functions of the fully differntiated cells. Its administration stimulates myelopoiesis.

These agents are given SC or slow IV

infusion. Filgrastim is infused at a dose of 1-20 microgm/kg/day over 30 min while molgramostim is given as 125-500 microgm/m²/day over 3-6 hours. Half life of filgrastim is 3.5 hrs and that of molgramostim is 2-3 hours. Dosages are adjusted based on the response and duration and will depend on the specific application. Generally 7-14 days' therapy is needed.

Adverse reactions: Both are well tolerated but bone pain, fever, myalgia and lethargy, pain and reddening at the site of injection, hypersensitivity reactions including skin rashes and hypotension, flushing, nausea, vomiting and dyspnoea (especially after IV infusion) have been reported. Filgrastim rarely causes dysuria and reversible abnormalities in liver function. It also produces mild to moderate splenomegaly on chronic administration. These agents stimulate growth of cells of tumors with myeloid characters; patients with such tumors should not be treated with these drugs.

Therapeutic uses:

(a) To reduce severity and duration of neutropenia induced by intensive cancer chemotherapy.

(b) To shorten duration of neutropenia in patients undergoing bone marrow transplantation after high dose intensive chemotherapy, with or without total body irradication and thereby reduce morbidity.

(c) To stimulate release of progenitor cells in circulation, which are harvested and infused (peripheral blood stem cell transplantation) instead of bone marrow cells after high dose intensive chemotherapy.

(d) To expand number of harvested progenitor cells ex vivo before infusing them.

(e) For persistent neutropenia in advanced HIV infection, or that induced by zidovudine.

It may be used in patients with aplastic anaemia and myelodysplasia.

Lenograstim is the glycosylated analog of filgrastim. It has similar properties, adverse reactions and uses.

Pegfilgrastim is filgrastim conjugated to polyethylene glycol (PEG). Its half life is 5-8 hrs and requires to be given as a single injection per chemotherapy cycle.

Some drugs causing neutropenia are given in Chapter 35.

Drugs used in Thrombocytopenia

Recombinat human IL-11 (Oprelvekin) is available for cancer-chemotherapy-induced severe thrombocytopenia. Given SC, it leads to thrombopoietic response within 5-9 days. Two forms of **r-thrombopoietin** are also available. However, platelet transfusions are commonly used to treat thrombocytopenia.

Drug-Induced Blood Dyscrasias 35

In addition to blood loss caused by NSAID and anticoagulants, various types of blood dyscrasias may occur following the use of certain drugs in toxic doses or sometimes even in therapeutic doses. These reactions can be grouped into :

- ***Those due to impaired production of blood cells*** e.g. aplastic anemia.
- ***Those due to increased destruction of blood cells*** e.g. hemolytic anemias, and
- ***Those due to derangement of blood cell functions*** e.g. methaemoglobinemia.

The important drug-induced blood dyscrasias are as follows :

Drug-induced anemias: Megaloblastic anemias following certain drugs have already been discussed in Chapter 34. Drugs responsible for this can be grouped as follows:

I **Folic acid inhibitors:**

- ***DHF reductase inhibitors or folic acid antagonists***: Methotrexate, Pyrimethamine, Triamterene, Trimethoprim and Diamidine compounds.
- ***Associated with impaired absorption and/ or utilization of folic acid***: Phenytoin, Primidone, Barbiturates, Cycloserine, Alcohol and probably Oral contraceptive agents.

II **Those which cause vitamin B12 malabsorption:** PAS, Colchicine, Neomycin and Alcohol.

Blood loss induced by anti-inflammatory drugs and anticoagulants can cause iron deficiency anemia.

Pyridoxine responsive anemia in humans is a hypochromic microcytic anemia with normal serum iron, and bone marrow showing normoblastic, erythroid hyperplasia. The anemia is probably due to inability of iron to get incorporated into hemoglobin.

The anti-tuberculous drug isonicotinic acid hydrazide causes such a type of anemia, which responds to the oral administration of pyridoxine.

Aplastic anemia: This is the most severe type of blood dyscrasia; fortunately, it is rare. The evidence that a given drug is responsible for aplastic anemia in a given patient is largely circumstantial and in many cases toxicity may occur 2 weeks to 6 months after cessation of therapy. It is associated with pancytopenia and hypocellular bone marrow. The mortality is very high (more than 50%) and recovery, if it takes place, occurs only after illness for many months. The important offenders in this group are phenylbutazone, oxyphenbutazone, amidopyrine, indomethacin, antineoplastic drugs and the antibiotic chloramphenicol. Other drugs reported to produce aplastic anemia are mephenytoin, gold salts, potassium perchlorate, benzene, insecticides like DDT, gamma benzene hexachloride, antithyroid drugs, sulfonamides and sulfonylureas. This reaction is probably not dose related and may represent some form of idiosyncratic phenomenon.

Cytotoxic drugs used in cancer chemotherapy may cause aplastic anemia as an extension of their pharmacological action.

The choice of therapy depends on the cause and the severity of the anemia, and the age of the patient. Apart from good supportive and nursing therapy, and blood transfusions, the main therapeutic choice is between allogenic bone marrow transplantation and immunosuppression with horse antithymocytic globulin (ATG), rabbit antilymphocytic globulin (ALG) or cyclosporine. Immunosuppression may be effective in 70-80% of the patients. ATG and ALG may cause anaphylaxis, serum sickness and temporary exacerbation of cytopenia. Immunosuppression is usually recommended in subjects for whom bone marrow transplantation is not available. Additional use of GCSF, erythropoietin and large doses of androgen may help some patients. Although glucocorticoids such as prednisolone (20-40 mg/day) do not induce a remission, they may control the hemorrhage.

Haemolytic reactions occur generally with the drugs which oxidize hemoglobin. Normally, the RBCs contain the enzyme glucose 6-phosphate dehydrogenase. Normal functioning of G-6-PD is necessary for maintaining glutathione in its reduced form, which in turn protects the red blood cells from the damage by oxidizing agents. The drug-damaged red cells show precipitated denatured hemoglobin, identified as Heinz bodies in an appropriate blood smear preparation.

Individuals whose RBCs are deficient in G-6-PD, reduced glutathione (GSH) or glutathione reductase are more susceptible to drug induced hemolysis. Such deficiency is hereditary. It is known to occur predominantly in Negros, and is relatively rare in white population. Its presence has also been noted in Indians.

A hemolytic reaction with oxidant drugs can occur even in normal individuals without G-6-PD deficiency, if the concentration of the drug is sufficiently high. Drugs which are known to cause hemolytic reactions in G-6-PD deficiency are listed in Table 35.1. Similar reactions can also occur due to improper functioning of phosphogluconate dehydrogenase and glutathione reductase.

Table 35.1: Some drugs causing hemolysis in G6PD deficiency

Antibacterial agents :
Sulfonamides, Furazolidone, Nitrofurantoin, Chloramphenicol, Fluoroquinolones

Antileprosy drugs (sulfones) :
Diaminodiphenyl sulfone, Sulfoxone

Antimalarials :
Primaquine, Pamaquine, Mepacrine, Quinine

Miscellaneous drugs :
Acetanilid, Salicylates, Phenacetin, Naphthalene, Water soluble analogues of vitamin K, Methylene blue, Niridazole

Drugs can also cause hemolysis by an immune mechanism, where the RBC destruction is caused by circulating antibodies. Drugs which can cause immune hemolytic anemia are methyldopa, quinine, quinidine, stibophen and phenacetin. Patients with abnormal hemoglobins may develop hemolysis if they are given sulfonamides or 8-aminoquinoline drugs. The treatment of hemolytic reactions is essentially symptomatic. Glucocorticoids such as hydrocortisone may produce beneficial effects in blood dyscrasias caused by immune mechanisms.

Methemoglobinemia: The oxygen carriage by red cell hemoglobin is dependent on the availability of haemoglobin iron in the ferrous form. Drugs such as phenacetin, sulfonamides, bismuth subnitrate, ammonium nitrate and nitrites are known to oxidize the hemoglobin iron from ferrous to ferric state and thus cause methemoglobinemia. Infants below 6 months are more susceptible to this reaction, probably on account of a low concentration of the erythrocyte enzyme nicotinamide adenine dinucleotide (NADH) which normally reduces methemoglobin

Table 35.2: Some drugs causing neutropenia and agranulocytosis

Tranquillizers:
Chlorpromazine and related drugs, Meprobamate
Analgesics:
Amidopyrine, Phenylbutazone, Oxyphenbutazone, Analgin, Indomethacin
Antibacterial agents:
Chloramphenicol, Sulfonamides, Streptomycin, Cotrimoxazole
Antithyroid drugs:
Propylthiouracil, Methimazole, Potassium perchlorate
Miscellaneous:
Troxidone, Procainamide, Thiacetazone, Gold preparations, Impiramine.

to hemoglobin. This enzyme is also genetically deficient in certain subjects who are more prone to develop drug-induced methemoglobinemia.

Treatment consists of stoppage of the drug and the administration of methylene blue, an effective antidote. 50 ml. of 1 per cent solution is administered intravenously.

Neutropenia: In this condition, specific depression of leucocytes, particularly granulocytes, occurs. Drugs known to produce this condition do so relatively frequently, in 1 in 1000 to 1 in 100 of patients. Certain drugs like amidopyrine and dipyrone produce neutropenia by an immune mechanism, where patient's serum with specific antibodies lyses granulocytes in the presence of the drug. However, with drugs like phenothiazines and antithyroid compounds the exact mechanism is not known. Drugs that are commonly known to produce neutropenia are listed in Table 35.2.

Periodic blood counts may not necessarily predict impending neutropenia. Patients taking such drugs, therefore, should be warned about unexplained fever, or sore throat with ulceration, and should be instructed to report immediately. The mortality rate is more than 20 per cent, mainly as a result of infection, which needs prompt treatment. Blood transfusion may be necessary. Treatment with human granulocyte colony stimulating factor is discussed in Chapter 34.

Table 35.3: Some drugs causing thrombocytopenia

Antiarrhythmics : Quinidine, Procainamide
Antibacterials : Sulfonamides, Penicillin, Ampicillin, Rifampicin
Antiepileptics : Phenytoin, Carbamazepine, Valproic acid
Diuretics : Thiazides, Furosemide, Acetazolamide
H_2 receptor antagonists : Cimetidine, Ranitidine
Miscellaneous : Alpha methyldopa, Gold compounds, Danazol, Heparin, Quinine.

Thrombocytopenia: This is a less frequent complication and in most cases is due to immune mechanisms. This can be demonstrated by mixing fresh normal blood with the patient's serum containing an appropriate concentration of the drugs, where clot retraction is prevented. Drugs known to cause thrombocytopenia are listed in Table 35.3. Quinidine is most commonly involved in causing this reaction. In addition, all drugs causing aplastic anemia also cause thrombocytopenia.

Section IX
Water, Electrolytes and Drugs Affecting Renal Functions

Water, Sodium, Potassium and Hydrion Metabolism; Therapy of Dehydration

36

Correction of body water and electrolyte balance forms an important aspect of therapy in clinical practice, and on many occasion it is a life saving measure. Water accounts for 75% of body weight in humans. The most important determinants of the amount of body water (% of body weight) are age and gender. The water content of the newborn, the middle aged adult and the elderly are 75%, 60% and 50%, respectively. The females, because of their higher fat percentage, have lower water content. The gender differences develop after puberty.

Distribution of body fluids: Body fluid is broadly divided into:

- ***Intracellular fluid*** (ICF); and
- ***Extracellular fluid*** (ECF).

As pointed out by Robinson and McCance (1952), ECF is like the continuous phase while ICF is like the dispersed phase of an emulsion. ECF, being continuous, plays an important role as a transport medium for various substances moving into and from the cells, while the confinement of ICF in the cells provides the basis for individual cellular functions.

The extracellular compartment is divided anatomically, by the traversing blood vessels, into *intravascular* (plasma) and *extravascular* (or interstitial) moieties. Physiologically, however, these compartments are continuous in respect of their electrolyte composition, as small molecules and ions can easily cross the capillary walls, the main difference being their protein content which is lower in the interstitial fluid.

The fluid present in the CSF, tracheobronchial tree, aqueous humor, the lumen of the GI tract and certain glands, sometimes designated as the *transcellular* fluid, constitutes about 2.5 per cent of total body water.

In a healthy, 70 kg man, total body water (TBW) comprises about 40 litres. Table 36.1 gives the distribution of the body water in various body comparments in a young man.

Table 36.1: Distribution of body water (per cent of body weight)

Compartment		Per cent
Intracellular (ICF)		33.0
Interstitial	**(ECF)**	20.5
Intravascular	**(ECF)**	4.0
Transcellular	**(ECF)**	2.5
Total		60.0%

Body fluids contain various substances, some of which are vital for normal functioning of life. Some of these exist as ionized particles carrying a positive or a negative charge. When placed in an electrical field, they migrate to the cathode (**cation**) or the anode (**anion**); hence they are known as *electrolytes*. The electrolyte composition of ECF is different from that of ICF. Thus, sodium, chloride and bicarbonate are

Table 36.2: Electrolyte composition of plasma and ICF (m mol/l)

	Plasma	ICF
Cations		
Na	142	14
K	4.2	140
Ca	1.2	Negligible*
Mg	0.8	20
Anions		
Cl	108	4
HCO_3	24	10
PO_4	2	11
SO_4	0.5	1
Protein	1.2	4

* ICF contains 10,000 times less Ca than plasma.

mainly extracellular while potassium, magnesium, phosphate and sulfate are essentially intracellular. The electrolyte composition of plasma and ICF is given in Table 36.2.

The higher ionic concentration of the ICF than of ECF does not result in higher ICF osmolality, because 25% of the IC ions are bound to proteins and other cellular components, rendering them osmotically inactive. Thus, the osmolalities of both compartments are nearly identical despite their different total ionic contents.

There are, however, certain similarities between the ECF and the ICF. Thus, in each compartment the total cation concentration in milliequivalents (mEq) is almost same as the total anion concentrations in mEq (Table 36.2). Both fluids are, therefore, very nearly electrically neutral.

Functions of electrolytes:

• ***Maintenance of osmotic pressure*****:** The amount of water present in a given compartment is determined by the number of particles present, exerting an osmotic effect. Electrolytes play a major role in maintaining osmotic pressure. It is the number of molecules and ions per kg of water and not the mass of a solute per unit volume of fluid that determines its osmotic pressure. Substances with low molecular weight possess a larger number of molecules per unit mass than substances with high molecular weight. Hence, although the plasma protein mass is very much larger than the plasma sodium mass, the latter contributes far more to the osmotic pressure of plasma than the proteins. Thus, the biological functions of the electrolytes will be better understood, not by noting their concentration in mg. per cent but by some other unit which express the concentration in terms of molecules per unit weight of the solvent (i.e. molality). Molal solution is one which contains one mole of solute per 1000 g. of the solvent. One millimolal solution is also one milliosmolal. The osmotic balance between the ICF and the ECF is largely maintained by the electrolytes, whereas that between the ECF and the intravascular compartment is largely determined by the osmotic effect of the plasma proteins.

Normally, the volume, the total electrolyte concentration and the osmolality of ECF are maintained within narrow limits. The normal osmolality of the plasma is about 300 milliosmoles per kg. of water and most of it is due to the sodium. It is maintained constant by the kidneys. A rise in blood urea or glucose in some diseases, however, may increase the plasma osmolality significantly. Potassium is mainly responsible for maintaining intracellular osmolality.

• ***Maintenance of electroneutrality*****:** Electroneutrality of the body fluids is maintained by the concentrations of positively charged ions (Cations) and negatively charged ions (Anions) being nearly equal. In order to emphasize the concept of electroneutrality of the body fluids, it is customary to express the concentrations of electrolytes in terms of their chemically reactive units viz. milliequivalents rather than mg. per cent. The concentration in mg./100 ml. can be converted to mEq./1. by the formula :

$$\frac{\text{mg./100 ml. x 10}}{\text{Equivalent weight}} = \text{mEq./1.}$$

As per International System of Units (SI), the electrolyte concentration is expressed as mmol./1 instead of mEq/1.

- ***Production of energy*****:** Energy at the cellular level is produced by anaerobic and aerobic glycolysis and is stored in available form in high energy phosphate bonds. Intracellular potassium and magnesium are essential for the function of various enzymes necessary for this process. Inorganic phosphorus is necessary for ATP synthesis. Potassium depletion is known to affect various metabolic processes such as utilization of carbohydrates and synthesis of proteins. Weakness in chronic diarrhoea is attributed partly to potassium depletion. For effects of phosphorus depletion, see Chapter 68.

- ***In impulse transmission*****:** The neuronal and the muscle activities are associated with transmembrane shift of the electrolytes, with reversal of these during recovery period. Some drugs like dilantin sodium, quinidine and digitalis modify these shifts of electrolytes and thus alter the cell signalling.

- ***Miscellaneous*****:** Electrolytes also have certain specialized functions to perform, e.g., calcium in blood clotting and bone formation.

Water Metabolism

In health, the TBW content is usually maintained within normal limits, although the water and electrolyte output varies from day to day. Water intake varies widely in subjects from different climates and even among the individuals from the same region. The daily water intake includes that taken as water and beverages (≈1200 ml), and that in food (≈ 500 ml). Approximately 300 ml. of water is produced daily in the body during oxidation of food. The output (about 1500 ml./day) is mainly in the urine; in addition, about 100 ml. is lost in feces and about 1000 ml. (insensible loss) in the expired air and through sweating. Considerable loss of water in sweat can occur in tropical countries like India. Under basal conditions, water balance can be calculated as follows : (24 hours intake + 400 ml. produced by oxidation of food) - (24 hours urinary volume + 1000 ml. lost from skin and lungs). This obviously gives only a gross assessment but is useful in clinical practice. In normal subjects, the water balance is zero.

In individuals from the tropics, the TBW on body weight basis and the water turnover are more than in those from the temperate zones. The amount of water lost by insensible perspiration is also likely to be more, particularly in *hot and dry* climate where the heat loss occurs mainly by evaporation of water from the skin. Water lost in *hot but humid* climate is somewhat less because of less evaporation from the skin.

The rate of sweating in terms of body mass is greater in children upto age of 9 months than in adults, owing to higher metabolic rate.

Acclimatization to heat reduces the volume of sweat produced at a given temperature, probably increases the threshold for the onset of sweating and also reduces the volume of sweat produced for a given heat load. The local inhabitants of tropics, therefore, produce 30 per cent less sweat from a unit skin area in a saturated hot environment than unacclimatized Europeans.

In health, water balance is maintained by:

- ***Intake as regulated by thirst*****;** and
- ***Output in the urine as regulated mainly by antidiuretic hormone (ADH).***

The exact stimulus for the production of thirst is not known. However, thirst can be induced by:

(a) Increase in ECF osmolality, leading to cellular dehydration;

(b) Significant ECF volume depletion; and

(c) Increase in the CNS angiotensin II, a potent stimulus to thirst.

It is known that one feels thirsty after eating excessively sweet or salty food. Water depletion increases ECF sodium level. An increase in extracellular solute concentration causes extraction of water from the cells. Thus, the cellular dehydration caused by water deficit or an increase in extracellular solute concentration acts as an effective stimulus to thirst.

Osmoreceptors responding to changes in the plasma osmolality have been demonstrated in the basal forebrain and the hypothalamus. Further, hypovolemia stimulates stretch/volume receptors which elicit thirst through vagal afferents reaching the hypothalamus. Hypovolemia also increases angiotensin II levels.

The output of water in the urine is controlled mainly by the ADH. Increased plasma osmolality caused by water depletion activates the osmoreceptors in the hypothalamus, which in turn stimulates the release of ADH. The threshold for ADH secretion is a plasma osmolality of about 280 mosm/kg. of plasma water; below this level, such secretion is shut off. ADH promotes water absorption in the distal tubules and the collecting ducts of the kidney, thus reducing the urine volume and increasing its osmolality. The body thus tries to conserve water. Other stimuli like pain, decreased blood volume, mental stress, and drugs like morphine, nicotine and barbiturates also increase ADH release.

Both the mechanisms, thirst and ADH activity, are very sensitive even to small changes in the osmolality of body fluids. They are, however, less influenced by changes in the volume alone. In the natural stress of water deprivation, these two mechanisms act synergistically and protect the body from water depletion. Water excess is countered by inhibition of ADH release, resulting in a decrease in renal water resorption and water diuresis.

Water metabolism is intimately connected with the changes in solute content of the body. Thus, an increased intake of solutes necessitates increased water intake, and increased retention of sodium is associated with retention of water causing edema. Similarly, an excessive loss of solutes in the urine causes an increased water loss (**osmotic diuresis**).

Aldosterone, the mineralocorticoid hormone, influences the water balance by modifying the sodium metabolism. Physiologically, hydrocortisone, another hormone of the adrenal cortex, is essential for eliminating an extra load of water from the body. In its absence as in case of Addison's disease, patients are unable to excrete the water load adequately.

Water depletion: The clinical syndrome of water depletion is usually associated with disturbances of electrolyte metabolism as well; selective water deficiency is uncommon. Relative water deficiency, however, can occur:

- Due to reduced water intake in patients with extreme lethargy or coma.
- In GI disorders with defective water absorption.
- Due to excessive sweating as in fever; hypotonicity of the sweat causes a greater loss of water than of sodium.
- In certain cases of chronic renal failure.
- In diabetes insipidus; and
- After damage to thirst centre.

Infants, in general, are more prone to develop water depletion than adults, as the kidneys of infants are unable to concentrate the urine adequately. This is also partly due to lack of water.

In **mild water depletion**, the osmolality of body fluids increases as their volume is decreased. This decrease in the volume is initially spread evenly over all the fluid compartments. Marked ECF contraction however, stimulates the secretion of aldosterone causing sodium retention which conserves the ECF volume in preference to ICF. (Fig. 36.2).

Clinical history helps to suspect water depletion. Such a patient is usually apathetic and confused. The urine volume is markedly reduced except in conditions like diabetes insipidus or chronic renal failure. *The plasma sodium, proteins and blood urea levels are raised*; but as the loss of fluid from the plasma is associated with a corresponding loss of fluid from the erythrocytes the hematocrit is not significantly raised. A conscious patient usually complains of thirst, dryness of mouth and difficulty in swallowing. Severe water depletion causes unconsciousness and finally even respiratory failure. *In practice, the clinical picture of water depletion is usually complicated by the associated sodium depletion (dehydration).*

The treatment is to give enough water, which, in the presence of normal kidney function, is well tolerated. In patients who are vomiting or unconscious, water in the form of 5 per cent glucose is given IV, as the solution is isotonic with blood. This also supplies calories and prevents ketosis. Associated disturbances in electrolyte concentrations should be corrected. Patients with fever and polyuria, and those on high protein intake need higher water intake.

In the absence of thirst, the water requirement can be judged by noting the 24 hour urinary volume and plasma sodium concentration. Free water deficit can be calculated by

$$\text{Water deficit} = \left\{\frac{\text{Plasma Na}^+(\text{mEq}) - 140}{140}\right\} \text{X TBW(L)}$$

After adequate water supplementation, the plasma Na^+ concentration decreases to normal levels.

Water excess: This is not so commonly seen as water depletion, but can occur following unrestricted administration of fluids in the presence of inadequate urinary output and in patients with cortisol deficiency. In mild cases, the patient may develop headache, nausea, vomiting and mental confusion. Body weight increases and edema may occur. Severe water intoxication can produce convulsions and coma. The plantar response may be extensor and pupils unequal. The symptomatology of water intoxication is probably due to hypotonicity of body fluids with resultant cerebral edema.

The presence of oliguria, in spite of adequate hydration of subcutaneous tissues, low serum sodium level, and an awareness on the part of physician that such a possibility may exist, help to diagnose the water excess.

The treatment of water intoxication consists of restriction of intake of non-saline fluid. In severe cases with convulsions and coma, 50 to 100 ml. of 5% saline is given IV, repeatedly, till the plasma Na^+ is raised to about 130 mEq./1. *Isotonic saline is not useful in water*

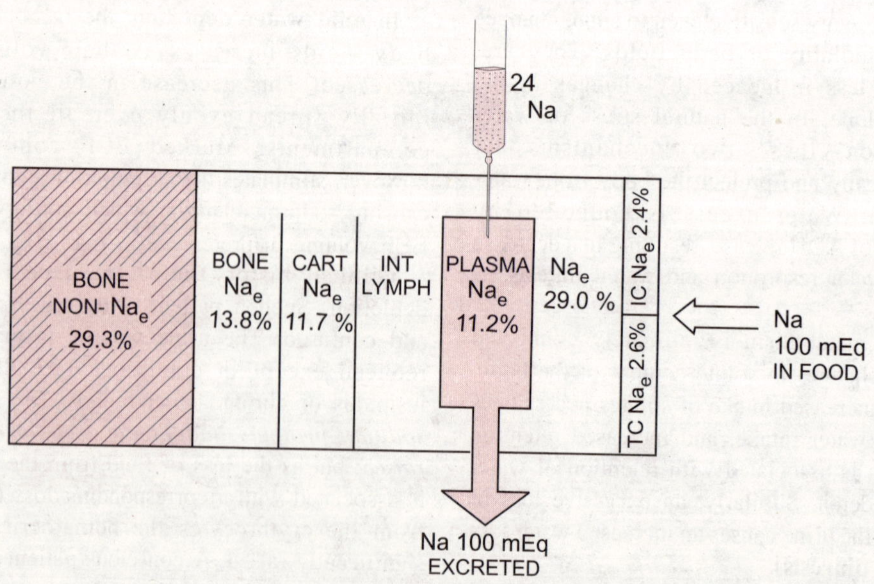

Fig. 36.1: Distribution of body sodium. Note that a considerable amount of sodium is in the bone and is not exchangeable with radiosodium within 24 hours of equilibrium
T.C.: Transcellular; I.C.: Intracellular; Cart.: cartilage.

intoxication as it does not help to raise the serum sodium level. In patients with renal disease with oliguria, water intoxication must be avoided by restricting the water intake as guided by the urinary output.

Sodium Metabolism

The study of sodium metabolism is fundamental to the understanding of electrolyte physiology and ECF volume regulation.

Sodium distribution: The distribution of body sodium is shown in Fig. 36.1. Sodium is present principally in ECF, though this is not its only location. There is a considerable amount of sodium in bones, which act as a sodium reservoir. The total body sodium can be measured by (i) direct carcass analysis and (ii) isotope dilution technic using radioactive sodium. The radioactive sodium, when injected IV, gets uniformly distributed in all the body fluids and tissues containing stable sodium, except some portion of the bone; the distribution is proportional to the sodium content of various body compartments and tissues. This process is known as 'sodium exchange'. Since plasma represents the ECF, by noting the dilution of injected radiosodium, total *body exchangeable sodium* can be calculated.

Body sodium calculated by the isotope dilution method is approximately 45 mEq./kg. in Indian males and about 43 mEq./kg. in Indian females. Thus, an average Indian male weighing 60 kg. will have 2700 mEq. of exchangeable sodium. This value, however, is less than 'actual total body sodium', as part of the bone sodium is not estimated by isotope dilution technique, using 24 hours equilibrium period. Estimation of exchangeable sodium is commonly used in studying the sodium metabolism in preference to elaborate sodium balance studies which are more laborious and may involve cumulative errors. Although the exchangeable sodium may vary over a wide range, the serum sodium level is maintained remarkably constant in health at 140.9 ± 4.8 (SD) mEq./litre.

Body content of sodium over a long period depends on the balance between intake and output. The daily intake of sodium varies considerably between 50 and 500 mEq. Unlike the phenomenon of thirst, no craving for salt is generally observed in sodium depletion; and hence, excessive sweating in tropics can easily cause salt depletion producing the symptoms of 'heat exhaustion'. Sodium loss in stools is very small. This may, however, be very marked in watery diarrhoea. The major output of sodium occurs in the urine and varies considerably, even on a constant diet. In tropical countries, the loss of sodium in sweat can be considerable, particularly with occupations that involve heavy labour. Sweat contains less sodium per litre than plasma. The sodium content of sweat in infants is 2.5 mEq./1, while in adults, not acclimatised to hot weather, it is 90 mEq./1. With acclimatisation, it is reduced to 10-15 mEq./1. *Excessive sweating thus causes proportionately more water loss than sodium loss.*

Although the rate of absorption of sodium and water from isotonic saline solutions is probably very similar in the human jejunum and ileum, there are important differences. It appears that the sodium absorption in the jejunum occurs mainly by passive process. Experiments with human *proximal jejunum* suggest that;

- ***Concurrent glucose or fructose absorption stimulates water absorption*** and that water movement across the mucosa stimulates passive absorption of sodium by 'solvent drag'.
- ***Glucose also stimulates active sodium absorption.***
- ***Fructose, unlike glucose, stimulates active potassium absorption.***
- ***The sodium absorption increases with rising intraluminal sodium concentration;*** and
- ***Bicarbonate absorption is an active process*** and increases with increasing intraluminal bicarbonate concentration; however, it is minimally affected by concurrent glucose or fructose absorption.

In contrast to jejunum, *in the ileum* sodium can be absorbed against large concentration gradients and it is not affected by water flow nor by the addition of glucose or bicarbonate. Thus, *sodium absorption in the ileum occurs mainly by active transport process.* These findings have an important clinical application in oral fluid therapy (see management of dehydration).

About 1000 mEq. of sodium are secreted daily into the GI tract. This is totally reabsorbed. Aldosterone promotes the sodium absorption from the intestines and the colon.

Urinary excretion of sodium: Normally, about 13-20 mEq. of sodium is filtered out every minute at the glomeruli. Of this, over 98 per cent is reabsorbed by the renal tubules and only 2 per cent is excreted in the urine. Hence, even a slight interference with the tubular reabsorption can produce a marked increase in the urinary sodium loss. Increasing the amount of sodium filtered at the glomeruli has a less marked effect on urinary sodium. A decrease in the filtered load of sodium as in congestive heart failure, however, leads to sodium retention and edema. On the other hand, failure of the tubules to reabsorb sodium due to lack of aldosterone causes marked sodium loss as in Addison's disease.

Urinary excretion of sodium is regulated by:

- ***Renal blood flow***, which depends upon cardiac output, local condition of the kidney vessels, and plasma and ECF volumes; and
- ***Hormonal control*** particularly by aldosterone, which influences tubular reabsorption of sodium.

Hormonal control of sodium metabolism: The bulk of sodium filtered by the glomeruli is reabsorbed in the proximal tubules independently of hormonal control. However, the adrenal salt retaining steroids are involved in the final control of sodium balance. Aldosterone promotes sodium reabsorption and potassium excretion, by acting on distal renal tubule. It also modifies the sodium concentration of sweat, saliva and intestinal juices and the movement of sodium and potassium across the cell membrane (Chapter 64).

The aldosterone secretion is regulated by :

- ***A reflex pathway with a regulatory centre in the brain*** which responds to changes in serum electrolytes such as sodium depletion, potassium loading and to ECF volume changes such as blood loss or reduction in body water. With respect to volume receptors, two have been clearly established and stimulation of either the right atrial wall or the juxta-glomerular apparatus in the kidneys can alter the secretion of aldosterone; and
- ***A humoral mechanism related to renin-angiotensin-aldosterone system*** (RAAS) with its trigger in the kidney plays an important role in the maintenance of salt and water homeostasis through the formation of angiotensin II and aldosterone (Chapter 64).

In normal man, sodium depletion increases while sodium loading decreases the plasma renin levels. The Yanomamo Indians inhabiting the tropical rain forests of Brazil, who do not use salt in their diet and thus have life-long very low levels of sodium intake, show elevation of plasma aldosterone and renin. Interestingly, their BP does not rise with age unlike in the developed world consuming a lot of salt. Chronic elevation of renin without hypertension indicates the importance of the level of body sodium in affecting BP in man. Total body exchangeable sodium is increased in hypertensive subjects, and it correlates *positively* with BP. Conversely, the exchangeable potassium correlates *negatively* with BP in essential hypertension. Sodium retention decreases the synthesis of nitric oxide, a potent vasodilator, by the endothelial cells. The RAAS, however, does not fully account for the physiological mechanisms involved in the renal handling of sodium.

NATRIURETIC PEPTIDE (NP) : This vasoactive natriuretic peptide hormone, released from the myocardium and the brain, plays an important role in sodium homeostasis. Three NPs have been identified :

(1) **Atrial NP (ANP),** released mainly from the atrium.

(2) **B-type NP (BNP),** released mainly from the ventricles of the heart; and

(3) **C-type NP (CNP),** released mainly from the brain and the vascular tissue.

ANP and BNP are released from the myocardiac tissue following atrial/ventricular myocyte stretch. They have similar chemical structures and actions. Apart from the myocyte stretch, their synthesis is also increased by glucocorticoids, tachycardia, thyroxine, angiotensisn II and endothelin I.

Three NP receptors have been indentified. ANP and BNP bind to specific receptors situated on the surface of target cells and cause generation of cyclic guanosine monophosphate (cGMP). CNP binds to the third specific receptor (the clearance receptor) to block the clearance of ANP and BNP, thus prolonging their action. These peptides are inactivated by the enzyme neutral peptidase (**vasopeptidase**). It is present on the surface of endothelial cells, cardiac myocytes, smooth muscle cells, kidney epithelium and in the brain. This enzyme is nonspecific and also catalyses the breakdown of other peptides such as bradykinin and angiotensin II.

Both ANP and BNP exert almost identical actions. They act on:

- ***Kidneys*** to increase the renal blood flow and GFR, and decrease sodium reabsorption, causing natriuresis.
- ***Vascular smooth muscle,*** causing vasodilatation, and reduce blood pressure and ventricular preload.
- ***Renin-angiotensin-aldosterone system,*** which they inhibit by direct action, reducing the release of angiotensin II and aldosterone.
- ***ANS,*** decreasing the activity of the sympathetic nervous system and increasing the vagal tone; and they possibly exert.
- ***Antiproliferative and antifibrotic*** actions in the vascular tissue.
- ***Inhibit the production of the vasoconstricor endothelin.***

Unlike ANP and BNP, CNP acts locally as a vasodilator; it does not function as a circulating hormone. The blood concentration of BNP is consistently raised in patients with cardiac dysfunction, and this may be of diagnostic and prognostic significance in heart failure.

Recombinant human BNP (Nesiritide) and vasopeptidase inhibitors which inhibit the metabolic degradation of BNP are under evaluation for their therapeutic application in CHF (Chapter 30).

Centrally released ANP suppresses pituitary ADH release and angiotonsin II mediated thirst.

Other Hormones such as hydrocortisone, oestrogens and testosterone can produce sodium retention. Adrenaline and noradrenaline may affect sodium metabolism indirectly by their actions on blood vessels. ADH has no direct effect on sodium metabolism. However, in the syndrome of inappropriate ADH secretion (SIADH), expansion of plasma volume leads to natriuresis, probably through inhibition of aldosterone secretion. The marked sodium loss that occurs in diabetic ketoacidosis is due to hyperglycemia with resultant polyuria.

The usual salt intake in humans (100-400 mmol of Na^+/day) is generally not a true reflection of salt requirement. The customary quantities of salt in contemporary diets far exceed the amount necessary to maintain sodium balance in health and this results in depressed levels of renin and aldosterone.

Sodium Depletion

True sodium depletion is one in which there is actual loss of sodium from the body. This must not be confused with the 'low salt syndrome' characterised by low plasma sodium concentration (hyponatremia). In *low salt syndrome* the total body sodium may not necessarily be low.

The effects of pure sodium depletion are distinctly different from those of pure water depletion. During the early stages of sodium depletion, the filtered sodium is almost completely reabsorbed. In addition, an excess of water is excreted by the kidneys, producing

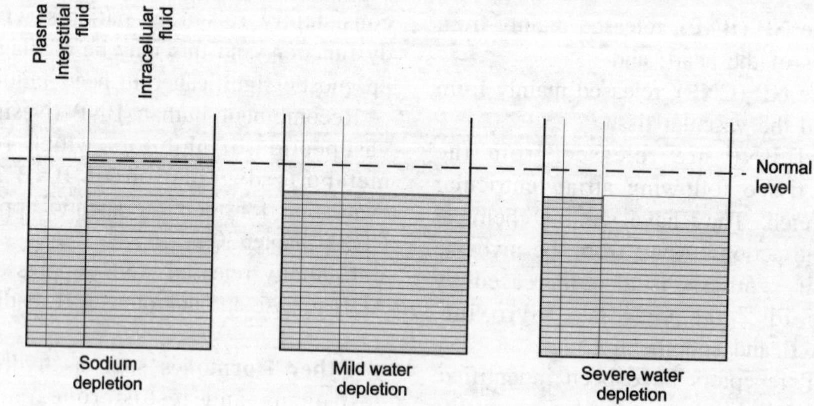

Fig. 36.2 : Effect of sodium depletion and of mild and severe water depletion on the partition of fluid between ECF and ICF (Black D.A.K., Essentials of Fluid Balance, 4th Ed. 1967, Blackwell Scientific Publications. The figure is reproduced by the courtesy of the author and the publishers)

dilute urine. The body, thus, conserves sodium concentration at the cost of ECF volume which contracts. Bones release some of their sodium which helps to maintain the serum sodium level; such release is more marked in younger and sodium depleted acidotic animals. With further losses of sodium, the serum sodium level falls. This causes further loss of ECF water, partly into urine and partly by a shift of water into the cells resulting in increased volume and decreased osmolality of ICF. This is in contrast to changes observed in severe water depletion, where the ECF and plasma volumes are maintained at the cost of ICF volume, which diminishes (Fig. 36.2).

Sodium depletion thus causes decrease in ECF and plasma volumes resulting in a rise in the hematocrit and the serum protein concentration.

Causes of sodium loss:

- ***GI loss***: as in diarrhoea and discharge from fistulae. Sodium loss can be severe in watery diarrhoea eg. in cholera or acute bacillary dysentery. In such cases, it is also associated with loss of bicarbonate causing acidosis.
- ***Renal loss***: Urinary loss of sodium is observed following diuretics, in diabetic coma, and during starvation or increased catabolism of proteins. A primary renal disease like acute tubular necrosis during its recovery phase and salt losing nephritis may produce marked sodium loss. Sodium loss is not directly linked with the urine volume. It can occur even in the absence of polyuria (e.g. Addison's disease); on the other hand, sodium excretion may be normal in the presence of polyuria (e.g. diabetes insipidus).
- ***Cutaneous loss***: Considerable cutaneous losses of sodium can occur in people working in hot climate like deserts and in patients with burns.
- ***Miscellaneous***: Draining of ascitic fluid can also produce marked sodium loss.

Symptomatology of sodium depletion: The clinical findings depend on:

- ***Amount of volume loss.***
- ***Rate of volume loss.***
- ***Nature of the fluid lost*** (blood or water); and
- ***Response of the vasculature to volume loss.***

Mild sodium depletion (100-200 mEq.) is common in tropical countries. Patients usually complain of loss of appetite, lethargy and cramps and have tachycardia. Since sweat is hypotonic, drinking water without correcting the sodium loss would cause body fluid dilution, which is partly responsible for these symptoms.

Massive sodium loss such as 1000-1500 m.

Eq. is usually accompanied by shock leading to **extrarenal uremia**. Limbs are cold. Cardiac output is low and pulse rate is high, due to hypovolemia. There is a fall in BP, with marked vasoconstriction in the skin and kidney vessels. Loss of tissue elasticity and turgor is characteristic of sodium depletion and is due to a decrease in the interstitial fluid content. Eyeballs appear 'sunken'. Symptoms like muscle cramps, anorexia and vomiting are probably due to relative body fluid dilution, as these are also seen in water intoxication.

It is vitally important to distinguish this extrarenal uremia from that due to renal tubular necrosis and acute renal failure secondary to acute severe sodium depletion with volume contraction; the former is reversible with proper treatment. In case of doubt, a therapeutic trial with saline infusion is justified. Primary sodium depletion can cause albuminuria but the presence of hematuria and casts is suggestive of intrinsic renal disease.

In sodium depletion, the serum sodium may be low but presence of normal serum sodium level does not rule out sodium depletion. Blood urea rises out of proportion to serum creatinine. The urine volume decreases, the urine sodium falls and the specific gravity rises. Sodium depletion following GI losses is obvious. In other conditions, history and symptoms help to suspect it. The possibility of sodium loss from the kidney itself should be borne in mind.

Sodium depletion and kidneys: A variety of mechanisms in the body operate to protect the body against the deleterious effects of sodium depletion and the resulting extra cellular volume (ECV) contraction.

- ECV contraction is sensed by ***extrarenal baroceptors*** located in the high (carotid body and aortic arch) and low (atria and thoracic veins) pressure areas of the circulation. Their activation results in increased sympathetic nerve activity, leading to tachycardia and rise in BP due to increased peripheral arteriolar resistance.
- Within the kidney, increased arteriolar resistance brings about ***renal hypoperfusion;*** this and the direct stimulation of the renal sympathetic nerves causes more complete sodium reabsorption by the proximal tubules.
- Activation of the extrarenal baroceptors also causes non-osmotic release of ***ADH*** which in turn causes renal water conservation, and reduces renal perfusion by vasoconstriction.
- Sympathetic nerve stimulation of the juxta-glomerular (JG) apparatus within the kidney (an ***intrarenal baroceptor***) enhances renin release. Renin, in turn, accelerates the formation of angiotensin II.
- ***Angiotensin II*** (i) is a potent pressor agent; (ii) causes release of aldosterone, which stimulates sodium reabsorption by the distal renal tubules; (iii) within the CNS, is a potent stimulus to thirst. Finally, (iv) *in low concentrations*, it has a selective constricting effect on efferent renal glomerular arterioles, and thus maintains GFR; *in higher concentrations*, however, it constricts afferent renal glomerular arterioles as well, leading to decrease GFR and renal ischemia.
- ***In mild to moderate ECV contraction***, beneficial peripheral vasoconstriction and renal sodium conservation occur; renal blood flow, GFR and osmoregulation are unaffected.
- ***When ECV contraction becomes severe***, the vasoconstrictive effect of high levels of noradrenaline and angiotensin II reduces both GFR and rate of sodium excretion. Further, nonosmotic ADH release, angiotensin II mediated thirst and reduction in salt delivery to the loop of Henle, all cause hyponatremia. Finally, excessive noradrenaline and angiotensin II cause renal blood flow to be compromised, leading to renal ischemia and **prerenal azotemia.**

Table 36.3: Agents which modulate renal circulation

Vasoconstrictors	Vasodilators
Noradrenaline	PGE_2
ADH	Natriuretic peptide(s).
Angiotensin II	
Endothelin 1	
Thromboxane A_2	

The other **vasoconstrictors** that may play a role in modulating systemic hemodynamics are endothelin 1 and thromboxane A_2 (Table 36.3).

As against the vasoconstrictors, **PGE_2 and NP act to protect the renal hemodynamics against the onslaught of excess vasoconstrictors.** They are the negative feedback elements of the renal, volume regulatory response.

PGE_2 is produced in the renal glomeruli, where angiotensin II activates eicosanoid production and release, as well as by the renal medullary interstitial cells. It :

- ***Is a natriuretic***, causing direct inhibition of tubular sodium reabsorption;
- ***Is a vasodilator*** and protects the kidney against the injurious effects of noradrenaline and angiotensin II; and
- ***Antagonises the renal tubular effect of ADH directly.***

Table 36.4: Principles of treatment of sodium depletion

- Introduce a good IV line.
- Start with 0.9% (normal) saline. This is the fluid of choice with isotonic fluid loss.
- In severe cases, a rapid rate of infusion (2-3 litres/2-3 hours) may be required.
- Add potassium and bicarbonate, depending upon the type of fluid lost. Excessive use of normal saline alone aggravate acidosis, if present, because of its chloride content.
- In case of diarrhoea, 40 mEq of potassium (40 ml. of 7.5% KCl) and 45 mEq of bicarbonate (50 ml. of 7% sodium bicarbonate) may be added to each litre normal saline.
- Monitor the therapy in severe cases by measuring the CVP, which should be maintained at 6-12 cm of water.
- If the urine output does not rise in spite of adequate fluid replacement, renal failure should be suspected.

Treatment of sodium depletion: The aim of therapy is to maintain the urine output at 30-50 ml./hour and the BP within normal limits. The principles of treatment are shown in Table 36.4.

Mild degrees of volume depletion can be corrected by giving about 10 g. of sodium chloride and 2-3 litres of oral fluid daily. This can be done by administering adequate amounts of 0.9 per cent saline. The amount needed would vary, but moderately depleted cases usually require about 3 litres. Overfilling of the neck veins indicates overloading with saline which should be avoided as it may cause pulmonary edema. Deficiency of other electrolytes, particularly potassium and bicarbonate, if present, should be corrected.

In patients with *severe sodium and water depletion*, the amount of isotonic saline needed is so large that if injected quickly, it may overload the circulation. Serum sodium levels below 110 mEq/1 may precipitate convulsions and coma. In such severe hyponatremia, slow IV infusion of hypertonic (3-5 per cent) sodium chloride solution is used for restoring plasma volume and renal circulation, particularly in patients with extrarenal azotemia. The **hypertonic saline** injected gets diluted by a shift of the water (which has entered into the ICF during severe sodium depletion) back to ECF. As severe sodium depletion is generally associated with acidosis, sodium bicarbonate has to be administered to correct the acidosis. Severe hyponatremia with marked sodium depletion should be corrected slowly to serum Na^+ of 125 mEq/L (no more) over 24 hours. Further rise in serum Na+ to normal level should take several days.

For subjects working in hot environment and in diseases like Addison's disease, where continued sodium loss occurs, prophylactic addition of sodium chloride to the diet is necessary.

Hyponatremia: Hyponatremia, defined as serum sodium concentration of < 135 mmol/litre is quite common in hospitalized patients. It is associated with high morbidity and mortality in patients with chronic heart failure, cirrhosis and neurological diseases. It must be emphasized that although serum sodium may be low in cases with sodium depletion, not all patients with low serum sodium levels (hyponatremia) are suffering from body sodium depletion. In some of these cases with *hyponatremic syndrome* where plasma sodium level is low, the total body sodium may be normal or even high.

It has been observed that serum sodium correlates well with the osmolality of serum which is related to

$$\frac{\text{Exchangeable sodium + Exchangeable potassium}}{\text{Total body water}}$$

This observation in man provides a rational basis for the classification of hyper and hyponatremic states.

Hyponatremia may be caused by:

- ***Primary sodium loss.***
- ***Primary potassium loss.***
- ***Primary water excess***; or
- ***Combination of these.***

In practice, hyponatremia can be classified as **hypovolemic, euvolemic** and **hypervolemic**. Hyponatremia in diarrhoea is due to loss of Na^+ and K^+ while that observed in CHF and cirrhosis is due to loss of K^+ and gain in body water. In these patients, water retention is mediated by vasopressin-V_2 receptors in the renal collecting tubules. In some cases, it is associated with inappropriate ADH secretion (SIADH).

The treatment of hyponatremic syndrome depends upon the cause. However, its management is not always easy. Serum sodium concentration can be temporarily raised by water deprivation in mild cases, and by administration of saline in symptomatic patients. Recently, selective, vasopressin V_2 receptor antagonists such as tolvaptan have been shown to be useful in maintaining serum Na^+ concentration in euvolemic or hypervolemic hyponatremic patients (Chapter 38).

Sodium Excess

Sodium retention is always associated with water retention and may manifest as pitting edema. Sodium excess due to increased intake is most unlikely in the presence of normal kidney function. The main cause of sodium retention is the failure of the kidneys to excrete the sodium load. This may be due to :

- ***Intrinsic kidney disease*** e.g. acute nephritis, nephrosis.
- ***Excessive reabsorption of sodium by the tubules*** e.g. in aldosteronism.
- ***Decreased renal blood flow*** such as in CHF and acute hypotension and
- ***Iatrogenic, following certain drugs*** e.g. NSAID, hydrocortisone.

Estimation of serum sodium levels is not of much help in the diagnosis of body sodium excess and in fact, in some cases the levels may be even subnormal.

The treatment of sodium excess depends upon the cause which should be corrected, if possible. Therapeutically, sodium depletion can be brought about by:

- ***Restricting the daily dietary sodium intake*** to 20-50 mEq.
- ***Increasing the sodium output in urine*** by using diuretics (Chapter 38); and
- ***Improving renal perfusion*** e.g., digoxin in CHF or IV infusions in oligemic shock.

Usually, these methods are combined.

Hypernatremia or increased serum sodium level is not necessarily associated with increased total body sodium. Hypernatremia may be due to:

- ***Primary sodium excess.***
- ***Primary potassium excess.***
- ***Primary water deficit***; or
- ***Combination of these.***

In practice, it is commonly due to excessive loss of total body water as in diabetes insipidus. It may cause mental impairment in the adults.

Hypernatremia has been reported in a patient

with perphenazine poisoning who was given 10 per cent hypertonic saline as emetic but failed to vomit, and in infants who were given feeds prepared with salt instead of sugar by mistake; half of these infants died. The clinical picture showed pyrexia, hyperpnea, hyper-reflexia and coma. Brain damage has been reported to be associated with hypernatremia due to heat stroke.

The treatment is directed towards reducing the serum sodium level. In patients with severe dehydration and contraction of blood volume, hypernatremia should be corrected slowly at the rate of 12-13 mEq/1/24 hours for the first 48 hours. This is best brought about by initial infusion of normal saline followed by infusion of ½ strength saline. Infusion of 5% dextrose in water in this condition has two disadvantages :

(1) It lowers the plasma osmolality too fast for the brain to keep pace; the brain which remains hypertonic then swells up by transfer of water from ECF; and

(2) It can cause hyperglycemia with osmotic diuresis; the latter can aggravate hypernatremia. In children the best solution is 2.5% dextrose in ½ normal saline.

Potassium Metabolism

The body potassium in man, as measured by isotope dilution, amounts to about 45 mEq./kg. in males and 38 mEq./kg. in females. These figures are lower than the actual total body potassium as estimated by cadaveric analysis by about 15 per cent.

Distribution of potassium: Potassium is essentially a cation of the cells and hence its distribution is related to the cell mass. It is predominantly (98%) restricted to the IC space. About 70 per cent of the total potassium is in the muscles, about 20 per cent in the brain and large viscera while 10 per cent is present in the skin and subcutaneous tissues. As compared to sodium, the amount of potassium in the bone is small, estimated at about 218 mEq.

The mean serum level of potassium is 4.5 mEq/1 ± 0.46 (S.D.). Although this is considerably lower than the mean serum sodium level, changes in serum potassium concentration can produce profound effects on body functions. Disturbances due to altered potassium metabolism can, therefore, be studied by noting the effects following changes in (a) total body potassium and (b) serum potassium levels.

Potassium intake and excretion: The daily potassium intake varies considerably and is estimated to be about 50-150 mEq. It is more in vegetarians than in non-vegetarians as vegetables and fruits (citrus fruits, tomatoes, bananas) contain large amounts of potassium. Processed foods are usually high in sodium and low in potassium.. Kidney is the major regulator of long term potassium homeostasis. The major loss (90%) of potassium occurs in urine by tubular secretion. That which is filtered by the glomeruli is totally reabsorbed. The kidney reabsorbs sodium and, in exchange, excretes H^+ and K^+ ions into the distal tubules (Berliner mechanism). The normal urine is, thus, acidic in reaction. Because of this tubular secretion of potassium, the urinary loss of potassium would continue and may even be greater than the intake, when daily intake of potassium is markedly restricted. *Increased sodium intake increases the potassium loss because it makes more sodium available for exchange with potassium while low sodium intake reduces the urinary loss of potassium.*

Normally, about 10% of potassium is excreted in the feces. As in the case of urine, a part of this is secreted by the colon in exchange for sodium which is reabsorbed. This part of potassium loss in stools would continue even in subjects on very low potassium intake. This is in contrast to body sodium which is conserved by achieving its complete reabsorption by the renal tubules and the intestines, when sodium intake is markedly reduced.

The potassium concentration of sweat in infants is 3.9 m.Eq. as compared to the sodium concentration of 2.5 mEq/1. In nonacclimatised adults it is 10 mEq/1. Thus, *proportionately more potassium is lost per unit volume of sweat than sodium, with respect to their plasma levels.* Excessive sweating, as occurs during dry heat or during fevers, may cause significant potassium depletion.

The requirement of infants and growing children for potassium is relatively higher than that of adults.

The Institute of Medicine, USA, recommends a *daily intake* of 65-70 mmol of sodium (3.8 g of sodium chloride) for normal adults younger than 50 years of age and 50 mmol for those over 70 years. Their recommendation for daily intake of potassium is 100-120 mmol (4.7 g of potassium), thus maintaining a dietary K^+/Na^+ ratio at about 2. As per current estimate, industrialized nations which consume lots of processed foods ingest as much as 100-400 mmol of sodium and 50-70 mmol of potassium, with a dietary K^+/Na^+ ratio of less than 0.4.

Factors affecting plasma potassium: Estimation of plasma potassium gives information about ECF potassium changes.

- ***Potassium intake:*** With normal intake of sodium, reduction of potassium intake would cause a fall in plasma potassium on account of continued loss of potassium in urine and feces, leading to potassium depletion. Hyperkalemia may occur in older patients with renal insuffeciency. *Salt substitutes which may contain as much as 200 mmoles of potassium per tablespoonful are a hidden source of ingested potassium.*
- ***Total body sodium increase*** causes loss of body potassium. Part of the retained sodium shifts into the cells, thus displacing some amount of potassium which is excreted. Conversely, in severe sodium depletion, as in diabetic coma, the serum potassium may be raised. It appears, therefore that changes in the ECF volume may cause a rise or a fall in serum potassium levels. In CHF, where sodium retention is marked and ECF volume is increased, the serum potassium is usually low.
- ***Acidosis and alkalosis*:** Normally, the kidney compensates for *metabolic acidosis* by secreting more H+ ions than K+ ions in exchange for sodium. This leads to potassium retention. Acidosis also reduces the potassium uptake by the cells. This may cause hyperkalemia. If the plasma potassium level is high to begin with, acidosis will cause further rise in plasma potassium with resultant toxicity. Acidosis, in the presence of marked potassium depletion, however, will cause severe cellular derangement as it will aggravate the fall of intracellular potassium.

Alkalosis is associated with lowering of plasma potassium level.

- ***Changes in the cell metabolism*:** Increased uptake of glucose by the cells is associated with a shift of potassium into the cell. This may cause a transient fall in serum potassium. In the presence of potassium depletion, such a shift may cause marked hypokalemia. This phenomenon occurs in patients recovering from diabetic coma where, as the tissue glycogen is repleted following insulin and glucose, potassium shifts into the cells thus causing a fall in serum potassium level. *Protein anabolism* is also associated with increased potassium uptake by the cells while *protein catabolism* would cause cellular potassium loss.
- ***Hormones* :** Potassium is a major stimulus to aldosterone roduction.Aldosterone secretion is integral to potassium homeostasis,controlling its excretion in the urine, feces, sweat and saliva.The normal physiological regulators insulin and catecholamines are stimulated by the ingestion of foods containing glucose and potassium.They are essential in shifting potassium intracellularly, mainly into the liver and the muscles.
- ***Drugs:*** See below.

Potassium Depletion and Hypokalemia

Hypokalemia is usually defined as plasma potassium less than 3.5 mEq/litre. However, body potassium depletion can exist in the presence of normal serum potassium. As much as 100 to 200 mEq of potassium loss is necessary in adults before the serum potassium falls below 3 mEq/1.

Causes of potassium depletion: These can be grouped as follows:

- ***Decreased Intake:*** Potassium deficiency due to decreased intake can occur but is more likely in old people who may have inadequate dietary intake (less than 1 g/day).
- ***GI loss*** (urinary K^+ equal to or less than 20 mEq/day) : This occurs in such conditions as excessive vomiting, copious discharge from a fistula, aspiration of intestinal contents and diarrhoea. In diarrhoea, both sodium and potassium are lost. In formed bulky stools, however, sodium loss may not be much but the loss of potassium could be considerable e.g. in steatorrhea and following chronic use of purgatives.
- ***Renal loss*** (urinary K^+ more than 30 mEq./l day): Perhaps the commonest cause of hypokalemia is diuretics. Increase in plasma potassium level due to intracellular potassium loss in such conditions as sodium overload, starvation, acidosis or protein catabolism increases renal loss of potassium. In addition, renal loss of potassium also occurs in:

(a) The presence of excessive aldosterone, hydrocortisone.

(b) Extra-renal states like diabetic acidosis.

(c) Magnesium depletion can cause severe hypokalemia by increasing K^+ excretion.

(d) Certain primary renal diseases such as renal tubular acidosis (Fanconi syndrome) and nephrotic syndrome.

Patients with glomerular diseases do not lose potassium; in fact, they generally retain potassium. However, potassium loss may be severe in some patients with renal tubular dysfunction. *It must also be borne in mind that potassium depletion, in itself, may cause renal tubular dysfunction.*

- ***Transcellular shift:*** Transient hypokalemia occurs in patients with diabetic ketoacidosis following treatment with insulin and glucose. Metabolic alkalosis is always associated with hypokalemia.
- ***Drug induced :*** Apart from diuretics, laxatives, $beta_2$ adrenergic agonists such as salbutamol, theophylline, exogenous insulin and rarely calcium channel blockers can cause hypokalemia.
- ***Excessive sweating*** is also likely to be an important cause of potassium loss in the tropics.

Clinical manifestations: Since potassium is the major intracellular cation, its depletion is expected to produce widespread dysfunction.

- ***Mild potassium depletion,*** (serum K^+ 3.0 – 3.5 mEq/l) about 10 per cent of the total body potassium, does not produce any dramatic symptoms. Many vague symptoms such as lethargy, malaise, weakness of muscular activity, anorexia and thirst have been attributed to but not definitely proved to be due to mild potassium deficiency. On average, a reduction of serum K+ by 0.3 mEq/l suggests a total body deficit of about 100 mEq.
- ***Marked hypokalemia*** (serum K^+ less than 2.5 mEq/l) impairs neuromuscular function leading to paralysis, causes conduction defects in the heart, intestinal dilatation and even paralytic ileus, and lowers the BP. Clinically, hypokalemia is associated with arrhythmias and tachycardia. Tetany can occur on account of ECF alkalemia.
- ***Excessive potassium depletion*** causes reduction in the capacity of the kidneys to concentrate urine. Loss of potassium in amounts greater than 30 per cent of the total body potassium causes widespread damage to cell function.
- ***Chronic cumulative potassium loss*** may cause nonspecific symptoms like muscular pain, abdominal distension and nocturia. If such a deficiency is not suspected, these symptoms may lead to the erroneous diagnosis of neurosis and may even result in death, if left untreated. It must be pointed out that there is no consistency in the symptoms for any given level of plasma potassium. In general, in severe potassium depletion plasma potassium level is below 2.5 m. Eq./1. except in cases with acidosis and associated sodium depletion.

Hypokalemia in humans can cause sodium retention, phosphate reabsorption and increased renal ammonia production. By impairing renal urine concentrating mechanism,it can cause nephrogenic diabetes insipidus.

Other changes: The normal activity of both skeletal and smooth muscles is impaired. The neuromuscular abnormality is probably due to alteration in the excitability. The skeletal muscle fibres may show rhabdomyolysis, and the heart muscle, degenerative changes. Excess of sodium and deficit of potassium in the diet has been correlated with the development of high BP and tissue injury in rats. Current evidence suggest that a potassium deficit has an important role in hypertension and its cardiovascular sequelae in man (Chapter 29). In moderate to severe hypokalemia, ECG changes may show prominent U wave, ST depression, prolonged QT and inversion of T wave.

Potassium depletion inhibits insulin secretion and is associated with glucose intolerance. Chronic potassium deficiency causes metabolic alkalosis by bringing about a shift in H^+ ions from the extracellular space into the intracellular space in exchange for K^+ ions. The ability to form gastric acid and to absorb electrolytes from the bowel is impaired. Animals with chronic potassium depletion fail to grow.

Treatment of potassium depletion: Normally, potassium deficiency can be prevented by taking diet rich in vegetables and fruits, and avoiding processed foods. Fruit juices and tender coconut water contain good amounts of potassium in palatable form; in addition, these also supply some calories. Fresh, green, coconut water contains about 70 mEq/1 of potassium. A single orange gives 6-8 m.Eq. of potassium, a tomato 16-20 mEq and a banana 18-22 mEq. In the presence of normal kidney function, oral administration of adequate amounts of potassium (50-100 mEq/day) is usually effective in controlling chronic potassium depletion with low serum level.

Drug of choice is potassium chloride although potassium citrate is less unpalatable than potassium chloride. Potassium bicarbonate is used to prevent metabolic acidosis. *Three grammes of potassium chloride gives 40 mEq of potassium.* The bad taste of the salt can be masked by adding a small quantity of ginger extract. Usually, a mixture is preferred to tablets as the latter can cause intestinal ulcerations.

In acute cases, potassium depletion is associated with other electrolyte disturbances such as sodium depletion and acidosis. These, along with the water depletion, should be corrected as discussed elsewhere. *A vigorous correction of acidosis should be avoided as potentially lethal hypokalemia may be precipitated.*

In emergency, potassium can be given by IV infusion; 40 mEq of potassium per litre are recommended as a safe limiting concentration, with a drip-rate of one litre in 2-3 hours. Such a concentration can be prepared by adding 20 ml. of potassium chloride injection BP to one litre of saline or glucose drip. During the IV infusion, the serum potassium level and ECG should be monitored as a sudden marked rise in serum potassium may cause cardiac arrest.

Potassium should never by administered as an IV bolus or injected into the tubing of an intravenous infusion as this may cause sudden rise in serum K^+ level and death from cardiac arrest. Further, the serum K^+ level must be known and adequate urine output established before treatment.

Potassium salts can also be used prophylactically in patients receiving digitalis and certain diuretic drugs that cause K^+ loss. In such cases, a daily supplement of 25-50 mEq. is adequate. Table 36.5 summarises the treatment of hypokalemia.

Alkalosis due to hypokalemia cannot be corrected except by potassium administration.

Hyperkalemia and Potassium Excess

Hyperkalemia or the serum potassium more

Table 36.5 : Treatment of hypokalemia

(1) **Oral potassium:**
- Potassium chloride KCl 40-100mEq/day in divided doses.
- Potassium phosphate in patients with concurrent hypophosphatemia.
- Potassium bicarbonate in acidotic patients.

(2) **IV Potassium chloride :** This is usually reserved for patients with K^+ level less than 2.6 mEq/l. It is administered under monitoring, at a rate not exceeding 20 mEq/hour.

than 5 mEq/l is fairly common and may often cause fatal complications.

Causes of hyperkalemia: In the presence of normal kidney function, increased oral intake of potassium causes only a transient hyperkalemia. Usually, dangerous blood levels are not reached, unless potassium is injected IV, rapidly and in large quantities.

The most important cause of hyperkalemia is decreased renal excretion following acute or chronic renal insufficiency. Occasionally, it can occur following tissue injury, due to increased catabolic processes, diabetic and chronic respiratory acidosis, in patients with Addison's disease due to lack of aldosterone, and following certain drugs like spironolactone, triamterene, ACE inhibitors, NSAID and trimethoprim. Hyperkalemia due to transcellular shift of K+ may be observed following insulin deficiency, acidosis and the use of beta-blockers.

It should be noted that the plasma potassium in newborn is high and levels upto 8 mEq./l. may be observed without any obvious toxic effects.

Pharmacological effects of high serum potassium: Mild hyperkalemia (less than 5.5 mEq/l) is often asymptomatic. Severe hyperkalemia affects both cardiac and skeletal muscles. It may cause various arrhythmias, idioventricular rhythm and finally, cardiac arrest in diastole, if the serum level exceeds 7 mEq./l. The ECG shows peaking or tenting of T wave, depression of ST segment and widening of QRS complex. PR interval may be prolonged.

Skeletal muscles may show paralysis. Ascending paralysis involving respiratory muscle has been described in hyperkalemia; this is probably due to a block in transmission in the muscle membrane as direct application of potassium to the muscle causes contraction.

Treatment of hyperkalemia: Hyperkalemia with ECG changes is a medical emergency and requires immediate treatment; the detailed work-up is postponed till the K+ level is brought down to safe a level.The treatment is directed at:

(a) **Minimizing the membrane depolarization** over 2-3 minutes, thus reducing the membrane excitability:
- IV Calcium gluconate 10%, 10 ml, over a few minutes.

(b) **Promoting an intracellular shift of K^+**
- Plain insulin, 5-10 units, in 25-50 g of dextrose in water, over 5 minutes.
- A beta-adrenergic agonist, either parenterally or by nebulization.

(c) **Promoting K^+ loss from the body**
- Dialysis in patients with chronic renal failure.
- Cation exchange resin (Chapter 38)
- The mineralocorticoid fludrocortisone (Chapter 64).
- A loop diuretic in combination with a thiazide, in patients with normal renal function.

(d) **Minimizing the entry/retention of K^+.**
- Cessation of K^+ rich foods and drugs.
- Cessation of K^+ retaining drugs such as spironolactone and ACEI..

(e) **Treatment of associated infection and acidosis**

Acidosis and Alkalosis

The regulation of the reaction of the body fluids is mainly influenced by their 'hydrogen ion' concentration designated by the term **"hydrion"** [H^+].

An acid is a proton donor molecule or ion which provides a proton (hydrion H^+) a positively charged particle, and thus lowers the pH of a solution into which it is placed. Apart from conventional acids like HCl, other agents like ammonium ion which can split into a proton + ammonia or even water which can split to give a hydrion + a hydroxyl ion can be considered as acids. By this definition, chloride, sulfate and phosphate ions are not acids but considered as the conjugate bases of a true acid. On the other hand, a molecule or an ion which can accept a proton (hydrion) is termed as a base; it thus raises the pH of a solution into which it is placed. Thus, ammonia (NH_3) and hydroxyl (OH) ions are bases as they can accept a proton and produce ammonium (NH4) and water respectively.

Water can act as an acid as well as a base, depending upon the circumstances. As an acid, it gives up a hydrion to yield OH ion, while as a base it can accept a hydrion to produce hydronium (OH_3) ion.

Unlike the concentration of sodium and potassium, the body fluid concentration of hydrion is very small and can be measured using a pH meter.

In the plasma, CO_2 is present as carbonic acid ($H.HCO_3$) whereas bicarbonate (HCO_3) is present in combination with cations as $B.HCO_3$. Hence CO_2/HCO_3 ratio may also be expressed as $H.HCO_3/B.HCO_3$ ratio. If the concentrations of both carbonic acid and bicarbonate in the blood were fixed, the [H+] of the blood would also be fixed. Thus, in health the [H+] of blood is remarkably constant. The changes in the [H+] of the body fluids are resisted by three mechanisms:

- ***Buffer systems.***
- ***Renal mechanisms***; and
- ***Respiratory mechanisms.***

Buffer mechanisms merely minimize disturbances when strong acids or bases are added to the blood but the blood [H^+] is maintained constant at its normal value mainly by the combined efforts of kidneys and lungs. The respiratory mechanisms fix the carbonic acid concentration in the blood at 1.4 mEq./1. and the kidneys maintain the blood bicarbonate level at 28 mEq./1. The ratio of $H.HCO_3/B.HCO_3$ is thus fixed at 1.4: 28 resulting in a [H^+] of 40 nanoEq./1. Normally, the arterial plasma [H^+] varies between 36-44 n. Eq./1. Since the pH of the solution is the negative logarithm of [H^+] expressed in g. Eq./1., the normal pH of arterial plasma is calculated to be between 7.44-7.36. The remainder of the buffer systems in plasma then adjust the ratios of their acids to bases in keeping with this pH.

Unlike with sodium and potassium one cannot measure 'hydrion balance', as hydrion does not maintain its identity in the body; it is constantly disappearing or is constantly produced during various complex reactions of energy metabolism. Major portion of the body hydrion is produced during the oxidation of food and tissue metabolism; the contribution made by the actual intake of hydrion is very little.

Metabolically, hydrion is produced in the body in two forms:

- ***Potential hydrion*** or as CO_2, which is produced by the combustion of foods. This can normally be eliminated by the lungs. In the presence of respiratory diseases, however, retention of CO_2 raises the $H.HCO_3/B.HCO_3$ ratio and hence, increases hydrion concentration in the plasma, although the total body production of hydrion is not raised; and
- ***Non-volatile hydrion*** which is derived from:

(i) Incomplete oxidation of carbohydrates and fats, giving organic acids,

(ii) Sulfuric acid, produced following the oxidation of sulfur containing amino acids, and

(iii) Phosphoric acid, produced following the oxidation of phosphoprotein residues.

The nonvolatile hydrion is normally excreted by the kidneys, mainly in the form of ammonium ion NH_4 (H^+ buffered by NH_3) and titratable acidity (H^+ buffered by HPO_4). Very little acid is excreted as free H ions.

The plasma concentration of hydrion being regulated mainly by the lungs and the kidneys is proportional to the plasma ratio CO_2/HCO_3; the level of plasma CO_2 is regulated by the lungs and the respiratory centre while HCO_3 level is regulated by renal conservation. Physiologically, effect of a sudden rise in plasma hydrion is countered by the action of blood and tissue buffers and to a certain extent by exchange of hydrion with bone cations. The renal adjustment, though important, is rather slow to occur.

The ratio $H.HCO_3/B.HCO_3$ and thus the blood $[H^+]$ can be disturbed by factors that change either the carbonic acid or bicarbonate levels in the blood. Thus, a fall in carbonic acid or a rise in bicarbonate level will decrease the ratio and the $[H^+]$ in the blood, leading to *alkalosis.* Similarly, a rise in carbonic acid or a fall in bicarbonate will increase the ratio leading to rise in the $[H^+]$, causing *acidosis.* In all the cases of $[H^+]$ disturbances, when the fault is primarily respiratory the compensation is primarily renal and vice versa.

Table 36.6 gives the normal values of acid-base parameters in arterial blood. In modern instruments, pH, PO_2 and pCO_2 are determined and SaO_2 and HCO_3 are calculated. The pH gives a quantitative idea of the acid-base balance of the extra-cellular space but only a qualitative idea of the total body acid-base balance. To obtain the latter an additional parameter called *'bicarbonate deficit'* is calculated.

Table 36.6: Normal values of acid base parameters in arterial blood

Parameter	Normal range
pH	7.38 - 7.42
pCO_2 (mm Hg)	37 - 42
HCO_3 (mMol/L)	24 - 28
pO_2 (mm Hg)	85 - 100
SaO_2 (%)	98

Bicarbonate deficit = (body weight kg x 0.6) x (Normal HCO^-_3 — Actual HCO^-_3)

The **anion gap** represents anions which are not normally measured in acid-base studies: proteins, phosphate, sulfate and organic acids.

Anion gap = $(Na^+ + K^+) — (Cl^- + HCO^-_3)$, all in mMol/1.

Normal anion gap is 10 - 18 mMol/1.

The anion gap is used to divide metabolic acidosis into those with **normal anion gap** and those with **high anion gap**.

Metabolic acidosis with normal anion gap is due to bicarbonate loss from the GI tract or the kidneys. *Anion gap is widened in* ketoacidosis, lactic acidosis, uremic acidosis and salicylate poisoning.

Acidosis

Acidosis is defined as an increase in either potential and/or nonvolatile hydrion *content* of the body. Increase in the hydrion *concentration* of the plasma is termed as *acidemia* and is manifested by a fall in pH of the blood. In certain instances, although excessive potential hydrion is produced in the body, the plasma level of hydrion may remain normal due to a compensatory increase in the ventilation. Such a state of acidosis without acidemia is known as 'compensated acidosis', which could become 'decompensated' if the metabolic cause remains uncorrected. Similarly in lung diseases, retention of potential hydrion CO_2 can be compensated by renal conservation of bicarbonate, thus maintaining the plasma ratio of $H.HCO_3/B.HCO_3$ constant. But this too would become 'uncompensated' if respiratory failure is not corrected.

Acidosis can occur as:

Metabolic acidosis: This is due to excess production of hydrion in the body because of:

- Acceleration of the normal metabolic processes as during excessive catabolism in fever, starvation, dehydration and during diabetic ketoacidosis.
- Excessive loss of alkaline fluids from the intestines, as in diarrhoea which causes a relative loss of hydroxyl (OH) ions.
- Ingestion of toxic doses of agents which are hydrion-donors e.g. salicylates and methanol.

- Administration of large quantities of normal saline.
- A high level of plasma potassium which results in a fall in plasma bicarbonate by interfering with the reabsorption and manufacture of bicarbonate by the kidneys; and
- Accumulation of lactic acid. This is seen in conditions like severe circulatory failure or following extracorporeal circulation where tissue hypoxia is present. Lactic acidosis is also seen following oral hypoglycemic agents, biguanides, which inhibit aerobic glycolysis.

The rise in hydrion and fall in blood pH in metabolic acidosis are to a certain extent compensated by the buffering action of the blood and tissues, by increased ventilation and by increased renal excretion of the hydrion. Although hyperpnea and the buffering systems reduce acidemia they do not help to eliminate the excess of hydrion, which is solely excreted by the kidneys.

The net effect of metabolic acidosis is that the plasma bicarbonate and pCO_2 fall and urine becomes strongly acidic and has a high ammonium content.

Renal acidosis: This is associated with increase in body hydrion due to its defective renal excretion, either as titratable acid or as ammonium ion. This is observed either in selective tubular disorders (renal tubular acidosis) or in diseases primarily damaging the glomeruli (glomerulonephritis and diabetic nephropathy). Renal acidosis is also seen in Addison's disease where ammonia formation is inadequate. Carbonic anhydrase inhibitor drugs like acetazolamide which interfere with tubular secretion of hydrion can cause renal acidosis.

In renal acidosis the excretion of titratable acid and ammonium is impaired. The plasma bicarbonate and pCO_2 concentrations are low. The urine, however, may be alkaline.

Respiratory acidosis: This is due to increased retention of the potential hydrion (CO_2) in the blood leading to a rise in plasma carbonic acid content. It usually occurs in chronic lung diseases with cor pulmonale, in diseases with respiratory muscle paralysis and following the respiratory centre depression.

Unlike in metabolic or renal acidosis, the plasma bicarbonate and pCO_2 are raised. The urine is strongly acidic. The associated hyperpnea may be difficult to differentiate from that due to original respiratory pathology.

Clinical manifestations of acidosis: The clinical picture is usually complicated by the associated electrolyte disturbances such as sodium depletion. Uncomplicated acidosis causes hyperpnea, muscle twitching and mental confusion. Patients with renal and metabolic acidosis may have Kussmaul breathing although they may not complain of dyspnoea. Ultimately, coma may result, which occurs more frequently in patients with respiratory acidosis; in such cases, the blood pH value is below 7.25. The diagnosis of acidotic coma is important as it is reversible following appropriate treatment. In patients with chronic acidosis, mental or respiratory changes may not be so prominent but the patient may complain of bone pains and tenderness due to demineralization of bones. This is usually seen in chronic renal acidosis.

Treatment of acidosis: In acute cases, other electrolyte disturbances like sodium and potassium depletion should be corrected and in many cases, this, along with the treatment of the cause, is the major form of therapy, e.g., in diabetic acidosis and in diarrhoea. In severe cases (pH 7.1 or less, or HCO_3 less than 10 mEq/l) acidosis can be corrected by a slow infusion of 7.5% sodium bicarbonate in quantities sufficient (1 mEq/kg over 20-30 minutes) to raise the plasma bicarbonate concentration to about 15-20 mEq./1. No attempts should be made to correct the acidosis rapidly or fully. *When sodium bicarbonate solution for injection is available, the use of sodium lactate (1/6 molar) to correct acidosis is not justified* for two reasons: (a) it depends upon the body oxidative mechanisms for conversion to bicarbonate; and (b) it can cause lactic acidosis.

Administration of excessive alkali in the

presence of marked kidney damage may cause tetany and pulmonary edema. Acidosis associated with renal failure, therefore, may be better managed by peritoneal dialysis or by hemodialysis. Chronic renal acidosis responds to alkaline mixture containing sodium citrate and citric acid. Shohl's mixture which is commonly used contains 140 gm. of citric acid and 90 gm. of sodium citrate per litre of water. The adult dose is 50-100 ml. per day.

Respiratory acidosis is often a terminal event in patients with extensive lung damage or respiratory centre failure. In general, it is difficult to treat. Oral/IV sodium bicarbonate should be tried as an emergency measure. Treatment of respiratory infection, use of bronchodilators and intermittent oxygen may be useful.

Alkalosis

Alkalosis is defined as a reduction in the total hydrion *content* of the body. *Alkalemia* is a reduction in the hydrion *concentration* of the plasma, manifested as an increase in the blood pH. Alkalosis without alkalemia is called compensated alkalosis, that accompanied by alkalemia is called decompensated alkalosis.

Metabolic alkalosis: Normally, in the presence of healthy kidneys an individual can tolerate large daily doses (140 g.) of sodium bicarbonate for about 3 weeks, without any gross disturbances. Alkali ingestion in the presence of renal damage, however, may cause alkalosis. Excessive vomiting or gastric suction can cause a marked loss of body hydrion and chloride, producing alkalosis. Excessive milk and alkali ingestion can also cause alkalosis of the **milk-alkali syndrome**.

The blood pH and plasma bicarbonate show a rise. The urine is usually alkaline, containing excess of bicarbonate. In patients with severe electrolyte depletion, however, urine may be scanty and acidic; this is probably due to accompanying potassium depletion which leads to increased renal tubular secretion of hydrion.

Hypokalemic alkalosis as observed with diuretics such as thiazides (Chapter 38).

Respiratory alkalosis: Excessive ventilation which washes away large amounts of carbon dioxide causes lowering of the arterial pCO_2 and reduction in the ratio $H.HCO_3/B.HCO_3$ with a fall in hydrion content. This is commonly seen following hyperventilation, involuntarily carried out by certain individuals probably in response to anxiety. Physiologically, it can occur at high altitudes during climbing. A similar phenomenon can occur in fever, encephalitis, hypothalamic tumors and following drugs like salicylates.

Excessive washing out of potential hydrion would tend to raise the blood pH. This is initially countered by transfer of cation (B) from ECF to ICF, release of chloride into ECF by red cells and lactate from the muscles. This causes decrease in B and replacement of HCO_3 by chloride, resulting in correction of the $H.HCO_3/B.HCO_3$ ratio. Later, kidneys eliminate more cation and bicarbonate, the urine becoming alkaline. In contrast to metabolic alkalosis, the plasma bicarbonate is decreased. In later stages, the urine may become acidic, particularly in patients with marked depletion of sodium and potassium.

Clinical manifestations of alkalosis: In functional cases, respiratory alkalosis is episodic and is associated with feeling of tingling and muscle cramps; sometimes tetany can occur. Tetany in alkalosis is due to lowering of plasma ionized calcium and responds to IV calcium gluconate; increased neuromuscular irritability due to raised blood pH also contributes to this phenomenon. *Tetany following hyperventilation needs no treatment* other than reassurance about its harmless nature.

Chronic metabolic alkalosis causes anorexia, apathy and mental disturbances. Kidney function may be impaired and attacks of tetany can occur.

Treatment of alkalosis: This is aimed at removal of the cause and correction of the body fluid disturbances. Acute loss of chloride due to vomiting can be corrected by IV normal saline. In chronic cases, similar treatment given orally is adequate, except that occasionally an associated potassium loss needs to be rectified.

Management of Dehydration due to Diarrhoea

Massive diarrhoea with watery stools causes marked depletion of sodium, potassium and bicarbonate and metabolic acidosis resulting in high mortality. Hence, immediate replacement of the fluid and electrolyte losses forms the most important therapeutic aspect of dehydration. It is ideal to tailor-make the fluid and electrolyte therapy in a seriously ill patient by monitoring the blood chemistry. This, however, may not always be possible.

Management of dehydration: The extent of dehydration in cholera and severe diarrhoea can be estimated by noting the quality of pulse, BP, condition of the neck veins and skin turgor. The plasma protein concentration and plasma specific gravity can be reliable guides, in judging the degree of dehydration. Normal plasma specific gravity is 1.025. It has been estimated that for each 0.001 increase in the plasma specific gravity, an adult patient requires about 4 ml. of fluid per kg. body weight.

In an emergency, isotonic saline along with isotonic sodium bicarbonate, should be used in the proportion of 2:1. This would correct sodium loss and acidosis. If IV sodium bicarbonate is not available, 5 per cent solution of sodium bicarbonate may be given orally ad lib. Potassium should be given, preferably orally. About 15 mEq. of potassium is needed to correct the potassium loss in a litre of stools. The quantity of stools passed should, therefore, be noted. Potassium can be conveniently administered as 200 ml. of tender coconut water for each litre of stools passed. Alternatively, potassium salts such as potassium citrate and bicarbonate may be given orally or by IV infusion.

Coma and convulsions during diarrhoea often indicate hypoglycemia and need for IV glucose.

In a collapsed patient the IV fluids are given rapidly initially, at the rate of at least 100 ml. per minute, to correct hypovolemia and to avoid irreversible shock. Later on, the infusion may be adjusted according to the loss of fluids in stools and sweat. In practice, IV therapy is monitored by noting the state of the neck veins and the urine output. Usually IV fluid therapy is continued until the shock state is corrected and the patient is strong enough to drink the *oral glucose-electrolyte solution.*

- ***Oral rehydration therapy (ORT):*** In severe diarrhoea, water, sodium and chloride are not retained adequately during oral administration of an isotonic electrolyte solution that does not contain glucose. The sodium and water absorption by the small bowel is very much enhanced by the addition of glucose to the oral fluid. Dehydration can therefore be successfully treated with oral fluids containing glucose, once the initial hypovolemia is corrected by 2-4 litres of IV fluid replacement. Moderate dehydration and acidosis due to diarrhoea can be corrected in 3-6 hours by oral therapy alone. In many cases it is a life-saving measure. The treatment should continue even when diarrhoea is not controlled. The ORT has many advantages:

(1) It is far less expensive than IV fluids.

(2) No expertise is needed to administer the fluid.

(3) The solution need not be sterile and can be prepared on spot with components purchased from the local bazar.

(4) It can be given by family members and non-professionals as well as by health workers.

Patients strong enough to drink generally take the solution avidly. They may continue to vomit and in some cases the stool volume may increase. Inspite of this, there is a net absorption of water and electrolytes. Moreover, vomiting which is probably caused by acidosis and volume depletion is likely to be corrected by the oral therapy itself. One teaspoonful given to a child every minute can provide 200-300 ml. per hour. A conscientious mother can work wonders. Adults can take 750-1000 ml. per hour for several hours until signs of dehydration disappear and abundant pale urine is produced. If the patient needs rest, the same fluid may be given by a nasogastric tube.

Table 36.7: Composition of oral rehydration solution (ORS)

Substance	Weight (g)	Home measure	Components (mMol/1)
Sodium chloride (Table salt)	2.6	¾ teaspoon	Na^+ 75
Potassium chloride	1.5	½ teaspoon	K^+ 20
Trisodium dihydrate citrate*	2.9	¾ teaspoon	HCO_3 equivalent 10
Glucose** (Anhydrous)	13.5	1½ tablespoon	Glucose75
Water	1000	1 litre	Total osmolarity 245

* Citrate in ORS diminishes stool output in high output diarrhoeas.
** Glucose 20 g. can be replaced by 40 g. of sucrose. Alternatively, it can be replaced by 50 g. of cooked rice powder.
Cl^- content is 65 mMol/L

The composition of WHO-recommended, modified ORS is shown in Table 36.7. Earlier ORS recommended by WHO, when used in acute diarrhoea and dehydration, occasionally caused hypernatremia in some children. The newly recommended ORS has lower osmolarity. This ORS has also been found effective and safe in adults with cholera, though a few patients might develop hyponatremia. As some commercially available ORS contain less sodium and glucose than the WHO recommended ORS, their use should be avoided.

Immediate institution of ORT would avoid shock from continuing dehydration in cholera and other diarrhoeas. Children under five years should be given plain water in addition to above solution in quantities approximately 1/3rd of the total volume administered.

- ***Cereal-based oral rehydration solution (CORS)***: The correct concentration of Na+ and glucose in the ORS is critical for optimal effect and safety. The ORS administered cannot greatly exceed plasma in osmolality without the risk of increased diarrhoea and hypernatremia. Fortunately, nature has provided foods containing starches such as cereals and roots which have low osmolality in solution. Studies have indicated that ORS in which rice and other food sources of starch are substituted for glucose effectively replace lost fluids, decrease vomiting, and reduce the severity of diarrhoea. Although glucose based ORS effectively replaces the fluids lost in the stool by patients with diarrhoea, it does not decrease and may slightly increase the stool volume. Several studies have now shown that cereal (rice) based solutions are equally effective in reducing volume losses, and may also shorten the duration of illness. Rice has been shown to contain a low molecular weight fraction which has a direct effect on the chloride channel. It inhibits the response of the crypt cell chloride channel to cAMP. This suggests a cellular basis for the well documented beneficial effect of rice based ORS in patients with cholera, since it is this ion channel that is the target of such toxigenic secretory states. Addition of sodium bicarbonate and potassium chloride is not critical to success of cereal based ORS. The use of **rice conjee** is traditional in India for ages. Cereal-based ORS, however, needs to be prepared by boiling and is not available ready-to-use. Further, as such preparations ferment in 8-12 hours, they need to be prepared fresh for use.

Physiologically, cereal-based ORS are identical to their glucose based counterparts. The dominant component in the cereals is starch from rice, corn, wheat, potato, sorghum, millet or even plantain. Starch is a large polymer of glucose that, on exposure to amylase in the intestine, is digested into smaller polymers that are then split by maltase into glucose at the intestinal brush border. This digestive process supplies a larger number of glucose molecules for transfer sodium ions from lumen into the blood, while generating less luminal osmotic "back drag" than would the direct ingestion of an equivalent amount of glucose. The cereal proteins also provide small peptides and amino acids which also facilitate the absorption of additional sodium ions. Of course, the presence of sufficient digestive enzyme is essential to the success of such solutions. In the vast majority, this is not the problem, except perhaps in infants under 4 months in whom intestinal glucoamylase is not fully developed.

Nutritional Supplementation Therapy

37

Nutritional supplementation therapy is an important part of the total therapeutic planning, and without it, pharmacotherapy and surgery may not be optimally effective. In fact, there are diseases (e.g., phenylketonuria) in which nutritional therapy is the only treatment available. Complete coverage of nutritional therapy is, however, beyond the scope of this book. This chapter outlines the principles of nutritional supplementation in adults, mainly in acute medical and surgical illnesses.

Nutritional Requirements in Healthy Adults

Energy: The *total daily requirement* (TDR) for energy must be met every day. Ideally, energy intake equals energy requirement unless weight gain or weight loss is desired. The best way of assessing whether a person is in energy balance (Intake - Requirement = zero) is to weigh him daily. TDR can be calculated as the sum of

- ***Basal metabolic rate.***
- ***Energy expenditure on physical activity;***

and

- ***Specific dynamic action.***

Basal metabolic rate (BMR) is the energy requirement at rest and is related to the body surface area.

Basal energy requirement in persons above the age of 20 years can be calculated by Wilmore's formula:

$$\text{BMR (KCal/M}^2\text{/day)} = 24 \times \left(37 - \frac{\text{Age} - 20}{10}\right)$$

A more rough and ready formula is :

BMR (KCal/day) = 24 x 0.9/kg. (i.e. 22/kg/day) People in tropics have relatively low BMR as compared to those from the temperate climate.

Because the second formula does not include a term for age, it tends to overestimate the basal requirement in older people.

Energy expenditure on activity (EEA) values for different physical activities are available from textbooks of physiology.

Specific dynamic action (SDA) refers to the additional calories required to metabolise and utilise the consumed foods. It is estimated at 10% of the sum of BMR and EEA.

Proteins: Unlike with fats and carbohydrates, the body has very little mobilizable protein store. All the proteins in the body are either structural or functional. Repair of damaged tissue and recovery from an illness are critically dependent on readily available protein. In the absence of external supply of protein, there occurs breakdown of endogenous protein and hence damage to tissues. Therefore, negative protein balance can be harmful even in the short run. The average protein requirement in adults is 0.6g./kg./day, out of which at least 25-30%

Table 37.1: Daily requirement of minerals

Mineral	Daily requirement
Sodium	1.4 - 2.0 mEq/kg
Potassium	1.2 - 1.5 mEq/kg
Calcium	0.2 - 0.3 mEq/kg
Magnesium	0.3 - 0.45 mEq/kg
Iron	10 - 20 mg/day
Phosphorus	7 - 9 m mol or 14-18 m Eq/1000 KCal/day.

should be animal protein including milk. Protein requirement is often stated in terms of nitrogen requirement, where 1 g. of nitrogen = 6.25 g. of protein.

Water: Water requirement in healthy adults is around 40 ml./kg./day. This will allow the excretion of about 1000 ml. of urine. In hot and dry climates, upto 800 ml./day should be added, especially in summer, to offset the insensible losses.

Minerals: Table 37.1 gives the daily mineral requirements.

Various trace elements are also required, e.g., zinc, iodine, chromium, copper and manganese.

Vitamins: Recommended daily allowances (RDA) for vitamins are given in Chapter 75. Those not mentioned in that table are: panthothenic acid 4-7 mg., biotin 100-400 mcg and vitamin K 70-140 mcg.

Essential fatty acids (EFA): The RDA for linoleic acid is 2-4% and that for linolenic acid 0.5% of the total daily calorie intake. The polyunsaturated fatty acid (linoleic + linolenic) content of the commonly used edible fats is as follows (all figures are in g per tablespoonful i.e. 15 ml): safflower oil 10, soyabean oil 7.4, cottonseed oil 6.8, maize (corn) oil 6.1, til oil 5.7, rice bran oil 4.7, groundnut oil 3.9, mustard oil 3.4, olive oil 1.35, palm oil 1.2, vanaspati 0.8, ghee 0.55 and coconut oil 0.3. Weekly ingestion of 50-100 ml of safflower oil, soyabean oil, cotton seed oil or corn oil satisfies the requirement for EFA.

Alterations in Nutritional Requirements in Acute Illness

Energy :

- ***Fasting and undernutrition*** decrease the BMR by about 25%.
- ***Fever*** increases the BMR by about 13% for every degree rise of body temperature above 37°C. *Rigors* raise the BMR further. Secretion of catecholamines in acute stress also elevates BMR. On the other hand, these conditions reduce the appetite and food intake (and hence SDA), as well as physical activity (and hence EEA).
- ***Illness***: In addition to fever and its consequences, the hormonal response of the body to physical trauma and infection, as well as the losses from the body (e.g., protein in burns), increase the TDR. In illness, the calculations of energy requirement are based on BMR; EEA and SDA are ignored. Thus, in mild illness (elective hospitalization or mild infection) TDR=110% of BMR; in moderate illness (fracture or severe infection) TDR = 125% of BMR; and in severe illness (severe burns or a combination of stresses) TDR=150 to 200% of BMR. Thus, *TDR does not exceed twice the BMR even in the most severe illness.*

Protein: During acute illness, the protein requirements rise: 0.6-0.8 g./kg./day in mild illness, 0.8-1.0g./kg./day in moderate illness and 1-1.5g./kg./day in severe illness. For optimum utilization of protein, about 150 total KCal must be supplied per day per 6.25 g of protein consumed.

Water: The water requirement increases because of insensible sweating, visible sweating, vomiting, diarrhoea, burns or fistulae. At the same time, the intake is likely to be poor because of apathy, obtundation of consciousness, or damage to the thirst centre as in head injury. Electrolyte-free water (as 5% dextrose in water) must be made available to the patient parenterally under these circumstances.

Electrolytes: Their requirements go up if

there are excessive losses from the body such as sweating, diuresis, vomiting, diarrhoea, aspiration or fistulae. They must be calculated and must be made good.

Iron requirements must be considered carefully in the presence of trauma and bleeding. Further, some patients may be anemic to begin with.

Vitamins: During acute illness, especially if it is prolonged, the requirements for vitamins go up because of the catabolic state. If the patient is unable to ingest a normal diet, water soluble vitamins should be supplemented daily and fat soluble vitamins once a week.

Sequelae of Malnutrition

Malnutrition has several deleterious effects which may impair patient's ability to recover from an acute illness:

- ***Weight loss :*** Reduction in body fat and in muscle mass, and weakness.
- ***Hypoproteinemia and edema.***
- ***Impairment of cellular and humoral immunity.***
- ***Delayed wound healing.***
- ***Deficiencies of vitamins and minerals.***
- ***Deficiency of EFA:*** This is known to arise during the course of prolonged total parenteral nutrition. The deficiency causes dry, scaly cracked skin, coarse hair, hair loss, and may impair wound healing.
- ***Malaise and poor morale;*** and
- ***Increased mortality.***

Assessment of Nutritional Status

A detailed history and physical examination, together with selected laboratory tests, help in the nutritional assessment of the patient. Deficiencies are commonly multiple; evidence of one deficiency should make one look carefully for other deficiencies. A nutritional assessment helps in estimating the overall nutritional impact of the disease; it helps to decide whether intensive nutritional support is necessary and if so how urgently; lastly, it helps to predict organ dysfunction which may dictate that elective surgery should be postponed.

Table 37.2 gives a protocol for assessment for protein-calorie status. Laboratory estimations of haemoglobin and of serum Na^+, K^+, Ca^{++}, P^{---} and Mg^{++} are other helpful parameters.

Table 37.2: Assessment for protein-calorie status

Parameter	Result which suggests significant malnutrition
Weight loss in adults*	
% loss in past 1 month	> 5
% loss in past 6 months	> 10
Serum albumin	< 2.8 g%
Serum transferrin from TIBC**	< 150 mg%
Total lymphocyte count	< 1200/cumm.

* It is necessary to distinguish between weight loss due to dehydration and that due to loss of fat or muscle.

** Transferrin (mg %) = (0.83 x TIBC) - 43 where TIBC is the total iron binding capacity.

Nutritional Supplementation: Aims and Indications

Nutritional supplementation therapy aims at establishing or maintaining good nutritional status; establishing positive nitrogen balance and increasing weight in the malnourished; and overcoming the effects of malnutrition.

Nutritional intervention to prevent malnutrition or to replenish the malnourished patient improves recovery and increases survival from many diseases.

Table 37.3: Indications for nutritional supplementation

- To correct existing malnutrition.
- To prevent malnutrition that will occur unless there is intervention (e.g., in patients in coma; in those with severe burns, serious intestinal obstruction, trauma or sepsis).
- When bowel rest is required (as in acute symptomatic inflammatory bowel disease, acute pancreatitis, intestinal fistulae).
- When serious GI symptoms occur during cancer chemotherapy or radiotherapy.
- When mechanical problems exist (e.g., dysphagia, surgery of head or neck; and
- After massive bowel resection or other disorders causing malabsorption.

Indications for nutritional supplementation are listed in Table 37.3.

Enteral Nutrition

Nutritional supplementation may be done :

- ***Orally.***
- ***By enteral tube feeding*** (forced enteral feeding); or
- ***Parenterally.***

In the last case, it may be partial or total (Total Parenteral Nutrition, TPN). Wherever possible, oral or enteral tube feeding is the preferred method.

Enteral feeding, advantages :

- Oral and enteral tube feeding use a physiological route, and are safe and inexpensive.
- They can provide almost any nutrient that is required.
- Calorie supplementation can be done easily and completely by these methods.
- Luminal nutrition which :

(a) Maintains the structural and functional integrity of the small intestine.

(b) Is a stimulus to hormonal homeostasis, to adaptation of the gut in patients with short bowel syndrome, and to maintenance of immunocompetence of the gut. This last factor permits the gut to maintain its normal secretion of IgA into the gut lumen and to minimise bacterial translocation from the gut into the systemic circulation, as occurs during TPN.

- They are the methods of choice, whenever possible, if supplementation is going to last for more than a week.

Contraindications to enteral nutrition:

- Severe malabsorption in which tube feeding is liable to cause uncontrollable diarrhoea.
- Total bowel obstruction.
- Persistent and uncontrolled vomiting; and
- Tendency to aspirate, especially in the presence of serious pulmonary disease.

Oral supplementation requires satisfactory appetite, intact deglutition and the conscious co-operation of a patient; it also requires that the oral supplements must be palatable; *it has no disadvantages.*

Enteral tube feeding circumvents the need for adequate appetite and deglutition; it requires less cooperation from the patient and can be carried out even in an unconscious patient. Its disadvantages are:

- Less acceptability than oral feeds.
- Nasopharyngeal irritation by the tube.
- Erosion of the esophagus.
- Infection of the nose, paranasal sinuses and ears; and
- Incompetence of the gastroesophageal sphincter with regurgitation of gastric contents into the esophagus followed by their aspiration into the tracheobronchial tree. To prevent the risk of regurgitation of gastric contents and pulmonary aspiration, the patient should be kept in a semi-sitting position (head of the bed elevated 30°) during feeding and for one hour thereafter. Such a position should be maintained all the time in the elderly, infants and comatose patients.

Enteral tube feeding should be done cautiously in patients with loss of gag reflex, hiccuping, a tendency to vomit or significant pulmonary dysfunction; under these circumstances bolus feeds and feeding by the nasogastric tube should be avoided; slow drip feeding by a nasoduodenal tube may be done with caution.

Types of enteral feeding:

- ***Oral supplementation*** with high calorie, high protein 'table foods' (milk; milk products such as cheese and ghee; meat; and groundnuts) is the most pleasant form of supplementation in patients who can tolerate it and will cooperate in consuming them. Vegetables, fruits, fruit juices, dal, cereals and a multivitamin capsule would complete the list. Medium chain triglyceride (MCT) preparations (Precision LR, Pregestimil) containing 8-10 carbon, fatty acid residues are valuable in patients with steatorrhoea; these medium chain fatty acids are absorbed directly into the portal circulation without the help of bile salts. MCT preparations, however, are expensive.

The oral route can also be used to supplement the intake of water and electrolytes.

- ***Enteral tube feeding*** can be carried out either by nasogastric or by nasoduodenal route in patients with intact GI tract, who are unconscious or who are not sufficiently cooperative to take all the calculated daily requirement by mouth. Local irritation and erosion can be minimised by using a small diameter tube, preferably made of plastic. Larger diameter tubes, however, permit the administration of an almost normal meal, blenderized to the consistency of a thick soup.

A problem with *nasogastric* feeding is the gastric distension, especially when bolus feeds are used. The *nasoduodenal* tube is more difficult to position properly, and diarrhoea is more likely to occur with nasoduodenal feeding; however, the problem of gastroesophageal reflux and its consequences are less troublesome. The other problems with enteral tube feeding are: electrolyte disturbances, volume overload, lactose intolerance, diarrhoea and hyperosmolality syndrome. They can be minimized by :

(a) Proper adjustment of the composition of the feeds.

(b) Not using too much of milk but using buttermilk, instead; and

(c) Not being overambitious with tube feeding.

Bolus feeding: This is used only with nasoduodenal tube. Begin with 50-100 ml. of a half strength feed every 3-6 hours; aspirate the gastric contents before each feed; flush the tube with water after each feed; and gradually increase the volume of a feed to 250-300 ml. to be given every 3-4 hours. Finally, increase the concentration of the feed gradually to the full strength.

Continuous infusion: This can be employed with either nasogastric or nasoduodenal tube. The initial rate of 25-50 ml. per hour is gradually increased, once in 24 hours, to 100 - 150 ml. per hour. Additional water may be given to prevent hyperosmolality. A variety of foods can be used by this route: soups; fruit juice; milk, buttermilk, eggnog; blenderized normal meals (rice, chapatti, dal, vegetables, meat, etc.); commercially available protein powders (Casilan, Protinex, Protinules, Trophox, etc.).

During enteral feeding by any method, it must be remembered that some patients have lactose intolerance and may not tolerate large quantities of milk (equivalent to more than 8 g. of lactose per day); others may be intolerant of sucrose.

Strict intake output charts must be maintained in patients on enteral tube feeding. Unfortunately, the enteral route is not available in patients with medical or surgical abdominal diseases.

Parenteral Nutrition

Partial parenteral supplementation: Maintenance therapy with water and electrolytes is indicated in a patient who is temporarily not able or not allowed to ingest food and fluids e.g. a postoperative patient. No pre-existing deficit or excess of water or electrolytes or altered renal function should be present. Such therapy should not be extended beyond 7 days, if it can be avoided. The daily maintenance requirement in an adult can be provided by 1000 ml. of 0.9% NaCl in 5% dextrose in water (=170 calories); 1000 ml. of 5% dextrose in water with 20 m Eq of KCl added; and 1000 ml. of 5% dextrose in water. It is customary to avoid infusing NaCl solution for 24-48 hours after surgery as the stress of surgery produces intense salt and water retention during this period. It must be remembered that even healthy postoperative patients tend to have glucose intolerance and can develop hyperglycemia while receiving 5% dextrose in water. Water soluble vitamins should be given daily, particularly thiamine as prolonged parenteral glucose supplementation without thiamine can precipitate acute thiamine deficiency and Wernicke's encephalopathy. Fat soluble vitamins should be administered once a week. Calcium, magnesium, phosphorus and protein supplements become necessary if parenteral supplementation is continued beyond 1 week. Strict intake output chart should be maintained in these patients. Table 37.4 shows the composition of some fluids for intravenous use.

Table 37.4: Composition of some fluids for intravenous use

Solution	Dextrose (g/L)	Na^+ (mEq/l)
5% Dextrose in water	50	-
5% Dextrose in saline	50	145
0.85% Saline (isotonic)	-	145
0.9% Saline	-	154
Ringer lactate*	-	130
5% Saline	-	855
1/6th Molar lactate	-	167

* Also contains potassium 4 mEq/l, chloride 109 mEq/l (as against 154 mEq/l of 0.9% saline), calcium 3 mEq/l and lactate 28 mEq/l.

All these solutions can be administered through a peripheral vein. Table 37.5 shows the composition of some parenteral additives.

Table 37.5: Composition of some parenteral additives

Solution	Volume ml per ampoule	Cation (mEq/amp)	Anion (mEq/amp)
7.5% Sodium bicarbonate	50	44.6	44.6
15% Potassium chloride	30	60.0	60.0
10% Calcium gluconate	10	4.6	4.6
50% Magnesium sulfate	10	40.6	40.6
42% Disodium hydrogen phosphate	15	36.0	36.0
46% Potassium dihydrogen phosphate	15	100.0	100.0

* equal to 18 mMol ** equal to 50 mMol.

Phlebitis is a well recognized complication of intravenous infusion therapy. Such phlebitis may be either infective or noninfective. Contamination of the fluid to be infused during manufacturing process, frequent manipulations of the intravenous system, and entry of bacteria at the cannula-skin junction account for the infective phlebitis. However, most phlebitis following intravenous infusions is non-infective. Many factors contribute to it; they all seem to operate through mechanical and physicochemical interaction at the cannula-vein junction. These factors are:

- ***Type of cannula***: Metal cannulae cause less phlebitis than plastic ones and short cannulae less than long ones.
- ***Duration of cannulation***: The longer the cannulation, the greater the risk of phlebitis.
- ***Location of the cannula***: Veins in the upper extremity and the large central veins are less liable to develop phlebitis than those in the lower extremity and the periphery; and
- ***Type and composition of the infusateand the presence of additives*** in it. Certain drugs are more liable to produce phlebitis than others. Fluids with non-physiologic pH, hypertonic

fluids and fluids which contain particulate matter are prone to produce phlebitis. Particulate matter is often present in solutions that appear clear to the naked eye, and comprises glass, cotton fibres, precipitated proteins, microcrystalline drug particles, and degradation products of interaction between fluids and glass, plastic or even rubber stoppers. The above list of causes of phlebitis suggests possible ways of preventing it.

Catheter sepsis can be a serious complication during prolonged intravenous infusion therapy. Methods of preventing catheter sepsis are listed in Table 37.6.

Table 37.6: Prevention of catheter sepsis

- Insertion of the catheter under aseptic conditions.
- Subcutaneous tunneling of the catheter.
- Use of transparent polyurethane dressings over the site of cannulation.
- Changing of dressings by experienced staff.
- Change of the infusion set every 2-3 days; and
- Administration of blood products or drugs via separate set from the one used for the main infusate.

Catheter sepsis should be the uppermost in the physician's mind when a patient receiving an intravenous infusion develops fever or any metabolic deterioration. A special in-line filter in the infusion line is available to intercept any particulate matter in the fluid.

Total Parenteral Nutrition (TPN)

TPN is used to supply all the essential nutrients without using the gastrointestinal tract.

Indications for TPN: These are given in Table 37.7.

TPN has also been used in other situations such as for routine preoperative support and as an adjunct to cancer chemo-/radio-therapy.

Table 37.7: Indications for TPN

- Short bowel syndrome.
- Prolonged ileus, such as that following visceral trauma.
- Pancreatic abscess/fistula.
- Intestinal fistula.
- Hypermetabolic states, such as severe burns, major sepsis.
- Alimentary tract cancer causing mechanical obstruction.
- Severe vomiting or anorexia, such as anorexia nervosa, hyperemesis gravidarum; and
- Crohn's disease with malabsorption and retarded growth in children.

TPN has been used in the hospital setting as well as at home. It has been shown to achieve positive nitrogen balance, and to promote growth in children. One of the aims of TPN is to ensure complete bowel rest which minimises the intestinal motor and secretory activity and encourages the healing of bowel lesions.

Composition and requirements:

- ***Calories***: These are provided by means of 20 - 25% dextrose in water through a central vein, as it is hypertonic. *Water* is provided in the quantity of 40ml/kg/day.
- ***Protein***: This is supplied in the form of specially prepared mixtures (Hermin, Astymin-3, Aminoplasmal)) of synthetic, essential amino acids. They contain 8 - 9% of the amino acids in 200 ml bottles for intravenous use. The calories provided by the amino acids are not taken into account in the daily calorie calculation. These mixtures are used as a source of protein as the endogenous protein breakdown is less when some protein is made available than when only carbohydrate is supplied. Further, the protein prevents fatty infiltration of the liver which is likely to occur when only carbohydrate is supplied to the patient. Patients who are losing protein in exudates need infusion of human

serum albumin in the dose of 10-25 g/day; they and anemic patients also benefit from blood transfusions. Amino acid mixtures and albumin solutions, however, are expensive.

- ***Fats***: Milky emulsions of soyabean oil (Intralipid 10% and 20%) and safflower oil (Liposyn 10% and 20%) in combination with glycerol and emulsifying agents are available for intravenous administration. The 10% emulsions supply 1.1 calorie per ml. Both are good sources of linoleic acid; the soyabean oil preparations are a good source of linolenic acid as well. A weekly injection of 500-1000 ml of a 10% emulsion is used to provide the necessary essential fatty acids to prevent the development of a deficiency syndrome. As the fat emulsions are isotonic, they can be administered by a peripheral vein. In the usual doses, intravenous fats are metabolised in the same manner as the natural chylomicrons.

- ***Minerals***: Mineral requirements are as per Table 37.1. In addition, trace elements are supplied as follows: zinc 2.5-4 mg/day; copper 0.5-1.5 mg/day; iodine 75-150 mcg/day; manganese 0.15-0.8 mg/day; chromium 10-15 mcg/day; and selenium 50-200 mcg/day. They are added to the intravenous infusion.

- ***Vitamins***: The recommended vitamin supplements during TPN are

Daily: Thiamine 3 mg, riboflavin 3.6 mg, pantothenic acid 15 mg, pyridoxine 4 mg, niacin 40 mg, biotin 60 mg, folacin 400 mcg, cyanocobalamin 5 mcg, ascorbic acid 100 mg; and vitamin D 200 IU. Prolonged use of larger doses of vitamin D has been reported to cause a reversible form of metabolic bone disease.

Weekly: vitamin A 3300 IU, and vitamin E 10 IU.

Technique of TPN: The base solution for TPN is a mixture of an amino acid solution and dextrose solution (final concentration of dextrose 20-25%); it is prepared daily by mixing an amino acid solution and a dextrose solution in a laminar flow hood in the hospital pharmacy. The minerals and vitamins are added to this base solution. The calorie content of dextrose solution is calculated on the basis of 3.4 KCal per gramme as the dextrose used is not anhydrous (=4 KCal/g) but in the form of monohydrate. The calorie contribution of amino acids is ignored. The total calories supplied should bear a ratio of 125-190:1 to nitrogen (in g) supplied, in order to optimise the utilization of the aminoacids for anabolic purposes. *As the base solution is hypertonic, it must be infused through a central vein,* taking all the precautions datailed above. The rate of dextrose infusion should not exceed 5-7 ml/kg/min in adults. The lipid emulsion is administered separately through a peripheral vein.

In order to prevent cracking, nothing should be added to the fat emulsion.

Insulin (soluble) in the dose of 10 units per 250 g of dextrose is added to the base solution to prevent hyperglycemia. **Heparin** may be added to the infusate to prevent fibrin plugging of the central venous catheter. If corticosteroids are required for the patient's primary condition, they (preferably those with little mineralocorticoid activity, such a dexamethasone) may be added to the base solution.

TPN is generally initiated with one litre of the base solution (containing about 250 g of dextrose and about 40 g of amino acids) per 24 hours. If this amount is tolerated, the quantity infused is increased by ½-1 litre per day till the desired amount of calories and protein are being delivered. This concentrated glucose solution is infused in 18 hours and 5% dextrose infused during the remaining 6 hours of the day; the latter helps to prevent rebound hypoglycemia. Further, when TPN is being discontinued, the amount of glucose infused should be tapered gradually for the same reason.

Physical therapy is a valuable adjunct for restoring muscle function and muscle mass in patients on TPN.

Monitoring of TPN: Patients on TPN need close clinical and laboratory monitoring. A strict intake output chart must be maintained. The daily physical examination of the patient should include weighing, looking for signs of fluid overload and for TPN related sepsis. Daily examination of urine for glucose and acetone, and daily estimation of plasma glucose, urea nitrogen, creatinine, Na, K, Ca, Mg and P should be done till the patient stabilizes. The appearance of hyperglycemia during apparently stable TPN suggests a catabolic stress such as catheter sepsis. Serum bilirubin and liver enzymes should be done once in 3-4 days to detect hepatic dysfunction.

A weekly weight gain of about 1.5 kg. indicates successful TPN. Improvement in muscle strength is a good indication of improved skeletal muscle function. Improvement in plasma albumin and transferrin occurs only gradually. Growth is known to be normalised in children with retarded growth due to inflammatory bowel disease and malabsorption.

Complications of TPN: A variety of complications can occur in a patient on TPN. An attempt should be made to prevent them; at the same time they should be carefully looked for and treated promptly and vigorously, if they occur. The complications are listed in Table 37.8.

Table 37.8: Complications of TPN

- Hyperglycemia.
- Rebound hypoglycemia on cessation of TPN.
- Electrolyte abnormalities.
- Azotemia.
- Liver dysfunction.
- Volume overload.
- Metabolic bone disease.
- A variety of non-metabolic complications such as adverse reactions to lipid emulsions; sepsis; allergic reactions; and complications due to the physical trauma by the catheter in the vein.

TPN is more expensive, and requires more careful monitoring than enteral nutrition. Therefore, it should not be instituted unless it is absolutely necessary. Further, an attempt should be made to re-establish enteral supplementation as soon as possible in all patients who are treated with TPN.

Diuretic and Anti-Diuretic Drugs 38

The kidney is not just a simple excretory organ but it plays an important role in regulating the volume and the composition of the body fluids. The functional unit of the kidney is termed as the nephron. Drugs can modify the renal functions:

- ***Indirectly by modifying its circulation;*** or
- ***Directly by affecting the nephron function.*** Most of the therapeutically useful agents act mainly by modifying various functions of the nephron.

Physiology of urine formation : Diagrammatic representation of a nephron is shown in Fig. 38.1. The volume and composition of urine are essentially determined by:

- ***Glomerular filtration.***
- ***Tubular reabsorption;*** and
- ***Active tubular secretion.***

Urine formation begins in the glomerular capillary tufts by the process of ultrafiltration. The composition and the volume of fluid filtered out from the plasmá depend upon the composition of the plasma, the condition of the glomeruli and the blood pressure within them. The glomerular filtrate is a protein free ultra filtrate of the plasma. Both the renal plasma flow and glomerular filtration can be affected by

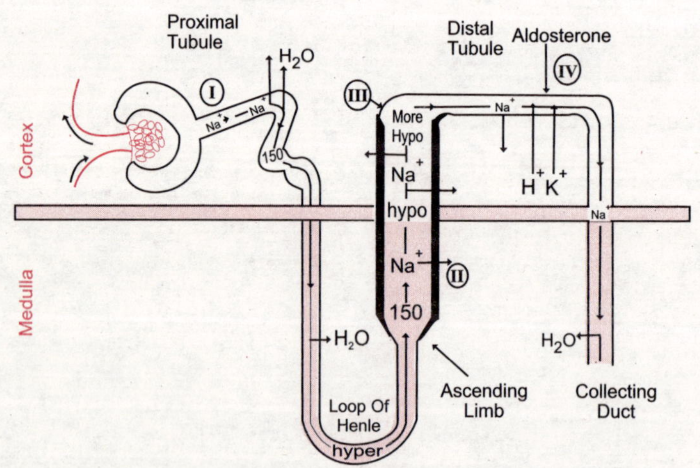

Fig. 38.1: The simplified schematic diagram showing functional subdivisions of a mammalian nephron and sites of diuretic action on sodium reabsorption--(I) Proximal tubule, (II) Ascending limb of Henle's loop, (III) Early distal tubule and (IV) Distal tubular Na+/K+ exchange site.

factors which may cause sodium retention and edema; e.g. chronic heart failure, renal vascular disease etc. The GFR is directly related to the cortical blood flow since 90-95% of the renal blood flow passes through the cortex. The medullary blood flow is of importance in the concentrating ability of the kidney.

The transport of sodium and other solutes across the tubular epithelial cells involves several mechanisms: (1) solute movement with bulk water flow; (2) simple diffusion; (3) channel mediated diffusion; (4) carrier mediated or facilitated diffusion (**uniport**); (5) primary ATP mediated transport; (6) secondary ATP mediated transport which is either in the same direction (co-transport or **symport**) or in opposite directions (counter transport or **antiport**). Sodium is actively transported from the tubular lumen, involving Na^+-K^+-ATPase pump. The type of transport in a particular nephron and its location (luminal or basolateral) determine the electrolyte transport across that segment.

Nearly 70-80 per cent of the filtered sodium, most of the protein, potassium, amino acids and glucose are reabsorbed in the **proximal tubule**. Proportionate quantities of water are absorbed along with sodium (obligatory reabsorption), so that the tubular fluid remains isotonic with plasma. Reabsorption of sodium in the proximal tubule varies with changes in ECF and GFR; it is enhanced markedly in response to contraction of ECF volume and acute reduction in GFR from any cause, whereas it is depressed following ECF expansion which causes the release of a natriuretic hormone (ANP). Reabsorption of sodium from the tubular fluid into the peritubular capillaries makes the tubular fluid electrochemically negative to the tubular cell and establishes an *electrochemical gradient* which determines the reabsorption of chloride. This then establishes an *osmotic gradient* along which water is reabsorbed. Removal of water from the tubular lumen sets up a *concentration gradient* for urea which is then reabsorbed. Thus, reabsorption of sodium is the event of primary importance in tubular reabsorption; chloride is absorbed passively.

Quantitatively less (25%) of filtered sodium is absorbed from the next portion of the nephron, the **loop of Henle** (Fig. 38.1). Juxtaglomerular apparatus (JG) is located at the vascular pole of the glomerulus and contains modified smooth muscle cells called the myoepithelial cells, which secrete renin. The JG apparatus is responsible for tubulo-glomerular feedback which regulates the glomerular hemodynamics via altering the renin secretion.

The loop is of considerable interest since it acts as a counter-current multiplier. According to the counter-current concept, the descending and the ascending limbs of the loop (Fig. 38.1) have relatively different permeabilities to water and sodium. In the thick segment of the ascending limb of the loop, sodium and chloride are actively transported (symport) from the tubular lumen to the interstitium by ion transporter system. The tubular epithelium at this site is impermeable to water and hence, the tubular fluid becomes dilute (hypotonic) and the interstitium becomes hypertonic. In contrast, the tubular epithelium in the descending limb is permeable to water, which is absorbed readily into the hypertonic interstitium. Thus, the tubular fluid, which is isotonic with plasma at its entry into the descending limb of the loop of Henle, becomes progressively more hypertonic as it approaches the tip of the loop. From then on, its osmolality diminishes progressively because of passive reabsorption of Na^+ from the ascending thin limb and active extrusion of chloride (accompanied by sodium) from the ascending thick limb of the loop; the fluid entering the distal convoluted tubule (Site III) thus is hypotonic to plasma. This circular and repetitive transfer of sodium across the loop is called the 'hairpin counter-current multiplier system'. It is largely responsible for creating a hypertonic medullary interstitium. Preferential transport of sodium by the ascending limb of Henle's loop with its low water permeability is important in the process of concentration of the urine.

The active reabsorption of sodium along with chloride through specific sodium channels continues in the **distal convoluted tubule** and the **collecting tubule**. This is the driving force for secretion of K^+ into the lumen of the tubule. In the collecting tubules there is a H^+ ATPase pump on the luminal site which secretes H^+ into the lumen. Most of the potassium filtered by the glomeruli (80%) is reabsorbed in the proximal tubules and the fluid presented to the distal tubule probably does not contain any potassium. *The potassium that appears in the urine is, therefore, secreted by the distal tubule in exchange for sodium which is reabsorbed.* The exchange of potassium with sodium in the distal tubule is largely but not completely under the influence of aldosterone, excess of which causes sodium retention and potassium depletion. PGE synthesized in the renal medulla participates in the autoregulation of renal blood flow and glomerular filtration, and also regulates the sodium handling by the renal tubules.

Most of the filtered calcium (70%) is reabsorbed in the proximal tubule;about 25% is reabsorbed in the thick descending limb.The rest is reabsorbed in the distal convoluted tubule.About 25% of the filtered magnesium is reabsorbed in the proximal tubule whereas 70% is reabsorbed in the thick ascending limb.

In the proximal tubule, H^+ ion is transported from the tubular cell cytoplasm to the tubular lumen in exchange for the Na^+ ion which is absorbed into the tubular cell *(antiport)* and is pushed out into the interstitium by Na^+–K^+–ATPase pump. (Fig. 38.2). In the lumen,H^+ reacts with the filtered HCO_3^- to form $H_2CO_3^-$; the latter in the presence of **carbonic anhydrase** in the luminal membrane of the cell splits into CO_2 and water. Carbon dioxide (CO_2) diffuses across the luminal membrane into the tubular epithelial cell where it forms H_2CO_3, a reaction that is catalysed by cytoplasmic carbonic anhydrase; within the cytoplasm, H_2CO_3 splits into HCO_3^- and H^+. The hydrogen ion then repeats the above cycle and exchanges with luminal Na^+ which is reabsorbed into the tubular cell and again pushed out into the interstitium.The HCO_3^- in the tubular cell cytoplasm is also pushed out into the interstitium and there combines with Na^+ to form $NaHCO_3$. In this manner, Na^+ and HCO_3 from the lumen are transferred by the tubular cell into interstitium and $NaHCO_3$ formed reabsorbed into the systemic circulation for conservation.

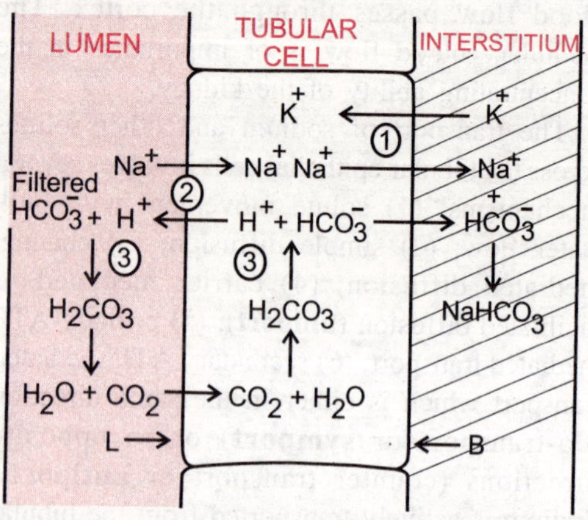

1 = Na^+K^+ ATPase. 2 = Na^+/H^+ exchanger.
3 = Carbonic anhydrase. L = Luminal cell membrane.
B = Basolateral cell membrane.
L, B and cytoplasm are rich in carbonic anhydrase

Fig. 38.2 : Carbonic anhydrase action in renal tabules

Addition of H^+ ion to the luminal fluid in the distal tubule makes the normal urine acidic. The presence of bicarbonate and phosphate buffers in the filtrate prevents the tubular fluid from becoming excessively acidic. Renal tubular cells also produce ammonia (NH_3) which diffuses and reacts with hydrogen ion in the urine to form NH4 which cannot be reabsorbed. The acidification of urinary buffers and formation of ammonium ion are thus necessary for the reabsorption of sodium bicarbonate.

The final volume and composition of the urine to be excreted are regulated by the **collecting duct** which runs from the relatively isosmotic cortex through the hyperosmotic renal medulla to the papilla. The urine entering the collecting tubule is isotonic with plasma. Under the influence of ADH, collecting ducts are relatively permeable to water which passes freely to hyperosmotic renal medulla, thus concentrating the urine further. In addition, collecting ducts also reabsorb sodium actively and secrete H^+ and ammonium ions.

Since tubules normally absorb over 99 per cent of the glomerular filtrate, marked diuresis can be achieved by interfering with the tubular reabsorption of sodium. The distal convoluted tubule, the collecting duct and the ascending limb of the loop of Henle have reserve capacity for reabsorption of sodium. This is utilized when sodium reabsorption is decreased in the proximal tubule. Hence, a diuretic acting on the proximal tubule alone may not cause increased sodium excretion since its effect would be counterbalanced by increased distal reabsorption.

Diuretics

Diuretic are the drugs which increase the rate of urine formation together with natriuresis.

Only a few drugs produce diuresis by increasing the GFR, and these are relatively weak in action. Most of the diuretics used therapeutically act by interfering with sodium reabsorption by the tubules.

Diuretics can be classified therapeutically as:

I **Weak diuretics :**

- ***Osmotic diuretics***: Sodium and Potassium salts.
- ***Xanthine derivatives*** such as Aminophylline.
- ***Carbonic anhydrase inhibitors*** such as Acetazolamide.

II **Moderately efficacious diuretics :**

- ***Osmotic diuretics*** such as Mannitol, Isosorbide, Sucrose and Glycerol.
- ***Benzothiadiazines and related compounds*** such as Chlorthalidone, Chloroxozone and Clopamide. They inhibit Na^+–Cl^- symport. These drugs have a moderately rapid onset of action, lead to excretion of 5-10% of the filtered NaCl and have a wide spectrum of duration of action (8-72 hours). They are ineffective with GFR below 30 ml./minute.

III **Very efficacious diuretics (High ceiling diuretics)** e.g. Furosemide, Mefruside, Bumetamide and Ethacrynic acid. They are called **loop diuretics.** They inhibit Na^+–K^+–$2Cl^-$ symport. These drugs have a rapid onset and short duration of action. They cause excretion of 15-20% of the filtered NaCl and tend to be effective when drugs from group II, given in maximum doses, fail to act. They are effective even in the presence of markedly reduced GFR.

IV **Potassium sparing diuretics :**

(a) **Aldosterone antagonists :** Spironolactone, Potassium canreonate and Eplerenone.

(b) **Renal epithelial sodium channel inhibitors :** Triamterene and Amiloride.

By themselves, they are weak diuretics. But, they are useful adjuncts because of their potassium sparing effect.

Classification of diuretics according to the site of action is given in Table 38.1.

Water, given in excess, acts as a physiological diuretic. During water diuresis the influence of ADH remains inhibited and the ADH responsive portion of the nephron becomes impermeable to water. The urine consists of water that is excreted along with the electrolytes (osmolar clearance) as well as the solute free portion (free water clearance). In edema, the basic problem is sodium retention, the water retention being secondary. In such cases, water does not act as a diuretic. Conversely, in patients with sodium retention, there need not be a rigid restriction of water intake when sodium intake is restricted. **Water diuresis** is used to wash out certain drugs which irritate the urinary tract or are of limited solubility in the urine, e.g. salicylates or sulfonamides. It is also useful in urinary tract infections.

Osmotic Diuretics

Osmotic diuretics are solutes which have the following properties. They are:

- ***Pharmacologically inert.***

Table 38.1: Site of action of diuretics and their effects

Site of action	Drug group	Mechanism of action	Effect on ions
I **Proximal tubule**	Carbonic anhydrase inhibitors	Inhibition of carbonic anhydrase	Inhibition of $Na^+ – H^+$ exchange indirectly
II **Loop of Henle and Proximal tubule**	Osmotic diuretics	Osmotic effect to reduce medullary tonicity	Limits passive reabsorption of Na^+
III **Thick ascending limb of loop of Henle**	Furosemide	Inhibition of $Na^+ – K^+ – 2\,Cl^-$ symport	Inhibition of reabsorption of Na^+ and Cl^- and increased excretion of K^+
IV **Site in distal tubule before Na/H^+ exchange**	Thiazides	Inhibition of $Na^+ – Cl^-$ symport	Inhibition of reabsorption of Na^+ and Cl^- and increased excretion of K^+
V **Late segment of Distal tubule (site of Na^+/H^+ exchange) and collecting duct**	Aldosterone antagonist	Blockade of mineralocorticoid receptors	Inhibition of Na^+ reabsorption and reduced excretion of K^+
	Triamterene	Inhibition of renal epithelial sodium channels	

- ***Generally non-metabolizable.***
- ***Increase osmolality of plasma and tubular fluid.***
- ***Freely filtered at the glomerulus***; and
- ***Not significantly reabsorbed by the renal tubules.***

Mechanism of action: In the proximal tubule, sodium is actively absorbed from tubular lumen, dragging water passively along with it. In the presence of a non-absorbable solute such as mannitol, diffusion of water is reduced relative to that of sodium. As a consequence the net absorption of sodium diminishes. There is an enhanced urine flow with a relatively smaller increase in the sodium excretion. However, this action is of secondary importance; the main site of action of the osmotic diuretics is the loop. They expand the ECF and increase the renal blood flow, thereby reducing the medullary tonicity, which inhibits water extraction from the descending limb. This limits the passive reabsorption of sodium from the ascending limb.

The other osmotically active solutes are urea, glucose, isosorbide, and urographic and angiographic contrast agents. In case of glucose, this mechanism becomes operative when the tubular maximum for reabsorption of glucose is exceeded because of hyperglycemia.

When GFR is acutely reduced (as in hypotension or dehydration), solutes undergo more complete reabsorption in the proximal tubule, so that there is a marked fall in the urine flow and solute excretion. Diuretics that act by directly inhibiting tubular resorption may also be ineffective in these circumstances. However, the osmotic diuretics retain their effectiveness. Although the GFR is reduced, a substance like mannitol is filtered at the glomerulus and is excreted in the voided urine, dragging water (and sodium) with it.

MANNITOL: It is a sugar (polyhydroxy aliphatic alcohol) which, when injected IV, is not metabolized and is rapidly filtered by the glomeruli. Being nonreabsorbable, it exerts marked osmotic activity, causing osmotic diuresis. It increases excretion of all the electrolytes including magnesium and calcium.

To be effective, mannitol has to be administered in sufficiently large doses. It is not a suitable diuretic to treat cardiac edema with sodium retention. This is because administration of mannitol increases the ECF volume by extracting water from the cells, thus increasing further the load on the already decompensated heart. When the renal tubules are damaged in addition to reduction in GFR (as happens with nephrotoxic agents or with prolonged, severe, renal ischemia), they become permeable to mannitol, which then loses its capacity to induce diuresis.

Adverse reactions: It can cause headache, nausea, chills, polydipsia, confusion and pain in the chest. Excessive amounts or rapid infusion of mannitol can cause cellular dehydration; pulmonary edema in patients with CHF and hyponatremia. Extravasation of mannitol may cause thrombophlebitis. It can cross the blood-brain barrier, though less readily than urea, and may occasionally cause rise in intracranial tension. Mannitol should not be mixed with whole blood because agglutination and irreversible crenation of RBCs may occur.

Contraindications to mannitol are given in Table 38.2.

Mannitol is supplied as 25 per cent solution in ampoules of 50 ml. for intravenous use.

Therapeutic uses:

- ***Barbiturate poisoning***: It is useful in *barbiturate poisoning* to increase the urinary elimination of barbiturate. In such cases, it is

Table 38.2: Contraindications to mannitol

- Pulmonary congestion/edema.
- Intracranial bleeding, except during craniotomy.
- Congestive heart failure.
- Metabolic edema with abnormal capillary fragility; and
- Established acute renal failure with anuria.

infused as a 5-25% solution. However, the loop diuretic furosemide is preferred.

- ***Threatened acute renal failure***: It is also useful in any condition of threatened acute oliguric renal failure from pre-renal causes (e.g. severe gastroenteritis) which result in hypovolemia and hypotension. In such cases, after initial correction of hypovolemia with adequate IV fluids, 200 mg. of mannitol per kg. may be infused rapidly in 10-15 minutes. If the urine flow rate increases to 100 ml. per hour further mannitol is given to maintain the high urine flow rate. This may prevent the establishment of acute renal failure. If no diuresis occurs after the initial mannitol infusion, established acute renal failure is diagnosed and no more mannitol is given.

Mannitol is also given pre-operatively during certain surgical procedures (aortic surgery or surgery in a deeply jaundiced patient) which are known to increase the risk of acute renal failure. It is also useful in preventing acute oliguric renal failure after severe trauma and hemolytic transfusion reactions.

- ***Raised intraocular pressure (IOP)*** : Mannitol infusion is used in the dose of 1.5-2 g./kg. (in 30-60 minutes) to reduce IOP in acute congestive glaucoma (see Chapter 70).
- ***Cerebral edema*** : See later.
- ***During rapid dialysis,*** to maintain osmolality of ECF.

GLYCEROL: Glycerol is used orally in the dose of 1 to 1.5 g./kg. (maximum dose 120 g./day), as a 50 - 75% solution, prior to ophthalmological procedures. Palatability is increased by chilling the solution and adding either lemon juice or instant coffee. Glycerol 10% in normal saline or in 5% dextrose, given IV in the dose of 1.2 gm. per kg. body weight, has been claimed to have certain advantages over mannitol; it is claimed to avoid the 'rebound edema' said to be common after mannitol. Moreover, it can be used in the presence of dehydration and cardiac failure where mannitol cannot be used. It has been used in the treatment of acute cerebral infarction, given IV daily 10% in 500 ml. saline for 6 days. Rapid infusion of high concentrations (30%) can cause hemolysis. It also causes hyperglycemia.

Xanthines as Diuretics

Xanthines (Chapter 12) act by increasing the renal blood flow by both cardiac and vascular action, as well as by inhibiting the tubular reabsorption of sodium. The diuretic action is not much affected by changes in acid-base balance and the loss of potassium is usually small.

Theophylline is the most effective xanthine diuretic and is generally used as theophylline ethylene diamine (aminophylline), a weak diuretic; to be effective, it must be given IV, slowly, over 20 minutes, in the dose of 0.25-0.50 g, diluted in 10-20 ml of 5% glucose solution. The drug may cause marked diuresis when given 3-4 hours after a thiazide or ½ hour after fresemide in a previously refractory patient.

Carbonic Anhydrase Inhibitors

ACETAZOLAMIDE (Diamox): This drug, a weak diuretic, is unique because of its mechanism of action.

$$CH_3-CO-NH-C \overset{N-N}{\underset{S}{\diagup\!\diagdown}} C-SO_2-NH_2$$

Fig. 38.3: Acetazolamide

Mechanism of Action: The enzyme carbonic anhydrase is present in the renal cortex, gastric mucosa, pancreas, eyes, CNS and RBC. It catalyses the reactions :

$$H_2O + CO_2 \rightleftharpoons H_2CO_3$$

$$H_2CO_3 \rightleftharpoons H^+ + HCO^-_3$$

Acetazolamide acts by inhibiting the enzyme carbonic anhydrase; carbonic acid is not formed, resulting in unavailability of H^+ for Na^+ exchange.

Pharmacological actions:

• ***Kidney and electrolytes***: The enzyme carbonic anhydrase plays an important role in the tubular reabsorption of sodium and bicarbonate (Fig. 38.2).

Normally, the secreted H ion combines with HCO_3 ion provided by the glomerular filtrate to form H_2CO_3. This is converted to water and carbon dioxide, which latter diffuses into the tubular cell.

$$H^+ + HCO_3^- \longrightarrow H_2CO_3$$

Acetazolamide inhibits both membrane-bound and cytoplasmic enzyme so that carbonic acid (H_2CO_3) is not formed and hydrogen ion is not made available for sodium exchange, leading to excretion of sodium along with water.

It must be noted that major portion of the sodium in the distal tubule is reabsorbed by an active process and K^+, H^+/Na exchange mechanism controls only a small amount of sodium that accompanies a less diffusible anion, bicarbonate. Following acetazolamide, due to lack of H^+ ion, bicarbonate will remain in the poorly diffusible form and hence excreted in large amounts. The urine becomes alkaline. Since exchange of potassium and hydrogen ions with sodium occurs along the same pathway, the decrease in available hydrogen ion may promote more loss of potassium. Acetazolamide, therefore, causes loss of sodium, potassium, bicarbonate and phosphate ions but has no effect on calcium and magnesium. The resulting decrease in the ECF base may cause metabolic acidosis which is accompanied by the loss of diuretic activity. Acetazolamide is thus a self-limiting diuretic. Its action is markedly decreased by acidifying salts while it is enhanced in the presence of metabolic alkalosis.

• ***Eye***: Carbonic anhydrase present in the ciliary processes is important in the production of aqueous humor, which has a high bicarbonate content. Acetazolamide reduces the intraocular tension by inhibiting this enzyme.

• ***CNS***: Acetazolamide decreases the CSF formation. For its antiepileptic action, see Chapter 7.

Absorption, fate and excretion: Acetazolamide, given orally, is well absorbed. It is not metabolized but is actively secreted into the urine by the proximal tubular cells through the organic acid pathway.

Adverse reactions: It can cause metabolic acidosis and hypokalemia. In fact, sometimes it produces excessive potassium loss without causing significant sodium loss. Occasionally, it can cause drowsiness and paraesthesiae. It can precipitate renal calcium and phosphorus calculi formation. Being structurally related to sulfonamides, rarely, it can cause other adverse effects like skin rashes, blood dyscrasias, crystalluria and kidney damage. Salicylates enhance the toxicity of acetazolamide by inhibiting its plasma protein binding and by interfering with its renal tubular secretion.

Preparation and dosage: Acetazolamide 0.25 g. tablet; dose : 1-2 tablets daily in divided doses. Sodium acetazolamide can be given parenterally.

Therapeutic uses: *It is no more used as a sole diuretic but is used as an adjunct in selected patients resistant to other diuretics.* Its use is restricted to:

• ***Prophylaxis and treatment of high altitude illness***:This term is used to describe the cerebral and pulmonary syndromes that can develop in unacclimatized persons after ascent to high altitude. The *cerebral syndrome* comprises acute mountain sickness and cerebral edema; the *pulmonary syndrome* is high altitude non-cardiogenic pulmonary edema.These conditions are caused by rapid ascent to heights of 8000 feet or more. At these heights, the low partial pressure of atmospheric oxygen causes marked hypoxemia, resulting in tissue hypoxia. The latter results in neurohumoral and hemodynamic responses which lead to hyperperfusion of microvascular beds, capillary leakage and consequent local edema.

Early symptoms of the cerebral syndrome are headache, and impairment of memory, judgement and ability to perform complex calculations. More advanced manifestations are anorexia, malaise and insomnia. The most serious symptoms are due to cerebral edema, noncardiogenic pulmonary edema with pulmonary arterial hypertension and retinal hemorrhages. Coma and death can occur.

The early symptoms of the pulmonary syndrome are decreased performance and dry cough. Later manifestations are respiratory distress, resting tachycardia, tachypnoea, fever, and pink or frankly bloody sputum. Manifestations of the cerebral syndrome may be superimposed in severe cases.

The principles of prevention and treatment of these conditions are:

(a) ***For acute mountain sickness and cerebral edema***:

(i) Gradual ascent to high altitude to promote acclimatization.

(ii) Avoidance of over-exertion at high altitudes.

(iii) Descent to lower altitude at the first appearance of sytmptoms.Descent may be simulated by stay in a portable hyperbaric chamber (Chapter 73).

(iv) Supplementary oxygen.

(v) Drugs : Prophylactic **acetazolamide** is the drug of choice. It is given in the dose of 250 mg q 8 hourly, the day before, during and for 5 days after the ascent. Lower doses may not be effective. Acetazolamide probably helps by causing mild metabolic acidosis; the latter increases the respiratory drive, prevents hypoxemia and pharmacologically produces an acclimatization response. *Acetazolamide ameliorates symptoms but does not reduce the* *risk of cerebral edema, pulmonary edema or retinal hemorrhages.* Hence, *acetazolamide is no substitute for slow ascent.* **Dexamethasone,** in the dose of 4 mg. every 6 hours, begun on the day of the ascent, continued for 3 days at high altitude, and then tapered quickly, may be useful in reducing the incidence and early symptoms of acute mountain sickness. *Acetazolamide and dexamethasone are useful for both prevention and treatment of these condition.*

(vi) Adjunct drugs used are **NSAID** and **antiemetics**, when necessary. *Sedative hypnotics are avoided for fear of causing respiratory depression.*

(b) ***For pulmonary edema***: The non-pharmacological measures are the same as those for the cerebral manifestations. **Nifedipine** is the preferred drug for prevention and treatment of pulmonary manifestations of high altitude illness. It probably acts by lowering pulmonary arterial pressure,which is critical in the development of pulmonary edema in this condition.The other drugs recommended are **beta adrenergic agonists** which clear the fluid from the alveolar space and may lower pulmonary arterial pressure. **Dexamethasone** is indicated if cerebral symptoms develop. *Prophylactic nifedipine should be considered before a future ascent in a person with a history of high altitude pulmonary edema.*

- ***Treatment of glaucoma*** (Chapter 70)
- ***Treatment of resistant epilepsy*** (Chapter 9).
- ***Prevention of attacks of periodic paralysis.***

DICHLORPHENAMIDE and METHAZOLAMIDE are the other carbonic anhydrase inhibitors, related to acetazolamide, used orally in the treatment of glaucoma (Chapter 70).

Benzothiadiazines

Introduction of **thiazide diuretics** revolutionized the oral diuretic therapy, since before chlorothiazide, no effective and reliable oral diuretic was available. Synthesis of thiazides stems from the original observation by Southworth (1937) that sulfanilamide, an antibacterial drug, possesses a mild diuretic activity. This was later shown to be related to its carbonic anhydrase inhibiting action. Interestingly, chlorothiazide, synthesized as one of the carbonic anhydrase inhibitor, revealed marked diuretic activity in doses that did not significantly inhibit the enzyme carbonic anhydrase. Since then, many thiazide-like diuretics have been introduced.

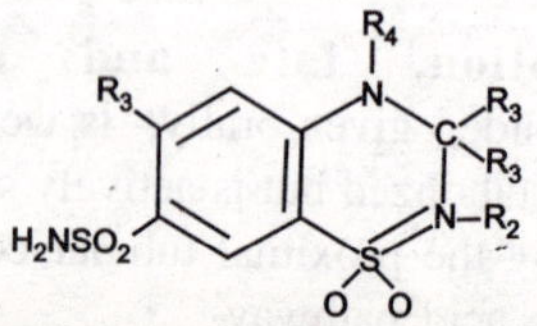

Fig. 38.4: Benzothiadiazine nucleus.

Pharmacological actions:

Kidney and electrolytes: Like acetazolamide, these drugs are secreted into the tubular fluid and block the electroneutral sodium and chloride transport (symport) in the distal convoluted tubule by competing with Na^+ and Cl^- for the binding sites. They primarily act on the site proximal to the sodium and potassium exchange region in the distal tubule (site III, Fig. 38.1). Hence, they are sometimes known as *early distal diuretics*. The GFR is not affected.

- Thiazides increase Na^+ and Cl^- excretion but as almost 90% of the filtered load of sodium is reabsorbed before reaching the distal tubules, they exert only a moderate diuretic effect.
- Chlorothiazide has a weak carbonic anhydrase inhibitory activity and hence it can cause some loss of bicarbonate. The newer thiazides, however, do not significantly increase the bicarbonate loss.
- Because of the marked inhibitory action on sodium reabsorption, a large amount of sodium is made available to the distal segment where exchange of K+ with Na takes place. This causes increased potassium loss, particularly in the presence of excessive aldosterone which stimulates this exchange mechanism.

● Excessive renal loss of sodium and chloride may cause hyponatremia and hypochloremia; excessive potassium loss can cause hypokalemia, thus leading to *hypokalemic hypochloremic alkalosis.* Long term use causes hypomagnesimia.

● Initially, the drug causes a diminution in sodium reabsorption in the distal tubule and a gradual reduction in the ECF volume. When the ECF volume falls to slightly below normal, the reabsorption of sodium from the proximal tubule is stimulated, resulting in diminished amount of sodium delivered into the distal tubule. This decreases its diuretic activity and causes resistance. Thiazides are less effective when GFR falls below 30-40 ml/min.

Antihypertensive action: Thiazides produce a mild antihypertensive effect partly due to their action on sodium metabolism and partly due to their direct action on blood vessels (Chapter 29).

Metabolic actions: Thiazide may cause:

- ***Hyperglycemia***
- ***Hyperuricemia***
- ***Hypercalcemia***
- ***Hyperlipidemia***

The mechanism by which thiazides cause hyperglycemia is not known. Catecholamine release, secondary to volume depletion, a direct inhibition of insulin release and hypokalemia are the possible mechanisms. These drugs can unmask or aggravate the pre-existing diabetes mellitus. Diazoxide, a thiazide derivative with potent hyperglycemic action, has been used in the treatment of hypoglycemia.

However, during long-term therapy of hypertension, thiazides do not significantly increase the incidence of diabetes mellitus.

Thiazides also decrease the excretion of uric acid, thus raising plasma uric acid level. Usually, this is asymptomatic but, occasionally, it can precipitate attacks of gouty arthritis.

Unlike loop diuretics (see later), *thiazides reduces urinary calcium loss and* **promote calcium retention**; *they are useful in treating idiopathic hypercalciuria.*

Serum cholesterol and triglycerides may increase slightly; however, this has hardly any significance as the elevation is not persistent beyond 6-12 months of treatment.

In patients with diabetes insipidus, especially the nephrogenic type, thiazides decrease urinary volume. This is discussed later.

Absorption, fate and excretion: Thiazides are well absorbed from the intestine and the effect starts within one hour. They are distributed throughout the ECF and are relatively concentrated in the kidney. They can cross the placental barrier. Like other organic acids, thiazides are secreted into the tubules and excreted in urine. The excretion rate varies with the individual drug. The slowly excreted compounds like polythiazide and bendroflumethiazide have prolonged action.

The long acting thiazides are long acting because of their greater plasma protein binding and greater lipid solubility. Bendroflumethiazide, polythiazide and indapamide are primarily metabolized in the liver; whereas chlorothiazide, hydro-chlorothiazide, hydroflumethiazide and chlorthalidone are excreted in the urine. Plasma half life of thiazides is sufficient to permit their use once or twice daily.

Adverse reactions: Apart from electrolyte disturbances such as hypokalemic and hypochloremic alkalosis, these drugs have remarkably few serious toxic effects. Hypokalemia increases the risk of fatal toxicity of certain arrhythmias (Chapter 27) and drugs like digoxin (Chapter 30). Because of structural similarity, they may rarely cause sulfonamide-like allergic reactions such as dermatitis and thrombotycopenia.

In the presence of renal and hepatic insufficiency, these drugs may precipitate renal failure or hepatic coma. This is attributed to the development of hypokalemia and alkalosis.

Preparations and dosage: Table 38.3.

Therapeutic uses:

● ***As diuretics***: Thiazides produce effective diuresis in most of the patients with sodium retention and edema. Since there is no special advantage in using any particular preparation, the cheapest of these should be the drug of first

Table 38.3: Commonly used benzothiadiazine and related diuretics

Name	Tablet mg.	Daily dose as antihypertensive mg.	Daily dose as diuretic mg.	Duration of diuretic action hours
Chlorothiazide (Chlorotride)	250, 500	125-250	500 to 1000 Children: 20 mg./kg.	6 to 12
Hydrochlorothiazide (Hydrothiazide)	25, 50	12.5-25	25 to 200 Children: 2 mg./kg.	12 or more
Hydroflumethiazide (Naclex)	50	12.5-25	25 to 200	18 to 24
Benzthiazide (Fovane)	25	12.5-25	50 to 200	12 to 18
Cyclopenthiazide (Navidrex)	0.5	0.25-0.5	0.5-1	18 to 24
Bendroflumethiazide (Neo-NaClex)	2.5, 5	1.25-2.5	2.5 to 5	18 to 24
Polythiazide (Nephril)	1, 2, 4	2	1 to 4	24 to 48
Chlorthalidone (Hythalton)	100	12.5-25	50 to 200	48 to 72
Quinethazone (Hydromox)	50	25	50 to 200	18 to 24
Metolazone (Zaroxylin)	5	1.25-2.5	5 to 10	18 to 24

choice. Dosage has to be adjusted in individual cases depending upon the response. Occasionally, patients may develop resistance to these drugs. In majority of such cases, hypokalemia may be present which needs correction; for this purpose, potassium chloride is commonly used. *Enteric coated thiazide tablets containing potassium chloride should not be used as they can cause intestinal ulcerations.* Excessive potassium loss can be prevented by combining thiazide drugs with spironolactone or triameterene.

As the maximum diuretic effect of all thiazides is similar, a patient resistant to the maximum dose of one thiazide is unlikely to respond to another.

- ***As antihypertensives***: See Chapter 29.
- ***In the prevention of recurrent renal calculi***: In patients with idiopathic hypercalciuria, hydrochlorthiazide (50 mg. twice a day) reduces the frequency of stone formation.
- ***In nephrogenic diabetes insipidus***: See later.

Thiazide-like diuretics : These drugs, structurally similar to thiazides, have similar mechanism but longer duration of action. As diuretics, they offer hardly any advantage over thiazides.

CHLORTHALIDONE (Hythalton): This phthalimidine derivative is absorbed slowly, and is not significantly metabolized. It remains preferentially bound to renal tissue for prolonged periods. Hence, its duration of action is upto 48 hours or more. *It may be preferred in the treatment of hypertension.* It is more liable to cause hypokalemia than the thiazides. It has been reported to be useful in the treatment of hypoparathyroidism where it corrects hypocalcemia without the danger of causing hypercalcemia which is inherent in vitamin D therapy of this condition.

Chlorexolone (Nefrolan): This long action phthalimidine derivative is claimed to be more effective than chlorothiazide on weight basis.

Indapamide (Natrilix, Lorvas) and xipamide, (Xipamid) are used in the treatment of hypertension (Chapter 29).

Clopamide (Brinaldix) is administered in a single daily dose of 20 to 60 mg. in the morning, on alternate days. It has longer duration of action (18-24 hr.). Blood urea levels are not affected during treatment.

QUINAZOLINONES: **Quinethazone** and **Metolazone** belong to this group. These compounds have diuretic characteristics similar to those of benzothiadiazines.

Loop Diuretics

FUROSEMIDE (Frusemide, Lasix, Kinex): It is a potent, oral, diuretic, possessing a halogenated sulfamoyl benzene ring common to thiazide diuretics (Fig. 38.5).

Fig. 38.5: Furosemide. Note the sulfamoyl benzene ring.

Mechanism of action: Like thiazides, the loop diuretics are secreted into the tubular fluid via the organic acid pathway. The drug acts along the entire nephron (sites II and III in Fig. 38.1), primarily on the thick ascending limb of the loop of Henle with the exception only of the distal site where Na^+ is exchanged for K^+ and H^+. It blocks the Na^+– K^+– $2Cl^-$ symport. Hence *unlike thiazides, urinary excretion of Na^+ may continue uninterruptedly even when the patient's ECF volume has been severely depleted.* It also inhibits the reabsorption of Ca^{++} and Mg^{++}. The drug has little effect on carbonic anhydrase.

Intravenous administration in addition increases the renal blood flow. Further, it increases PGE_2 synthesis in the kidneys, which has a locally protective, vasodilator effect. Under normal circumstances, this PG system is dormant, but it becomes operative in times of physiological or pharmacological stress and counters the intrarenal vasoconstriction which would otherwise occur.

Pharmacological actions:

Kidneys :

- Intense diuretic action starts within an hour of oral administration and is completed in 4-6 hours. It has a steep dose-response curve without a ceiling effect. Because of its short duration of action, furosemide is administered twice a day when sustained diuresis is desired.
- It causes marked sodium, potassium, chloride and phosphate loss. The bicarbonate loss is not marked.
- Excessive chloride loss can cause hypochloremic alkalosis. The associated potassium loss leads to hypokalemia. However, the free water clearance is larger and the hypokalemia less marked with furosemide than with thiazides.
- Furosemide causes little change in the urinary pH and its diuretic action does not appear to be particularly limited by the prevailing state of electrolyte or acid-base balance.
- Loop diuretics, in general, are potent renin releasers.

Blood vessels and blood pressure: Intravenous furosemide dilates the peripheral vasculature, lowers the arterial BP, and causes rapid venous pooling of blood, thus reducing the cardiac preload and afterload. This action of bringing about a re-distribution of blood from the congested pulmonary circulation into the systemic, capacitance vessels is more rapid than its diuretic effect; it may be more important than the latter in the treatment of acute LVF with pulmonary edema.

Its effects on the BP on oral administration are comparable to those of thiazide diuretics.

Metabolic actions : Like thiazides, furosemide can cause an increase in blood uric acid and disturbances of glucose tolerance; rise in blood urea has also been reported. Calcium and magnesium excretion is increased.

Absorption, fate and excretion: The drug is rapidly absorbed from the GI tract to the extent of 60-100%. Food reduces its bioavailability. It is excreted within 4 hours by glomerular filtration and tubular secretion. The onset of action is quick and the duration short. Given IV, the diuresis begins within 2 minutes and lasts for 2-3 hours. It is best given in a single dose. Fifty per cent of the dose is excreted unchanged in urine; the rest is conjugated with glucuronide in the kidney. Hence, in patients with renal insufficiency the plasma t½ is prolonged.

Adverse reactions: As it is a potent diuretic, its unintelligent use can precipitate serious electrolyte and water disturbances due to excessive loss of sodium, potassium, chloride and water. A patient may complain of weakness, fatigue, dizziness, and cramps; orthostatic hypotension can occur. Excessively rapid diuresis in elderly patients may precipitate acute urinary retention. Cardiac arrest following IV frusemide and sudden death following its IM administration have been reported. The drug can precipitate hepatic coma in the presence of liver disease. Other less common reactions include skin rashes, nausea, diarrhoea and rarely acute pancreatitis, thrombocytopenia and neutropenia. It can produce hyperuricemia and hyperglycemia, and unmask latent diabetes mellitus. It increases plasma triglycerides, total and LDL cholesterol.

Hearing loss, usually transient, with or without tinnitus, has been reported following *very large doses* in patients with renal failure. Furosemide can enhance the toxicity of lithium, aminoglycosides and cephalosporins. Cross reaction with sulfonamides can occur. Its action is inhibited by NSAID such as indomethacin. It should be avoided in pregnancy.

Preparations and dosage: Furosemide tablet 40 mg., Furosemide injection, 20 mg. in 2 ml. Dose: 40-100 mg. daily depending upon the severity of the edema.

Therapeutic uses:

- ***As a diuretic***: Furosemide is a very effective, potent and usually safe diuretic. However, it has no distinct advantage over thiazides, in the treatment of moderate edema. It is more useful in severe edema resistant to thiazides.
- ***Pulmonary edema***: *Given IV, it can be life saving in patients with pulmonary edema.*
- ***Chronic renal failure***: The dose response curve with furosemide shows a steep rise and very large single doses (2000 mg.) have been used in patients with advanced renal failure. It is sometimes effective in the presence of marked decrease in GFR (as low as 2 ml./minute). *Since the drug continues to act even in the presence of electrolyte and acid-base disturbances, close monitoring of the therapeutic response and blood chemistry is very essential.*
- ***As an antihypertensive***: Furosemide cannot be recommended for long term antihypertensive therapy because of high dose requirements, short duration of action and its high diuretic potential. In this respect, thiazides are to be preferred.
- ***Acute renal failure***: see later.
- ***Barbiturate poisoning***: It is used to induce forced diuresis (Chapter 8).
- ***Hypercalcemia***: Intravenous furosemide, together with normal saline infusion, is valuable in the emergency management of hypercalcemia.

TORSEMIDE: This congener is as active as furosemide in similar doses. However, it is absorbed completely and 80% of the drug is metabolized in the liver. Hence, its plasma half life is prolonged in liver disease.

BUMETANIDE (Burinex, Bumet): This diuretic is chemically 3-n-butylamino-4-phenoxy-sulphamoyl benzoic acid. Its onset and duration of action and its effects on electrolyte excretion are similar to those of furosemide. Its absorption is nearly 80% and is more predictable than that of furosemide. It is metabolized in the liver and its half life is not prolonged in renal insufficiency. One mg. of bumetanide equals 40 mg. of furosemide in its diuretic potency.

Axosemide, tripamide, piretanide are the other diuretics belonging to the furosemide group.

ETHACRYNIC ACID (Edecrin): Ethacrynic acid, an unsaturated ketone derivative of phenoxyacetic acid, is a potent oral diuretic like furosemide. Chemically, it is unrelated to other diuretic drugs.

The diuretic and metabolic effects of ethacrynic acid are similar to those of furosemide. Given orally, the maximum diuresis occurs within 2-3 hours while on IV administration the effect starts within a few minutes and is complete within 1-2 hours. Like furosemide, it can be used in edematous states, especially in patients allergic to sulfonamides. It is now less used because it is more prone to cause adverse effects which are similar to those of furosemide.

Potassium Sparing Diuretics

These agents inhibit sodium absorption in the later part of distal tubule, collecting ducts and concomitantly, indirectly suppress the secretion of K^+ and H^+. Spironolactone acts as a competitive aldosterone antagonist; whereas triamterene and amiloride directly inhibit sodium reabsorption by inhibiting sodium channels. Both drugs can cause hyperkalemic, hyperchloremic, metabolic acidosis. However, they do not affect renal hemodynamics.

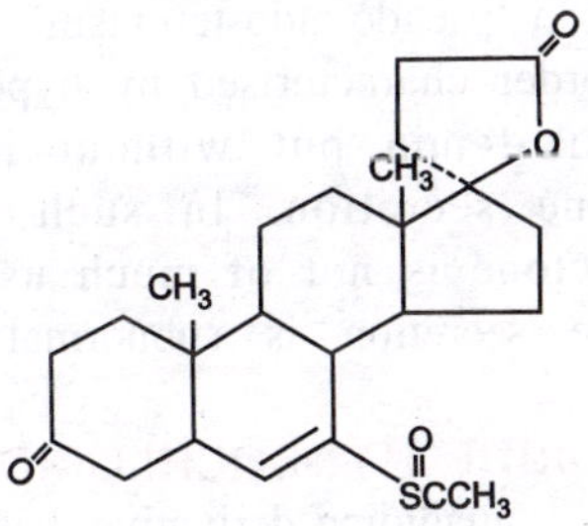

Fig. 38.6: Spironolactone

SPIRONOLACTONE (Aldactone): Spironolactone, with structural similarity to aldosterone, is a commonly employed **aldosterone antagonist**. It acts by competitive antagonism of aldosterone, in the distal part of the nephron, (**late distal diuretic**); it prevents potassium secretion and decreases sodium reabsorption. It does not produce significant natruresis in normal individuals or in those cases of edema, not associated with rise in aldosterone. Even in edema associated with an excess of aldosterone, its action is weak.

Given orally, it has a cumulative effect and full response is observed after 3-5 days of therapy. Given alone, it may cause a weak diuretic response but along with other diuretic agents such as thiazides, it causes diuresis without producing significant loss of potassium. It is metabolized to several inactive compounds.

Adverse reactions: No serious toxic effects have been reported even after long term use.

- ***Hyperkalemia*** : In the presence of renal insufficiency, it can cause dangerous hyperkalemia and metabolic acidosis. Simultaneous use of ACEI, or a beta blocker with spironolactone increases the risk of hyperkalemia.
- ***Endocrine effects:*** Occasionally, it may cause decreased libido, gynecomastia, impotence and menstrual irregularity. The drug has antiandrogenic activity at the receptor level and has been shown to affect both gonadal and adrenal steroidogenesis.
- ***Miscellaneous effects:*** Spironolactone may cause lethargy and drowsiness. It may increase blood urea nitrogen and serum uric acid levels. It can cause gastritis and is avoided in patients with acid-peptic disease. NSAIDs may inhibit the excretion of this drug.

Preparation and dosage: Spironolactone is supplied as a microcrystalline preparation, 25 mg. tablet. Dose : 100-200 mg. per day (maximum 400 mg. per day) in divided doses.

Therapeutic uses: It is used

- ***In the treatment of hypertension,*** as an adjunct to thiazide diuretics (Chapter 29).
- ***In the treatment of edema*** particularly cirrhotic edema. (see later)
- ***In severe congestive heart failure*** (Chapter 30).
- ***In patients with hirsutism due to polycystic* ovarian disease :** (Chapter 67); and
- ***In the treatment of its specific use primary hyperaldosteronism*** (Conn syndrome),

where it has been used as an alternative to adrenalectomy. It corrects the electrolyte abnormalities and lowers the BP in this disorder.

POTASSIUM CANREONATE (Spiroctan-M): This prodrug gets converted to canrenone in the body, which is an active metabolite of spironolactone and has similar uses as spironolactone but can be given parenterally. It is available as injections containing 20 mg./ml. in 10 ml. ampoules and is given IV, slowly, upto 400 mg. per day, in divided doses.

EPLERENONE (Inspra): blocks the mineralocorticoid receptors in the kidney, heart, blood vessels and brain more selectively than spironolactone; it has very little affinity for the androgen and progesterone receptors.

It is metabolized by the liver and has a t ½ of 4-6 hours. Its adverse reactions include GI intolerance, dizziness, hyperkalemia and hypertriglyceridemia.

It is used to treat:

(a) Hypertension, in the dose of 50 mg OD, increased to 100 mg OD (maximum dose) within 4 weeks, as required,

(b) Post-MI CHF, in one half of the above dosage. Its clinical efficacy is similar to that of spironolactone. Its probable advantage over spironolactone is the lower incidence of endocrine side effects. It is also used in the combined oral contraceptive pill, Yasmin. The drug is expensive.

TRIAMTERENE (Dytac): This drug, increases the excretion of water, sodium, chloride and bicarbonate but unlike other diuretics, it depresses the excretion of potassium. In this respect, it resembles the aldosterone antagonist spironolactone.

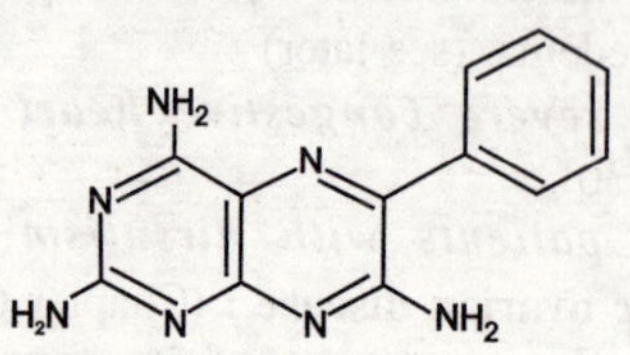

Fig. 38.7: Triamterene

Mechanism of action : It acts on the late distal tubule and collecting duct. It blocks renal epithelial Na^+ channels competitively. Combination of triamterene and spironolactone produces more marked natriuretic effect than the maximally effective dose of triamterene given alone. It also spares magnesium loss. *Triamterene has no antihypertensive action.*

After oral administration, the peak effect is reached in about 2 hours and the action is over in about 10 hours. It has an active metabolite which is secreted into the renal tubular fluid.

Adverse reactions: No serious toxic effects have been noted. Besides causing hyperkalemia, the drug may cause troublesome diarrhoea. Occasionally, skin rash and dryness of mouth have been noted. It may cause a decrease in glucose tolerance and a rise in blood urea level. Chronic administration causes a decrease in the uric acid excretion and renal calculi.

Preparation and dosage: It is administered orally in the dose of 100-200 mg.

Therapeutic uses:

- ***Potassium sparing diuretic*:** Triamterene itself is a weak diuretic. However, it is usually combined with a thiazide to prevent the potassium loss.
- ***Pseudo-aldosteronism*:** The drug has also been used in 'pseudo-aldosteronism', a familial renal disorder characterised by hypertension, and hypokalemia but without increased aldosterone secretion. In such patients, spironolactone is not of much use as the aldosterone secretion is subnormal.

AMILORIDE HYDROCHLORIDE : This compound, a guanidine derivative, has a weak diuretic activity, and is given orally in the dose of 10 mg. Its action is similar to that of triamterene. It prevents potassium loss. The plasma half life is about 6 hours. It is excreted unchanged in the urine. It is used:

- ***As a diuretic,*** in the dose of 10-20 mg daily, in combination with other diuretics. On weight basis, it is more potent than triamterene.
- ***In lithium-induced diabetes insipidus*** as

it blocks lithium reabsorption from the collecting tubules.

- ***In cystic fibrosis:*** An aerosolized preparation facilitates mucociliary clearance by blocking bronchial epithelial sodium channels. Reduced reabsorption of Na^+ increases the hydration of bronchial secretions.

Indications for diuretic therapy are given in Table 38.4. The **non-diuretic uses of diuretic drugs** are given in Table 38.5. These are discussed in the respective chapters.

Table 38.4: Indications for diuretic therapy

- Edema associated with sodium retention such as cardiac, hepatic and renal edema.
- Pulmonary and cerebral edema.
- Drug poisoning such as due to barbiturates or salicylates (see Chapter 6).
- Acute oliguric renal failure.
- Edema of pregnancy and idiopathic edema.

Table 38.5: Nondiuretic uses of diuretic drugs

- Hypertension (hydrochlorothiazide).
- Idiopathic calcium urolithiasis (hydrochlorothiazide).
- Diabetes insipidus (hydrochlorothiazide).
- Hypercalcemia (furosemide).
- Hyponatremic states due to water retention (furosemide).
- Glaucoma (acetazolamide).
- Mountain sickness (acetazolamide)

Management of Edema

Increase in extracellular sodium and fluid volume leads to the development of edema. This could occur due to either an excessive intake or decreased excretion of sodium and / or water. The edematous states observed in practice are mostly due to decreased rate of renal excretion of sodium and water.

Factors involved in promoting excessive sodium retention by the kidneys are:

(a) Decreased cardiac output and GFR as in CHF.

(b) Increased levels of aldosterone as in edema due to hepatic cirrhosis.

(c) Intrinsic renal disease such as acute nephritis; and

(d) Reduction in plasma colloids as in hypoproteinemic states (nutritional edema and nephrotic syndrome).

In a given case, more than one factor may be involved.

Although the treatment of underlying pathology is important in all such cases, great relief can be obtained by using proper diuretics.

Edema can be treated by :

- ***Ensuring adequate renal perfusion,*** by improving cardiac efficiency, as in cardiac edema,
- ***Restricting sodium intake or preventing its absorption from GI tract*** by using ion exchange resins; and
- ***By promoting sodium and water excretion*** by using diuretics and aldosterone antagonists.

Usually, these approaches are combined.

CATION EXCHANGE RESINS: Ion exchange resins are synthetic, macro-molecular compounds. Two types of resins are available: (a) the anion exchange resins which contain a basic group and were once used as gastric antacids; and (b) the cation exchange resins which contain an acidic group and their cations can be exchanged for ions with a positive charge.

The cation exchange resins, given orally, exchange their H^+ ions for Na^+ ions. The resultant compound is not absorbed, thereby preventing the absorption of sodium from the small intestine. Potassium is also exchanged along with sodium, resulting in a significant loss of potassium in feces along with sodium.

Prolonged therapy with cation exchange resins results in a significant absorption of H^+ ions from the GI tract leading to metabolic acidosis. Besides hypokalemia and metabolic acidosis, the resins often produce nausea, vomiting and diarrhoea and may cause fecal impaction. The dose needed is very bulky. Hence, they are rarely used in therapy.

The cation exchange resins available are:

(i) Sodium polystyrene sulfonate, used for removal of potassium, dose 15 to 60 g. daily.

(ii) Carbacrylamine resins, used for removal of sodium, dose 40 to 65 g. daily.

Cardiac edema: This is due to the failure of the heart as a pump, leading to a fall in the cardiac output and an inadequate renal perfusion (Chapter 30). Hence, unless the cardiac function is improved and adequate renal perfusion is restored, diuretics cannot cause worthwhile diuresis. Adequate GFR is ensured by :

- ***Complete rest***
- ***Improving the cardiac output by using ACE inhibitors and/or digoxin***; and by
- ***Treating the underlying cause*** such as hyperthyroidism, anemia, or hypertension.

Restriction of sodium intake and induction of diuresis are usually combined with the primary therapy of the cause.

In mild CHF, one should aim at diuresis which causes a weight reduction of not more than 1 kg per day, and a thiazide is preferred to a loop diuretic for this purpose. The latter causes abrupt diuresis with contraction of plasma volume. This results in secondary hyperaldosteronism. For the same reason, intermittent use of a diuretic (2-3 times a week) is preferred to daily administration. When planning continuous diuretic therapy, ACEI ± spironolactone may be combined with the primary diuretic right from the beginning with advantage, instead of waiting for diuretic resistance due to hyperaldosteronism.

As the disease progresses, the use of furosemide is inevitable. With **single-daily-dose of furosemide**, intense sodium retention post-diuresis can limit the efficacy of the drug. This can be overcome by increasing the daily dose of furosemide and administering it in 2-3 divided doses per day. In severe CHF, therapy may be started with larger oral/parenteral dose of furosemide; the latter may be reduced once diuresis is established. *However, the routine use of the very potent diuretics in all cases of cardiac failure from the beginning is not recommended* (Chapter 30), as over-enthusiastic treatment with diuretics may worsen the patient's condition.

Cirrhotic edema and ascites: This is due to:

- ***Increased portal venous pressure.***
- ***Decreased plasma colloid osmotic pressure following hypoalbuminemia;*** and
- ***Secondary rise in aldosterone secretion.***

The treatment, therefore, would be bed rest, salt restriction, use of spironolactone and, use of diuretics only *in severe cases.*

Compared to cardiac edema, the danger of precipitating hypokalemia and azotemia (volume contraction) with diuretic therapy is higher in cirrhotic edema; the chances of precipitating hepatic encephalopathy are also high. Hence, the diuretic therapy in a cirrhotic edema should be undertaken under supervision with checks on serum electrolytes. The dose used should be the smallest possible one and oral potassium supplements should be given. The regime recommended is as follows: (1) Begin with bed rest, restriction of sodium intake (to 20 mEq/day) and provided the blood urea is normal, oral potassium supplements in large doses (100 mEq/day). (2) After 4-5 days, spironolactone is added. Unlike in edema due to other causes, potassium supplement is continued in cirrhotic patients. (3) If adequate diuresis does not occur in 5 days, furosemide in doses 40-80 mg./day is added.

This is preferable to using spironolactone after the patient has become resistant to furosemide.

Seriously ill cirrhotic patients with ascites should not be treated too vigorously, as this may precipitate hepatic coma, azotemia and death.

Renal edema: Diuretics are ineffective

in treating edema due to **acute glomerulonephritis.**

The treatment of **nephrotic syndrome** depends on the underlying cause; in patients with diabetic nephrotic syndrome, furosemide is the diuretic of choice. In the 'idiopathic' nephrotic syndrome due to 'minimal change disease' in children, the treatment comprises (1) salt restriction; (2) dietary protein supplementation, unless concurrent renal insufficiency is present; (3) prednisolone (a glucocorticoid) in adequate doses (2 mg./kg./day); and (4) judicious use of diuretics; furosemide is the drug of choice. The response in children is very satisfactory, and remission without any permanent renal damage occurs in a high proportion of patients. The same disease in adults is less responsive to treatment. *It must be remembered that the concurrent use of large doses of furosemide and a glucocorticoid in a nephrotic child who has secondary hyperaldosteronism may cause severe hypokalemia.* In such circumstances spironolactone may be added.

Edema in patients with **chronic renal failure** may be due to salt loading or to congestive heart failure. In either case, the thiazide diuretics are ineffective in the presence of elevated serum creatinine. Furosemide is effective in such patients; but increasingly large doses, sometimes given IV as a bolus (100-200 mg), may be required. Concurrent salt restriction is necessary.

Nutritional edema: This is due to hypoalbuminemia and it responds to increased protein intake. Diuretics are usually not necessary. In severe cases, diuretics may be used to obtain temporary relief from the edema; *vigorous diuretic therapy is, however, dangerous and should be avoided.*

Pulmonary edema of cardiac origin : See Chapter 30.

Cerebral edema : See Table 38.6.

Drug-induced edema: Table 38.7.

Table 38.6 Treatment of cerebral edema

- ***Mannitol*** 25-50 g IV every 3-5 hours to a maximum of 2 g/kg/day.
- ***Furosemide*** IV in doses of 20-80 mg every 4-12 hours to supplement the effect of mannitol.
- ***Replacement of fluids*** to maintain serum osmolality.
- ***Glucocorticoids*** (dexamethasone 8 mg by injection every 6-8 hours) in intracranial neoplasms. Also see Chapter 64.
- ***Mechanical hyperventilation*** to achieve a CO_2 partial pressure of 25-30 mm Hg.
- ***Oral glycerine*** 30 ml TID
- ***Magnesium sulfate,*** saturated solution, 50-200 ml rectally.
- ***Surgical decompression*** if all above measures fail.

Table 38.7: Drugs causing fluid retention

NSAIDs
Fludrocortisone
Cortisone and hydrocortisone
Calcium channel blockers and certain other antihypertensives
Testosterone and estrogen
Danazol
Glitazones

Choice of a diuretic: The choice of a diuretic in the treatment of edema would depend on:

- ***Nature of the disease.***
- ***Potency of the drug.***
- ***Biochemical changes associated with its use.***
- ***Possibility of development of tolerance.***
- ***Convenience of administration.***

Majority of the patients with edema respond satisfactorally to relatively small doses of any moderately effective diuretic, and thiazides, being orally effective, safe and cheap, are to be preferred for routine use. Only in severe cases where quick and vigorous response is needed, loop diuretic like furosemide is employed. The thiazide diuretics are ineffective once the GFR has fallen below 30 ml./min. Furosemide and other loop diuretics remain effective until the GFR has fallen below 3 ml./min, but they often have to be used in very large doses that could be toxic. With such potent diuretics, the likelihood of serious electrolyte disturbances is greater. *Vigorous treatment with potent diuretics, coupled with strict restriction of sodium intake to clear the edema, may lead to rapid development of serious electrolyte disturbances and even death.*

Combination of diuretics: There is no advantage in routinely combining diuretics, especially drugs from the same group. In majority of cases, a single drug given in adequate doses is all that is necessary. However, *sequential nephron blocking* is an important principle in diuretic therapy, and the addition of diuretic drugs acting at different sites in the nephron in resistant cases is logical. Thus,

(a) A potassium sparing diuretic is commonly added to a thiazide or to furosemide, to prevent hypokalemia. Two potassium sparing diuretics should not be combined for fear of causing dangerous hyperkalemia.

(b) When fluid retention is refractory to furosemide, the addition of a thiazide may promote diuresis (see below).

(c) The concurrent use of furosemide and mannitol, both given by separate IV infusions, is effective in minimizing the dose of furosemide in patients with acute oliguric renal failure.

Diuretic tolerance/resistance : This can occur in two ways:

(a) A short term form may occur from second dose onwards (**early braking**). The decrease in the response can be prevented by restoring the diuretic-induced loss of volume. Its mechanism is not clear.

(b) Sometimes, long term administration of loop diuretics is followed by tolerance (**resistance**). In that case, the solute that escapes the loop of Henle floods the more distal segments of the nephron. The increased exposure to the solute causes hypertrophy of the distal nephron segments. This leads to reabsorption of sodium at more distal sites, decreasing the overall diuretic effect. Thiazide diuretics block the nephron sites at which hypertrophy occurs and this accounts for the synergistic effect of the combination of a thiazide and a loop diuretic.

In practice,when diuretic resistance occurs it can be due to:

- ***Drug related factors*** such as the choice of the diuretic; its dose; or interfering drugs such as NSAID, lithium or probenecid.
- ***Patient related factors*** such as non-compliance with instructions about bed rest or salt and fluid intake.
- ***Disease related factors*** such as markedly low GFR; severe hypokalemia, hyponatremia, hypovolemia, or hypomagnesemia; or severe CHF.

Correction of the underlying factors will often restore the response.

Complications of Diuretic Therapy

Diuretic therapy, no doubt, is very effective and many times life saving. However, it can produce various complications. These are:

Allergic reactions: These include various types of skin eruptions, uriticaria, occasional blood dyscrasias and rarely interstitial nephritis. Such reactions are usually confined to a single drug or class of drugs. In such circumstances, a drug from another group may be substituted.

Disturbances of electrolyte balance (see Table 38.8): These occur more commonly and are usually predictable. These include:

- ***Acute sodium depletion and hypovolemia*:** This is a relatively common complication especially following the loop diuretics and may be pronounced in hot weather, in patients on sodium restriction and in those with undetected renal disease. The patient

Table 38.8: Electrolyte excretion pattern following diuretics

Drug	Urinary electrolytes Na^+	K^+	Cl^-	HCO_3^-	Urine pH
Acetazolamide	++	+	–	+ +	8.2
Thiazides	+++	++	+	±	7.4
Furosemide	++++	++	++++	±	6.0
Spironolactone	+	*	+	±	7.2
Triamterene	++	*	++	+	7.2
Mannitol	+++	+	++	+	6.5

* denotes potassium retention. — denotes no change.

who improves dramatically initially with a diuretic suddenly becomes lethargic and sleepy. Signs of dehydration are present. Increasing the sodium intake reverses this condition. In severe cases, parenteral sodium chloride may be necessary (Chapter 36).

• ***Chronic sodium depletion*:** This is less common and is characterised by lethargy, weakness and disorientation. Absence of demonstrable edema along with a low serum sodium is the cardinal requirement for its diagnosis. This condition should be distinguished from the more severe condition of dilutional hyponatremia.

• ***Potassium depletion and hypokalemia*:** This occurs during long term use of thiazides and loop diuretics. It is especially liable to occur (a) when these drugs are used in large doses continuously rather than in small doses, intermittently; (b) when the diuresis is very brisk rather than gentle and the resultant contraction of plasma volume causes secondary hyperaldosteronism; (c) when the patient receives glucocorticoids at the same time; (d) in diabetics; (e) in elderly patients and the chronically sick who may have anorexia and may not eat properly; and (f) in states (such as cirrhosis of liver) with high circulating levels of aldosterone to begin with.

By itself hypokalemia can impair renal function and is dangerous to patients receiving digitalis. Diuretic induced hypokalemia can cause life threatening arrhythmias in patients taking drugs which prolong QT interval (quinidine, procainamide and amiodarone).

It can be prevented or corrected by :

(1) **Increased dietary intake of potassium**; this is a pleasant method of supplementing potassium; however, it must be remembered that potassium rich foods are also high in calorie content (9 KCal/mEq of K^+)

(2) **Potassium chloride supplement**; this is an effective method and 20-40 mEq of potassium should be given per day to groups (a) to (e). Patients from group (f) need 100 mEq/day as they lose much of the potassium supplement in the urine. This last group benefits from concurrent administration of spironolactone. Routine administration of supplemental potassium is probably not necessary when diuretics are used to treat hypertension and in young, ambulatory patients with good appetite.

(3) **Potassium sparing diuretics**; They are valuable but *when they are given, potassium supplements should be omitted except in cirrhotic patients* to avoid hyperkalemia.

• ***Hyperkalemia*:** This is less common. It occurs in cases with uremia and with drugs like triamterene. It is sometimes seen following massive diuresis with any potent drug; this is probably due to failure of potassium secretion by kidney tubules because of less availability of sodium at potassium secretory sites, after initial marked loss of sodium. (Chapter 36).

• ***Hypochloremic alkalosis*:** This occurs following thiazides and loop diuretics. It is caused by excessive loss of chlorides.

• ***Metabolic acidosis*:** This is seen following carbonic anhydrase inhibition (acetazolamide), and is discussed earlier.

• ***Chronic dilutional hyponatremia*:** This state is sometimes seen in patients with CHF where serum sodium is persistently low in spite of severe edema. This is because there is relatively more water retention than sodium retention by the kidneys resulting in extreme dilution of ECF; its mechanism is not clear. Although it is not a direct consequence of diuretic therapy, it may be aggravated following most of the diuretics. Such patients usually have severe myocardiac impairment and are unresponsive to the diuretics. The prognosis is usually poor, the treatment is difficult and replacement therapy with salt to correct hyponatremia is seldom successful. Rigid restriction of water intake (less than 700-800 ml. daily) is recommended. Glucocorticoids may be useful in some cases.

When serum sodium concentration approaches the normal value, the patient may exhibit responsiveness to a diuretic.

Selective adverse effects: These are discussed under each individual drug.

Thiazides and loop diuretics can cause magnesium deficiency which can give rise to ventricular arrhythmias. It can be corrected by 4 ml. of 50% magnesium sulfate given IV infusion over 10-15 min. followed by a small maintainance dose of 72 mmol over next 24 hrs.

With proper use of diuretics, there would be only a few patients who show refractoriness. In many such cases, correction of underlying electrolyte disturbances restores the responsiveness. Treatment of extra-renal factors such as pulmonary infection, adequate bed rest and proper use of other drugs like digoxin may help in some patients. However, in terminal cases, where the underlying pathology is continuously progressing and not correctable, no treatment is likely to prove useful.

Acute Renal Failure (ARF)

Acute renal failure (ARF) may be defined as a state in which the kidney's ability to maintain homeostasis has declined suddenly, with resultant retention of metabolic waste products as well as electrolyte, acid-base and volume disturbances. The causes of ARF are many and may be classified into prerenal, intra-renal and postrenal (obstructive). It is important to distinguish among these three types as:

• ***Prerenal ARF*** is largely due to a reduction in effective blood volume with resultant in reduction in glomerular filtration; *it is totally reversible with restoration of the effective blood volume;* if unrecognized and untreated, it can deteriorate into the intra-renal type.

• ***Intra-renal type of ARF*** due to intrinsic renal damage poses the maximum challenge to the clinician. Further, ARF may be oliguric (urine output less than 500 ml./day in adults) or non-oliguric. The distinction between oliguric and non-oliguric ARF is important because the larger urine output and diuretic-responsiveness in the latter permit more liberal administration of fluids, facilitating the general management of the patient and improving the prognosis of ARF.

• ***Postrenal ARF*** is reversible with the relief of obstruction.

The aims of therapy are (i) to treat the cause (if possible); (ii) to maintain the urine output at 30-50 ml./hour in adults without causing fluid overlaod; (iii) to maintain the BP normal; nutritional care; and (iv) prevention and treatment of infection, hyperkalemia, metabolic acidosis, hyperphosphatemia and other complications; all this while awaiting spontaneous recovery of renal function.

The principles of management, **when ARF is suspected**, are:

• ***Fluid challenge in oliguric patients,*** if the patient is not volume overloaded; typically 500-1000 ml. of normal saline is infused over

30-60 minutes while watching for signs of fluid overlaod. If the urine output increases, prerenal ARF is diagnosed and appropriate fluid administration is continued.

- ***IV furosemide :*** If there is no increase in the urine output in response to the above fluid challenge, 100-400 mg. of *furosemide* is infused to promote diuresis; this may accompanied by an infusion of 20% *mannitol* at the rate of 10-20 ml./ hour, in order to minimize the dose of furosemide needed. If these manoeuvres are successful in inducing a diuresis, they are continued in order to maintain the high rate of urine flow.

Table 38.9: Principles of management of established ARF

- Isolation and barrier nursing to prevent infection.
- Clinical monitoring (weight; B.P.; urine output; signs of dehydration or over hydration).
- Laboratory monitoring for anemia; electrolyte and acid base balance.
- Ensuring an intake of 30-50 Kcal/kg/day.
- Restriction of protein intake.
- Restricting fluid intake to (urine output + insensible losses from the skin and the lungs + visible losses such as sweat, vomit, stool) – 300 ml.
- Restricting sodium chloride intake to 2-4 g./ day.
- Restricting potassium intake to 40 mEq/ day.
- Restriction of phosphorus intake to 800 mg./day.
- Phosphorus binding antacids such aluminium hydroxide.
- Avoid magnesium containing drugs.
- Adjusting doses of drugs to renal status.
- Maintain blood pressure.
- Detection and treatment of acidosis, hyperkalemia and hypo- or hyper-natremia.
- Treatment of infection, anemia and G.I. bleeding.
- Hemodialysis.

If these manoeuvres fail, an established ARF is diagnosed; the further management is conservative with the purpose of maintaining the body homeostasis till there is spontaneous recovery of renal function. Hemodialysis may be needed and can be life-saving.

Table 38.9 outlines the principles of management of **established ARF.** Usefulness of frusemide in established ARF is doubtful.

Antidiuretic Agents

ANTIDIURETIC HORMONE (ADH, Vasopressin): The antidiuretic hormone is released from the posterior lobe of the pituitary along with oxytocin. Given in pharmacological doses, it also has a vasopressor action and hence, is also called **vasopressin.**

The hormone is formed by the supraoptic and paraventricular nuclei of the hypothalamus and travels to the posterior pituitary where it is stored. The rate of secretion of ADH is mainly determined by the plasma osmolality. Thus, dehydration stimulates whereas hydration inhibits ADH secretion. An increase or a decrease in the circulating blood volume may also influence the secretion through ill-defined 'volume receptors' found in the heart and the pulmonary veins and postulated in the hypothalamus. In addition, pain,nausea,hypoxia and some endogenous hormones and neurotransmitters can modify its secretion. Angiotensin is known to be a potent stimulator of vasopressin release. Some drugs that can stimulate or inhibit vasopressin release are given in Table 38.10.

Chemically, vasopressin is a polypeptide. The amino acid sequence of the hormone varies from animal to animal. Human antidiuretic hormone is **arginine vasopressin (AVP).**

Mechanism of action:Vasopressin acts on two receptors,V_1 (V_{1a} and V_{1b}) and V_2. Receptors V_1 are located in the vascular smooth muscle, the bladder and uterine smooth muscle, the platelets and the CNS. *Activation of* V_{1a}

Table 38.10: Drugs and vasopressin release

Stimulants	Inhibitors
Tricyclic anti-depressants	Alcohol
Nicotine	Phenytoin
Adrenaline	Chlorpromazine
Morphine(high doses)	Haloperidol
Barbiturates	Promethazine
Cyclophposphamide	Morphine(low dose)
Vincristine	Butorphanol
	Glucocorticoids

increases intracellular calcium and causes vasoconstriction, including that of the coronary vessels. Vasopressin acts directly on the cardiac myocytes which hypertrophy. It may also potentiate the synthesis of endothelin . In patients with CHF plasma vasopressin may rise early during the disease. ***V_{1a}*** *usually are not stimulated by physiological concentrations of the hormone.* ***V_{1b}*** *receptors are involved in vasopressin-stimulated secretion of ACTH.*

Receptors **V_2** are found predominantly in the renal collecting duct where they promote the reabsorption of water (**Antidiuretic action**). *Their effects are mediated by activation of adenylyl cyclase.* ***V_2*** *receptor activation* may also increase the Na^+ and Cl^- transport in the thick ascending limb.

Physiological and pharmacological actions: The predominant actions of vasopressin are

- ***Kidney***: Under the influence of vasopressin, the distal tubule and the collecting duct of the nephron become permeable to water, leading to water reabsorption and a reduction in the urine volume. In addition, activation of **V_{1a}** receptors reduces the renal medullary blood flow. Production of PGE_2 is stimulated. Absence of vasopressin causes diabetes insipidus.

The anti-diuretic response to vasopressin is enhanced by NSAID, chlorpropamide and carbamazepine; it is inhibited by lithium and demeclocycline.

- ***Cardiovascular system***: In large doses, AVP raises the BP by direct stimulation of the vascular smooth muscle. It also constricts the coronary and cerebral blood vessels. The hormone causes an initial tachycardia, probably secondary to coronary insufficiency and resultant hypotension, followed by bradycardia.
- ***Other smooth muscles***: Vasopressin stimulates the GI smooth muscle.
- *CNS*: AVP is believed to play a role as a neuromodulator/neurotransmitter.
- *Miscellaneous*:Stimulation of V_2 receptors increases the level of coagulation factor VII and von Villebrand factor.Vasopressin , stored in the platelets, plays a role in platelet aggregation.

Absorption, fate and excretion: It is given parenterally. When administered SC or IM, the drug remains in the body for a few hours; given IV, it is rapidly destroyed. However, vasopressin tannate in oil, administered SC or IM, produces an effect lasting for 24 to 48 hours.

Vasopressin is rapidly metabolized in the body, largely during passage through the liver and the kidney. Its plasma t½ is 20 minutes or less.

Adverse reactions: It may produce nausea, biliary colic and abdominal cramps due to increased peristaltic activity. Hypotension and shock are serious adverse effects probably due to coronary spasm.

Preparations and dosage:

(i) Vasopressin injection (Pitressin) 20 units per ml; dose 5-10 units every 4-6 hours SC or IM. It has a short duration of action.

(ii) Vasopressin tannate injection an oily suspension contains 5 pressor units per ml. Dose 0.5 to 1 ml. once in 24-72 hours. On standing, the drug settles down at the bottom of the ampoules as a yellow residue. The ampoule, therefore, should be warmed gently and shaken vigorously before administration.

(iii) Synthetic vasopressin analogue, DAVP (1-deamino-8-D-arginine-vasopressin, Desmopressin, Adiuretin), administered intranasally 5-10 mcg. bid, is a preparation with greater antidiuretic and decreased pressor activity. Its action lasts for 13-22 hours. It can also be given by SC or IM (Minirin, dose 1-4 mcg/ day) and orally (300-600 mcg/day as tablets).

(iv) Lysine-8-vasopressin (Syntopressin) is more stable and has activity of 50 units per 0.185 mg. (per ml). It is used intranasally by spray. Each squeeze delivers about 2 units. The dose is 1-4 squeezes 3-7 times a day.

Therapeutic uses:

I **Those related to vascular and smooth muscle (V1 receptor) actions:** These are treated with AVP.

- ***Postoperative ileus and abdominal distension.***
- ***Esophageal varices due to portal hypertension:*** **Vasopressin,** infused IV in the dose of 20 units within 30 minutes, produces a marked splanchnic vasoconstriction, reducing thereby the portal flow and venous pressure. It can also be given by continuous infusion. **Triglycyl lysine vasopressin** (Glypressin), an analogue, has practically no activity by itself on smooth muscle but *in vivo* it results in a slow release of active hormone. The effect, therefore, lasts for 10 hours after a single bolus injection as compared to the vasopressin which is active only for 30-40 minutes.
- ***Acute hemorrhagic gastritis.***
- ***Vasopressin IV has been found effective in the treatment of asystolic cardiac arrest. It may be given in a single dose of 40 IU, IM.***

II **Those related to antidiuretic action and release of blood coagulation factors (V_2 receptors).** These are treated with **desmopressin.**

- ***Diabetes insipidus:*** Desmopressin is the treatment of choice. It is administered intranasaly or by SC/IM injection. If desmopressin is not available, AVP may be used. As this is replacement therapy, it is lifelong in most cases. *It is effective in central but not in nephrogenic diabetes insipidus.*
- ***Nocturnal eneuresis:*** Desmopressin intranasally or orally (as tablet) at bedtime has been used effectively in short term treatment of this condition.
- ***Bleeding disorders***, Hemophilia A (factor VIII deficiency) and von Willebrand's disease (Chapter 34).

BENZOTHIADIAZINES: Surprisingly, benzothiadiazines are effective in controlling central as well as nephrogenic diabetes insipidus. The mechanism of action is not known. Various possibilities have been suggested; they probably act by causing a negative sodium balance and reducing the GFR. This leads to a decrease in volume and an increase in concentration of urine. A long acting drug such as polythiazide is usually preferred. Since symptomless hypokalemia is commonly associated with this therapy, a potassium sparing diuretic may be added to this regimen. In nephrogenic diabetes insipidus, where there is renal unresponsiveness to the action of vasopressin, thiazides are the most effective form of therapy.

In both idiopathic and nephrogenic diabetes insipidus, the beneficial effect of benzothiadiazines is reduced by liberal salt intake.

CHLORPROPAMIDE: This drug, used in the treatment of diabetes mellitus (Chapter 63), is effective in the treatment of diabetes insipidus. Interestingly the closely related compounds tolbutamide and glibenclamide are not effective. It probably acts by increasing the sensitivity of renal tubules to low and otherwise ineffective concentrations of vasopressin. Unlike thiazide diuretics, the response to chlorpropamide is not reduced by high sodium intake or steroid administration. *It is not useful in nephrogenic diabetes insipidus.* It is usually given in the dose of 500 mg. daily orally. If hypoglycemia supervenes the dose is reduced to 250 mg. daily.

Carbamazepine (400-600 mg./day) is effective in patients with partial diabetes insipidus. It probably acts by stimulating vasopressin release from the neurohypophysis. Action of carbamazepine and chlorpropamide is overcome by ethanol, which inhibits the release of ADH.

Vasopressin Receptor Antagonist

CONIVAPTAN: This is a combined vasopressin – V_1/V_2 receptor antagonist which causes decreased permeability of the renal collecting ducts to water, leading to excretion of free water (aquaresis). It is 99% protein bound and is metabolized in the liver. It has been used for short term treatment of euvolemic hyponatremia, usually caused by SIADH, hypothyroidism and adrennocortical insufficiency. In general, the drug is well tolerated but may cause headache, thirst, dry mouth hypokalemia, orthostatic hypotension, vomiting or diarrhoea in 5% of cases. It is not recommended during pregnancy.

Tolvaptan, another benzazepine derivative, has selective V_2 antagonistic action. It is effective orally and has been used to treat hyponatremia in patients with CHF, cirrhosis and SIADH, with encouraging results. Adverse effects reported are similar to those of conivaptan. It is under evaluation.

Drugs and Nephrotoxicity

Among the various body organs the kidney is particularly vulnerable to the toxic actions of drugs. Kidney has a rich blood supply and further, it can concentrate the drugs and their polar metabolites locally, thus exposing the renal tubules to very high concentrations of the drugs. Hence, in the presence of renal insufficiency drugs tend to accumulate.

Table 38.11: Drugs causing nephrotoxicity

Site of action	Drugs	Nature of Toxicity
Extra-renal	Tetracyclines, Corticosteroids. via increased protein breakdown.	Aggravation of azotaemia probably
Arteries and arterioles	Heavy metals e.g. Arsenic, Bismuth and Gold salts, Horse serum, Long acting sulfonamides, Iodides, Thiazides.	Vasculitis.
Glomeruli	Hydralazine, Long acting sulfonamides.	Vasculitis with glomerulopathy.
Convoluted tubules	Aminoglycoside antibiotics, e.g. Kanamycin, Gentamicin, Organic Mercurials, Colistin, Amphotericin B, Polymyxin B, Cephaloridine.	Necrosis of proximal and/or distal tubular epithelium.
Interstitium	Phenacetin, NSAID, Phenytoin, Sulfonamides	Interstitial nephritis with papillary necrosis. May cause acute renal failure or chronic nephropathy.
Collecting ducts	Acetazolamide, Sulfonamides, Antineo-plastic drugs.	Crystalluria, Calculi, Hyperuricaemia.
Ureters	Methysergide.	Obstruction due to retroperitoneal fibrosis.

Drugs can cause nephrotoxicity :

- ***Directly,*** e.g. NSAID, aminoglycosides, heavy metals.
- ***Indirectly,*** e.g., Vitamin D causing hypercalcemia leading to the formation of renal calculi; diuretics causing hypokalemia may cause renal tubular damage.
- ***By immunological mechanisms*** e.g., interstitial nephritis, vasculaitis, SLE.

Nephrotoxicity can be 'acute' leading to acute renal failure or may be 'chronic' and responsible for chronic renal disease. Drugs can damage the kidney at various sites from renal arteries to the ureters. Drugs can also cause the renal damage by crystal or calculi formation. From among the many compounds incriminated in producing such renal damage, only some of the better known nephrotoxic agents are included in Table 38.11. These drugs are discussed elsewhere.

Chronic nephropathy due to prolonged ingestion of analgesics has received considerable attention. Patients suffering from this syndrome may present with hematuria, renal colic, urinary infection and finally hypertension and renal failure. The lesions are reversible if the syndrome is detected early and the offending drug stopped. Although the blame is mainly levelled against phenacetin, all other NSAID can cause this syndrome (see Chapter 11).

Drug-induced nephrotic syndrome has been observed following therapeutic use of drugs like tolbutamide, probenecid, penicillamine, perchlorate and gold salts. It is characterised by marked proteinuria. Its mechanism is not known. Compounds like antiepileptic drugs, sulfonamides, phenylbutazone, tetracyclines, antihypertensive agents like hydralazine; and methyldopa can induce systemic lupus erythematosus (SLE) and affect the kidney. The damage may be reversible on discontinuation of the offending drug.

Apart from the therapeutic agents, **many chemicals** also cause nephrotoxicity. These include such compounds as aniline, carbon tetrachloride, phenol, ethylene glycol, phosphorus, arsenic and mercuric chloride.

In patients with impaired renal function it is necessary to reduce the doses of certain drugs to avoid toxicity. This is discussed with individual drugs elsewhere. In general, the srum creatinine is a useful rough guide to the severity of impairment of renal function. In mild failure, with a GFR of 25-50 ml/min., it is 1.8-2.8 mg%. With GFR of 10-25 ml/min., it is 2.9-7.9 mg% while in severe renal failure when the GFR is less than 10 ml/min. serum creatinine is 8 mg% or higher. Renal function deteriorates with age but this reduction, until marked, is not reflected in the serum creatinine level. *It should be noted that many apparently healthy elderly subjects also may have a GFR of less than 50 ml./min. and therefore, caution is needed in prescribing certain drugs in the elderly.*

Section X
Drugs Used in Disorders of the Gastrointestinal Tract

Appetite Stimulants, Digestants, Antiflatulents, Appetite Suppressants and Hypolipidemic Agents 39

Appetite, a desire to eat or drink, is a complex phenomenon influenced by several factors. The final outcome is achieved by the release of various hypothalamic peptides which are integrated with catecholaminergic, serotoninergic and opioid signaling pathways. Dopamine and 5-HT mediated processes in the CNS , and ghrelin, a gut-brain peptide, probably play an important role in appetite control.

Loss of appetite (anorexia) is a common complaint in clinical practice. Its etiology varies from prolonged, debilitating illnesses to purely psychological disturbances such as depression. It is common in patients with widespread cancer. It is imperative, therefore, to investigate thoroughly an individual complaining of anorexia for the underlying cause.

Temporary anorexia due to short illnesses usually needs no treatment. **Symptomatically**, appetite can often be improved by varying the diet and by use of such simple preparations as lemon pickles, bitters such as bitter orange peel and soups. The aromatic bitter appetite stimulants combine the property of bitterness with that of an aromatic volatile oil e.g. orange, ginger and cardamom. Use of costly **appetite stimulants** and 'tonics' for this purpose is unnecessary.

Alcohol: Alcohol (10%) in small quantities, given before a meal, can augment the gastric secretion both reflexly by stimulation of the taste buds and by a direct action.

It is a major constituent of popular 'tonics'. Various tonics dispensed in fancy bottles contain 10-15 per cent of alcohol. Repeated ingestion of alcohol, however, causes chronic gastritis and a diminution in appetite. The use of alcohol containing 'tonics' in children is to be condemned. Their prolonged use even in adults is to be discouraged.

Megestrol acetate and **glucocorticoids** are useful in increasing the appetite but not necessarily weight in patients with cancer-induced cachexia. **Insulin** augments gastric secretion by producing hypoglycemia; however, its use is irrational and hazardous. Similar claims have been advanced for **vitamin B_{12}** and **anabolic steroids** but whether appetite stimulation is a primary action of these compounds or secondary to their metabolic effects remains to be established. The 5-HT antagonist **cyproheptadine**, has also some appetite stimulating property; however, used in large doses, it inhibits the release of ACTH and depresses the circulating cortisol level (Chapter 23). *Thus there is no safe and reliable appetite stimulant.*

Anorexia nervosa is a chronic disorder characterised by loss of appetite and self induced weight loss, accompanied by psychological and physiological alterations such as amenorrhoea. Hypothalamic abnormalities are believed to play a role in its pathogenesis. Currently, no pharmacological agent of proven value is available for its treatment. Olanzapine, an atypical antipsychotic acting on multiple receptors, and reboxitine, an antidepressant, have been tried as adjuncts.

Digestants

The digestants are the drugs that are claimed to aid digestion in the gastrointestinal tract. The commonly used digestants are:

PEPSIN: This is a proteolytic enzyme, obtained from the glandular layer of the fresh stomach of the hog. It is administered orally in the dose of 0.5-1 g. It is of doubtful value except perhaps in patients with gastric achylia, a condition characterized by defective acid and pepsin secretion. Gastric achylia is often encountered in patients with carcinoma of the stomach and pernicious anemia.

Another enzyme, **papain**, obtained from vegetable source (papaya), also has proteolytic properties.

RENNIN: This is a partially purified milk-curdling enzyme, obtained from the glandular layer of calf stomach. It is used in the preparation of cheese.

PANCREATIN (Creon) : This contains the enzymes amylase, trypsin and lipase and is obtained from hog or ox pancreas. It has been employed as a replacement therapy in chronic pancreatitis, obstruction caused by the cancer of the head of pancreas, cystic fibrosis, and after total gastrectomy and pancreatectomy. It is not useful in GI disorders unrelated to pancreatic enzyme insufficiency. It is administered orally in enteric coated capsules, to prevent its gastric inactivation. However, this preparation contains very small amounts of enzymatic activity per tablet or capsule, compared to quantities necessary for efficient digestion. Hence, even with large doses, total correction of steatorrhoea may not occur. It may be used only as an adjunct to reduction in dietary fat intake. Prolonged use of pancreatin may cause fibrosing colonopathy.

BILE AND BILE ACIDS: Normally, about 1000 ml. of bile is secreted by the liver per day. It contains bile acids, cholesterol and bilirubin. Bile acids are important in emulsifying the fats in the intestine. Cholecystokinin (CCK), the polypeptide secreted by the duodenal mucosa, is the main stimulant to biliary secretion; it is not available for therapeutic use. Bile salts and bile acids increase the flow as well as the concentration of bile and are termed **choleretics.**

The bile salt preparations have been employed to facilitate surgical drainage, as replacement therapy in biliary fistulae, and for their choleretic effect in conditions like liver cirrhosis and functional hepatic insufficiency. Their usefulness, however, is doubtful.

The available preparations include:

(i) Dehydrocholic acid available as 250 mg. tablet. Dose: 500 mg. thrice daily, and

(ii) Sodium dehydrocholate injection, available as 20 per cent solution in 3 and 10 ml. ampoules. Dose: 3 to 5 ml. IV.

CHENODEOXYCHOLIC ACID (CDCA, Chenodiol, Chenofalk): This normal constituent of bile reduces biliary cholesterol concentration by depressing hepatic cholesterol secretion. Further, it increases the secretion of bile acids in some patients. *It dissolves radiolucent gallstones but is ineffective with the radioopaque ones.* The results are poor in the presence of a nonfunctioning gall bladder, in very obese persons, in persons with high dietary cholesterol intake and in those receiving clofibrate or octeotride. It has to be administered over a long period, 3-24 months, depending on the size of stone. The drug causes diarrhoea, increase in the LDL cholesterol and rarely hepatotoxicity. It has been replaced by ursodeoxycholic acid.

URSODEOXYCHOLIC ACID (Ursodiol, Udiliv) an analogue of CDCA is formed from chenodiol by colonic bacteria. It has similar actions but unlike chenodiol, it does not increase the secretion of bile acids into bile. Given orally, it is absorbed rapidly and taken up by the liver. It is better tolerated than chenodiol.

Ursodiol, given orally in the dose of 13-15 mg/kg/day, in divided doses, has been reported to cause clinical, biochemical and histological improvement in primary biliary cirrhosis. It acts by modifying the composition of bile acids in the liver, thereby hindering the progression of the pathological process. It also lowers the serum cholesterol levels in these patients. It is also used in the treatment of Non-Alcoholic-Steato-Hepatitis (NASH); however, its therapeutic usefulness needs confirmation.

Gallstones are common, and although they are blamed for many digestive symptoms they are probably innocent in most cases. Asymptomatic gallstones are often an incidental finding on ultrasonography. In most cases, they need little treatment. True symptoms of gallstone disease include acute cholecystitis, biliary colic, jaundice and acute pancreatitis. When they are proved to be the cause of severe symptoms, cholecystectomy is the best treatment. However, this may not guarantee improvement in all digestive symptoms of the patient. Bile acid therapy may be considered as another option for radiolucent cholesterol stones, 5 mm or less in diameter. **Ursodeoxycholic acid**, 750 mg/day for upto 2 years, may be used. This therapy, however, is unsuitable in patients with (1) non-cholesterol stones; (2) non-functioning gall bladder; or (3) severe recurrent symptoms. *Gallstones in the bile duct are more serious and need surgical treatment.*

Antiflatulents and Carminatives

These are the drugs used to expel gas from the stomach or the intestines in the treatment of flatulence and colics. Most of these drugs are aromatic volatile oils. They act by mild stimulation thereby increasing the GI motility and causing relaxation of sphincters. They produce a feeling of warmth in the stomach. They do not affect the gastric acid secretion significantly. Indian food contains enough carminatives in the form of various spices and condiments. The common ones are cardamom seeds, ginger, fennel seeds, asafoetida, cinnamon bark, cloves, coriander and anise. Along with sodium bicarbonate, they form important constituents of various 'gripe water' mixtures commonly used in infants to reduce griping. Usually, these volatile oils may be used in the form of tinctures Cardamom and Zingiber.

Although carminatives may afford some quick symptomatic relief and audible satisfaction, *it must be remembered that flatulent dyspepsia may be associated with disorders such as peptic ulcer, biliary tract disease, the irritable bowel syndrome, alimentary tumours and even IHD.*

DIMETHYLPOLYSILOXANE (Dimol): This silicone derivative has been advocated in symptomatic treatment of postprandial and postoperative flatulence and abdominal distension. It is believed to act as a defoaming agent, allowing the gas to escape from the GI tract, providing comfort to the patient with 'gases.' However, evidence to support these claims is not convincing. It eliminates mucus-embeded bubbles that interfere with visualization during gastroscopy, but is not particularly effective in reducing gas that may interfere with radiologic or ultrasound examination of the abdomen. It is available as 40 mg. tablets.

Anorexiants and Treatment of Obesity

Obesity is often simply defined as "a condition of abnormal or excessive accumulation of adipose tissue, to the extent that health may be impaired." People with abdominal fat distribution or **android** obesity are at greater risk to its consequences than those with the less serious **gynoid** fat distribution where fat is more evenly and peripherally distributed around the body.

Sedentary lifestyle of modern living, combined with the abundant availabililty of tempting, high fat (junk) foods has caused almost an epidemic of obesity in the affluent nations. The current estimate indicates that the number of 'overweight' individuals in the world is almost the same as that of 'underweight' ones. However, not everyone who partakes of such foods becomes obese. *The tendency to become obese is definitely inherited.* The mortality rises exponentially with increasing bodyweight and the incidence of heart disease, sleep apnoea, osteoarthritis and bowel cancer is higher in the obese than in the non-obese.

Regulation of energy balance : Obesity is a disorder of energy balance. Hypothalamus is a major centre that regulates food consumption by modulating hunger and satiety. It integrates neural, hormonal and nutrient messages from elsewhere and sends signals to the higher centres, leading to the feeling of hunger or satiety. Hypothalamus also controls the energy expenditure via the adrenergic nervous system and the pituitary hormones.

The central control of the bodyweight is a complex phenomenon regulated by multiple brain nuclei and many neurotransmitters. Some of the neurotransmitters known to control energy balance and body weight are listed in Table 39.1. Of these, neuropeptide Y is the most potent appetite stimulant and is abundantly present in the hypothalamus. It also suppresses sympathetic activity and thus reduces energy expenditure.

Recently, **ghrelin**, a 28 amino acid, gut-brain peptide which is a potent inducer of growth hormone release has been shown to have powerful appetite stimulating (orexigenic) properties. It is produced mainly by neuroendocrine cells in the gastric fundus and acts on the hypothalamus. Given in human volunteers, it stimulates appetite, induces hunger and increases food consumption.

Leptin is a peptide hormone synthesized in the fat cells; it acts on the hypothalamus to signal adequacy of body fat stores, suppress food intake and increase the calorie expenditure through inhibition of neuropeptide Y. Plasma leptin concentration is high in the obese persons and falls with weight reduction, which probably indicates resistance to the central effects of leptin in obese subjects.

Leptin acts as a signal from the adipose tissue to the CNS that the body is ready/ mature enough for reproductive functions such as entering into puberty in adolescents, and fertility in adults. It is not a trigger but a permissive factor for LHRH release in both the situations. Leptin has been used successfully in overcoming amenorrhoea in females with anorexia nervosa and those participating in vigorous sports.

Table 39.1: Neuropeptides affecting energy balance

- ***Increase food intake :***
  Noradrenaline, GHRH
  Neuropeptide Y, Ghrelin, Opioids,
  Endogenous cannobinoids
- ***Inhibit food intake :***
  5-HT, Dopamine
  Cholecystokinin (CCK), CRH
  Neurotensin, Bombesin and
  Glucagon-like peptide, α MSH

Normally, body weight is tightly regulated and a small excess of food consumption over burning of calories is all that is required to cause weight gain. Daily excess of 100 Kcal (a small chocolate bar or one chapati) would result in 4-5 kg weight gain in one year! Even modest weight loss of 10% improves physical performance and glucose tolerance. What is most important, however, is maintenance of the reduced weight for long term benefit.

Clinically, overweight and obesity are most simply assessed in terms of **Body Mass Index** (BMI = Body weight in Kg/ Height in meter^2). The normal value in adults is 18.5 to 24.9; overweight is BMI of 25 to 29.9; and obesity is 30 or higher. BMI of 35 or more means severe obesity. With the new Asian criteria, obesity is diagnosed with a BMI of over 23. *The perils of* *obesity, diabetes, hypertension and hyperlipidemia, are known to increase from a BMI of 23.*

Alternatively, obesity is diagnosed even with normal BMI if the waist circumference exceeds 102 cm in men and 88 cm in women in the western countries; for Asians, the corresponding figures are 90 cm and 80 cm, respectively.

Many of the co-morbidities of obesity present themselves in the form of the so-called **metabolic syndrome.** The latter is related to an excess of intra-abdominal rather than subcutaneous fat. (Chapter 63).

Many obese individuals show psychological disturbances and a compulsive desire to eat, though such individuals may not derive satisfaction from the act of eating.

Treatment of obesity is essentially medical. Surgical treatment (on the GI tract) may be useful only in severe, resistant cases. The general principles of treatment are outlined in Table 39.2. In an obese individual, if an organic cause such as an endocrine disease is present, it should be treated. Commonly, obesity is due to excessive eating and lack of adequate exercise and not due to 'glands'. The patient must be made to appreciate this at the beginning of the treatment and explained that *diet is the mainstay of the treatment of obesity;* he/she must be adequately motivated by the concept of 'positive health'. It must also be emphasized that dietary treatment of obesity consists of a lifelong reorientation of his eating habits (and often those of his family) and not merely of a 'course' of dieting. Those who look upon dieting as a course of treatment are bound to regain the lost weight.

Table 39.2: Principles of treatment of obesity

- Nutritionally adequate, low calorie diet, containing at least 1 gm of protein/kg of desirable body weight.
- Fat intake below 25% of total calories prescribed.
- Liberal use of fibre-containing foods.
- Regular exercise.
- Behavioural therapy for change in life-style.
- Restriction of alcohol.
- Anorectic drugs – as adjunctive therapy.

There are many diets for obesity. It has, however, been convincingly shown that *nothing about the diet matters except its calorie content.* Hence, the best diet is one which is low in calorie content (1000-1500 per day), contains all the essential nutrients, provides a variety and is simple for the patient to follow for prolonged periods. Such drastic one-step calorie reduction may not be tolerated by patients; a better plan is to reduce the daily calorie intake progressively in steps of 500 calories. The diet should also conform to the patient's pocket.

Diet rich in fruits, vegetables and whole grain, especially pulses, is to be preferred. Proprietary slimming foods are expensive and ineffective, though many patients believe that they can lose weight by consuming them in addition to their normal diet. Prolonged fasting is a drastic measure to be used rarely, only in resistant cases and that too under close medical supervision. The age-old Indian religious custom of fasting on certain days of the month has, however, much to recommend it, as it can atone for the minor sins of the palate indulged in at other times and thus, help to keep good health. If the patient realises the importance of dieting and exercise and if he has the necessary will, then the treatment of obesity is not that difficult and can easily be carried out at home without the help of 'obesity clinics', and fashionable 'health clubs'.

The results of therapy are likely to be more satisfactory in **hypertrophic** obesity (enlarged, distended fat cells, with usual onset in adult life) than in the **hyperplastic** variety (more numerous fat cells, with usual onset in childhood).

The patient should be told at the onset of therapy that an average weekly loss of 0.5 kg. is adequate and would result in annual loss of about 25 kg.

Sometimes, even with the best of motivation, drastic reduction in the customary food intake is initially a trying experience. In such cases, **appetite suppressants (anorexiants)** may help the patient to adjust to the prescribed diet. However, *these drugs only supplement and are not a substitute for the dietary restrictions.*

The drugs used in the treatment of obesity are classified as:

I **Centrally acting, appetite suppressants (Anorexiants)**

- ***Adrenergic agents*** e.g. Amphetamine, Mephenteramine, Benzphenteran, Mazindol.
- ***5-HT agonists*** e.g. Fenfluramine, Dexfenfluramine, Fluoxetine.
- ***Agents acting on both adrenergic and 5-HT systems*** e.g. Sibutramine
- ***Cannabinoid receptor antagonists*** *e. g.* Rimonabant.

II **Drugs acting in the GI tract**

- ***Bulk anorexiants*** e.g. Dietary fibre, Methylcellulose, Guar gum.
- ***Non-absorbable fat substitutes*** e.g. Olestra
- ***Lipase inhibitors*** e.g. Orlistat

III **Miscellaneous** e.g. Biguanides

I **Anorexiants :**

Amphetamine and related compounds: Their anorexiant effect appears to be related to the central release of DA and NA from the adrenergic cells. They also inhibit the reuptake of NA and DA. Their major drawback is the development of tolerance to the anorexiant effect and drug dependence. Withdrawal after their prolonged medication may cause drowsiness, sleep, tremors, fatigue and muscular weakness. Hence, *amphetamine and dexamphetamine (dexedrine) are no more recommended in the treatment of obesity* (Chapter 17). **Methylamphetamine is a highly addictive drug and is extensively used as a drug of abuse.**

Other compounds : Examples are phenteramine, phendimetrazine, benzamphetamine, mazindol and diethylpropion. Of these, the first three are suspected to produce dependence and could be abused. **Mazindol** is chemically unrelated to amphetamine, and probably acts through dopaminergic mediators. *None of these drugs is safe for long term use.*

SIBUTRAMINE (Splenfig, Reductil): This drug. acting cenrally, inhibits the neuronal reuptake of NA and 5-HT and increases satiety. Given in the single daily dose of 10-15 mg orally, it causes 4-5% reduction of weight in a year. The drug undergoes extensive first pass metabolism, as well as hepatic metabolism by CYP3A4 to active metabolites. It is mainly excreted (77%) in the urine. The main ADR are dry mouth, constipation, insomnia, nausea, tachycardia, a slight rise in BP and rarely cardiac arrhythmias. Hepatic, microsomal, enzyme inhibitors increase its toxicity. Its use is contraindicated during and within two weeks of MAO inhibitors, in patients with uncontrolled hypertension, and in those with history of heart disease, stroke, liver failure, and obesity of endocrine origin and that due to psychiatric disorders.

Fenfluramine (Ponderax): This drug, once used extensively, acts by increasing the brain synaptic 5-HT by accelerating its release and reducing its re-uptake. However, it was found to be toxic and caused cardiac valvular injury and primary pulmonary hypertension. It has been withdrawn from the market.

It took over 30 years to detect the serious adverse reaction to fenfluramine. This emphasises the vital importance of continued and vigilant post-marketing adverse drug reaction surveillance. Similar long term toxicity is likely to occur during the use of other drugs acting as 5-HT agonists.

Fluoxetine : This 5-HT reuptake inhibitor antidepressant, in the dose of 60 mg/day, is associated with weight loss; but its long term use should be avoided in view of the experience with fenfluramine. (Chapter 13).

Rimonabant (Amipiza): This drug is a central neurokinin-3 and selective, CB1 receptor antagonist (Chapter 20). Peripherally, it inhibits lipogenesis, enhances thermogensis, and promotes adiponectin production as well as vagally mediated CCK-induced satiety. Thus, it decreases food intake and causes weight loss. It also causes elevation of HDL cholesterol and improvement in HbA_{1c}. It prevents weight gain in persons trying to quit smoking. It is highly (99%) protein- bound and is metabolized by hepatic CYP3A4. The metabolites are largely excreted in bile and some in feces. It has a long duration of action. It is generally well tolerated but may cause dizziness, nausea, insomnia and diarrhea. *Its major drawback is neuropsychiatric disturbances, mainly depression in 6-7% of the patients.* Hence it has not been approved for the treatment of obesity.

Table 39.3: Limitations of centrally acting anorexiants

- Short term efficacy.
- Relapse of weight gain.
- Possible toxicity during long term therapy;
- Weight cycling as a result of drug holiday, leading to adverse outcomes such as coronary heart disease; and
- Inability to prevent obesity-related illnesses and to prolong life.

Table 39.3 summarises the limitations of the centrally acting anorexiants. As obesity is a chronic disease and as relapse is common after cessation of drug therapy, prolonged, and even lifelong, drug therapy may be desirable. However, none of the currently available drugs is safe enough for prolonged use. Hence, irrespective of the drug used, if significant weight loss does not occur within 4-6 months of therapy, the durg is discontinued. *For the same reason, drugs should not be used simply for cosmetic weight control.* Currently, there is no evidence to suggest that combined drug therapy is any better than drug monotherapy.

II Drugs acting in the GI tract :

Bulk anorexiants: **Methylcellulose,** a non-digestible polysaccharide, when ingested, swells and adds to the bulk in the diet. Though used as an appetite satiator, it is no more effective than the high residue low caloric diet for the obvious reason that an obese person is interested in eating good food and not something that would merely distend the stomach. It forms an important, cheap constituent of many 'costly', commercial preparations advertised for the treatment of obesity. **Guar gum** (Carbotard), **karaya gum** (Sterculia gum, Kanormal) and **glucomannan** (Dietmann) are the other bulking agents.

Digestion inhibitors :

OLESTRA : This is a mixture of sucrose-fatty-acid esters that is neither digested nor absorbed from the GI tract. When used as a component of diet, it increases the bowel function and stool bulk. It is recommended as a fat substitute in cooking. Long term effects on the health are yet not fully known. It is expensive.

ORLISTAT : Orlistat (Tetrahydrolipostatin, Xenical)) acts by inhibiting pancreatic and other lipases. It is not absorbed and the effects are confined to the GI tract, where it prevents the lipase-catalysed breakdown and subsequent absorption of about 1/3 of the dietary fat. The additional benefit is a modest reduction in the plasma levels of total cholesterol and LDL cholesterol but not of plasma triglycerides. It is almost completely excreted unchanged in feces. The common adverse effects are abdominal pain, increased defecation of oily/fatty stools with anal leaking, which can be inconvenient and socially embarrassing. It should be avoided in chronic diarrhea. It is used in the dose of 120 mg 2-3 times daily, with meals, for a maximum of two years.

III **Miscellaneous** : The antidiabetic, **metformin** induces weight loss in some nondiabetic obese individuals (Chapter 63).

Table 39.4: Some drugs causing anorexia

- Aminophylline
- Amphetamines and related drugs
- Antimicrobials : Metronidazole, Fluoroquinolones, Erythromycin, Nitrofurantoin, Tetracycline
- Antimalarials
- Metformin
- Digitalis
- Levodopa

None of the currently available drugs satisfies all requirements viz. efficacy, safety and affordability. *Therefore, the treatment of obesity mainly depends on permanent lifestyle modifications such as change in eating habits and regular physical exercise, supported by behavioral therapy.* Experts recommend that drugs may be considered in adults with a BMI of over 27 in the presence of an obesity-related complication,and in those with a BMI of over 30 even in the absence of such a complication. For persons with a BMI of over 40, bariatric surgery may be considered.

In practice, many drugs may cause some degree of anorexia as their side effect. Common among these are listed in Table 39.4.

Table 39.5 lists some of the commonly used drugs which may cause weight gain as a side effect.

Table 39.5: Drugs which may cause weight gain

- **Antipsychotics**, especially Olanzapine
- **Antidepressants:** tricyclics, SSRI, MAOI, Mirtazapine
- **Hormones:** Glucocorticoids, Insulin Progestogens, Oral contraceptives and Danazol
- **Beta blockers**
- **Oral hypoglycemic agents:** Sulfonylureas, Glitazones
- **Anticonvulsants:** Phenytoin, Sodium valproate
- **Antihistaminics**, especially the first generation agents
- **Pizotifen**

Atherosclerosis and Hyperlipidemia

Atherosclerosis, a disease which affects large and medium sized arteries, is now a leading cause of death in many developed countries. The lesion atherosclerotic is a localised plaque in the intima and is composed of cholesterol esters, proliferation of smooth muscle, deposition of fibrous proteins (predominantly collagen) and calcification. Such plaques:

- ***Narrow the arterial lumen causing distal ischemia.***
- ***Ulcerate into the arterial lumen, with thrombosis of the artery and distal embolization***; or,
- ***Weaken the arterial wall, leading to formation of aneurysms.***

The coronary and the cerebral circulations are common sites of atherosclerosis.

The cause of atherosclerosis is not known although several factors have been blamed. Experimental and epidemiological evidence suggests a relationship between atherosclerosis and elevated levels of plasma lipids (cholesterol and triglycerides). Although there is no diagnostic abnormal pattern of the plasma lipids in atherosclerotic subjects, an increase in plasma LDL cholesterol and triglycerides has been observed in such patients. The risk of ischemic heart disease (IHD) in hypercholesterolaemic subjects is about thrice that in those with normal plasma cholesterol. Hence, a reduction of plasma lipids by either dietetic restriction or drugs may prevent the development/progression of atherosclerosis. *Studies have shown that a reduction in elevated plasma cholesterol does in fact reduce the risk of MI.*

Being water insoluble, the plasma lipids are transported in several classes of lipoproteins.

Table 39.6: Serum lipid levels (mg/dl) and the risk of IHD*

Lipid	Desirable level (Low risk)	Borderline level (Moderate risk)	Abnormal level (High risk)
Total cholesterol	< 200	200-240	> 240
LDL cholesterol	< 130	130-160	>160
HDL cholesterol	> 60	40-60	< 40
Triglycerides	< 200	200-400	> 400

* The risk increases further with other risk factors such as smoking, diabetes and hypertension.

These classes are:

- ***Chylomicrons***.
- ***Chylomicron remnants***.
- ***Very low density lipoproteins (VLDL)***.
- ***Intermediate density lipoproteins (IDL)***.
- ***Low density lipoproteins (LDL)***.
- ***High density lipoproteins (HDL)***; and
- ***Lipoprotein (a)***.

The lipoproteins contain a non-polar core of triglycerides and cholesterol esters, surrounded by a polar coat made up of phospholipids, unesterified cholesterol and apoproteins. The lipid in the chylomicrons and VLDL is mostly TG whereas that in the LDL is mostly cholesterol. *High serum LDL and VLDL levels are considered as atherogenic while high HDL* (over 60 mg/dl) *has a protective effect.* Asians commonly have low HDL levels (<35 mg/dl), probably because of high carbohydrate diet.

The normal fasting plasma is clear and contains about 700 mg. of total lipids, comprising TG, cholesterol and phospholipids. About 70 per cent of cholesterol is in ester form. The plasma shows opalescence due to chylomicrons after ingestion of a fatty meal. This lipemia is rapidly cleared by a heparin-activated lipoprotein lipase.

Table 39.6 shows the risk of IHD associated with different levels of serum lipids. Recent work has incriminated folic acid deficiency leading to elevated plasma levels of homocysteine, and chronic infection with *Chlamydia pneumoniae* in the pathogenesis of atherosclerosis.

Hyperlipoproteinemias which are incriminated in the pathogenesis of atherosclerosis are divided into five Fredrickson's types (I to V) depending on the class of lipoprotein(s) elevated (Table 39.7). In practice, determination of the total triglycerides (TG), total cholesterol and HDL cholesterol levels also allows to (a) diagnose hyperlipidemia, and (b) to type the hyperlipoproteinemia. The commonest hyperlipidemias are secondary to dietary excess, uncontrolled diabetes mellitus, hypothyroidism, alcoholism, chronic renal failure and drugs such as etretinate, glucocorticoids used for prolonged periods and protease inhibitors. Therefore, every patient with hyperlipidemia (defined as elevation of cholesterol and/or TG) should be investigated for these factors.

The much rarer primary hyperlipoproteinemias are either (a) **monogenic** (strictly hereditary); the sufferer may be heterozygous for the defect with moderate elevation of plasma lipids, or homozygous with marked elevation; or (b) **polygenic** (like hypertension) where the heredity forms a background against which environmental factors (diet, alcohol etc.) produce hyperlipidemia.

Type I hyperlipoproteinemia is due to a defect in lipoprotein lipase and is induced by dietary fat. Type II is hereditary (see above). Type III is due to hereditary dysbetalipoproteinemia. Types IV and V are carbohydrate induced and are associated with insulin resistance as well.

Table 39.7: Fredrickson's classification of hyperlipoproteinemias

Phenotype	I	II a	II b	III	IV	V
Lipoprotein elevated	Chylo	LDL	LDL & VLDL	IDL	VLDL	VLDL & Chylo.
Total cholsterol mg%	N to slightly↑	300 - 600	300 - 600	300 - 600	N to slightly↑	250-500
LDL cholesterol	N	↑	↑	↑	N	N
Triglycerides mg%	Usually >2000	N	<400	200-1000	500-1500	500-1500
Relative frequency %	<1	10	40	<1	45	5
Atherogenicity	None	+++	+++	+++*	++	±

Chylo = Chylomicrons * = Especially for peripheral vascular disease

Elevation of plasma LDL cholesterol, especially when combined with reduced HDL, is associated with increased risk of atherosclerotic arterial disease. Extreme elevation of plasma TG can lead to pancreatitis.

Management : Stress reduction, weight reduction, modification of diet, abstinence from alcohol and smoking and treatment of the causative disease, if any, such as hypothyroidism and diabetes mellitus, are more important than lipid-lowering drugs. The cornerstone of the current therapy is **improvement in the lifestyle** for the primary and secondary prevention of coronary heart disease. It has been claimed that existing coronary artery disease can be reversed by appropriate non-surgical and even non-pharmacological regimens such that of Dean Ornish. The non-pharmacological treatment comprises :

- ***Dietary modification.***
- ***Increased physical activity.***
- ***Elimination of associated risk factors,*** e.g. smoking.

Dietary modification implies:

- ***Decreasing the consumption of foods rich in total and saturated fats and cholesterol*** e.g. high-fat meats, butter, eggs and whole milk; and
- ***Increasing the consumption of poultry, low fat fish and skimmed milk, together with large helpings of vegetables and fruits.*** In fact, the traditional Indian vegetarian diet has much to recommend in this respect.

The principles of dietary modification for treating hyperlipidemia are outlined in Table 39.8.

Basically, a single type of dietary modification is appropriate for the prevention and treatment of all types of hyperlipidemia, except primary chylomicronemia (Type I). In this last condition, the dietary fat needs to be reduced to the lowest possible level (10% of the total daily calories), and medium chain triglycerides substituted for other varieties in the diet. In all other varieties, the diet recommendation is as follows:

- ***Reduce the body weight to the ideal level.***
- ***Decrease the consumption of total fats to 15-20% of the daily caloric intake.*** Only one third of these fat calories should be supplied by saturated fats (fats of animal origin and coconut oil), one third by mono-unsaturated fats (olive oil, mustard oil, til oil and groundnut oil), and the rest one third by polyunsaturated fats (sunflower, corn and safflower oils).

Saturated fatty acids (SFA) are straight

Table 39.8: Principles of diet therapy in hyperlipoproteinemia

- Restriction of fat calories to less than 20% of total calories.
- Saturated, monounsaturated and polyunsaturated fats should form 1/3rd each of the total dietary fat.
- Restriction of cholesterol consumption to < 300 mg/day; not more than 4 eggs a week; minimize milk and milk products.
- Increased consumption of vegetables, fresh fruit, cereals, nuts especially walnuts and almonds (in moderation) and whole grain products.
- Increased consumption of fish, where possible/permitted.
- Drastic reduction in alcohol consumption.

The above principles may need to be modified in the case of children, pregnant women and old people.

chained and vary in the chain length. Uansaturated fatty acids (UFA), on the other hand, also vary in the number and the position of their double bonds. In natural products, the double bonds are in *cis* form; while in the case of commercial products, they are converted into *trans* form (TFA) following partial hydrogenation. These *trans* forms are more stable and have higher melting points; further, though unsaturated, they decrease HDL cholesterol and increase LDL cholesterol, triglycerides and lipoproteins. *Trans* fatty acids can also cause endothelial dysfunction, promote abdominal fat accumulation, and insulin resistance in animals. Further, their consumption is associated with increased risk of IHD in humans. Deep-fried and bakery food products are the major dietary sources of TFA and should be avoided. In fact, some countries have made it mandatory to keep the TFA content of all commercial food products to less than 2% of the total fat present.

Excessive use of polyunsaturated fats in diet is also no longer recommended as they are known to lower the protective HDL cholesterol levels; further, they are susceptible to hydroperoxidation, thus leading to the generation of the tissue damaging free radicals in the body. Use of hydrogenated fats and prolonged heating of fats should be avoided as these practices have deleterious effects similar to those of saturated fats.

With the reduction in the total fat content of the diet, carbohydrates become a major source of calories. Provided the excessive use of simple sugars (not to exceed 10% of the total daily calories) is avoided, the fear of hypertriglyceridemia with liberal carbohydrate consumption (65-70% of the daily calorie intake) is unfounded. Use of complex carbohydrates such as starchy foods (cereals, beans, pulses) should be encouraged.

Traditional approaches to prophylaxis of atherosclerosis have focused on one aspect of its pathogenesis viz. platelet function or blood lipids. Coastal Eskimos who eat a traditional diet of fish and seals have a low incidence of cardiovascular diseases, chronic inflammatory diseases such as psoriasis, and asthma. This is believed to be due to consumption of fatty fish rich in the two **omega-3-fatty acids**, icosapentaenoic acid and docosahexaenoic acid, as against omega-6 fatty acids (linoleic acid), present in vegetable oils, which is converted to arachidonic acid (Chapter 24). Studies indicate that the administration of omega-3-polyunsaturated fatty acids in the form of salmon or cod liver oil results in reduction in platelet responsiveness, lowering of blood lipids and improvement of blood flow. Long term intake of cod liver oil promotes the formation of the PGI_2. Further, exogenous eicosapentaenoic acid dose-dependently suppresses formation of leukotriene- B_4. Omega-3-fatty-acid-rich fish oil reduces the blood TG levels; it has little effect on cholesterol levels. Omega-3-fatty acids cannot be synthesized in humans and deficiency syndromes have been described. These fatty acids may play a role in the prophylaxis of atherosclerosis (see Chapter 24).

Drug therapy is indicated in those:

- ***In whom the above dietary measures are not successful.***
- ***Who find the dietary restrictions irksome;*** and
- ***Who are at risk of pancreatitis*** because of very high levels (1000 mg%) of TG.

Drug therapy should be started with the understanding that it will have to be continued **life-long.** The drugs do not cure the basic disorder of lipoprotein metabolism but symptomatically control only one aspect of the disease process. However, *used judiciously drugs are capable of retarding the atherosclerotic process and prolonging life.*

Antihyperlipidemic Drugs

These drugs act predominantly on:

- ***Elevated cholesterol,*** e.g., HMG-CoA reductase inhibitors (Statins), Cholestyramine resin, Ezetimibe, Fibre;
- ***Elevated triglycerides,*** e.g., Fibric acid derivatives (fibrates), Fish oil or,
- ***Both,*** e.g., Nicotinic acid.

Antihyperlipidemic drugs are most beneficial to those at greatest risk, including those with symptomatic atherosclerotic disease such as angina and many cardiovascular risk factors, as well as to those with the high plasma cholesterol levels.

STATINS (HMG-CoA-reductase inhibitors): Drugs belonging to this class are structural analogues of HMG-CoA. They are listed in Table 39.9.

Mechanism of action: Normally, about 70-75% of plasma LDL is removed by hepatocytes, by receptor-mediated endocytosis. Cholesterol esters from LDL molecules are hydrolysed in the liver to free cholesterol. The liver also produces cholesterol by *de novo* synthesis by a pathway involving formation of mevalonic acid by the enzyme hydroxymethylglutaryl co-enzyme A-reductase (HMG-CoA reductase); statins inhibit this rate-limiting enzyme. The resulting decrease in hepatic cholesterol synthesis leads to increased synthesis of high affinity LDL receptors on the surface of liver cells and increased clearance (uptake) of cholesterol-rich plasma LDL. This causes reduction in plasma LDL cholesterol (Fig. 39.1). The hypolipidemic effect is dose dependent and is observed in 10 days.

Table 39.9 : Doses of commonly used statins

Drug	Starting / Max. dose (mg/day)
Lovastatin	10 / 80
Pravastatin	20 / 40
Simvastatin	10 / 80
Fluvastatin	10 / 80
Atorvastatin	10 / 80
Cerivastatin	0.4 / 0.8
Rosuvastatin	10 / 40

Atorvastatin may be given at any time of the day; pravastatin and fluvastatin at bedtime; others with evening meal.

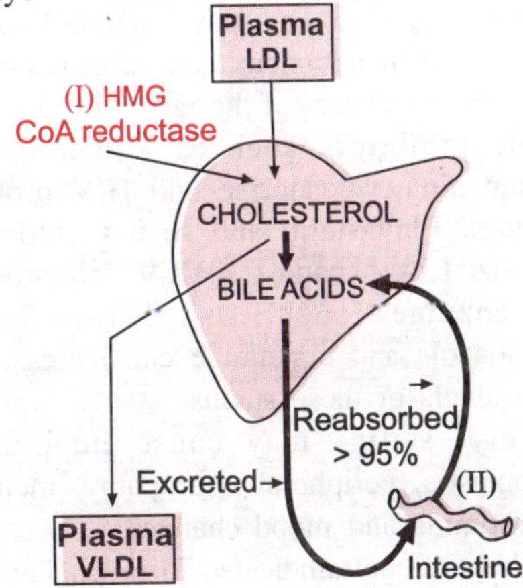

(I) Site of action of statins
(II) Site of action of resins and ezetimibe

Fig. 39.1 : Hepatic regulation of synthesis of cholesterol and bile acids

Simvostatin and atorvastatin, in addition, raise HDL level in some patients and lower the triglyceride levels.

Absorption, fate and excretion : Given orally, the absorption of all the statins (except fluvastatin) varies between 40% and 90%. Fluvastatin is absorbed almost completely. Lovastatin and simvastatin are prodrugs which are hydrolysed in the GI tract to the active metabolites. Atorvastatin, fluvastatin and rosuvastatin are fluorinated compounds that are active as such. All undergo first-pass metabolism and most of the dose is excreted in the bile; only about 5-20% is excreted in the urine.

Adverse reactions: Lovastatin and other statins may cause reversible rise in hepatic aminotransferase levels. Small rise in the plasma creatine kinase level is not uncommon. Rarely, it may be marked, and accompanied by muscular pains (myositis) and even myopathy. Rhabdomyolysis is still rarer. Combination of a statin with a fibric acid derivative, nicotinic acid or cyclosporine has potentiating effect on the rise in plasma CPK level. These effects are dose-dependent. Doses used do not seem to induce deficiency of other important steroids derived from cholesterol.

Lovastatin, simvastatin and atorvastatin undergo extensive first-pass metabolism by CYP3A4 and their toxicity can be increased by the concurrent use of hepatic microsomal enzyme inhibitors such as ketoconazole, erythromycin, cyclosporine and HIV protease inhibitors. Fluvastatin and rosuavastatin are metabolized by hepatic CYP2C9. Inhibitors of this enzyme such as ketoconazole, metronidazole and cimetidine can increase the plasma levels of these statins.

Rarely, statins may cause impotence, gynecomastia, peripheral neuropathy, memory loss, insomnia and mood changes.

Statins are contraindicated in pregnancy and in a woman planning to become pregnant, during breast-feeding, in children and in patients with severe liver disease.

Therapeutic uses: Statins are useful in both primary and secondary prophylaxis of hypercholesterolemia. They have been shown to reduce :

(a) Progression of atherosclerotic lesions;

(b) Occurrence of myocardial infarction; and

(c) Total mortality from all causes in men upto 70 years of age, with known IHD.

Statins, used alone in maximum doses, can lower LDL level by 40-60%. Addition of cholestyramine resin further lowers the LDL level (Table 39.10). Addition of nicotinic acid lowers the LDL level by more than 70%. Statin therapy can reduce the 5 year incidence of major coronary events, coronary revascularization and stroke significantly, largely irrespective of the initial lipid level or the other presenting characters. Hence, they should be considered for prolonged treatment in all patients at high risk for any type of major vascular events.

The statins may have several non-lipid beneficial effects. These are:

- ***Decrease in platelet aggregation and in fibrinogen levels.***
- ***Improvement in endothelial function and increase in local NO production.***
- ***Decrease in macrophage infiltration into the vessel wall.***
- ***Decrease in the arterial muscle proliferation.***
- ***Retardation of the progression of hypertrophy of the vessel wall; and***
- ***Decrease LDL oxidation in the vessel wall.***

However, their clinical implications are not known.

The choice of the statin depends upon the degree of LDL elevation, pharmacokinetics of the drugs, drug interactions, presence of hepatic/renal disease and cost. Atorvastatin and simvastatin are more efficatious than others, and therefore may be preferred in patients who require more than 35% reduction in LDL-C. Atorvastatin and fluvastatin need no dose adjustment in patients with renal impairment. Pravaststin and fluvastatin are not metabolized by CYP3A4 and are likely to cause few drug interactions. Atorvastatin and rosuvastatin have long t½ (14 and 19 hours, respectively) and can be taken at any time of the day. Since most cholesterol synthesis occurs during the night, the short t½ compounds are best administered at night as a single dose.

EZETIMIBE: This drug, 2-azetidinone, inhibits absorption of cholesterol by the small intestinal mucosa by binding to a mucosal transporter, leading to decreased delivery of dietary and biliary cholesterol to the liver. Reduction of hepatic cholesterol stores causes increase in LDL receptors on the hepatocytes and an increased cholesterol clearance from the blood. The plasma total and LDL cholesterol decrease and HDL cholesterol increases. A beneficial effect on the clinical outcome (reduced cardiovascular mortality and/or prevention of MI) is, however, yet to be documented. It is 90% bound to plasma proteins and its plasma t½ is 22 hours. It forms an active metabolite and may undergo enterohepatic circulation. It is largely excreted in the feces.

Adverse reactions are fatigue, dizziness, headache, abdominal discomfort, diarrhoea, arthralgia and hypersensitivity reactions.

Therapeutic uses : It can be combined in the dose of 5-10 mg./day with a statin in patients unable to achieve the desired LDL level with the maximum tolerated dose of the statin. It is contraindicated in severe renal insufficiency. It should not be used in children and in pregnant/ lactating women.

CHOLESTYRAMINE RESIN (Questran): Cholestyramine resin, an insoluble chloride salt of a basic anion exchange resin, has a strong affinity for bile salts (cholates) in the intestine. It binds the cholates into an insoluble complex which is excreted in faeces (Fig. 39.1). The result is decreased absorption of exogenous cholesterol and increased metabolism of endogenous cholesterol into bile acids in the liver. This leads to increased expression of LDL receptors on liver cells and increased removal of LDL from the blood. It causes a slight increase in HDL cholesterol. The drug, however, does not significantly lower the plasma levels of triglycerides (Table 39.10). It is given in the dose of 12-24 g. per day in a single or divided doses.

Adverse reactions: These include nausea, vomiting, heartburn and constipation. Large doses may interfere with absorption of fats and fat-soluble vitamins, causing steatorrhoea. It also interferes with the absorption of thyroid hormones, tetracyclines and organic acids such as phenobarbitone.

Therapeutic uses : The use of cholestyramine resin has declined with the documented efficacy of statins. However, it can be used in children and pregnant women.

In addition to its use in hyperlipidemia, it may be useful in relieving pruritus associated with biliary cirrhosis and cholestatic jaundice.

Colestipol (Colestid), like cholestyramine, is a bile acid sequestrant.

GUGULIPID (Guglip): This is the steroidal fraction derived from the plant *Commiphora mukul* and has variable hypocholesterolemic activity. It seems to be well tolerated. It is available as 25 mg. tablets.

FIBRE: Soluble fibres (pectins in citrus fruits, mucilages in psyllium seeds, gums in oat products and in beans) have a modest effect in lowering serum cholesterol. Psyllium seeds (Isapgol) is administered in the dose of 2.5-5 g. twice a day; oat bran is used in the dose of 50-150 g. a day. Insoluble fibre such as is present in wheat bran is not effective in lowering serum cholesterol (Chapter 41).

FIBRATES are the derivatives of fibric (isobutyric) acid and include **gemfibrozil** (Lopid, Normolip), **bezafibrate** (Bezalip) and **fenofibrate** (Lipantil). Clofibrate is no more used. Fibrates are effective in lowering plasma VLDL and triglycerides and in elevating plasma HDL levels. They may elevate LDL cholesterol (Table 39.10). They are claimed to reduce plasma fibrinogen levels, to increase fibrinolysis and to reduce abnormal platelet stickiness.

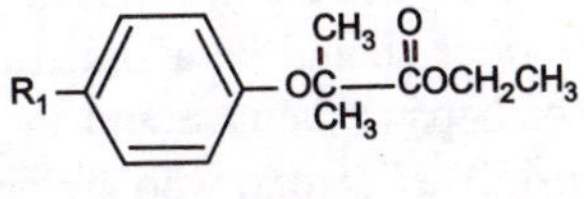

$R_1-C_6H_4-OC(CH_3)_2-COCH_2CH_3$ (with C=O)

Fig. 39.2: Fibrate nucleus. R differs with the analogue

Table 39.10: Effects of lipid lowering agents on lipid fractions

Drug	Total cholesterol	LDL cholesterol	HDL cholesterol	Triglycerides (TG)
Statins △	↓	↓↓	↑	↓
Ezetimibe	↓	↓	–	–
Fibrates	↓	↑	↑	↓↓
Nicotinic acid (NA)	↓	↓	↑↑	↓

↑/↑↑ = Increases; ↓/↓↓ = Decreases. Physical exercise increases HDL cholesterol.
△ Lovastatin and simvastatin may reduce the risk of osteoporotic fractures

Mechanism of action: These drugs stimulate the nuclear transcription receptor, Peroxisome Proliferator Activated Receptor alpha (PPAR-α) that controls the expression of genes that mediate TG metabolism. They increase lipoprotein lipase (LPA) activity and the hydrolysis of TG and promote HDL production; they reduce the incorporation of fatty acids into VLDL in the liver, thus inhibiting the synthesis and secretion of VLDL. The plasma TG decline by 50%, cholesterol by 10-15% and HDL increases by 20%.

Absorption, fate and excretion: They are almost completely absorbed from the gut, are highly protein bound (more than 90%). They are largely excreted unchanged in the urine.

Adverse reactions: Fibrates are generally well tolerated although, they occasionally produce allergic reactions, nausea and diarrhoea. An increase in the body weight occurs in some patients. These drugs displace acidic drugs from their plasma protein binding and may enhance the action of warfarin and sulfonylureas. Serum transminase levels sometimes show a rise. Though rare, potentially serious effects on the skeletal (myositis) and cardiac muscle have been reported. Fibrates should be avoided in patients with renal or hepatic damage and in alcoholics (with hypertriglyceridemia) who are predisposed to myositis. Long term therapy is associated with an increase in gallstone formation. *The combination of a fibrate and a statin increases the chance of rhabdomyolysis and myopathy.*

Preparations and dosage:

i) Gemfibrozil 300 mg. capsules. Dose: 600 mg. twice a day 30 minutes before meals.
ii) Bezafibrate: 200 mg. tablets. Doses: 200 mg. three times a day with meals.
iii) Fenofibrate: 67, 134, 200 mg. single dose capsules. Dose: One capsule OD with a meal.

Therapeutic uses: These drugs are effective in reducing plasma TG in both genetic and secondary hypertriglyceridemias. They may be useful in mixed hyperlipidemias.

Fish oil: Epidemiological evidence suggests that fatty-fish-eating communities have a lower incidence of IHD than non-fish-eaters. **Omega-3 PUFA** in the fish oil can reduce plasma TG but have little effect on HDL and LDL cholesterol and can sometimes increases total cholesterol upto 50%. They also lead to synthesis of leukotrienes and prostaglandins of series 1 and 3, which are less pro-inflammatory than those of series 2 (Chapter 24). Unlike gemfibrozil and niacin, omega-3 PUFAs do not interact with statins to enhance the incidence of myositis. They may decrease the risk of cardiac dcath in recent MI. But, in chronic IHD there is a possibility of a proarrhythimic effect. Eating fatty fish may be beneficial in healthy people but

Table 39.11: Choice of lipid lowering drugs

Drug	Hypercholesterolemia (Elevated LDL-C+ TG<200 mg/dl)	Combined hyperlipidemia (Elevated LDL-C+ TG 200-400 mg/dl)	Hypertriglyceridemia (TG>400 mg/dl)
Statins	Drugs of choice	Effective	—
Fibrates	—	Effective in high doses	Drugs of choice
Nicotinic acid (N)	Effective; usefulness limited by adverse effects of full doses	Drug of choice	Effective but poorly tolerated

Statins can be combined with (a) incotinic acid, or (b) a fibrate in resistance cases.

there is no evidence currently supporting prevention of cardiovascular disease in the general population. The dose is five 1 g capsules bid. The drug is contraindicated in patients with type IIa hyperlipidemia.

Omega-3 fatty acids are also present in nuts (especially walnuts), dark green leafy vegetables, soya beans, flax seeds and flax seed oil, and hemp seeds.

NICOTINIC ACID: This vitamin in large doses effectively and rapidly reduce plasma TG by lowering VLDL levels; LDL levels diminish more slowly, whereas HDL levels rise during therapy. *Nicotinamide does not have this action.*

Mechanism of action: In the adipose tissue, nicotinic acid inhibits adenylyl cyclase, and consequently lipolysis by hormone sensitive lipase. This reduces the transport of fatty acids to the liver. In the liver, niacin reduces both synthesis and esterification of fatty acids. The end result is reduction in the hepatic production of VLDL and reduction in plasma TG, VLDL cholesterol and LDL cholesterol. (Table 39.10).

Adverse reactions: In pharmacological doses, nicotinic acid produces intense cutaneous flushing and pruritus by increasing the local prostaglandin levels. They can be minimized by starting with a small dose and gradually building it up to the full dose, and by taking the drug with meals; further, one tablet of aspirin, taken 30 minutes earlier, markedly reduces the flush. Other adverse reactions are nausea, vomiting, diarrhoea; abnormalities of liver function, clinical jaundice; hyperuricemia, hyperglycemia; and potentiation of hypotension caused by antihypertensives.

Therapeutic uses: Nicotinic acid is useful in all forms of hyperlipoproteinemias except type I and is drug of choice in type V hyper-lipoproteinemia.

The usual dose is 2-8 g/day, in divided doses, with meals. It is advisable to start with 100 mg. tid with meals and to build up the dose in 2-4 weeks. Nicotinic acid in pharmacological doses probably reduces the incidence of recurrent MI.

Folic acid supplements are used to prevent homocysteinemia (Chapter 34).

Choice of lipid lowering drugs : This is outlined in Table 39.11. The current evidence indicates that the statins are the lipid lowering drugs of choice for most patients at risk of CHD. Full effect is generally observed within six weeks, when lipid response, ADR, liver and muscle enzymes should be reviewed and neccessary changes in doses of drugs made.

Emetics, Drug Therapy of Vomiting, Vertigo and Diarrhoea 40

Vomiting, though unpleasant, is a protective reflex, and is associated with upper GI motor activity, which helps to rid the stomach of noxious material. Vomiting also occurs in physiological situations such as pregnancy, but often it is an indication of ill health and needs to be treated.

Physiology of vomiting: The act of vomiting is accompanied by a complex series of movements, controlled by the **vomiting centre** in the medulla oblongata. The vomiting centre is the final common pathway for the act of vomiting. It receives afferent impulses from:

- ***Higher centres in the brain.***
- ***Chemoreceptor trigger zone*** **(CTZ).**
- ***Vestibular apparatus;*** and
- ***Peripheral structures including the GI tract and nucleus tractus solitarius.***

Figure 40.1 shows the mechanism of vomiting and the receptors involved.

A major sensory relay station in the afferent vomiting pathway is the chemoreceptor trigger zone (CTZ), situated in the lateral border of the area postrema of the medulla oblongata. Histologically, CTZ resembles the carotid body and is not a part of the brain. It is in direct contact with the circulating blood and is outside the BBB. A variety of drugs like morphine, apomorphine, alkylating agents and digitalis stimulate the CTZ while the phenothiazines and certain antihistaminics depress it. However, the CTZ being a purely sensory relay station, is incapable of initiating vomiting in the absence of vomiting centre, while direct stimulation of the latter evokes vomiting irrespective of the CTZ. Vomiting due to irritation or overdistension of the GI tract and delayed gastric emptying does not involve the CTZ but is directly mediated by stimulation of the vomiting centre via visceral vagal afferents. Similarly, it is likely that vomiting of central origin due to emotions, nauseous odors, and similar factors does not involve the CTZ but is due to impulses directly reaching the vomiting centre. On the other hand, vomiting of vestibular origin is mediated by the pathway: vestibular nuclei, cerebellum, CTZ and the vomiting centre.

Gastrointestinal reflux (GER) is not true vomiting; it occurs as a result of failed normal esophageal function. GER is effortless and generally not associated with autonomic symptoms.

Apart from 5-HT, DA, neurokinins (NK) and histamine probably play an important role in the process of vomiting. Three different NKs have been identified — substance P, neurokinin A and neurokinin B which are believed to act as neurotransmitters/ neuromodulators. Substance P has been identified in the nucleus tractus solitarius and the area postrema of the brainstem, and also with 5-HT within the enterochromaffin cells of the GI tract. It is excitatory in nature and can induce vomiting. It may be involved at various stages of the emetic pathway (Fig. 40.1).

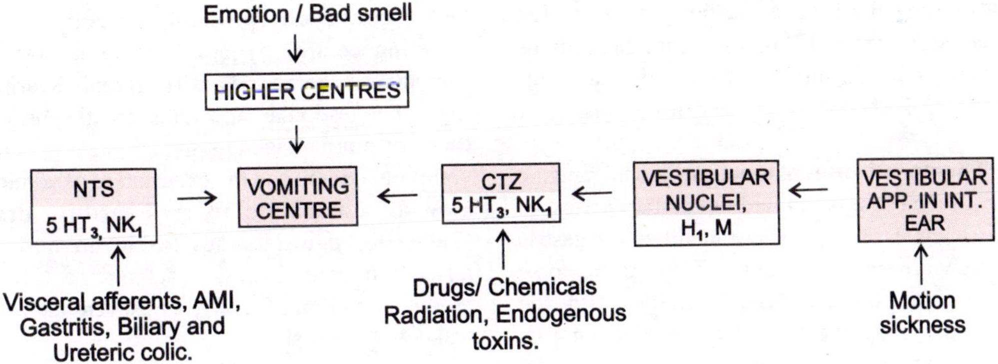

Fig. 40.1 : Mechanism of vomiting

Vomiting is usually preceded by the feeling of nausea and increased secretion of saliva, bronchial fluid and sweat. The muscles involved in the act of coughing take part in the act of vomiting, and the vagal, vomiting, and cough centres have a close functional relationship. Vomiting can also be induced voluntarily.

Emetics

The drugs that produce vomiting are termed emetics. These can be classified as:

I **Centrally acting**, by stimulation of the CTZ e.g. Apomorphine and Morphine.

II **Peripherally acting** e.g. Mustard, Antimony – potassium tartrate (tartar emetic) and Hypertonic sodium chloride.

III **Both peripherally and centrally acting** e.g. Ipecacuanha.

I Centrally acting emetics:

APOMORPHINE: This drug (Chapters 10 and 14), given SC, causes vomiting within 15 minutes. In hypersensitive individuals, however, even a subtherapeutic dose may elicit severe emesis. Vomiting is often accompanied by sedation. Apomorphine induced vomiting is effectively suppressed by chlorpromazine. Large doses often produce restlessness, tremors, occasionally convulsions, and respiratory depression. The drug may cause hypotension, syncope and coma. The adverse effects can be treated by a specific antidote, nalorphine, 5-10 mg. IV.

Although apomorphine is a highly effective emetic, syrup of ipecac is safer.

II **Peripherally acting emetics:** These cause vomiting reflexly by irritating the gastric mucosa; vomiting will not be induced if the vagi are cut. The drugs are :

MUSTARD: This acts by virtue of its volatile oil which is formed as a result of a reaction between a glycoside and an enzyme, in the presence of water. Although it is uncertain in action, it is safe and easily available. Hence,it forms one of the common household remedies. Dose: 1 teaspoonful in water.

SODIUM CHLORIDE (hypertonic): Given orally, it withdraws fluid from the cells lining the stomach and thus causes irritation which causes reflex emesis.

III **Both peripherally and centrally acting emetics: Ipecacuanha syrup** which contains, an alkaloid emetine is a safe emetic. It can be administered relatively safely in children. The drug can evoke emesis in poisoning with drugs that depress the CTZ e.g. chlorpromazine. The usual adult dose is 15 ml. by mouth and may be repeated after 20 minutes if the individual fails to vomit. It should be avoided in infants.

Therapeutic uses of emetics: The therapeutic use of emetics is limited to certain cases of poisoning, especially where facilities for gastric lavage are not available. This is because aspiration of the gastric contents into the respiratory passage may occur during emesis. Further, in case of a caustic poison, emesis may cause gastric perforation. The central depressant action of emetics like apomorphine may sometimes make the patient's condition worse. Severe emesis can cause collapse.

Emetics should generally be avoided in:

- ***Children and the elderly.***
- ***Pregnant women;*** and
- ***Patients with cardiac decompensation, hypertension, hernia, peptic ulcer and pulmonary tuberculosis.***

Drug Therapy of Vomiting

In many situations nausea and vomiting seem to serve no discernibly useful purpose and need treatment. Similar stimuli in progressively increasing intensity produce successively anorexia, nausea, and vomiting.

There appear to be wide differences in individual susceptibility to 'become sick' e.g. infants are less susceptible to motion sickness than older children and adults (among whom again there are wide individual differences); women are more susceptible than men and the aged are less susceptible than young adults to postanaesthetic vomiting. Estrogens are believed to lower the threshold of the CTZ, thus possibly explaining the vomiting of pregnancy and the nausea during combination OC therapy.

Vomiting may be psychic in origin and initiated by sights or bad smells. Secondly, it may arise reflexly from the GI tract, the impulses being conveyed (probably directly to the vomiting centre) by both the vagus and the sympathetic nerves. Thirdly, impulses arising from the vestibular apparatus are the primary cause of motion sickness though sight of others vomiting, odours and the expectation of vomiting may all contribute to it. Fourthly, drugs (Table 40.1), metabolites (as in uremia) and raised intracranial tension act on the CTZ to produce vomiting. Finally, any severe pain may make a person 'sick'.

Table 40.1: Some drugs which cause vomiting

- Anticancer drugs
- Amiodarone
- Apomorphine; Morphine
- Chloroquine; Quinine
- Diltiazem
- Emetine
- Ergot derivatives
- Antimicrobials : Erythromycin; Tetracyclines, Fluroquinolones Metronidazole

The treatment of vomiting consists of:

- ***Treatment of the cause,*** e.g., relief of pain, treatment of intestinal obstruction and colic, reduction in the intracranial tension or correction of metabolic acidosis.
- ***Symptomatic treatment*** with antiemetics.
- ***Supportive therapy,*** e.g., correction of dehydration and associated electrolyte disturbances.

Antiemetic agents are drugs used specifically to prevent or relieve nausea and vomiting. They can be classified as:

I **Antidopaminergic,** e.g., Chlorpromazine and related drugs (Chapter 13) Metoclopramide, Domperidone;

II **Antihistaminic,** e.g., Cyclizine, Meclizine, Promethazine, Dimenhydrinate (Chapter 22);

III **Antimuscarinic,** e.g., Scopolamine;

IV **Anti-5HT** e.g., Ondansetron, Granisetron,

Dolasetron and Palonosetron; and Ginger (Chapter 23);

V **Antagonist of the NK1 receptors for substance P :** Aprepitant.

VI **Miscellaneous** such as Nabilone (a cannabinoid), Trimethobenzamide, Benzquinamide, Dexamethasone.

Clinically, the antiemetics are grouped according to their potency as:

- ***Most potent*:** Ondansetron, Granisetron and high dose Metoclopramide.
- **Moderately potent :** Low dose Metoclopramide, Phenothiazines (Prochlorperazine), Butyrophenones (Droperidol), and Cannabinoids.
- **Weak:** Anticholinergics, Antihistaminics and Benzodiazepines (Lorazepam).
- **Adjunctive:** Glucocorticoids such as dexamethasone given parenterally in large doses, are used as adjuncts in the management of resistant nausea and vomiting induced by cancer chemotherapeutic agents.

Antihistaminic-antiemetic drugs like dimenhydrinate, cyclizine, promethazine and meclizine act on the vomiting centre and also have mild sedative effect. They are effective in motion sickness, in vomiting due to labyrinthine disorders (vestibular neuronitis, Meniere's disease etc.) and in vomiting of pregnancy. **Phenothiazines** like chlorpromazine, a dopamine D2 antagonist, selectively depress the CTZ but have no action on the vomiting centre. Hence, they are ineffective in motion sickness. They are however, the drugs of choice in nausea and vomiting due to uremia, carcinomatosis, radiation sickness and that due to drugs. Among the phenothiazines, triflupromazine and the piperazine phenothiazines are more effective than others. However, their extrapyramidal adverse effects must be remembered. In general, the phenothiazines are preferred when vomiting is severe and hazardous but is of short duration e.g. postoperative vomiting. On the other hand, the antihistaminic antiemetics, though less effective than the phenothiazines, are safer and preferred for long term use.

Vomiting due to gastroenteritis does not respond well to antiemetic drugs. Cyclizine may, however, be tried in nausea due to hepatitis.

Dopamine present peripherally in the upper GI tract has inhibitory effect on the GI motility and intragastric pressure.These effects are believed to be due to the suppression of ACh release from the primary motor neurons in the myenteric plexus, the activity of which is modulated by inhibitory dopaminergic-D_2 neurons. The drugs that act as D_2 antagonists peripherally, therefore, would be useful in the treatment of GI motility disorders, and are known as **prokinetic drugs** eg., metoclopramide and domperidone. By acting as antagonists of dopamine in the CTZ, they also act as central antiemetics. Since 5-HT plays an important role in GI motility and is present in the neurons of the myenteric plexus, prokinetic action can also be achieved by the action of 5-HT_4 receptor agonists, on the excitatory interneurons. In fact, cisapride and metoclopramide are believed to act as prokinetic drugs by acting as 5-HT_4 receptor agonists (Chapter 23).

METOCLOPRAMIDE (Maxolon, Maxeron, Perinorm): This antiemetic, chemically related to procainamide, acts predominantly as a **dopamine antagonist**. It also has 5-HT_4 agonist properties. Its antiemetic effect has two components :

- ***Promotion of forward propulsion of the contents of the upper GI tract, particularly the stomach (prokinetic action)*** due to 5-HT_4 action. The cholinomimetic effect of metoclopramide is restricted to the proximal gut and is due to enhancement of the action of acetylcholine at the muscarinic receptor; and
- ***Central inhibition of vomiting*** due to action on the DA receptors in the CTZ.

Pharmacological actions: The drug increases the resting tone of the gastroesophageal sphincter and stimulates coordinated gastric motility to speed up gastric emptying. An injection of 20 mg. produces gastric emptying within 90 minutes in most patients. It also increases the activity of the pyloric antrum and duodenal peristalsis, and accelerates transit along the small bowel. It has no significant action on the biliary tract and the large bowel motility.

Centrally, metoclopramide blocks the dopaminergic receptors in the CTZ and reduces post-operative vomiting and vomiting due to morphine and pethidine.

The drug stimulates prolactin secretion.

Adverse reactions: It is a relatively safe drug. The common adverse effects are drowsiness and dystonic or extrapyramidal (EP) reactions. The others include diarrhoea, lassitude, skin rash, hyperprolactenemia, gynecomastia and galactorrhoea. It should not be used to treat vomiting in patients with breast cancer. It may aggravate sodium retention and hypokalemia in patients with edema. EP reactions and malignant neuroleptic syndrome following metoclopramide are dose related; and the daily intake of this drug should not exceed 0.5 mg/kg.

Preparations and dosage: It is available as 10 mg. tablets, as syrup and as an injection. Dose 5-10 mg. tid. orally; 10-20 mg. IM or IV.

Therapeutic uses:

- ***As an antiemetic***, especially in post-operative vomiting, in *low doses* (10 mg IM or IV three times a day).
- ***Before and during cancer chemotherapy*** to prevent nausea and vomiting, *in high doses* (0.5-3 mg./kg. IV over 15 minutes).
- ***To accelerate gastric emptying*** before induction of general anaesthesia for emergency surgery; prior administration of atropine can, however, block this effect of metoclopramide.
- ***To assist the passage of tubes (including an endoscope) into the duodenum; and***
- ***To treat gastroparesis and upper GI motility disorders*** with retention from a variety of causes: vagotomy, diabetes, gastritis and gastric ulcers.

Its efficacy in **reflux esophagitis** and persistent hiccup is equivocal.

DOMPERIDONE (Motilium, Domstal): This agent acts as a selective DA receptor antagonist. However, unlike metoclopramide it does not cross the BBB easily and, therefore, causes fewer EP reactions. It causes hyperprolactinemia. It enhances the gastric motility and increases the rate of gastric emptying. Its peripheral dopamine antagonistic action is responsible for its antiemetic effect. The drug is effective orally as well as parenterally. The oral dose is 10-20 mg. 3-4 times a day.

CISAPRIDE (Alimax, Ciza, Cisapid): This drug is a GI motility stimulant **(prokinetic).** It has no direct antiemetic action. It acts as a 5-HT_4 receptor agonist and modulates the activity of the primary motor neurons in the myenteric plexus. It also has an action on the colon.

Adverse reactions include increased urinary frequency, abdominal cramps and diarrhoea. EP reactions are rare. It prolongs the QT interval and can enhance the toxicity of drugs which prolong QT interval. Drugs which inhibit hepatic microsomal enzymes such as macrolides, azole antifungal drugs and cimetidine increase its plasma levels and enhance its toxicity. *Serious cardiac arrhythmias and sudden death have been reported. Because of its cardiotoxicity, cisapride may be used only when a safer drug cannot be* used for some reason. It has been withdrawn from the market in some countries.

Therapeutic uses :

- ***Impaired gastric motility*** due to diabetes mellitus or autonomic neuropathy. It may produce some symptomatic relief in GERD, but is not useful in esophagitis (Chapter 42);
- ***Symptoms of dyspepsia,*** after exclusion of peptic ulcer disease and other known causes.

Mosapride is another selective 5HT_4 agonist claimed to have fewer side effects. **Itopride** has actions similar to those of metoclopramide.

Table 40.2 compares the actions of the three prokinetic drugs.

Erythromycin: This macrolide antibiotic causes diarrhoea as a major side effect.This has been shown to be due to activation of motilin receptors. Motilin is a peptide hormone, found in the GI tract; it increases the smooth muscle

Table 40.2: Actions of prokinetic drugs

Action	Metoclo-pramide	Domperi-done	Cisa-pride
• $5\text{-}HT_4$ agonist	+++	—	+++
• Antidopami-nergic	++	+++	—
• CNS	++	+	—
• Hyperpro-lactinemia	++	+++	—
• Antiemetic	++	++	—
• Prokinetic	Upper GI tract	Upper GI tract	Upper GI tract and colon

contractibility. Erythromycin has been used as a prokinetic drug in patients with diabetic gastroparesis.

NABILONE: This is a synthetic cannabinoid used to treat nausea and vomiting caused by cancer chemotherapy, unresponsive to conventional antiemetics. The adverse reactions are mainly neurological and comprise drowsiness, vertigo, visual disturbances, headache, dysphoria, confusion, hallucinations and psychosis. Hypotension, tachycardia and abdominal pain may also occur. Its use is contraindicated in severe hepatic impairment, pregnancy and breast-feeding. The adult dose is 1 mg bid, increased to a maximum of 2 mg tid (Chapter 13).

DRONABINOL (Marinol): is D-9 tetra-hydrocannobinol (D-9 THC), a natural ingredient of cannabis, now manufactured synthetically. It acts on CB_1 receptors to exert its antiemetic action. It is used orally to prevent and treat cancer-chemotherapy-induced nausea and vomiting. It acts synergistically with phenothiazine antiemetics. The adverse reactions are wider than those of nabilone and include drug abuse. For selective $5\text{-}HT_3$ antagonists, see Chapter 23.

Therapy of vomiting of pregnancy: The exact etiology of vomiting of early pregnancy is not established and the treatment, therefore, is purely empirical.

The patient is advised to take frequent small meals and more fluids. Psychotheraphy including reassurance and placebo therapy are often beneficial. Though it is ideal to avoid drugs in the first trimester, some women are severely nauseated and need drug therapy. Drugs usually employed are **vitamin B_6** (pyridoxine), **antiemetic antihistaminics** (dimenhydrinate, doxylamine, cyclizine and meclizine) and **metoclopramide.** Promethazine may be used *except* near delivery time and during labour, when it may cause adverse effects in the newborn. The relative usefulness of pyridoxine alone as an antiemetic is not known. Usually, **doxylamine** 40 mg + pyridoxine 40 mg combination bid is considered safe and effective. **Dimenhydrinate** (50-100 mg) is safe and rapid in onset, and can be used as a suppository. Prochlorperazine, a phenothizine, 5-10 mg is reported to be safe and can be given IV in severe cases. **Ginger**, a kitchen item, in palatable form, is safe and effective remedy in mild cases. Its active components are $5\text{-}HT_3$ antagonists. *Finally, vomiting due to an unrelated but associated condition such as peptic ulcer, hepatitis, drug reaction or gall bladder disease should not be forgotten.*

Therapy of motion sickness: Motion sickness is a syndrome characterized by vertigo and nausea resulting from body motion. The word 'nausea' is derived from Greek word 'nautical' as it usually occurs at sea.

The receptors for motion sickness are located in the vestibular apparatus. Other stimuli such as visual, proprioceptive and emotional, may facilitate or enhance motion sickness. Children are more susceptible to motion sickness and the vulnerability diminishes with advancing age. Deaf persons with disease of the inner ear and infants, however, do not get motion sickness.

The susceptibility to motion sickness is determined by the balance of activation between the ACh and NA sensitive neurons in the reticular activating system adjacent to the vestibular nuclei. Drugs that block ACh in the CNS e.g. scopolamine, and those which activate the central sympathetic areas e.g. d-amphetamine are highly effective in its treatment.

SCOPOLAMINE : The belladonna alkaloid, scopolamine (hyoscine), was among the first drugs to be used in the treatment of motion sickness. *A central muscarinic antagonism of ACh may be the basis of its therapeutic efficacy.* Scopolamine is more effective when used prophylactically than during an attack. A single oral dose of 0.3 to 0.6 mg. in an adult, 15 minutes before food and 30 minutes before a journey, gives satisfactory protection. The onset of the effect usually coincides with the development of dryness of mouth. The drug action persists for 2 to 3 hours and in the event of a prolonged journey, an additional dose of 0.1 to 0.2 mg. is given after 2 hours. The drug may cause drowsiness, dizziness, blurring of vision, dry mouth and urinary retention.

Scopolamine is also available in transdermal delivery system, as an adhesive unit, for placement behind the ear (Scopoderm). The drug is released at a uniform rate for 72 hours.

ANTIHISTAMINICS: A number of H_1 receptor antagonists have been used in the treatment of motion sickness. These include the phenothiazine antihistaminics, promethazine and its chlorotheophyllinate, dimenhydrinate, and the piperazine antihistaminics cyclizine, buclizine, meclizine and cinnarizine (Chapter 22). Some of these have antimuscarinic action as well.

The number of individuals protected by these agents varies from 60 to 70 per cent. They are administered orally, 30 minutes before the journey. The piperazine antihistaminics have a prolonged action, a single dose providing relief for 6-12 hours. The action of meclizine is claimed to persist for 24 hours.

Table 40.3 lists the applications of antiemetics in vomiting from different causes.

Antiemetics should not generally be used, especially in children, without establishinlg the cause of vomiting, as they may mask the underlying disease and delay the diagnosis.

Table 40.3 : Antiemetics in different types of vomiting

GI irritation : Anticholinergics; in severe cases, a Phenothiazine.
Motion sickness : Scopolamine; Dimenhydrinate; Cyclizine, Meclizine.
Pregnancy: Doxylamine, Pyridoxine, Dimenhydrinate.
Uremia, radiation sickness, carcinomatosis, anticancer chemotherapy: Phenothiazine and Butyrophenone Antipsychotics; Metoclopramide; Ondansetron; Nabilone; Dexamethasone (as adjunctive drugs during cancer chemotherapy).
Gastroperesis: Prokinetic drugs.
Postoperative: Prokinetic drugs, Antihistaminics.

Therapy of Vertigo and Dizziness

Vertigo is a **hallucination of movement**, generally spinning, caused by a disturbance of the orientation-detecting system of a person.

Orientation in space is achieved by integrating information mainly from :

- ***Vestibular apparatus.***
- ***Vision; and***
- ***The proprioceptors in the muscles and joints.***

The collected information is processed in the sensory integrating areas of the reticular formation. Such processing occurs at the subconscious level in normal persons; when the information contains a new or an unusual element, vertigo can occur. *Dizziness* is less specific than *vertigo* and comprises all symptoms of disequilibration including lightheadedness, giddiness, swimminess, floating etc; its pathogenesis is similar to that of vertigo. Individual patients may not be able to differentiate between vertigo and dizziness. Both are caused by different pathological processes including CNS, CVS and metabolic disease. If a definite cause for vertigo can be established, it may be amenable to specific treatment. **Cawthorne-Cooksey exercises** help to induce a compensation mainly in vertigo due to peripheral vestibular disorders. The principle is to retrain the eye, neck and body musculature to generate visual and proprioceptive input to compensate for the lost vestibular information. The movements that cause vertigo must be especially practised, since the more often vertigo is induced, the more quickly compensation occurs.

Table 40.4 lists the drugs used in the symptomatic treatment of vertigo.

Table 40.4: Drugs used in vertigo

Vestibular sedatives, e.g., Antihistaminics.
Central sedatives, e.g., Scopolamine, Benzodiazepines, Antidepressants.
Betahistine
Diuretics
Glucocorticoids

Antihistaminics suppress the vestibular end organ receptors and thus inhibit the activation of the central muscarinic receptors. Of the antihistaminics, cinnarizine (Stugeron) (15 mg. three times a day) is the most effective antivertigo agent. The other antihistaminics used include flunarizine, dimenhydrinate, hydroxyzine and promethazine (Chapter 22).

Phenothiazines and **central anticholinergics** (scopolamine) suppress the cenral vestibular nuclei and pathways. All centrally acting sedative drugs interfere with the integration of vestibular with other sensory information; they might delay the compensatory mechanisms which alleviates vertigo induced by peripheral vestibular disease. Chronic use of central sedatives (and even their withdrawal after prolonged use) can be associated with dizziness. However, benzodiazepines are likely to be helpful when anxiety is a feature in the response to vertigo. When depression is a major response, amitryptiline may be useful (Chapter 13).

Betahistine, a vasodilator, is useful in some cases of Meniere's disease (Chapter 22). **Diuretics** have been used on the assumption that vertigo is in some cases due to endolymphatic hydrops. **Glucocorticoids** (methylprednisolone 40 - 80 mg/day for 4-5 days, followed by 20 mg/day for 4 days) have been used to suppress intralabyrinthine edema due to virus infection.

An acute attack of vertigo is best treated with parenteral prochlorperazine; an oral antihistaminic should be started when the acute symptoms have subsided.

Cawthorne-Cooksey exercises should be started as soon as possible after an acute attack due to a peripheral vestibular disorder. **Meniere's disease** is initially treated with low salt diet and a thiazide diuretic. If this is not effective, an antihistaminic or betahistine should be used. Chronic persistent vertigo due to central or peripheral cause may be helped by small doses of an antihistaminic.

Drug Therapy of Diarrhoea

Diarrhoea is a very common problem in the tropical and subtropical countries and like vomiting, it can be caused by a variety of conditions varying from infections and allergy to emotional disturbances. It is defined as the frequent passage of liquid or unformed stools with or without blood or mucus; in the case of former it is usually due to a known cause such as amoebic or bacillary dysentery.

Table 40.5 outlines the pathophysiology of diarrhoea.

In nearly all forms of acute infectious diarrhoeas, the abnormally formed stools reflect small bowel hypersecretion of fluid and electrolytes and not increased intestinal motility. Most water absorption occurs in the jejunum by passive transport in response to the osmotic pressure generated by the absorption of soluble products of digestion. An excess of

Table 40.5: Pathophysiology of diarrhoea

Osmotic diarrhoea due to poorly absorbable, osmotically active substances as after ingestion of osmotic laxatives, in lactase deficiency and in malabsorption syndromes.

Secretory diarrhoea due to active ion secretion by the small intestinal epithelium as in cholera, enterotoxigenic *E.coli* diarrhoea and carcinoid syndrome.

Deranged intestinal motility as in irritable bowel syndrome, thyrotoxicosis and diabetic neuropathy.

Altered mucosal morphology as in viral gastroenteritis, bacterial infection with tissue invasion and radiation enteritis.

Allergic diarrhoea as in food allergy.

Drug induced diarrhoea (see later).

Miscellaneous such as in neurological and endocrine disease.

unabsorbed material in the gut may cause osmotic diarrhoea.

In coeliac disease, the mucosal permeability to water and small solute is decreased. Some invading infections can damage intestinal villi to cause marked reduction in absorption of fluids. Finally, prostaglandins, 5-HT and bacterial toxins can cause hypersecretion and diarrhoea.

Not all diarrhoeas need drug treatment. For example, irritant diarrhoea can be self-limited.

Treatment of diarrhoea consists of:

I **Specific treatment.**

II **Treatment of dehydration;** and

III **Symptomatic and protective treatment.**

I **Specific treatment** of the diarrhoea depends upon the cause. The common pathogens responsible for acute diarrhoea are listed in Table 40.6. A number of drugs are now available to treat bacterial and protozoal infections but no specific antiviral agent is available for viral diarrhoea.

The initial clinical evaluation of the patient with acute diarrhoea should include assessment of its severity, the need for rehydration and the likely cause, based on history, clinical findings and stool examination. Specific therapy of diarrhoea would be easy if the responsible pathogen could be identified quickly. However, in practice this is many times not possible and the physician has to decide largely on the basis of his clinical judgement.

Many patients suffer from **simple diarrhoea** manifested by watery stools, low grade fever, malaise, nausea and sometimes vomiting. *In developed countries*, it is most often of viral origin and could be treated without using antibacterials. On the other hand, *in developing countries*, this syndrome is more often due to a bacterial pathogen. The pathogen most commonly involved is enterotoxigenic *E. coli*, which is a major cause of infant diarrhoea. The other pathogens involved are: the enteropathogenic *E. coli*; enteroinvasive *E. coli*; shiga-toxin producing *E. coli*; shigella; salmonella; campylobacter; *Entamoeba histolytica*; cyclosporidium and others. Such patients tend to have more severe diarrhoea, fever and blood in stools (**dysentery**). Cyclosporidiasis causes marked fatigue in most patients. Although classical cases such as those of amoebic or bacillary dysentery can be diagnosed relatively easily by microscopic examination of stool, in the vast majority of cases with diarrhoea this is not possible. Such diarrhoea with "negative stool" could be due to the presence of *E. coli* endotoxin, staphylococcal endotoxin, *Campylobacter jejuni*, yersinia or viruses such as rotavirus or atypical adenovirus. **Travellers' diarrhoea** can be either simple diarrhoea or dysentery.

Regardless of the causative agent (documented or putative), the initial therapy should always include rehydration (Chapter 36) and nutritional support (soft rice, ripe bananas and cooked apple). Milk and milk products should be avoided since transient lactase deficiency may occur. Continued feeding improves the outcome in children. Antimotility drugs may be used in simple diarrhoea but

Table 40.6 : Clinical features and drugs recommended in acute infective diarrhoeas

Organism	Blood in stool	Polymorphs in stool	Vomiting	Drugs recommended
I **Bacterial :**				
Shigella	+	+ + +	+++	Ciprofloxacin; Norfloxacin; Cotrimoxazole; Nitazoxamide
Salmonella (non–typhi species)	+	+ + +	+	Cotrimoxazole; Fluoroquinolone or Ceftriaxone in several cases
E.coli	+ +	+ +	+	Fluoroquinolone; Cotrimoxazole
E.coli (Shiga toxin producing)	+ + +	±	+	Avoid antimotility drugs
Vibrio	±	±	±	Doxycycline; Fluoro quinolone
Campylobacter	+	+ +	+	Erythromycin
Cl. difficile	+	+ + +	–	Metronidazole
II **Protozoal :**				
E.histolytics	±	±	±	Metronidazole
Giardia	–	–	±	Metronidazole
Cryptosporidium	–	–	–	Azithromycin; Nitazoxamide
Cyclospora	–	–	+	Cotrimoxazole
III **Viral :**	–	–	++	No antimicrobial

should be avoided in infective diarrhoea and in children.

Antimicrobials are ineffective in viral diarrhoea. Some antibiotics (e.g. neomycin, polymyxin B, furazolidine and some cephalosporins) have potent antimicrobial activity in vitro but show no efficacy in vivo. Hence, their reckless use is not only wasteful but may be harmful.

Antibiotics are of value in the infective diarrhoeas (Table 40.6). Co-trimoxaozole is effective against all the strains of *E. coli* mentioned above. It is also effective in shigellosis with diarrhoea; such patients may also respond to tetracycline, either 500 mg qid for 5 days or 2.5 gm as a single dose; ampicillin and amoxicillin are equally effective. Bacterial resistance to co-trimoxazole, ampicillin and nalidixic acid has been reported. Hence, a fluoroquinolone is now considered the drug of choice in patients with inflammatory diarrhoea due to bacterial dysentery; they are now considered safe in children. Most patients show a rapid response but those infected with *Campylobacter jejuni* may not respond; such patients are best treated with azithromycin, 1 gm as a single dose or 500 mg tid for 3 days. Travellers' diarrhoea has been treated with

rifaximin, a new nonabsorbable rifampin derivative, as an alternative to quinolones, in the dose of 200 mg tid for 3 days; it is well tolerated but is ineffective in patients with fever or blood in stool and in those infected by *Campylobacter jejuni.* It should be avoided in pregnancy.

Patients with cholera or cholera-like gastroenteritis should be treated with a tetracycline e.g. doxycycline in a single dose of 300 mg; it is effective in reducing stool volume and eradicating Vibrio cholerae within 48 hours.

If diarrhoea persists for more than 5-7 days despite treatment, the causative organism is likely to be a protozoon. Lack of evidence of a pathogen should arouse the suspicion of IgA deficiency or irritable bowel syndrome. Table 40.6 summarises the salient features and choice of the antimicrobial drug in acute diarrhoea.

II **Correction of dehydration and electrolyte disturbances** *is the most important aspect of treatment of diarrhoea* and in many cases, it may be the only treatment needed (Chapter 36).

III **Symptomatic and supportive therapy:** Symptomatic treatment includes (a) GI protectives, and (b) drugs acting on GI motility.

Agents useful in symptomatic treatment of diarrhoea may act:

- ***Locally, as protectives by coating the gut.***
- ***By decreasing the propulsion of the intestinal contents,*** e.g., morphine like compounds.
- ***Directly on mucosal transport processes,*** reducing fluid accumulation in the intestinal lumen (*anti-secretory action*). Aspirin-like drugs and morphine-like drugs which inhibit the synthesis or the action of PG have anti-secretory action. Phenothiazines have similar antisecretory effect in some patients; and
- ***On intestinal microcirculation;*** some drugs may lower the hydrostatic pressure thus favouring water absorption.

Temporary reduction in the intake of foods rich in fibre (unrefined cereals, fruits and vegetables) is desirable in acute diarrhoea.

(a) **GI protectives and adsorbents:** These agents may be useful predominantly because of their ability to adsorb noxious substances such as gases, bacteria and bacterial toxins. In addition, some of these possess an astringent action, while others protect the GI mucous membrane from the irritants by coating it physically. They are cheap, and devoid of adverse effects but their usefulness is limited to the treatment of mild diarrhoea. However, they may adsorb simultaneously administered anti-infective agents and anticholinergics. The drugs employed are :

BISMUTH SALTS: The commonly employed bismuth salts are bismuth subcarbonate and bismuth subsalicylate. They have an astringent, protective and adsorbent effect. They are devoid of serious toxicity. They also act on *Helicobater pylori* (Chapter 42).

Bismuth subsalicylate binds toxins produced by *V. cholerae* and *E.coli;* an antimicrobial action has been demonstrated both *in vitro* and *in vivo*. In case of subsalicylate salt, it is possible that the liberated salicylic acid may inhibit the PG synthesis responsible for intestinal inflammation and hypermotility. Salicylate may also exert an antisecretory action and stimulate fluid and electrolyte absorption.

Bismuth subcarbonate is insoluble in water and administered as a constituent of a binding mixture; the dose of subcarbonate being 0.6 to 2 g. Other bismuth salts used are bismuth subgallate and bismuth subnitrate.

PECTIN: It is a purified carbohydrate obtained from the extract of the inner portion of citrus fruits or from apple pomace. It consists chiefly of partially methoxylated polygalacturonic acids. The mechanism of its antidiarrhoeal effect is not clear. When ingested, it passes into the intestinal tract where it probably acts by physical coating. It helps to produce formed stools. It is decomposed in the colon by bacterial action.

It forms a viscous, colloidal solution with 20 parts of water. The solution is tasteless; it is administered either as a colloidal suspension alone or with kaolin. Pectin can also be given in the form of cooked apple or overripe banana.

ACTIVATED WOOD CHARCOAL: This preparation is the residue from the destructive distillation of vegetable matter such as saw dust, cellulose residue and coconut shells, treated with zinc chloride to increase its adsorptive power. It is employed in the treatment of flatulence, nonulcer dyspepsia and various types of diarrhoeas, as a suspension in water for gastric lavage and for the emergency treatment of poisoning with alkaloids like morphine, strychnine and atropine. (See Chapter 2).

Other preparations employed are **prepared chalk**, a native form of calcium carbonate (often used as an antacid); and **light kaolin**, which is hydrated aluminium silicate. Both these agents are insoluble in water and form a protective coating on the intestinal mucosa.They may also have some adsorbent properties.They are administered as suspension, and form an important constituent of 'over-the counter' (OTC) andiarrhoeal remedies. *There is no rigourous demonstration that these GI protectives and adsorbents help in diarrhoea, although their administration may result in more formed stools.*

(b) **Drugs affecting GI motility and secretion :**

• ***Opioids*** : Morphine-like compounds act by inhibiting the first phase of the peristaltic reflex, the acetylcholine dependent contraction of the longitudinal muscle, followed by a depression of rapid PG sensitive phase. In addition, they also produce anti-secretory effect by acting on intestinal opiate receptors. They may provide symptomatic relief. However, *opioids and other nonspecific agents (eg. adsorbents) are not recommended for use in children under 2 years. They should be avoided in infective diarrhoeas at all ages.*

The preparations used are:

(i) Codeine phosphate, 15 to 60 mg. at 8-12 hourly.

(ii) Tincture of opium (1 ml = 10 mg of morphine) in the single adult dose of 0.6-1.5 ml

(iii) Diphenoxylate, a pethidine substitute in the dose of 5 mg. along with 0.25 mg. of atropine (Lomotil) 3 to 4 times a day. *This combination is contraindicated in children as well as in the elderly as it may cause paralytic ileus.*

(iv) Paregoric (Chlorodyne, Embedyne): This is camphorated tincture of opium (10 ml = 5 mg of morphine). Dose: In adults 4 ml.

LOPERAMIDE (Imodium): It has a structural resemblance to pethidine. It acts directly on intestinal opiate receptors. The action is prompt and prolonged. Naloxone is a much poorer antagonist of loperamide than of morphine.

Loperamide has a characteristic tissue distribution and almost 85% of the drug can be recovered from the gut. It does not easily cross the blood-brain barrier, has high antidiarrhoeal specificity as compared to morphine and is devoid of CNS toxicity.

Although the drug has been used to treat diarrhoeas, its routine use to stop diarrhoea is debatable. *Loperamide has been reported to cause paralytic ileus in children and in the elderly.*

RACECADOTREIL (Redocil; Zedott) : Given orally, this antisecretory prodrug is hydrolysed to the active compound thiorphan. In the peripheral tissues, including the intestines, membrane-bound encephalinase enzymes degrade endogenous opioids/encephalins. Thiorphan inhibits encephalinase, thus increasing the availability of local encephalins which acts on the opioid delta receptors in the GI tract. Its efficacy is claimed to be as much as that of loperamide. It may be used to treat acute diarrhoea in children below the age of 2 years, in whom loperamide is contraindicated.

• ***Atropine and its substitutes*** such as propantheline, are useful to relieve colic associated with diarrhoea. They are particularly useful in controlling "intestinal hurry" following gastrectomy. Their use in chronic diarrhoeas, however, is not without danger and they may precipitate paralytic ileus in patients with regional enteritis and fulminating ulcerative colitis. The preparations used are atropine sulphate 0.25 to 1 mg. and hyoscine butylbromide 10-20 mg (Chapter 18).

- ***PG Inhibitors:*** Prostaglandins are known to stimulate intestinal fluid secretion and intestinal motility, thus causing diarrhoea. It is possible that PGF_{2a} release is involved in the genesis of certain diarrhoeas. PG inhibitors such as aspirin and indomethacin have been shown to be effective in diarrhoeas induced by bacterial toxins in animals, and in certain diarrhoeas in humans. In contrast to opiates, aspirin like drugs produce reduction in diarrhoea by acting on PG sensitive phase, without much decrease in total water excretion (Chapter 11).

Nutmeg, in combination with ginger, jaggery and ghee, is an age-old Indian household remedy for diarrhoea. It has been demonstrated that nutmeg often works where other drugs have failed. PG inhibition is suspected to be the mechanism of this antidiarrhoeal effect.

Miscellaneous agents:

Probiotics: These are live, nonpathogenic bacteria or yeasts which have been used for centuries in the form of home-made curd (yogurt), whey and buttermilk for health benefits. They contain variable lactobacillus species and *Saccharomyces boulardi.* Acetic, lactic and propionic acids produced by these bacilli lower the intestinal pH and inhibit the growth of certain pathogenic intestinal bacteria. e.g. *E. coli.* Probiotics may also act physically to prevent colonization by pathogenic organisms and may also enhance immune responses. Clinically, they may be beneficial in infectious (rota-virus induced) or antibiotic associated diarrhoea, IBS and inflammatory bowel diseases.

Probiotics are pleasant to take but may occasionally produce flatulence. Commercially, they are available as powders, liquids and capsules.

Energy and nutrient intake is impaired during acute diarrhoeal disease and in the catabolic state that may persist afterwards. It is recommended that adults and children be discouraged from fasting and that they resume their usual diet (nonirritant, non oily) with frequent small snacks. Drinks and foods containing caffeine and lactose should be avoided as they may prolong diarrhoea. Fluid and electrolyte balance can be maintained by drinking boiled water, fruit juice and buttermilk and by eating salted biscuits. Intake of starchy foods (rice conjee) will reduce diarrhoeal fluid output. **Rice powder** is cheaper than glucose and sucrose, and may increase absorption further by supplying aminoacids and di- and tri-peptide (Chapter 36).

Chronic Diarrhoea

Chronic diarrhoea, lasting more than 3-4 weeks, needs detailed evaluation. The drug therapy of chronic diarrhoea depends on its cause.In many cases, it is non-infectious e.g. irritable bowel syndrome (IBS), osmotic, diarrhoea, steatorrhoea, inflammatory bowel disease such as ulcerative colitis, and drug-induced diarrhoea (Table 40.7).

Drugs used in the treatment of chronic diarrhoea include the 5-HT antagonist cyproheptadine employed in dumping syndrome; glucocorticoids used in the treatment of ulcerative colitis; H_2 receptor blocking agents

Table 40.7: Drugs causing diarrhoea

- Magnesium antacids
- Antibiotics : Erythromycin, Ampicillin, Tetracyclines.
- GI prokinetic drugs, e.g., Cisapride.
- Quinidine
- Prostaglandin analogues.
- Anticholinesterases.
- Colchicine.
- Emetine.
- Cytotoxic drugs
- Lithium.

used in Zollinger-Ellison syndrome; and folic acid in the treatment of tropical sprue.

Irritable bowel syndrome (IBS): As per Western criteria, IBS is diagnosed when the subject complains of recurrent abdominal pain or discomfort at least three days a month in the past three months, associated with two or more of the following: (a) relief after defecation; and (b) onset associated with change in frequency of stools or the form of the stools. Thus, the disorder can be subdivided into (1) IBS with constipation; (2) IBS with diarrhea; and (3)the mixed type with both hard and soft stools. Thc symptoms are worse after meals, and one third of the patients also have functional dyspepsia/ gaseous abdominal distension. Some patients may also complain of non-GI somatic symptoms such as lethargy, backache and bodyache.

In India, IBS is more common in middle aged men. Majority of patients (90%) have combination of upper abdominal discomfort and lower abdominal fullness, relieved by defecation. Nearly 70% have feeling of inadequate evacuation. Diarrhea or constipation diagnosed as per Western criteria is uncommon and stool frequency is usually within normal limits (1-2 per day) for most of the patients.

IBS is often associated with anxiety or depression. General examination is usually normal. There is no known cure and the treatment is symptomatic. Education of the patient about the benign nature of the ailment is essential. Avoidance of fried spicy and pungent food is likely to be helpful; so is avoidance of stress. Patients with predominant diarrhea should be tested for gluten (wheat) sensitivity and milk intolerance.

Currently, pain in these patients is considered to be due to visceral hypersensitivity to physiological and noxious stimuli. Serotonin appears to be involved in this syndrome of visceral hyperalgesia. The patients in whom constipation is predominant benefit from bulk forming agents such as isapgol; while those in whom 'gas' is the predominant symptom are likely to benefit from a reduction in consumption of unrefined fibre products. Mild antimuscarinics like dicyclomine and isopropamide are helpful in those who complain of postprandial abdominal pain and distension.

Alosetron is a potent and selective 5-HT$_3$ receptor antagonist. Given in the dose of 1 mg b.i.d., it decreases intestinal motility, secretion and pain significantly. Thus, it relieves abdominal pain and discomfort and may control diarrhoea. Commonly, it causes constipation; rarely it can cause dangerous ischemia of the bowel. It is recommended only in women with IBS not responding to other therapy.

Tegaserod, a 5-HT$_4$ receptor agonist, reported to be useful in patients with predominant constipation, has been withdrawn due to its cardiovascular toxicity (MI, stroke).

Tricyclic antidepressants such as amitryptiline have also been reported to be useful in some case with diarrhoea.

Inflammatory bowel disease (IBD): See Chapter 44.

Intestinal malabsorption: Some of the diarrhoeas associated with fat malabsorption improve with substitution of medium chain triglycerides in place of long chain fatty acids. Similarly, osmotic diarrhoea due to intestinal disaccharidase deficiency improves on reducing consumption of milk and dairy products which contains lactose. Diarrhoea due to carcinoid syndrome responds to 5-HT antagonists while that due to blind loop syndrome responds to antibacterial therapy.

Drugs causing diarrhoea: Physicians should be made aware that many self administered OTC remedies for a variety of ailments, including hyperacidity and alleged constipation, may contain substances with laxative action e.g. magnesium salts and herbal products. *This awareness will help to reduce the need for extensive and expensive evaluation of patients with chronic diarrhoea, whose initial evaluation is unrevealing* (Table 40.7).

Pharmacotherapy of Constipation 41

People have been very particular about the 'regular bowel habit' from the earliest times and purgation, believed to be the panacea for many diseases, formed an important part of medieval therapeutics. At one time it was almost fashionable to take a regular purge or an enema to keep the bowels clean. "Fashionable seventeenth century France was a trendsetter. Louis XIII had 212 enemas, 215 purgations and 47 bleedings in one year. With Louis XIV, the enema came into its own. It became a household ritual and most upper-crust people had one every day. A celebrated legal case concerned payment for the administration of 2,190 enemas, all within two years to a Canon of Troyes." The fashion also spread to England and America and in the Victorian era constipation was treated with every conceivable concoction. Even today, many people have wrong notions about the quantity, consistency and frequency of stools in health and 'ritual purgation of children and the obsessional catharsis of adults' is still not uncommon. Purgatives are widely advertised for the treatment of constipation and are extensively used by lay people as they are easily available over-the-counter without a prescription. Almost half of the patients suffering from digestive tract disorders complain of 'constipation' and often drugs are self-prescribed.

Drugs which are used to promote defaecation are called **laxatives.**

The effect of drugs on the motility of the GI tract can be studied in a variety of *in vitro* preparations like isolated guineapig ileum, rat fundal strip, rat colon and rabbit duodenum. The human methods include radiological examination after administration of barium meal, use of food markers like charcoal, colouring agents, beads and radioactive isotopes, and radiotelemetry.

Regulation of GI motility: Orderly movement of ingested material through the gut is essential for adequate absorption of fluids, electrolytes and nutrients. The CNS (via the sympathetic and the parasympathetic nerves), local neuronal reflexes and the circulating, enteric peptide hormones play an important role in regulating the neurohumoral control of the GI smooth muscles. The enteric neurons contain both excitatory and inhibitory neurotransmitters. When stimulated, many nerve cells release more than one neurotransmitter (Table 41.1). The complex interactions among the excitatory and the inhibitory neurotransmitters coordinate the intestinal movement. The enteric nervous system (ENS) integrates information from the periphery and the CNS, and modulates the effector function.

After eating, various enteric peptides are released from the gut mucosa into the blood. These peptides act as hormones and affect gastric, small intestinal and colonic smooth muscle contractions. They are either **stimulatory** or **inhibitory** (Table 41.1). Unlike the enteric

Table 41.1: Some enteric neurotransmitters and peptide hormones which control GI motility

Excitatory	Inhibitory
Acetylcholine	Vasoactive inhibitory polypeptide (VIP)
Gastrin	Noradrenaline
Neurokinins	Nitric oxide
Cholecystokinin	ATP
5-Hydroxytryptamine	Somatostatin (in large doses)
Somatostatin (in small doses)	Peptide YY
Motilin	Enteroglucagon
Enkephalin	

neurotransmitters which affect the function immediately, the peptide hormones may mediate a delayed GI response to eating. Since the CNS plays an important role in controlling the activity of the GI smooth muscle, psychological disturbances also cause GI motility disorders.

Physiology of defaecation: Intestinal movements are mainly of three types :

- ***Pendular***, due to annular contraction of longitudinal muscles.
- ***Segmental***, due to contraction of circular muscles; and
- ***Peristaltic.***

The first two are responsible for mixing of the food while peristalsis helps in propulsion. Normally, food leaves the stomach in about ½ to 2½ hours and its residue reaches the caecum by about 5 to 6 hours. It takes approximately 18 to 24 hours before the process of evacuation starts and the total time necessary for complete clearance of the ingested material is approximately 5 to 6 days. After ingestion of barium sulfate, the barium shadow can be first seen in the caecum at about 4½ hours, in the descending colôn at about 11 hours and in the pelvic colon at about 18 hours. The global transit time (the time after ingestion to complete clearance from the G.I. tract) of a radio-opaque marker, such as barium sulfate, is about 5 days. If it is normal, the patient is probably not constipated. Usually, the peristaltic waves occur frequently upto ileum while they are very irregular in case of transverse, descending and pelvic colon, except during the gastrocolic reflex.

The Asians have relatively shorter colonic transit time (CTT) of 15-24 hours than the mean CTT of 30.7 hours in the Americans. The normal frequency of stools (1-2/day) among Indians is higher than that (3 or more times a week) in the western populations. These differences could be due to differences in the diet, especially its fibre content.

Normally, most of the ingested water and fluids secreted by various gastrointestinal glands are reabsorbed and only about 100 ml. of fluid is excreted with the faecal matter. Most of the absorption takes place in the small intestine and caecum. Hence, a laxative which acts mainly in the small intestine is likely to produce considerable loss of fluids, electrolytes and nutrients from the gut. Furthermore, the absorption of food is also interfered with. On the other hand, laxatives which act only on the colon produce relatively less fluid loss and do not interfere with the absorption of food. Absorption of water continues even in the colon and contents which are normally fluid upto ascending colon become semisolid during their passage through transverse and descending colon and are then stored as faecal matter in pelvic colon. The act of defaecation is initiated by distension of the rectum. If this sensation is ignored habitually, it may lead to the development of constipation.

The rate of intestinal passage of food depends on the nature of the diet and its fluidity. The greater the indigestible residue and water content, the more rapidly it reaches the rectum and produces its distension. Diminished intake of both water and indigestible residue can lead to constipation. Further, constipation, though commonly due to a lax, atonic colon, may also be associated with a hypersegmenting, high pressure bowel. Although emotional stress and physical exercise can modulate the GI transit, they are not its primary regulators.

Table 41.2: Drugs and GI contractility

Drugs	Stomach	Small intestine	Colon
Cholinergics : Carbachol, Neostigmine	E	E	E
Dopamine antagonists : Metoclopramide, Domperidone	E	E	–
5-HT$_4$ agonist : Cisapride	E	E	E
Antimuscarinic : Atropine	I	I	I
CCB : Verapamil, Nifedipine	I	I	I
Macrolide antibiotic*: Erythromycin	E	E	?
Opioids	I	I	–
Nitrates	?	I	I
Peppermint oil	?	I	I

E = excitatory; I = inhibitory; * = probably act on the motilin receptors. ? = Not clear

Most diarrhoeal diseases act through multiple mechanisms and affect many types of cells in the intestinal tract, including neurons, endocrine cells, inflammatory cells and epithelial cells. **The mechanisms include:**

- ***Increasing the adenylate cyclase and cAMP content of the intestinal epithelial cells,*** resulting in a decrease in sodium absorption and stimulation of chloride secretion.
- ***Stimulation of enteric nerves and 5HT-containing neuroendocrine cells;*** and
- ***Initiation of intestinal metabolism of arachidonic acid by the cyclo-oxygenase pathway with the formation of PGs.***

Laxatives act through multiple mechanisms affecting the epithelial transfer, directly or indirectly, leading to decreased sodium absorption and increase in chloride secretion by intestinal epithelial cells. Similarly, increase in fecal concentration of PGs has been observed following some laxatives.

Table 41.2 lists the effects of other drugs on GI contractility.

Classification of laxatives: These drugs are classified according to the intensity of action as **mild**, **moderate** or **drastic**. Laxative effect suggests the elimination of soft, formed stool without griping and without much loss of water. In large doses,many laxatives promote **catharsis** which means purgation, the passage of fluid stools and griping. Laxatives can also be classified according to their mechanism of action as follows:

I **Stimulant or irritant laxatives:**

- ***Anthraquinone*** group e.g. Cascara sagrada and Senna.
- ***Irritant oils,*** e.g., Castor oil.
- ***Miscellaneous,*** e.g., Phenolphthalein, Bisacodyl, Sodium picosulfate.

All these drugs can cause some amount of griping, mucus production and fluid loss.

II **Osmotic laxatives** e.g. Magnesium sulfate, Milk of magnesia, Magnesium citrate, Potassium sodium tartrate, Lactulose and Polyethylene glycol (PEG).

III **Bulk laxatives,** e.g. Methyl cellulose, Agar agar, Plantago seeds and Bran.

IV **Emollient laxatives,** e.g. Liquid paraffin and Dioctyl sodium sulfosuccinate.

V **Chloride Channel activator,** e.g. Lubiprostone.

VI **Prokinetic agents,** such as e.g. 5-HT$_4$ receptor agonist e.g. Tegeserod (now withdrawn).

They may also be classified clinically

according to the onset of laxative effect following the therapeutic doses into those with:

- ***Slow onset*** which soften the stool after 1 to 3 days of daily use : Bulk laxatives, Mineral oil, Dioctyl sodium sulfosuccinate, Lactulose.
- ***Intermediate onset*** which cause soft or semifluid stool in 6-12 hrs. of a single dose : Saline laxatives (low dose), Bisacodyl (oral), Anthraquinone group;
- ***Rapid onset*** which produce watery evacuation in 2-6 hrs. of a single dose: Saline laxatives (high dose), Castor oil, Bisacodyl (rectal).

Anthraquinone Group

The two most commonly used agents are **Cascara sagrada** and **Senna.** The active constituent anthraquinone is present as an inactive precursor glycoside in the leaves, pods and roots of these plants. Anthraquinone is also present in a variety of other plants in the vegetable kingdom. On oral administration of extracts from these plants, the active anthraquinone derivatives, mainly oxymethyl anthraquinones, are liberated in the small intestine, where they are partly absorbed. These agents do not act on the small intestine, probably because the release of the active principle is too slow. However, sufficient quantity reaches the large intestine, via the blood as well as by intestinal propulsion of the unabsorbed portion.

Anthraquinone acts by stimulation of the large bowel, and also probably by inhibiting NaCl and water absorption in the colon.

Pharmacological actions: As these drugs act mainly on the large bowel, evacuation occurs 6-8 hours after their ingestion. Stools are usually semisolid and the incidence of griping is low. There are no other important actions of the absorbed anthraquinone derivatives. However they are excreted in milk during lactation and this may produce diarrhoea in breast-fed infants. Some of the constituents are excreted in urine and colour the acid urine yellowish brown and alkaline urine reddish violet. The patient should be informed about this.

Cascara is more bitter in taste while senna produces more griping.

Adverse reactions: The only important toxicity is excessive purgation and griping. Chronic use may lead to benign melanotic pigmentation of the colonic mucosa.

Preparations and dosage: Cascara sagrada is obtained from the bark of a tree *Rhamnus purshiana.* The available preparations are:

(i) Cascara sagrada liquid extract. Dose: 2-5 ml.

(ii) Cascara sagrada extract in powdered preparation. Dose: 300 mg.

(iii) Cascara sagrada tablets: one to two tablets at bed time.

Both the dried senna fruits (Senna pods) and dried senna leaves, obtained from the plants *Cassia acutifolia* and *Cassia angustifolia* respectively, are employed as cold water decoction in India as home remedies for their laxative effect. The dose in each case is 0.6 to 2 g. at bedtime. Other unofficial preparations are senna fluid extract, dose 2 ml. and senna syrup, dose 8 ml. Laxative preparations containing standardized, purified concentrates (Senocot) and those containing purified senna glycosides (Glaxenna) are also available.

Aloe and **rhubarb**, used as vegetable foodstuffs, also have a mild laxative effect.

Irritant Oils

CASTOR OIL: It is a fixed oil obtained from the seeds of *Ricinus communis* Linn. Chemically, it is a triglyceride of ricinoleic acid, an unsaturated hydroxy fatty acid. Castor oil itself is non-irritant and is used as hair oil or applied to skin as emollient. When ingested, it is hydrolysed in the intestine by pancreatic lipase to glycerol and ricinoleic acid. Ricinoleic acid acts as an irritant and produces purgation.

Pharmacological actions: As ricinoleic acid acts on the small intestine, it produces copious, liquid stools, with associated fluid loss. Colonic emptying may be so complete that the patient may not pass a stool for several days. The action is quicker than that of anthraquinone and is evident within 2-3 hours. It causes griping. Ricinoleic acid that is absorbed is metabolized like any other fatty acid. The drug interferes with the absorption of various nutrients. It may stimulate uterine contraction in pregnant women.

Castor oil is a pale yellowish or almost colourless oil with peculiar odour and an initially bland but a nauseating after-taste.

Miscellaneous Stimulant Laxatives

PHENOLPHTHALEIN: The discovery of phenolphthalein as a laxative was purely accidental. In order to identify cheap wines, the Hungarian government ordered addition of this compound to such wines, since on the addition of alkali it turns brilliant red. The procedure was considered to be harmless. Those who took such sparkling drinks freely, obviously could not enjoy them as they suffered from diarrhoea.

Pharmacological actions: The drug acts as a stimulant mainly on the large bowel after 6-8 hours, and produces soft, semi-liquid stools, with a little griping. About 15 per cent of the dose is absorbed, some of which is re-excreted in the bile. This **enterohepatic circulation** of the drug causes prolongation of its effect. A part of the absorbed portion is excreted by the kidney, mainly in the conjugated form. The alkaline urine and faeces may get a reddish colour.

Adverse reactions: Phenolphthalein can cause excessive purgation. Allergic skin rash with colourful lesions may persist for long time.

Phenolphthalein is no more recommended because of its potential carcinogenicity.

BISACODYL (Dulcolax): This drug, structurally related to phenolphthalein, is used orally and as rectal suppository. It is rapidly converted by intestinal enzymes and bacteria to **its active desacetyl metabolite which directly stimulates the large bowel.** It is not absorbed from the gut and is less toxic. It is supplied as 5 mg. enteric coated tablets for oral use and as 10 mg. rectal suppositories. The suppository is effective within 15 minutes to 1 hour. Prolonged use (more than 10 days) may cause local irritation.

SODIUM PICOSULFATE (Cremalax): Like bisacodyl, this drug is hydrolysed by colonic bacteria, **acts on the large bowel** and results in a soft, formed stool in 10-14 hours. The oral, adult dose is 5-15 mg as a single bedtime dose.

Osmotic Laxatives

Certain salts, non-absorbable disaccharides and higher alcohols, given orally, are not much absorbed and are retained in the GI tract. Such preparations exert an osmotic effect and hold considerable amounts of water, thus increasing the intestinal bulk. This acts as a mechanical stimulus causing an increase in the intestinal motor activity and evacuation. Release of cholecystokinin-pancreozymin with consequent stimulation of intestinal secretory and motor activity has been proposed as an additional mechanism of action of the magnesium salts.

The commonly employed saline laxatives are magnesium, sodium and potassium salts.

Pharmacological actions: These compounds act in the small as well as the large intestines and, therefore, produce a watery evacuation within 3 to 6 hours. Because of their quick onset of action, they are given early in the morning before breakfast. They do not cause irritation and there is very little griping. Patients should be instructed to take plenty of water along with these drugs since administration of a hypertonic solution may produce dehydration.

Small amounts of these drugs may get absorbed into the circulation and may cause occasional toxicity, in the presence of kidney damage. Thus, the absorption of magnesium may cause CNS depression while that of sodium may worsen the existing CHF. This is most unlikely in normal subjects, as the small amount absorbed is rapidly excreted by the kidneys.

Preparations and Dosage:

(i) Magnesium sulfate, $7H_2O$. (Epsom salt)- bitter salt, soluble in water. Dose 5-10 g. Hypertonic solution is sometimes used rectally to reduce increased intracranial tension.

(ii) Dried magnesium sulfate, Dose 2 to 12 g.

(iii) Milk of Magnesia is a 7.0 to 8.5 per cent acqueous suspension of magnesium hydroxide. Dose: 20 ml.

(iv) Magnesium carbonate, heavy or light. Dose : 2 to 4 g.

(v) Magnesium citrate is pleasant to take but expensive.

(vi) Magnesium oxide. Dose: 2 to 4 g.

(vii) Sodium potassium tartrate (Rochelle salt) is administered in the dose of 8 to 16 g. Tartrate ion, not being absorbed from the GI tract, does not produce systemic toxicity.

(viii) Seidlitz powder is a mixture, in which 2.5 g. of sodium bicarbonate and 7.5 g. of Rochelle salt are dispensed together in a blue paper while 2.5 g. of tartaric acid is dispensed in a white paper. The user dissolves the contents of two papers separately in 30 ml. of water and drinks the mixture after the effervescence begins to subside. *The powders must not be taken separately.* Carbon dioxide evolved acts as a carminative and masks the unpleasant saline taste.

LACTULOSE (Livoluk): This is a synthetic non-absorbable disaccharide which acts by its osmotic effect. It is converted to lactic acid which can bind ammonia. Because of this property as well as its laxative effect, lactulose is used in the dose of 30-50 ml. of the solution (3.5 g. of lactulose per 5 ml.) with plenty of water, three times a day in the treatment of hepatic coma; the dose is adjusted to produce 2-3 soft stools per day. The primary osmotic effect may be aided by lactate and other organic acids to which it is metabolized by bacterial action in the distal ileum and colon.

Lactitol: This synthetic disaccharide is more palatable than lactulose.

GLYCERIN: Glycerin is used in the form of rectal suppositories (3 g. for adults and 1 to 1.5 g. for children). It acts by its osmotic effect to soften and lubricate the dried up feces. It may also stimulate rectal contractions. Glycerin is also used as a glycerin-edible oil (30-50 ml. of each) enema, introduced into the rectum with a syringe. Other uses of glycerine are:

Oral glycerin:

- Treatment of acute congestive glaucoma (Chapter 70) and cerebral edema (Chapter 38).
- As a sweetening / flavouring agent.

Topical glycerin:

- As a hygroscopic agent along with magnesium sulfate as dressing for wounds, ulcers and abscesses (Chapter 68).
- As an emollient.

In-vitro uses:

- As a vehicle for drugs.

Polyethylene glycol (PEG)-electrolytes: (Osmolax, Pegleg) is supplied as a powder or as a ready-to-use electrolyte solution. It is administered orally in the dose of 4 litres, 250 ml every 15-20 minutes, over a period of 4 hours. It can also be given by nasogastric tube at the rate of 25 ml/minute. Since the solution is isotonic, dehydration does not occur. It can be used for bowel cleansing before bowel surgery, colonoscopy, radiological examination, and to treat acute poisoning. The dose to treat constipation is 250-500 ml orally once a day. After reconstitution, the solution should be stored in a fridge, and used within 24 hours. It is not recommended in patients weighing less than 20 kg.

Bulk Laxatives

These are natural or semisynthetic polysaccharides and cellulose derivatives, which are not absorbed and increase the indigestible residue. They absorb water and swell up, thus providing the stimulus of mechanical distension for evacuation. Generous amounts of water are prescribed with all bulk laxatives.

Pharmacological actions: These agents act because of their physical property. Their action is mild and is usually seen 12-36 hours after ingestion. They produce evacuation of solid or semisolid stools without irritation or griping. Some of these agents also have lubricating properties. Usually, these drugs are administered at bed time, with plenty of water.

These drugs are not absorbed and do not have any systemic toxicity. Intestinal obstruction has been reported very rarely.

Because these agents help to produce formed stools, they are also recommended in the treatment of diarrhoea. As many of these agents, when administered in a palatable form, can increase the bulk of indigestible material in the food, they have also been recommended in the treatment of obesity for satisfying appetite.

Preparations and Dosage:

AGAR: It is a mucilagenous substance extracted from marine algae. It contains indigestible hemicellulose. With water, it forms a gel which has emollient or lubricating properties. The dose is 4 g.; occasionally, however, a large dose 40 g. may be required.

ISAPGOL: consists of dried seeds of *Plantago ovata Forsk.* The seeds, which are hard and pinkish-grey to brown in colour, contain a large amount of natural mucilage. Many OTC preparations contain Psyllium husk derived for plantago seeds. Dose: 5 to 15 g.

SABZA: This consists of the dried seeds of *Ocimum basilicum* Linn, a plant belonging to the *tulasi* family. The seeds are rich in mucilage and can be used as a substitute for isapgol.

BRAN: It is the byproduct of the milling of wheat and contains almost 40% of fibre. Processed bran is palatable as such and it may be mixed with flour for preparing chapatis/bread. Dose : 12-24 g. daily, in divided doses.

METHYL CELLULOSE, AND SODIUM CARBOXYMETHYL CELLULOSE are hydrophilic, semisynthetic derivatives of cellulose. The latter is insoluble in hydrochloric acid. Methylcellulose is administered in the dose of 1 g., 1 to 4 times daily, while sodium carboxymethyl cellulose is administered in the dose of 1.5 g., 1 to 4 times a day. The preparations should be taken with 30 to 40 ml. of water to minimize the risk of oesophageal obstruction.

Bulk forming laxatives are especially useful in patients with:

- ***Irritable bowel syndrome.***
- ***Hemorrhoids and anal fissures.***
- ***Chronic diarrhoea*** associated with diverticular disease and ulcerative colitis; and
- ***Colostomy or ileostomy.***

Dietary fibre and bowel disorders: Unrefined plant products (fruits, vegetables, pulses, nuts and especially wholegrain products such as 100% whole-wheat flour and unpolished rice) are rich in indigestible cell wall materials. This material, known in the past as 'roughage' or 'residue' is now called 'fibre'. Chemically, this consists mainly of cellulose, hemicelluloses, pectins and lignin. Following ingestion, they hold water, form gels, exchange cations and bind bile acids. **In the colon, they are mainly broken down to short-chain fatty acids, which may influence the colonic function favourably.** Thus, the stool becomes bulkier and softer so that the need for straining is decreased. Occasionally, frequency of defaecation is increased. Increased intake of such fibre has been found useful not only in simple constipation but also in spastic colon, irritable bowel syndrome, colonic diverticular disease, and in anal fissures and piles. Higher consumption of fibre rich food (vegetables and fruits) may decrease the duration of contact of locally (in the colon) formed carcinogens with the colonic wall and may be helpful in preventing colonic cancer.

The best way of increasing the fibre-intake is to include fibre-rich foods in the diet. In persons who cannot or will not consume sufficient fibre-rich food, wheat bran may be added to food or taken with water. Eating of raw fruits and certain raw vegetables may however, often cause abdominal discomfort, bloating, griping and diarrhoea and should be avoided. A daily intake of 20-60 g. of dietary fibre would appear to be sufficient for easy bowel movements. Bran and other similar substances such as gum have been claimed to be useful in reducing hyperglycemia in diabetics, as well as plasma cholesterol.

Emollient Laxatives

LIQUID PARAFFIN: This mineral oil is the most widely used emollient laxative. It consists of a mixture of hydrocarbons obtained from petroleum. Given orally, it is not significantly absorbed and exerts a softening and lubricating effect on faeces.

Pharmacological actions: It is mild in action and in itself **does not initiate peristalsis**. Because of its **lubricant action**, the straining during defaecation can be avoided. It is usually given at bed time, but can be taken at any time of the day.

It is almost non-toxic but used repeatedly, it may interfere with the absorption of essential fat soluble substances and may cause a deficiency of vitamins A, D and K. The small amount which is absorbed from the intestinal tract may get deposited in the intestinal mucosa, liver and spleen and may, therefore, interfere with their functions. Its chronic use can cause granulomatous fibrosis in the intestinal wall and more diffusely in the reticuloendothelial system. Rarely, it can cause lipoid pneumonitis, if it gets into the lungs during its administration in bedridden patient and in old people. *It should not be used in children under three years of age.*

Preparation and dosage: Liquid paraffin is a colourless, oily liquid. Dose: 10 to 30 ml. It is also available in emulsified form (Cremaffin).

Edible oils like coconut oil, ground nut oil, cotton seed oil and corn oil are employed as lubricant laxatives. However, they are digested and hence, fairly large doses are needed for lubricant effect. The usual dose is 30 ml.

DIOCTYL SODIUM SULFOSUCCINATE (Docusate, Cellubril) : This drug, which is used in pharmaceutical industry as a dispersing agent, **acts by its physical property of lowering surface tension.** It does not stimulate peristalsis but promotes softening of faeces. It is slow acting and takes 1-2 days to act.

Dose: 100-200 mg. three times a day. It should not be combined with liquid paraffin as it may enhance the absorption of the latter.

5-HT$_4$ Receptor Agonists

TEGASEROD : This prokinetic drug acts as a 5-HT$_4$ agonist in the entire GI tract. It has been withdrawn from the market in the USA for reasons of safety (Chapter 40).

Chloride Channel Activators

Lubiprostone (Amipizo) : This drug acts locally in the GI tract by opening chloride channels, resulting in secretion of chloride rich intestinal fluid. This **accelerates small intestinal and colonic transit.** The drug also delays gastric emptying. The adverse effects are nausea (31%), headache and diarrhoea. It is contraindicated during pregnancy. It is used in chronic idiopathic constipation. It is expensive.

Therapeutic uses of laxatives:

- ***In constipation due to diminished intestinal tone*** as in old age and pregnancy.
- ***In food or drug poisoning*** to flush the intestinal tract. Saline laxatives are generally preferred.
- ***To provide a fresh stool*** for parasitic examination.

• ***Following anthelmintic therapy,*** to eliminate the parasites; saline laxatives are preferred.

• ***Preoperatively in abdominal surgery or prior to radiological examination of the abdomen (bowel cleansing action).***

• ***In patients with painful anal conditions (fissure, thrombosed piles), and in cardiac disease (acute myocardial infarction),*** in order to spare the patient straining during defecation. In these conditions, a lubricating laxative such as liquid paraffin is preferred.

• ***In patients with severe neuromuscular disease*** who have poor muscle strength.

• ***In drug induced constipation*** such as that during the use of opioids or drugs with antimuscarinic property.

• ***In patients with hepatic encephalopathy***, to reduce the colonic absorption of ammonia and other unknown toxins.

• ***In patients with an ileostomy or colostomy***, to modify the effluent; and

• ***In children with encopresis (passage of normal stools in socially unacceptable places; it is normal in the first 3 years of life) and congenital/acquired megacolon.***

It must be pointed out that laxatives are more often misused than used properly. Such misuse can lead to serious consequences.

Irritant laxatives should be avoided during pregnancy as these may cause pelvic congestion, although abortion following therapeutic doses of laxatives is most unlikely. Similarly, these drugs should also be avoided in case of typhoid fever and in very ill cardiac patients; in such patients, if satisfactory evacuation fails to occur following lubricant laxatives, simple enema or a suppository may be employed.

Laxatives are absolutely contraindicated in patients with undiagnosed acute abdomen and in cases with intestinal obstruction as violent contractions may lead to intestinal rupture and subsequent peritonitis.

ENEMAS: See Chapter 1 for general information on enemas. Their use for bowel evacuation is discussed here; the use of retention enemas for other purposes is discussed in appropriate chapters.

Evacuant enemas cause fragmentation, liquefaction or lubrication of the feces. Fluid distention of the bowel wall causes reflex evacuation. They act locally and may be preferred to laxatives in some situations. As an enema, one may introduce into the rectum plain tap water (this should be used only in adults but not in infants or children); soapsuds (only neutral but not alkaline soap should be used for this purpose); isotonic sodium chloride (one level-teaspoon common salt per half litre of water); mineral or vegetable oil; glycerine; a surfactant (docusate sodium); or a stimulant laxative (bisacodyl).

The enema should be administered very gently to prevent local injury to the bowel. Tap water enema may cause water intoxication, especially in infants and children. Irritant substances such as hot water, household detergents and strongly hypertonic salt solutions should not be used.

The indications for evacuant enema are:

• ***Fecal impaction.*** This may have to be treated intially by introducing a mineral or vegetable oil, followed by digital rectal evacuation.

• ***To empty the colon and the rectum before radiologic or endoscopic examination.***

• ***To cleanse the large bowel prior to surgery or childbirth.***

• ***In patients with incontinence or colostomies; and***

• ***As substitutes for glycerine suppositories and oral laxatives to re-establish the rectal reflex in constipated patients.***

Constipation and Laxatives

Constipation may be defined as "functional impairment in the inherent capacity of the colon to produce normally formed stools at regular intervals." Individuals are known to differ widely in the 'normal' habits concerning the frequency, quantity and consistency of stools, and missing a bowel movement does not necessarily affect the health adversely. Failure to realise this may lead to self medication and to laxative habit. In most cases, 'constipation' is functional and can be corrected by simple measures such as increasing the roughage and water intake, exercise and by treatment of emotional factors, if any. The proper 'habit time' (conditioned effect) should be developed and the natural reflex, when it occurs, should not be ignored habitually.

The bulk residue can be increased and stools can be softened by simple measures such as increasing bran or leafy vegetables in the diet or by using bulk laxatives like isapgol, methyl cellulose or agar agar. Food fibre is more effective as a laxative than synthetic fibre. Cereal fibre (bran) is more effective in this respect than fruits and vegetables. Such measures are particularly useful in patients with irritable bowel syndrome, who may complain of constant or intermittent symptoms with the passage of small, round 'rabbit' or 'sheep' stools and abdominal pain aggravated by fatigue, smoking and mental tension. The pain could be related to the ingestion of certain foods such as coffee, spices, fried foods, certain vegetables and fruits and even milk. Only in a few cases of chronic constipation, mild stimulant laxatives from the vegetable group may be necessary in initial stages. In old or obese individuals and in convalescing patients who find it difficult to strain, lubricant drugs or suppositories are useful, while in those in whom spastic colon is suspected, use of antimuscarinic preparations may be beneficial. Constipation associated with diseases like vitamin B deficiency or hypothyroidism will be corrected following vitamin B or thyroxine therapy. The presence of a painful anal condition should be enquired into in patients with constipation. Retraining of bowel habits is important. Encouraging patients to drink plenty of water, to do abdominal muscle exercises and avoidance of excessive use of laxatives are helpful. In elderly patients with chronic constipation, the use of senna along with a bulk laxative may be effective and economical.

Constipation in infants and children sometimes poses a problem. In many cases, however, it is exaggerated by the anxious parents who believe that a daily good evacuation is necessary for good health. It is essential, therefore, that parents, particularly mothers, should know that the dire consequences of constipation are mostly imaginary. It is known that breast fed babies may have infrequent stools, sometimes once every four days, without any abnormal symptoms. This obviously needs no treatment. In artificially fed babies, hard stools are often produced because of under-feeding or deficient intake of water and sugar in the feeds; the water requirement in warm countries like India is usually more than that in the temperate zones. In such cases, increasing the water intake and adding more sugar to feeds corrects the constipation. Daily consumption of a few black resins or a fig or two is known to help children with constipation. Occasionally, however, one has to prescribe a laxative particularly in those children in whom passing of hard stools is associated with considerable discomfort. The drug usually advocated is magnesium hydroxide mixture (Milk of magnesia). Suppositories containing glycerine may be prescribed when other methods are not helpful. It acts by its hygroscopic action within 10-20 minutes. It is reliable, safe and cheap. In some cases with really formidable constipation, enemas are necessary to clear the bowel.

Laxatives used occasionally are not harmful but their repeated administration may produce:

- ***GI disturbances*** like dyspepsia, anorexia, nausea and spastic colitis.
- ***Nutritional deficiency*** of calories, vitamins, and minerals due to interference with their absorption.
- ***Loss of fluid and electrolytes***, particularly potassium and calcium, giving rise to hypokalemia and osteomalacia.
- ***Complete dependence on drugs*** and later even resistance to all the mild laxatives, due to the development of spastic colon.

- *Selective toxicity* due to certain drugs.

After a thorough evacuation following a laxative, it may take some days to normalise the bowel movement and individuals should be told about this. Otherwise, they may feel that the constipation is continuing and continue to take the purgative.

It is important that family physicians should counter the false notions created in the minds of lay people, many times by commercial advertisements, and must emphasize the limitations of laxatives rather than prescribe them readily, whenever the patient complains of 'constipation'.

In the clinical management of persistent constipation, it is very essential to carry out an abdominal and rectal examination to exclude any local rectal or anal lesion to exclude possible local organic disease. In patients with primary intestinal pathology and secondary constipation, attention to primary disease is of utmost importance.

Table 41.3: Drugs causing constipation

- Those with antimuscarinic action (atropine-like agents, antihistaminics with H_1 blocking effect, antiparkinsonian agents, tricyclic antidepressants and phenothiazines).
- Prostaglandin inhibitors (NSAIDs).
- Opioids
- Calcium carbonate and aluminium hydroxide used as antacids.
- Sympathomimetic amines.
- Antidiarrhoeal agents.
- Miscellaneous : Clonidine, iron, MAO inhibitors, verapamil and phenytoin.

Table 41.3 gives the commonly used drugs which may cause constipation.

Treatment of Hemorrhoids and Anal Fissure

Perianal pruritus, soreness and excoriations are common symptoms in addition to bleeding in hemorrhoids; and acute anal pain due to spasm of the anal sphincter occurs in anal fissure. Avoidance of hard stools by the use of bulk laxatives and/or liquid paraffin and a high fibre diet are helpful in these conditions. Local application of a bland, zinc salt containing ointment relieves these local symptoms. Application of an ointment containing a local anaesthetic such as nupercaine before passing a stool helps to relieve the local pain and ease the sphincter spasm. There is evidence that relaxation of the anal sphincter is mediated by nitric oxide NO (Chapter 28). Nitroglycerine ointment (0.2%, Myovin) or isosorbide dinitrate 1% ointment is used for local application in cases of anal fissure, with relief of spasm and pain, and healing of the fissure. While prescribing the preparations, the patient should be warned that headache might follow their application. Similarly, botulinum toxin by local injection (Chapter 21) into the anal sphincter has been used in resistant cases. It acts by preventing the release of acetylcholine locally.

Preparations for local application containing antibiotics and corticosteroids have little rationale and may even be harmful. For sclerosant therapy of bleeding hemorrhoids see Chapter 32.

Pharmacotherapy of Peptic Ulcer Disease 42

Peptic ulcer disease is one of the common GI disorders in clinical practice. The common forms of peptic ulcer are:

- ***Duodenal ulcer (DU).***
- ***Gastric ulcer (GU).***
- ***Stress ulcer(s)***; and
- ***NSAID induced ulcer.***

Of these, the DU is largely a disease of adult males. Women are relatively immune to DU during the child-bearing age. Gastric ulcers occur most frequently in the older age group and in the lower socio-economic class of individuals. DU, on the other hand, occur commonly in younger individuals and are evenly distributed among various socio-economic groups.

Peptic ulceration occurs mostly in areas which are bathed by the acid juice. Although the exact etiology of ulceration is not known, a high association between *H. pylori* infection of the stomach and duodenum and peptic ulcer disease has now been established. It was Dr. Warron, a pathologist who, by chance, first noticed "numerous curved bacilli lying below the stomach's protective mucus in a gastric biopsy sample" (1979). Later work by Warrron and Marshall conclusively showed the association of these bacilli, now known as *Helicobacter pylori*, with chronic gastritis and ulceration. They were awarded the Nobel Prize in 2005. *H. pylori* is a Gram negative bacillus that colonises the stomach and the duodenum. The infection is acquired by fecal-oral route in early childhood and is mainly transmitted within families. The organism does not invade the mucosa but attaches itself to the epithelial cells. It secretes (a) a urease which hydrolyses urea into carbon dioxide and ammonia; the latter permits the bacilli to survive in the acid environment of the stomach; and (b) an exotoxin which directly damages the epithelial cells. Although *H. pylori* is present in the G I tract of 50% of the adult population, only 10-20% of the latter develop DU. Therefore, there must be a *host factor* in the pathogenesis of peptic ulcer disease.

H. pylori causes chronic gastritis in majority of the persons whose GI tract it colonises. Nearly all patients with DU and almost 80% of patients with GU show colonization of the stomach by *H. pylori*. *H. pylori* are also strongly implicated in the pathogenesis of gastric carcinoma and gastric lymphoma. Those with infection of the gastric antrum have hyperacidity and develop DU; those with infection of the body of the stomach develop low acidity and GU. Eradication of *H. pylori* benefits patients with all these clinical entities. Once the infection is eradicated, reinfection is rare (less than 1% per year) and hence, the benefit is lasting.

Factors modifying gastric acid secretion: The gastric juice is a mixture containing hydrochloric acid, pepsin, renin (in children), neutral chlorides, mucus, intrinsic factor and traces of potassium, ammonium and calcium.

The gastric acid and pepsin are secreted by the

main gastric glands, containing highly specialized cells, present all over the body and fundus of the stomach. The rate and the composition of the secretion of main gastric glands vary considerably, depending upon the number of acid-secreting cells (the parietal cell mass), emotional factors, digestive state, hormonal status and the presence of extrinsic chemical stimuli such as caffeine and histamine.

The **parietal (oxyntic) cells** are located in the walls of the midsection of the oxyntic glands, the secretory unit of the gastric mucosa. The parietal cell has prominent cytoplasmic turbulo-vesicles. In addition, these glands contain chief, mucous, ECL and somatostatin cells.

Gastric acid secretion is regulated by intricate central and peripheral mechanisms. The central mechanism acts through the vagus nerve. In addition, ACh liberated from the postganglionic nerve fibres directly stimulates the parietal cells.

Three distinct but interdependent pathways deliver chemical messengers that stimulate acid secretion by parietal cells (Fig. 42.1) :

- ***The neurocrine pathway***, that acts through the transmitter acetylcholine.
- ***The endocrine pathway*** which delivers hormone gastrin from antral G cells; and
- ***The paracrine pathway*** which delivers tissue factors, such as histamine from enterochromafin like (ECL) cells.

The tubulovesicular and canalicular structures of the parietal cells possess a specific hydrogen-potassium-ATPase enzyme **(proton pump)**. When stimulated, it causes the transport of H^+ ions across the parietal cells in exchange of K^+ ions. The final process of acid transport *per se* rests with this enzyme. Hydrogen ions combine with Cl^- ions to form HCl. The proton pump is activated by protein kinases, histamine, acetylcholine and gastrin.

The fundic mucosa also contain several paracrine cells, secreting somatostatin, histamine, and serotonin (5-HT). They possess receptors that may regulate acid secretion by modulating the release of the paracrine transmitters. Thus, ACh may enhance the secretion of acid not only by stimulating the parietal cell directly, but also by reducing the level of somatostatin, a potent inhibitor of acid secretion.

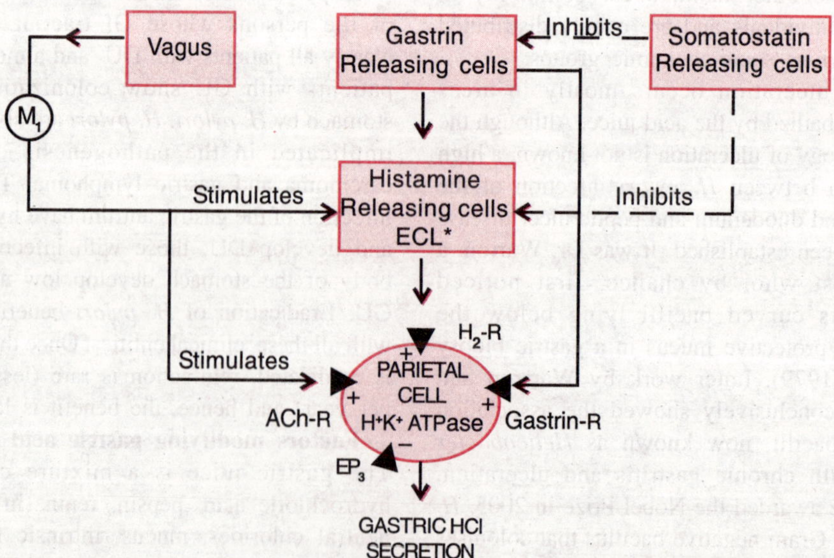

Fig. 42.1 : Mechanisms involved in regulation of gastric acid secretion by the parietal cells. R = Receptors. * Enterochromaffin like (cells). Gastrin acts mostly indirectly by releasing histamine. EP_3–R = PG receptor for PGE_2; M_1 = Muscarinic

Prostaglandin E (PGE) is produced by cells throughout the GI tract. PGE, inhibits the secretion of gastric acid in humans, particularly food and NSAID stimulated acid secretion.

The **pyloric glands**, present in pyloric antrum, secrete:

- ***Gastrin, directly into the blood;*** and
- ***An alkaline, viscid, mucous-rich juice, into the stomach.***

Gastrin stimulates acid secretion mainly by causing the release of histamine from the ECL cells which are the sole source of gastric histamine involved in acid secretion (Fig. 42.1). The *chief cells* of the gastric glands secrete pepsinogen, which is activated at acidic pH below 5 to the enzyme pepsin. Optimal activation occurs at pH 2.

Normal gastric acid secretion acts as a chemical barrier to bacterial invasion and is important for the maintenance of optimum pH at 1.5 to 4, necessary for the activity of pepsin, which is markedly reduced at pH above 4 and almost ceases at pH 5.

Phases of gastric secretion: Gastric acid secretion is generally divided into four phases:

- ***Interdigestive or basal.***
- ***Cephalic.***
- ***Gastric;*** and
- ***Intestinal.***

During the first three phases, acid output is stimulated when food is first encountered and it continues as nutrients traverse the small intestine. During the fourth phase, acid is secreted in the absence of an external stimulus.

Basal secretion: This follows a circadian rhythm, reaching its peak around midnight and its nadir at approximately 7 a.m. Measured as nocturnal acid secretion, it is high in some patients with DU but may be normal or low in patients with GU.

Secretion in response to food: Gastric secretion in response to food may be divided into two phases, neurogenic and hormonal.

- ***In neurogenic* or *cephalic phase,*** the secretion occurs as a result of sight, smell, taste or even simple thought of food. The juice secreted is highly acidic and rich in pepsin. It is mediated by the vagus and is abolished by vagotomy and antimuscarinic drugs. The gastric secretion induced by emotions are also mediated centrally. In man, depression and fear result in a suppression of gastric secretion, whereas anger and resentment result in increased production. Violent emotions cause gastric congestion and hyperemia rendering it more susceptible to traumatic ulceration.
- ***In hormonal phase (gastric and intestinal phases),*** the gastric secretion is increased due to stimulation of the parietal cells by *gastrin*. Gastrin-containing cells are stimulated by food in the stomach and by neuronal input to release gastrin. Gastrin is carried to the ECL (Entero Chromaffin Like) cells where it stimulates the release of histamine, which then activates the H_2-receptors in the parietal cells (Fig. 42.1). In addition, acid secretion is stimulated chemically, specifically by an increase in intraluminal pH and by certain substances in the food, principally proteins and individual amino acids. A cocktail or a protein broth soup before a meal stimulates acid secretion and prepares the stomach for the main dish! Digested protein in the duodenum enhances the output of acid.

After a meal, the secretion of acid is modulated by a *negative-feedback* mechanism in which antral acidification inhibits the further release of gastrin. As the luminal pH approaches 3.5 to 3.0, inhibition of gastrin becomes apparent and at pH 1.5 gastrin release is completely inhibited. **Somatostatin** and its analogue **octreotide** inhibit the antral release of gastrin and also decrease acid secretion directly. In addition, like gastric motility, gastric secretion is inhibited by reflexes initiated in the duodenum by distension, hypertonic contents, fatty acids, amino acids and acid in the duodenum. Thus, a highly fatty meal delays gastric emptying to 4-6 hours, whereas a meal rich in carbohydrate and proteins leaves the stomach in 2-3 hours. Fat in the duodenum stimulates the release of gut hormone *cholecystokinin* (CCK) whereas acid in the duodenal chyme is an effective chemical stimulus for the release of another gut hormone *secretin*. Both secretin and CCK act via circulation to inhibit the stomach motility and glandular secretion. *The hormonal phase is inhibited only partially by antimuscarinic drugs but substantially by H_2-receptor antagonists.*

Natural gastrin is a polypeptide containing 17 aminoacids. A synthetic pentapeptide, **Pentagastrin,** containing five amino acids (alanine, tryptophan, methionine, phenylalanine and aspartic acid) produces secretory and other biological effects similar to those of the gastrin.

Histamine-stimulated gastric secretion is highly acidic but poor in pepsin content. This is similar to gastrin-induced secretion since gastrin acts through the local liberation of histamine. Histamine directly stimulates the parietal cell H_2-receptors that are linked to adenylyl cyclase. Acetylcholine and gastrin may also stimulate the parietal cells directly through different receptors. *Thus, H_2 receptor antagonists inhibit not only gastric secretion elicited by injected histamine but also that elicited by various physiological stimuli, mediated by the vagus or by gastrin.*

Factors which are postulated to protect the gastric and duodenal mucosa against the effects of the 'aggressive factors' are summarised in Table 42.1.

No abnormalities have been consistently demonstrated in *all* patients with either DU or GU, although various abnormalities have been demonstrated, each in *some* peptic ulcer patients. These are:

- ***Acid hypersecretion*** found in 30-40% of patients with DU; it is seen only in patients with GU due to Zollinger-Ellison syndrome.
- ***Hereditary factors*** such as rapid gastric emptying and a larger than normal parietal cell mass found in peptic ulcer patients with rare genetic syndromes.
- ***Diminished gastric mucosal blood flow*** believed to be responsible for the acute gastric erosion occurring during serious medical or surgical illnesses (**stress ulcers**).
- ***An incompetent pyloric sphincter*** found in some patients with peptic ulcer; and
- ***High gastric acid output in stressful situations*** (such as an interview or an examination) and during certain emotions such as hostility, resentment, guilt or frustration.

Table 42.1: Factors protecting the gastric and duodenal mucosa

- ***Mucus*** produced by the cells of the gastric mucous glands.
- ***Bicarbonate*** secreted by the surface epithelial cells, which protects the gastric mucosa from the effects of the highly acidic gastric luminal contents.
- ***Rich Mucosal blood flow*** which removes the acid that might diffuse through the mucosa.
- ***Prostaglandins*** which enhance all the normal gastroduodenal protective mechanisms.
- ***Various growth factors such as epidermal growth factor, and transforming growth factor;***
- ***A competent pyloric sphincter*** which prevents the regurgitation of the aggressive factors (bile acids and pancreatic enzymes) into the stomach.

Principles of peptic ulcer therapy: These are

- ***Controlling gastric acidity, hypermotility and promoting ulcer healing*** (Table 42.2).
- ***Treament of H.pylori infection;*** and
- ***Prevention of complications and recurrence.***

Exogenous factors such as cigarette smoking, NSAID, glucocorticoids and alcohol have been strongly associated with ulcerogenesis, and non-healing of peptic ulcers.

Gastric Antacids

Gastric antacids are substances which, on ingestion, react chemically with gastric acid and

Table 42.2: Measures to control gastric acidity

- Inhibiting the gastric acid secretion and protecting the gastric mucosa:
  (a) H_2 receptor antagonists.
  (b) Proton pump inhibitors; and
  (c) Mucosal protectives.
- Neutralizing gastric acid using antacids.
- Cessation of smoking.
- Withdrawal of gastric acid secretion stimulants such as alcohol, caffeine and soft cola drinks.
- Avoiding acid - inducing drugs.

lower the acidity of gastric contents. They produce symptomatic relief of pain, mainly by reducing the acidity and partly by the consequent relief of muscle spasm. Reduction in acidity inhibits the action of pepsin. It also increases the tone of the esophagogastric sphincter and reduces the reflux of the acid, gastric contents into the esophagus.

If adequate relief of symptoms in DU is to be brought about without seriously interfering with peptic digestion of food, the gastric pH must be raised from the usual level of 1-2 to between 3.5 and 4.5. Although this is possible with antacids, it is difficult to maintain it continuously. Hence, to achieve even a reasonable control of gastric acidity regular and frequent administration of an antacid round the clock would be necessary, which is its main disadvantage.

In spite of their limitations, antacids are valuable as they produce considerable, immediate, symptomatic relief in patients with DU, gastritis and reflux esophagitis. They are often used for the symptomatic treatment of dyspepsia as OTC drugs.

Antacids – Classification:

I **Non-systemic antacids:** Such as aluminium hydroxide gel, magnesium trisilicate, magnesium hydroxide, calcium carbonate.

II **Systemic antacids:** Sodium bicarbonate is absorbed and may cause alkalosis; hence, it is called 'systemic antacid'. A combination of sodium citrate and citric acid, modified Shohl's solution, is equally effective.

Mechanism of action: These drugs acting as weak bases neutralise the gastric HCl. They raise the gastric pH to above 4. Antacids like sodium bicarbonate can theoretically raise the gastric pH above 7. Because of the varying rates of acid neutralization by various antacids, comparison of the amount of acid neutralized per gramme of the antacid does not give valid information about its relative clinical efficacy. The figures of mEq of acid neutralized per gramme or per ml. of the antacid' represent the number of mEq of 1 N HCl that can be brought to pH 3.5 in 15 minutes (Acid Neutralizing Capacity, ANC).

Non-Systemic Antacids

These are water insoluble and largely unabsorbable preparations. In the stomach, the cation e.g. Mg^{++} of the antacid forms a chloride during neutralization of the acid. In the alkaline pH of the small intestine, the chloride salt reacts with the bicarbonate from the intestinal juices to regenerate the original salt (hydroxide or carbonate). There is, thus, no net gain or loss of H^+ or HCO_3— ions to the body. Hence, systemic alkalosis is avoided. In the case of calcium and magnesium salts, formation of soaps may also help to prevent alkalosis by binding organic acids in the intestinal lumen.

Non-systemic antacids are insoluble till they come into contact with the gastric acid. The antacid which escapes this reaction remains in the stomach and reacts with the acid subsequently secreted. Hence, their duration of action of is, longer than that of soluble antacids.

ALUMINIUM HYDROXIDE GEL: This is available either as a white, colloidal, viscous suspension or as dried gel in the form of powder or tablets. It reacts with gastric acid to form aluminium chloride.

Each ml. of 4 per cent gel suspension neutralizes 1.2 to 2.5 mEq of acid. The neutralizing action is slow. The gastric pH is raised to 4. The acid neutralizing capacity differs according to the process of manufacture and age of the product and to vary from batch to batch. Pepsin activity is not significantly inhibited. It has, however, astringent and demulcent properties by which it forms a protective coating over the ulcer crater. It may also adsorb toxins, gases and bacteria.

In the intestines, $Al(OH)_3$, is regenerated from $AlCl_3$ and chloride liberated is reabsorbed.

Adverse reactions: Constipation is the major adverse effect. This is countered by combining it with magnesium trisilicate. Aluminium hydroxide may prevent the absorption of phosphate from the intestines. This may rarely cause osteomalacia. In patients with chronic renal failure, high plasma aluminium may rarely cause encephalopathy and deposition of aluminium in the bone with resultant osteodystrophy.

Preparations and dosage: (i) Aluminium hydroxide gel 4-8 ml. every 2-4 hours. (ii) Aluminium hydroxide 0.5 g tablets; 1-2 tablets to be chewed qid.

ALUMINIUM PHOSPHATE GEL : It is sometimes preferred to aluminium hydroxide gel, as it does not interfere with phosphate absorption.

MAGNESIUM TRISILICATE : It is a fine, white, tasteless powder, insoluble in water. In the stomach, it reacts with acid to form hydrated silicon dioxide. As it becomes gelatinous in consistency, it provides a protective coating to the ulcer crater.

The neutralizing action of magnesium trisilicate is slow in onset but prolonged. In the intestines, magnesium chloride reacts with the bicarbonate to form magnesium carbonate, which is excreted in feces; about 7 per cent is absorbed and excreted in the urine.

Hydrated silica gel has adsorbent properties similar to those of aluminium hydroxide gel.

One gramme of magnesium trisilicate neutralizes about 9-11 mEq of gastric acid.

Adverse reactions: It may cause mild diarrhoea which can be countered by combining it with aluminium hydroxide. A small amount of magnesium absorbed may produce CNS depression in the presence of impaired renal function.

Dose: 2-4 g. every 1-4 hours. The tablet should be chewed before it is swallowed. The drug can also be used in powder form.

MAGNESIUM OXIDE AND HYDROXIDE: Magnesium oxide, on contact with water, is converted to magnesium hydroxide which combines with gastric acid. It is a quick acting antacid with prolonged action. In small intestine, $Mg(OH)_2$ is regenerated and excreted in feces.

Magnesium oxide is a light, colourless, water insoluble powder. One gramme neutralizes 50 mEq of the acid. The dose is rather bulky.

Magnesium hydroxide is available as 'Milk of magnesia' containing 7 to 8.5 per cent of magnesium hydroxide. It is more palatable than other formulations of magnesium salts. One ml. of milk of magnesia neutralizes 2.7 mEq of acid.

Adverse reactions : These are similar to those of other magnesium salts.

Dose: Milk of magnesia as an antacid 4 ml; as a laxative 15 ml.

MAGNESIUM CARBONATE: This antacid has properties similar to those of magnesium hydroxide except that carbon dioxide is liberated during neutralization of the acid. One gramme neutralizes 20 mEq of acid. It has been shown to be an excellent antacid in clinical practice.

CALCIUM CARBONATE: It occurs as a white, powder with a chalky taste. In the stomach, it reacts with gastric acid to form calcium chloride. In the intestine, $CaCl_2$ reacts with bicarbonate to regenerate $CaCO_3$ which is excreted in feces. Calcium carbonate acts quickly and has a high neutralizing capacity. One gramme neutralizes 21 mEq of the caid. Its action is prolonged and it is inexpensive.

Magnesium salt can counteract its constipating effect. Calcium carbonate increases serum gastrin level and gastric acid secretion above the basal level. Prolonged therapy may cause hypercalcemia.

Dose: It is given as powdered precipitated chalk or as tablets containing 1 g. of calcium carbonate. Dose: 2-4 g.

Systemic Antacids

SODIUM BICARBONATE: Sodium bicarbonate is a white, water soluble and completely absorbable antacid. It reacts with the gastric acid to form sodium chloride, water and carbon dioxide. One gramme of the drug neutralizes 12 mEq of acid. In the intestine, sodium chloride remains unchanged.

Excess of bicarbonate of the intestinal contents is absorbed, causing systemic alkalosis.

It is an effective and rapidly acting antacid. Its duration of action, however, is short. Eructation of the carbon dioxide liberated during the process of acid neutralization often gives the patient a sense of relief from abdominal discomfort. This is the basis of its reputed carminative action. During its repeated administration in sufficient quantities, the output of the gastric juice and acid far exceeds the basal secretion. This is probably because the continuous maintenance of raised pH in pyloric antrum stimulates gastrin liberation.

Adverse reactions: The release of carbon dioxide with resultant belching, flatulence, feeling of fullness, nausea and exacerbation of esophageal reflux are the common side-effects. Systemic alkalosis and edema due to sodium retention are rarely encountered.

Therapeutic Uses:

- ***As an antacid***: Dose 1-5 g. in water, repeated as required.
- ***Metabolic acidosis*** (see Chapter 36).
- ***Alkalinization of urine***: To render urine alkaline in the treatment of certain urinary tract infections and to prevent precipitation of substances such as sulfonamide and uric acid.
- ***Topical use***: Sodium bicarbonate solution is used as an antipruritic lotion, as an eye wash, mouth wash, douche and to loosen ear wax.

Antacid Therapy

Being advertised to the laity and sold OTC, antacids are among the most abused drugs. Their indiscriminate use without an attempt to establish the cause of 'dyspepsia' can sometimes lead to masking of the warning symptoms of a serious condition like cancer of the stomach. However, when used properly and in adequate doses, they help to relieve the pain of gastritis and peptic ulcer and promote healing.

While using antacids, it is necessary to remember that :

- ***They should be prescribed in optimal dose at 1 and 3 hours after each meal, at bed time and as needed for pain.*** In the fasting state antacids have only a transient intragastric buffering effect, about 15-30 minutes. When ingested 1 hour after meal, however, they have a much longer effect, about 3-4 hours.
- ***The in vitro buffering effect of an antacid may not necessarily correlate with its in vivo effect.***
- ***The quantity of an antacid required to produce optimal buffering varies from one patient to another.*** As a general rule, the hypersecretors, such as DU patients, need larger quantities than the non-hypersecretors.
- ***Antacid tablets, though more convenient than liquids, are less effective buffers,*** unless they are chewed; hence, liquid formulations are to be preferred.
- ***Antacids may interfere with absorption of other drugs.*** (Table 42.3).
- ***Persistent reduction in gastric acidity by antacids may increase susceptibility to intestinal pathogens.***

Choice of the antacid: Adequate dosage and

Table 42.3: Drug interactions of antacids

Antacids	Decrease in bioavailability of
Aluminium compounds	Phosphate, iron salts, tetracyclines, antimuscarinic drugs, phenothiazines, digoxin, indomethacin (but not aspirin), prednisolone, ranitidine, sulfadiazine and fat soluble vitamins.
Calcium carbonate	Antimuscarinic agents, iron, phenothiazines, quinidine and tetracyclines.
Magnesium salts	Digoxin and tetracyclines.

While the clinical significance of the above drug interactions is uncertain, it is prudent to avoid simultaneous administration of antacids and drugs intended for systemic absorption.

frequency of administration are more important than the actual antacid chosen. Cost is also a major consideration. In general, systemic antacids should be avoided. Magnesium trisilicate, is more effective than aluminium hydroxide. *It can be prescribed as a non-proprietary, powder form which is cost-effective and acceptable to many patients.* Antacid mixtures do not necessarily produce better results than individual antacids, but may counter the mutual adverse reactions. *The commercially available, liquid preparations of antacids may vary by as much as 7 fold in their acid neutralizing capacity, a fact not indicated on the product label.*

Antisecretory Agents

These drugs reduce the gastric acidity by acting as : (Fig. 42.1)

I **Histamine (H_2) receptor antagonists.**
II **Proton-pump inhibitors (PPI)**; or
III **Antimuscarinics.**

I **H_2-receptor antagonists:** Because of their structural similarity to histamine (Fig. 42.2), these drugs act selectively by competitive blockade of parietal cell H_2 receptors

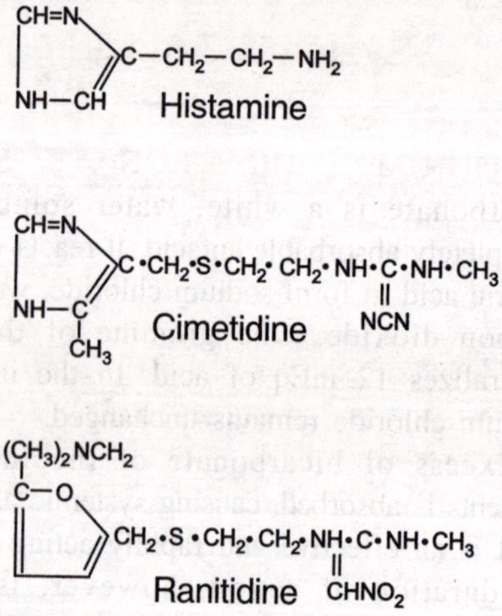

Fig. 42.2: Histamine and H2 receptor antagonists

CIMETIDINE (Tagamet): Cimetidine inhibits markedly (80-90%) histamine, pentagastrin, caffeine and vagus stimulated gastric acid secretion. It also inhibits the basal and meal-stimulated gastric secretion in normals and in DU patients. Given orally, it reduces the gastric secretion of acid to about 20 per cent within an hour. The effect is on both volume and acid content of the gastric juice; the pepsin secretion is much less affected. Food does not interfere with its action. It has minimal action on intrinsic factor secretion, gastric emptying and gastroesophageal sphincter pressure.

Absorption, fate and excretion: It is well absorbed (60-80%) orally but its bioavailability is reduced to 1/3rd when it is given with sucralfate or large doses of antacids; the latter two should not be given within 2 hours of cimetidine and other H_2 receptor antagonists. It has a plasma t½ of 1.5-2.3 hours. Therapeutic effect of a single dose lasts for 5-8 hours. It is largely excreted unchanged in the urine within 24 hours. It can cross the placenta and is secreted in milk.

Adverse reactions: The drug is generally well tolerated. The adverse effects include rashes, diarrhoea, muscle pain, fatigue and bradycardia. It must be noted that histamine and H-receptors are widely distributed in various areas such as brain, heart, blood vessels, bone marrow and so on (Chapter 22). Blockade of cerebral H_2-receptors can cause drowsiness, mental confusion, delirium and hallucinations in the elderly and in those with hepatic or renal failure. On long term use, hepatotoxicity, gynecomastia, hyperprolactinemia, sexual dysfunction and blood dyscrasias have rarely been reported.

It is a CYP450 inhibitor and reduces the clearance of drugs which are metabolized by oxidation e.g. phenobarbital, phenytoin, propranolol, warfarin, theophylline and diazepam; the hepatotoxicity of INH and paracetamol is enhanced.

Preparations and dosage: The drug is available as 200 mg. tablet and as injection 100 mg/ml for IM or slow IV use. In cases with DU, it is usually given in the dose of 400 mg. twice or thrice daily after meals, or 800 mg. at bed-time. A single night-time dose of cimetidine (and other H_2receptor antagonists) is more effective in bringing about ulcer healing than the split dose regimen, as suppression of the day-time acidity contributes to ulcer healing less than that of nocturnal acid secretion. With this treatment, 70-80% of the DUs heal in 6-12 weeks. In resistant cases, larger doses (maximum 2-4 g/day) may be needed. Dosage should be reduced in patients with impaired renal function.

Therapeutic uses:

- ***Duodenal and gastric ulcers*:** Cimetidine is valuable in the treatment of DU. It appears to be less effective in promoting the healing of GU.
- ***Zollinger-Ellison Syndrome*:** It has also been used successfully to treat multiple peptic ulcers due to gastric hypersecretion from excessive circulating gastrin (Zollinger-Ellison syndrome). It is useful in treating stress induced ulcers; in this condition, prophylaxis with intensive antacid regimens and/or cimetidine is recommended during the period of risk.
- ***Gastroesophageal reflux disease (GERD):*** It is effective but less so than proton pump inhibitors (see later).
- ***Prevention of acute erosive gastritis in acutely stressed patients*** (see later).
- ***NSAID induced ulcers*:** It is useful in treating ulcers induced by NSAID therapy but not in the prevention of this condition.

RANITIDINE (Zantac, Zinetac): This nitroethane derivative of furan is 5-10 times more potent than cimetidine, is adequately absorbed and has similar pharmacokinetic properties. Its plasma t½ is 1.6-2.4 hours. Its action is more selective and longer lasting than that of cimetidine. A single oral dose of 150 mg. controls gastric acid secretion for upto 8-12 hours. An IV preparation is also available.

Adverse reactions: It may give skin rash, constipation and fecal concretions. However, it:

- ***Does not inhibit hepatic drug metabolism.***
- ***Has less antiandrogenic effes and is less likely to cause gynecomastia and sexual dysfunction; and***
- ***Causes little, if any, central effects.***

The dose is 150 mg 12 hourly or 300 mg once daily at bed time.

FAMOTIDINE (Famocid, Famotin): Unlike cimetidine and ranitidine it has a thiazole ring. On weight basis, famotidine is 30 times more potent than cimetidine and 7.5 times more potent than ranitidine. Its plasma t½ is 3-4 hours, and therapeutic effect lasts for 24 hours. A single oral dose of 40 mg. at night for 8 weeks, produces healing of DU in most cases, while a dose of 20 mg. reduces the relapse considerably. IM or IV preparations are also available. It is well tolerated but may cause headache, dizziness and GI symptoms. *It does not interfere with drug metabolising enzymes in liver.* It is most cost effective and is preferred.

Nizatidine (Axid) and **roxatidine** (Rotane) are other drugs with similar properties, and have no significant advantages over ranitidine and famotidine.

Tolerance can develop to the action of H_2 receptor blockers, in contrast to the PPI.

II **Proton pump inhibitors (PPI):** These drugs irreversibly inhibit the gastric H^+-K^+-ATPase proton pump which is the final common pathway for acid secretion in response to all stimuli (Fig. 42.1). PPIs are prodrugs and require activation at an acid pH. After absorption, they diffuse from the blood into the parietal cells, are secreted into and become ionized at the acid pH around the canaliculi, and irreversibly inactivate the enzyme H^+-K^+-ATPase. All of them have short plasma t½, 0.5-2 hours but the action lasts much longer. *All PPIs are acid labile and the tablet should be swallowed unbroken/ uncrushed; or the drug should be given as enteric coated granules.*

Fig. 42.3: Omeprazole

OMEPRAZOLE (Omezole, Lomac): This is a substituted benzimidazole with potent and prolonged action. As the concentration of the proton pump molecules in the parietal cells is highest after a prolonged fast at night, the PPIs act best when taken about ½ hour before the breakfast. If a second dose is required, it should be taken ½ hour before the dinner. Further, as only a fraction of the PP molecules are activated at a given time, a single daily dose takes 4-5 days to achieve the maximum reduction of acid secretion (65-90 per cent). A second dose before dinner daily is required to achieve a faster result. Its action is independent of the type of the stimulus. It also selectively inhibits gastric mucosal carbonic anhydrase. Acid secretion does not show a rebound increase after the drug effect wears out. It has negligible effect on pepsin content. With once a day regimen, 90% DU heal in 2 weeks and almost all heal in 4 weeks. Gastric ulcers require larger doses for 8 weeks. It is highly effective in Zollinger-Ellison syndrome with severe gastric acid hypersecretion and DUs resistant to H_2 receptor blockers, and in reflux esophagitis. It has also been used to treat *bleeding peptic ulcers* in the dose of 40 mg twelve hourly.

Adverse reactions: The drug is generally well tolerated. GI disturbances, dizziness and drowsiness may occur. The main concern about this drug is that it causes marked hypergastri-naemia due to prolonged achlorhydria. Carcinoid-like lesions in the stomach have been observed in rats. The drug has now been widely used and appears to be safe. However, use for more than 5 years may be associated with increased incidence of osteoporotic fractures.

It inhibits the hepatic microsomal enzymes and can prolong the half life of drugs such as diazepam, phenytoin, carbamazepine and warfarin.

Table 42.4 : Proton pump inhibitors

Drug	Bioavailability %	Dosage* mg/day
Omeprazole	40-65	20-40
Pantoprazole	77	40
Lansoprazole	80-90	30
Rabeprazole	52	20-40
Esomeprazole	50-89	20-40

* For peptic ulcer and GERD.
In single or two-divided doses.

Lansoprazole, **pantoprazole**, **esomeprazole and rabeprazole** are the other analogues of omeprazole. Pantoprazole and rabeprazole are available for IV use and the former is more acid stable than other PPIs. (Table 42.4).

III **Antimuscarinic drugs:** Atropine and its substitutes were used for their antimuscarinic effect on the gastric acid and pepsin secretion and gastric motility, in the hope of relieving pain and promoting ulcer healing (Chapter 19). Experimentally, antimuscarinic drugs inhibit the basal and maximum gastric acid secretion by up to 40%. Clinical evidence indicates that tension type of ulcer pain which is relatively uncommon may be relieved but the commoner pain related to the food ingestion is little affected. Further, they also cause various side effects.

Antimuscarinic drugs prolong the gastric emptying time, which increases the stay of an antacid in the stomach and increases its effectiveness; in the absence of antacids, they would prolong the contact of the acid secretion with the ulcer. This may lead to aggravation of the symptoms. In the presence of pyloric stenosis, these drugs may cause gastric retention. They are no more recommended in DU.

Antimuscarinics are contraindicated in the presence of concurrent reflux esophagitis, which they aggravate by relaxing the lower esophageal sphincter.

Pirenzepine (Gastrozepin): This drug has selective antimuscarinic action on M_1 muscarinic receptors in the stomach and has been shown to reduce gastric acidity.

Mucosal Protective Drugs

BISMUTH SALTS : The preparations commonly used are: colloidal bismuth subcitrate and bismuth subsalicylate. They are not absorbed and the white precipitate (Bismuth chelate) formed in the gastric acid (pH less than 3.5) coats the ulcer crater with bismuth-glycoprotein complex; the latter is relatively impermeable to the H+ ion and acts as a diffusion barrier to gastric acid. It is also toxic to *Helicobacter pylori.* They are used as tablets before each of the three main meals and at bed time. The drugs may cause constipation, black stools and rarely neurotoxicity (see later).

SUCRALFATE (Carafate): This drug is a complex of sulfated sucrose and aluminium hydroxide. Its acid neutralizing capacity is very poor; and it has no antisecretory property. However, in the acid environment of the stomach, it forms a gel which coats the ulcer crater for more than 6 hours, thus forming a physicochemical barrier which may act as a mucosal defence. This coating is not disturbed by food and is relatively impermeable to the H+ions of the gastric acid. It also binds pepsin and bile acids. It is well tolerated. It is given as 1 g tablets, taken 1 hour before a meal and at bed time (four times daily) for 4-8 weeks. An antacid should not be taken for ½ hour before or after sucralfate. Unlike H_2 receptor antagonists, it needs to be given in multiple, daily doses. The drug may cause constipation, dryness of mouth and abdominal discomfort. Rarely, it may cause aluminium toxicity and hypophosphatemia. It interferes with the absorption of ciprofloxacin, phenytoins, digoxin and aminophylline.

It is of no value in the treatment of reflux esophagitis.

PROSTAGLANDIN E: Both the gastric and intestinal mucosa synthesise large amounts of prostaglandins (PG). PGE and PGI reduce the secretion of gastric acid and at lower concentrations may promote cytoprotection by acting on EP_3 receptors. Analogues of PGE_1 (**Misoprostol**,15-deoxy - 16-hydroxy - 16 methyl PGE_1, Cytotec) and of PGE_2 (**Enprostil, Arbaprostil, Rioprostil**), given orally, produce similar effects. The protective effect lasts for hours. These drugs may cause dose related diarrhoea and oxytocic effects. Their main clinical value is due to their ability to prevent ulceration and bleeding from the gastric mucosa in patients who take large doses of aspirin or NSAID for chronic pain. They are inferior to H_2-receptor antagonists in the treatment of DU. Misoprostol is administered in the dose of 200 mcg qid. *They should not be used in pregnant women and those contemplating pregnancy.* It is very expensive.

Rebapimide, a new drug, is claimed to act as a gastric mucosal cytoprotectant; it acts by stimulation of gastric PG generation. It has been used to treat gastric ulcers and acute gastritis. It is under evaluation.

Management of Peptic Ulcer

The management of peptic ulcer is essentially medical. It has undergone a major change with the discovery of the association of DU with *H.pylori* infection. *H.pylori* infection can be confirmed by:

(a) Detection of IgG antibody against *H.pylori* in the serum and antigen in the stool.

(b) Carbon labelled urea breath test; and

(c) Rapid urease test and histopathological examination of the biopsy of gastric antral mucosa at endoscopy.

The principles of medical treatment of peptic ulcer are shown in Table 42.5.

Table 42.5: Principles of medical treatment of DU and GU

- Rest and sedatives in acute stage.
- Withdrawal of offending agents such as NSAID, smoking, alcohol and caffeine.
- Dietary modification.
- Antisecretory drugs.
- Antacids; and
- Treatment of *H.pylori* infection.

- ***Rest***: Clinical studies have clearly shown that bed rest promotes ulcer healing. An initial period of bed rest, therefore, may be useful in patients with recent ulcers and in those with severe symptoms.

- ***Withdrawal of the offending agents***: Cessation of smoking, avoidance of NSAID, alcohol and caffeine containing beverages are definitely helpful in promoting ulcer healing.

- ***Diet***: Contrary to common belief, there is no special merit in frequent, small meals nor in the additional night feeds. In fact, peptic ulcer disease can be effectively treated with the usual 3-4 meals a day. Night feeds only stimulate further gastric acid secretion at a time when a patient is asleep; hence they should be avoided. However, irritants such as chilly, other spices and fried food should be avoided. Edible vegetable oils, ghee and butter taken as such are helpful, as these have an inhibitory effect on gastric acid secretion.

- ***Antisecretory drugs and antacids***: In humans, the mean diurnal gastric pH is about 1.4-2.0; low pH is mainly found at night. For the treatment of DU, the pH has to be elevated to a level higher than 3.0 for about 16-18 hours a day. For the treatment of reflux esophagitis, it must be raised to at least 4.0 for 16-18 hours per day. Hence, a course of therapy with an H_2-receptor blocker or a proton pump inhibitor should be given for 8-12 weeks. PPIs are the most potent antisecretory drugs available. They may be prescribed twice daily for 3-5 days; after that a single prebreakfast dose may be prescribed for 8-12 weeks. If the ulcer recurs, another course of full therapy is indicated. Patients with Zollinger-Ellison syndrome who are resistant to H_2-receptor blockers should be treated with PPI.

H_2 receptor antagonists, as a class, are remarkably free from adverse reactions. The total daily dose of these drugs is usually given after the evening meal. Cimetidine 800 mg is equivalent to 300 mg of ranitidine, 40 mg of famotidine and 300 mg of nizatidine. Therapeutically, there is little to choose from among the various drugs of this class. The difference is mainly in the potency as on mg basis and the cost; famotidine is perhaps the most cost-effective. Antacids can be used as adjuncts for quick pain relief.

- ***Treatment of H.pylori infection***: Eradication of *documented H. pylori* infection is now considered the mainstay of treatment of *documented* DU and GU. For that purpose, antibiotics are used in combination regimens using 3 or 4 drugs. Although no perfect regimen exists, some of those which are currently

Table 42.6: Suggested antimicrobial regimens for *H.pylori* infection

1 Clarithromycin 500 mg bid + amoxicillin 1 g bid + PPI bid
2 Tetracycline 500 mg qid + Metronidazole 200 mg qid + Bismuth subsalicylate 2 tablets qid + Omeprazole 20 mg bid. ranitidine 150 mg bid.
3 Clarithromycin 500 mg bid + Metronidazole 400 mg bid + Omeprazole 20 mg bid.

Tetracycline can be substituted for metronidazole or amoxycillin.
Other PPI or H_2 blocker can be used instead of omeprazole.
Duration: 10-14 day.

recommended are shown in Table 42.6. *The concurrent administration of a PPI or an H_2 receptor antagonist enhances the eradication of H.pylori.* PPIs are superior in this respect. The organism may develop resistance to metronidazole in 20-30% of cases.

The drug regimens mentioned in the table are effective in 75-90% of patients. Some side effects occur in 20-30% of patients. For ulcer healing and cure, antisecretory and antimicrobial therapy is usually given together for the first 10-14 days, followed by anti-secretory therapy (PPI or an H_2 blocker) alone for 6-8 weeks to ensure complete ulcer healing. Efficacy of the antimicrobial therapy is assessed by a negative urea breath test. *Once H.pylori infection is eradicated, long term maintenance anti-secretory therapy is not needed.* Less than 10% of the ulcers may recur after *cure* following eradication of *H. pylori* infection. However, recurrence may be precipitated by NSAID or some other ulcerogenic factor.

Some workers feel that a course of antimicrobial therapy is justified in all patients with documented DU even without demonstrating *H.pylori* infection. *However, patients with GU must have malignancy ruled out before any treatment is started.*

Table 42.7: Current guidelines for treatment of *H. pylori* infection

(1) **Strongly recommended in:**
- ***Duodenal and gastric ulcer*** (whether active or not, including complicated peptic ulcer disease)
- ***Gastric lymphoma.***
- ***Atrophic gastritis;*** and
- ***Recent resection for gastric cancer.***

(2) **May be used in:**
- ***Functional dyspepsia.***
- ***First degree relatives of patients with gastric cancer (prophylaxis)***

Table 42.7 summarises the current guidelines for treatment of *H. pylori* infection.

- ***Adjuvant therapy:*** A sympathetic discussion of the patient's problems may be useful in relieving the anxiety and tension. A tranquillizer or an antidepressant may be needed in some cases. Tricyclic antidepressants also possess antimuscarinic action (Chapter 13). Formal psychotherapy, however, has not been shown to produce any dramatic effects.

With adequate drug therapy, relief of symptoms occurs within 7-10 days. This does not, however, necessarily mean that ulcer has healed, and treatment has to be continued for some weeks after relief of symptoms. With PPIs, complete healing occurs within 4-6 weeks whereas it takes 8-12 weeks with H_2 receptor antagonists. Failure to respond to medical treatment indicates chronicity or the presence of some complication. A gastric ulcer may undergo

Table 42.8: Drugs to be avoided in peptic ulcer disease

- Salicylates and other NSAID.
- Caffeine, theophylline.
- Glucocorticoids in pharmacological (but not in replacement) doses.
- CCB
- Some iron salts; and
- Alendronate.

malignant change.

- ***Prevention of recurrence***: In the absence of documented *H. pylori* infection (which is curable), no treatment available at present, however meticulously carried out, can permanently guarantee against a recurrence of the peptic ulcer. However, cimetidine (400 mg daily) and ranitidine (150 mg daily), used prophylactically reduce ulcer recurrence and prevent complications in resistant cases. Patients should be advised moderation in living and in eating, and to avoid smoking, drinking and certain drugs (Table 42.8). *Up to fourfifths of gastric ulcers have been attributed to smoking and use of NSAID.* Many elderly persons with osteoarthritis often receive potent *antiinflammatory* drugs in full doses, whereas all that they require is an *analgesic* such as paracetamol or low dose ibuprofen (200 mg).

Table 42.9: Prevention and treatment of acute erosive gastritis

- Prevention of hypovolemia, systemic acidosis, sepsis and hypoalbuminemia.
- Maintenance of intragastric pH above 5.0 with the use of antacids, an H_2 receptor blocking agent or PPI; the latter is more convenient.
- Ranitidine: 50 mg. IM or IV every 6-8 hours; or 6.25 mg/hour by IV infusion. Famotidine: 20 mg. every 6-12 hours IM or IV. Pantoprazole repeated as bolus or by continuous infusion over 24 hours.
- Antacid in liquid form: 15-30 ml/hour by a nasogastric drip.

Surgery is indicated when

- ***Malignancy is suspected in a GU.***
- ***A DU becomes chronic and refractory to adequate medical management.***
- ***A complication such as organic obstruction or perforation is present***; and
- ***The patient suffers from repeated attacks of GI bleeding.***

Acute erosive gastritis (Table 42.9) with bleeding occurs as a complication of a serious medical or surgical illnesses and is common in intensive care units. Compromise in the gastric mucosal blood supply appears to be an important aetiological factor. As such bleeding doubles or even triples the mortality, patients at risk must be given prophylactic treatment; and

Table 42.10: Current guidelines for treatment of GERD

- ***Non-pharmacological measures:*** Reassurance and advice about lifestyle; elevation of the head of the bed by 15-20 cm; weight reduction in obese patients; avoidance of tight garments, large meals, and lying down for 3 hours after a meal; cessation of smoking; avoidance of reflux-inducing foods (such as spicy/fatty foods, chocolates and coffee), alcohol, NSAID, CCBs, theophylline and antimuscarinics.
- ***PPI (high dose)*** are the most effective drugs for promotion of healing of the *erosive esophageal lesions*. Maintenance therapy upto 1 year may be needed.
- ***H_2 receptor antagonists*** are less effective than PPIs in erosive esophagitis but may be cost-effective in long term maintenance therapy. In non-erosive GERD, they are almost as effective and PPIs and much less expensive.
- ***Antacids*** help to relieve mild reflux symptoms promptly.
- ***Prokinetic drugs*** have only slight efficacy in esophagitis and are not recommended for routine use. However, they may be used as add-on drugs with antisecretory agents in refractory cases.
- ***On demand therapy*** is a cost effective alternative to continuous maintenance therapy in case of mild, non-erosive GERD,
- When symptoms have resolved, an attempt should be made to stop therapy. Relapse is, however, very common.
- ***Routine anti-H. pylorie therapy is not indicated in GERD.***

any patient who has begun to bleed deserves aggressive management. Efforts to improve volume status, cardiac output and respiratory function are critical to both prevention and treatment. The incidence of bleeding is reduced if the gastric pH is maintained above 5.0.

Gastroesophageal reflux disease (GERD): This is a chronic, unremitting, essentially incurable disease that quickly relapses on cessation of drug therapy. It is characterized by "the reflux of gastric contents into the esophagus, leading to esophagitis and reflux symptoms sufficient to impair the quality of life." It is subdivided into non-erosive GERD and erosive GERD. The commonest symptoms is heartburn; and about half the patients have erosive esophagitis. Incompetence of the lower esophageal sphincter (LES) its transient, repeated relaxation not associated with swallowing, and delayed gastric emptying seem to be the important factors in its pathogenesis. The current guidelines for the treatment of GERD are outlined in Table 42.10. Acid suppression is the key aspect in both acute and long term therapy of GERD. It is advisable to start the therapy with PPI given bid and once the symptoms are relieved substitute it with H_2 receptor blockers/antacids in non-erosive but not in erosive GERD.

Patients with infrequent heart-burn and dyspepsia (less than three times a week) can be managed with an H_2 antagonist such as famotidine 20 mg bid as needed.

NSAID-induced ulcers: Aspirin and other non-selective NSAID are known to cause dyspepsia and symptomatic gastric ulcers, particularly when given in large doses and for prolonged periods (Chapter 11). Among the various drugs used for prophylaxis, misoprostol, a PG analogue, given concurrently with NSAID, daily, in divided doses, appears to reduce such complication by about 40%. The drug, however, causes diarrhoea and is expensive. H_2 receptor antagonists such as ranitidine may offer some protection against NSAID-induced dyspepsia but their prophylactic value in prevention of ulceration is doubtful. PPI are being marketed in combination with non-selective NSAID, with the hope of preventing the ulcerogenic action of NSAID. There is no convincing evidence that such a combination prevents the GI complication in the long term. These combinations are not recommended while prescribing the conventional doses of NSAID for short term therapy. (Chapter 11).

Section XI
Oxytocics and Uterine Relaxants

Pharmacology of Ergot Alkaloids, Oxytocin, other Oxytocics and Uterine Relaxants 43

Oxytocics are the drugs which stimulate uterine contractions (ergot alkaloids, oxytocin and prostaglandins), and are used to:

- *Minimise the placental blood loss.*
- *Induce or augment labour;* and
- *Induce abortion.*

Ergot Alkaloids

Ergot is obtained from a fungus *Claviceps purpurea* which grows mainly on rye and occasionally on other grains. Ergot spores, carried by insects or wind, are deposited on the ovaries of young rye where they germinate. Their hyphal filaments penetrate deep into the rye, and destroy the entire grain substance with formation of a hardened, black purple body termed the sclerotium, which serves as the commercial source of ergot. Consumption of ergot-infested rye was the cause of the disease termed *St. Anthony's fire,* observed in the middle ages and characterised by dry gangrene of extremities and a high incidence of abortions and stillbirths; a visit to St. Anthony's shrine was thought to be curative and hence the name.

Chemistry of ergot : Ergot has been termed a treasure house of pharmacological constituents. The most important of these are the alkaloids. In addition, active components like histamine, tyramine and acetylcholine are also present. Other constituents include steroids, acids, quaternary ammonium bases and inorganic compounds. Only the levorotatory forms of the alkaloids are active. They can be divided into:

I **Amino acid alkaloids :** Ergotamine, Ergosine and Ergotoxin. Ergotoxin is a mixture of three alkaloids, ergocornine, ergocristine and ergokryptine.

II **Amine alkaloid :** Ergometrine (ergonovine).

III **Semisynthetic dihydrogenated amino acid alkaloids :** Dihydroergotamine (DHE) and Hydergine, the latter being a mixture of dihydroergocornine, dihydroergocristine and dihydroergokryptine.

Pharmacological actions: (Table 43.1).

- ***Uterus* :** All the natural ergot alkaloids cause contraction of the uterine smooth muscle (***oxytocic action***). The response depends upon the alkaloid employed, the dose used, the degree of uterine maturity and stage of gestation. Thus, the amino acid alkaloids elicit a delayed but powerful response; their dihydrogenated derivatives, however are active only on pregnant uterus at term. Ergometrine and its derivative methylergometrine elicit an immediate and powerful response. Small doses produce an increase in the force of contraction, with normal relaxation in between consecutive contractions. With larger doses, the contractions become more powerful, tetanic, and frequent and the resting muscle tone increases markedly; this precludes the use of ergot preparations for induction of labour. Still higher doses cause a sustained contracture. Both amino acid and the amine alkaloids are capable of stimulating the uterus during any phase of estrous cycle or gestation; and even an immature uterus is stimulated. In general the uterus at full term and immediately after delivery is highly sensitive.

The amine alkaloid **ergometrine** has several advantages over the amino acid alkaloids such as ergotamine, viz.:

(a) It is effective orally and elicits a prompt contractile response.

(b) In small doses, it produces marked contraction of the uterus with minimum ADR.

(c) It is devoid of significant adrenergic blocking, vasoconstrictor and emetic activity; and

(d) It is less toxic.

Compared to oxytocin, ergot alkaloids increase the tone of the cervix. Oxytocin decreases it. Further, the frequency of contractions is increased more with ergot alkaloids than with oxytocin.

● ***Vascular actions***: The a-adrenergic blocking action of the amino acid alkaloids has been discussed in Chapter 17. In addition, they possess direct vasoconstrictor effect. Peripheral vasoconstric-tion is accompanied by damage to the capillary endothelium, particularly with large doses. Ergotamine is the most potent vasoconstrictor. The dihydrogenated amino acid alkaloids are powerful alpha adrenergic blocking agents and their direct vasoconstrictor effect is minimal, except in the case of DHE, which, in addition to alpha adrenergic blockade, also produces significant vasoconstriction. In contrast to the amino acid alkaloids, the amine alkaloid ergometrine has no adrenergic blocking activity and causes minimal vasoconstriction (Table 43.1)

● ***Gastrointestinal tract***: Ergotamine increases peristaltic activity and can potentiate the action of neostigmine on the gut.

● ***Miscellaneous***: The amino acid as well as the amine ergot alkaloids are partial 5-HT agonists on certain blood vessels and selective antagonists on various smooth muscles. Methysergide, a clinically useful 5-HT antagonist, is a derivative of ergometrine. They all can cause nausea and vomiting due to a direct action on emetic centre.

Absorption, fate and excretion: Ergotamine and the dihydrogenated derivatives are erratically absorbed from the gut, and have poor bioavailability. Ergometrine and methyl-ergometrine, on the other hand, are rapidly and completely absorbed; their oxytocic effect is seen within 10 to 15 minutes of oral, 3 to 5 minutes of SC and 1 to 2 minutes of IV administration. They are metabolized in the liver and the degradation products eliminated in urine. Liver damage enhances the toxicity.

Adverse reactions: Toxicity of amino acid

Table 43.1: Pharmacological actions of ergot preparations

Preparation	Uterus (contraction)	Alpha adrenergic blocking action	Vaso-constriction	5-HT* antagonism
Ergotamine	+++ (delayed)	+++	++++	+++
Ergometrine	++++	±	+	+++
DHE	++ (on pregnant uterus)	++++	++	+

* All are also partial 5-HT agonists

alkaloids and their dihydrogenated derivatives has been discussed in Chapter 17. Ergotamine and erogotoxin are more toxic than the dihydro derivatives. Toxicity is mainly due to direct vascular actions leading to thrombosis and gangrene. Treatment consists of : (1) immediate withdrawal of the drug; (2) use of antiemetics; (3) administration of heparin; and (4) vasodilator agents like tolazoline and sodium nitroprusside, for the treatment of peripheral vascular insufficiency. Good nursing care is imperative if gangrene of an extremity develops.

Ergometrine and methylergometrine may produce nausea and vomiting but serious toxic effects are rare. Their use during the 1st and 2nd stage of labour may, however, result in death of foetus in utero or rupture of the uterus.

Preparations and dosage :

(i) Preparations of ergotamine and dihydroergotamine (Chapter 17).

(ii) Ergometrine tablet. Dose: 0.5 to 1 mg.

iii) Ergometrine maleate injection contains 0.5 mg. of the drug per ml. Dose : 0.2 to 1 mg. intramuscularly and 0.1 to 0.5 mg. intravenously.

(iv) Ergotamine tartrate 0.25 mg. with ergometrine maleate 1.25 mg. injection (Neogynergen). Dose: 1 ml. IM.

(v) Methylergometrine maleate tablet (Methergine) 0.125 mg. Dose : 0.125 mg tid.

(vi) Methylergometrine injection 0.2 mg. per ml. Dose: 0.2 mg. SC, IM or IV.

(vii) Dihydroergotamine mesylate (DHE) 1 mg./ml. for injection.

Therapeutic uses:

- ***Postpartum hemorrhage***: Ergometrine and methylergometrine are extremely useful in both prophylaxis and treatment of postpartum hemorrhage. For prophylaxis, *they are administered after the expulsion of the placenta*, in the IM dose of 0.2 to 0.3 mg. If immediate action is desired, an IV dose of 0.2 mg. is given. However, IV administration may result in dangerous hypertension. In abortion, where the loss of foetus is inevitable, ergometrine may be employed to control bleeding.

- ***Migraine***: Ergotamine is used to treat acute attacks of migrane (Chapter 23).

- ***Uterine involution***: Ergometrine, in the dose of 0.2 mg. orally thrice daily, is employed for 7 days after childbirth to hasten the process of uterine involution, although the beneficial effect of this agent on the normal process of involution is not yet established. It is, however, useful in the same dose in cases of delayed involution where it hastens involution, prevents bleeding and checks the spread of infection.

- ***Orthostatic hypotension***: Severe orthostatic hypotension can be disabling and its management is unsatisfactory. The first step is to establish that the condition is persistent and find out whether there is a remediable cause. Drug therapy (diuretics, nitrates, phenothiazines, antiparkinsonian drugs, tricyclic antidepressants and antihypertensives) is by far the commonest correctable cause. When other causes are excluded, the most likely cause is chronic orthostatic hypotension due to autonomic failure secondary to diseases such as diabetes mellitus. *It is important to treat the symptomatic orthostatic hypotension and not the blood pressure reading alone.* Patients with starting systolic BP as low as 70 mm Hg. may be completely symptom-free. Orthostatic hypotension is often most troublesome on rising in the morning and after meals.

Initially in mild cases, simple nonpharmacological measures should be tried : advice to rise slowly, high salt diet, sleeping with the head of the bed elevated 10 cm and use of 'support tights'. Drug therapy is used for those who remain disabled or have severe faintness, syncopal episodes or inability to stand. The patient may be advised to drink two cups of coffee (250 mg. of caffeine) before breakfast. Oral DHE may be tried, provided there is no contraindication; a single dose in the morning may be sufficient. In severe cases, fludrocortisone probably remains the drug of choice despite its shortcomings. The main problem with this drug is the occurrence of supine hypertension (Chapter 17).

BROMOERGOCRYPTINE: This synthetic ergot derivative is discussed in Chapter 65.

Oxytocin

The posterior pituitary extract shows two distinct pharmacologically active principles:

- ***Vasopressin*** which acts on the kidney and the blood vessels (Chapter 37); and
- ***Oxytocin***, which has a dominant action on the uterus and the myoepithelium of the mammary gland.

OXYTOCIN: This is an nonapeptide usually represented in the following simplified form:

```
GLU(NH2)—ASP(NH2)—CYS—PRO—LEU—GLY(NH2)
 |                 |
ILEU ——— TYR ——— CYS
```

Fig. 43.1: Oxytocin

The polypeptide is freely water soluble and acid stable. A synthetic preparation with identical structure and pharmacological actions is also available.

Formation and release of oxytocin: Oxytocin and vasopressin are synthesized in hypothalamic nuclei. They travel along the hypothalamo-hypophyseal tract to the posterior lobe of the pituitary where they are stored and from where they are released under a variety of stimuli, such as dehydration, hemorrhage, dilatation of the cervix and uterus and emotional stimuli. As both oxytocin and vasopressin are bound to a common protein, such stimuli cause a simultaneous release of both the hormones.

Pharmacological actions:

- ***Uterus***: The oxytocic activity of oxytocin varies according to the dose, the species, the stage of estrous cycle, and in a pregnant animal, according to the stage of gestation. These effects are highly dependent on the presence of estrogen. In the early period of pregnancy in humans only very high doses are effective. However, as the pregnancy advances, from 5th to 6th month onwards, the sensitivity of pregnant uterus to oxytocin increases rapidly.

Oxytocin, given in small doses by IV infusion, exerts a physiological action on the pregnant uterus. The effect is the result of a direct stimulation of the uterine smooth muscle. The upper uterine segment, consisting of the fundus and body, is contracted while the lower uterine segment, consisting of the cervical portion, is dilated. This results in an expulsion of the fetus from the uterine cavity. The contractions also squeeze the maternal blood out of the placenta into the maternal inferior vena cava. The periods of relaxation which intervene between the two successive contractions allow refilling of the placental blood vessels by the maternal arterial blood and thus prevent asphyxial injury to the foetus. *Oxytocin, therefore, can be used by slow IV infusion for inducing labour at term* in contrast to ergot preparations which are contraindicated.

With high doses of oxytocin, the uterine tone increases, the contractions become more powerful and frequent, and asphyxial injury to the fetus may develop due to direct compression and ischemia caused by inadequate filling of the placental blood vessels.

- ***Mammary gland***: The myoepithelium, a modified smooth muscle, which surrounds the alveolar ramifications of the mammary gland is stimulated by oxytocin, resulting in expulsion of milk from the alveolar lumen and ducts into large cisterns and sinuses. This is termed milk ejection or milk 'letdown'. The milk ejection reflex is initiated by the stimulus of suckling, which results in the release of oxytocin.
- ***Cardiovascular system***: In small doses, it produces a vasodilator effect by direct relaxation of the vascular smooth muscle. Transient hypotension and flushing accompanied by tachycardia are usually observed. The usual infusion rates employed in obstetrics do not modify the BP. The vasodilator effect of oxytocin can be readily blocked by small amounts of vasopressin. The hypotensive

phase is followed by a rise in BP, probably due to an increase in the cardiac output.

• ***Kidney*:** Synthetic oxytocin possesses antidiuretic activity in man and a dose of 100 milli-units causes a definite antidiuresis in postpartum women; this is associated with a diminution in the renal plasma flow and the GFR. The renal effects of oxytocin may be due to constriction of renal cortical vessels.

Absorption, fate and excretion: Oxytocin given orally is inactivated by trypsin. The aqueous solution, on IM administration, is absorbed rapidly. The t½ *in non-pregnant women* is about 10 to 15 minutes. The removal from the circulation is mainly by kidneys and the liver. Plasma from men and nonpregnant women does not inactivate oxytocin but the plasma, the uterine tissue and the placenta in pregnant women contain an enzyme termed 'oxytocinase' which probably inactivates oxytocin. The t½ of oxytocin *in pregnant women* at term is approximately 3 minutes.

Besides the parenteral route, oxytocin is absorbed from the nasal and buccal mucous membranes. Absorption from these routes, however, is erratic.

Adverse reactions: Oxytocin given by IV infusion may occasionally cause water retention leading to water intoxication. It is characterised by nausea, vomiting, anorexia, weight gain and lethargy. Injudicious use of oxytocin during labour may result in premature birth, foetal death, too rapid a delivery or uterine rupture.

Preparations and dosage:

(i) Oxytocin injection (Pitocin, Syntocinon) contains 10 units of synthetic oxytocin per ml. It is devoid of vasopressin activity.

(ii) Oxytocin (Syntocinon) nasal spray, 40 units per ml. It facilitates breast feeding and is used 2-5 minutes before a breast feed.

Therapeutic uses:

• ***Induction and augmentation of term labour*:** For the induction of labour, oxytocin is administered by IV infusion, 5 units in 500 ml. of 5 percent dextrose solution. Initially 0.1-0.2 ml. of the solution, (1-2 milliunits) should be given per minute; the rate is then gradually increased to a maximum of 2 ml. (20 milliunits) per minute. During the whole procedure, the uterine response should be closely observed.

Before using oxytocin, cephalopelvic disproportion must be ruled out. Multiparous patients (para 4 and over), those with malpresentation or complete placenta previa and those with uterine scars should not receive oxytocin for induction for fear of uterine rupture. In all cases, the dose should be regulated by foetal heart rate monitoring.

• ***Hypotonic uterine dysfunction*** (Uterine inertia) : Oxytocin is occasionally employed to initiate uterine contractions in cases of prolonged, stubborn and hypotonic uterine inertia.

• ***Postpartum hemorrhage (PPH):*** Oxytocin is routinely administered either SC or IM in the dose of 2 to 5 units *after the delivery of placenta* to produce a firm contraction of the uterus and thus prevent PPH. The drug may also be administered in the same dose after delivery of the anterior shoulder of the foetus to produce a prompt expulsion of the placenta and to prevent PPH. The same dose may also be injected directly into the uterus, after delivering the foetus by caesarean section.

• ***Miscellaneous*:** Oxytocin may be given intranasally in the dose of 40 units 2-5 minutes before breast feeding to promote milk ejection when this component of lactation appears to be deficient in nursing mothers. It is often used in veterinary practice to increase the milk yield.

Oxytocin is no more employed to induce therapeutic abortion.

Other Oxytocics

PROSTAGLANDINS (PG, Prostin) : Prostaglandins are C20 fatty acids containing a cyclopentane ring. Prostaglandins are described in Chapter 24; only the actions on uterus are discussed below.

Apart from human seminal fluid, PGs are found in the ovary, myometrium and menstrual fluid. Their physiological significance, however, is not well understood. Majority of PGs in varying doses inhibit the spontaneous activity of isolated non-pregnant human myometrium. However, PGF_2 and PGE in low doses stimulate both the tone and amplitude of the uterine contractions. Four PGs have been isolated from human amniotic fluid, obtained during normal labour and during spontaneous abortion. Experimentally, they are shown to sensitize the uterus to oxytocin as well as causing oxytocin release. Furthermore, PGF_2 was also found in samples of blood obtained during normal spontaneous labour but not during other stages of gestation. Since PGF_2 has smooth muscle stimulating action it is possible that it participates in the process of labour.

PGs act during pregnancy in at least three different ways:

- ***As uterine smooth muscle stimulants***, causing uterus to contract;
- ***As cervical primers***, thus hastening the process of softening and dilation of the cervix, sometimes referred to as 'cervical ripening'. Unlike oxytocin, $PGF_{2\alpha}$ and $PGE_{2\alpha}$ actually decrease cervical stiffness and PGs are being used for cervical priming at the time of delivery and before inducing abortion; and
- ***As luteolytic agents***, inhibiting the secretion of progesterone by corpus luteum. This effect has not been observed in humans.

PGs are most effective in the second trimester (13th-20th weeks). Doses required to produce abortion in the first trimester may result in serious systemic effects whereas in the third trimester PGs are less effective than oxytocin. Prior administration of mifepristone (Chapter 66) sensitizes the uterus to the action of PGs.

Adverse reactions: These are not troublesome with smaller doses but could be severe with larger doses. They include nausea, vomiting, abdominal cramps, diarrhoea, headache, fever and vasodilatation. PGs should be used cautiously in the presence of raised intraocular pressure, hypertension, diabetes, angina or epilepsy. They are contraindicated in the presence of cardiac, renal, pulmonary or hepatic disease. Smoking and alcohol should be avoided during their use and for 48 hours afterwards.

Preparations and dosage:

(i) Dinoprost (Prostin $F_{2\alpha}$) 5 mg per ml for intraamniotic use to induce abortion.

(ii) Dinoprostone (Prostin E_2, Primiprost) 500 mcg tab for oral or intravaginal use for induction of labour.

(iii) Carboprost (Prostin/15 m, Prostodin) is 15-15 dimethyl $PGF_{2\alpha}$ analogue with a longer duration of action. Dose 250 mcg/ml deep IM.

(iv) Dinoprostone 0.5 mg per syringe (Cerviprime) for endocervical injection for cervical ripening.

(v) Misoprostol, PGE_1 (Chapter 66) has been used orally/intravaginally to bring about medical abortion. The intravaginal administration is also used to cause cervical dilatation.

Therapeutic uses:

- ***Therapeutic abortion***: *PGs are not so useful for terminating early, first trimester pregnancies* because of the high incidence of incomplete abortions and consequent need for surgical procedures. Further, the procedure takes a relatively long time, and the dose needed usually causes pain and adverse GI reactions. Many clinicians, therefore, prefer suction evacuation to PGs (Chapter 66).

PGs are now widely used to terminate the pregnancy in the second trimester. Gemeprost, administered vaginally as pessaries, is the preferred PG for this purpose. Alternatively, oral or intravaginal misoprostol may be used. They are combined with mifeprostone (Chapter 66).

The analogue $PGF_{2\alpha}$ (Carboprost) is probably more effective and safer. It can also be given IM or as suppositories and is useful over a wide range of gestational ages.

All methods of abortion using PGs alone cause a high incidence of adverse effects and there is a possibility of delivering a live fetus. Some of them may also cause bronchospasm.

- ***Cervical priming***: Dinoprostone has been used extra-amniotically for cervical priming. Endocervical gels, suppositories and oral tablets containing PGs may also be useful.

- ***Post-partum hemorrhage*** : The newer PG analogues such as carboprost, given IM, are effective in managing PPH due to uterine atony in patients unresponsive to ergometrine and oxytocin. The drug, however, loses its potency unless stored at 2-4°C. This is a disadvantage. Further, current evidence indicates that PGs are no better, only more expensive, than ergometrine.

- ***Induction and augmentation of term labour***: Dinoprostone may be preferred to oxytocin for this purpose in the presence of chronic renal failure or pre-eclampsia because of its diuretic action. Apart from this, it offers no significant advantage, it is more expensive. Dinoprostone (Primiprost) is given orally as 0.5 mg. tablets at 30-60 min. intervals upto a maximum of four tablets. It can also be administered vaginally. The PGs can cause hyperstimulation of the uterus which compromises uteroplacental blood flow, and they have a longer duration of action than oxytocin. *Signs of uterine hypertonus and foetal distress should therefore be watched for.*

As the obstetric regimens of PGs are complicated, the manufacturer's literature should be consulted before using these drugs.

ETHACRIDINE LACTATE (Emcredil, Vecredil): This acridine compound has been used extra-amniotically for second trimester abortion. GI adverse effects may occur but serious toxicity is claimed to be rare. It is instilled in the dose of 10 ml. of 0.1% solution for each gestational week upto a maximum of 150 ml. On an average, it takes 30 hours to effect abortion.

Intra-amniotic hypertonic saline and urea, once used for terminating pregnancy, are not recommended because of the high failure rate and the risk of increased plasma volume.

Medical termination of pregnancy is discussed in Chapter 66. There is really no absolutely safe method of terminating pregnancy in the second trimester. Introduction of various irritants into the uterine cavity for this purpose, as done by quacks, is usually associated with serious complications and cause death.

Uterine Relaxants (Tocolytics)

Tocolytics are the drugs which inhibit myometrial contractions.Although they are uterine relaxants, not all uterine relaxants are effective tocolytics e.g. ephedrine and atropine. Tocolytics are used to prevent spontameous preterm births.

The spontaneous preterm birth (before the conclusion of 37 weeks of gestation), may involve several contributing factors. Important among these are: myometrial and fetal membrane over-distension, decidual hemorrhage, precocious fetal endocrine activation, and intrauterine inflammation and infection. The major goal in preventing preterm birth is to eliminate the risk of neonatal complications and death. Since the contracting uterus is the most commonly recognized mechanism, stopping the contractions by using the tocolytics constitutes the major therapeutic approach.

Tocolytics can be classified as:

I Calcium channel blockers e.g. Nifedipine.

II COX (cycloxygenase) inhibitors e.g. Indomethacin.

III Beta-2 adrenergic agonists e.g. Ritodrine and Salbutamol.

IV Oxytocin receptors antagonist e.g. Atosiban.

V Magnesium sulfate; and

VI Nitric oxide (NO) donors e.g. Nitroglycerine.

Before starting tocolytic therapy, accurate estimation of gestational age, and clinical plus laboratory evaluation for the possible cause of preterm labour should be done.

Calcium channel blockers: Nifedipine (Chapter 28) may be administered sublingually/ orally in the loading dose of 10 mg, and the dose repeated every 20 minutes for 3 doses. Maintenance dose of 10 mg may be given orally every 4-6 hours. It is effective in reducing neonatal complications and is relatively safe. It can be used at any gestational age.

COX inhibitors: Human decidua, myometrium and fetal membranes express COX-1 enzyme. During labour, there is a dramatic increase in COX-2 in the decidua and the myometrium. **Indomethacin** (Chapter 11), given early, inhibits COX non-selectivily and hence PG synthesis, and thus reduces the chance of birth before 37 weeks. It is avoided in gestation more than 32 weeks to prevent *in utero* closure/narrowing of the ductus arteriorus.

Beta$_2$-adrenergic receptor agonists: These drugs can be used as alternatives to nifedipine and indomethacin. Although they delay preterm delivery for 24-72 hours and reduce the immediate risk, a significant reduction in perinatal morbidity and mortality has not been convincingly demonstrated. Further, their adverse effect profile is less favourable than that of CCB. **Salbutamol**, **terbutaline** and **ritodrine** (selective beta-2 agonists, Chapters 17, 26) have been used to delay preterm delivery in uncomplicated labour. They are contraindicated in pre-eclampsia.

Salbutamol is used by IV infusion in the dose of 10 mcg. per minute, gradually increased to 45 mcg. per minute until contractions cease; then, the dose is reduced gradually. It can also be given by IM injection in the dose of 100-250 mcg, repeated as necessary. The adverse reactions include nausea, vomiting, tremor, tachycardia; hypokalemia, pulmonary edema; increased tendency to uterine bleeding; and hyperglycemia.

Ritodrine is used by IV infusion in the dose of 50 mcg/minute, increased by the same amount once every 20 minutes, until the uterine contractions are controlled and then maintained for an hour thereafter. Then, the lowest dose that maintains uterine quiescence is continued for about 12 hours.

Nitric oxide donor: Nitroglycerine IV (Chapter 28) can delay preterm labour for 48 hours. Transdermal NTG can prolong gestation to 37 weeks.

Oxytocin receptor antagonist: Atosiban acts as a competitive antagonist of oxytocin. Evidence indicates that the drug does not reduce the incidence of preterm birth or improve neonatal outcome as compared with the placebo. The drug was associated with excess fetal and infant mortality following its use before 28 weeks of gestation. Hence it is not used.

Magnesium sulfate: Experimentally, this agent inhibits the contraction of and decreases the intracellular calcium in myometrial strips obtained from pregnant women. However, clinically magnesium sulfate as a tocolytic showed no benefit over placebo with respect to the risk of preterm birth.

Tocolytics may not always prevent preterm birth. Thus, there is no first line tocolytic; however, these drugs offer other benefits. A delay of 24-48 hours in labour can be utilized (a) for administering a glucocortidoid (beta-, dexa-methasone) to bring about maturation of the fetal lungs and thus decrease the occurrence of neonatal respiratory distress syndrome (Chapter 62); and (b) to transfer the patient to a centre where neonatal ICU is available. Ideally, tocolytics should not be given for more than 48 hours, and the treatment should be individualized.

In a pregnant woman with a history of preterm delivery the treatment of asymptomatic bacteriuria during early pregnancy may reduce the occurrence of preterm birth and low birth weight. However, routine use of broad spectrum antibiotics for eradication of asymptomatic colonization of the vagina is not conclusively shown to be useful. Similarly, the usefulness of 17-alpha hydroxyprogesterone caproate prophylaxis for prevention of preterm delivery is controversial.

Section XII
Chemotherapy

Sulfonamides, Trimethoprim, Cotrimoxazole, Nitrofurans and Quinolones

44

The word **Chemotherapy** can be defined as the use of chemical compounds in the treatment of infectious diseases, so as to destroy offending organisms and parasites without damaging the host tissues. The evolution of chemotherapy can be traced through three distinct periods :

- ***A pre-Ehrlich era before 1891.***
- ***The period of Paul Ehrlich; and***
- ***The period after 1935, highlighted by the discovery of sulfonamides and antibiotics.***

In the long pre-Ehrlich era, many compounds were employed in therapeutics empirically, occasionally with beneficial and often with disastrous consequences. Thus, the usefulness of Cinchona bark in the treatment of malaria and of mercury in syphilis was known for many years. With the advances in chemistry and microbiology, a variety of infective organisms were identified and isolated.

Paul Ehrlich (1854-1915), an organic chemist, was struck by the fact that certain vital dyes like methylene blue specifically killed and stained certain bacterial cells and he reasoned that chemical substances might be produced that could unite with and destroy the parasitic agents of disease without in any way injuring the host cells. He aptly called them "magic bullets". In 1891, he demonstrated the efficacy of methylene blue in the treatment of human malaria. He also synthesized a series of arsenical compounds effective against spirochaetal infections. To express the therapeutic utility of these compounds he introduced the term **chemotherapeutic index**, a ratio of the maximum tolerated dose of a drug to its minimum curative dose. This index has now been replaced by the **therapeutic index**.

Ehrlich postulated that the cell membrane contained specific chemical groups or 'receptors' which combined with essential materials like oxygen and caused their uptake by cells. He visualised a drug as containing a chemical grouping or '*heptaphore*' that enabled the drug to get attached to the cell receptor and another grouping termed '*toxophore*' which enabled the drug to produce its specific pharmacological effect. A drug could exert either a curative or a toxic effect depending upon its affinity for the parasite or the host. Thus, a compound with a high affinity for the host tissue, an *organotropic* compound, could be toxic while one with high affinity for parasites, a *parasitotropic* compound, might be curative. Based on this hypothesis, Ehrlich introduced arsephenamine, the first really effective chemotherapeutic agent in man, in the treatment of syphilis.

The pioneering work of Ehrlich established the importance of cellular chemistry in drug action and inspired many workers to synthesize newer antibacterial substances. Ehrlich is aptly called 'the Father of Modern Chemotherapy'. He was awarded the Nobel Prize in 1909.

The next major contribution to chemotherapy came from Domagk, Mietsch and their colleagues (1938), who, while working on azo dyes, demonstrated the efficacy of 'Prontosil', a dye with a sulfonamide side chain, in inhibiting the growth of Streptococci both *in vitro* and *in vivo.* Nitti, Bovet and Fuller proved that prontosil owed its therapeutic efficacy to its conversion into sulfanilamide in the body. Since then, a variety of sulfonamides were synthesized. It is interesting to note that sulfanilamide was prepared by Gelmo as early as 1908 but 30 years elapsed before its therapeutic value was discovered!

The idea of using one micro-organism to cure the infection caused by another was repeatedly suggested during the last century. Thus, Pasteur and Joubart in 1877 demonstrated that 'common bacteria' prevented the growth of anthrax bacilli in urine, and Babes in 1885, using solid culture media, established that one bacterium could elaborate a substance that would stop the growth of another. Emmerich and Low in 1899, while working on the organism *Pseudomonas aeruginosa,* discovered that extracts of this organism in high dilutions could destroy a variety of pathogenic cocci, as well as diphtheria, cholera, typhoid and plague organisms.

In 1928, Sir Alexander Fleming, while studying staphylococcal variants, found one of his culture plates contaminated by a fungus (eventually identified as *Penicillium notatum)* which prevented the growth of surrounding bacterial colonies. He cultivated the fungus in a broth and showed that the filtrate, which he named penicillin, inhibited the growth of a number of Gram positive organisms. This compound was not toxic to animals. The discovery of penicillin, however, remained for a long time more or less a scientific curiosity. The work of Chain, Abraham and Florey in 1941 during the 2nd World War established penicillin as the most potent anti-infective agent. In 1945, Fleming, Chain and Florey were awarded the Nobel Prize for the revolutionary contribution. The isolation of 6-aminopenicillanic acid nucleus of penicillin led to the development of a variety of semisynthetic penicillins.

In 1944, after more than ten thousand micro-organisms had been screened, Schatz, Bugie and Waksman reported the isolation of streptomycin from *Streptomyces griseus.* Waksman also defined an **antibiotic** as *"a chemical substance produced by micro-organisms having the property of inhibiting the growth of or destroying other micro-organisms in high dilution".* This was a major advance, as streptomycin, unlike penicillin, was found to be effective against Gram negative organisms, and also against *Mycobacterium tuberculosis.* The above definition has now been widened to include the antibacterial chemotherapeutic agents such as sulfonamides and quinolones.

Majority of antibiotics are obtained from fungi but some like bacitracin, colistin, polymyxin B and tyrothricin are obtained from bacteria. Some are now entirely synthesized by chemical methods, e.g., chloramphenicol, imipenem etc. The important factors in determining the efficacy of chemotherapeutic agents are outlined in Table 44.1. Of these, the host plays an important part in the curative action of most of the specific remedies.

Table 44.1: Factors determining the efficacy of chemotherapeutic agents

- Host defence.
- Source of infection.
- Tissue(s) affected.
- Margin of safety; and
- Bacterial susceptibility / resistance to the agent being used.

An antimicrobial agent may act by destroying the organism **(bactericidal)** *or by inhibiting its growth* **(bacteriostatic).** The selective toxic action on the infecting organism is the key to beneficial actions of antibiotics. These drugs can hit multiple targets in bacteria:

- ***The cell wall.***
- ***The cytoplasmic membrane.***
- ***The ribosomes***
- ***The RNA molecules involved in transcription of genetic information.***

- ***Enzymes required for DNA synthesis/ replication;*** and
- ***Metabolic pathways.***

The cell wall of bacteria is a thick rigid envelope, mainly composed of sugar and peptides called mucopeptide or murein. The mucopeptide is much thicker in Gram-positive cells than in Gram-negative cells. Underneath the rigid cell wall is a cytoplasmic membrane which encloses the cytoplasm. This membrane has lipoprotein structural elements, which account for selective permeability to water, ions and nutrients. Antimicrobials attacking this membrane may alter the permeability of the cell or may disorganize the lipoproteins leading to cell death.

Inside the cytoplasm are ribosomes, spherical particles, which are concerned with protein synthesis. Ribosomes act as an assembly line where aminoacids are joined together into peptide chains and proteins. The process is directed by messenger RNA (mRNA), which carries the code for such synthesis from the nuclear DNA. Messenger RNA becomes attached to ribosomes where the transcribed code is translated into appropriate protein synthesis. Antimicrobials can bind to ribosomes and may interfere with peptide chain formation in bacteria or with the transcription mechanisms.

Mechanisms of action of various antimicrobials are summarized in Table 44.2.

Table 44.2: Mechanism of action of antimicrobial drugs

- **Interference with cell wall synthesis:** Penicillins, Cephalosporins, Bacitracin, Vancomycin, and Cycloserine.
- **Damage to the cytoplasmic membrane:** Polymyxins, Colistin, Polyene antibiotics and Detergents.
- **Inhibition of protein synthesis and impairment of function of the ribosomes:** Aminoglycosides, Tetracyclines, Chloramphenicol, Macrolide antibiotics and Lincomycin.
- **Interference with transcription/ translation of genetic information:** Quinolones, Metronidazole and Rifampicin.
- **Antimetabolite action:** Sulfonamides, Sulfones, PAS and Trimethoprim.
- **Inhibition of viral enzymes:** Protease Inhibitors, Acyclovir, Zidovudine and Nevirapine.

Classification of antibiotics: The organisms susceptible to the inhibitory or lethal effect of an antibiotic constitute its 'spectrum'. According to their spectra, antibiotics may be classified as:

I **Antibiotics mainly effective against Gram-Positive bacteria :**

- ***For systemic infections,*** e.g., Penicillins, Macrolides (Erythromycin), Lincomycin, Vancomycin, Novobiocin and Fucidin.
- ***For topical use,*** e.g., Bacitracin.

II **Antibiotics mainly effective against Gram-negative bacteria:**

- ***For systemic infections,*** e.g., Streptomycin, and other aminoglycosides.
- ***For local use*** in the intestines, e.g., Neomycin.

III **Antibiotics effective against both Gram-positive and Gram-negative bacteria:**

- ***For systemic infections***, e.g., Ampicillin, Amoxycillin, Carbencillin, Cephalosporins, Rifamycins, Imipenem.
- ***For topical use,*** e.g., Neomycin, Tyrothricin and Framycetin.

IV **Antibiotics effective against both Gram-positive and Gram-negative bacteria, rickettsiae and chlamydia (broad spectrum),** e.g., Tetracyclines and Chloramphenicol.

V **Antibiotics effective against acid fast bacilli (*M. tuberculosis*),** e.g., Aminoglycosides (Streptomycin), Rifampicin, Viomycin, and Quinolones.

VI **Antibiotics effective against fungi,** e.g., Nystatin, Amphotericin B, Griseofulvin.

VII **Antibiotics effective against protozoa,** e.g., Paromomycin, Tetracyclines, Fumagillin.

VIII **Antimalignancy antibiotics,** e.g., Actinomycin D., Mitomycin and Azaserine (Chapter 59).

Sulfonamides

SULFONAMIDES are the antimicrobial compounds containing a sulfonamido (SO_2NH_2) group (Fig. 44.1). This group is also present in other non-antibacterial compounds like the antidiabetic sulfnonylureas, diuretics like thiazides and their congeners furosemide and acetazolamide, and the anticonvulsant sulthiame.

NH_2 (4) — benzene ring — SO_2-NH_2 (1)

Fig. 44.1: Basic structure of a sulfonamide.

N_1–Nitrogen of the sulfonamido group.

N_4–Nitrogen of the para-amino group.

The sulfonamides are white powders, mildly acidic in character. They form water soluble salts with bases. The pH of the sodium salts, with some exception, eg., sodium sulfacetamide is very high; given IM, their marked alkalinity causes damage to the tissues.

Classification: The sulfonamides can be classifed according to their therapeutic utility as:

I **Those employed for the treatment of systemic infections.** Depending upon their duration of action, they are subdivided into:

- ***Short acting***: Sulfadiazine, Sulfadimidine (sulfamethazine), Sulfacetamide, Sulfafurazone (sulfisoxazole), and Sulfamethizole.
- ***Intermediate acting***: Sulfamethoxazole.
- ***Long acting*** : Sulfadoxine, Sulfamethoxypyridazine, Sulfadimethoxine, Sulformethoxine.

Their use as single agents in therapy is discouraged because of their association with severe allergic reactions such as Stevens-Johnson syndrome. However, some of them are used as combination drugs in malaria (Chapters 54)

II **Those employed orally for the treatment of ulcerative colitis:** Sulfasalazine.

III **Those used topically:** Mafenide; Silver sulfadiazine; Sulfacetamide.

Mechanism of action: The compound sulfanilamide exhibits a structural similarity to para-aminobenzoic acid (PABA) (Fig. 44.2). Sulfonamides, because of their structural similarity to PABA, compete with and substitute for it in the bacterial metabolism (Woods-Fields theory).

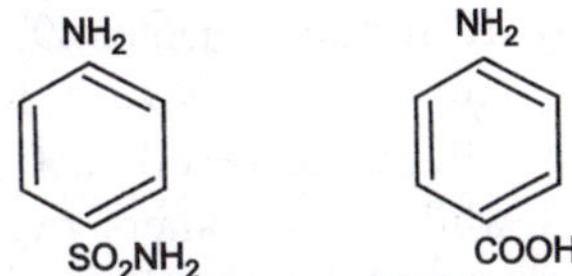

Fig. 44.2 : Sulfanilamide PABA

Folic acid derived from PABA is important in bacterial metabolism. Sulfonamides compete with PABA for the enzyme folic acid synthase which is involved in the conversion of PABA to folic acid. (Fig. 44.3). Inhibition of folic acid synthase by sulfonamides causes folic acid deficiency resulting in injury to the bacterial cell. Such an injured or disrupted bacterial cell can be easily phagocytosed.

Sulfonamides are ineffective in the presence

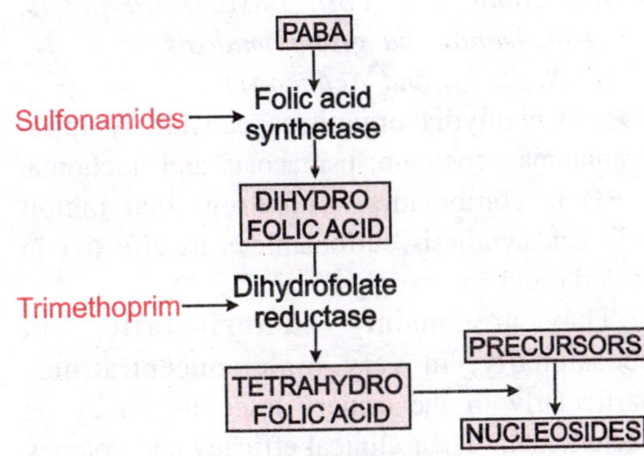

Fig. 44.3 : Mode of action of sulfonamides – trimethoprim combination

of pus and tissue breakdown products which contain large amounts of PABA. Their bacteriostatic action can be countered by PABA; sulfonamide resistant microorganisms often show enhanced PABA synthesis.

This theory, however, cannot explain the antibacterial action of mafenide hydrochloride. The antibacterial action of this compound is not antagonized by PABA.

Sulfonamide resistance: A variety of micro-organisms, such as *Staphylococci, Streptococci, Pneumococci, Meningococci, Gonococci* and *E. coli* can acquire resistance to sulfonamides. Resistance in all enterobacteria is now common, and in *Shigella sonnei* it is almost invariable. Resistance can be chromosomally mediated or transferred by 'R' factors (Chapter 49). Some of the resistant strains synthesize a folic acid synthetase with a lowered affinity for sulfonamides while some others overproduce PABA. Widespread bacterial resistance to sulfonamides now limits their clinical usefulness.

Pharmacological actions: They are effective against a variety of Gram positive and Gram negative organisms and certain chlamydia; these are:

(a) *Streptococci, Staphylococci* (some strains), *Gonococci, Pneumococci* and *Meningococci. Streptococcus fecalis* is resistant.

(b) *Clostridia, Bacillus anthracis.*

(c) *Haemophilus influenzae, H. ducreyi, Vibrio comma, E. coli, Pastuerella pestis, Shigella, Donovania granulomatosis.*

(d) *Nocardia and Actinomyces.*

(e) Chlamydia organisms causing lymphogranuloma venereum, psittacosis and trachoma.

(f) In combination with drugs that inhibit folic acid synthesis, sulfonamides are effective in malaria and in toxoplasmosis.

They are mainly **bacteriostatic**, but occasionally, in very high concentrations, particularly in the urinary tract, they may be bactericidal. Their clinical efficacy and potency are much less than those of other antibiotics. Thus, the minimum inhibitory concentration of sulfonamides for a highly susceptible bacterial strain is 1 : 10,000 to 1 : 20,000, in comparison to 1 : 50 million observed with penicillin.

Absorption, fate and excretion: Sulfonamides intended for systemic use are rapidly absorbed from the GI tract, and 70 to 90 per cent of the oral dose reaches the blood stream. The main site of absorption is the small intestine. The absorption of sulfonamides from other sites like the abraded skin, respiratory tract and vagina is variable, but sufficient amounts may be absorbed to produce sensitization and even toxicity.

In the blood, these drugs are bound to plasma proteins, particularly albumin. The degree of binding differs among the various compounds. In general, at least 50 per cent of the compound is bound to plasma proteins.

Protein binding of sulfonamides is important for several reasons:

- ***The bound sulfonamide has much less of bacteriostatic activity*** and cannot normally pass into tissue fluids or cross the blood brain barrier.
- ***Since the bound form is not available for renal excretion, protein binding helps to prolong the action of sulfonamides.*** The long acting sulfonamides are long acting because they are extensively bound to plasma proteins and are excreted slowly.
- ***The highly protein bound sulfonamides are not so effective in the treatment of acute infections because of low plasma levels of free sulfonamide.***

The free form of sulfonamides is uniformly distributed throughout all the tissue fluids although the concentration in the tissue fluids is usually lower than in the plasma. Sulfadiazine, with lower degree of binding with plasma proteins, achieves a CSF concentration 50 to 80 per cent that of the plasma levels and, therefore, is used in the treatment of meningococcal meningitis. These drugs readily cross the placental barrier and are also secreted in milk.

Sulfacetamide and sulfadiazine readily penetrate into the aqueous humour.

After a single oral dose of a short acting sulfonamide, the peak plasma concentration is usually reached within 2 to 4 hours. The effective blood levels vary between 6 and 12 mg. per 100 ml. As they are concentrated by the kidney, lower plasma levels of sulfonamides are adequate to produce therapeutic benefits in urinary tract infections.

They are metabolized in the liver by acetylation of the nitrogen of the para-amino group (N_4). Sulfadiazine is much less acetylated than sulfadimidine, while sulfamethoxypyridazine is acetylated to the extent of 10 to 15 per cent.

Individuals can be differentiated into two distinct groups according to their capacity to acetylate sulfonamides.

- ***Rapid acetylaters*** acetylate 62-90 per cent of sulfadimidine while
- ***Slow acetylaters*** acetylate only 40-53 per cent of it.

The acetylated form:

(a) Is devoid of antibacterial activity.

(b) Possesses the toxic potentialities of the parent drug.

(c) In addition, certain acetylated products are poorly soluble in acidic urine and may cause crystalluria and renal complications.

The urinary solubility of acetylated derivatives of sulfadiazine is increased in alkaline urine; the acetylated as well as the free forms of compounds like sulfafurazole, and sulfamethizole are, however, soluble even in acid urine. The free and the acetylated sulfonamides are mainly eliminated in urine, mostly by glomerular filtration. The urinary concentration of sulfonamides is higher than their plasma levels. The excretion of the intermediate and the long acting sulfonamides is slow. They are also present, in small amounts, in sweat, bile and saliva.

Preparations and dosage:

I **Short acting** (5-6 hours)

Sulfisoxazole (Sulfafurazole, Gantrisin): Highly soluble;urinary concentration greatly exceeds the plasma concentration and may be bactericidal. Dose : Initial 1-2 gm, then 0.5-1 gm 12 hourly.

II **Intermediate acting (10-12 hours)**

(i) Sulfadiazine : Good penetration into CSF. Can cause crystalluria. Tab 500 mg. Dose: 150 mg/kg/ 24 hrs. in 4-6 divided doses. Injection 250 mg/ml in 10 ml ampoules.Dose (in adults) by slow, IV injection, 100 mg/kg body weight, 2gm initially,then 30-50 mg /kg 6-8 hourly.The solution is strongly alkaline.

(ii) Sulfadimidine: Acetyl derivative relatively more soluble in urine. Dose: similar to that of oral sulfadiazine.

(iii) Sulfamethoxazole (Gantanol): Used only as a component of cotrimoxozole.

III **Long acting (7-9 days)**

Sulformethoxine (Sulfadoxine): Plasma t½ 150-200 hrs. Used in combination to treat malaria.

IV **Used in inflammatory bowel disease:**

Sulfasalazine (Salazopyrine): See text.

V **Used topically**

(i) Mafenide propionate (Marfanil): Prevents colonization of burns by Gram positive and Gram negative bacteria. It is used in 1% methyl cellulose and as 10% cream.

(ii) Silver sulfadiazine (1% cream): Silver is released slowly and has wide antibacterial spectrum.

(iii) Sulfacetamide (Albucid):Sodium salt has almost neutral pH and better tissue penetration. Used as 6% eye ointment and 10% eye drops.

Adverse reactions: *Unfortunately, there is a tendency to exaggerate the ill-effects of sulfonamides which are still valuable in therapeutics.* However, the toxic potential of these drugs should be remembered and their indiscriminate use avoided.

- ***Allergy***: This can occur at any time during therapy. The commonest allergic symptoms are drug fever, skin rash and eosinophilia. Rarely, severe exfoliative dermatitis and high fever may develop. Serum sickness, characterised by fever, joint pains, urticaria, bronchospasm and leucopenia sometimes develops within the first two weeks of therapy.

The uncommon allergic manifestations include cutaneous photosensitization, a fatal necrotizing arteritis resembling polyarteritis nodosa, acute toxic hepatitis and rarely fatal hepatic necrosis, toxic nephrosis, and acute haemolytic anemia.

A severe exudative type of erythema multiforme, associated with widespread lesions of the skin and mucous membranes, termed **Stevens Johnson syndrome,** has been reported with long acting sulfonamides. The syndrome, which is fortunately rare, is usually self-limiting but can occasionally be fatal.

Cross sensitivity among various sulfonamides and between sulfonamides and other drugs containing the sulfonamido (SO_2NH_2) group is known. Local application of sulfonamides to skin can sensitize the patient.

- ***GI symptoms*:** They commonly produce nausea and vomiting, but these are rarely troublesome. *Unlike the broad spectrum antibiotics, sulfonamides do not usually produce troublesome disturbances in the gut flora.*

- ***Renal toxicity*:** In the presence of acid urine, the acetylated form of the drug may be precipitated, mainly in the collecting tubules and the calyces. This may cause urinary obstruction and may precipitate renal colic. Crystalluria, albuminuria and haematuria can occur. These can be minimised by :

(i) Ensuring an adequate fluid intakes to maintain urine output of 1200 ml per day.

(ii) Making the urine alkaline to increase the solubility of the conjugation products.

(iii) Use of sulfonamides with acetylated metabolites soluble in acid urine e.g. sulfisoxazole

Renal damage with tubular necrosis and vasculitis can also occur as an allergic reaction.

- ***Haemopoietic toxicity*:** This includes thrombocytopenia, agranulocytosis and rarely aplastic anemia. Sulfonamides tend to oxidize hemoglobin to methemoglobin. In patients with G6PD deficiency, they may cause intravascular hemolysis.

- ***Bilirubin metabolism*:** Sulfonamides compete with serum bilirubin for albumin binding sites. Administered during late pregnancy, they may displace bilirubin from albumin binding sites in the foetus. The free bilirubin, by crossing the blood-brain barrier, which is permeable to bilirubin only in foetuses and infants, causes kernicterus. Sulfonamides may also cause kernicterus when administered to new born and premature infants. They should not be given to neonates, and to pregnant women.

- ***Nervous system toxicity*:** These include CNS disturbances like confusion, depression, ataxia, tinnitus, fatigue and acute psychotic episodes. These disturbances are commoner in children than in adults. Rarely, peripheral neuritis may occur.

- ***Miscellaneous*:** Endocrinal disturbances such as goitre and hypothyroidism have been reported after prolonged use.

Drug interactions: Table 44.3 lists the common interactions of sulfonamides.

Table 44.3: Interactions of sulfonamides

Interfering drug	Result
Sulfonylureas	ID displaced from plasma protein binding, with possible hypoglycemia
Coumarin anticoagulants, Methotrexate, Phenytoin, Thiopental	ID activity enhanced
Phenylbutazone, Salicylate, Probenecid	S displaced from plasma binding, with enhancement of S activity
Methenemine	Certain S are precipitated in urine
PABA-containing local anaesthetics e.g. Procaine	Direct inhibition of S activity

ID = Interfering drug; S = Sulfonamide

Therapeutic uses: Sulfonamides are relatively cheap, broad spectrum chemotherapeutic agents. However, *their importance in therapeutics has diminished because of the development of resistance by a variety of organisms.*

For routine systemic use, **sulfadimidine, sulfadiazine** and similar other short acting compounds are as good as each other. As these drugs are bacteriostatic, effective blood levels must be maintained by a regular dose regimen.

The therapeutic uses are:

- ***Urinary tract infections***: See Chapter 50.
- ***Meningococcal meningitis*** (used as cotrimoxazole) **:** See Chapter 47.
- ***Inflammatory bowel disease*** **(IBD) :** IBD results from a "dysregulated inflammatory response to the commensal, microbial flora residing in intestinal lumen". It shows a genetic predisposition. Ulcerative colitis is an IBD affecting mainly the rectum and the colon. Clinically, it causes diarrhea with blood in the stools, weight loss and may cause systemic symptoms. Generally, it is mild but sometimes it can develop into toxic colitis with severely ulcerated mucosa. This condition and another IBD, Crohn's disease, are due to an immunological response to bacterial antigens of intestinal luminal origin. In contrast to ulcerative colitis, Crohn's disease affects the small intestine and the colon. The lesions in ulcerative colitis are superficial whereas those in Crohn's disease are transmural.

The mainstay of therapy for mild and moderate ulcerative colitis is sulfasalazine and other aminosalicylic acid (ASA) compounds (Table 44 .4). They can induce and maintain a remission in ulcerative colitis; but their beneficial effect in Crohn's disease is less predictable. Acute exacerbations may respond to glucocorticoid therapy. Cases resistant to both mesalazine and glucocorticoids may be treated with either an immunosuppressant drug or infliximab (Table 44.4). Favourable response to azathioprine is seen in two-third of the patients. Mesalazine and glucocorticoids may be used during pregnancy and are generally safe.

SULFASALAZINE (Salazopyrine) is sulfapyridine linked to 5-aminosalicylic acid (5-ASA, **mesalazine**) by an azo bond; it was one of the first drugs, which, when given orally, reach the colon unaltered; and it is split there by the colonic bacteria into its constituents. Sulfapyridine is absorbed rapidly, is acetylated in the liver and excreted in the urine. It has no therapeutic action in ulcerative colitis.

Table 44.4: Drugs used in ulcerative colitis

Drugs	Doses/day (in divided doses)
Antiinflammatory	
*Oral**	6
Sulfasalazine	2-4 g
Olsalazine	1-2 g
Mesalazine	1.5-4.8 g
Prednisolone	40-60 mg
Topical	
Mesalazine enema	1-4 g
Hydrocortisone enema	100-200 mg
Intra venous	
Hydrocortisone	300 mg
Antimicrobials**	
Metronidazole; Ciprofloxacin; Co-trimoxazole; Clarithromycin	In severe cases.
Immunosuppressants	
6-Mercaptopurine	50 - 150 mg
Azathioprine	50 - 150 mg
Methotrexate	15-25 mg***
Anti-TNF α antibody	
Infliximab (Chapter 71)	

* Used for maintenance.
** More useful in Crohn's disease.
*** Parenterally once a week

Mesalazine which is poorly absorbed induces remission in ulcerative colitis.

Adverse Reactions to sulfasalazine include nausea, malena, headache, myalgias and sulfa-induced allergic reactions. Folate deficiency can occur, and folic acid administration (1mg/day) is recommended during long term treatment. Table 44.5 summarises the mesalazine preparations.

Mesalazine is rapidly absorbed from the jejunum, and hence is marketed as delayed release forms (Table 44.5). The drug may cause nausea, abdominal pain, diarrhea, and rarely interstitial nephritis.

Glucocorticoids: Moderate and severe acute *exacerbations* of ulcerative colitis and Crohn's disease respond to additional oral or IV

Table 44.5: Mesalazine (MS) preparations

Preparation	Chemical / pharmaceutical form	Delivery of MS	Distribution of MS	Dose
Sulfasalazine (Salazopyrine)	MS linked to sulfapyridine	Bacterial cleavage	Colon	2-6 g/day in divided doses
Balsalazide (Colazide)	MS linked to an inert molecule	Bacterial cleavage	Colon	2.25 g (three 750 mg capsules) tid
Olsalazine (Dipentum)	MS linked to MS	Bacterial cleavage	Colon	1.5-3.g/day in divided doses
MS (Pentasa)	Time release preparation	Time release	Ileum and colon	3-4 g/day in divided doses
MS(Asacol)	pH-sensitive coated MS	Release at pH > 7	Distal ileum and colon	2.4-4.8 g/day in divided doses
MS suppository	MS	Direct	Rectum	0.5-1 g OD/bid
MS enema	MS	Direct	Left colon	4 g in 60 ml

Linkage is by azo bond. Preparation without a sulfonamide are better tolerated than sulfasalazine, and therefore are preferred.

glucocorticoid therapy, which can induce a remission. Glucocorticoids, however, have no role in the maintenance therapy. The patients with IBD may be classified as: glucocorticoid responsive (40 %), glucocorticoid dependent and glucocorticoid unresponsive (20 %). The therapeutic response is generally observed in 1-2 weeks, whereas the unresponsive patients do not improve even with prolonged, high dose therapy. After remission, the dose is tapered over six to eight weeks. In ulcerative colitis restricted to the rectum or the left hemicolon, glucocorticoid suppositories or enemas may prove useful.

Glucocorticoid therapy may sometimes lead to intercurrent, opportunistic infections and sepsis. Reactivation of pulmonary tuberculosis is another dreaded complication Patients not responding to steroids are given immunosuppresants (Chapter 75).

Antibiotics: Antibiotics (Table 44.4) are used (a) as adjuncts to the above drugs in active IBD; (b) as treatment for a specific complication of Crohn's disease such as an intra-abdominal or perianal abscess.; and (c) for prophylaxis of postoperative recurrence in Crohn's disease.

- ***Toxoplasmosis and Malaria:*** Sulfonamides in combination with pyrimethamine are used in the treatment of resistant malaria and toxoplasmosis (Chapters 54, 56).
- ***Acute bacillary dysentery***: Used as co-trimoxazole. See Chapter 48.
- ***Chancroid***: See Chapter 51.
- ***Trachoma and inclusion conjunctivitis***: Though effective, it is no more the drug of choice. See Chapter 70.
- ***Miscellaneous***: Sulfadiazine, in the dose of 4 to 6 g. daily, in combination with an antibiotic, for several months, is of some value

in nocardiosis. Sulfasalazine therapy has been found useful in rheumatoid arthritis (Chapter 71).

- ***Use in prophylaxis***: Sulfadimidine in the dose of 1 g. twice daily has been used to prevent attacks of streptococcal tonsillitis in patients who have recovered from rheumatic fever, but are allergic to penicillin. *Sulfonamides should not be used to treat established streptococcal pharyngitis* because they fail to eradicate the bacteria, and late sequelae may develop.

Although sulfonamides are mainly bacteriostatic, they do not antagonize the bactericidal effects of penicillin and can be combined with it for treating susceptible infections.

Co-trimoxazole

TRIMETHOPRIM / COTRIMOXAZOLE: Trimethoprim is a pyrimidine derivative which is effective against many common pathogenic bacteria. It is slightly soluble in water. Given alone, it is either bacteriostatic or bactercidal. In *in vitro* studies it is highly effective against *Staph, aureus, Streptococci, C. diphtheria, E. coli, Salmonella, Shigella, H. influenzae, K. pneumoniae, Proteus* and *V. cholerae.* It is somewhat less effective against *N. gonorrhoeae, N. meningitidis, Cl. welchii* and *B. pertusis.* Mycobacteria and pseudomonas, however, are not affected. Its action may be inhibited in necrotic wounds containing pus and other cellular debris, as the pus contains thymine and thymidine.

Mechanism of action: Bacteria and protozoa synthesize folic acid from para-aminobenzoic acid (PABA), which is necessary for their growth (Fig. 44.3). Trimethoprim inhibits the enzyme dihydrofolate reductase, which converts dihydrofolate to tetrahydrofolic acid. It is known that the bacterial and mammalian cells differ, resulting in a greater susceptibility of the bacterial enzyme to trimethoprim. Since higher animals and man utilize preformed folic or folinic acid from the diet they are relatively immune to the harmful effect of trimethoprim. Further, any depressant effect of this drug on human folate metabolism can be countered by feeding exogenous folate.

Since sulfonamides act by inhibiting the incorporation of PABA into dihydrofolate by organisms, a combination of trimethoprim and sulfonamide acts sequentially in the same metabolic pathway in the synthesis of nucleotides (Fig. 44.3). Hence, trimethoprim which is 20-100 times more potent than the sulfonamide is combined with sulfamethoxazole. This combination, known as **Co-trimoxazole,** is synergistic and acts as bactericidal. Bacterial resistance to this combination develops less frequently than when either drug is used alone.

Absorption, fate and excretion: Trimethoprim is rapidly and almost completely absorbed from the intestines. The peak plasma level is achieved in 1 ½ to 3 ½ hours.

To achieve optimum synergism, trimethoprim is combined with sulfamethoxazole which has absorption and excretion characteristics very close to those of trimethoprim. Co-trimoxazole contains trimethoprim 80 mg. with sulfamethoxazole 400 mg. (1 : 5). Given orally it has been shown to give the optimum synergistic ratio in the plasma against common pathogens.

Trimethoprim is distributed more widely than sulfamethoxazole which essentially remains in the ECF. This explains the higher optimum (20:1) sulfonamide: trimethoprim ratio in the plasma than that (5:1) in the tablets. Because of the differences in the distributions of these two drugs, different ratios may be observed in different tissues. Adequate concentration is reached in CSF and in bile. Vaginal secretions contain substantially more drug than the plasma. Trimethoprim is a weak base and hence, its excretion increases markedly with acidification of urine, due to its ionization.

The half lives of trimethoprim and sulfamethoxazole are 16 and 10 hours respectively. About 70% of the oral dose of trimethoprim is excreted in the urine within 24 hours; about 80% of this is in an unchanged form.

Adverse reactions to cotrimoxazole: These are due to

- ***Sulfonamide component;*** and
- ***Trimethoprim.***

The combination can cause nausea, vomiting, abdominal pain and diarrhoea. Skin reactions are three times more common with the combination than with individual agents. Glossitis and stomatitis are relatively common. Trimethoprim may precipitate megaloblastic anemia in persons with pre-existing folic acid deficiency. Serious toxicity appears to be more common in patients with AIDS.

When creatinine clearance falls below 30 ml/min. the interval between doses of 2 tablets should be increased from 12 to 24 hours and when it is below 15ml/min, the drug should not be used.

Bacteria can develop resistance to such combination. Further, *its use in pregnant women should be avoided because of the teratogenicity of large doses of trimethoprim in animals.*

Preparations and dosage:

(i) Cotrimoxazole contains trimethoprim 80 mg. + sulfamethoxazole 400 mg. (Septran, Methoxaprim, Bactrim); dose 2 tablets (3 tablets in severe infection) twice daily for 10-14 days for the management of most infections. The drug can also be used IM or IV in the dose of 960 mg. (equivalent to 2 tablets) every 12 hours. The large fluid volumes required for IV cotrimoxazole may complicate the care of cardiac and renal patients. Paediatric tablets contain trimethoprim 20 mg. + sulfamethoxazole 100 mg. Suspension of 40 mg. trimethoprim + 200 mg. sulfamethoxazole per 5 ml. is also available.

(ii) Trimethoprim (Trimopan, Ipral, Soloprim) 200 mg. tablets; 1-1½ tablets every 12 hours.

Therapeutic uses of co-trimoxazole:

- ***Urinary tract infection*** due to *E.coli* and *Proteus* group of organism (Chapter 50).
- ***Prostatitis*** **:** It is the therapy of choice. Trimethoprim alone has been used in treating UTI and prostatitis.
- ***Respiratory tract infections such as bronchitis, sinusitis and otitis media.***
- ***GI infections such as shigellosis.***
- ***Typhoid fever*** (Chapter 48).
- ***STD such as Gonorrhoea, Chancroid*** (Chapter 51).
- ***Serious infections*** such as meningitis and osteomyelitis due to susceptible Gram negative organisms.
- ***Infection by Pneumocystis carinii:*** It has been used in high doses (15-20 mg/kg/day of trimethoprim plus 75-100 mg/kg/day of sulfamethoxazole) to treat *Pneumocystis carinii* infection in immunocompromised patients where it is the drug of choice. Intravenous administration of cotrimoxazole plus carbenicillin has been used to treat infections in neutropenic patients. Low dose therapy (150 mg/m²/day of trimethoprim plus 750 mg/m²/day of sulfamethoxazole) has been used for prophylaxis of *P. carinii* in severely neutropenic patients.
- ***Miscellaneous:*** Plague, brucellosis and nocardiosis. (Chapter 48).

Advantages of cotrimoxazole are that it is:

- ***A broad spectrum antibacterial drug***
- ***Relatively safe and well tolerated;*** and
- ***Highly cost-effective in many common infections in practice.***

Nitrofurans

The antibacterial activity of the nitrofuran compounds was demonstrated by Dodd and Stillman in 1944.

Mechanism of action: They undergo enzymatic reduction, resulting in a highly reactive intermediate that damages the DNA. They also possess radiomimetic and mutagenic properties.

Pharmacological actions: Nitrofurans exert antimicrobial action against a variety of Gram positive and Gram negative organisms including *Staphylococci, Streptococci, E. Coli, Salmonella* and *Shigella* organisms. Some of these compounds, particularly furazolidone, inhibit the growth of *Trichomonas vaginalis,* a protozoal organism, while another compound nifuroxime is effective against *Candida albicans* and other fungi. Though usually bacteriostatic, the nitrofurans can be bactericidal in high concentrations. The presence of heavy bacterial infection, plasma or blood reduces the antibacterial activity. Bacterial resistance can develop and cross resistance among the various compounds is also known.

Adverse reactions: These include abdominal discomfort, nausea, vomiting and rashes of various types. Rarely, haemolytic anemia may develop in individuals with G6PD deficiency. Immunological reactions such as pulmonary infiltration and fibrosis, chronic active hepatitis, and SLE-like reaction have been reported. The drug may precipitate antabuse-like reactions in alcoholics. Polyneuritis is an important adverse effect which particularly occurs in the presence of impaired renal function. These compounds are avoided during pregnancy and infancy.

Preparations: Nitrofurans are yellow, crystalline compounds, sparingly soluble in water. They should be protected from light. The drugs available are:

NITROFURANTOIN (Nifran): It is rapidly and completely absorbed from the GI tract. Food increases its bioavailability. It does not achieve a bacteriostatic concentration in the plasma but approximately 40 per cent of the drug is excreted unchanged by the kidney, achieving a bactericidal concentration in the urine. The drug is effective against many common urinary pathogens, including *E. coli* and *Aerobacter,* and is used exclusively as a urinary antiseptic (Chapter 50). Its activity is considerably less at pH 8 than at pH 5.5. *Therefore, the urine should not be alkalinised during therapy with nitrofurantoin.* The plasma half life is 0.3-1 hour. It is bactericidal to some anaerobic bacteria. The low plasma levels achieved by oral route make such treatment useless for systemic infections. It interferes with the therapeutic action of some quinolones.

It is administered orally with food in the dose of 50-100 mg. six hourly. The comparable dose in children is 50 mg. upto 1 year, 75 to 100 mg. from 1 to 5 years and 150 to 200 mg. from 6 to 12 years in 3 or 4 divided doses. The drug should not be continued in this dose for more than 2 weeks. The dose for long suppression of susceptible urinary tract pathogens is 100 mg once a day. *It does not appear in the urine in severe renal failure and in azotemic patients, and hence should be avoided.* The drug colours the urine brown.

FURAZOLIDONE (Furoxone): This compound has been employed effectively in the treatment of gastrointestinal infections such as bacterial enteritis, bacillary dysentery and giardiasis; and locally in trichomonal vaginitis. The drug does not significantly depress the normal intestinal flora. It is bactericidal. It is administered orally; the adult dose is 100 mg. 4 times daily for 5-7 days. It is used locally, along with nifuroxime, in the treatment of bacterial, trichomonal and monilial vaginitis.

NIFUROXIME: The compound is effective against the fungus *Candida albicans,* a common vaginal pathogen, and is employed locally usually along with furazolidone.

NITROFURAZONE (Furacin) is available as 0.2 per cent solution and ointment for topical application for the treatment of superficial wounds and skin infections. It is used systemically in trypanosomiasis (Chapter 56).

Quinolones

Quinolones, particularly the fluoroquinolones are an important therapeutic advance. These agents have broad antimicrobial activity and are effective orally. (Table 44.6).

Mechanism of action: Quinolones inhibit (a) DNA gyrase and (b) DNA topoisomerase IV. The former action is direct and leads to an arrest of DNA replication. The latter action also arrests DNA replication but by blocking the enzyme's normal function of delinking the daughter DNA molecule. The activity of quinolones against Gram negative bacteria is primarily due to their action on DNA gyrase, whereas that against Gram positive bacteria is primarily due to their action on topoisomerase IV. This may explain the differences in the antibacterial spectra of the various quinolones. They are more active against Gram negative than against Gram positive bacteria. Bacteria can develop resistance to quinolones by mutation.

NALIDIXIC ACID (Neg-Gram, Gramoneg): It is a 4-quinolone derivative. As suggested by its trade name, nalidixic acid is effective against certain Gram negative bacteria, especially *E. coli* and shigella. The most important action, however, is its efficacy against many strains of Proteus. It is relatively ineffective against Gram positive organisms. Bacteria can develop resistance to it fairly rapidly *in vitro.*

Nalidixic acid is readily absorbed from the GI tract. The serum levels of the drug are low, but approximately 80 per cent of it is eliminated in the urine within 8 hours. It is present in the urine in both active (20 per cent) and inactive, conjugated forms.

Adverse reactions include allergic reactions, nausea, vomiting and diarrhoea. Allergy is manifested by pruritus, rash, urticaria, fever, eosinophilia and photosensitivity. The CNS manifestations include headache, malaise, drowsiness and myalgia. Convulsions may appear with overdosage, particularly in children. It may cause hemolytic anemia which has been reported in a two week old baby fed on breast milk, due to the presence of the drug in the breast milk. It may cause increase in intracranial pressure (pseudotumour cerebri) in young children. Erosion of weight bearing joints has been reported in growing animals. Because of its toxicity, limited utility and availability of fluoroquinolones, its use has now diminished.

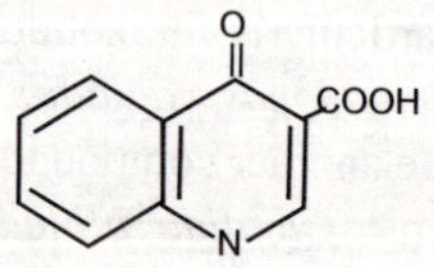

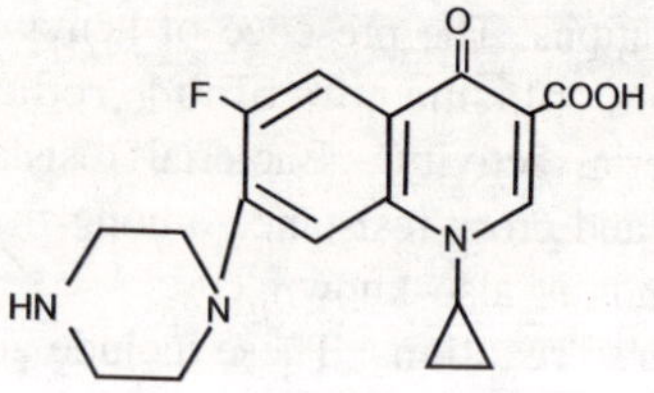

Fig. 44.4 : Fluoroquinolones

FLUOROQUINOLONES: These drugs are chemically related to nalidixic acid and are called fluoroquinolones because of the fluorine in their chemical structure. They are :

- ***Highly effective orally.***
- ***Rapidly bactericidal with broad antibacterial spectrum.***
- ***Effective against bacteria resistant to beta-lactam and aminoglycoside antibiotics.***
- ***Relatively safe;*** and
- ***Relatively immune to the development of resistance by bacteria.***

Antibacterial Activity: They are effective against both Gram positive and Gram negative organisms, in a concentration dependent manner. Thus, these compounds have excellent activity against the Enterobacteriaceae (*E.coli, Klebsiela* and *Proteus mirabalis*) including many organisms resistant to penicillins, cephalosporins and aminoglycosides.

They are highly effective against Shigella species, salmonellae (including those resistant to chloramphenicol), *H.ducrei. H. influenzae, B. catarrhalis* and Neisseria species including penicillinase producing gonococci. *Pseudomonas aeruginosa* is inhibited in the urinary tract but not in other tissues/sites due to inadequate concentrations available in the latter sites. Staphylococci including methicillin resistant *Staph. aureus* are well inhibited. They have high activity against streptococci including *Strept. pneumoniae*. Intracellular pathogens such as legionella, brucella, chlamydia and mycoplasma pneumoniae are inhibited to variable degrees. However, they are highly effective against *Mycobacterium tuberculosis* and *M.avium complex.*

Bacteria, including pseudomonas and staphylococci, can develop resistance to fluoroquinolones, generally by genetic mutation.The activity of fluoroquinolones diminishes in acid urine.

Absorption, fate and excretion: The oral bioavailability of fluoroquinolones is excellent and the plasma levels after oral administration are similar to those after IV administration. Hence, their IV administration is rarely indicated. However, the simultaneous administration of compounds of aluminium, magnesium (antacids), zinc, iron and calcium leads to formation of complexes in the GI tract, and a reduction in their bioavailability. Food delays their absorption. They are concentrated in urine, kidney, prostatic tissue, and achieve therapeutic levels in lungs and bones. There is substantial excretion and reabsorption in the colon. They are concentrated within macrophages and polymorphonuclear neutrophils. Newer fluoroquinolones have larger volumes of distribution than the older analogues.

Metabolism of the fluoroquinolones varies considerably. Thus, levofloxacin, ofloxacin and lomefloxacin are entirely eliminated by the kidneys, and a dose adjustment is a must even with minor reductions in renal function. On the other hand, pefloxacin, gemifloxacin and sparfloxacin are mostly eliminated by the liver. Ciprofloxacin is eliminated by both liver and kidneys.

Quinolones such as ciprofloxacin are potent liver enzyme inhibitors and can reduce the metabolism of warfarin, theophylline and sulfonyluereas.

Due to differences in the pharmacokinetic properties, norfloxacin is effective in infections of the urinary and GI tracts; serum levels of norfloxacin are relatively low and therefore, it is not recommended for systemic infections. Other fluoroquinolones are useful for infections at other sites as well.

Preparations and dosage : See Table 44.6.

Nadifloxacin is available as 1% cream for topical application to the skin.

Adverse reactions: In general, these drugs are well tolerated.

- ***GI toxicity***: Anorexia, nausea, vomiting, abdominal discomfort and diarrhoea are the commonest side effects. Trovafloxacin can cause severe hepatotoxicity.
- ***CNS toxicity***: They cause CNS toxicity such as mild headache, dizziness, nervousness and insomnia. Confusion, agitation, hallucinations and rarely seizures are seen especially in patients receiving INH, theophylline and NSAIDs.
- ***Tendon and cartilage damage***: Rupture of shoulder, hand and Achilles tendons that require surgical repair have been reported with these drugs. Treatment should be discontinued if the patient experiences pain, inflammation and rupture of a tendon. Because of the cartilage damage in weight bearing joints of young animals, they should be avoided in pregnant and nursing mothers and in young children.
- ***Cardiac toxicity*** : Sparfloxacin and rarely gatifloxacin and moxifloxacin can prolong QTc interval in patients on class III or class Ic antiarrythmic drugs.
- ***Miscellaneous toxicity***: Allergic reactions such as skin rash, arthralgia and photosensitivity have been reported. Rarely, leucopenia and renal damage with acute renal failure can occur. Rupture of tendo achillis has been reported in elderly persons, especially those on glucocorticoids. Gatifloxacin has been reported to cause both hyperglycemia and hypoglycemia.

Therapeutic uses: Because of their pharmacokinetic properties (superior bioavail-

Table 44.6: Quinolone generations: Pharmacokinetic features, doses and indications

Name	Oral bioavailability %	t½ (hours)	Metabolism/ Clearance	Dose	Indications
			Second generation: Class I		
Norfloxacin (Norflox)	30-40	3-4	R/H	400 mg. bid	UTI, prostatitis
Lomefloxacin* (Lomaday)	About 90	6-8	R	400 mg. OD IV 400 mg.	
			Second generation: Class II		
Ciprofloxacin *(Cifran)	60-70	3.3-4.9	R/H	250 mg OD 250 - 750 mg. bid 200 - 400 mg. by IV infusion (over 30-60 min) bid	UTI, Typhoid, Gonorrhoea, Gastroenteritis, skin, soft tissue, bone and joint infections especially Gram negative
Ofloxacin* (Tarivid)	About 95	5-7	R	200-400 mg. OD	
Pefloxacin *(Pelox)	About 90	8-13	H	400 mg. bid; 400 mg. by IV infusion (over 1 hour) bid	
			Third generation		
SparfloxacinrΔ (Sparlox)	>90	21	H	200-400 mg. in one or two divided doses per day	Like Class II Preferred in community acquired pneumonia.
LevofloxacinrΔ (Tavanic)	> 90	6 -8	R	500 mg. OD for 7-14 days	
GatifloxacinrΔ (Tequin)	95	7	R/H	400 mg OD	
MoxifloxacinrΔ (Avelox)	90	12	R/H	400 mg OD	
GemifloxacinΔ (Factive)	70	7	H	300 mg OD	
			Forth generation		
Trovafloxacin	88-90	7-8	H	100-200 mg OD	Treatment of intra-abdominal infection

Nalidixic acid and conoxacin are first generation quinolones.

* Also available for IV infusion. R = Renal. H = Hepatic.

Δ These are termed **respiratory fluoroquinolones** because of their excellent antipneumococcal activity.

Table 44.7: Conditions in which fluoroquinolones are preferred

- ***Complicated urinary tract infections*** (Chapter 50), especially those caused by *Ps.aeruginosa* or other drug resistant Gram negative pathogens.
- ***Bacterial gastroenteritis*** in patients ill enough to merit empiric therapy, especially salmonella gastroenteritis.
- ***Typhoid fever resistant to chloramphenicol,*** and of the fecal carrier state of *S.typhi* (for which they are the drugs of choice).
- ***Invasive otitis media*** by *Ps.aeruginosa.*
- ***Gram negative osteomyelitis.***
- ***Respiratory infections*** including acute pneumonias and acute exacerbations in chronic bronchitis.
- ***Multidrug resistant tuberculosis.***
- ***Atypical avian complex.***
- ***Leprosy.***
- ***Empiric treatment of septicemia.***

ability, tissue distribution and penetration) broad spectrum, and bactericidal activity against most aerobic Gram negative and many aerobic Gram positive bacteria, fluoroquinolones are useful in treating a wide variety of infections in many anatomical sites. Table 44.7 lists the conditions for which the fluoroquinolones are preferred.

Although they may be highly effective in gonorrhoea and chancroid, the need to exclude syphilis diminishes their value as primary agents in sexually transmitted diseases. **Ofloxacin** and **sparfloxacin** are effective against acid fast bacilli and are used to treat tuberculosis and leprosy. (See Chapters 52 and 53).

Though effective, fluoroquinolones *are not recommended* for the routine treatment of uncomplicated UTI, mild to moderate GI infections and skin infections. Because of drug toxicity and cost, they are the drugs of first choice only in a limited number of situations (Table 44.7). Their routine use in all and sundry infections, where a cheaper and equally effective drug such as co-trimaxazole is available, is to be discouraged.

Penicillins and Other Antibiotics Effective Mainly Against Gram Positive Organisms

45

PENICILLIN, the most important of the antibiotics, was first extracted from the mould *Penicillium notatum.* Subsequently, a mutant of a related mould, *P. chrysogenum,* was found to give the highest yield of penicillin and is employed for its commercial production.

Pencillins belong to a group of antibiotics called as **beta-lactam antibiotics;** the other members include **cephalosporins, cephamycins, monobactams** and **carbapenems.**

The basic structure of the penicillins consists of a thiazolidine ring fused with a beta lactam ring which is essential for antibacterial activity. The two rings constitute the fundamental nucleus of all the pencillins, namely, 6-amino-penicillanic acid (6-APA). A variety of semi-synthetic penicillins are produced by altering the composition of the side chain attached to 6-APA nucleus (Fig. 45.1). Both the 6-APA nucleus and the side chain are essential for the antibacterial activity, but the side chain, in addition, determines the stability of the penicillin against degradation by gastric acid and by the enzyme **penicillinase (betalactamase)** produced by certain micro-organisms such as *Staphylococcus aureus, Pseudomonas, Enterobacter* and some strains of *H. influenzae* and *N. gonorrhoea.*

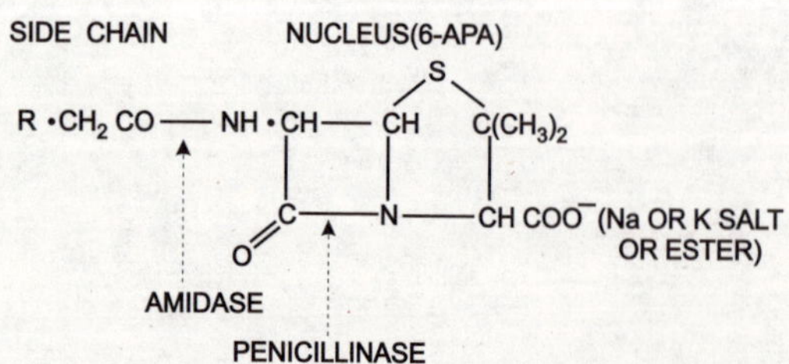

Fig. 45.1: Basic structure of penicillins

Mechanism of action: Penicillins are bactericidal drugs. The effect continues for a period of 3 to 8 hours after withdrawing penicillin G and a bacteriological cure is assured if penicillin is present in patient's plasma for a total period of 6 hours per day. The best effect is achieved by a concentration 5-20 times greater than the minimum concentration which inhibits growth.

The action of penicillins requires the presence of a cell wall that contains peptidoglycans. Peptidoglycan is a major structural component of the bacterial cell wall that is cross-linked into a net like structure that surrounds the bacterial cell to provide it with strength and rigidity. Penicillin binding proteins are bacterial enzymes located on the cell membrane (which is inside the cell wall) and are responsible for the biosynthesis and cross linkage of the peptidoglycans in the cell wall. Penicillins bind to these proteins and inactivate them, thereby preventing the synthesis of peptidoglycans. This weakens the bacterial cell wall and makes the organisms vulnerable to rupture by solutes in the surrounding medium (viz, plasma). As cell wall synthesis occurs during the growth phase, the antibiotic is most effective against actively multiplying organisms. Although human cells have cell membrance, they lack a cell wall. In addition to the above action, penicillins activate the bacterial, endogenous, autolytic system and initiate cell lysis and death.

The cell-walls of Gram-negative bacilli are chemically more complex. Although some inhibition of cell-wall synthesis has been demonstrated in these organisms with penicillin, a relatively high concentration of the drug is required to achieve this effect. These cell walls contain betalactamases in small amounts that are enough to inactivate penicillin.

Bacterial resistance: Bacterial resistance to penicillin can be

- ***Natural or***
- ***Acquired.***

Fortunately, bacteria do not acquire resistance to penicillin easily and sensitivity of many of the susceptible pathogens has so far remained unchanged. The resistance develops stepwise. Staphylococci resistant to penicillin are common. *Streptococcus viridans* also develops resistance but to a lesser extent. Partially resistant strains of gonococci, meningococci and pneumococci are also encountered.

The most important mechanism of bacterial resistance to the beta-lactam antibiotics is bacterial production of beta-lactamases, that hydrolyse the beta-lactam ring and render the drug inactive. Penicillin-resistant strains of staphylococci elaborate an enzyme a beta-lactamase (penicillinase). Staphylococci that do not produce beta-lactamase may, however, also develop resistance to penicillin *in vitro.* Many other microorganisms such as *E. coli, M. tuberculosis, B. anthracis* and *A. aerogenes* also produce beta-lactamases. Presence of beta-lactamase elaborating bacteria in a mixed infection may lead to a rapid destruction of penicillin with a consequent reduction in its therapeutic efficacy. Thus, penicillin may not be effective in the treatment of *Strep. pyogenes* pharyngitis if beta-lactamase-elaborating staphylococci are also present in the throat.

BENZYLPENICILLIN: Benzylpenicillin is available in the form of its water soluble sodium and potassium salts. These salts in a dry state are stable at room temperature for years; the aqueous solution, however, requires refrigeration and deteriorates considerably within 72 hours.

The Oxford international unit for benzylpenicillin is equivalent to the activity contained in 0.6 micrograms of sodium salt of benzylpenicillin. One mg. of sodium salt is thus equivalent to 1667 units of penicillin. A mega unit of penicillin is 1 million units.

Antibacterial activity: Benzylpenicillin is one of the most potent antimicrobial agents and inhibits the growth of susceptible organisms *in vitro* in a concentration as low as 1 in 50 million.

It is effective mainly against Gram-positive and Gram-negative cocci and some Gram-positive bacilli. Gram-negative bacilli are usually resistant. Thus, majority of *Streptococci* with the exception of D strains (enterococci) are highly susceptible. *Staphylococci,* initially highly sensitive to penicillin, have acquired resistance on a large scale. *Gonococci, Pneumococci* and *Meningococci* are sensitive to penicillin. *Bacillus anthracis, Corynebacterium diphtheriae* and most anaerobic microorganisms, including the *Clostridium* species, are highly sensitive; *Bacteroides fragilis,* however, needs very high concentration to inhibit its growth. Among the spirochaetes, *Treponema pallidum* is extremely sensitive to penicillin while leptospira infection responds moderately. Although penicillin is effective in actinomycosis, it is not useful against other fungi.

Absorption, fate and excretion: Given orally, benzylpenicillin is largely inactivated by the gastric acid. The drug is mainly absorbed from the duodenum. Only a small proportion of the oral dose is detected in feces as a large amount is inactivated by the intestinal bacterial flora. Because of inadequate (15-30%) and irregular absorption, the oral dose of benzylpenicillin required to achieve an effective therapeutic plasma level is 4 to 5 times larger than the equivalent IM dose. *As food interferes with its absorption, it should be given at least 30* *minutes before or 2 to 3 hours after a meal.* In infants, gastric acidity is low and hence, higher blood levels can be achieved on oral administration.

Benzylpenicillin in aqueous solution is rapidly absorbed after SC or IM administration. Peak plasma level of 8 to 10 units per ml. is reached within 15 to 30 minutes and the drug disappears from the plasma within 3 to 6 hours. Absorption of penicillin from mucous membranes is erratic and variable. Moreover, a high risk of sensitization accompanies the use of penicillin in such forms as lozenges and troches which are, therefore, not recommended.

Penicillin is widely distributed in the body after absorption. Very high concentrations are detected in the kidneys. However, the drug penetrates poorly into the serous cavities, the concentrations in ocular, pericardial, pleural and peritoneal fluids being low. In the presence of inflammation, its concentration in these fluids is higher. Subconjunctival injection results in high concentration in the ocular fluid. The drug does not readily cross the BBB, but therapeutically adequate CSF concentration is achieved in the presence of meningeal inflammation. It crosses the placental barrier.

Approximately 60 per cent of plasma penicillin is bound to albumin; the remainder is present in the free form.

Nearly 30 per cent of a single parenteral dose is metabolized. Small amounts appear in bile, milk and saliva. *The major portion is eliminated by the kidneys.* About 50 per cent of the drug elimination in urine occurs within the first hour, resulting in a rapid decline in the plasma level. The elimination half-time is about 30 minutes. Nearly 80 to 85 per cent of urinary excretion occurs by tubular secretion and only 10 to 15 per cent by glomerular filtration. It is important to note that *doubling the dose does not double the duration of effect, and that for continuous effect, large and frequent doses are essential.* Neonates and infants in whom renal function is not adequately developed, and individuals with renal insufficiency show prolonged and higher plasma levels. In anuria the plasma half life of penicillin is increased to about 10 hours. Thus, in an adult with anuria an adequate dose for the treatment of a highly sensitive infection would be only 2000 units per dose.

Rapid urinary elimination of benzylpenicillin necessitates its parenteral administration at 4 or 6 hourly intervals. Repository preparations overcome this drawback. They are relatively insoluble and release benzylpenicillin slowly when injected. They thus produce relatively low but prolonged plasma concentration. These agents, however, are not useful for treating severe infections where an immediate, high plasma concentration of benzylpenicillin is desirable. In contrast to adults, neonates and infants excrete penicillin slowly and require 12 hourly administration.

Preparations and dosage:

(i) Benzylpenicillin (Penicillin G) (sodium and potassium salts) injection 500,000 units per ml.

(ii) Benzylpenicillin tablet (Pentids) contains 50,000 to 500,000 units of benzylpenicillin. Dose: 200,000 to 400,000 units 4 hourly. Peak plasma level of 0.2 to 0.3 units/ml. is reached within 1 to 2 hours after oral ingestion.

The **repository preparations** are:

(i) Procaine benzylpenicillin available in powder form, to be suspended in distilled water, prior to injection. Dose : 600,000 to 1,200,000 units daily by IM injection. After a single dose, the peak plasma level of 0.3 units per ml. is reached within 1 to 3 hours. This level is 25 times lower than that attained by parenteral aqueous benzylpenicillin. The drug, however, remains in blood for 8 to 12 hours, and in some patients for 24 hours. Aqueous solutions are stable for many months at temperatures below 25^{0}C.

(ii) Fortified benzylpenicillin injection contains a mixture of 300,000 units of procaine benzylpenicillin and 100,000 units of benzylpenicillin per ml. Such a preparation achieves a quick and high serum penicillin concentration and the effective concentration persists in the plasma for 12 to 24 hours.

(iii) Benzathine penicillin (Penidure, Benapen) is a dibenzylethylenediamine salt of benzylpenicillin. It has a very poor water solubility and is administered by IM injection in the dose of 600,000 to 2,400,000 units. With the IM dose of 600,000 units, blood levels of 0.03 to 0.1 units per ml. are reached which persist for 10 days and the drug is detected in the plasma for 2 weeks. A dose of 1.2 million units produces detectable blood levels for 3 weeks. Benzathine penicillin should be used only in conditions where the infecting microorganism is exquisitely sensitive to low concentrations of penicillin viz, (a) for treatment and prophylaxis of pharyngitis due to group A beta-hemolytic streptococci; (b) for treatment of pyoderma due to group A beta-hemolytic streptococci; and (c) for treatment of syphilis *not involving the CNS.*

Probenecid, a uricosuric agent, competes with penicillin for tubular transport and delays its excretion. Administered orally in the dose of 2 g. per day, in divided doses, along with penicillin, it raises its plasma level twofold to fourfold which is maintained for approximately twice as long as without probenecid; hence it is sometimes used for this purpose. Probenecid is not recommended in children under two years of age (Chapter 71).

Adverse reactions: Penicillin is a remarkably safe drug. The only important reaction to be feared in practice is anaphylaxis.

● ***Minor reactions*:** Oral use of penicillin may rarely produce nausea, vomiting and diarrhoea. Benzathine penicillin IM may cause local pain erythema and induration; occasionally pyrexia may develop.

Prolonged administration of IV benzylpenicillin may lead to thrombophlebitis; accidental IV administration of procaine benzylpenicillin can cause anxiety, mental disturbances, paraesthesiae and seizures, due to procaine.

Benzylpenicillin, even in large doses, is almost devoid of toxic manifestations provided kidney function is normal. However, when given by intrathecal route, the drug may cause arachnoiditis, convulsions and encephalopathy. Hence, *penicillin should not be administered intrathecally*. Large doses may also cause neurotoxicity in uremic patients.

● ***Allergy and anaphylaxis*:** The risk of allergic reactions is 5 to 10 per cent with benzathine penicillin, 2 to 5 per cent with procaine pencillin and 1 to 3 per cent following benzylpenicillin, when these are administered parenterally. The mortality in severe reactions has been assessed at 9 to 13 per cent. As a generalization, the incidence of these reactions is considerably greater when benzylpenicillin is used either topically or in an aerosol form, and it least when the drug is taken orally. However, fatalities have occurred following ingestion.

Some individuals are so sensitive that the mere handling of a tablet of penicillin or even a skin test dose may precipitate immediate severe reaction. Further, severe reactions have been recorded following first dose of penicillin, in persons who had never received the drug before. This is probably because many of us are exposed and slightly sensitized to various common airborne moulds that readily grow on and elaborate penicillin and penicillin-like substances in foodstuffs such as bread, fruit, and oil, with or without decay. Penicillin sensitization can also occur from the presence of the drug in the environment of patients using penicillin aerosols, and by ingesting milk containing penicillin.

Metabolites of penicillin form covalent bonds with serum and tissue proteins and are highly immunogenic. It is believed that **penicilloic acid**

Table 45.1: Important allergic reactions to penicillin

- Skin rashes.
- Arthritis
- Serum sickness like syndrome.
- Renal disturbances.
- Hemopoietic disturbances.
- Angioedema; and
- Anaphylaxis.

either alone or linked to a plasma protein is responsible for allergic reactions. *A person known to be allergic to one penicillin will also be allergic to other penicillins.*

The important allergic reactions are:

- ***Skin rashes*** of various types associated with pruritus are the most common reactions.
- ***A serum sickness like syndrome***, characterised by rash, fever, eosinophilia lymphadenopathy, angioneurotic edema, bronchospasm and arthralgia.
- ***Renal disturbances*** like hematuria and albuminuria.
- ***Hemopoietic disturbances*** like hemolytic anemia and neutropenia, very rarely.
- ***Anaphylaxis*** is the most serious reaction but occurs in fewer than 0.01 per cent of patients. The symptoms of anaphylaxis usually begin within a few minutes after penicillin administration. Anaphylaxis can develop even with a minute quantity of penicillin and irrespective of the route of administration. It is characterised by an acute cardiovascular collapse, bronchospasm, and angioedema, particularly edema of the larynx. For details, see Chapters 2 and 20.

Tests for detection of penicillin allergy: A reliable method of detecting penicillin allergy is not available. History of allergy or even a positive skin test is not in itself a complete evidence of allergy, nor does a negative history or negative skin test indicate the safety of penicillin administration. Estimation of IgE antibodies in the serum may be helpful.

Skin tests: One method of skin testing is to scratch the skin through a drop of solution containing 10,000 units of benzylpenicillin per ml. If a central wheal due to local edema (not diffuse erythema) occurs after 15 minutes, it is considered a positive reaction. A positive skin reaction is a relatively reliable indicator of potentially serious penicillin allergy. Unfortunately, fatal anaphylactic reactions have been reported though rarely even in persons with negative skin response, whereas some patients with a positive reaction have accepted penicillin without serious allergic reactions. Furthermore, even the small amount of penicillin used for the test may itself rarely produce severe reaction.

Another skin test involves the administration of 0.05 ml. of **penicilloyl-polylysine intradermally** and subsequent observation of the inflammatory response. This test is often combined with benzylpenicillin scratch test. Combination of these two tests will predict virtually all reactions to penicillin. Scratch test should precede the intradermal test to avoid any dangerous reaction following the latter. However, such elaborate testing is not feasible in clinical practice.

If a person with a positive skin test has to be administered penicillin for a life-threatening infection, penicillin desensitisation should be carried out under cover of corticosteroid and antihistaminic therapy in a closely monitored setting. Benzylpenicillin should be administered in doses of 1, 5, 10. 100 and 1000 units ID at 60 minute intervals. If that is well tolerated, then progressively larger doses such as 10000 units and 50000 units and so on may be given SC. Desensitization may also be done with oral administration of penicillin. When full doses are reached, penicillin must not be discontinued and then restarted because an immediate allergic reaction may occur. The above procedure is dangerous and its efficacy is unproven. Further, corticosteroids may have to be administered in very large doses (50 to 100 mg. of prednisolone per day) to prevent the developement of anaphylaxis. Such large doses of steroids may affect the host resistance and this must be weighed against the beneficial antiallergic effect desired. *Antihistaminics do not decrease the incidence of penicillin anaphylaxis;* they are, however, valuable in controlling the commonly occurring minor allergic reactions.

Even in patients in whom the skin test is negative, most physicians administer a small dose of 1000-2000 units of penicillin and proceed to higher doses if no reaction occurs.

- ***Jarisch-Herxheimer reaction*** is a rare reaction reported in patients with syphilis treated with penicillin (Chapter 51).
- ***Superinfection***: Use of penicillin may

suppress the sensitive coccal members of the bacterial flora, and encourage superinfection in the form of bacteremia, urinary infection or pneumonia owing to overgrowth of such resistant microorganisms as *Klebsiella, Aerobacter, Pseudomonas* and *Candida.*

Stomatitis, glossitis and a black hairy tongue are known to develop after local use of penicillin troches and lozenges and may occasionally occur even after systemic therapy.

- ***Hyperkalemia***: Each 15 million units of potassium benzylpenicillin supplies 975 mg. (25 mEq.) of ionic potassium, and the drug administered repeatedly in such doses to patients with impaired renal function may cause hyperkalemia.

- ***Acute non-allergic reactions***: Intramuscular aqueous procaine penicillin sometimes produces acute non-allergic reaction, which could be serious. It is characterized by transient palpitation, hypertension, twitchings, auditory and visual disturbances, headache, and dizziness. In addition, psychiatric symptoms like fear of imminent death and acute depersonalization may occur. The mechanism of this reaction is not clear.

Therapeutic uses:

The various penicillin regimens can be summarised for practical purposes as shown in Table 45.2. These regimens cover the methods of administration of penicillin in majority of penicillin responding infections.

Table 45.2: Penicillin regimens

- ***Regimen 1 (oral):*** Penicillin V 250-500 mg or benzylpenicillin 400,000-800,000 units orally every six hours.
- ***Regimen 2 (IM small dose, repository penicillin):*** Fortified benzylpenicillin (procaine benzylpenicillin 600,000 units + benzylpenicillin 200,000 units) IM once a day.
- ***Regimen 3 (IM, large dose benzylpenicillin):*** Benzylpenicillin 1-2 megaunits IM every 4-6 hours (4-12 megaunits per day).
- ***Regimen 4 (IV, large dose benzylpenicillin):*** Benzylpenicillin 2 megaunits IV every 2 hours (24 megaunits per day).

Regimens 1 or 2 is used in mild infection such as streptococcal pharyngitis. Regimens 3 and 4 are needed in severe infections such as severe pneumonia empyema, meningitis and bacterial endocarditis. The choice of the regimen in each individual infection is indicated in Table 45.3.

- ***Pneumococcal infections***: Most strains of pneumococci are extremely susceptible to benzylpenicillin and hence, it continues to be the drug of choice for these infections.

Pneumococcal pneumonia: (Table 45.3). The therapeutic response to penicillin becomes apparent within 48 to 72 hours. In milder cases and in patients known to be allergic to penicillin, an oral macrolide such as erythomycin or azithromycin may be used. Unfortunately, 15-30% of *S.pneumoniae* show resistance to penicillin. Some of them are multi-drug resistant. Hence, in hospitalised patients who are seriously ill, cefotaxime or ceftriaxone is to be preferred.

Pneumococcal empyema and pericarditis: (Table 45.3). In addition to regimen 4, half to one mega unit of benzylpenicillin in 50-100 ml. of isotonic saline should be instilled intrapleurally daily for several days. If the pleural fluid is thick and viscous, the proteolytic enzymes streptokinase and streptodornase may be injected intrapleurally along with penicillin, in the dose of 200,000 to 400,000 units and 50,000 to 100,000 units respectively. Several injections may be necessary, particularly when the empyema becomes loculated. By the use of these enzymes combined with daily aspiration and the local injection of penicillin, cure of empyema can be obtained. When these measures do not show definite signs of being effective, surgical intervention is indicated.

Pneumococcal meningitis : Chapter 47.

- ***Streptococcal infections*** :

Infections due to Strep pyogenes that respond satisfactorily to penicillin, are listed in Table 45.3.

Table 45.3: Choice of penicillin regimen in the common infections

Organisms	Regimens 1 and 2	Regimens 3 and 4
S. pneumoniae	Pneumonia (mild-moderate), until afebrile for 4 days	Empyema, pericarditis, osteomyelitis, arthritis* (2-4 weeks), meningitis (10-14 days)
S. pyogenes, S.viridans, Group A beta hemolytic streptococci	Pharyngitis**, erysipelas, pyoderma (7-10 days), otitis media (2 weeks)	Mastoiditis (2weeks) osteomyelitis, arthritis* (2-4 weeks), meningitis (10-14 days), SBE (4-6 weks)
Type D streptococci (enterococci)	—	Meningitis (14-21 days with gentamicin)
Staph. aureus	—	Meningitis (14-21 days with gentamicin)
N. gonorrhoeae	Gonorrhoea (uncompli cated) single injection; complicated (14 days)	—
Treponema pallidum	Syphilis (single dose or weekly for 3 weeks)	—
Actinomyces israeli	Actinomycosis (2 weeks with sulfadiazine 4 g)	—
Nocardia brasilliensis	Nocardiasis	—
Corynebactrium diphtheriae	Diphtheria (10-12 days)	—
Clostridium tetani	Tetanus (10-12 days)	—
Clostridium species		Gas gangrene (1-2 weeks)
Fusospirochetal infection	Gingivostomatitis (trench fever) and pharyngitis (Vincent's angina)	Lung abcess
Pasturella multocida	—	2-4 weeks
Listeria monocytogenes	—	Listeriasis (2 weeks)
Streptobacilli: Actinobacillus muris and Spirilum minus	—	Rat-bite fever (7-10 days)

SBE = Subacute bacterial endocarditis. * Intracavitary local injection
** = Single injection of 1.2 megaunits, benzathine penicillin

In suppurative arthritis 50,000 to 100,000 units of penicillin may be instilled into the joint cavity.

Streptococcal subacute bacterial endocarditis (SBE) : The alpha-hemolytic streptococci *(Strep. viridans)* account for the majority of cases of subacute bacterial endocarditis whereas in a few cases the enterococci (*Strep. fecalis*) and coagulase negative staphylococci may be the causative organisms.

Therapeutic response in bacterial endocarditis depends upon the proper selection of antibiotics, the stage at which treatment is begun and its thoroughness. If the diagnosis and consequently the treatment are delayed, irreversible cardiac damage occurs. Again, the disease, once firmly established, becomes more difficult to eradicate. In all cases it is imperative that therapy be continued for a minimum period of 4-6 weeks and monthly blood cultures be done for at least 3 months to detect a recurrence.

Before institution of therapy, isolation and identification of the causative organism are necessary. During the therapy, its efficacy is determined by a simple serum bactericidal test using the serum of the patient receiving the antibiotic and his own organisms, isolated before starting the antibiotic. If the serum exhibits a bactericidal activity in 1:8 dilution, good correlation between therapy and cure is usually assured.

Regimens for the treatment of the common forms of bacterial endocarditis are given in Table 45.4. The choice of the antibiotic(s) and duration of therapy depend upon the type of organism and the nature of underlying lesion (whether rheumatic valve disease or prosthatic valve).

If the appropriate cephalosporin and vancomycin as mentioned in Table 45.4 are not available, a regimen comprising erythromycin

Tabel 45.4: Antibiotic regimens for the treatment of bacterial endocarditis

Organism		Antibiotic regimen
Strepto. viridans (Alpha–hemolytic)	1.	Penicillin G 10-20 million units/day IV, in six equal doses, plus gentamicin 1 mg/kg IV or IM 8 hourly. Avoid gentamicin in patients over 65 years and in presence of renal failure or eighth nerve damage. Penicillin alone may be used for 4 weeks or combination for two weeks
	2.	In patients allergic to penicillin : Ceftriaxone 2 g IV or IM once daily or Vancomycin 30 mg/kg (not to exceed 1 g) IV 12 hourly. Duration : 4 weeks.
Strepto. pyogenes (Beta-hemolytic, Group A)	1.	Pencillin G 2 million units IV 6 hourly.
	2.	Cefazolin 2 g IV 8 hourly Duration : 2 - 4 weeks.
Strepto. fecalis (Entero. fecalis) (Beta-hemolytic, Group D)	1.	Ampicillin 2 g IV 4 hourly *plus* gentamicin 1 mg/kg I.V. 8 hourly for 4-6 weeks.
	2.	Vancomycin 30 mg/kg (not to exceed 1g) IV 12 hourly *plus* gentamicin as above. Duration : 4 - 6 weeks.
Staph. aureus	1.	Nafcillin 2 g IV 4 hourly, for 4-6 weeks.
	2.	In complicated cases, nafcillin as above *plus* gentamicin 1 mg/kg IV 8 hourly for the first 3 - 5 days.
	3.	In patients allergic to penicillin, cefazolin 2 g IV 4 hourly *OR* vancomycin as above for. 4-6 weeks.

plus gentamicin may be substituted in patients allergic to pencillin. Streptomycin may be used instead of gentamicin. If the diagnosis is well established on clinical grounds and blood cultures are negative, the patient may be treated with the same regimen as for *Strep. fecalis* (ampicillin + gentamicin for 4-6 weeks).

• ***Staphylococcal infections*** : A major therapeutic problem is the development of penicillin resistant staphylococci. It has been estimated that 70-90 per cent of staphylococcal infections due to hospital strains and 15 to 20 per cent of those acquired in the community are resistant to penicillin. Table 45.5 lists the drugs recommended in community-acquired staphylococcal infections.

Table 45.5: Drugs for community-acquired staphylococcal infections

- Antistaphylococcal penicillins and cephalosporins.
- Co-trimoxazole.
- Minocycline.
- Gentamicin; and
- Fluoroquinolones.

As penicillin penetrates poorly into abscesses, surgical treatment is indicated. Topical application of penicillin for cutaneous infections is discouraged because of the risk of sensitization. For serious systemic staphylococcal infections, see Table 45.3. For infections caused by staphylococci producing beta lactamase, one of the new semisynthetic penicillins or a cephalosporin may be employed.

• ***Meningococcal meningitis*** : See Chapter 47. Penicillin is the drug of choice in meningococcal meningitis (Table 45.3). But, penicillin and its derivatives do not effectively eradicate this organism from the nasopharynx with short courses, and hence they are not recommended for prophylaxis in close contacts of patients with meningococcal infections.

• ***Sexually transmitted diseases (STD)***: Penicillin is the drug of choice in the treatment of gonorrhoea and syphilis (Chapter 51).

• ***Actinomycosis*** : Penicillin is the agent of choice in this condition (Table 45.3). Other antimicrobial agents employed include the tetracyclines, chloramphenicol, clindamycin and erythromycin

• ***Anthrax***: Benzylpenicillin is the drug of choice. It is given in the dose of 0.5 mega units (500,000 units) IM every 4-6 hours (2-3 mega units per day) for 8-10 days. Alternative drugs include the cotrimoxazole, erythromycin and the tetracyclines.

• ***Diphtheria, tetanus and gas gangrene***: (Table 45.3) Diphtheria and tetanus in addition to penicillin, require the administration of the specific antiserum. This helps to eliminate the bacilli from the lesions (Chapter 76).

• ***Miscellaneous infections***: These are shown in Table 45.3.

Erysipeloid, caused by the Gram positive bacillus, *Erysipelothrix insidiosa* responds to a single injection of 1 to 2 million units of benzathine penicillin. The organism may also cause endocarditis, which is treated in a similar fashion as viridans endocarditis.

• ***Penicillin prophylaxis*** :

(a) **Rheumatic fever** : Antibiotics neither modify the course of rheumatic fever nor influence the subsequent development of carditis. Yet, it is customary to give antibiotics to eradicate rheumatogenic group A streptococci in the tonsils and the pharynx, in order to prevent the spread of the organism to close contacts. The preferred regimens are (a) Inj. benzathine penicillin 1.2 mega units I.M., single dose; or (b) erythromycin 40 mg/kg/day, orally, in divided doses, for 10 days.

It is important to prevent recurrence of rheumatic fever by penicillin prophylaxis. benzathine penicillin IM 1.2 million units every 3 weeks provides the best protection. Oral penicillin V may also be used in the dose of 125 mg. 12 hourly in cooperative patients. In patients allergic to penicillin, erythromycin 250 mg twice daily may be used. The prophylactic therapy is continued for 5 years in children without evidence of carditis. In those who develop carditis, it is continued till the age of 20 years. *In patients with valvular disease, it should preferably be life long.*

(b) **Streptococcal infections:** Oral benzylpenicillin in the dose of 200,000 units twice daily for 5 days or a single injection of 1.2 mega units of benzathine penicillin affords satisfactory protection from repeated infections due to *Strep. pyogenes.*

(c) **Bacterial endocarditis:** Prophylactic penicillin is indicated in individuals with rheumatic or congential heart disease, who have to undergo surgical procedures like tooth extraction, dental scaling, surgery involving the gums, and procedures involving the lower genitourinary tract. Recommended drug for this purpose is amoxycillin 2 g in adults and 50 mg /kg in children to be given *orally* 1 hour before the procedure. The alternatives are: (i) azithromycin or clarithromycin 500 mg in adults and 15 mg/kg in children; or (ii) clindamycin 600 mg in adults and 20 mg/kg in children; and (iii) cephalexin 2 g in adults or 50 mg/kg in children, given similarly. In each case, ½ the dose is repeated once, 6 hours after the procedure.

When **parenteral administration** is indicated, give IM or IV (½ hour before the procedure): (i) ampicillin 2g in adults and 50 mg/kg in children; or (ii) clindamycin 600 mg in adults and 20 mg / kg in children; or (iii) cefazoline 1 g in adults and 25 mg/kg in children. In multi-drug-resistant cases and those allergic to penicillin, a combination of vancomycin and gentamicin is used. *These regimens should be used even in patients on rheumatic fever prophylaxis with penicillin.*

Daily oral penicillin for rheumatic fever prophylaxis may favour the growth of viridans streptococci relatively resistant to penicillin; in such patients, azithromycin should be used.

(d) **Gonorrhoea and syphilis :** Chapter 51.

(e) **Recurrent lymphangitis:** Benzathine benzylpenicillin, 600,000 units, administered IM once a month is effective in preventing recurrent lymphangitis and consequent lymphedema in patients who have congenital abnormalities of the lymphatic system and in filariasis.

Semisynthetic Penicillins

The major drawbacks of benzylpenicillin are:

- ***Inactivation by the gastric acid.***
- ***Short duration of action.***
- ***Poor penetration into the CSF.***
- ***Narrow spectum of activity.***
- ***Development of resistant organisms, especially staphylococci;*** and
- ***Possibility of anaphylaxis.***

Attempts, therefore, have been made to synthesize penicillins free from such drawbacks. The problem of its short duration of action has been effectively overcome by the development of repository preparations.

P. chrysogenum which produces the natural penicillins produces 6-APA nucleus before the attachment of the side chains. This process of attachment of the naturally occurring side chains can be inhibited, and instead, various organic radicals can be substituted to produce a variety of semisynthetic penicillins (Table 45.6). *These synthetic penicillins, however, are capable of producing allergic reactions similar to those caused by penicillin G.*

I **Acid resistant penicillins:** These penicillins are relatively resistant to inactivation by gastric acid and hence, can be given orally.

POTASSIUM PHENOXYMETHYLPENICILLIN (Penicillin V): Its antibacterial spectrum is like that of benzylpenicillin. It is rather more active against resistant staphylococci because it is more slowly destroyed by betalactamase. On an equivalent oral dose basis, the plasma levels achieved by this compound are 4 to 5 times higher than those with benzylpenicillin. Approximately 50 to 70 per cent of the drug is bound to the plasma proteins and nearly 25 per cent is eliminated in the urine.

Potassium phenoxymethylpenicillin is freely soluble in water. It is available as 65 and 125 mg. tablets. The drug is usually administered in the dose of 250 to 500 mg. at 4 to 8 hourly intervals, at least 30 minutes before food.

Table 45.6: Classification of the penicillins

I **Penicillin G and its esters**
Penicillin G (Benzyl penicillin)
Procaine penicillin G
Benzathine penicillin G

II **Acid resistant penicillins:**
Phenoxymethlypenicillin (penicillin V)
Phenoxyethylpenicillin (phenethicillin)

III **Penicillinase-resistant penicillins***
(a) **Acid labile:** Methicillin, Nafcillin Cloxacillin, Dicloxacillin
(b) **Acid resistant:** Flucloxacillin

IV **Penicillins effective against Gram-positive and some Gram-negative organisms:**
Ampicillin, Amoxycillin
Talampicillin, Pivampicillin

V **Extended spectrum penicillins:**
1) **Antipseudomonal penicillins**
a) **Carboxypenicillins**
Carbenicillin, Ticarcillin
b) **Ureidopenicillins**
Piperacillin, Mezlocillin, Azlocillin
2) **Amidinopenicillins**
Mecillinam, Pivmecillinam

VI **Penicillins with betalactamase inhibitors:**
Amoxycillin-clavulanic acid (Augmetin)
Ticarcillin-clavulanic acid (Timentin)

Groups other than III are not resistant to penicillinase (beta lactamase) and not effective against Staph. aureus.
* Antistaphylococcal penicillins, not effective against MRSA.

Therapeutic Uses: Penicillin V may be employed in less serious infections due to pneumococci and streptococci, in conditions that have been brought under control by parenteral therapy, and in infections which require a prolonged treatment. It is much less active than benzylpenicillin against gonococci; hence it is not used to treat gonorrhoea. It may be used prophylactically for similar purposes as benzylpenicillin.

A dose of 250 mg. of penicillin V 4 times daily for 4 days, with sulfafurazole 26 to 30 mg. per kg. upto 2 g. maximum per day for 3 days, has been used for prophylaxis against meningococcal infection in contacts and in school children during an epidemic. However, oral rifampicin 10 mg/kg per day for three days, is preferred.

Penicillin V has no place in the management of severe infections and should not be used for the treatment of meningitis, syphilis or actinomycosis.

POTASSIUM PHENOXYETHYL PENICI-LLIN (Phenethicillin): is similar to phenoxymethylpenicillin, and weight for weight, there is no difference in its antibacterial activity.

AZIDOCILLIN: This drug is acid resistant and is well absorbed orally. It has properties similar to those of penicillin V.

II **Beta-lactamase (Penicillinase) resistant penicillins:** These are penicillins effective in the treatment of infections due to beta-lactamase producing staphylococci.

METHICILLIN: It is given IM or by slow IV infusion in the dose of 1 g. every 4-6 hours. Over 70% of the community acquired *S.aureus* strains (*coagulase positive staphylococci*) are sensitive to methicillin, whereas less than 30% of the hospital acquired strains are sensitive to methicillin. Over 70% of the *coagulase negative staphylococci* are resistant to methicillin.

The term *methicillin resistant Staphylococcus aureus* (MRSA) is used to refer to beta-lactam-antibiotic-resistant (i.e., penicillinase producing) staphylococci. Most of MRSA strains are resistant to cloxacillin, flucloxacillin and all beta-lactam antibiotics (penicillins, cephalosporins and imepenam) and often to other classes of antimicrobial agents (multiresistant). These need special attention (see later).

CLOXACILLIN (Klox): This drug has a weaker antibacterial activity than benzylpenicillin but is 5 to 10 times more active than methicillin against resistant staphylococci. Food interferes with its absorption.

After a single oral dose, peak plasma levels are attained within an hour and persist for 4 to 6 hours. The drug is distributed throughout the body, with the highest concentrations in the kidney and liver. Nearly 30 per cent of a single dose is excreted in the urine; over 95 per cent of the 24 hour urinary excretion occurs within the first 6 hours. Significant amounts are excreted in the bile.

The initial oral dose of cloxacillin varies from 0.5 to 1 g. 6 hourly, and the maintenance dose is 250 mg. given at the same intervals. In children, the dose varies from 50 to 100 mg. per kg. daily (according to severity of infection) divided into 4-6 portions. The drug should be administered 1 hour before or 2 hours after a meal to ensure adequate absorption. It can also be given IM and by slow IV bolus, 250-500 mg. 4-6 hourly.

DICLOXACILLIN: This derivative of cloxacillin is absorbed better (60%) and gives blood levels twice those of cloxacillin on oral administration. It is, however, very highly (95%) protein bound and does not cross the placenta significantly; it is excreted slowly. It has similar properties as cloxacillin. It is administered orally in the dose of 0.25 to 1 g. at 6 hourly intervals.

Flucloxacillin (Floxapen) is similar to dicloxacillin but is relatively less protein bound, and hence may be preferred to dicloxacillin.

NAFCILLIN (Unipen): In *in vitro* studies, this drug has been shown to be more active than methicillin and cloxacillin, but less active than benzylpenicillin, against susceptible organisms. On oral administration, its absorption is slow, irregular and incomplete. IM injection yields quicker and higher plasma levels. Approximately 87 per cent of the drug is bound with plasma proteins. It is predominantly excreted by the liver in bile and may be preferred in patients with renal damage. Its toxicity is similar to that of cloxacillin.

The oral doses are similar to those of cloxacillin. The IM dose is 0.5 to 1 g. 4 to 6 hourly and 25 mg. per kg. twice daily, respectively, in adults and in children. It can be given IV.

Initial treatment of a severe staphylococcal infection should always be with one of the beta-lactamase resistant penicillins or a cephalosporin. Staphylococci resistant to the above penicillinase-resistant penicillins have been reported. This resistance is based on the chromosomally mediated production of a new penicillin-binding protein with decreased affinity for these penicillins.

III Penicillins effective against Gram-positive and Gram-negative organisms:

AMPICILLIN (Roscillin, Ampilin): Ampicillin is water soluble and acid resistant. Its antibacterial activity is generally similar to that of benzylpenicillin; in addition it is highly effective against a variety of Gram-negative bacteria. The Gram-positive cocci are less sensitive to ampicillin than to benzylpenicillin. The drug is effective against *H. influenzae, Strep. viridans, Proteus mirabilis, Neisseria gonorrhoea, Salmonella typhosa,* many strains of *E. coli* and several strains of *Shigella.* It is moderately effective against *Klebsiella,* certain strains of *Aerobacter* and *Enterococci. Pseudomonas* and indole positive *proteus,* however, are resistant. Ampicillin is inactivated by beta lactamase and, therefore, is ineffective against staphylococci resistant to benzylpenicillin. Bacteria can develop resistance to ampicillin, and many strains of salmonella, shigella, E. coli and proteus resistant to this drug have been isolated.

Absorption, fate and excretion: It is readily but incompletely absorbed on oral administration. *Food does not significantly interfere with its absorption.* The portion not absorbed is inactivated by penicillinase of the colonic bacterial flora and hence, the drug rarely produces superinfection in contrast to tetracyclines.

Peak plasma levels are reached within 2 hours and 1 hour respectively after administration of a single oral or IM dose. The levels are considerably higher and more prolonged on IM administration. The drug persists in the plasma for 6 to 8 hours, and only 20 per cent of it is bound to plasma proteins. About 1/3rd of the dose is excreted unchanged in urine and high concentrations are also present in the bile. In premature and very young infants, excretion of ampicillin is delayed. The drug crosses the placental barrier and achieves therapeutic concentrations in the amniotic fluid.

Adverse reactions : These are similar to those of penicillin G; however, skin rashes are more common. Ampicillin rash is usually maculopapular and not urticarial like that caused by benzylpenicillin. The onset is delayed. Diarrhoea is common with oral ampicillin and its derivatives. It is sometimes associated with *Clostridium difficile* infection. Interstitial nephritis is an uncommon adverse effect.

Preparations and dosage: The ampicillin capsule contains ampicillin hydrate equivalent to 250 mg of the base. The usual adult dose of ampicillin by all routes is 250 to 500 mg. 6 hourly; doses as large as 1 g. 6 hourly may be required for more refractory Gram-negative infections. In children below 13 years, the daily oral dose of the drug is 50 to 200 mg. per kg. while parenterally, 25 to 50 mg. per kg. may be given per day in divided doses. High doses are used in the treatment of meningitis and bacterial endocarditis. Ampicillin 500 mg. dissolved in 5 to 10 ml. normal saline may be injected intrapleurally or intra-articularly.

Stability of sodium ampicillin in solution decreases markedly and storing of solutions even at refrigeration temperature results in deterioration of activity. The presence of dextrose and lactate may further accelerate the loss of potency.

Therapeutic uses:

- ***Urinary tract infections*** caused by *E. coli, P. Mirabilis,* non-hemolytic *streptococci* and *enterococci.* It is also useful for prophylaxis against recurrent UTI (Chapter 50).
- ***Respiratory tract infections*:** Particularly in mixed infections with *H. influenzae* and *D. pneumoniae.*
- ***Meningitis and subacute bacterial endocarditis*:** See Chapter 47 and Table 45.3.
- ***Biliary tract and intestinal infections*:** Ampicillin can be used against intestinal infections due to *E. coli, enterococci, salmonella* and *shigella.* Although the drug is effective in typhoid fever, chloramphenicol and ciprofloxacin appear to be superior. However, it is claimed that the relapse rate after ampicillin is low. The drug has been used to treat the typhoid carriers. Good results have been obtained in shigella dysentery.
- ***Miscellaneous*:** Ampicillin is preferred to tetracyclines in pregnant women and in infants to avoid tetracycline deposition in bones and teeth. It can also be used as an alternative to tetracyclines in the management of intestinal malabsorption and is preferred in the treatment of whooping cough. The other drugs useful in whooping cough are erythromycin (the drug of choice) and co-trimoxazole.

Because of increasing resistance by bacteria, ampicillin has lost its status as a drug of choice for the empiric treatment of childhood meningitis, salmonellosis, shigellosis and gonococcal infections.

TALAMPICILLIN: This is a carboxylic ester of ampicillin. It is rapidly absorbed from the gut and is hydrolyzed by tissue esterases in the intestinal wall to release ampicillin into the circulation. It has no intrinsic antibacterial activity and hence is not likely to have direct effect on the bacterial flora of the gut. It is given in the dose of 250-500 mg. 3-4 times a day.

Pivampicillin has properties similar to those of talampicillin.

AMOXYCILLIN (Mox, Lamoxy, Novamox): This structural analogue of ampicillin (amino-p-hydroxy-benzylpenicillin) has properties and uses similar to those of ampicillin. It has certain advantages over ampicillin:

(a) Its absorption is not influenced by food.

(b) The blood levels on oral administration are twice as high as those after similar dose of ampicillin.

(c) It is less protein bound and the urinary excretion is higher than that of ampicillin.

(d) The incidence of diarrhoea is less.

It is, however, much more expensive. It is available as 250 mg. capsules. The usual oral dose in adults is 250-500 mg. 8 hourly. In severe or recurrent purulent, respiratory infections doses as large as 3 g. 12 hourly are recommended. It can also be given IM or IV. It is preferred for preventing the carrier state in typhoid fever.

IV Extended Spectrum Penicillins :

(1) The **carboxypenicillins** and the **ureido penicillins** (Table 45.6) are considered extended-spectrum penicillins, because they inhibit a wide variety of aerobic Gram negative bacilli, including *Ps. aeruginosa.* They have the following properties:

- ***They are highly active against anaerobes.***
- ***They are most useful in infections caused by P.aeruginosa and other Gram negative rods.***
- ***They act synergistically with aminoglycoside antibiotics, particularly against P.aeruginosa and the Enterobacteriaceae.***
- ***They are much less active than penicillin G against Gram positive organisms and are not reliable for treating staphylococcal infections.***
- ***The CNS penetration of the carboxy- and the ureido-penicillins is about 10% of their serum levels, and hence they are not recommended for the treatment of meningeal infections.***
- ***They may inactivate the aminoglycoside antibiotics in vitro when mixed together in the same bottle and in vivo in patients with renal failure.***
- ***They are acid labile and susceptible to beta-lactamase.***

P.aeruginosa may develop resistance to these drugs, which is prevented by concurrent administration of an aminoglycoside (but see above).

CARBENICILLIN (Pyopen, Carbelin): This penicillin has a similar spectrum as but weaker antibacterial activity than ampicillin. Its important advantage over ampicillin is that it is effective against all strains of *Proteus* and *Pseudomonas aeruginosa.*

Carbenicillin has to be administered IM or IV. When given IM, the peak plasma levels are reached within 2 hours and the drug is eliminated in urine within 6 hours. The dose is 2 g. 6 hourly IM. It can also be given IV slowly or by rapid infusion in severe systemic infections in the dose of 5 g. 4-6 hourly. In such patients, it is generally combined with an aminoglycoside, commonly gentamicin.

The drug can cause CHF because of its large sodium content, and bleeding due to abnormal platelet aggregation.

TICARCILLIN (Ticar): This thienyl analogue of carbenicillin has spectrum similar to that of carbenicillin but is but is twice as active against *Ps. Aeruginosa.* Some anaerobes, including many forms of *Bacteroides fragilis,* are also sensitive to it. It is, however, much less active than ampicillin against streptococci, pneumococci and penicillin sensitive staphylococci. A combination of ticarcillin with an aminoglycoside is synergistic against the pseudomonas species. It is excreted by the kidneys and diffuses well into the CSF, pleural fluid and sputum. The dose recommended in severe infections is 15-20 g./day, given as 5 g. diluted in 20 ml. and injected IV over 3-4 minutes every 6-8 hours. It can also be given IM (1-2 g. 6 hourly) in less severe infections. It can be used in the treatment of severe UTI.

PIPERACILLIN (Pipril): Like ampicillin, it has a broad spectrum of activity against Gram negative bacilli, particularly *Ps. aeruginosa* (against which it is three times as active as ticarcillin). It is regarded as one of the most broadly active of the currently available penicillins with regard to other bacterial species especially *Proteus, Klebsiella, Bacteroides fragilis, H. influenzae* and *Gonococci.*

Piperacillin is given parenterally. It is mainly eliminated in the urine (70-90%) by glomerular filtration and tubular secretion. Hence, adjustment of its dose is needed in the presence of renal damage. Piperacillin crosses the BBB and may be useful in neonatal meningitis. Adverse effects are similar to those of other penicillins. The dosage regimen is identical to that of ticarcillin. The recommended pediatric dose is 100-300 mg/kg/day in two divided doses for infants under 2 months of age and in 4 divided doses for older infants and children.

Although it is useful in a variety of infections, its use should be reserved for serious infections, especially those due to *Ps. Aeruginosa.*

Azlocillin and **mezlocillin** have similar indications as piperacillin.

(2) **Amidinopenicillins**

MECILLINAM (Selexidin): Mecillinam, an amidinopenicillin, has no therapeutic activity against gram positive organisms but is highly effective against Gram negative organisma such as *E. coli,* (including those resistant to ampicillin), *Klebsiella* species, *Shigellae* and *Salmonellae. Proteus* is less susceptible; *it has no action on Pseudomonas.* It is poorly absorbed orally and is given I.M. Its ester **pivmecillinam** (Selexid) is better absorbed orally and is hydrolysed to mecillinam. These compounds have been used in UTI and in typhoid fever, but do not appear to be superior to the other commonly used antibacterial drugs.

CLAVULANIC ACID: This penicillin analogue produced by *Streptomyces clavuligerus* has the following properties:

- ***It is well absorbed on oral administration but has only a weak antibacterial activity.***
- ***It is a potent and irreversible inhibitor of many betalactamases and protects betalactam antibiotics from inactivation, when combined with them.***
- ***When combined with amoxycillin, it widens the antibacterial spectrum of the latter to include betalactamase producing strains of Staph. aureus, H. influenzae, N. gonorrhoea, E. coli, Proteus, Klebsiella, M. catarrhalis*** **and** ***Bacteroides species.***

It is used in combination with amoxycillin (Augmentin) or ticarcillin (Timentin).

Sulbactam is another betalactamase – inhibitor penicillin analogue similar in action to clavulanic acid, and it is combined with ampicillin (Dicapen). **Tazobactam** is a penicillanic-acid-sulfone, beta lactamase inhibitor. It is combined with piperacillin (Zosyn).

The betalactamases produced by Ps.aeruginosa and by Enterobacter species are resistant to clavulanic acid and sulbactam. Further, methicillin resistant staphylococci are not susceptible to antimicrobials containing clavulanic acid or sulbactam.

Macrolides

Erythromycin, oleandomycin, triacetyloleandomycin and **spiramycin** constitute the macrolide group of antibiotics, so named because of the presence of a large lactone ring in their chemical structure. These drugs have similar antibacterial spectra, erythromycin being the most effective of all.

Mechanism of action: Macrolides act by inhibiting the protein synthesis by binding to the 50s ribosomal subunits. Depending upon its concentration, the antibiotic can be bacteriostatic or bactericidal. Bacteria can develop resistance to macrolides by mutation.

ERYTHROMYCIN is a fermentation product of the fungus *Streptomyces erythreus.* Its antibacterial spectrum resembles that of penicillin. It is mainly effective against the Gram-positive cocci including the *streptococci, staphylococci* and *pneumococci. Neisseria,* some strains of *H. influenzae, C. diphtheriae, Campylobacter jejuni, Listeria, P. multocida, Mycoplasma pneumoniae, Rickettsiae* and *Treponemas* are also inhibited by low concentration. The drug is effective against penicillin resistant staphylococci. Staphylococci and hemolytic streptococci can develop resistance to erythromycin. Its activity increases with an increase of pH upto 8.

Absorption, fate and excretion: Erythromycin is mainly absorbed from the small intestine. The drug is partially destroyed by the gastric juice and, therefore, has to be administered in the form of enteric coated tablets. The ester form, erythromycin estolate, is more resistant to inactivation by the gastric acid and is absorbed better than the base.

Peak plasma levels are reached within 2 to 4 hours after a single oral dose and the levels decline within 6 to 8 hours; hence, it is given 6 hourly.

Erythromycin readily diffuses into the body fluids but the penetration into the CSF is poor. It is concentrated in the liver, and the levels of the active form in bile are significantly high. Most of the drug is metabolized in the liver and only about 2-5% is excreted in the urine in active form. It can pass into the foetal circulation.

Adverse reactions: Serious adverse effects are uncommon. Allergic reactions include fever, eosinophilia, urticaria, dermatitis and lymphadenopathy. Nausea, vomiting, epigastric pain and diarrhoea are common. Hepatic dysfunction, particularly cholestatic hepatitis and jaundice, has been described following of erythromycin estolate. It is probably an allergic manifestation though a direct hepatotoxic action cannot be ruled out. It usually clears up within a few days after discontinuation of therapy. Hepatic dysfunction is a relative contraindication for erythromycin therapy. Superinfection with Gram-negative organisms and Candida may develop.

Drug interactions: Important interactions between erythromycin and other drugs are shown in Table 45.7. Some of them have been documented for other macrolide antibiotics as well. Erythromycin is a potent inhibitor of hepatic microsomal CYP3A4, thereby interfering with the metabolic degradation of number of drugs such as terfenadine, cisapride, ketoconazole and cimetidine.

Table 45.7: Drug interactions of erythromycin

- ***Reduction in plasma clearance with increased plasma levels and increased toxicity of:*** Ketoconazole, Theophylline, Carbamazepine, Cyclosporine, Digoxin, Warfarin, Disopyramide, Methylprednisolone.
- ***Interference with the action of chloramphenicol and clindamycin*** as these drugs compete for the same bacterial binding sites.
- ***Physical/chemical incompatibility (in solution) between parenteral forms of Erythromycin*** and Vitamin B complex, Ascorbic acid, Tetracycline, Colistin, Chloramphenicol, Heparin, Metaraminol and Phenytoin.

Preparations and dosage:

(i) Enteric coated tablets contain 250 mg. of erythromycin base. Dose: 1 to 2 g. per day in divided portions, administered 6 hourly. Food should not be given immediately after its administration. The dose in children is 5 mg. per kg. 6 hourly in children below 1 year, 10 mg. per kg. 6 hourly in children upto 8 years and 15 mg. per kg. in children between 8 and 12 years.

(ii) Erythromycin estolate (E-mycin, Althrocin) tablets contain the equivalent of 125 and 250 mg. of erythromycin base. It is administered in similar dosage. It is tasteless and resistant to gastric acid. Food does not interfere with its absorption. It is hydrolysed in the body to the active base. Because of its hepatotoxicity, it should not be used for prolonged periods.

(iii) Erythromycin stearate (Erythrocin), filmtabs, contain 100 and 250 mg. of the base; cherry flavoured granules for syrup containing 100 mg. per 5 ml. for children. Dose in children: 30-50 mg/kg. per day in divided doses.

(iv) Erythromycin ethylsuccinate for IM injection 2 ml. containing 100 mg. of the base.

Therapeutic uses:

- ***As a substitute for penicillin*:** Erythromycin is valuable in patients who are allergic to penicillins and in those in whom microorganisms have developed resistance to penicillin. Its antibacterial activity, however, is weaker than that of benzylpenicillin. As erythromycin (bacteriostatic) may interfere with the action of penicillin (bactericidal), the combination of these two drugs should be used only when it has been documented to be beneficial. For subacute bacterial endocarditis due to *Strep. viridans,* in a penicillin allergic individual, 1 g. of the drug is administered at 4 to 6 hourly intervals for 4 to 6 weeks, along with gentamicin 1 mg/kg 8 hourly. The drug eradicates the diphtheria carrier state in the dose of 250 and 500 mg. every 6 hours for 10-12 days in children and adults respectively. The drug can be used for prophylaxis against streptococcal infection and rheumatic fever.

***Mycoplasma and chlamydial infection* :** *It is the drug of choice in the treatment of mycoplasma pneumoniae.* It should be used in chlamydial pneumonia in infancy and in urogenital infections during pregnancy, situations where tetracyclines are avoided.

***Whooping Congh* :** Erythromycin is the drug of choice in the treatment of whooping cough (*B.pertusis*). It is given in the dose of 50 mg/kg/ day in four divided doses for 14 days. Alternatively co-trimoxazole may be used. Although these drugs are useful in clearing *B.pertussis*, no drug has been shown to alter the course of the illness, once frank paroxysms have supervened.

- ***Diarrhoea due to Campylobacter jejuni.*** It is the drug of choice (Chapter 40).
- ***Legionnaries disease*** is caused by legionella, an intracellular pathogen. Erythromycin and tetracycline achieve high intracellular concentration and are effective in its treatment; newer macrolide azithromycin may be preferred. Fluoroquinolones are also highly effective.
- ***STD*:** See Chapter 51.

Oleondomycin, triacetyloleandomycin and **spiramycin** (Rovamycin) have much weaker actions than those of erythromycin; hence, are now rarely used. Spiramycin is effective in the treatment of toxoplasmosis.

New macrolides (azalides) have a similar spectrum of activity as erythromycin. However,

- ***They are resistant to acid hydrolysis.***
- ***They are absorbed better and give higher tissue levels***; and
- ***They have longer duration of action and can be given once daily.***

Examples are **roxithromycin, azithromycin** and **clarithromycin.** The latter two are also active against *H.influenzae, M.catarrhalis, T.gondii and M.avium complex.*

ROXITHROMYCIN: This substituted erythromycin has antibacterial spectrum and therapeutic uses similar to those of erythromycin. It is rapidly absorbed from the gut with a bioavailability of 50%; food interferes with its absorption. Most of the drug is excreted in the feces, either unchanged or as metabolites. Its adverse effects are similar to those of erythromycin but it is claimed to be better tolerated. The adult dose is either 150 mg bid or 300 mg OD, taken before meals, for 10 days. It is used in ear, throat, respiratory tract and non-gonococcal genitourinary infections.

AZITHROMYCIN (Azithral, Aziwok): This azalide antibiotic differs chemically from the macrolide group in that the lactone ring contains a nitrogen atom. It has similar activity as erythromycin but in addition, it acts against certain Gram negative bacilli including *H.influenzae* and *C.trachomatis*. It also shows activity against *M.avium* complex. Compared to erythromycin, it penetrates the tissues better, concentrates in polymorphs and has a longer half life (68-72 hours). It can be used in respiratory tract infections, cervicitis and urethritis, all due to chlamydial infections. In NGU (Chapter 51) the drug is given in a single 1 g dose. In trachoma, three oral doses of 20 mg/kg each, given at weekly intervals, are highly effective. It is used for prophylaxis and treatment of avian complex in AIDS patients.

CLARITHROMYCIN (Clarimac): This azalide differs from erythromycin only in methylation of the hydroxyl group in 6th position. It has good activity against *H.influenzae*, *N.gonorrhoea, L.pneumophiliae* and chlamydia. It is better than azithromycin against MAC (Chapter 52) and *H.pylori.* The drug is absorbed rapidly from the gut, has a short half-life (3-7 hours) and has better tissue penetrability than erythromycin. It is metabolized to 14-hydroxy-clarithromycin (which is active), and is excreted by renal and extrarenal mechanisms. Clarithromycin is administered orally in the dose of 500 mg bid.

TELITHROMYCIN : This first ketolide antibiotic is related to erythromycin with similar antibacterial spectrum. However, it is also effective against macrolide resistant pneumococci. It is given 800 mg OD for 5-10 days. Dose adjustment is necessary in the presence of severe renal damage. The drug is a potent inhibitor of CYP3A4. Adverse reactions include GI disturbances, hepatotoxicity, blurred vision, diplopia and QTc prolongation. It can cause exacerbation of myasthenia gravis.

Among the newer macrolide antibiotics, clarithromycin and azithromycin have much better activity against *H.influenzae* and *M. catarrhalis* and hence they may be preferred for the treatment of community aquired preumonia. Clarithromycin is the macrolide of choice for the treatment of *H.pylori* while azithromycin is preferred for the treatment of *Clamydia trachomatis* infections.

Lincosamide Antibiotics

LINCOMYCIN (Lincocin): Lincomycin, elaborated by *Streptomyces lincolenesis,* is an orally effective antibiotic. It is mainly bacteriostatic with spectrum of activity similar to that of penicillin and erythromycin. It inhibits the growth of many Gram-positive organisms, especially *Staphylococci* (including those producing penicillinase), *Pneumococci,* certain *Streptococci* and *C. diphtheriae.* It also has activity against anaerobes such as B. fragilis. *B. anthracis* is moderately sensitive. *Enterococci, meningococci, hemophillus* and *gonococci*, however, are little affected. Many clostridia are also resistant. Development of resistance by staphylococci has been reported. Like erythromycin, the drug acts by interfering with protein synthesis. Cross resistance with macrolide antibiotics may occur.

Absorption, fate and excretion: On oral administration, approximately 20 to 35 per cent of lincomycin is absorbed. Food interferes with its absorption. Injection of 600 mg. IM produces within 30 to 60 minutes peak plasma levels which are twice as high as those obtained on oral administration; detectable antibacterial activity persists in the plasma for 24 hours. It can also be given IV.

After absorption, the drug is distributed throughout the body and is concentrated in the liver, spleen, kidneys, lung and bone. Most of the drug is metabolized in the liver. As with erythromycin, high concentration occurs in bile. CSF and brain concentrations are low. Nearly 4 to 13 per cent of the orally administered and 17 to 47 per cent of the IM administered lincomycin is excreted in the urine within 24 hours.

Adverse reactions: The drug is free from serious adverse effects. Nausea, vomiting, abdominal pain and diarrhoea may occur. Rarely, it may cause pseudomembranous colitis. A few patients may experience dizziness, headache, rash, bodyache, pruritus, proctitis and vaginitis. A few instances of jaundice, leucopenia or neutropenia have been reported. Monilial superinfection may occur.

Preparations and dosage: The oral adult dose of lincomycin hydrochloride monohydrate is 500 mg. 3 to 4 times daily. Children are given 30 to 60 mg. per kg. daily in 3-4 divided doses. The IM and the IV doses are 600 mg. given at 12 and 8 to 12 hourly intervals respectively. The comparative doses in children are 10 mg. per kg. and 10 to 20 mg. per kg. respectively.

Therapeutic uses: Lincomycin has been employed clinically in staphylococcal, pneumococcal and streptococcal infections resistant to penicillin or erythromycin and in individuals allergic to these antibiotics. The drug is claimed to be more effective in the treatment of acute and chronic osteomyelitis probably because of its better penetration into bones.

CLINDAMYCIN (Clinimycin): This is 7-chloro-7-deoxylincomycin, a semisynthetic derivative of lincomycin. It is bacteriostatic at low concentrations and bactericidal at slightly higher ones. It has antibacterial spectrum similar to that of lincomycin. However, it is much better absorbed orally and the absorption is not significantly affected by food. It is more protein bound than lincomycin and is mostly metabolized in the liver (t½ 3hours). Like lincomycin, it also gives high levels in bone and bile. Blood levels are not affected by hemodialysis, and anuria increases the blood level only slightly. It, however, should be used with caution in liver disease.

Adverse reactions : The toxicity is similar to that of lincomycin, including the diarrhoea due to pseudomembraneous colitis. The latter is due to superinfection with *Cl. sordellii* and *Cl. difficile* which secrete exotoxins with a necrotizing effect on the colonic mucosa. The organisms are sensitive to vancomycin. However, metronidizole 250 mg tid for 10-14 days is equally effective and cheaper.

Therapeutic uses: They are similar to those of lincomycin. It is also useful in prophylaxis and treatment of anaerobic infections, particularly along with an aminoglycoside, in the treatment of peritonitis due to fecal contamination or mixed infection. Its usual dose varies between 150 and 450 mg. four times daily, depending upon the severity of the disease.

In children and infants, it is given orally in the dose of 10-20 mg./kg. daily in 3 to 4 divided doses. Intramuscularly or by IV infusion, dose is 600 mg. 8-12 hourly.

For severe infections in adults, doses upto 4.8 g. by IV infusion have been used.

The drug has also been used in combination to treat malaria and toxoplasmosis (Chapter 54).

There is cross resistance between clindamycin and lincomycin.

Glycopeptide Antibiotics

VANCOMYCIN: Vancomycin, obtained from the fungus *Streptomyces orientalis,* is highly effective against Gram positive cocci, MRSA and *Enterococcus fecalis.* The drug is bactericidal and acts by inhibiting cell wall synthesis.

Vancomycin is not absorbed orally and IM administration is very painful. It is given IV in the dose of 2 g. daily, in divided doses. Approximately 80 per cent of the drug is eliminated in urine within 24 hours. Bacteria (enterococci and staphylococci) can develop resistance to vancomycin.

Adverse reactions: These include local thrombophlebitis, generalised cutaneous reactions (Red Man Syndrome) and renal/ auditory damage. As the drug is mainly eliminated by the kidney, it should be used with caution in patients who have renal damage.

Therapeutic uses: Vancomycin may be used in penicillin and cephalosporin resistant infections. It is used to treat multi resistant staphylococcal and *E.fecalis* infections. It is given IV in the dose of 500 mg. over 60 minutes every 6 hours or 1 g. every 12 hour.

Vancomycin, when given orally in the dose of 125 mg. 6 hourly, adequately controls acute staphylococcal enterocolitis, and pseudomembranous colitis caused by the toxins of *Clostridium difficille*. However, metronidazole is equally effective and cheaper.

Teicoplanin (Targocid) : It is produced by *Actinoplanes teicomyetius*. It is structurally related to vancomycin and has similar properties. Staphylococci can develop resistance to this drug. Unlike vancomycin, it can be given safely by IM injection. It is highly (90%) protein bound with elimination t½ of 50 hours.

It is used in preference to vancomycin in the dose of 6-30 mg/kg/day to treat infectons caused by multi-resistant staphylococci and other organisms such as streptococci and enterococci. However, it is not as efficacious as antistaphylococcal penicillins for treating severe infections caused by methicillin-susceptible organisms.

Other Related Antibiotics

DAPTOMYCIN : This bactericidal antibiotic belongs to a new class, **cyclic lipopeptides**. It binds to the bacterial plasma membrane causing membrane depolarisation and release of intracellular ions. This causes cell damage. Its spectrum is similar to that of vancomycin and includes MRSA and VRSA, penicillin resistant *S.pneumoniae, VR E.faecalis*. It has plasma t½ of nine hours. It is largely excreted by the kidney. Adverse effects reported so far include GI disturbances, rash, headache and rarely muscle discomfort/weakness. The drug appears to be similar to vancomycin in efficacy against vancomycin sensitive organisms, but is also useful to treat vancomycin resistant skin and soft tissue infections. It is usually administered in the dose of 4 mg/kg. IV O.D.

SODIUM FUSIDATE (Fucidin): Fucidin, the sodium salt of fucidic acid, is obtained from the parasitic fungus *Fusidium coccineum*. It has a steroidal structure. The drug is effective mainly against Gram-positive organisms, though streptococci and pneumococci are relatively resistant. Nearly all the strains of *Staph. aureus* are sensitive regardless of their sensitivity to other antibiotics. It is bactericidal. The antibiotic exerts a synergistic effect when administered in combination with penicillin and erythromycin. Staphylococci rapidly develop resistance to this antibiotic by mutation.

After an oral dose of 500 mg., peak plasma levels are obtained at 2 hours, and antibacterial activity can be detected in the plasma upto 24 hours (t½ 5 hours). Milk considerably retards its absorption. Very little fucidin is excreted in urine; significant amounts are present in bile. CSF concentration is low.

Adverse reactions: These include skin reactions, nausea, vomiting, epigastric pain, diarrhoea and hepatic dysfunction. Generally, it is well tolerated.

Therapeutic uses: In resistant staphylococcal infections, sodium fusidate may be administered orally in the dose of 500-1000 mg. 8 hourly. It can also be given by IV infusion as diethanolamine fusidate in the dose of 580 mg. 8 hourly. It is employed locally as 2% sodium fusidate in a neutral ointment base.

BACITRACIN: Bacitracin is a polypeptide antibiotic obtained from *Bacillus subtilis*. It resembles penicillin in antibacterial activity and is effective against Gram-positive organisms like *streptococci, staphylococci, pneumococci* and *enterococci. Corynebacterium, gonococci, meningococci, Cl. tetani, treponema* and *H. influenzae* are highly sensitive. Microorganisms do not readily develop resistance to bacitracin. It probably acts by inhibiting the bacterial cell wall synthesis.

Bacitracin is not much absorbed orally. Given parenterally, it is nephrotoxic. Acute tubular necrosis and anuria may occur. Allergic manifestations on topical use are uncommon. It is used topically as an antiseptic.

MUPIROCIN (Pseudomonic acid, Bactroban): This is an antibiotic obtained from the cultures of *Pseudomonas fluorescens*. It is bactericidal.

It is most active against Gram-positive bacteria but also has activity against Gram-negative aerobic organisms. It is used as 2% ointment to treat localized superficial skin infections caused by staphylococci and streptococci, and for eradication of nasal colonization by *Staph. aureus.* Its application to large areas should be avoided because the PEG in the ointment may get absorbed and cause toxicity (Chapter 6).

Streptogramins

QUINUPRISTIN (Q) / DALFOPRISTIN (D) (Synercid): is a combination of streptogramin B with streptogramin A in the ratio of 30 : 70. They are semisynthetic derivatives of pristinamycin which has been in use for 30 years in France. They act synergistically on the bacterial ribsome to disrupt protein synthesis. The combination is bactericidal. It is active against *E.faecium, S, aureus, S.epidermidis, S.pneumoniae, N.meningitidis, Moraxella catarrhalis, Legionella, Mycoplasma pneumoniae and Cl.perfringens.* It has no activity against Enterococcus faecalis. The combination is administered by IV infusion in 5% dextrose (not in saline) and both have elimination half life of about one hour. They are metabolised in the liver and excerted mainly in bile. Bacteria can develop resistance to these drugs.

Adverse reactions : Locally, the combination causes inflammation, pain and thrombophlebitis. Other adverse reactions reported are arthralgia and myalgia. Both the drugs are potent inhibitors of the liver cytochrome enzymes CYP3A4 and hence may increase the blood levels of drugs such as nifedipine, midazolam, cisapride and cyclosporine during co-administration.

Therapeutic uses : Currently the combination is used to treat the Vancomycin resistant *Enterococcus faecium* (VREF) and complicated skin infections caused by multi- resistant *Staph.aureus* and *Strep. pyogenes*, nosocomial pneumonia with *S. pneumoniae*. Because of high incidence of ADR, drug interactions and very high cost, their use to treat other conditions should be severely restricted.

Oxazolidinones

LINEZOLID (Zyvox) : This new antibacterial drug belongs to a new chemical class called oxazolidinones. It is bacteriostatic against staphycocci and enterococci and bactericidal against streptococci. Its main advantage is that it is active against *E. faecium*, MRSA and those resistant to vancomycin. It also acts against penicillin-resistant pneumococci. However, *it has no action against Gram-ve organisms.* It acts by preventing the formation of 70S ribosome complex which initiates protein synthesis. Because of its unique binding sites, there is no cross-resistance with other drug classes. Bacteria can develop resistance to this drug by mutation.

Given orally, the drug is rapidly and completely absorbed. It undergoes nonenzymatic oxidation in the liver and excreted in urine, 30-35% being in an active form. It has a half life of about 5 hours. It can also be given IV. Adverse reactions reported so far include diarrhoea, nausea, vomiting, headache, rash, leukopenia and rarely bone marrow suppression. The drug is an MAO inhibitor.

As linezolid and its metabolites are eliminated by dialysis, the drug should be administered following dialysis. No dose adjustment is recommended in chronic renal failure.

Currently, the drug is expensive and should be reserved for the treatment of well documented serious VREF and VRSA infections. It is given in the dose of 400-600 mg 12 hourly.

Aminoglycosides and Other Antibiotics Effective Mainly Against Gram Negative Organisms

46

Aminoglycosides form an important group of antibiotics, useful mainly against aerobic Gram-negative bacteria. They are protein-synthesis inhibitors, interfering with ribosomal function (Table 46.1). Compounds derived from Streptomyces are called 'mycins' (e.g., streptomycin) whereas those derived from Micromonospora are called 'micins' (e.g., gentamicin). The aminoglycosides have certain features in common :

- ***Chemically, they are polycations containing aminosugars in glycoside linkage.***
- ***They are bactericidal and their activity is maximum in an alkaline medium.***
- ***They are highly polar (water soluble) and are not absorbed orally. Their distribution is essentially extracellular, and penetration into the"CSF (except in the neonate) and into the eye is poor on systemic administration.***
- ***High concentrations are found in the renal cortex and in the endolymph and the perilymph of the inner ear.*** This perhaps contributes to their nephrotoxicity and ototoxicity.
- ***They are excreted unchanged relatively rapidly by the kidneys by glomerular filtration.***
- ***Bacteria develop resistance to them fairly rapidly and may even exhibit cross resistance among different aminoglycosides.***
- ***They have similar spectrum of activity.*** They are highly effective in infections caused by Gram negative microorganisms, and are not effective in infections due tó anaerobes.
- ***They exhibit synergism when combined with a beta lactam antibiotic such as penicillin or cephalosporin***; however, they should not be added to an infusion containing these drugs, as aminoglycocides tend to be inactivated by them.
- ***They are toxic to the neuromuscular junction, kidney and 8th nerve.***

Table 46.1: Aminoglycosides in therapeutic use

For topical use in the eye and on the skin: Neomycin, Framycetin, Gentamicin.

For GI infections and gut sterilisation: Neomycin, Paromomycin.

For systemic use: Streptomycin, Gentamicin, Kanamycin, Amikacin, Tobramycin, Netilmicin.

Mechanism of action: Aminoglycosides diffuse through the outer cytoplasmic membrane and are transported to ribosomes. Ribosomes manufacture enzymes under the directions from messenger RNA (mRNA). Aminoglycosides bind to 30S ribosomes and interfere with initiation of protein synthesis, block the translation of mRNA and prematurely terminate the synthesis. Incorrect amino acids are incorporated in the protein chain, leading to production of abnormal proteins. These proteins get inserted into the cell membrane, causing its disruption. They exhibit concentration-dependent killing and also have a post-antibiotic effect, depending on concentrtion.

Aminoglycoside resistance: The microorganisms readily develop resistance to aminoglycosides. Some important examples are *D. pneumoniae, M.tuberculosis, Proteus, E. coli, Aerobacter, H. influenzae, Brucella, Staph. aureus* and *Strep. fecalis.*

Resistance to aminoglycosides arises from several different mechanisms.

- ***Low level resistance*** is due to decreased cell permeability to the antibiotic. Thus, the bacterial cell becomes impermeable, preventing the drug reaching the drug sensitive ribosomes.
- ***High level resistance*** results from a single step mutation which affects the ribosomal proteins. This is relatively uncommon and is specific for streptomycin.
- ***'R' factor mediated resistance*** (see Chapter 48) is clinically significant. The genetic material transferred during conjugation confers on the recipient cell the capacity to synthesize specific enzymes which destroy the aminoglycoside. There is cross resistance among various aminoglycosides.

STREPTOMYCIN: This antibiotic, obtained from *Streptomyces griseus,* is an organic base. It is stable in dry state at room temperature. The aqueous solution of the salt retains its activity at pH 3 to 7 for 3 months, if kept at 28°C or below.

Antibacterial activity: The organisms usually sensitive to streptomycin are *M.tuberculosis, Shigella* species, *E. Coli, Proteus, Pseudomonas aeruginosa, Aerobacter aerogenes, H. influenzae, H. ducreyii, P. Pestis, P. tularensis, Brucella, Actinobacillus mallei, Listeria* and *Nocardia.* The moderately sensitive organisms include *Staphylococci, Strep. pyogens, Strep. faecalis, Strep. viridans, D. pneumoniae, Vibrio comma* and the *Salmonella* organisms. The *Gonococci* and *Meningococci* exhibit a variable response.

The drug is more effective at alkaline (7-8) than acidic pH. Streptomycin is bacteriostatic in low and bactericidal in high concentrations. Its bactericidal action increases progressively with rise in concentration.

Absorption, fate and excretion: Given orally it is poorly absorbed from the intact GI tract and is entirely excreted in the feces.

Given IM, peak plasma level is reached within 30 to 60 minutes and the activity persists for 6 to 8 hours. The drug is well absorbed when instilled intrapleurally. It is distributed extracellularly and does not readily penetrate into bone cells. About 30 to 35 per cent of the drug is bound to plasma proteins. It diffuses into the synovial, pericardial and peritoneal fluids but repeated systemic administration is necessary to produce a high concentration in the pleural fluid. It does not readily cross the BBB; however, in the presence of meningeal inflammation, higher CSF concentrations are usually achieved. It is concentrated mainly in kidneys, liver and skeletal muscles. It crosses the placental barrier and the cord blood concentration of the drug is similar to that of the maternal blood.

Streptomycin is excreted mostly unchanged by glomerular filtration. Approximately 50 to 60 per cent of the drug is eliminated in urine in an active form within 24 hours. Renal impairment retards its excretion.

Adverse reactions:

- ***Local irritation*:** Pain at the site of injection is common. Intrathecal injection can result in a shock like state with respiratory depression, nystagmus and convulsions.
- ***Allergy*:** The manifestations include various skin rashes, eosinophilia, drug fever and lymphadenopathy. Serious manifestations like angioedema, pericarditis, exfoliative dermatitis and blood dyscrasias are rare.
- ***Central nervous system*:** The most important and serious adverse effect of streptomycin is the damage to the 8th nerve (ototoxicity). Streptomycin is more prone to impair the vestibular function; this is not so calamitous as the deafness caused by dihydrostreptomycin, since the symptoms of vestibular damage are usually reversible as the equilibrium is partly restored by ocular and deep proprioceptive sensations. The incidence of this complication is dependent on the dose and

duration of therapy. The likelihood of ototoxicity is greater in infants, elderly patients who are dehydrated and in those with impaired renal function.

The labyrinthine dysfunction presents itself with a moderately severe headache which precedes the acute illness in which nausea, vomiting, giddiness, ataxia and nystagmus develop. These persist for 8 to 15 days. The acute stage is usually followed by chronic labyrinthitis and ataxia which persist for 40 to 60 days. With stoppage of the drug, full recovery occurs within 12 to 18 months, but in some cases residual dysfunction may persist.

Streptomycin also causes deafness. It is usually preceded by tinnitus. A few cases of congenital loss of hearing have been reported following its administration during pregnancy.

Other rare toxic effects include optic neuritis and peripheral neuritis. As chloramphenicol is also capable of producing optic neuritis, the two drugs should generally not be combined.

- ***Neuromuscular blockade***: All aminoglycosides have a potential curarimimetic action, producing neuromuscular block and respiratory arrest on intrapleural or intra-peritoneal instillation. It probably acts by inhibition of ACh release at the neuromuscular junction through competition with calcium ions. The blockade can be antagonized by calcium salts and by neostigmine.

- ***Kidney***: Mild albuminuria, cylindruria or acute tubular necrosis may occur in patients receiving streptomycin, but azotemia is rare. In patients with inadequate renal function aminoglycosides can accelerate the development of azotemia. Hence, dosage adjustment must be made in patients with renal insufficiency,

- ***Superinfection***: Superinfection with *Staph. aureus* and *Candida* has been reported.

Preparations and dosage: Streptomycin sulfate injection: Dose: 0.5 to 1 g. of the base daily by deep intramuscular injection.

Therapeutic uses: The important therapeutic uses of this antibiotic are :

- ***Tuberculosis***: Chapter 52.

- ***Plague***: Streptomycin is highly specific and the drug of choice in the treatment of plague. The specific therapy must be instituted within first 15 hours of overt illness, particularly in plague pneumonia, to ensure a favourable response. It is administered in the dose of 30 mg/kg/day IM in 2 divided doses for 10 days. Streptomycin may be used in pregnant women, old people and children with pneumonic plague. For optimum results, tetracycline may be combined with streptomycin, in the dose of 30 mg/kg/day, preferably IV (or orally), in four divided doses per day, for 5 days. In meningitic plague, chloramphenicol-streptomycin may be the preferred regimen; chloramphenicol is administered in the dose of 40-50 mg/kg/day IV in four divided doses, for 10 days. Supportive care includes the use of IV fluids, oxygen and vasopressor drugs to combat hypotension.

Contacts of a case of pneumonic plague should be treated with either tetracycline (250 mg. q.i.d. orally) or cotrimoxazole (250 mg. q.i.d. orally) for 5-10 days.

Doxycycline, amoxycillin, fluoroquinolones beta-lactams and newer aminoglycosides are effective *in vitro* and in experimental plague in animals; but, the clinical experience is inadequate.

- ***Tularemia***: This infection is highly sensitive to streptomycin and most cases respond to IM dose of 1 to 2 g. daily for 7 to 10 days.

- ***Brucellosis***: Brucellosis is transmitted to humans from the cattle and camel through contaminated dairy products, especially fresh cheeses. In several Eastern Mediterranean countries, serious outbreaks of *B. mellitensis* infection in the sheep are causing epidemics in people. Till recently, tetracycline was used in the dose of 0.5 g. 6 hourly for upto 6 weeks, usually in combination with streptomycin (1.0 g. daily) for the first 3 weeks. Currently, doxycyclin 200 mg. plus rifampicin 600 mg. once daily for 6 weeks is recommended as the treatment of choice; it causes rapid clinical improvement with only few relapses. Cotrimoxazole can also be used if doxycyclin is contraindicated.

- ***Enterococcal infections***: Streptomycin is

sometimes used in serious infections with susceptible enterococci. It exhibits synergistic effect with penicillin G.

KANAMYCIN (Kancin): This aminoglycoside is derived from *Streptomyces kanamyceticus*. Its antibacterial spectrum, pharmacokinetics and toxicity are similar to those of streptomycin. However, it is much more toxic and is now rarely used.

GENTAMICIN (Garamycin, Primicin, Genticin): This aminoglycoside antibiotic is produced by *Micromonospora purpura*.

Antibacterial activity: Gentamicin is highly effective against *Pseudomonas, E. coli, Proteus, A. aerogenes, K. pneumoniae, salmonellae* and Group A *beta hemolytic streptococci. Staphylococci* are also highly sensitive including those resistant to penicillin. It is 5-10 times more effective than kanamycin against *Pseudomonas aeruginosa. M. tuberculosis* and *Mycoplasma pneumoniae* are also highly sensitive. Resistance develops slowly. It exerts synergistic action with β-lactams and metronidazole.

Absorption, fate and excretion: Gentamicin is not significantly absorbed on oral administration. Given IM, the peak plasma levels are reached within 60-90 minutes and therapeutically effective concentration persists for 6-8 hours. Diffusion of the drug into the body fluids is inadequate. Approximately 25 to 30 per cent of the drug is bound to plasma proteins. It is excreted largely unchanged by glomerular filtration and its urinary concentration ranges from 50 to 100 times that in the plasma. High plasma levels are seen in patients with impaired renal function.

Adverse reactions: Allergic skin reactions and possibly photosensitivity reactions have occurred following topical gentamicin. Parenteral therapy, particularly in the presence of renal impairment, may produce vestibular damage and ototoxicity. Dizziness is the main presenting symptom. A transient rise in blood urea nitrogen has also been reported in some patients. The drug however is much less toxic than kanamycin and streptomycin. It should be avoided in pregnancy.

Preparations and dosage: It is available as sulfate. The IM or slow IV dose of the drug is 2-5 mg/kg/day in divided doses, for patients with normal renal function. The dose should be reduced in the presence of renal damage.

Administration of entire dose (5.5 mg/kg over 30-60 min) once daily appears to be less toxic and is as effective. High concentration achieved by the single dose accounts for higher efficacy and may be cost effective. It is preferred in clinical practice except in pregnancy, neonates and low dose combination therapy of bacterial endocarditis. The single dose regimen is also avoided if creatinine clearance is less than 20-25 ml per min.

A 0.3% cream, ointment or eye drops is used for topical application.

Therapeutic uses:

- ***Topical use***: Gentamicin has been employed in a variety of skin infections. It is useful in treating cases of burns infected with pseudomonas, bed sores, the nasal carriers of staphylococci, and ocular infections.
- ***Urinary tract infections***: Chapter 50.
- ***Systemic infections***: Although several Gram-positive bacteria are susceptible to gentamicin, safer and equally or more effective agents are available for treating infections caused by these bacteria. However, gentamicin is a valuable adjunct to penicillin G and ampicillin in the treatment of bacterial endocarditis caused by *Streptococcus viridans* and *Streptococcus fecalis*, respectively. Gentamicin, along with a carbenicillin or a cephalosporin, is valuable in treating serious Gram negative bacillary infections especially those caused by *P. aeruginosa, enterobacter, Klebsiella* and *Serratia* and by other species resistant to other antibiotics. The infections so treated include urinary tract infections, peritonitis, meningitis, osteomyelitis, septic burns, otitis, pneumonia and septicemia. In pseudomonas infections, the gentamicin plus

carbenicillin or piperacillin combination has been shown to be particularly effective. *Tetracyclines and chloramphenicol should not be used together with gentamicin as they reduce its therapeutic efficacy.* However, the effect of ampicillin is additive and it can be used together with gentamicin.

Netilmicin (Netromycin) has activity similar to that of gentamicin but is effective against a number of Gram negative bacilli except enterococci, resistant to gentamicin and tobramycin. It is less active than gentamicin against pseudomonas. It is available as sulphate for IM and IV use.

TOBRAMYCIN (Nebcin): This aminoglycoside antibiotic, belonging to the **family of nebramycins**, is derived from the actinomycetes *Streptomyces tenebrarius.* Its antibacterial spectrum, pharmacodynamic properties and toxicity are similar to those of gentamicin. However, clinically, it is four times as active as gentamicin against Pseudomonas and is relatively less toxic. It is active against a number of bacterial strains with acquired resistance to gentamicin. It is, however, less active against proteus. It is administered IM or IV in the dose of 3-5 mg./kg./day in 3-4 equal doses. Like other aminoglycoside antibiotics, it should be used in smaller doses in patients with impaired renal function.

AMIKACIN is a semisynthetic derivative of kanamycin A with pharmacokinetic properties similar to those of kanamycin. It has the broadest spectrum antibacterial activity among the aminoglycosides. Its therapeutic use and adverse effects are similar to those of gentamicin. It is little or not affected by the great majority of enzymes that degrade gentamicin and tobramycin. Hence, the drug is active against gentamicin-resistant organisms such as *P.aeruginosa, Klebsiella, E. Coli* and *Proteus.* It is much more expensive than gentamicin and should be reserved for hospital-acquired Gram-negative infections and in multi-drug resistant (MDR) tuberculosis. It is given IM or by slow IV drip in the dose of 15 mg./kg./day in two divided doses.

From among gentamicin, amikacin and tobramycin, gentamicin is the most active against all gentamicin sensitive bacilli except *Ps. aeruginosa* which is more sensitive to tobramycin.

NEOMYCIN: This antibiotic obtained from *Streptomyces fradiae,* is a polybasic, water soluble substance relatively stable to heat and changes in pH. The crude material contains neomycins A, B and C. The commercial preparation is an isomeric mixture of neomycins B and C. It is used as a sulfate complex which is stable at room temperature.

Antibacterial activity: Neomycin is effective against a wide variety of Gram-positive and Gram-negative organisms including *Enterococci, Streptococci, Staphylococci, B. anthracis, C. diptheriae, H. Influenzae, H. pertusis, Proteus, Pasteurella, Vibrio comma, Salmonella* and *Shigella.* Resistance to the antibiotic is known and the resistant organisms show cross resistance to kanamycin and streptomycin.

Neomycin is poorly absorbed orally. It is used mainly as an intestinal antiseptic. It is administered orally in the dose of 1g. 4-6 hourly. Dermatological and ophthalmic ointments (5 mg. per g.) are applied twice or thrice daily.

Adverse reactions: Its toxicity on parenteral administration is qualitatively similar to but more severe than that of streptomycin. Hence, it is not used systemically.

Therapeutic uses:

- ***For topical application to the skin and eye***, it is usually combined with other antibiotics like bacitracin or polymyxin to prevent the emergence of resistant strains and to widen the spectrum;
- ***As an intestinal antiseptic*** prior to colonic surgery and for suppression of intestinal flora in hepatic failure.

FRAMYCETIN (Soframycin): This antibiotic, produced by *Streptomyces decaris,* is used as the water soluble sulfate salt. Its antimicrobial spectrum and toxicity are similar to those of neomycin. The uses of this antibiotic are identical with those of Neomycin B.

Framycetin sulfate, as a 0.5 per cent ointment, cream or solution is used for staphylococcal skin infections and in the treatment of nasal carriers of staphylococci.

PAROMOMYCIN (Aminocidin, Humatin): This antibiotic, obtained from a strain of *Streptomyces rimosus,* has a similar spectrum of activity and toxicity as neomycin. It also shows considerable activity against *E. histolytica.* The drug is not absorbed orally. Adverse effects of oral therapy include headache, emesis, diarrhoea and skin rashes; superinfection with Candida may occur after prolonged oral therapy. The drug was used in amoebic dysentry, for sterilization of the bowel before surgery and in hepatic coma. It has been reported to be effective in treating visceral leishmaniasis (Chapter 56).

Non-aminoglycoside Agents

COLISTIN (Polymyxin E) : This polypeptide antibiotic is obtained from the bacterium *Aerobacillus colistinus.* It acts by causing disruption of the phospholipids of the cell membrane because of its detergent property.

Antibacterial activity: Colistin is bactericidal to many Gram-negative organisms, e.g., *H. pertussis, Pseudomonas, E. coli, A. aerogenes, K. pneumoniae, H. influenzae* and Shigella. Most strains of Proteus, Gram-negative cocci, Gram-positive organisms and fungi are resistant to it. Resistance to the antibiotic appears slowly. There is a complete cross-susceptibility as well as cross resistance between colistin and polymyxin B.

Absorption, fate and excretion: Colistin is not significantly absorbed orally. It is given parenterally for systemic infections. It is largely excreted unchanged by the kidneys.

Adverse reactions: These occur in a large proportion of patients and include local pain, circumoral and lingual paraesthesiae, nausea, skin rash, pruritus, vertigo, ataxia, nystagmus (neurotoxicity) and renal damage. Other serious toxic effects include partial deafness, neutropenia, hepatotoxicity and transient disturbances of vision and speech. The drug has a curariform effect. Because of its toxicity, its use is now restricted to topical purposes and sometimes for bowel sterilization.

POLYMYXIN B (Aerosporin): Polymyxin is the generic name for a group of closely related polypeptide antibiotics elaborated by various strains of *Bacillus polymyxa.* Polymyxin B, initially thought to be the least toxic of these antibiotics, is used as a sulfate. The antibacterial spectrum, absorption, metabolism and toxicity of polymyxin are similar to those of colistin. The development of bacterial resistance is rare; and the drug does not interfere with wound healing. It is prescribed as spray, cream or powder for local application, for skin, ear and eye infections.

TYROTHRICIN: This antibiotic, obtained from *Bacillus brevis,* is in fact a 80:20 mixture of two antibiotics, **Tyrocidine** and **Gramicidine**, respectively. Tyrothricin is bacteriostatic. It is particularly effective against *Pneumococci, Streptococci, Staphylococci* and *C. diptheriae.* In addition, it exhibits a mild antibacterial action against certain Gram-negative organisms. Tyrothricin is ineffective orally and is too toxic parenterally. It is employed only for topical therapy to treat infected superficial ulcers and pyodermas, and as troches in throat infections.

CYCLOSERINE: This antibiotic, obtained from *Streptomyces orchidaceus* is mainly used as a second line drug in the treatment of tuberculosis (Chapter 52) and in UTI due to resistant *E.coli* (Chapter 50).

SPECTINOMYCIN: This antibiotic derived from *Streptomyces spectabillis* has moderate *in vitro* activity against many Gram-positive and Gram-negative bacteria. Although it is not an aminoglycoside, like streptomycin it contains a cyclic amino polyol (aminocyclitol) group. Resistance tends to develop rapidly by certain microorganisms, particularly the staphylococci. It is bactericidal for both penicillin sensitive and penicillin resistant strains of gonococci. Hence, it is mainly used to treat uncomplicated gonorrhoea, as an alternative to penicillin. It is usually administered in the dose of 2-4 g. deep IM as a single dose. Adverse effects reported include nausea, insomnia and allergic reactions.

FOSFOMYCIN: This antibiotic has bactericidal action against many urinary pathogens-*E.coli, E.fecalis,* klebsiela, *P.aeruginosa,* enterobacter, enterococci including VREF, and staphylococci. Combination with beta lactam antibiotics, aminoglycosides or fluoroquinolones acts synergistically against Gram positive and Gram negative organisms.

Mechanism of Action : As a phosphonic acid derivative, fosfomycin inhibits bacterial cell wall synthesis (bactericidal) by inactivating the enzyme, pyruvyl transferase, which is critical in the synthesis of cell walls by bacteria.

Absorption, fate and excretion : It is well absorbed orally and high concentrations are achieved in the urine. Antacids or calcium salts may decrease its absorption. Protein binding is minimal. Half life is 4-8 hours. It is excreted unchanged in the urine and high urinary levels (100 mcg/ml) persist for more than 48 hours.

Adverse reactions: These are headache, rash, diarrhea, nausea, vomiting, abdominal discomfort, anorexia, dizziness, drowsiness, fatigue, pruritus. No dosage adjustment is required in hepatic impairment.

Therapeutic uses : It is available as a powder to be mixed with water. It is administered as single dose of 3 g in 100 ml of water. It is currently used in the therapy of uncomplicated UTI in women. Multiple doses, 3 g every 3 days for 3-7 doses, are used in complicated UTI.

For **extended spectrum penicillins** effective against Gram negative organisms, see Chapter 45.

Monobactams

AZTREONAM (Azactam): This synthetic antibiotic belongs to the class of beta lactam antibiotics, referred to as monobactams. The monobactams are naturally occurring and, unlike penicillins and cephalosporins, are not produced by moulds or fungi but by bacteria in the soil. The word monobactam is derived from *mono* (a single ring), *bact* (produced by bacteria) and *am* (a beta lactam). Aztreonam is produced in nature by *Chromobacterium violaceum.* Like other beta lactam antibiotics, it acts on the bacterial cell wall and is bactericidal. It has activity only against aerobic Gram negative species; *E. coli, Klebsiella, H. influenzae* and *Proteus* are highly sensitive. Higher concentrations are effective against *Pseudomonas.* It has negligible activity against anaerobes.

Absorption, fate and excretion: It is not absorbed orally. It is resistant to hydrolysis by most beta-lactamases and does not induce production of beta-lactamase. It is largely excreted unchanged by glomerular filtration.

It is administered IM or by IV infusion in the dose of 1-2 gm. every 8-12 hours. Higher doses are used in systemic *Ps.aeruginosa* infection and in lung infection in patients with cystic fibrosis.

Adverse reactions: Toxicity reported so far is mild and includes skin rashes, GI upset, neutropenia and rarely hepatotoxicity. Its advantage is lack of cross allergenicity with penicillins and cephalosporins. It lacks the ototoxicity and the nephrotoxicity of aminoglycosides.

Therapeutic uses:

- ***As an alternative to aminoglycosides*** in severe infections caused by susceptible **Gram negative organisms** e.g. complicated UTI (Chapter 50).
- ***In neonatal Gram negative infections,*** in conjunction with ampicillin; and,
- ***In patients who are allergic to penicillin and cephalosporins.***

Antibiotics Effective Against Both Gram Positive and Gram Negative Organisms

47

Antibiotics which are effective in both Gram-positive and Gram-negative infections are: semisynthetic penicillins, e.g., ampicillin, and carbenicillin; rifamycins (see later); cephalosporins; tetracyclines and chloramphenicol. The last two are also effective against certain protozoa and rickettsiae and hence are called 'broad spectrum antibiotics'. They are discussed in Chapter 48.

Cephalosporins

The discovery of cephalosporins is as fascinating as that of penicillin. In 1945, Professor G. Brotzu of Sardinia made cultures from sea water at a sewage outfall on the assumption that this might contain organisms antagonistic to intestinal pathogens. He succeeded in isolating a fungus, identified as *Cephalosporium acremonium.* The crude extract prepared from its culture was demonstrated to be active in humans against certain pathogens. He published the original findings of this brilliant work in a local Sardinian journal. But for Dr. Blyth Brook, a public health officer in Sardinia who wrote to Florey about Dr. Brotzu's work, it might have remained unknown to the rest of the world. The culture was received by Florey in 1948, and in 1955 he described the amazing initial findings that the fungus produced not one but seven antibiotics.

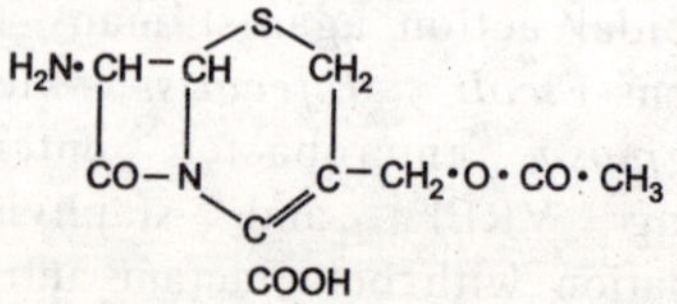

$H_2N \cdot CH - CH$ — S — CH_2; CO — N — C — $C - CH_2 \cdot O \cdot CO \cdot CH_3$; COOH

Fig. 47.1 : 7-Amino cephalosporanic acid

Cephalosporins have 7-amino cephalosporanic acid nucleus which bears close resemblance to the 6-APA nucleus of penicillins. Structurally, they contain beta lactam and dihydrothiazine rings. They are water soluble and stable to changes in pH and temperature. The various cephalosporins, however, differ in their antibacterial spectrum and their resistance to betalactamases.

Cephamycins are similar to cephalosporins but they are derived from an actinomycete. Examples are cefoxitin and cefotetan.

Antibacterial activity: Cephalosporins possess a wide range of activity against Gram-positive and Gram-negative bacteria. They are effective against pneumococci, *C. diphtheriae* and *Group A* and *beta hemolytic streptococci.* The older cephalosporins (cephaloridine and cephalothin) are active against staphylococci. No cephalosporin available at present exhibits useful activity against *Streptococcus fecalis.* Although cefotaxime is active against *Bacteroides fragilis,* its activity against this species is not superior to metronidazole.

The Gram negative organisms susceptible to these antibiotics include *E. coli, Proteus mirabilis, K. pneumoniae, N. gonorrhoea* and *Paracolobacterium* species. Cephaloridine shows good activity against *S. typhi* and *paratyphi,* and is also effective against some strains of Shigella. The newer derivatives are effective against *Pseudomonas aeruginosa,* Enterobacter, indole positive Proteus and Bacteroides, and against many strains of *E. coli* and Klebsiellae resistant to the older cephalosporins. They have a limited activity against *H. influenzae.*

Mechanism of action : Cephalosporins act by inhibiting bacterial cell wall synthesis in a manner similar to penicillins, and are bactericidal. Resistance to cephalosporins develops slowly and is mediated either by bacterial betalactamases or by lack of bacterial permeability to the drug. Cross resistance for other betalactam agents also occurs. Therefore, their use should be restricted to selective indications.

Some of the newer cephalosporins are much more resistant than the older ones to the action of betalactamases, and consequently have a broader anti-bacterial spectrum.

Absorption, fate and excretion: Cephalosporins are administered either orally or IV; IM administration is painful. There are significant differences among the various cephalosporins regarding their pharmacokinetics. Their body distribution is similar to that of penicillin but the concentration in the eye and the CSF is poor.

Cephalosporins are eliminated mainly by renal tubular secretion and high concentrations are achieved in the urinary tract. As with penicillins, renal tubular blocking with probenecid increases the plasma levels significantly. The renal excretion is markedly reduced in renal insufficiency. Therefore their dose should be appropriately reduced in case of renal impairment. Concentration in the bile is similar to that in the plasma. Unlike other cephalosporins, cefotaxime is partly metabolized by the liver before excretion by the kidneys.

Adverse reactions: In general, cephalosporins are well tolerated.

- ***Local reactions*:** IM injections are painful and IV injections can cause thrombophlebitis.
- ***Allergy*:** Skin rash, fever, serum sickness, anaphylactoid reaction (rare), eosinophilia, neutropenia, transient splenomegaly and increased SGOT levels.
- ***Drug fever:*** Cephalosporins are among the common causes of drug fever.
- ***Superinfection*:** Superinfection with resistant organisms can occur during therapy, generally with broad spectrum third generation agents.
- ***Nephrotoxicity*:** Large doses can cause nephrotoxicity. It is probably dose related and is potentially reversible on drug withdrawal; it is enhanced by loop diuretics such as furosemide.
- ***CNS toxicity*:** Signs of cerebral irritation, nystagmus and hallucinations may occur following intrathecal administration.
- ***Blood toxicity*:** Impairment of normal hemostasis may result from hypoprothrombinaemia and abnormalities in platelet aggregation. Parenteral vitamin K therapy will correct the abnormality and is recommended prophylactically when moxalactam, cefaperazone, cefotetan and cefamandole are used for prolonged periods. A false positive Coomb's test may occur in as many as 60 per cent of patients on cephalothin therapy. Thrombocytopenia, neutropenia and hemolytic anemia may rarely occur.
- ***Disulfuram like reaction*:** Some of the newer cephalosporins cause disulfiram-like effect when combined with alcohol.

Cross reactivity with penicillin does occur and cephalosporins should not be used in patients who have history of anaphylactic reaction to penicillin or in patient with skin-test reactivity to antigen of penicillin metabolite.

Several cephalosporins give a positive glucose test with copper reduction reagents.

Preparations and dosage: Table 47.1 shows various available cephalosporins.

Therapeutic uses: The cephalosporins have added substantially to the therapeutic

Table 47.1 : Cephalosporins – bacterial sensitivity, pharmacokinetics and doses

	Staph. aureus	*H.influenzae*	*Enterobacter*	*Ps.aeruginosa*	*B.fragilis*	Protein binding %	Plasma half life (hr)	Disposal	Urinary excretion %	Dose
					I Generation					
Oral										
Cefalexin (Sporidex)	++	0/+	++	0	0	18-20	0.9	R	88	0.25-1.0 g q 6-8 h
Cefadroxil (Droxyl)	++	0/+	++	0	0	18-20	1.6	R	88	0.5-1.0 g q 12 h
Parenteral										
Cefazolin (Azolin)	+++	+++	++	0	++	80	1.8	R	90	0.5-1.0 g IM/IV q 6 - 8 h
					II Generation					
Oral										
Cefaclor (Distaclor)	++	++	++	0	0	40	0.6	R	60	0.25-0.5 g q 8 h
Cefuroxime axetil (Ceftum)	++	+++	+++	0	+	40	1.3	R	50	0.25-0.5 g q 12 h
Parenteral										
Cefamandole (Kefadol)	++	+++	+++	0	+	70	0.8	R	75	0.5-2.0 g IM/IV q 4 - 8 h
Cefoxitin (Mefoxin)	++	++	+++	0	+++	75	0.7	R	90	1-2 g IM/IV q 6 - 8 h
Cefuroxime (Supacef)	++	+++	+++	0	+	35	1.4	R	80	0.75-1.5 g IM/IV q 8 h

(Table 47.1 contd.)

	Staph. aureus	*H.influenzae*	*Enterobacter*	*Ps.aeruginosa*	*B.fragilis*	Protein binding %	Plasma half life (hr)	Disposal	Urinary excretion %	Dose
				III Generation						
Oral										
Cefixime (Suprax)	+	+++	+	+	+	67	3.5	H/R	18	200-400 mg/day in 1-2 div. doses
Cefpodoxime Proxetil (Monocef-O)	+	+	++	+++	+++	25	2.2	H/R	30	200-400 mg q 12 h
Parenteral										
Cefotaxime* (Omnatax, Claforan)	+	+++	+++	++	+	40	0.9	H/R	90	1-2 g IM/IV q 8 h
Ceftriaxone * (Oframax, Rocephin)	+	+++	+++	++	+	95	8.5	H/R	60	1-2 g IM/IV q 12-24 h
Cefaperazone (Cefobid)	+	+++	++	+++	+	90	1.7	H/R	25	1-2 g IM/IV q 8-12 h
Ceftazidime* (Fortum)	0	+++	+++	++++	0	17	1.8	R	85	1-2 g IM/IV q 8-12 h
Ceftizoxime* (Cefizox)	+	+++	+++	++	+	30	1.6	R	80	1-2 g IM/IV q 8-12 h
				IV Generation						
Cefepime (Maxipime)	+	+++	+++	++	0	17	2.0	R	80	2 g IV q 8-12 h

q 6-8 h = every 6 - 8 hours. R= Renal. H = Hepatic. * Good CNS penetration. *Penetration of others is not enough to treat meningitis.*

armamentarium of the physicians, but the physicians find their multiplicity confusing. For the generalist, it is enough to remember a few guiding principles about using cephalosporins, and to learn in detail how to use a few of the latter. The guiding principles are shown in Table 47.2.

Table 47.2 : Guiding principles for the use of cephalosporins

- Cephalosporins are expensive and should not be used where an equally effective, alternative antibiotic is available.
- None of them is effective against infections by enterococci (*Strep. fecalis).*
- None of them is the agent of choice against anaerobic infections.
- Except for cefotaxime, ceftriaxone, ceftazidime, ceftizoxime and cefepime, the CNS penetration of cephalosporins is poor. However, these five are the drugs of choice in Gram negative bacillary meningitis (see Tables 47.1 and 47.3).

First generation cephalosporins predominantly act against Gram positive organism such as staphylococci, pneumococci, streptococci, but also against (though less effectively) the common Gram negative pathogens such as *E.coli,* Klebsiella and Proteus. However, they are not effective against salmonella, shigella, *B.fragilis* and pseudomonas. Further their efficacy against beta lactamase producing organisms is poor. Cefalexin and cefadroxil have been useful in treating community acquired, respiratory and urinary tract infections, and in surgical prophylaxis. However, *they are not considered the agents of choice for any serious systemic infections.*

Cefazolin is considered the agent of choice for antimicrobial prophylaxis in most surgical procedures because of its activity against most pathogens that cause infection of wounds. It is given IM/IV.

- ***Second generation cephalosporins*** offer a wider coverage against Gram negative bacilli than the first generation cephalosporin. They are also more resistant than the first generation drugs to beta lactamases. Their main use would appear to be in the Gram negative infections, especially those caused by beta lactamase producing organisms, including *H.influenzae.* They have less activity than the first generation drugs against the Gram positive cocci and are inactive against anaerobes and *Pseudomonas aeruginosa.* Only cefoxitin and cefotetan are active against *B.fragilis.*

- ***Third generation cephalosporins*** are more active against the Gram negative bacilli than the first and second generation cephalosporins. In addition, they possess anti-pseudomonal activity. They have poor activity against the gram positive cocci. The CNS penetration of these drugs is better than that of the first two generation drugs. Ceftriaxone has sufficiently long half life to permit once a day administration in some infections. These agents are not indicated for routine surgical prophylaxis.

The potential indications for these drugs include aminoglycoside resistant or multi-resistant Gram negative bacillary systemic infections. They have almost replaced the second generation cephalosporins for this purpose.

In serious Gram negative infections, a third generation cephalosporin is combined with gentamicin or amikacin.

- ***Fourth generation cephalosporin:*** **Cefepime** has properties like those of the third generation cephalosporins, but it is more resistant to some beta-lactamases. It is active against streptococci and methicillin-sensitive staphylococci, but not against MRSA. Its main use is in serious Gram negative infections (especially enterobacter, citrobacter and serratia groups of organisms), including infections of the CNS into which it has excellent penetration. It has a half life of about 2 hours. It is administered in the dose of 2 gm IV every 12 hours.

Cefpirome is a new fourth generation cephalosporin with properties and therapeutic uses similar to those of cefepime. It gives CSF concentration many times in excess of the minimum bactericidal concentration required to eliminate susceptible organisms.

Carbapenems

This group of betalactam antibiotics are obtained by modification of a parent antibiotic thienamycin, derived from *Streptomyces cattleya*. Thienamycin itself is chemically unstable. Like penicillin, carbapenems act by inhibiting cell wall synthesis. They are bactericidal and have a wider antibacterial spectrum than cephalosporins. *They are not active against MRSA and Enterococcus fecium.*

IMIPENEM: This carbapenem is highly active against Gram negative aerobes including *Ps.aeruginosa,* Gram positive aerobes and many anaerobes. It is not easily hydrolysed by bacterial beta lactamase. It is not active against chlamydia and mycoplasma species.

Absorption, fate and excretion: It is not absorbed orally and must be administered parenterally. It does not penetrate intracellularly and therefore is inactive against intracellular organisms. It is hydrolysed by a dehydropeptidase in the kidney and therefore the concentration of the active drug in the kidney is less than that in the plasma. It is commonly combined with **cilastatin**, an inhibitor of the renal dehydropeptidase. Cilastatin has no anti-microbial activity.

Adverse reactions: Imipenem has most of the adverse effects of other beta lactam antibiotics. They include nausea, vomiting, allergic reactions and transient elevation of liver enzymes in the blood. It can cause pseudomembranous colitis. In high doses, it can cause convulsions. Leucopenia and granulocytopenia have been reported. It has not been associated with renal toxicity or coagulation abnormalities. Cross allergy with penicillin can occur.

Therapeutic uses: Imipenem + cilastatin combination (Primaxin) is highly effective in infections due to Gram positive and Gram negative aerobes and anaerobes (including all subspecies of *B.fragilis).* It should not be used in meningitis because of its epileptogenic properties. Its use should be restricted to the treatment of (a) seriously ill and/or hospitalized patients with mixed bacterial infections, and (b) multi-drug resistant Gram negative infections including those due to pseudomonas. It is administered in the dose of 500-750 mg. (in terms of imipenem) by deep IM injection 8-12 hourly; it can also be administered by IV infusion in the dose of 1-2 g. daily, in 3-4 divided doses. Bacteria can develop resistance to this drug.

Meropenem (Zenece) is a dimethy-lcarbamoyl derivative of thienamycin. It is not susceptible to renal dipeptidase and does not require co-administration with cilastatin. Its antibacterial spectrum is similar to that of imipenam, but it is effective against imipenam-resistant *P.aeruginosa.* It is less likely than imipenen to cause convulsions.

Ertapenem (Inbanz) is once daily IV carbapenem, not active against pseudomonas and acinobacter species. It has longer t½. Its spectrum includes Gram+ve organisms, enterobacter and anaerobes, which allows its use in intraabdominal and pelvic infections.

Doripenem is a parenteral carbopenem with properties and uses similar to those of meropenem.

A carbapenem is the reasonable first choice for empiric monotherapy of serious, complicated, intra-abdominal infections. Other alternatives are: piperacillin + tazobactam; a fluoroquinolone + metronidozole; or tigecycline.

Rifamycins

These are a group of antibiotics derived from

Table 47.3: Drug therapy of specific forms of bacterial meningitis (adult doses)

Organism	Preferred regimen	Other regimens
• *Meningococci**	a) Penicillin G 4 million units I.V. q 2 h for 5-7 days after the patient becomes afebrile. b) In patients allergic to penicillin, chloramphenicol 4-6 g IV q 6 h. for 5-7 days	Cefatoxime or ceftriaxone, with or without ampicillin. A fluoroquinolone. Vancomycin.
• *Pneumococci*	Same as for meningococcal meningitis If multidrug resistant, vancomycin for 10-14 days.	Vancomycin + rifampicin.
• *H.influenzae*	Cefotaxime 2 g IV q 4 h or ceftriaxone 2 g IV q 12 h Duration : 10 days.	Ampicillin + sulbactam.
• *Enterococci* **	Penicillin G as above plus gentamicin 1 mg/kg IV q 8 h. for 14-21 days	Vancomycin + gentamicin.
• *Staphylococci*	Nafcillin or oxacillin 2 g. IV q 4 h for 14 days	Vancomycin 1 g. IV q 12 h (in penicillin allergic patients). Rifampicin may be used in MRSA.
• *Gram negative bacilli (other than Ps. aeruginosa)*	Cefotaxime 2 g. IV q 4 h or ceftriaxone 2 g. IV q 12 h for 21 days	Cotrimoxazole or (ampicillin + sulbactam).
• *Ps. aeruginosa* **	Ceftazidime 2 g. IV q 8 h + gentamicin 1 mg/kg IV q 8 h. for 21 days	Piperacillin + gentamicin/amikacin Aztreonam.

* Close contacts and family members should receive prophylaxis with rifampicin 600 mg. orally b.i.d. for 2 days; alternatively ceftriaxone 250 mg single IM dose or ofloxacin 400 mg. single oral dose may be used. These drugs, in short courses, achieve long term (3-4 weeks) eradication of meningococci from the pharynx. The index case should also be treated with rifampicin before discharge.

** 2 g. I.V. q 4 h = 2 g. intravenously every 4 hours.

Penicillin should not be injected intrathecally.

a strain of *Streptomyces mediterranei*. **Rifampicin** (Rifampin) is a semisynthetic derivative of rifamycin B while **rifabutin** is a derivative of rifamycin S. Both these drugs act by inhibiting RNA polymerase and have action against certain Gram positive and Gram negative bacteria and mycobacteria. They are mainly used in the treatment of tuberculosis, leprosy and infections with *Staph. aureus* (Chapters 52 and 53).

Rifaximin is an oral, non-absorbed rifampin derivative, used to treat infective diarrhoeas (Chapter 40).

Drug Therapy of Bacterial Meningitis

Acute bacterial meningitis is a medical emergency. **In adults** the commonest organisms are *Strep. pneumoniae* and *N.meningitidis*, with gram negative bacilli, staphylococci and streptococci following suit. **In the neonates**, the vast majority of infections are due to Gram negative bacilli and streptococci, commonly non-haemolytic. **In children under the age of 15**, the majority of cases are due to *Strep. pneumoniae, N. meningitidis,* and *H.influenzae.* Gram negative meningitis should also be thought of in the setting of head injury, neurosurgical procedures, diabetes mellitus, cirrhosis of the liver and renal failure. It is important to keep this in mind because to be effective, the appropriate antibiotic treatment must be started immediately, before the full identification of the causative pathogen is available.

The antibiotics which penetrate the CSF well are penicillin G, ampicillin, chloramphenicol and the third generation cephalosporins. These drugs should be administered parenterally in high doses. The recommended drug regimen for initial empirical therapy of severe meningitis is : a third generation cephalosporin + vancomycin ± ampicillin (all given IV).

Drug therapy, recommended after identification of the offending organism, is outlined in Table 47.3.

Initial treatment before identification of the pathogen or when the CSF culture is negative (although the diagnosis of bacterial meningitis appears to be reasonably certain) is based on the probability of the offending pathogen as mentioned earlier. In adults IV penicillin G 2 million units every two hours or a third generation cephalosporin IV is recommended for initial treatment.

In children the initial treatment should be with a third generation cephalosporin or with ampicillin + chloramphenicol. **In the neonate**, the preferred initial regimen is (ampicillin + cefotaxime) with or without gentamicin.

Tetracyclines, Chloramphenicol and Antifungal Agents 48

Tetracycline antibiotics were discovered as a result of a systematic plan by the American Pharmaceutical Industry for screening a multitude of soil microorganisms for potential antibiotic activity. The first member chlortetracycline, isolated from *Streptomyces aureofaciens,* was introduced in 1948. This was followed by oxytetracycline derived from *Streptomyces rimosus* in 1950 and tetracycline prepared by catalytic hydrogenation of chlortetracycline in 1953. Many other semi-synthetic tetracyclines have since been introduced into therapy.

Tetracyclines

The tetracyclines are naphthacene derivatives, made up by fusion of four partially unsaturated cyclohexane radicals and hence the name tetracyclines (Fig. 48.1). The various tetracyclines differ only slightly in structure. The crystalline bases of these compounds are pale yellow, slightly bitter and sparingly soluble in water. However, they form water soluble sodium salts. Tetracyclines are more stable at acid pH.

Antibacterial activity : Various tetracyclines have similar antibacterial spectrum. They are bacteriostatic and along with chloramphenicol are termed **broad spectrum antibiotics**, as in addition to their antibacterial activity against a number of Gram-positive and Gram-negative organisms, they also inhibit the growth of certain actinomyces (fungi), rickettsiae and chlamydia organisms. Gram-positive organisms in general respond better than Gram-negative organisms.

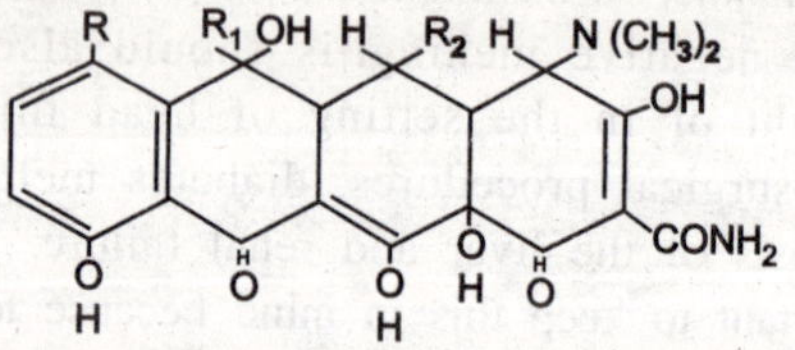

	R	R_1=	R_2=
TETRACYCLINE	H	CH_3	H
CHLORTETRACYCLINE	C1	CH_3	H
OXYTETRACYCLINE	H	CH_3	OH
DEMETHYLCHLORTETRA-CYCLINE	C1	H	H

There is no OH attached to the carbon atom to which R is attached.

Fig. 48.1 : Basic structure of tetracyclines

The Gram-positive and Gram-negative organisms inhibited by tetracyclines include Pneumococci, Gonococci, some strains of *alpha* and *beta hemolytic Streptococci, Clostridia, H. Influenzae, H. Pertussis, H. ducreyi, Brucella, K. pneumoniae, Vibrio comma* and *Donovania granulomatis.* The moderately sensitive organisms include *E. coli, Aerobacter, Salmonella, Shigella, B. anthracis, P. tularensis, P. pestis, Fusobacterium, Listeria monocyto-genes* and *M. tuberculosis. Pseudomonas* is relatively resistant. Other organisms which respond satisfactorily are *Borrelia recurrentis, Mycoplasma pneumoniae (PPLO), Leptospira icterohaemorrhagiae* and *T. pallidum.* Actinomyces and Nocardia also respond but less than to penicillin. Amongst the protozoa, it has action against *E. histolytica* and plasmodia. Tetracyclines are highly effective against rickettsial organisms and chlamydia. They are, however, ineffective against the viruses.

Mechanism of action: The susceptible bacteria accumulate the antibiotic by an active transport system which is absent in the mammalian cells. Tetracyclines bind to 30S ribosomes and interfere with protein synthesis by blocking the attachment of aminoacyl transfer RNA to the acceptor site on the MRNA-ribosome complex. Tetracyclines chelate cations like calcium and magnesium. As these are essential for the functional integrity of various enzyme systems and ribosomes, chelation may be its basic mechanism of action.

Tetracycline resistance: This has been demonstrated by many organisms including Staphylococci, Group A Steptococci, *H. influenzae, Pneumococci,* and *E. coli.* Resistance develops slowly *in vitro* and cross-resistance within the group is usually complete. Resistance may occur through several mechanisms and can be passed from one organism to another by transfer of plasmids called R-factors that contain genetic information for the development of resistance. In resistant organisms, accumulation of the drug is absent. Gram-negative organisms resistant to tetracyclines are usually resistant to chloramphenicol as well, but the tetracycline resistant Gram-positive organisms are usually susceptible to chloramphenicol.

Absorption, fate and excretion: The absorption of oral tetracyclines is variable but adequate (Table 48.1). They are not destroyed by the gastric acid or the intestinal flora. The tetracyclines form insoluble complexes by chelation with calcium, magnesium and aluminium and hence, substances like milk that contain calcium, and antacids reduce their absorption. Ingestion of food and iron also interferes with the absorption of tetracyclines.

The tetracyclines are mainly absorbed from the duodenum and the upper small intestine. With larger doses, proportionately more of the drug escapes absorption and may cause gastro-intestinal disturbances.

After oral administration of a single therapeutic dose of tetracycline and oxytetracycline, peak plasma level is reached within 3 to 4 hours. They are usually administered at 6 hourly intervals in order to maintain their therapeutic concentration in plasma. Oxytetracycline and tetracycline, given IM, produce peak plasma levels within 1 hour and adequate levels are maintained for 12 hours; the injection, however, is painful.

The tetracyclines are widely distributed in the body and their diffusion into various body fluids and glandular secretions is very much like that of penicillin. Concentrations in the bile are 5-20 times those in the plasma and a closed enterohepatic circulation has been demonstrated. The compounds are concentrated in liver, bone marrow, enamel of unerupted teeth and lungs. They cross the placental barrier and are also secreted in milk. Their concentration in the ocular fluids, however, is poor.

The tetracyclines are metabolized in the liver and metabolites excreted mainly in the urine by glomerular filtration. In anuria, the plasma $t^1/_2$ of tetracycline is 4 to 5 days and that of oxytetracycline 2 to 3 days. Doxycycline and minocycline are eliminated by non-renal route.

Adverse reactions: Used in recommended dosages, tetracyclines, in general, have a low toxicity. The adverse effects are:

- ***Allergy*:** Skin rashes may develop mainly on topical application of these agents. Severe allergic reactions, however, are rare.

Photosensitivity manifested by marked erythema and even vesicular exanthema has been reported. A brown-black discoloration of nails accompanied by marked loosening may also occur. In some cases, simultaneous yellowish brown discoloration of the teeth has been observed.

Table 48.1: Properties of commonly used tetracyclines

	Tetracycline	Oxytetracycline	Doxycycline	Minocycline
Stability	Less	Less	More	More
Absorption	77%	58%	>90%	> 90 %
Plasma protein binding	65%	35%	90%	76%
Urinary recovery	60%	70%	42%	6%
CSF level	+	+	++	+++
Half-life (hours)	8	9	18	16
Effect on bone	+++	+++	++	+
Relative *in vitro* activity*	100	80	110	200 #
Usual oral dose	250 to 500 mg. 6-8 hourly		200 mg. loading 100 mg. daily	100 mg b.i.d.

* Against *S. aureus.* # Active against organisms resistant to other tetracyclines.
Ref.: A.M.A.Drug Evaluation, 6th Ed., 1986.

● ***GI tract***: Nausea, vomiting, epigastric distress and loose stools are relatively common. Nausea and vomiting may be prevented by taking these drugs after meals. Mild diarrhoea appears to be dose-dependent and is more commonly observed following daily doses of 2 g. or more.

Diarrhoea secondary to irritation is not accompanied by RBCs or pus cells in feces, and can thus be differentiated from diarrhoea secondary to GI superinfection.

● ***Superinfection***: Suppression of the normal intestinal flora with resultant superinfection is liable to occur after prolonged tetracycline therapy, particularly in patients with diabetes mellitus, leukemia or leucopenia and when steroid therapy is being given simultaneously.

Infection with *Candida albicans* is especially common and may cause in diarrhoea or soft, bulky, odourless stools, soreness and redness of the mouth (thrush), glossitis, black hairy tongue and inflammatory lesions of the vulva, vagina and perianal region causing troublesome pruritus. Treatment with antifungal agents is only indicated in serious cases or if the lesions persist even after stoppage of tetracyclines. Nystatin is effective locally in oropharyngeal, vaginal and perineal lesions. Serious systemic infections need systemic antifungal therapy. Most of the yeast infections are generally limited to the duration of therapy and routine prophylaxis with antifungal agents is unnecessary.

Superinfection with resistant S. *aureus* occurs more frequently in hospitalized patients. Serious staphylococcal enteritis is heralded by sudden loss of appetite, abdominal discomfort, distension and a profuse watery diarrhoea; the stools show the presence of blood. It carries a mortality rate of 40%. Immediate stoppage of tetracyclines, institution of appropriate antibiotic therapy and correction of dehydration and electrolyte imbalance are recommended.

Pseudomembranous colitis characterised by profuse diarrhoea and fever may occur due to superinfection with *Clostridium difficile.* The stools contain shreds of mucous membrane and blood (also see Chapter 45).

● ***Antianabolic effect***: Since tetracyclines inhibit protein synthesis, their prolonged use produces an antianabolic effect leading to weight loss.

● ***Liver***: Fatal hepatic dysfunction with pancreatitis may occur in patients receiving large doses of tetracyclines over short periods, particularly by IV route. Such patients develop jaundice, azotemia, acidosis, hemorrhagic diathesis, hypotension and coma. Pregnancy, hepatic damage, renal impairment and concurrent use of other hepatotoxic drugs may enhance the hepatotoxic action. *Tetracyclines should be avoided in pregnancy in the interest of both mother and foetus.*

- ***Teeth and bones***: Tetracyclines chelate calcium, forming a tetracycline-orthophosphate complex and are deposited in areas of calcification in bones and teeth. Administration of these antibiotics to pregnant women may lead to yellow staining of the teeth of the infant; defective formation of enamel and hypoplasia of the teeth may also occur. Pigmentation of permanent teeth and increased risk of caries may occur in children. Even a short course given after the 14th week of pregnancy can be damaging.

Tetracyclines administered during pregnancy are deposited in foetal bones and may reduce their linear growth. For similar reason, they should also be avoided in infants and in children upto the age of 12 years. Tetracyclines are also deposited in nails, and fluorescence of the nails may be demonstrated after prolonged tetracycline therapy.

- ***Kidney*** : In patients with significant renal impairment, tetracyclines may cause an aggravation of azotemia and exaggerated antianabolic effect.

A reversible 'Fanconi-like' syndrome, characterised by nausea, vomiting, proteinuria, glycosuria, acidosis and gross aminoaciduria may develop after ingestion of outdated tetracycline capsules. It is attributed to a degradation product, epianhydrotetracycline. The formation of this toxic product is promoted by warmth, moisture and an acidic pH, with change of colour from yellow to brown.

- ***Benign intracranial hypertension***: Some patients may develop increased intracranial pressure. This causes bulging of the anterior fontanelle in infants and headache, photophobia and papilloedema in adults.

- ***Miscellaneous***: IV tetracyclines may cause local thrombosis. They may interfere with blood coagulation. This effect is probably secondary to chelation of calcium.

Jarish-Herxheimer reaction has been reported very rarely following IV tetracycline. It is characterized by sudden rise of temperature, rigors, hypertension, hyperventilation and tachycardia, followed by hypotension. This is probably due to release of large quantities of endotoxin – like material.

Uremic patients may develop peptic ulcers. Tetracyclines have been observed to inhibit urease of gastric mucosa which breaks down urea into ammonia. Ammonia serves to reduce gastric acidity and hence, lowering of ammonia concentration by tetracyclines may lead to hyperacidity with ulceration.

Steatorrhea and deficiency of vitamin K may occur after prolonged tetracycline therapy.

Drug interactions: See Table 48.2.

Table 48.2: Drug interactions of tetracyclines

- ***Decreased bioavailability of tetracyclines***: Divalent or trivalent cations (Ca^{++}, Mg^{++}, Fe^{++}, Zn^{++}, Al^{+++}); milk and milk products; antacids, vitamin or mineral products and cathartics containing divalent or trivalent cations; bismuth subsalicylate.
- ***Decreased half life of tetracyclines***: Carbamazepine; Phenytoin; Barbiturates; Chronic ethanol ingestion.
- ***Interference with the bactericidal action of penicillin.***
- ***Potentiation of the anticoagulant action of coumarin drugs,*** eg. warfarin

Preparations and dosage:

(i) *For oral administration*: Oxytetracycline hydrochloride (Terramycin), Tetracycline hydrochloride (Alcyclin, Resteclin, Achromycin, Tetracyn) capsules or tablets contain 250 mg., as paediatric syrup contain 125 mg/5 ml. and paediatric drops contain 100 mg/ml. The adult dose varies between 1 and 2 g. per day in 3-4 divided doses; for children 15 - 25 mg/kg. body weight, daily, in divided doses.

(ii) *For parenteral administration*: Oxytetracycline and tetracycline are available for IM and IV administration. The usual IM dose is 100 mg at 8 hourly intervals. Because of the local pain and irregular absorption, IM administration is generally not satisfactory. The total daily IV dose of oxytetracycline and tetracycline for most acute infections in adults is 1-2 g. in two equal doses at 12 hourly intervals. For this, 250 mg. of the drug is dissolved in 10 ml. sterile water and is further diluted with 5% dextrose or normal saline so as to achieve the concentration of 1 mg/ml. It is given slowly at the rate of 5 ml. per min.

The tetracyclines are never administered intrathecally.

(iii) Ophthalmic ointments and eye drops containing tetracyclines (0.5-1%) are available.

Semisynthetic Tetracyclines

These compounds have better absorption, longer duration of action or greater facility of parenteral administration than the older tetracyclines. Whereas tetracycline and oxytetracycline are short acting, demeclocycline and methacycline are intermediate acting, and doxycycline and minocycline are long acting.

Demethylchlortetracycline (Demeclocycline, Ledermycin): Given orally, it is well absorbed (66%); is 90 per cent protein bound and has t½ of 12 hours. The concentration in the CSF is poor. As the drug is slowly excreted by kidneys the therapeutic blood levels are maintained for at least 24 hours after cessation of treatment.

Demethylchlortetracycline shares all the adverse effects of the tetracyclines.

It is available as 150 mg. and 300 mg. capsules and as a syrup. The usual adult dose is 600 mg. daily in 2 or 3 divided doses. It is now used for SIADH (See later).

Methacycline (Rondomycin) shows almost identical *in vitro* activity as demethylchlortetracycline. It gives higher and more sustained blood levels than the older tetracyclines. **Lymecycline** (Lymesal) is a tetracycline made soluble by combining it with the amino acid lysine. It is claimed to be almost completely absorbed on oral administration, and is also preferred for IM use as it is less irritant.

DOXYCYCLINE (Doxy, Vibramycin, Vivocycline): It is well absorbed from the gut and is more slowly excreted than other tetracyclines (Table 48.1). With a single dose of 500 mg. serum level of 1 mcg. per ml. has been reported to be present upto 4 days. It is excreted in feces as an inactive conjugate. Its plasma half life is not significantly affected by renal insufficiency and the drug does not seem to aggravate azotemia in this condition.

Doxycycline has similar toxicity as the conventional tetracyclines. However it has many advantages over other tetracyclines. These are:

- ***Better GI absorption*** and hence smaller doses.
- ***Longer half life***, (t ½ 16 hours), permitting less frequent dosing schedule.
- ***Higher lipid solubility,*** leading to higher tissue concentrations.
- ***Elimination independent of renal function***; hence it can be used in patients with impaired renal function; and
- ***Less propensity to cause diarrhoea.***

The drug is available in 100 mg. capsules. The recommended dose in adults is 200 mg. (single dose) on day one and then 100 mg. once a day. In severe infections a dose of 100 mg. every 12 hours is recommended. For children, a dose of 3-4 mg. per kg. daily is given initially in 2 divided doses. In severe infections a larger dose may be given. Subsequently, a maintenance dose of 1-2 mg. per kg. is administered either as a single dose or divided into 2 doses. Doxycycline can also be given IV by infusion.

MINOCYCLINE (Minocin): This tetracycline is absorbed completely from the GI tract and exhibits greater antibacterial activity than older tetracyclines. It is retained in fat; hence it is long acting with t½ of 16 hours. It is excreted in bile and faeces and does not exacerbate azotemia. The drug has better tissue penetration. It is effective against tetracycline resistant *Staph. aureus, Strep. pyogenes, enterococci, meningococci* and *E. coli* and exhibits a significant activity against nocardia, asteroides and *acid fast bacilli.* Among the available tetracyclines, minocycline achieves satisfactory levels in the CNS. However, unlike other tetracyclines it causes reversible vestibular toxicity such as vertigo, dizziness, ataxia, nausea and vomiting. Aural hyperpigmentation, autoimmune hepatitis, SLE-like syndrome have been reported rarely. The dose is 100 mg. b.i.d.

TIGECYCLINE is a glycylcycline, a derivative of minocycline. Its mechanism of action is similar to that of other tetracyclines. It is highly effective against methicillin-resistant staphylococci (MRSA), vancomycin-resistant enterococci (VRE), penicillin resistant *Streptococcus pneumoniae* and many Gram negative bacilli. It is given IV and has a t½ of 36 hours. About 85% is excreted unchanged via the biliary route into the feces. The IV dose is 50 mg every 12 hours. It is generally well tolerated but may cause nausea and vomiting. It should not be used in children and pregnant women. Its use should be restricted to life-threatening infections, and when resistant pathogens are suspected.

Therapeutic uses of tetracyclines: Although tetracyclines are effective against a wide range of organisms, they are not to be preferred routinely against the organisms that are highly sensitive to other equally safe and bactericidal agents like penicillin and cotrimoxazole. Tetracyclines are indicated in:

- ***Rickettsial infections*:** The tetracyclines are very effective in rickettsial infections like murine, epidemic and scrub typhus, Q fever and Rocky mountain spotted fever. Fever subsides within 24 to 72 hours and the rash disappears within 4 to 6 days. Relapses are rare. The dose is 2 to 3 g. during the first 24 hours, followed by 1-2 g. daily till the temperature subsides.

- ***Primary atypical pneumonia*:** This condition, caused by *Mycoplasma pneumoniae,* responds satisfactorily to tetracyclines, given in the daily dose of 2 g. for 6 to 7 days. However macrolides and fluoroquinolones are preferred.

- ***Cholera*:** Cholera is caused by strains of Gram negative *Vibrio cholerae* and is characterized by severe diarrhoea, leading to rapid and massive loss of Na^+, K^+, HCO^-_3 and water, and shock. *Hence, rapid rehydration is the mainstay of treatment.* Since the sodium loss is very high, ORS containing 90 mMol/litre of Na^+ is recommended (WHO). Being concentrated, its intake is alternated with that of milk or water. Commercial oral rehydration preparations may contain less glucose and Na^+ than the WHO formulation. Patients in shock will need IV fluids initially, given rapidly; acidosis can be corrected by giving IV Ringer lactate and oral potassium supplements (Chapter 36).

The organisms respond to a single oral dose of doxycycline 200 mg or tetracycline 2gm (above 8 years); ciprofloxacin 20-30 mg/kg as a single dose or 15 mg/kg bid for 3 days is also effective. For children, erythromycin 40 mg/kg/day in 3-4 divided doses, for 3 days or a single dose of azithromycin is useful; cotrimoxazole may also be used (Chapter 44).

In patients with multi-drug-resistant (MDR) cholera, azithromycin 1 g as a single dose is reported to be highly effective.

- ***Chlamydia infections*:** *Chlamydia trachomatis* causes trachoma, non gonococcal urrethritis (NGU), cervicitis, epidydimitis, inclusion conjunctivitis, lymphogranuloma venereum and infant pneumonia (Chapter 51). Like the viruses, these organisms are obligate intra-cellular parasites of very small size but unlike viruses and like bacteria they multiply by binary fission. Their cell walls resemble those of Gram-negative bacteria. Table 48.3 lists the drugs used in chlamydial infections.

In *psittacosis* caused by *C.psittaci* a dosage schedule of 2 g. daily for two weeks is usually recommended. Use of tetracyclines in *lymphogranuloma venereum* and NGU is discussed in Chapter 51.

Table 48.3: Drugs used in chlamydial infections

- Doxycycline/Tetracycline.
- Erythromycin, Azithromycin.
- Ofloxacin; and
- Sulfonamides.

The tetracyclines are generally preferred in *trachoma*. An ophthalmic ointment may be applied in the eye 3 to 4 times daily for 4 weeks, along with 3 to 4 g. oral sulfadimidine, given for 3 weeks. Adequate drug therapy early in the disease can lead to complete healing without any sequelae; but when it is started late, even though the infection is often controlled, pannus and scarring persist. In endemic areas, where adequate therapy is not possible, the antibiotic ointment may be applied twice daily on every alternate day for 6 months.

In children, azithromycin given as single dose is preferred to tetracycline.

Inclusion conjunctivitis responds to topical application of tetracycline ointment 4 times daily for a period of 2 to 3 weeks.

- ***Granuloma inguinale***: See Chapter 51.
- ***Bacillary infections***: Tetracyclines can be used in the treatment of traveller's diarrhoea, caused by enterotoxigenic *E.coli*. Although tetracyclines are effective in tularemia, streptomycin is usually preferred. They can also be used in infections due to *H. influenzae* but either ampicillin or chloramphenicol is preferred.
- ***Brucellosis***: See Chapter 46.
- ***Sexually transmitted diseases***: Although tetracyclines are effective in the treatment of gonorrhea, syphilis and chancroid, they are not preferred (Chapter 51).
- ***Urinary tract infections***: They are particularly useful in non-gonoccocal urethritis caused by chlamydia trachomatis. Doxycycline is often preferred for the empiric treatment of the acute urethral syndrome (Chapter 50).
- ***Plague***: See Chapter 48.
- ***Acne vulgaris*** : See Chapter 69.
- ***Drug resistant malaria*** (see Chapter 54).
- ***Amoebic dysentery***: (See Chapter 55).

Balantidium coli, a protozoon, causes a disease similar to amoebic dysentery in children. Tetracycline in the dose of 8-10 mg/kg. thrice daily for 10 days is highly effective.

- ***H.pylori infection*** in patients with peptic ulcer: (Chapter 42).
- ***SIADH*** : Demeclocycline is useful in the treatment of syndrome of inappropriate secretion (SIADH). Its action is dose dependent and reversible.
- ***Miscellaneous***: Other infections which respond to tetracyclines include anthrax, actinomycosis, yaws, relapsing fever, lyme disease and leptospirosis. In these conditions, penicillin is preferred. Tetracyclines are also useful in the treatment of tropical sprue and blind loop syndrome.

Chloramphenicol

Chloramphenicol is a broad spectrum antibiotic derived originally from *Streptomyces venezuelae*. The commercial preparation however, is entirely synthetic. It is a derivative of dichloroacetic acid, containing a nitrobenzene moiety (Fig. 48.2). The antibiotic is stable over the pH range of 2 to 9.

$$NO_2-C_6H_4-CH(OH)-CH(CH_2OH)-NH-CO-CHCl_2$$

Fig. 48.2: Chloramphenicol

Antibacterial activity: The antibacterial spectrum of chloramphenicol resembles that of tetracyclines. Thus, it is effective against Rickettsia, the chlamydia of the psittacosis-lymphogranuloma group, *Mycoplasma pneumoniae,* and against a variety of Gram-negative and Gram-positive organisms. *Salm. typhi, H. influenzae* and *H. pertussis* are more susceptible to chloramphenicol than to almost any other antibiotic. The other Gram negative organisms sensitive to it include *Shigella, E.*

coli, K. pneumoniae, A. aerogenes, certain strains of *Proteus, Pasturella, Brucella and Vibrio cholerae.* The bacteroides, some staphylococci resistant to penicillin and a few strains of streptococci are also inhibited. Chloramphenicol is less active against Gram positive cocci than penicillin. Essentially it is a bacteriostatic but can be *bactericidal against common meningeal pathogens—H. influenzae, N. meningitidis* and *Strep. pneumoniae.*

Mechanism of action: Chloramphenicol readily penetrates into the bacterial cell and acts by interfering with the synthesis of bacterial proteins by inhibiting 50S ribosomes. Resistance develops slowly to this antibiotic *in vivo.* However, resistant strains of *E. coli,* salmonella, shigella and other Gram negative bacteria have been reported; it is due to the presence of a specific resistance (R) factor.

Absorption, fate and excretion: Unlike tetracyclines, chloramphenicol is completely absorbed from the gut and is better diffusible into the tissues. *Blood levels of chloramphenicol after oral administration are superior to those after IM administration* because of the hydrolysis of its salt in the gut. Being poorly water soluble, its absorption depends to a great extent on particle size. Preparations containing large particles may give blood levels only ¼ to ½ of those containing small particles.

Given orally, peak plasma levels are reached within 2 hours; it has a plasma t½ of 1½-3½ hours. A 6 hourly administration of the drug is advocated to maintain a steady therapeutic level. Given IV, the peak blood level is attained immediately. About 60% of plasma chloramphenicol is bound to protein. The binding is reduced in cirrhotic patients and in neonates, giving high concentrations of the free drug.

The drug is found in effective concentrations in the pleural fluid and the bile, and it reaches the CSF in about half the blood concentration. Being lipid soluble, chloramphenicol concentrates in various tissues including the brain. It is also secreted in milk and crosses the placental barrier.

Chloramphenicol palmitate, the pediatric oral preparation, is inactive *in vitro,* but *in vivo,* it is slowly hydrolyzed by pancreatic lipases in the duodenum, which release free chloramphenicol for absorption. Hence, blood levels achieved are lower than those after chloramphenicol itself.

Chloramphenicol is largely inactivated by hepatic conjugation to glucuronide. Nearly 9/10 th is excreted as the inactive form by the kidney. *Hence, chloramphenicol can be relatively safely administered in patients with renal impairment but not in those with hepatic insufficiency.*

Adverse reactions :

- ***Allergy*** **:** This is relatively uncommon. However, skin rashes, drug fever, angioneurotic edema, exfoliative dermatitis, atrophic glossitis have been reported.
- ***Bone marrow toxicity*****:** Aplastic anemia, reported in all age groups, is an idiosyncratic reaction; its incidence is between 1 : 10,000 and 1: 100,000. Prolonged treatment and repeated courses with large doses appear to be more likely to cause this complication, although cases of aplastic anemia on ingestion of a few grammes of the drug and even after its prolonged intraocular instillation have been rarely reported. In some cases, the onset of clinical manifestations may be delayed for 2 to 6 months after treatment. Thus, menorrhagia or GI hemorrhage occurring several months after a course of treatment may be the first indication of aplastic anemia. Many patients may develop less pronounced hemopoietic changes which are dose dependent and reversible.

To prevent the deadly complication of aplastic anemia, indiscriminate, prolonged or repeated use of the drug should be avoided; peripheral blood smear is examined at least once weekly during therapy. The treatment should be stopped if the total leukocyte count drops below 4000 c.mm. or when the proportion of granulocytes is reduced below 40 per cent.

It must be noted that *the risk of this complication should not prevent the use "of chloramphenicol in life-threatening situations.*

- ***Gray baby syndrome*:** This complication with high mortality is observed in neonates and infants. The clinical manifestations appear within 2 to 9 days following the first dose. The initial manifestations are vomiting, lethargy, anorexia, abdominal distension and shallow irregular respiration. After 24 hours, the condition worsens, leading to hypothermia, flaccidity, peripheral vascular collapse, gray cyanosis, shock and finally death. The factors incriminated are (i) the deficient conjugation of chloramphenicol in the liver due to a low level of hepatic glucoronyl transferase enzyme activity in the first 2 or 3 weeks of life; and (ii) immaturity of the renal tubules leading to impairment of excretion of the free form.
- ***Superinfection*** during chloramphenicol therapy is uncommon as the drug is almost completely absorbed.
- ***Liver toxicity*:** Liver damage with chloramphenicol is rare.
- ***CNS toxicity*:** It may cause headache, peripheral neuritis, internal ophthalmoplegia, mental confusion, depression and delirium. Optic neuritis, probably secondary to drug induced pyridoxine deficiency, may occur rarely. The drug may also affect the cochlear function if used locally, for ear infections.
- ***Miscellaneous*:** A 'typhoid shock' syndrome may develop in patients having typhoid fever, on administration of a large loading dose. It is attributed to excessive release of endotoxin from the micro-organisms.

Drug interactions: Pre-treatment with phenobarbitone results in lower chloramphenicol blood levels, whereas chloramphenicol may increase the toxicity of phenytoin in epilepsy, and may cause hypoglycemia in diabetics on tolbutamide, by inhibiting the hepatic microsomal enzymes that metabolise drugs.

Preparations and dosage:

(i) Chloramphenicol (Chloromycetine) 250 mg. capsules. Dose: adults, 1 to 3 g. daily in divided doses. For children, 25 to 50 mg. per kg. daily in divided doses.

(ii) Chloramphenicol palmitate oral suspension contains 125 mg. of chloramphenicol base in each 4 ml. of the suspension. The preparation is tasteless and, therefore, employed orally for pediatric use.

(iii) Chloramphenicol monostearoylglycolate used in the form of a dry syrup.

(iv) Chloramphenicol sodium succinate has a high aqueous solubility in comparison to chloramphenicol base and is, therefore, the agent of choice for parenteral chloramphenicol therapy. A 10% solution is administered SC. A 25 to 40 per cent solution is used IM while a 10 per cent solution is injected slowly by IV route or administered through a saline drip. The doses are similar to those given orally. *Absorption from SC and IM sites is unreliable.*

(v) Chloramphenicol 1 per cent ophthalmic ointment, as applicaps and as eye drops 0.5 per cent.

Therapeutic uses: Chloramphenicol can be used for similar purposes as tetracyclines but because of its bone marrow toxicity, it should not be employed primarily as a broad spectrum antibiotic. The major therapeutic indications for chloramphenicol are :

- ***Typhoid fever*** is caused by *S.typhi*. After invading the intestinal mucosa (mainly terminal ileum) the organisms invade the regional lymph nodes and other tissues. Before the introduction of chloramphenicol (in 1948), the mortality due to typhoid fever was about 20%, which dropped to almost 1 % following its use. Drugs effective in treating typhoid fever are listed in Table 48.4.

Chloramphenicol is highly effective if the organisms are sensitive. For best results, early administration is desirable. It is given orally in the dose of 50 mg. per kg. daily (about 2 g. in adults) in 4 divided doses at 6 hourly intervals until the temperature is normal. The dose may then be reduced to 30 mg. per kg. per day. It should be continued for a total period of 14 days. The drug can also be administered IM or IV.

After institution of therapy, clinical improvment is seen within 48 to 72 hours. Temperature returns to normal within 3 to 5

Table 48.4: Drugs effective in typhoid fever

- Chloramphenicol.
- Ciprofloxacin, Ofloxacin and Pefloxacin
- Ampicillin; pivampicillin.
- Cotrimoxazole; and
- Third generation cephalosporins : Ceftriaxone, Cefoperazone.

days. Clinical cure is thus achieved before the GI ulcerations have healed and hemorrhage and perforation can occur during therapy even in an afebrile patient. *It is desirable, therefore, to advise bed rest for a period of 2 to 3 weeks to allow sufficient time for healing of the ulcerated bowel.* Relapses can occur but are amenable to similar treatment.

Resistance to chloramphenicol is well documented from many countries including India. In such cases, a fluoroquinolone such as **ciprofloxacin or ofloxacin** is most effective with cure rate of 98% when given twice a day for 10 days. Since they are bactericidal, relapse rate is lower and the occurrence of fecal carrier state is less than 2%. **Co-trimoxazole** in the dose of 2 tablets bid, continued for 5-7 days after defervescence, is also effective,

Ampicillin, has also been used to treat typhoid fever. The therapeutic response, however, is slower in onset and often inadequate.

Unfortunately, the emergence of multi-drug-resistant (MDR) *S.typhi*, resistant to chloramphenicol, ampicillin and co-trimoxazole, has been frequently observed in endemic areas. In such cases, fluoroquinolones such as ciprofloxacin (0.5 gm bid for 10 days) or a third generation cephalosporin such as **ceftriaxone** (1-2 gm IM/IV for 10-14 days) is recommended. **Ofloxacin** 10-15 mg/kg/day in two divided doses for 5 days has been found to be equally effective. Fluoroquinolone-resistant typhoid fever can be treated with a third generation cephalosporin such as ceftriaxone or cefixime, or with azithromycin. *Children with MDR organisms should be treated with a cephalosporin.* Patients with severe typhoid fever (diarrhea, persistent vomiting, delirium, obtundation, stupor, coma or shock) should receive parenteral therapy for 7-10 days, and total therapy for 14 days.

A glucocorticoid may be added to antibiotic therapy in severe typhoid fever and in those with shock-like syndrome. Prednisolone is given in the dose of 40 mg. in 4 divided doses on the first day, 30 mg. on the 2nd day and 20 mg. day subsequently. Patients unable to take orally may be treated with equivalent doses of a parenteral glucocorticoid. Treatment should be given for a total period of 5-6 days and withdrawal should be gradual and tapering; earlier cessation may result in a sharp recurrence. *Their routine use in all cases is, however, not recommended.*

The incidence of relapse following fluoroquinolones (1.5%) and broad spectrum cephalosporins (5%) is lower than that following chloramphenicol, co-trimoxazole and ampicillin (10%). Supportive therapy includes maintenance of adequate, nutrition and antipyretics. Either ibuprofen (superior) or paracetamol 6 hourly may be given till 36 hours after defervescence. They appear to be superior to tepid sponging. Irritant purgatives are contraindicated for fear of causing hemorrhage or perforation.

In addition to *S.typhi*, campylobacter and yersinia infections can progress to 'enteric fever' by penetrating the intestinal cells and causing systemic infection. *Thus, typhoid is an enteric fever but all enteric fevers are not typhoid.*

Treatment of carriers: Carriers are defined as patients who continue to excrete the organisms in the stool for more than 3 months after recovery. Chloramphenicol does not prevent or eliminate the carrier state. The treatment of choice in this condition is **ciprofloxacin** in the dose of 750 mg. twice daily for 28 days; the other drugs effective are ampicillin or amoxycillin (2 g qid for 4 weeks); and cotrimoxazole (2 tablets bid for 4 weeks). Patients with cholecystitis may need cholecystectomy.

Paratyphoid fever, though usually a milder disease, needs similar treatment.

- ***H. influenzae meningitis***: Chapter 47.
- ***Ricketssial infections and anaerobic infections*** including those due to *B.fragilis* are effectively treated with chloramphenicol; however chloramphenicol is not preferred in ricketssial infections because of its toxicity.
- ***Plague***: Chapter 46.
- ***Miscellaneous***: Because of its satisfactory penetration into the intraocular fluid on local and systemic administration, chloramphenicol is widely employed in the treatment of ocular infections and is also useful in trachoma. It is also used in chronic otorrhea, particularly due to Gram negative organisms. It may be effectively used in **brucellosis**, in the dose of 0.75 to 1 g. at 6 hourly intervals, in place of tetracyclines. However, rifampicin is preferred.

Pharmacotherapy of Bacillary Dysentery

Bacillary dysentery or shigellosis is usually a self-limited acute illness characterized by diarrhoea with blood and mucus in the feces, tenesmus, fever, intestinal colic and tenderness. Nausea and vomiting may occur to a variable degree. In many patients, the illness is characteristically short, for 12-24 hours, followed by constipation, and needs to be treated only with **Oral Rehydration Therapy (ORT)** (Chapter 36). The infection is usually localised to the GI tract but pneumonitis is not infrequent in children and bacteremia may occur rarely. *Shigella shiga* infection is often more severe than that due to other strains.

I **Specific treatment:** Cotrimoxazole or ampicillin is preferred for general use. *Amoxycillin should not be substituted for ampicillin* because it is not so useful against shigellosis. In cases of suspected multi-drug resistant shigellosis, norfloxacin or ciprofloxacin, given twice daily, for 5-7 days, is now preferred, particularly in cases where the drug susceptibility is unknown (Chapter 40). Neonates with shigellosis should be treated with parenteral antibiotic combination. The other drugs found useful are pivamipcillinam, azithromycin and ceftriaxone.

It must be emphasized that spontaneous clearance of stools is known to occur over a period of weeks irrespective of whether or not the patient has received antibacterial treatment. *Nonabsorbable drugs such as neomycin, kanamycin and colistin are clinically ineffective despite in-vitro activity.* Tetracyclines and chloramphenicol, though effective, are not recommended because of possible drug resistance.

II **Adjuvant treatment:**

- ***Correction of fluid and electrolyte imbalance*** is very important (Chapter 36); and
- ***Symptomatic treatment of diarrhoea:*** The role of antimotility agents in shigellosis is controversial; they may control the diarrhoea but delay the excretion of the infecting organisms and delay the recovery (Chapter 40).

In the post-diarrhoeal phase, the patient's constipation should not be interfered with because it represents the body's effort to splint the bowel and it usually clears up within 3 days.

Pharmacotherapy of Chronic Bronchitis

Chronic bronchitis is a symptom complex clinically characterised by chronic cough with production of sputum in the absence of an obvious cause such as acute inflammatory or neoplastic disease of the lung or bronchiectasis. In many elderly patients, it is progressive and incurable, terminating eventually in right heart failure. COPD comprises two distinct processes, emphysema and chronic bronchitis.

Patients with chronic bronchitis should receive a dose of pneumococcal vaccine (Chapter 75).

Pharmacotherapy of chronic bronchitis is directed primarily towards the inflammation and infection which are controllable. The pathological changes associated with emphysema, however, are irreversible.

The treatment can be divided into

I Treatment of exacerbations and

II Management of the chronic state.

I **Treatment of exacerbations:**

• ***Antimicrobial therapy*: *Patients with chronic bronchitis*** are extremely susceptible to acute attacks which usually develop during the monsoon months in India and during the winter in the Western countries. During such attacks, the sputum becomes purulent, more viscous or merely more profuse. The commonest pathogens involved are *H. influenzae, S. pneumoniae* and *Moraxella catarrhalis* although *Staph. aureus* or *K. pneumoniae* are not infrequent.

Acute exacerbations of chronic bronchitis should be treated promptly with an antibiotic. Microscopic examination and culture of the sputum should be carried out if the patient has a chill, fever or chest pain, and if purulence of the sputum fails to respond to the antibiotic. *The antibiotic regimens recommended in the absence of pneumonia* are (i) tetracycline 250 mg. q.i.d.; (ii) doxycycline 150 mg. once daily; (iii) ampicillin/amoxycillin 250 mg. q.i.d. ; and (iv) cotrimoxazole, 2 tablets bid. All these regimens are equally effective and any one may be selected. Some patients may need erythromycin, a newer macrolide, a respiratory fluoroquinolone (Chapter 44) or a cephalosporin, depending upon the causative organism.

Antimicrobial therapy should be continued for at least 7-10 days. If the patient fails to respond satisfactorily, bacteriological examination of the sputum is indicated and an appropriate change in the antibiotic therapy should be made. Prompt institution of antibacterial treatment at the beginning of illness minimises further bronchopulmonary damage.

Patients with pneumonia need amoxycillin (with or without clavulinic acid), co-trimoxazole, a fluroquinolone or a third generation cephalosporin, depending on the nature of the infecting organism.

• ***Control of symptoms*:** Bronchodilators counter the respiratory distress due to bronchospasm. If the asthmatic element is prominent, glucocorticoid may have to be employed. For liquefaction of thick and sticky secretions, mucolytic agents have been employed; their usefulness however, is doubtful. Steam, inhalation and expectorants may facilitate the expulsion of secretions. If the patient is expectorating large quantities of sputum, postural coughing is highly beneficial.

In severe respiratory distress with hypoxia and hypercapnia, oxygen has to be given intermittently. The administration of oxygen, however, removes the hypoxic stimulus to the respiratory centre and thus, can increase the carbon dioxide retention. The patient therefore, should be treated in an ICU.

II **Management of ch** Usefulness of routine antibacterial prophylaxis is questionable and it is expensive. Hence, a short course of therapy, started at the first sign of an exacerbation, is recommended. It is, however, important to avoid all irritants to the respiratory tract, especially smoke and dust, and environmental pollutants. Breathing exercises may be beneficial and patients should be trained and encouraged to take such exercises at home.

Antifungal Agents

Fungal infections are common, both as primary diseases, and secondary to oral antibiotics therapy. Individuals suffering from malignancy, diabetes mellitus, those on corticosteroids and immunocompromised subjects are more prone to fungal infections.

Fungi occur as either rounded budding forms (yeast-like) or hyphi (moulds). The common fungi are listed in Table 48.5.

Classification of antifungal agents:

I **Those employed topically:** These include many synthetic drugs such as Azoles, Tolnaftate, Undecyclenic acid and Ciclopirox.

Table 48.5: Types of fungi infecting the humans

Yeast/Yeast-like : Candida sp.,*Cryptococcus neoformans, Pityrias versicolor*

Moulds, fuzzy colonies : Aspergillus sp., Rhizopus sp., Dermatophytes (ring worm fungi).

Dimorphic spherical in tissues but growing like moulds : *Histoplasma capsulatum, Blastomyces dermatitidis, Coccidioides immitis, Sporothrix schenckii, Trichosporon sp.*

(Chapter 69). Only Nystatin, an antibiotic, is discussed here.

II **Those used systemically:**

- ***Antibiotics***: Griseofulvin and Amphotericin B.
- ***Antimetabolites***: Flucytosine.
- ***Azole derivatives***: eg. Clotrimazole, Ketoconazole, Itraconazole and Fluconazole.
- ***Miscellaneous***: Terbinafine, Echinocandins.

I **Agents employed topically:**

NYSTATIN (Mycostatin): This antibiotic, obtained from *Streptomyces noursei*, contains many double bonds in its chemical structure and hence, is called a polyene antibiotic. It is a pale yellow, water-insoluble substance, stable for several months in dry state at 4^{0}C; it rapidly loses its activity in the presence of water or plasma.

Antifungal activity: Nystatin shows inhibitory activity against several fungi *in vitro; Candida, Histoplasma, Blastomycoses, Trichophyton* and *Microsporum audouini* are sensitive. It combines with ergosterol present in the cell membrane of the yeast and creates pores/channels, thus increasing the membrane permeability. Depending upon concentration, it can act either as a fungistatic or a fungicidal.

It is not absorbed from the gut, the skin or the mucous membranes. On parenteral administration, it produces a variety of toxic effects including serious nephrotoxicity; its activity is reduced in the presence of plasma. Hence, it is not used for systemic infections. Resistance does not readily develop to this antibiotic *in vivo*.

Adverse reactions: Adverse effects encountered with nystatin used locally are usually mild. Oral administration may cause nausea, vomiting and diarrhoea.

Preparations and dosage:

(i) Nystatin tablet 500,000 units. Dose: 500,000 units 8 hourly in adults and in children over 6; 200,000 units 8 hourly in younger children; and 100,000 units 8 hourly below the age of 1 year.

(ii) Nystatin suspension 100,000 units per ml. for oral topical application.

(iii) Nystatin pessary or vaginal tablet 100,000 units twice or thrice daily.

(iv) Nystatin ointment 100,000 units per gram.

Therapeutic uses: Nystatin is effective in the treatment of localized candidiasis of vagina, mouth, skin and the gut. Nail involvement due to candida does not respond to it.

Monilial infection of the vagina responds to the insertion of 100,000 units twice daily for a minimum period of 2 weeks. Treatment of monilial vaginitis in pregnant patients reduces the possibility of thrush in the newborn. For the latter, a suspension containing 100,000 units of the antibiotic is dropped into the infant's mouth 4 times daily. The treatment should be continued for a prolonged period after all clinical lesions have subsided. For intestinal candidiasis, 500,000 units 6 hourly is the adult dose.

II **Agents employed systemically:**

GRISEOFULVIN (Grisovin, Idifulvin): Griseofulvin, isolated from *Penicillium griseofulvium* is the first oral compound to cure effectively infections due to the superficial dermatophytes (ringworm).

Antifungal activity: *In vitro*, the antibiotic inhibits the growth of various species of *Trichophyton, Microsporum* and *Epidermophyton*. It is not effective against bacteria, *C. albicans*, or any of the deep fungi. The antibiotic is mainly fungistatic.

Mechanism of action: The antibiotic exhibits mild cytotoxic properties similar to those of colchicine, and damages the microtubular protein, thus preventing mitosis. It acts mainly on the growing fungal cells and inhibits hyphal cell-wall synthesis. Dermatophytes specifically attack the keratinous tissue. Griseofulvin binds to the keratinocyte precursor cells and gets incorporated into keratin of the skin, hair and nails, making the new keratin resistant to fungal invasion. The already established fungus is not affected. Hence, the treatment takes a long time to ensure cure. It also has a weak anti-inflammatory action.

Absorption, fate and excretion: Small particles are better absorbed than large particles; divided oral doses achieve higher level than a single dose; and a diet rich in fat enhances its absorption. Of the oral dose, 50% get excreted in the urine as metabolites.

Adverse reactions: These are:

- Mild reactions such as headache, epigastric distress, nausea, vomiting and diarrhoea.
- Allergic and photosensitivity reactions. Cross allerginicity with penicillin, as griseofulvin is derived from a penicillium.
- Nervous system disturbances such as parasthesiae, peripheral neuritis, vertigo, psychomotor incoordination, lethargy, fatigue and blurred vision.
- Superinfection with candida albicans.
- Rarely, hepatotoxicity transient leucopenia, proteinuria, gynecomastia, pigmentation of the genitalia, increase in the urinary excretion of coproporphyrin and/or protoporphyrin are reported.

Drug interactions : Simultaneous administration of griseofulvin and phenobarbitone may retard the absorption of the former from the GI tract. It is hepatic microsomal enzyme inducer and hence it depresses the blood levels of warfarin and oral contraceptives. It can cause antabuse like reaction with alcohol.

Preparations and dosage: The adult dose is 500 mg. daily in 2 or 4 divided doses. In certain infections like *Tinea capitis*, a larger dose of 1.5 g. daily may be necessary. Children are given 10 mg. per kg. daily, administered as a single dose or in divided doses.

Therapeutic uses: Griseofulvin has made clinical control of some chronic resistant ringworm infections possible and has shortened the duration of treatment in others. Nevertheless, the narrow spectrum and the high cost of griseofulvin demand that it should not be used unless the cheaper and well established topical therapy fails or the lesion is known to be resistant to such topical therapy. The indications are :

- ***Tinea capitis*** (ringworm of the scalp) where clinical cure usually occurs within 4 to 6 weeks of therapy.
- ***Tinea barbae*** (fungus infection of the beard caused by *T. faviforme, T. mentagrophytes and M. canis*).
- ***Tinea cruris*** and tinea corporis (ringworm of the groin and the body).
- ***Tinea pedis*** and ***tinea manus*** (ringworm of the feet and hands). Griseofulvin is more effective in chronic fungal infections at these sites than in the acutely inflamed forms.

In all above conditions, the treatment is continued for some weeks after both clinical and microscopic evidence of infection has disappeared. Usually, this takes 4-8 weeks..

- ***Onychomycosis*** (fungus infection of the nails): Treatment with griseofulvin is more successful for fingernails than toenails which may respond minimally or not at all. Treatment for infection of the fingernails is given for 4 to 6 months, while an infection of the toenails is treated for 8 to 12 months. Since chronic fungal infections tend to cause hyperkeratosis, concomitant topical keratolytic therapy with salicylic acid is beneficial.

AMPHOTERICIN B (Fungizone): This polyene antibiotic, obtained from *Streptomyces nodosus*, is a yellowish powder relatively insoluble in water. Its mechanism of action is similar to that of nystatin. In addition, it also causes oxidative damage to fungi cells.

Antifungal activity: Amphotericin B has a wide antifungal activity. It inhibits the growth of *Histoplasma capsulatum, Cryptococcus* *neoformans*, *Sporotrichum schenkii*, *Coccidioides immitis* and *Blastomycosis brasiliensis* in low concentrations. Candida responds to a slightly higher concentration. Depending upon the concentration, it can be fungistatic or fungicidal. Candida may develop resistance to this antibiotic *in vivo*.

Absorption, fate and excretion: Amphotericin B is poorly absorbed from the gut and after topical application. The IM administration is painful. The drug, therefore, is given by IV infusion. On IV administration of a therapeutic dose, only 5 per cent of the drug is found in urine within 24 hours. It is concentrated in liver, spleen, kidney and lungs and remains in the body for several weeks. The drug does not achieve a satisfactory concentration in the CSF. Its metabolic fate is unknown.

Adverse reactions: Amphotericin B is highly toxic, especially nephrotoxic. Many patients develop impairment of renal function, hypokalemia, appearance of urinary casts and sometimes microscopic hematuria. Irreversible renal damage may occur.

Other reactions include phlebitis at the site of injection, nausea, anorexia, vomiting and profound generalized malaise. Chills, fever, flushing, headache, skin rash, diplopia, vertigo, convulsions, myalgia and peripheral neuritis are also seen. Intrathecal administration of the drug may result in arachnoiditis. The drug can cause hemorrhagic gastroenteritis, anemia, thrombocytopenia and hepatic failure. Hypotension, ventricular failure and cardiac arrest may develop rarely.

Preparations and dosage:

(i) Amphotericin B lotion 3 per cent.

(ii) Amphotericin B Deoxycholate (IV): A concentration of 0.1 mg./ml. in 5 per cent dextrose should be used. Therapy is initiated with 0.25 mg/kg/day, infused over 6-12 hours. If the drug is tolerated, the dose is gradually increased to 1 mg/kg/day. The maximum dose is 1.5 mg/kg/day on alternate days. *It is recommended that one litre of normal saline should be infused on the day of amphoterian therapy, to reduce the risk of nephrotoxicity.*

(iii) Other lipid formulations available are amphotericin B lipid complex, amphotericin B colloidal dispersion and liposomal amphotericin B (AmBisome). The drug is released slowly from these formulations and hence causes less nephrotoxicity. They are very expensive.

Therapeutic uses:

- ***Topically***, the antibiotic is useful in the treatment of candida lesions and as eyedrops to treat fungal corneal ulcers and keratitis.
- ***For systemic therapy***, the patient should be hospitalized. A course of treatment should not be embarked upon unless the diagnosis is certain. Though toxic, it could be life saving in many cases. Its toxicity could be reduced by using smaller doses of the drug in combination with certain other systemic antifungal agents.

Amphotericin IV is the treatment of choice in the primary, cutaneous and disseminated forms of blastomycosis, histoplasmosis, cryptococcosis, candidiasis, sporotrichosis, aspergillosis, chromoblastomycosis and occasionally in phycomycosis and maduramycosis. It may be administered intrathecally in fungal meningitis that does not respond to IV therapy. It is useful to treat mucormycosis in diabetics.

FLUCYTOSINE (Alcobon): This prodrug is a synthetic fluorinated pyrimidine, particularly useful in systemic infections with yeasts. It is taken up by fungal cells and converted to 5-fluorouracil. The antifungal activities are due to its conversion to antimetabolites which inhibit DNA and RNA synthesis. Human cells do not convert the drug to active metabolites. Given orally, it is well absorbed and reaches adequate concentrations in blood and CSF. It is almost entirely excreted unchanged by glomerular filtration.

Adverse reactions include GI disturbances, liver damage, neutropenia and thrombocytopenia and colitis. It is less toxic than amphotericin B.

Therapeutic uses : The drug is useful in cryptococcal meningitis and systemic candidiasis, including UTI. Used alone, it can lead to rapid emergence of drug resistance. Hence, it is usually combined with amphotericin

B. It is administered daily, in the oral dose of 100 200 mg/kg. in four divided doses. It can also be given by IV infusion.

Azole Derivatives

Therapeutically, drugs belonging to 'azole' group are classified as :

(1) **Antibacterial** and **anti protozoal agents** e.g. Metronidazole and Tinidazole.

(2) **Authelminitic agents** e.g. Mebendazole, Albendazole and

(3) **Antifungal azole agents.**

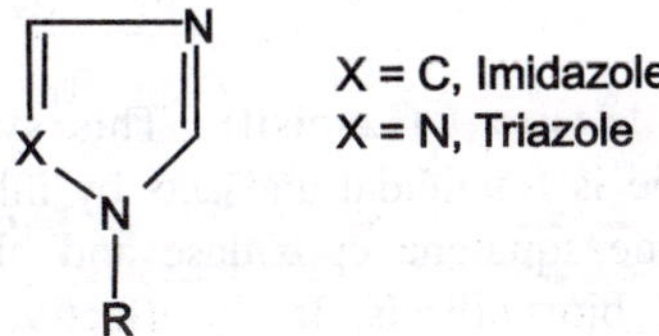

Fig. 48.3 : Azole nucleus

Azoles possess a five member azole ring that is attached by a carbon-nitrogen bond to other aromatic rings as their basic structural unit (Fig. 48.3) According to their chemical structure antifungal azoles are classified into:

I **Imidazoles** indicating two nitrogen atoms in the azole ring, e.g., Clotrimazole, Miconazole, Ketoconazole, Econazole and Sulconazole. Imidazoles are generally used topically to treat superficial mycoses, and cutaneous and vaginal candidiasis; and

II **Triazoles** with three nitrogens in the azole ring e.g. Itraconazole, Fluconazole. Triazoles in general, have greater volume of distribution, greater selectivity and better CNS penetrability than imidazoles. They are also considered to be less toxic and cause less endocrinal disturbances.

Antifungal activity: Azoles act by inhibiting synthesis of ergosterol in the fungal cell membrane, thereby disturbing the membrane. They also interfere with fungal enzymes and cause accumulation of hydrogen peroxide with lethal effect.They possess a broad spectrum antifungal and antibacterial activity. They are effective against Dermatophytes, Microsporum, Cryptococcus, Blastomyces, Coccidioides, Madurella, Nocardia, and candida.

All azoles are potentially embryotoxic and teratogenic, and should be avoided during pregnancy and lactation. The azoles used systemically are potent inhibitors of hepatic microsomal enzymes and can increase the blood levels and toxicity of several drugs.

CLOTRIMAZOLE (Candid, Imidil): Although this drug is effective against many fungi, it is not used for systemic fungal infections because of its toxicity. It is used as 1% cream or 100 mg tablets in vaginal candidiasis (Chapter 69), and locally to treat dermatophytosis and other fungal infections.

Econazole, **sulconazole**, **isconazole** and **fenticonazole** have similar actions and uses.

MICONAZOLE (Daktarin, Zole): This imidazole has a broad spectrum antifungal and Gram positive antibacterial activity. High concentrations are trichomonicidal. It is useful locally in mixed skin infections as 2-4% cream.

The drug is metabolized in the liver. For systemic fungal infections, it is given IV and sometimes intrathecally. Good results are reported in infections caused by Candida, Cryptococcus and Aspergillus.The drug may cause fever, chills, nausea and allergic reactions and rarely, leucopenia and thrombocytopenia.

KETOCONAZOLE (Nizoral, Fungicide): This imidazole derivative is water soluble and is well absorbed from the gut. Its spectrum is similar to that of miconazole but it is claimed to be more active against Coccidioides.

In large doses, ketoconazole inhibits several biosynthetic steps in the synthesis of adrenal and gonadal steroids. It can thus reduce the plasma levels of cortisol and testosterone.

Adverse reactions : The drug can cause headache, gastric irritation, allergic reactions, gynecomastia (due to impairment of testosterone synthesis) and acute hepatic necrosis. It is a CYP3A4 inhibitor and inhibits the metabolist of many drugs such as warfarin, phenytoin and combination OC pills.

Therapeutic uses:

- ***As a topical antifungal agent*** (Chapter 69).
- ***In Cushing's syndrome.***
- ***Familial testotoxicosis*** (gonadotropin independent activation of Leydig cells); and
- ***Prostatic cancer.***

Because of its poor efficacy and its toxicity it has now been largely replaced by itraconazole and fluconazole.

ITRACONAZOLE : This broad spectrum antifungal drug is related to ketoconazole. It is given orally or IV. Food increases its absorption whereas drugs that lower gastric acidity impair it. It is metabolized mostly in the liver (t½ 25 hours) to its active metabolite. It is both a substrate for and a potent inhibitor of CYP3A4. It does not appear in the urine or the CSF and unlike ketaconozole it does not inhibit the production of steroids. It exerts both topical and systemic activity. It is administered in the dose of 100-200 mg od for candidiasis. Larger doses for longer periods (6-12 months) are required to treat deep fungal infections. It may be preferred to treat infections with Cryptococcus, candida, histoplasma and aspergillus.

FLUCONAZOLE (Diflucan, Forcan): This triazole derivative is effective both orally and by IV infusion. It has plasma t½ of 31 hours and is given once daily. *It penetrates readily into the CSF.* Unlike itraconazole, almost 80% of the drug is eliminated in the urine unchanged. It is used in the treatment of local and systemic candidiasis and cryptococcal infections including meningitis. It is not active against aspergillosis or mucormycosis. The drug may cause nausea, GI disturbances, thrombocytopenia, and abnormalities of liver enzymes. It is given orally or by IV infusion as a single dose 150 mg.

POSACONAZOLE, an oral azole, is related chemically to itraconazole. It is particularly useful in prevention and treatment of invasive fungal infections, including aspergillosis, and oropharyngeal candidiasis refractory to fluconazole. It is now preferred to amphotericin-B for the treatment of zygomycete infection. It is well tolerated. Like itraconazole it inhibits CYP3A4. It is used in the dose of 200 mg qid initially, followed by 400 mg bid for 25 days.

The other, newer triazoles **ravuconazole** and **voriconazole** are claimed to be effective in aspergillosis.

Miscellaneous

TERBINAFINE (Lamisil) : This synthetic allyl-amine is fungicidal and acts by inhibiting the enzyme squalene epoxidase and blocking ergosterol biosynthesis. It is effective orally and topically. It is extensively metabolized in the liver. Oral treatment with 250 mg daily has been reported to cure onychomycosis in about 12 weeks as against 18 months required by griseofulvin. Topically, it may be used to treat dermatophyte infections of the skin. It is generally well tolerated. Adverse effects include GI distress, headache and rash.

CASPOFUNGIN : This agent belongs to a group of new antifungals called **echinocandins.** Unlike the azoles, it acts on the fungal cell wall to block the synthesis of deglucans. It is fungicidal and is effective in infections with *C. albicans* and *Aspergillus fumigatus.* It is not absorbed orally. Given IV, it is highly bound (97%) to albumin and is metabolized by the liver. Its plasma t½ is 10 hours. It is given once daily. The drug is well tolerated. The adverse reactions reported are local phlebitis, headache, nausea, fever and rash. It may cause hypercalcemia and is embryotoxic. Currently, it is used in the treatment of serious, invasive candidiasis and aspergillosis, and appears to be as effective as amphotericin B. It is very expensive.

General Principles of Chemotherapy of Infections

49

Infections still remain a major problem in medical practice; and their rational treatment with drugs is of prime importance. Since many therapeutically effective antimicrobials are now available and more are being added, it is necessary to lay down certain guiding principles for tailoring a rational therapeutic regimen for an individual patient.

Selection of Antimicrobial Agent

The choice of an antimicrobial agent is decided by:

I **Host-related factors :**

• ***Age of the patient***: Certain drugs like chloramphenicol may cause serious toxic effects in infants in whom liver enzymes/renal function are not fully developed.

• ***Pregnancy and neonatal period***: Most antimicrobial agents cross the placenta and can reach therapeutic concentrations in fetal tissues. Hence, they should, in general, be used during pregnancy only when it is a must. Penicillins, cephalosporins, erythromycin, (except estolate which is hepatotoxic), lincomycin, clindamycin, azithromycin, INH, ethambutol and probably sulfonamides (for short term use) can be safely used in pregnancy. As serious Gram-negative infections are common in the neonatal period, a bactericidal drug (a third generation cephalosporin) or a drug combination (gentamicin plus ampicillin) effective in Gram-negative infections is recommended for use during this period of life.

• ***Immunocompetency status of the patient.*** Bactericidal agents are always preferred in immunocompromised patients.

• ***Severity of the infection*** and general condition of the patient. Thus, a mild case of bacillary dysentery in an otherwise healthy individual will usually respond satisfactorily to oral rehydration therapy, while in severe cases, cotrimoxazole or a fluoroquinolone may be necessary, in addition. A combination of bactericidal agents effective against a wide variety of organisms (Gram-positive and Gram-negative organisms as well as the anaerobes) is commonly used in patients with neutropenia.

• ***History of previous allergic reaction or intolerance*** to the antimicrobial agent.

II **Pathogen-related factors :**

• ***The probable causative organism and the expected clinical course of the infection*** : One must decide whether the given illness is likely to be due to a microorganism susceptible to one of the available antimicrobials. *Antibiotics are not nonspecific antipyretics and their use in all cases of fever is to be deprecated.* It should also be appreciated that many cases of fever such as due to common cold are due to viruses that

Table 49.1: Commonly used bactericidal and bacteriostatic drugs

Bactericidal	Bacteriostatic
Penicillin	Sulfonamides
Aminoglycosides	Nitrofurans
Rifampicin	Erythromycin
Cephalosporins	Tetracyclines
Metronidazole	Chloramphenicol
Cotrimoxazole	Lincomycin
Fluoroquinolones	Trimethoprim

are not susceptible to antibiotics. Routine use of antibiotics in such cases is not justified.

The choice of the antibiotic based on expectation of a particular micro-organism has been illustrated by reference to meningitis. (Chapter 47).

- ***Identification of the causative micro-organism and its sensitivity to antimicrobial drugs:*** Though ideal, this may not always be possible owing to lack of facilities.
- ***Possibility of drug resistance :*** If the infection is due to Staphylococci, many strains of which are known to be resistant to penicillin, another antibiotic will have to be used.

III **Drug-related factors :**

- ***Nature of the drug,*** bacteriostatic or bactericidal (Table 49.1). Bactericidal drugs are always preferred to bacteriostatic agents. Carriers should be treated only with bactericidal drugs since bacteriostatic agents are not so effective in the absence of inflammation.
- ***Risk of drug toxicity***, particularly in the presence of liver or kidney damage. The risk involved in using a more toxic drug in preference to less effective but less toxic agent is justified only if the infection is severe.
- ***The cost of therapy*:** This is particularly important where many equally effective drugs are available for a given infection. An antibiotic should not be selected simply because it is 'the latest'. Newer drugs are always costly and not necessarily better than established ones.
- ***Pharmacokinetic properties of the drug*** e.g., oral/parenteral; tissue penetration; metabolism; duration of action; and
- ***Probability of drug compliance by the patient*** (Chapter 4).

Although bacterial sensitivity tests give important information, they are neither necessary nor practicable in daily practice. Sometimes, they can even be misleading and hence, the physician should use his clinical judgement in selecting the antibiotic and not depend blindly on the results of such tests. It must be realised that the organisms isolated by the bacteriologist may not be the prime cause of the disease under treatment. This is particularly so in case of organisms cultured from sputum and feces. Similarly, the sensitivity data obtained from *in vitro* studies do not necessarily hold true *in vivo.* Bacterial sensitivity tests, however, are useful in selecting a proper regimen in chronic diseases like respiratory or urinary tract infections, resistant Staphylococcal infections, endocarditis and chronic osteomyelitis.

Certain antimicrobial drugs are cleared from the blood by mechanisms not involving the kidneys (Table 49.2). These drugs are metabolized by the liver to inactive products and although these metabolic products accumulate in the presence of renal failure, they are not so harmful to the patient. In contrast to this, other antimicrobial drugs (see Table 49.3) are removed almost entirely by the kidney and accumulate in the blood in the active form in patients with impaired renal function. Many of these agents eg. aminoglycosides are highly effective against

Table 49.2: Antimicrobials cleared by non-renal mechanisms

- Erythromycin
- Chloramphenicol
- Doxycycline
- Rifampicin
- Cefaperazone and
- Ceftriaxone

Table 49.3: Antimicrobials eliminated by renal excretion

- Penicillins.
- Aminoglycosides.
- Most cephalosporins.
- Fluoroquinolones.
- Polymyxins.
- Colistin.
- Amphotericin B; and
- Amantadine.

Gram negative organisms but are also capable of producing nephrotoxic and neurotoxic effects. If these drugs are to be used in the presence of renal damage, they must be used in reduced doses, as guided by the plasma creatinine level.

The maintenance dose, in patients with impaired renal function, of drugs which are eliminated almost completely (> 90%) by renal excretion can be calculated as follows. The renal clearance of such drugs (penicillins, aminoglycosides, most of the cephalosporins and tetracycline) is reduced by the same proportion as the reduction from 100 ml per minute in the measured or calculated creatinine clearance. Creatinine clearance *in adults* can be calculated from serum creatinine by the formula:

$$\text{Creatinine clearance (ml/min) in males} = \frac{(140\text{-Age in years}) \times \text{Weight (kg)}}{72 \times \text{Serum creatinine (mg/dl)}}.$$

It is corrected to 1.73 square meter body surface area (BSA). In females, multiply the figure obtained by 0.85. Thus, if the serum creatinine is 2.5 mg/dl in a 50 year old male who weighs 60 kg, then his calculated creatinine clearance is 30 ml/min. It should be corrected to BSA of 1.73 square meter. The maintenance dose of the above drugs then equals corrected creatinine clearance/100 x the usual daily maintenance dose.

However, the first dose in such patients should be the same as the initial dose used in a patient with normal renal function (loading dose). In the case of penicillin G, no adjustment is required if the daily dose is 1.2 mega units or less; it is required in case massive doses are being used. *It is beyond the scope of this book to give detailed instructions about dose adjustment for each antimicrobial drug in renal impairment. The manufacturer's instructions should be consulted for this purpose.* However, the following generalizations can be made:

- Antibiotics like ampicillin, cloxacillin, carbenicillin and other penicillins can be used safely but need reduction in dosage, in patients with chronic renal failure.
- The tetracyclines increase protein catabolism. Further, accumulation of protein metabolites in the uraemic patient would make the condition worse. The disturbance in protein metabolism may result in liver failure. It is advisable, therefore, to avoid tetracyclines (except doxycycline) in chronic kidney disease.
- Sulfadimidine or sulfadiazine could be used in the presence of mild renal failure but should be avoided in moderate or marked impairment of renal function.
- The renal excretory mechanisms in neonates and in premature infants are not well developed. Hence, antimicrobials which are essentially excreted by the kidney tend to accumulate in such cases, leading to toxic effects. The doses of these drugs for newborns and premature infants should therefore be reduced and spacing between doses increased compared to those advocated for adults (See also Chapter 77).
- The elderly have diminished renal function, and antimicrobials which are disposed of largely by the kidneys should be administered in reduced doses.
- It takes longer to reach a steady state if the t½ is prolonged due to renal damage e.g. amoxicillin and gentamicin.

Antimicrobials of choice in various infections are given in Table 49.4.

The selected drug should be given in adequate doses for a sufficient period depending upon the type of case. In majority of the simple acute

Table 49.4: Antimicrobial drugs of choice

Organism	Antimicrobial Agents	
	First choice	Other effective drugs
Actinomyces israeli (bovis)	Penicillin G, ampicillin,	A tetracycline, erythromycin,
Anaerobes (other than clostridia)	Metronidazole, penicillin G.	Lincomycin, clindamycin chloramphenicol, cefoxitin
Bacillus anthracis	Penicillin G	Erythromycin, doxycycline
Bordetella pertussis	Erythromycin	Co-trimoxazole, ampicillin.
Brucella	Rifampicin + doxycycline	(Streptomycin or co-trimoxazole) + doxycycline, chloramphenicol.
Candida albicans	Nystatin or amphotericin B (locally applied)	Gentian violet.
Chlamydia trachomatis	Erythromycin, Azithromycin	Tetracycline ± Sulfonamide
Clostridium difficile	Metronidazole	Oral vancomycin
Clostridia tetani	Penicillin G, metronidazole	A tetracycline, chloramphenicol
Corynebacterium diphtheriae	Erythromycin, a cephalosporin, rifampicin	Penicillin G
Donovan bodies of granuloma inguinale	A tetracycline	Co-trimoxazole, chloramphenicol, ampicillin.
Enterococcus, (Streptococcus faecalis)	(Penicillin G or ampicillin) + gentamicin	Vancomycin, + gentamicin
Escherichia coli	Co-trimoxazole	Ampicillin, fluoroquinolones, gentamicin, a cephalosporin.
Fusospirochetes	Penicillin G	Erythromycin, clindamycin, metronidazole
Gardenela vaginalis	Metronidazole	Clindamycin.
Haemophilus ducreyi	Azithromycin, ceftriaxone	Fluoroquinolone, erythromycin
Haemophilus influenzae	Ampicillin, cephalosporin	Chloramphenicol, co-trimoxazole fluoroquinolones.
Klebsiella pneumoniae *In seriously ill patients*	Imipenem A cephalosporin,	Gentamicin, co-trimoxazole, Fluoroquinolone
Legionella pneumoniae	Erythromycin	Fluoroquinolone, Doxycycline, Cotrimoxazole.
Micrococcus catarrhalis	Cotrimoxazole	Amoxycillin, Erythromycin, Tetracycline, Cephalosporin.
Mycoplasma pnumoniae	Erythromycin	Fluoroquinolone, Tetracycline
Neisseria gonorrhoeae	(Penicillin G + probenecid), ceftriaxone, cefotaxime	Spectinomycin, fluoroquinolones,

Table 49.4 Continued

Organism	Antimicrobial Agents	
	First choice	**Other effective drugs**
Neisseria meningitidis (intracellularis)	Penicillin G or ampicillin	Third generation cephalosporin, fluoroquinolone.
Pasteurella pestis	Streptomycin ± tetracycline	Cotrimoxazole, Chloramphenicol.
Pasteurella tularensis	Streptomycin or gentamicin	A tetracycline, chloramphenicol.
Pneumocystis carinii	Co-trimoxazole	–
Proteus mirabilis	Ampicillin	Co-trimoxazole, gentamicin, fluoroquinolones, cephalosporin
Proteus vulgaris	Third generation cephalosporin	Gentamicin, co-trimoxazole, carbenicillin, fluoroquinolone
Pseudomonas aeruginosa	Ceftazidime, cefepime, aztreonam, imepenam	Gentamicin + (carbenicillin or piperacillin), A fluoroquinolone
Rickettsiae	Doxycycline	Chloramphenicol, fluoroquinolone
Salmonella typhi	Fluoroquinolone, Chloramphenicol	Co-trimoxazole, ampicillin, cefoperazone, ceftriaxone
Shigella	Co-trimoxazole, Norfloxacin.	Ampicillin, Azithromycin, Ceftriaxone.
Spirillum minus	Penicillin G	Streptomycin, a tetracycline.
Staphylococcus aureus	Penicillinase resistant penicillin eg. cloxacillin	Amoxycillin + Clindamycin Cephalosporin, Vancomycin, Rifampicin, Ciprofloxacin, Linezolid
Streptococcus pneumoniae	Penicillin G	A third generation cephalosporin, a fluoroquinolone, erythromycin, lincomycin
Streptococcus pyogenes	Penicillin G or V	A cephalosporin, erythromycin lincomycin
Streptococcus viridans	Penicillin G alone or with (gentamicin or steptomycin)	Cephalosporin, vancomycin,
Toxoplasma gondii	Sulfadiazine + pyrimethamine	Clindamycin + pyrimethamine Spiramycin
Trachoma	Doxycycline	Azythromycin, erythromycin,
Treponema pallidum	Penicillin G	Doxycycline, ceftriaxone
Vibrio cholerae	Doxycline	Co-trimoxazole, chloramphenicol, fluoroquinolone

infections and even in certain chronic conditions, orally effective, relatively nontoxic and inexpensive drugs should be preferred. Drugs such as chloramphenicol, rifampicin and co-trimoxazole have such reliable oral absorption that parenteral therapy is seldom indicated. Parenteral therapy is inconvenient to the patient, is more expensive, and needs medical supervision. It should be reserved for:

- ***Serious cases with bacteremia/ shock.***
- ***Patients who cannot take oral therapy or in whom the drugs are not likely to be absorbed orally; and***
- ***Those in whom the organisms have developed resistance to orally used drugs.***

In the management of obstructive lesions, necrotic and pyogenic infections, surgical intervention may be necessary for effecting a complete cure.

Drugs used commonly to treat infections with common Gram negative anaerobes are listed in Table 49.5.

Table 49.5: Drugs used to treat infections with common Gram negative anaerobes

Metronidazole
Fluoroquinolones
Ticarcillin-clavulanic acid
Piperacillin-tazobactam
Imipenem
Monobactams
Ampicillin-sulbactam

Antimicrobial Combinations

Simultaneous use of two or more antimicrobial agents is not routinely recommended. These drugs may, however, be combined under certain circumstances for the following reasons :

- ***To achieve an additive or synergistic effect against a single organism*:** True antibiotic synergism is rare and the enhanced therapeutic activity observed following certain combinations is usually an additive effect. Penicillin is combined with streptomycin in bacterial endocarditis due to streptococci. Brucellosis responds better to rifampicin + tetracycline combination than to tetracycline alone. A combination of gentamicin with carbenicillin acts synergistically against pseudomonas infection. It should be noted, however, that for a given antibiotic combination the dose of the individual antibiotic needed to accomplish synergism varies according to the type of organism.
- ***In mixed infections with bacteria sensitive to different drugs*:** Penicillin or metronidazole is combined with an aminoglycoside in peritonitis to control certain aerobes as well as anaerobes.
- ***To delay the development of or to overcome the drug resistance*** as in chronic infections like tuberculosis and malaria (see Chapters 52, 54).
- ***To decrease the adverse reactions*** to an individual drug, another agent may be added so that the doses of each drug can be reduced and possible dose-dependent toxicity avoided. e.g. flucytosine + amphotericin B.
- ***When etiological diagnosis is difficult, the infection is severe and the body defence is poor*** (as in malnourished patients, chronic alcoholics, patients with chronic renal failure, immunosuppressed patients and in neutropenic patients), combined antimicrobial therapy may be given in order to broaden the spectrum of antibacterial activity. However, in such cases, the appropriate regimen should be instituted once the organisms are identified.
- ***For reducing the chances of super-infection*:** Long term tetracycline therapy is sometimes combined with antifungal agents to prevent the superinfection due to fungi such as monilia. Unfortunately, not all fungi are eliminated and even when the fungal population is decreased, diarrhoea may persist.

It is not possible to predict which combination will have a synergistic effect and which will be antagonistic. The laboratory data are not always applicable to the disease processes in humans.

The bactericidal drugs more effectively attack the multiplying bacteria and hence, if a bacteriostatic drug is used along with a bactericidal agent, inhibition of bacterial multiplication may reduce the efficacy of the bactericidal agent. Combination of penicillin with chlortetracycline has been shown to produce antagonistic effect in pneumococcal meningitis. Significant antagonism occurs if patients are exposed to a broad spectrum bacteriostatic antibiotic before the institution of penicillin therapy. The presence of leucopenia may further compound the development of antagonism. Similar antagonism between chloramphenicol and gentamicin has been reported; however, with this combination the clinical results vary considerably, depending upon the organism studied and the status of host defence. Such antagonism between a bactericidal and a bacteriostatic drug is not always seen e.g., the action of penicillin is not antagonised but may be actually enhanced by addition of sulfonamides.

If a bacteriostatic drug is added to a bactericidal agent, one of the following things may happen:

- ***Drug antagonism:*** If the bacteria are highly sensitive to the bactericidal drug; or
- ***Additive effect:*** If the bacteria are relatively resistant to the bactericidal drug.

Combining bacteriostatic drugs usually leads to an additive effect; but the effect may sometimes be synergistic as with the combination of sulfamethoxazole and trimethoprim. Combination of bactericidal drugs among themselves may cause synergistic effect particularly with the drugs with different mechanisms of action. Thus, streptomycin or gentamicin added to pencillin has a synergistic effect in the treatment of enterococcal endocarditis. Further, a combination of either ampicillin or carbenicillin with an aminoglycoside has been shown to act synergistically against susceptible *E. coli, Klebsiella, Proteus, Providencia and Pseudomonas*. This is because penicillin promotes the entry of the aminoglycoside through the microbial cell wall. A combination of ampicillin and clavulanic acid acts synergistically since the latter drug inhibits beta-lactamase production by the organisms and thus protects ampicillin. However, data about such clinically useful combinations are sparse.

Combined antibiotic therapy involves certain risks. These are:

- ***Emergence of organisms resistant to the multiple drugs used,***
- ***Increased risk of adverse reactions,***
- ***Increased risk of superinfection by resistant organisms,***
- ***Sense of false security*** which may lead to incomplete evaluation and inadequate therapy of the patient; and
- ***Increase in the cost of therapy.***

As a rule, antimicrobials should not be combined for purpose of synergy unless therapeutic results with one of the drugs is known to be unsatisfactory or proven to be so in a given patient. When indicated, the best known combination should be selected. Readymade combinations should not be used routinely, as they do not allow adequate doses of the major drugs and it is difficult to adjust the doses according to the patient's need. Furthermore, one should be critical of the combinations recommended on basis of laboratory evaluation or inadequately conducted clinical trials.

Antimicrobial Prophylaxis

Use of antimicrobials in prophylaxis of certain diseases is well established. It must be remembered, however, that a drug which can cure a disease does not necessarily prevent it. Antimicrobials are not likely to be useful in chemoprophylaxis, if they are given as a blanket cover to prevent colonization by various organisms in the internal and external environments of a patient. They are, however, useful when used as single specific agents to prevent or destroy the infection due to specific organisms. Further, prophylaxis for short periods is more likely to be successful than prolonged prophylaxis because resistant organisms are likely to emerge during prolonged prophylaxis. Circumstances where such chemoprophylaxis may be useful are:

- For preventing meningococcal infection in healthy children during an epidemic; for prevention of diseases like syphilis, gonorrhea, malaria, filariasis and bacillary dysentery. Syphillis in newborn can be prevented by treating the mother during pregnancy. Immunocompromised patients with neutropenia as in AIDS benefit from chemoprophylaxis.
- For preventing endocarditis following minor surgical procedures like tonsillectomy or tooth extraction in patients with cardiac lesions, for preventing repeated attacks of streptococcal infection particularly in patients with history of rheumatic fever, and for preventing recurrent UTI.
- For preventing invasion of blood stream by pathogens during certain surgical manipulations, e.g., catheterization in patients with UTI, colonic surgery, open heart surgery. Routine prophylaxis in all ordinary operative procedures is unnecessary. Such prophylaxis is, however, useful in surgery of the GI tract, biliary tract, uterus, and vagina; in joint replacement; and in open heart surgery. Prophylaxis should be started not more than 2 hours before surgery and should not be continued for more than 48 hours after surgery in majority of cases.
- In patients with compound musculo-skeletal injury, penetrating wounds and skull injuries with rhinorrhea and otorrhea.
- For those puncture wounds that are at high risk for infection, e.g., contaminated wounds, deep wounds, wounds to the forefoot and wounds in individuals with diabetes mellitus or peripheral vascular disease.
- Animal and human bites, as they are at high risk for infection by the oral flora.
- To prevent microbial complications like bronchopneumonia, e.g., in severe cases of measles and tetanus.
- Given orally for preventing the development or worsening of coma in hepatic failure, where they act by inhibiting the intestinal organisms which produce ammonia.
- In comatose or paralytic states to prevent aspiration bronchopneumonia, e.g., in poisoning cases; it must be emphasised that routine use of prophylactic antibiotics in all unconscious patients is of no benefit and may cause complications.

Routine prophylactic antimicrobial therapy to prevent secondary infection in conditions like mild viral upper respiratory infections in children, in congestive heart failure and in the newborn delivered after prolonged labour, is not of any benefit. The indiscriminate use of antibacterial agents can be hazardous because such a procedure may cause adverse and allergic reactions, produce resistant organisms and cause superinfection due to other nonsusceptible pathogens. As pointed out in an editorial in the Lancet "the unwarranted use of antibiotics and particularly broad-spectrum antibiotics in a mistaken prophylactic attempt is a sin and it would be wise to 'avoid not only the sin but also the occasions of sin' by better understanding of the epidemiology of Gram negative bacteria and the application of aseptic and other methods designed to prevent these bacteria colonising or infecting patients."

Microbial Drug Resistance

Drug resistance is not a characteristic of all bacteria and many strains responsible for common infections have largely remained susceptible to antibiotics e.g. *pneumococci, Streptococcus pyogenes, meningococci, and Treponema pallidum.* The host defense, environmental factors and the properties of the drug used influence the development of bacterial resistance to a drug.

Bacterial resistance is often quantitative and not qualitative. Thus, an antibacterial substance which is not effective in small doses may inhibit the bacteria *in vitro* in large concentrations. This, however, is not of much clinical significance as such high levels can rarely be achieved *in vivo* owing to possible toxicity. High concentrations may, however, sometimes be used for treating resistant local infections.

Bacterial resistance is:

(1) **Natural;** or

(2) **Acquired.**

In organisms which are **naturally resistant**, the drug sensitive enzyme reactions may be absent. Some naturally resistant organisms may elaborate a substance which destroys the antibiotic e.g. *E. coli* produce beta lactamase which destroys penicillin. Following the use of an antimicrobial agent which destroys the sensitive strain, these naturally resistant variants multiply and become dominant.

The development of **acquired microbial resistance** can be demonstrated *in vitro* by serially culturing the organism in increasing concentrations of an antimicrobial drug. Organisms thus made resistant *in vitro* usually again become susceptible to the drug following their serial subculture in the drug free medium. On the other hand, the organisms which are naturally resistant or those which develop resistance after exposure to the drug *in vivo* usually retain this property.

Acquired antimicrobial resistance can arise in bacteria in several ways. Microbes acquire resistance after a change in their DNA. Such change may occur by

- ***Genetic mutation*** i.e. by alteration in the structure of their own DNA; or more commonly,
- ***Genetic exchange*** i.e. by acquisition of *extra-chromosomal DNA* from other bacteria.

In **genetic mutation,** the resistance is of a low level, to a single drug, and involves non-enzymatic mechanisms such as decreased permeability to the antibiotic e.g. methicillin resistance of *Staph. aureus.* Such resistance is not transferable to other bacteria. In some cases, the mutant bacteria even possess the capacity to multiply in the presence of higher concentrations of the drug concerned. Streptomycin is an important example where drug-resistant mutants are produced during drug therapy.

Genetic exchange is the most important cause of serious clinical drug resistance because it can produce epidemic resistance to multiple drugs. In genetic exchange, the resistance genes are transferred from one bacterial species to another by means of discrete, movable, extrachromosomal DNA elements called *plasmids.* The plasmids that encode for resistance to anti-microbial drugs are called *R-plasmids* or *R-factors.* A plasmid can reproduce itself and in the case of plasmid transfer, the replicating plasmid donates one copy to the new recipient cell while the donor plasmid retains its own copy. Transfer of R-plasmids between bacteria can occur by

- ***Conjugation,*** i.e., direct physical mating between bacteria;
- ***Transduction,*** i.e., through the agency of bacteriophages;
- ***Transformation*** where resistance genes from chromosomes may be transferred directly through a sex pilus without the mediation of a vector (plasmid or phage). Examples of microbes where such transfer is seen are streptococci, pneumococci, and some species of hemophilus, clostridia and bacteroids; and
- ***Transposition*** occurs independent of R-plasmids. Resistance determinants (transposons) have the ability to 'hop' from one plasmid to another plasmid, or to a chromosome, or to a bacteriophage. After entry into the host cell, the plasmid and the phage may be lost, leaving the transposons permanently in the plasmids or the chromosomes of the host cell. Since tansposons may carry multiple resistances, the recipient bacteria will acquire resistance to one or multiple drugs.

Plasmid (R-factor) and/or transposon mediated resistance results in:

- ***Decreased bacterial cell wall permeability*** to the antibiotic, e.g., resistance to penicillin and chloramphenicol.

- ***Active extrusion of the antibiotic from the bacterial cell,*** e.g., resistance to tetracycline.
- ***Extracellular inactivation of the antibiotic,*** e.g., enzymatic degradation or modification of penicillin, cephalosporins, aminoglycosides and chloramphenicol by resistant strains.
- ***Intracellular inactivation of a small amount of the antibiotic;*** this inactivated part then binds to the bacterial ribosomes and prevents them from taking up the active drug e.g., resistance to aminoglycosides.
- ***Change in the bacterial ribosomes which are no longer susceptible to the action of the antibiotic e.g.,*** resistance to macrolides.
- ***Synthesis of a drug-resistant enzyme*** in place of the drug-sensitive enzyme in the biosynthetic pathway of the bacterial cell e.g., resistance to sulfonamides and trimethoprim.

Fortunately, in the absence of further exposure to the drug involved, the R-factor mediated resistance is often spontaneously lost within weeks or months of its acquisition. In contrast, the resistance due to genetic mutation is liable to be permanent.

Plasmids are known to transfer resistance for aminoglycosides, penicillins and tetracyclines; the other examples of microbes where plasmid mediated transfer is known to occur are pneumococci, penicillin resistant *H.influenzae* and *N.gonorrhoeae.*

R factors are found in intestinal bacteria, especially in *E. coli, Enterobacter aerogenes, K. pneumoniae, Salmonella, Shigella, Proteus,* and *Pseudomonas.* Since R factors can be transferred from one bacterial species to another, regardless of pathogenicity, they can be transferred from resistant *E. coli* to *Salmonella* or *Shigella* within the human bowel. In the case of some bacteria the R-factor may carry up to 8-10 different R-determinants, each responsible for resistance to a different drug.

Clinically, resistant Gram negative bacteria carrying R factors present a serious problem because their resistance to multiple drugs can be spread in epidemic proportions. Widespread outbreaks of bacillary dysentery caused by multiple-drug-resistant (MDR) Shigellae have been reported from Japan, Bangladesh and South America; many of these Shigella strains carried R factors. In Mexico, MDR *Salmonella typhi* produced the worst epidemic of typhoid fever in modern history; and MDR resistant *S. typhi* strains have been isolated from India. Transferable drug resistance is frequent in Gram negative bacilli causing urinary infections.

Organisms that become resistant to one drug may exhibit cross resistance to other related compounds, e.g., cross resistance is seen between kanamycin and neomycin, between erythromycin and triacetyloleandomycin and between polymyxin B and colistin.

It is known that resistance genes and plasmids were present in bacteria even before the advent of antibiotics. They would appear to be one of the mechanisms of natural selection and survival of the bacteria. It is likely that in their struggle for survival in nature, the bacteria (those nonpathogenic to humans and even those which are naturally present in animals) may develop resistance genes. Unfortunately, these genes can then be transferred to the human pathogens with disastrous results. Further, the extreme and indiscriminate use of antimicrobials in humans in the hospitals and in the community outside the hospitals, and in animals, has encouraged the development of resistance. For example, many hospital strains of staphylococci, certain strains of *E. coli* and pseudomonas have become resistant to the commonly used antimicrobial agents. Tetracycline-resistant strains of beta-hemolytic streptococci are not uncommon either.

Table 49.6 lists the various ways of avoiding the development of antimicrobial resistance.

Dangers of Antimicrobial Therapy

Antimicrobials are the most useful life-saving agents in therapeutics. But, they are potentially harmful. The harmful effects are:

Table 49.6: How to avoid development of antimicrobial resistance

- Use antibiotics only when necessary.
- Select the appropriate antibiotic and use it for an adequate period of time.
- Use a drug combination when it is known to delay the development of drug resistance (e.g., treatment of tuberculosis). However, remember that incidence of bacterial resistance parallels the number of antibiotics used in a given patient.
- Regular monitoring of drug resistance pattern in hospitals and the community, and recommending changes in prescribing to avoid the spread of resistant organisms.
- Establishing hospital committee for prescription audit and suggesting guidelines for antimicrobial usage.

- ***Development of allergic and anaphylactic reactions.*** Hence, antibiotics such as penicillin which are very useful for systemic infections must not be used locally.
- ***Selective toxicity*** such as aplastic anemia or nephrotoxicity by certain antibiotics, the toxicity being more serious than the disease being treated.
- ***Development of superinfection,*** defined as the new infection that occurs during the chemotherapy of a primary infection.
- ***Development of multiple-drug-resistant organisms***, the infection due to which may be difficult to manage.
- ***Deficiency of certain vitamins,*** e.g., vitamins K and folic acid because of the destruction of nonpathogenic bacteria in the intestine which synthesize these vitamins.
- ***Fetal damage*** by transplacental passage of certain antimicrobials.
- ***A false sense of security in the patient as well as the physician,*** leading to the neglect of the need to establish the exact diagnosis. Similarly, strict asepsis may be neglected by a surgeon who relies too much on antimicrobials.

Superinfections are manifested by new clinical symptomatology usually related to intestinal, renal and respiratory tracts or to blood stream. Infants, patients with pulmonary diseases, and diabetics and immunocompromised patients (such as with AIDS) are more prone to get superinfections. The organisms most commonly encountered are *Staphylococci, C. albicans, E. coli, Proteus* and *Pseudomonas*. Some of the superinfections can be dangerous and may cause fatal results, e.g., resistant Staphylococcal enterocolitis and systemic fungal infections.

Superinfections are usually related to the dose and duration of antimicrobial therapy. Further, they occur more frequently when large doses of two or more drugs are given simultaneously and in immunocompromised patients, e.g. AIDS. The mechanisms are given in Table 49.7.

Table 49.7: Mechanisms of development of superinfection

- Eradication of susceptible organisms in a patient with a mixed infection leaving the resistant strains to multiply.
- Destruction of normal nonpathogenic bacterial flora, thus creating a bacterial vaccum leading to overgrowth of resistant organisms; and
- Colonization of the lesion with resistant exogenous organisms from the environment.

Failure to respond to antimicrobial therapy: When a patient does not respond to antibiotic therapy, the case should be reviewed with a view to answer the questions listed in Table 49.8.

Misuse of Antimicrobial agents

The present total consumption of antimicrobials in relation to the known incidence

Table 49.8 : Failure of antimicrobial therapy — why?

- Was an antibiotic really necessary?
- Is the right antibiotic being used?
- Is the bacterial strain isolated really responsible for the illness? Or, is a previously unsuspected infection present?
- Is the antibiotic being given in adequate doses and by proper route?
- Is the antibiotic reaching the site of infection?
- Is drainage necessary?
- Does the patient have resistant organisms or a superinfection?
- Is the fever due to the underlying disease, a drug reaction or an iatrogenic complication such as phlebitis?
- Is diabetes mellitus or AIDS present?

of infections is very much in excess, indicating that antimicrobials are many times misused. This obviously would create many problems as discussed above.

From the many antimicrobials now available, one needs to know only the important representatives of each class and know them well. The various conflicting advertised claims of superiority of one antibiotic over the older established drugs used for similar purpose should be critically evaluated before accepting the change in established prescribing practice. Thus, co-trimoxazole may work out to be as effective and safe as and cheaper than a cephalosporin or a fluoroquinolone in the treatment of uncomplicated urinary tract infection.

It is suggested that the family physician familiarises himself/herself thoroughly with the use of the following drugs for day-to-day practice: co-trimoxazole, penicillin, ampicillin, erythromycin, doxycycline, gentamicin/amikacin, ciprofloxacin and metronidazole.

Once started, the drug must not be changed without valid reasons and should be continued until both clinical and bacteriological cure are achieved. This may vary from a few days to many months. Too large or too low a dosage should be avoided as it may either produce toxicity or cause bacterial resistance. If any adverse effect is observed during the therapy, the drug should preferably be withdrawn instead of using another compound to suppress it. *Lastly, antibiotics should not be used routinely in all fever cases without understanding their nature, simply with the hope of giving 'quick benefits' of chemotherapy.*

Chemotherapy of Urinary Tract Infections

50

Urinary Tract Infection (UTI) is a common disorder at all ages and in both sexes. A healthy and normal urinary tract is generally resistant to infection. However, for anatomical reasons, the female lower urinary tract is more susceptible to infection. In at least 50 per cent of patients, a predisposing cause cannot be demonstrated inspite of adequate investigations. In every patient with recurrent UTI, it is essential to look for a predisposing cause, especially diabetes mellitus, congenital anomalies and obstructive lesions.

UTI may present itself in acute or chronic form.

Acute infection: Infection localized to the urethra and bladder (cysto-urethritis, *lower UTI*) causes increased frequency and urgency of micturition, dysuria and pain in the perineum. Fever, chills and leucocytosis are generally absent. Such infections are generally self limiting. If the kidneys are also involved (pyelonephritis, *upper UTI*), the patient may have loin pain, fever, chills and leucocytosis. Urine is usually loaded with pus cells. Urine culture is positive and shows 'significant bacteriuria' (see later). Clinical distinction between bladder and renal infection is difficult except by means of special tests, which are not available to all doctors. During pregnancy and puerperium, in patients on immunosuppressants and in those with lymphoproliferative disorders, septicaemia can occur.

Inadequately treated acute UTI may lead to chronic pyelonephritis, especially in patients with a predisposing cause. Many patients with chronic infection, however, may not give a history of acute UTI.

Chronic infection: Patients with chronic infection may have few urinary symptoms unless renal failure has supervened, when polyuria may be present. General loss of health and weight, anemia and hypertension are frequently present. It must be remembered that *chronic pyelonephritis is an important cause of hypertension and chronic renal failure.* The urine may show a few pus cells. *Significant bacteriuria* is demonstrable in most patients with active infection and is essential for diagnosis, which cannot be made only on the basis of pus cells in the urine.

Patients having classical symptoms related to kidney infection, fever and pyuria, have definite bacterial invasion of the kidney. However, *symptom-free patients with bacteriuria as well as those with symptoms related to the lower urinary tract may also have renal tissue involvement.*

In infants and children, UTI often masquerades as fever of unknown origin, failure to thrive, unexplained vomiting or as vague abdominal pain. Hence, the diagnosis can be easily missed unless it is constantly kept in mind. Unlike in adults, it is difficult to distinguish between cystitis and pyelonephritis in this age group and hence, *all urinary tract infections at this age should be treated as if they were pyelonephritis.*

Pathogenesis and bacteriology: The bacteria commonly found in UTI originate in the rectum. Bladder infection in females is often preceded by the establishment of the infecting organisms in the vaginal introitus. From here, the organisms ascend to the urethra and the bladder. The few bacteria that normally gain access to the bladder are :

(a) Washed out during urination.

(b) Inhibited in their growth by the low pH (5.5), the high urea content and the hyper-osmolality of the urine; and

(c) Destroyed by a direct antibacterial action of the bladder mucosa.

Ninety-five per cent of the UTI are due to Gram-negative bacilli. *E. coli* is the comonest offender (80%) and next to it are *Proteus mirabilis, Klebsiella, Aerobacter* and *Pseudomonas aeruginosa (pyocyanea). Enterococci, Streptococci* and *Staphylococci* account only for 5 per cent of cases. Mixed infections are likely to be present in chronic cases, in diabetics, in those with obstructive uropathies and in those with indwelling bladder catheters. Such mixed infections are more difficult to treat.

For chlamydia, see below.

Significance of bacteria in the urine: The normal urinary tract, except for the distal urethra, is sterile. A few bacteria may, however, be sometimes found even in properly collected urine of apparently healthy individuals. The most widely used method for identification of UTI is the quantitative culture (colony count) of urine. Colony counts above 10^5 per ml. are designated as **significant bacteriuria** and are considered diagnostic of infection. Those below 10^4 may be regarded as due to contamination. However, some women with acute cystitis may have more than 10^4 but fewer than 10^5 bacteria per ml. of urine. A few apparently healthy individuals with normal urinary tract or those on corticosteroid therapy excrete in their urine bacteria in excess of 10^5/ml. of urine. Such individuals are said to have **asymptomatic bacteriuria**. On the other hand women with frequency of urination, dysuria and pyuria due to urethritis (*acute urethral syndrome)* may have fewer than 10^5 bacteria per ml. of urine or even a sterile urine on *routine* cultures (**symptomatic abacteriuria**). Many of them have urethritis either due to gonococci or chlamydia (non-gonococcal urethritis).

Investigations of a case of UTI:

- ***Urine obtained by midstream technique or by suprapubic bladder puncture is examined bacteriologically*** and the organism tested for its sensitivity to various antibacterial drugs. However, the *in vitro* drug sensitivity of bacteria does not necessarily correlate with the clinical response.

The definition of significant bacteriuria applies to urine obtained by midstream technique. Any growth at all from urine obtained by bladder puncture is pathological.

Catheterization of the bladder for collection of urine is totally unjustified as it may lead to dangerous infection.

- ***Diabetes mellitus must be ruled out.***
- ***Men with UTI often have obstructive lesions or a focus of infection in the prostate.*** Children with UTI often have congenital lesions including vesico-ureteral reflux. Therefore, urological evaluation should be carried out in men and children with a single attack. In women, this is necessary only if the UTI is recurrent; such women tend to have renal parenchymal lesions as predisposing causes.

Even a single UTI infection is a potentially serious condition and failure to treat it may lead to development of serious chronic pyelonephritis, hypertension and renal failure.

Drug Therapy of UTI

Goals for the treatment of UTI are:

(a) Symptomatic relief by altering the pH of urine and/or giving phenazopyridine.

(b) Therapy of the infecting organisms.

(c) Prevention and treatment of recurrence; and

(d) Identification and treatment of predisposing factors.

General principles: These are:

- In acute cases, an appropriate drug may be started as soon as the urine has been collected for bacteriological examination. When the results of drug sensitivity of the pathogen grown are available, another drug may be substituted for the first one, if necessary. Although the symptoms are relieved quickly, the pyuria takes a longer time to clear.
- In chronic cases, mixed infection is more likely and concomitant renal failure may modify drug therapy. In such cases, there is no desperate hurry to start drug treatment before the case is thoroughly investigated.
- It must be noted that the significant infection is in the tissues and not in the luminal urine alone. *This means that for successful treatment, the drug must achieve adequate concentration in the tissues as well as in the urine*. Further, the effects of the antimicrobial agent on the vaginal flora are also important in the lasting eradication of bacteriuria. The concentration of trimethoprim and fluoroquinolones in the vaginal secretions is high enough to eradicate the *E. coli* while nitrofurantoin and beta-lactams are not effective. *Bactericidal drugs are to be preferred for treatment.*
- The drug must be used in adequate doses and for adequate periods. The last dose should be given immediately before retiring, having emptied the bladder completely; this is important because the diminished urinary flow and frequency at night encourage bacterial growth. Duration of treatment will differ with the stage of the disease. It may be as short as a single dose of an appropriate antimicrobial drug (see below) or as long as several months of chronic suppressive therapy.
- The growth of *E. coli* is optimum at pH 6.0 to 7.0 and is inhibited at pH below 5.5 and above 7.5. The pH of the urine must also be maintained at a level that would permit optimum antibacterial activity of the drug used and would prevent crystalluria in the case of sulfonamides. Adequate alkalinization (pH 7.5) is achieved by the administration of 2 g. (½ teaspoon) of sodium bicarbonate, sodium citrate or potassium citrate, 6-8 times a day. Alkalinization of urine enhances the antibacterial activity of penicillins, erythromycin and aminoglycosides.
- It must be emphasised that infections due to proteus and sometimes other coliforms, *Staph. albus* and some diphtheroids, give rise to alkaline urine. This is because these organisms produce urease, an enzyme which splits urea to form ammonia. In such cases, acidifying drugs will not only be ineffective but may cause fatality due to uncompensated acidosis.
- The fluid intake should be liberal as frequent emptying of the bladder (every 2-3 hours) helps to reduce the bacterial counts in the urine and as the growth of *E. coli* is reduced if the urine is very dilute.
- There is no satisfactory antibacterial drug to which all the strains of *E. coli,* the commonest causative organism, are invariably sensitive. Hence, the initial choice of the drug depends upon the relative cost and the known adverse effects of the drugs.
- ***All pregnant women should be screened for bacteriuria in the first trimester*** and should be treated, if found, to reduce their markedly increased risk of acute pyelonephritis, premature delivery and low birth weight newborn. In such cases, a 7-14 day course is recommended. After successful treatment, the subject should be followed in order to detect a recurrence.

Classification of drugs :

I **Bacteriostatic agents** such as Sulfonamides, Tetracyclines and Nitrofurantoin.

II **Bactericidal agents** such as Cotrimoxazole, Ampicillin, Extended spectrum penicillins, Aminoglycosides, Fluoroquinolones and Cephalosporins.

Urinary antiseptics are the drugs which act as antibacterial agents mainly in the urinary tract e.g. Nitrofurantoin, Methenamine mandelate and Nalidixic acid.

SULFONAMIDES: Sulfonamides exert bacteriostatic action against most of the common urinary pathogens including *E. coli.* They produce effective urine and tissue levels. However, development of bacterial resistance is the major problem (Chapter 44). Hence, cotrimoxazole, which is bactericidal, has replaced sulfanomides.

CO-TRIMOXAZOLE (Septran, Bactrim): This combination of sulfamethoxazole and trimethoprim (Chapter 44) is a potent and cost-effective bactericidal agent against many common urinary tract pathogens especially *E. coli* and Proteus species but not Pseudomonas. In acute uncomplicated UTI, it is used in the dose of 2 tablets bid for 7-10 days. In smaller doses (as low as one tablet twice a week) it has been claimed to be effective in eliminating chronic bacteriuria. As trimethoprim has been reported to be teratogenic in animals, it should be avoided during pregnancy. Renal insufficiency leads to retention of trimethoprim and can alter the optimum 1:5 ratio of trimethoprim to sulfamethoxazole in urine. The fixed dose combination is, therefore, likely to be rendered less effective in renal insufficiency. As trimethoprim concentrates in the prostate much better than most other drugs, cotrimoxazole has been used successfully in eradicating the prostatic focus of infection, often responsible for recurrent UTI in adult men.

AMPICILLIN: Ampicillin is effective both orally and parenterally. It is bactericidal to *E. coli, Aerobacter* and certain strains of Proteus. *Pseudomonas* is resistant to it and it is ineffective against penicillinase producing strains of *Staph. aureus.* It produces good tissue levels and is excreted unchanged in the urine in high concentrations. It is well tolerated.

When used in a dose of 0.5 g. six hourly for 7-10 days, it eradicates majority of UTI due to *E. coli.* It is useful for treatment of UTI in pregnant women. *However, many infections with E. coli, especially those acquired in the hospital, are resistant to ampicillin.* This has reduced its usefulness as the drug of first choice in UTI.

CARBENICILLIN: In the dose of 1 gm. four times a day, it is useful in *Pseudomonas pyocyanea* infection of the urinary tract in which it is combined with gentamicin. They must, however, not be mixed in the same vial or syringe because carbenicillin inactivates gentamicin. (Chapter 45)

PIPERACILLIN: It has a broad spectrum of activity against Gram negative organisms, especially *Ps. aeruginosa.* It is given IV in divided, daily, adult doses of 4-8 g. for moderate infections in persons with normal renal function; the dose is raised to 12-16 g/day in life threatening infections. It can be combined with gentamicin with synergistic effects. Its use should be limited to severe UTI with life threatening septicemia (Chapter 45).

AMINOGLYCOSIDE ANTIBIOTICS: Gentamicin and amikacin are the aminoglycosides commonly used in UTI. They are effective against *E. coli, Proteus* and *Pseudomonas*. They have to be given parenterally and can cause ototoxicity and renal toxicity. The nephrotoxicity can be considerably reduced by giving the entire daily dose as a single dose. Their use is reserved for complicated UTI.

FLUOROQUINOLONES: Fluoroquinolones are considered ideal agents for nosocomial pyelonephritis and complicated UTI. They are useful even if renal function is very subnormal. Although they are several fold less active at pH 5.5-6.0 than at pH 7.4, the concentrations in acid urine far exceed the bactericidal concentrations against most pathogens (Chapter 44).

CEPHALOSPORINS: These drugs are valuable in infections with *E. coli* and *Proteus* resistant to other antibiotics. *They are the drugs of choice in Klebsiella infections.* The third generation cephalosporins are particularly effective against multi resistant enterobacteria and Pseudomonas resistant to other antibiotics. Cephalosporins are particularly indicated in septicemic UTI. (Chapter 47).

FOSFOMYCIN: Chapter 46.

CARBAPENEMS: These compounds may be useful in complicated UTI. They can be combined with aminoglycosides (Chapter 47).

TETRACYCLINES: See Chapter 48.

NITROFURANTOIN (Nifran): This drug is rapidly absorbed from the GI tract. Its urinary concentration is high but it gives poor tissue levels due to extensive protein binding. It is, therefore, unsuitable for treatment of renal parenchymal infections. It has mainly a bacteriostatic effect against common urinary pathogens. Most strains of Pseudomonas and some strains of Proteus are resistant.

Although the drug is effective in acute UTI, it is not recommended as better drugs are now available to treat such cases.

Nitrofurantoin given in the dose of 50-100 mg/day can be administered for several weeks to months for 'chronic suppressive therapy'.

As nitrofurantoin is mainly excreted by glomerular filtration and tubular secretion, adequate urine levels of the drug are not obtained even on prolonged therapy in patients with kidney failure. *The drug, therefore, should not be used in cases of severe renal insufficiency (creatinine clearance 20 ml/minute or less).* It is mainly useful in infections which are resistant to other, more commonly used drugs and in patients with mixed infections or infection accompanied by obstructive uropathy.

Nitrofurantoin exhibits therapeutic antagonism with nalidixic acid.

METHENAMINE MANDELATE (Mandelamine): This drug is a salt of mandelic acid and methenamine, and combines the antibacterial properties of both the drugs.

It is rapidly absorbed from the GI tract and is excreted in urine. At an acid pH of less than 5.5, methenamine liberates formaldehyde which is active against many Gram negative pathogens and *C. albicans.* Mandelic acid helps to lower the urine pH.

The drug is not effective against:

- ***Upper urinary tract infections*** as it is washed down too rapidly for therapeutic amounts of formaldehyde to be generated;
- ***Proteus and Pseudomonas species;*** and
- ***Acute infections.***

However, it may be of some value in chronic suppressive therapy.

The drug is available as 500 mg. and 1 g. tablets. It is used in a dose of 1 g. four times a day. Larger doses can cause acute inflammation of the urinary tract.

Adverse reactions : Except gastric discomfort, they are rare. Bacteria do not develop resistance to it. It should not be used along with sulfamethizole as the latter drug forms an insoluble precipitate with formaldehyde.

NALIDIXIC ACID (Gram-O-Neg): This drug is available in 0.5 g. tablets. The dose is 4 g. per day in 4 divided doses for 7-10 days. It has no special advantages over the other drugs and its use is reserved for the occasional case where the organism (especially *Proteus)* shows resistance to other drugs. Even in such cases fluroquinolones are preferred (Chapter 44).

Choice of therapy: UTI is common in women and its frequency increases with age. It is uncommon in men under the age of 50 years in the absence of an underlying structural abnormality of the urinary tract.

Detailed urological investigation is mandatory in:

- ***Children, who often have underlying congenital abnormalities of the urinary tract***
- ***All men;*** and
- ***Women who get more than two recurrences in one year.***

The first attack is most often due to *E.coli.* Further, more than 80% of UTI in women are caused by *E. coli,* and a smaller percentage are attributable to *Staph. saprophyticus* and less often to other Gram negative bacilli. In men, Gram negative bacilli are responsible for about 75% of UTI, and *E. coli* causes less than half of the infections. Bacilli particularly involved include *Proteus* sp. and, to a lesser extent, *Providencia* sp. Gram positive organisms account for about a fifth of infections. Unusual microorganisms such as *H. influenzae, Gardneralla vaginalis* may be suspected when a urine culture is negative but the patient has pyuria or persistent symptoms.

Pre-treatment urine culture is not required in the first attack in young women with dysuria and pyuria, and without a known underlying abnormality of the urinary tract; such attacks can be treated straightaway as if they are due to *E.coli. Urine culture should be done in all other situations*. Successful treatment of an acute attack with an antibacterial agent leads to disappearance of bacteriuria within 24 hours; but pyuria and symptoms take longer to disappear. Post-treatment cultures are important in judging cure of the infection. Persistent chronic UTI may be obvious (pyuria in the presence of an indwelling catheter) or may present itself only with chronic ill health and even renal failure; children show stunted growth as well.

Choice of antibacterial thereapy of UTI is determined by:

- ***The site of the infection in the urinary tract.***
- ***Whether a predisposing cause such as diabetes mellitus or an abnormality of the urinary tract is absent (uncomplicated UTI) or present (complicated UTI); and***
- ***Whether the infection is caused by drug-sensitive or drug-resistant organisms.***

Other factors influencing the choice of therapy are shown in Table 50.1

Lower UTI is often an uncomplicated infection whereas upper UTI is commonly a complicated infection in this sense.

Table 50.1: Choice of therapy in UTI

- ***The patient***: Site of infection in urinary tract, symptomatic or not, age, sex, pregnancy, first attack or a recurrence, underlying abnormality of the urinary tract, renal function, and associated diseases such as diabetes mellitus.
- ***The organisms (expected or isolated):*** Their identity, single or multiple species and their drug sensitivity.
- ***The drug***: The route of administration, cost, and adverse effects.

Tetracyclines, cotrimoxazole and fluoroquinolones should be avoided during pregnancy (Chapter 77). Tetracyclines should be avoided in children.

Generally fluoroquinolones should be reserved for complicated and resistant UTI; they should not be used routinely in uncomplicated UTI for fear of emergence of drug resistance.

Treatment of Lower UTI

● ***Acute uncomplicated cystitis-urethritis in females***: The first attack in a young, healthy woman is treated by some physicians with a *single dose regimen* : sulfisoxazole 2 g orally; cotrimoxazole 6 tablets orally; or ampicillin/ amoxycillin 3 g orally. Although such therapy is effective, it gives low cure rates and leads to frequent recurrences especially with drugs such as amoxycillin and oral cephalosporins, which are excreted rapidly. A single dose antibiotic regimen fails to eradicate Gram negative bacteria from the rectum,the major reservoir for recruitment of ascending uropathogens. *The three-day therapy reduces the rectal carriage of Gram negative bacteria and is not associated with increased recurrence rate in UTI. Hence, a 3 day regimen appears optimum.* Co-trimoxazole is perhaps the best choice for empirical therapy.

Single dose therapy with fosfomycin tromethamine (3 g) has been advocated for uncomplicated, first attack of infection in a pregnant woman

In all other situations, a *7-14 day regimen* is indicated. These situations are:

- ***Failure of the 3 day regimen.***
- ***Symptomatic men.***
- ***Recurrences in both men and women.***
- ***Age more than 65 years.***
- ***Symptoms longer than 7 days.***
- ***Pregnant women.***
- ***Children; and***
- ***Patients with underlying renal disease and/or urinary tract obstruction/ abnormalities and diabetes mellitus.***

The regimens are shown in Table 50.2.

Table 50.2: Suggested oral antimicrobial regimens (for 3 days or 7-14 days) for acute uncomplicated cystitis

- Co-trimoxazole 2 tablets bid.
- Ampicillin 250-500 mg. qid;
- Cephalexin 500 mg. qid; or
- Trimethoprim 100 mg. bid.
- Nitrofurantom 100 mg bid. for 7 days.

A **Fluoroquinolone** such as norfloxacin 400 mg. bid, ciprofloxacin 250-500 mg. bid or carbenicillin indanyl 2 tab bid may be used in infections caused by *Ps.pyocyaneus* and other resistant organisms.

- ***Recurrent infection*** manifested by repeated bacteriuria usually within 2 weeks of apparently successful treatment, is caused by the same organism which caused the first infection. Hidden source of infection or a urological abnormality should be looked for in such patients. The use of diaphragm, spermicides and vaginal tampons has been associated with recurrences in some patients probably because spermicides encourage vaginal colonisation with *E.coli.* Recurrence should be documented by a culture at least once before starting treatment. Such women should receive treatment for at least 4-6 weeks with either co-trimoxazole or a fluoroquinolone. Other expensive alternatives would be : amoxacillin + clavulinic acid orally; a third generation cephalosporin such as cefixime or cefpodoxime proxetil. *It is important to eliminate the vaginal colonization by E. coli.*

In patients with suspected **prostatic focus of infection**, drugs like trimethoprim, erythromycin (for Gram positive bacteria), fluoroquinolones, doxycycline and aminoglycosides are recommended. Despite prolonged (6-12 weeks) therapy with these agents, failure rates in men with chronic bacterial prostatitis are usually 30-40%. *It should be remembered that non-bacterial prostatitis is far commoner than proven bacterial prostatitis.* The entity is defined by evidence of prostatic inflammation but negative cultures of urine and prostatic fluid in a man with genitourinary symptoms. Its cause is unknown.

Where bacteriuria cannot be eradicated, chronic suppressive therapy with 1 tablet of co-trimoxazole or 50-100 mg. of nitrofurantoin once daily can suppress symptomatic infection. *Trimethoprim alone should not be used for suppression for fear of development of drug resistance.*

- ***Chronic persistent infection*** with pyuria and bacteriuria commonly occurs in patients with indwelling catheters. In such patients, only acute symptomatic infections should be treated with one of the 7 - 14 day regimens given above. *Long term continued administration of antibacterial agents only leads to the emergence of drug resistant organisms.* Bladder washes with 1 : 10,000 chlorhexidine is a better alternative to the continuous long term use of systemic antibacterial agents. Further, the indwelling catheters should be used sparingly.
- ***Asymptomatic bacteriuria***: Asymptomatic bacteriuria is often transient and resolves without treatment. The available data do not support routinely treating all men with asymptomatic bacteriuria. Treatment is appropriate (i) before genitourinary instrumentation in patients with congenital or acquired abnormality of the genitourinary tract; (ii) in infection with microorganisms with special virulence such as urea-splitting

bacteria; and (iii) in immunocompromised host. Neutropenic patients with asymptomatic bacteriuria are treated for 6 weeks.

However, children and pregnant women with asymptomatic bacteriuria must be treated adequately to prevent chronic renal infection.

• ***Post-coital cystitis*:** Some women seem to get a lower UTI following every sexual intercourse and in some of them it may produce urgent symptoms. Such a patient should be initially treated by a full course of a suitable antibacterial drug. Following this, she should be advised to apply 0.5% cetrimide cream to the periurethral area before coitus and to empty her bladder immediately after the sexual act. This may be followed by a single dose of ampicillin 250 mg., nitrofurantoin 100 mg. or a co-trimoxazole tablet after each coitus.

Acute urethral syndrome occurs commonly in women and is often due to *chlamydial* infection (nongonococcal urethritis). Its treatment is discussed in Chapter 51.

Treatment of Upper UTI

This is usually due to the same pathogens that cause lower UTI but is a more serious condition.

• ***Acute pyelonephritis*** is commonly associated with a predisposing factor such as obstructive uropathy or diabetes mellitus (complicated UTI). The patient may be septicaemic and severely ill. *Urine and blood cultures are mandatory before starting the antibacterial therapy; the results of the tests may be helpful in modifying the initial therapy which is started without waiting for the culture report.* The drugs used are: ciprofloxacin 500 mg bid for 7-14 days; or a cephalosporin (Chapter 47) with or without gentamicin. Co-trimoxazole orally 2 tablets bid; ampicillin 1-2 g orally or IV (especially in infection due to enterobacter) can be given if the organisms are susceptible. Longer treatment may be required occasionally.

Ciprofloxacin or an extended spectrum penicillin has to be used in infections due to highly resistant organisms. If fever and flank pain persist after 3 days of therapy, urine culture should be repeated and ultrasonography should be carried out to rule out a perinephric or intrarenal abscess, or a urological abnormality. Follow up urine culture is recommended after 2 weeks of therapy. In pregnant women, a parenteral cephalosporin and/or an extended spectrum penicillin are indicated.

In severely ill hospitalized patients and in those with recurrent, complicated UTI, empirical treatment should be started with (a) a third generation cephalosporin; (b) a fluoroquinolone: (c) a carbapenem: or (d) piperacillin + tozabactam (Zosyn), sometimes together with gentamicin, for 10-21 days, to adequately control most of the common pathogens, including *Ps. aeruginosa.* This should be followed by therapy with a fluoroquinolone or co-trimoxazole for 10-14 days, guided by urine culture.

• ***Chronic pyelonephritis*** **:** This is a serious condition which can lead to chronic renal failure. An underlying cause such as obstruction must be carefully searched for in all cases. The antibacterial drug treatment must be prolonged and the choice of the drug is governed by the identity of the organisms and their drug sensitivity, and by the extent of renal impairment, if present (see below).

Complicated chronic UTI is difficult to treat. It is important to detect drug failure early so that an ineffective drug is discontinued; its continuation will only help superinfection with resistant microorganisms and add to the cost of the therapy. In such cases, it may be better to use antimicrobials only during acute episodes. Suppressive therapy is rarely effective.

• ***Renal impairment*:** Tetracyclines, except doxycycline, must be avoided in chronic renal failure. The dose of aminoglycosides and cephalosporins must be scaled down. Nitrofurantoin and nalidixic acid do not achieve adequate urinary concentration in patients with renal failure; further, their systemic toxicity is increased in such patients.

Follow up: Patients with acute UTI should be followed up for at least 6 months after treatment and urine cultures should be repeated at 1-2 month intervals. Cases with recurrent acute infection or with chronic infection need prolonged suppressive drug therapy (6-12 months) after the initial treatment; in these cases, follow up cultures at regular intervals should be done for about two years.

Unarrested or repeated kidney infection not only leads to chronic pyelonephritis but also prevents the kidney growth in children. Results in children with kidney infections indicate that daily sulfisoxazole (0.25 gm. at less than 1 year; 0.5 gm. at 1 to 5 years and 1 gm. at more than 5 years of age) or nitrofurantoin (2-4 mg./kg.), given for a prolonged period, reduces markedly the incidence of pyelonephritis and helps to restore the kidney growth. Ampicillin is probably better and safer for this purpose. Patients with vesicoureteral reflux should be taught the practice of 'double micturition' to minimize residual bladder urine.

Antibacterial Prophylaxis

This is indicated under the following circumstances:

- ***Following instrumentation of the urinary tract.***
- ***In patients with uncorrectable congenital anomalies of the urinary tract.***
- ***More than three symptomatic UTI attacks***; and
- ***Chronic prostatitis and pregnant women with asymptomatic bacteriuria.***

Co-trimoxazole, nitrofurantoin and ampicillin are the most commonly employed agents for this purpose. It must be remembered, however, that doses which are employed for long term suppressive therapy may not produce adequate tissue levels. Thus, although the urine may remain sterile, renal infection may continue to progress without being detected.

Short term catheterization may be covered by giving the patient nitrofurantoin or by washing the bladder with chlorhexidine 1:10,000 solution. Intermittent catheterization has been shown to cause a lower incidence of bacteriuria than long-term indwelling catheterization. During long term catheterization, measures such as closed drainage are far more important than drugs.

PHENAZOPYRIDINE (Pyridium, Pyridacil): This azo dye is used in the dose of 200 mg. three times a day to relieve pain, burning, urgency and frequency associated with lower UTI (cystitis, prostatitis and urethritis). *It does not act as a urinary antiseptic but can give symptomatic relief.* The drug colours the urine red or orange and can stain clothing. Therapy with this drug is generally limited to one week.

Chemotherapy of Sexually Transmitted Diseases

51

Sexually transmitted diseases (STD) comprise a group of infections most commonly transmitted by sexual contact; accidental infection through fomites and infection of laboratory workers are rare modes of transmission. In the case of syphilis and AIDS, transplacental transmission to the foetus can occur.

However desirable, total prevention of STD is an impossible goal. Survey by W.H.O. has indicated a worldwide rise in the prevalence of STD. Permissiveness, homosexuality and changing sexual practices, particularly among the adolescents, are responsible for such increase in all societies, rich and poor. Hence, chemotherapy will continue to play an important role in their treatment as in the past. However, the emergence of strains of gonococci and *H. ducrei* resistant to the commonly available drugs now poses problems, not the least of which is the need to use the more expensive drugs such as third generation cephalosporins and fluoroquinolones. Fortunately, the organisms causing other STD have retained their original drug sensitivity. The concurrent presence of AIDS (HIV infection) complicates the management of STD by suppressing the immune system. Since more than one type of STD may commonly be present in a person at the same time, it has been recommended that all patients with suspected STD should be screened for HIV, syphilis, gonorrhoea and chlamydia. However, the laboratory facilities required for this purpose are beyond the means of most third world countries; so are the fluoroquinolones and the third generation cephalosporins on the scale on which they are required.

The important STD are syphilis, gonorrhea, non-gonococcal urethritis (NGU), chancroid, lymphogranuloma venereum, granuloma inguinale, vaginitis, genital warts, genital herpes, AIDS (acquired immuno deficiency disease) and hepatitis B.

When concurrent, multiple, STD infection is suspected and laboratory facilities for making correct diagnosis are not available, it may be advisable to differentiate the disease into a few **"Clinical syndromes":**

- ***Anogenital ulcer***
- ***Urethral discharge, dysuria and increased frequency*** (urethritis).
- ***Vaginal discharge*** (vaginitis); and
- ***Lower abdominal pain / dyspareunia*** (pelvic inflammatory disease, PID).
- ***Warty lesion (genital warts).***

Each syndrome is then treated with multiple drugs to cover multiple pathogens.

Drug Therapy of Syphilis

Syphilis is caused by the spirochete *Treponema pallidum. Penicillin is the drug of choice for all stages of syphilis.* With adequate treatment of early cases, almost 90 per cent of cases can be cured. Penicillin resiatant *T. pallidum* is so far unknown.

Clinically, syphilis manifests as :

(a) **Primary syphilis,** characterised by genital or extra-genital, painless indurated ulcer (chancre), occurring within 3 weeks after the infection. This can be diagnosed easily by dark-field microscopy or direct fluorescent antibody test of the exudates.

(b) **Secondary syphilis,** characterised by skin and mucosal lesions occurring within 6 weeks to 6 months after the infection. This is diagnosed by serological tests (see below). Both these stages can resolve even without treatment.

(c) **Latent syphilis** is asymptomatic but with positive serological evidence. **Early latency** is diagnosed if the infection has been acquired within the preceeding 1 to 2 years (WHO classification). After that, it is considered as **late latency**.

(d) **Tertiary syphilis** which manifests 4-5 years after the infection, and includes neurosyphilis (GPI, tabes dorsalis), cardiovascular syphilis and gummatous syphilis. This is called **late syphilis.**

There are several reasons for distinguishing between early (upto 4 years after infection) and late disease:

'Late syphilis' is not contagious and needs more prolonged treatment with higher doses of penicillin. Even with such doses, complete cure may not be possible. Moreover, Herxheimer reaction could be more severe, even leading to death.

Reversal of positive serology to negative one is possible in early syphilis ; it may not occur in late syphilis. Finally, *syphilis is considered a great imitator, and almost every organ in the body can be affected.*

Principles of therapy: The spirochete is extremely sensitive to penicillin, plasma concentrations as low as 0.03 unit per ml. being spirocheticidal. The concentration must be continuously maintained for about 10 days in cases with **early syphilis** and about 14-20 days in cases with **late syphilis**. The antibiotic is always given IM because oral administration of penicillin has two dangers: patients may not take the tablets regularly as advised and may try to save some tablets for self administered chemoprophylaxis in future.

- ***Before starting treatment, the diagnosis must be established with certainty.*** Dark-field microscopy of material from surface lesions is a must in the case of primary chancre and secondary syphilis. When surface lesions are absent, one has to rely on serological tests such as (1) Treponemal-specific tests such as *T. pallidum* particle agglutination test, fluorescent antibody –absorbed test (FTA-Abs. test); and (2) Nontreponemal tests such as Venereal Disease Research Laboratory (VDRL) test and Rapid Plasma Reagin (RPR) test. These tests may be false positive in less than 1% of a non-infected population. A CSF examination is carried when neurological involvement is suspected.
- ***Treated cases should be followed up for adequate period.***
- ***It is necessary to trace and treat contacts.***

The recommendations for the treatment of different stages of syphilis are :

Primary and secondary syphilis (early syphilis) and early latent syphilis of less than one year's duration:

- Procaine penicillin 600,000 units IM daily for 10 days; or
- Benzathine penicillin 2.4 mega units IM (1.2 mega units in each buttock) in a single dose. Benzathine penicillin is likely to be painful. Further, some patients may distrust such a regime consisting of a single injection, whereas others may take the disease lightly, knowing that it can be cured by a single injection.
- Patients who are allergic to penicillin are treated with doxycycline 100 mg bid, or erythromycin 500 mg. qid, on empty stomach, for 15-20 days. Ceftriaxone may also be used.

All treated patients must be examined clinically and a quantitative serological test carried out at monthly intervals for three months, at three monthly intervals for one year, at six monthly intervals during the second year and at yearly intervals till the completion of four years from the beginning of the disease. The CSF must be examined at the end of the first year to rule out neurological involvement. If there is a relapse or a rise in the titre of the serological test, the penicillin course must be repeated.

Syphilis (except neurosyphilis) of more than one year's duration (late latent, and cardiovascular) :

(a) Procaine penicillin 600,000 units IM daily for 15 days; or

(b) Benzathine penicillin 2.4 mega units IM once a week for 3 weeks.

(c) Patients allergic to penicillin should be treated with doxycycline 100 mg bid or erythromycin, 500 mg. orally, four times a day, on empty stomach for 30 days.

Neurosyphilis: All clinical types of neurosyphilis are associated with CSF changes, and CSF cell count provides good monitoring for judging the effects of therapy. Ideally, penicillin G is given IV in the dose of 18-24 megaunits daily in 6 divided doses continuous or as infusion, for 12-14 days. Alternatively, it may be treated with procaine penicillin 2-4 million units IM once a day, together with probenecid 500 mg. daily, for 10 days. Patients with syphilis of more than one year's duration and those with neurosyphilis should be followed clinically, serologically and with CSF examination at frequent intervals. The optimum duration of penicillin therapy for neurosyphilis is unknown. *Persistently positive serology alone is not an indication for more treatment.* If, however, the test becomes positive in a higher titre or if CSF abnormalities persist, treatment should be repeated.

Syphilis in HIV positive patients usually progresses rapidly and has higher risk of neurological complications and treatment failure.

Pregnancy and syphilis: Congenital syphilis is a completely preventable disease. Hence, syphilis detected during pregnancy should be treated with any of the regimes of penicillin described above. *Patients allergic to penicillin should be treated with erythromycin or ceftriaxone but not with tetracycline.* Once a patient has received an adequate course of penicillin, she need not receive penicillin treatment during subsequent pregnancies.

Congenital syphilis detected in infants and children can be treated by injecting procaine penicillin 100,000 units daily for 10 days. Interstitial keratitis, a complication of congenital syphilis, needs additional treatment with local or systemic glucocorticoids.

Adverse Reactions and contraindications to penicillin treatment:

- ***Allergy*** to penicillin is the only known contraindication to penicillin (Chapter 45).
- ***Jarish-Herxheimer reaction***: *This consists of an initial exacerbation of lesions at any stage of syphilis following the first therapeutic dose of a quick acting spirocheticidal drug like penicillin.* Any reaction that occurs after second or subsequent injections of penicillin is unlikely to be due to Herxheimer phenomenon. This phenomenon is due to a rapid destruction of a large number of spirochetes with release of the endotoxin. It occurs in many cases of early syphilis, and leads to an aggravation of the mucocutaneous lesions and a mild systemic illness consisting of malaise, tachycardia and fever. Lymph nodes are enlarged and tender. It lasts for 2-6 hours and is harmless. The patient should, however, be forewarned about it as, otherwise, he might feel that wrong treatment was administered. Further, the treatment with penicillin must be continued despite the reaction.

A sharp febrile reaction occurring within 24 hours of the use of penicillin in gonorrhoea suggests the possibility of concurrent syphilis as Jarisch-Herxheimer reaction is known to occur even in the incubation period of syphilis.

In cardiovascular and neurosyphilis, however, a Herxheimer reaction may precipitate severe angina or CHF; and psychosis, convulsions, coma or optic atrophy respectively. Fatalities have been reported following laryngeal edema or coronary occlusion.

Herxheimer reaction is an *all or none* phenomenon and cannot be prevented by starting treatment with small doses of penicillin. The first spirocheticidal dose is likely to precipitate it. An attempt can be made to prevent it in cardiovascular and late neurosyphilis by starting prednisolone in the single, daily dose of 30 mg. in the morning, two days before starting penicillin. From the 7th day, the prednisolone dose can be tapered and the drug omitted with the end of penicillin therapy.

Other measures: In early syphilis, no other treatment than penicillin is required. Marriage is usually prohibited until four years have elapsed from the acquisition of the disease. In cardiovascular syphilis, treatment of CHF and surgical treatment of aortic lesion, if feasible, may be required in addition. Fever therapy, once popular for neurosyphillis is now rarely used.

Drug Therapy of Gonorrhea

Gonorrhoea is caused by gonococci, *most strains of which remain sensitive to penicillin;* however some strains are resistant to penicillin (penicillinase-producing *N.gonorrhoeae*, PPNG), to tetracycline (tetracycline-resistant *N.gonorrhoeae*, TRNG), or to penicillin, tetracycline, spectinomycin and/or others (chromosomally mediated resistant *N.gonorrhoeae*, CMRNG). Quinolone resistance has now increased considerably.

Eradication of acute, uncomplicated gonococcal infection caused by penicillin sensitive organisms is easy. When a local complication such as a periurethral abscess or prostatitis or a more distal complication such as salpingitis, parametritis or epididymoorchitis is present, or in case of penicillin resistant organisms, eradication of the infection is difficult.

Gonococcal infection is more difficult to diagnose and treat in females than in males. Further, **acute pelvic inflammatory disease** (PID) may be caused by other organisms (*Chlamydia trachomatis, Mycoplasma hominins,* vaginal flora including anaerobes, Gram negative organisms such as *E.coli*, and Group B streptococci) in addition to the gonococci; hence *the treatment of acute PID must be undertaken with multiple drugs covering all the above potential pathogens.*

Before starting chemotherapy, the diagnosis must be established by smear and culture of material obtained from the urethra and by prostatic massage in the males and the urethra, vagina, cervix or Bartholin's glands in the females. A quantitative gonococcal complement fixation test on patient's serum done at the beginning, serves as a guide to patient's progress after treatment.

Penicillin should be given first unless the patient is known to be allergic to it or harbours penicillin resistant gonococci. However, *benzathine penicillin which gives low but prolonged plasma penicillin levels should not be used to treat gonorrhoea.* Further, although doxycycline may be used to treat patients allergic to penicillin, it is ineffective against penicillin resistant gonococci.

Unlike other drugs, **ofloxacin** for 7 days is effective against both gonococcal and chlamydial infections. Emergence of multi-drug resistant organisms necessitates use of increasing doses of **ceftriaxone** or **cefixime**.

Acute uncomplicated cases: The various regimens used are given in Table 51.1. The response to treatment is usually prompt and dramatic. The patient should be advised abstinence from alcohol for about 2 weeks and sexual abstinence till he is cured.

As NGU is known to be commonly associated with gonorrhoea, it is now recommended that any of the above regimens should be followed by a 7 day course of doxycycline 100 mg. twice a day or azithromycin 1 g single dose.

Table 51.1: Antimicrobial regimens for acute uncomplicated gonorrhoea

- **Penicillin G** (aqueous) 4.8 mega units, injected in two divided doses, at two different sites, at one visit, 30 minutes after 1 g. of probenecid orally. The procedure is repeated in case of failure of the first treatment. *This is the regimen of choice.*
- **Ampicillin** 3.5 g. orally, a single dose preceded by 1 g. of probenecid.
- **Procaine penicillin** 1.2 mega units plus penicillin G 1 mega units IM, followed by two similar injections, 24 hours apart.
- **Co-trimoxazole** 2 tablets twice daily for 5 days, or 4 tablets twice daily for two days. It does not mask syphilis.
- **Ciprofloxacin** 500 mg orally, single dose.*
- **Levofloxacin** 250 mg. orally, single dose.
- **Ceftriaxone** 125-250 mg. IM, single dose.*
- **Cefixime** 400 mg. orally, single dose; and
- **Spectinomycin** 2 g. IM, single dose.

* Drug of choice for resistant gonococcal infection.

Table 51.2: Antimicrobial regimens for gonorrhoea complicated by acute PID

- **Procaine penicillin** 2 mega units daily for 10 days **plus doxycycline** 100 mg. BID for 14 days.
- **Cefoxitin** IV 2 g. every 6 hours **plus doxycycline** IV 100 mg. every 12 hours; continue drugs IV for at least 48 hours after substantial clinical improvement; then, continue doxycycline orally 100 mg. bid to complete 14 days of total treatment.
- **Gentamicin** IV or IM 2 mg/kg (loading dose) followed by 1.5 mg/kg every 8 hours (in patients with normal renal function) **plus clindamycin** 900 mg. IV every 8 hours; 48 hours after the patient shows substantial clinical improvement, change over to oral **doxycycline** 100 mg. 12 hourly, to complete 14 days of total treatment.
- **Ofloxacin** orally 400 mg. bid for 14 days **plus clindamycin** orally 450 mg. qid for 14 days (**or metronidazole** orally 500 mg. bid for 14 days). This regimen may be used in OPD patients.

Complicated cases: The regimens shown in Table 51.2 have been recommended in gonorrhoea complicated by acute PID.

The other measures that may be needed in these patients are : surgery, local irrigation with antiseptic lotions, local heat and prostatic massage.

Treated patients are followed up clinically, bacteriologically and serologically at frequent intervals for at least six months before they are declared as 'cured'. It must be remebered that, 'cure' is not synonymous with 'relief of symptoms'. The antibiotic course needs to be repeated if symptoms persist or recur or if the serum antibody titre rises during the follow up.

All patients treated for gonorrhea should be investigated regularly and frequently for the development of positive serological test for syphilis. This, however, is less practicable in practice where initial therapy with penicillin may mask the early manifestation of concomitant syphilitic infection. Therefore, *penicillin should be used in full doses as recommended for syphilis, in all cases.*

Drug Therapy of Non-Gonococcal Urethritis (NGU)

Non-gonococcal urethritis may be due to:

- ***Infection with Trichomonas vaginalis*** (Chapter 56) or ***Mycoplasma genitalium.***
- ***A generalized urinary tract infection***; or
- ***Nonspecific urethritis*** : This common STD is caused by *Chlamydia trachomatis* in about 50% of the cases. The cause in the remaining cases is obscure. The patients complain of dysuria and a variable amount of urethral discharge; the disease shows a tendency to frequent recurrences. The diagnosis is by exclusion of gonococcal and trichomonal

infections in cases of urethritis. The treatment of choice is doxycycline 100 mg. twice a day for 7 days. The newer macrolide, azithromycin, in the single oral dose of 1g. is highly effective and safe during pregnancy. The sexual partner of the patient should be treated at the same time to prevent a re-infection of the patient. During therapy, the patient should abstain from sexual intercourse and alcohol which may aggravate urethritis. For treatment of the newborn with conjunctivitis due *to C.trachomatis,* the drug of choice is systemic erythromycin for 14 Days.

Erythromycin 500 mg. six hourly for 7 days may also be effective but is likely to be inadequate for associated gonorrhoea. Azithromycin is also effective against *M.genitalium.*

Drug Therapy of Lymphogranuloma Venereum

This is a more invasive disease caused by chlamydia. Tetracycline 0.5 g. six hourly or doxycycline 100 mg bid for 21 days is effective in curing the acute inguinal disease. In the chronic hypertrophic type, surgery may be needed in addition to tetracyclines for 6-8 weeks. Alternatively, erythromycin may be used. The prognosis in chronic cases is poor.

Drug Therapy of Chancroid

Chancroid or soft sore is caused by *H.ducreyi* The diagnosis is made by clinical findings and a specific skin test.

The treatment of choice is erythromycin 500 mg. orally four times a day for 7-10 days. Azithromycin in the single, oral dose of 1 g is also effective. Alternative regimens are cotrimoxazole 2 tablets bid for 7 days; ciprofloxacin 500 mg. orally bid for 3 days; and ceftriaxone 250 mg. IM single dose. Ampicillin and tetracycline should not be used as resistance is likely to be present. If the patient is HIV positive, longer antibiotic courses are required.

Drug Therapy of Granuloma Inguinale

Granuloma inguinale is caused by *Donovania granulomatis.* This infection responds to doxycycline 100 ml bid. or co-trimoxazole 2 tablets bid. or ampicillin orally in the dose of 500 mg. 6 hourly for 3-4 weeks. Azithromycin 1 g. once a week for 4 weeks is also effective.

Vaginitis – Drug Therapy

This is a common condition predominantly caused by 3 types of organisms

- ***C. albicans*** (yeast)
- ***T. vaginalis*** (protozoon)
- ***Gardenella vaginale*** (bacteria)

Sexual transmission is important in trichomoniasis, unimportant in candidiasis and unclear in bacterial vaginitis.

Candida vaginitis responds to intravaginal therapy with triazole compounds (Chapter 48), once each night for 3 to 7 days. A single oral dose (150 mg) of fluconazole is as effective as several days of clotrimazole and miconazole locally. Asymptomatic carriers need no treatment.

Metronidazole is the drug of choice for **trichomoniasis** (Chapter 56).

Bacterial vaginitis also responds to metronidazole 500 mg bid for 7 days. Alternatively, clindamycin may be used. Similar regimens should be used to treat male partners, since 90% of them are urethral carriers of *G. vaginale.* Douches and local application of broad spectrum antimicrobials is not reliable for the treatment of vaginal infections.

Table 51.3 lists the single dose regimens for the various STDs.

Table 51.3: Single dose regimens for treatment of STDs	
Syphilis (early)	Benzathine penicillin 2.4 megaunits in two IM injections, one on each buttock once.
Gonorrhoea	See Table 51.1.
Chlamydial NGU	Azithromycin 1 gm orally.
Chancroid	Azithromycin 1gm or Ciprofloxacin 500 mg orally OR Ceftriaxone 250 mg IM.
Trichomoniasis	Metronidazole 2 gm orally.

Drug Therapy of Viral STD

Genital warts : This condition is due to local papilloma virus infection and is sexually transmitted in 60% of cases (condylomata acuminata). The warts grow rapidly in the presence of moisture and are inhibited by dryness. They are treated either by electric cautery under local anaesthesia or by applying **podophyllum resin** (20% suspension in liquid paraffin or alcohol) or trichloracetic acid weekly. The surrounding skin must be protected by application of soft paraffin. Cryotherapy with liquid nitrogen is also effective.

Podophyllotoxin (Podofilox) 0.5% solution or gel applied twice daily for 3 consecutive days each week for 10-15 weeks is also effective. It should be avoided in pregnancy.

Imiquimod 5 % cream, applied three times a week on alternate days for 10-15 weeks can eradicate about 50% of these anogenital warts. It acts by inducing the local production of interferon alpha along with pro-inflammatory cytokines interleukines 1, 6 and 8, and TNF alpha. It should be avoided during pregnancy.

Imiquimod (1% cream) applied three times a day for 5 days a week also resolves the lesions of molluscum contagiosum, a non STD disease.

Sinocatechines (Veregen), is a watery extract of green tea leaves (*Camellia sinensis*); 15% ointment is used locally for external genital and perianal warts. The drug may cause erythema, pruritus, rash and erosions.

Genital herpes: *Herpes simplex* 1 (HSV 1) and *Herpes simplex* 2 (HSV 2) are known to infect the anogenital areas. Of these, HSV 2 causes most of the recurrent infections associated with itching, parasthesiae, and maculovesicular eruptions. HSV is one of the important causes of genital ulcers. The drugs used are acyclovir 250 mg orally tid, or famciclovir 250 mg tid or valaciclovir 1 g bid, for 7-10 days. Similar treatment for 5 days is given for recurrences (Chapter 57).

AIDS (Acquired immunodeficiency syndrome): It is caused by a retrovirus, Human Immunodeficiency Virus (HIV) which is most commonly transmitted by sexual intercourse, either heterosexual or homosexual. The other modes of transmission are by contaminated syringes and needles, by blood transfusions and by blood products. It is also transmitted from an infected mother to the foetus during pregnancy and during childbirth. The virus is not spread by casual contact such as handshake with a sufferer, nor by aerial transmission, nor by fomites.

The virus infects the lymphocytes, the brain cells and macrophages. *The illness is due to a single defect, viz destruction of the helper T lymphocytes (CD_4) by the replicating virus particles, and impairment of functioning of the surviving CD_4 cells.* The patient, suffers from a specific defect in the cellular arm of the immune system. Impared CMI makes the patient susceptible to opportunistic infections.

The incubation period is estimated to be 1 to 7 years (mean 4.5 years). Antibodies to HIV develop in 2-8 weeks after infection. *Most of the subjects remain asymptomatic carriers for prolonged periods and can transmit the disease;* a few develop a short febrile illness. The next stage is the development of a persistent generalised lymphadenopathy with or without infections such as oral candidiasis and herpes zoster. In the final stage, the patient suffers from opportunistic infections (tuberculosis, candidiasis, *Pneumocystis carini* pneumonia, cryptococcal meningitis and toxoplasmosis of the CNS), repeated chronic GI infections and malignancies such as Kaposi's sarcoma, Burkitt's lymphoma and non-Hodgkins lymphoma. Severe neurological disorders such as dementia, encephalitis and meningitis can also occur. Death is inevitable.

None of the currently used drugs (Table 51.4) can eradicate HIV infection; but used in combination, they can decrease the viral replication, improve immunologic status and prolong survival.

Drug therapy of AIDS is still difficult, mainly because:

- ***It is difficult to eradicate HIV since the virus becomes an integral part of the T cells it infects;*** further, the virus can remain quiescent (non-replicating) in the affected cells for decades regardless of chemotherapy;
- ***It infects the brain cells and many antiviral drugs do not cross the BBB***
- ***The available drugs are toxic;*** and
- ***The virus can develop resistance when a single drug is used.***

The decision to start **antiretroviral therapy (ART)** is guided by CD_4 cell count (less than 200 cells/microlitre), severity of clinical symptoms, and the plasma viral load (greater than 100,000 copies/ml). The classification of the drugs used in AIDS is outlined in Table 51.4.

Table 51.4: Drugs used against the retrovirus in AIDS

I **Nucleoside reverse transcriptase inhibitors (NRTI) :** Azidothymidine, Didanosine, Zalcitabine, Stavudine, Lamivudine, Emtricitabine, Abacavir.

II **Non-nucleoside reverse transcriptase inhibitors (NNRTI) :** Nevirapine, Efavirenz, Delavirdine.

III **Protease inhibitors:** Saquinavir, Ritonavir, Indinavir, Amprenavir, Nefinavir, Lopinavir, Atazanavir.

IV **Nucleotide reverse transcriptase inhibitor:** Tenofovir.

V **Fusion inhibitors :** Enfuvirtide.

VI **Integrase strand transfer inhibitor (In STI)**: Raltegravir

VII **Miscellaneous** : Maraviroc.

I **Nucleoside reverse transcriptase inhibitors (NRTI):** All these drugs are 2' 3' dideoxyribonucleoside analogues and inhibit RNA-dependent **DNA polymerase (reverse transcriptase)** of HIV; they thus terminate DNA chain elongation. However, they differ in their intracellular action pathways and side effects. They block acute infection but are minimally active against chronically infected cells.

NRTIs can cause the potentially fatal syndrome lactic acidosis with hepatic steatosis due to mitochondrial toxicity. This is attributed to inhibition of human mitochondrial DNA polymerase. It is less common with the newer NRTI (lamivudine and abacavir).

AZIDOTHYMIDINE (AZT, Zidovudine): Given orally, 3'-azido-3'-deoxy thymidine gets incorporated into DNA of the HIV and terminates chain synthesis of viral DNA. The viral DNA polymerase is about 100 times more susceptible to inhibition by AZT, than the DNA polymerase of mammalian cells.

AZT is well absorbed when given orally; it can also be given IV. It is mostly metabolized in the liver and excreted by the kidneys. Its plasma t½ is about one hour. The drug appears to penetrate fairly well into CSF and amniotic fluid.

Adverse reactions include severe anaemia granulocytopenia due to bone marrow suppression in many patients. The anemia usually improves when the drug is stopped. In a few cases, it causes thrombocytopenia. It may also cause GI upset, headache, insomnia, agitation, seizures, hepatotoxicity and myopathy.

Therapeutic uses: The drug has been used in the dose of 200 mg. orally, tid. More recent studies have shown that a dose of 500 mg/day

(100 mg. every 4 hours, while the patient is awake) is equally effective and less toxic.

DIDANOSINE (Videx): This nucleoside analogue of deoxyadenosine has similar actions as AZT, but longer duration of action. It is rapidly but incompletely absorbed, and about 50% is excreted unchanged in the urine. It is non-toxic to the hemopoietic cells but can cause pancreatitis and peripheral neuropathy. The other ADR are headache, diarrhoea, nausea/vomiting, asthenia, insomnia, CNS depression, aches and pains, loss of taste, arthritis, alopecia, dizziness, retinal depigmentation and optic neuritis.

Zalcitabine is a cytosine nucleoside with less toxicity. It is combined with AZT in advanced HIV infection. The major side effects are peripheral neuropathy and stomatitis.

LAMIVUDINE (Empirir) is perhaps the best tolerated of the NRTIs. It is given in the dose of 150 mg bid. It causes malaise, fatigue, and GI disturbances. Rarely, it can cause serious lactic acidosis and liver failure. It is also active against hepatitis B virus. Lamivudine-resistance emerges rapidly and these strains may show cross resistance to zalcitabine, didanosine and abacavir.

Abacavir (ABC) is a well tolerated NRTI with low affinity for human DNA polymerase. The ADR include hypersensitivity reactions, sometimes fatal.

Emtricitabine is a fluorinated derivative of lamivudine. It is almost completely (93%) absorbed and has intracellular t½ of 39 hours. Hence, it is given once daily.

Stavudine has properties similar to those of didanosine, and should not be combined with it because of similar toxicity.

II **Nonnucleoside reverse trancriptase inhibitors (NNRTI):** These drugs, like NRTIs, inhibit reverse trancriptase but by a different mechanism. Hence, they are usually combined with an NRTI. They do not inhibit human DNA polymerase. HIV isolates resistant to NRTIs remain sensitive to these drugs. Used alone, organisms develop resistance rapidly. They are effective only against HIV_1. They are metabolized in the liver. They cause skin rash, hepatotoxicity and multiple drug interactions.

EFAVIRENZ (Sustiva): This NNRTI crosses the BBB, which most other anti-HIV drugs fail to do. The development of resistance to this drug is claimed to be slower than to the older drugs. It is given once a day (t½ 52 hours). The adverse reactions comprise dizziness, insomnia, impaired concentration, hallucinations and abnormal dreams. The drug is teratogenic in animals. It is a mixed inducer and inhibitor of CYP3A4.

NEVIRAPINE is more effective, and penetrates the CNS well. A single oral intrapartum dose to the mother, followed by a single dose to the newborn, is superior to AZT in preventing vertical transmission. It is a hepatic CYP3A4 inducer. It is the drug of choice for women during child bearing age and pregnancy.

Etravirine is effective against HIV resistant to efavirenz and nevirapine.

III **Protease inhibitors (PI)**: These drugs effectively arrest replication and block the infectivity of the nascent virions. They prevent subsequent waves of infection. They have no effect on cells already harbouring integrated proviral DNA. Given orally, they are well tolerated and metabolized by hepatic CYP450 (Table 51.5). Ritonavir and atazanavir inhibit CYP3A4 and this allows reduction in the dose of the other protease inhibitors used concurrently (saquinavir and lopinavir). This **booster PI regimen** is now preferred.

Adverse reactions: Commonly, they cause nausea, vomiting, diarrhea and parasthesiae. Hepatotoxicity, insulin resistance, hyperglycemia, dyslipidemia and lipodystrophy (buffalo hump) can occur. Indinavir may cause nephrolithiasis. Drug interactions are common.

Table 51.5: Currently available protease inhibitors

Drug	Dose
Amprenavir	1200 mg bid
Indinavir	800 mg tid
Nelfinavir	750 mg tid
Saquinavir	600 mg tid
Ritonavir	600 mg bid
Lopinavir	400 mg bid
Atazanavir	400 mg od

Preparations and dosages: Table 51.5.

IV **Nucleotide, reverse transcriptase inhibitor**

Tenofovir (Vired) is a prodrug. It is a potent inhibitor of HIV replication, and is given once daily.It appears to be effective against HIV strains resistant to other drugs. It is well tolerated; nephrotoxicity can occur in patients with pre-existing renal damage.

V **Fusion inhibitors :**

Enfuvirtide is a synthetic HIV-derived peptide which selectively inhibits membrane fusion of HIV with cells and prevents their entry into cells.. It is administered SC twice daily and is reserved for patients resistant to other drugs. Apart from local reactions, it induces lymphadenopathy and suppresses IL-12.

VI **Intergase strand transfer inhibitors (InSTI):**

Raltegravir: It blocks the enzyme HIV_1 integrase needed for viral DNA insertion into the host genome. It is used in combination to treat patients with MDR HIV-1 strains. It is given orally.

VII **Miscellaneous:**

Maraviroc: This drug acts by binding to the chemokine receptor-5 (CCR-5), a co-receptor needed for viral entry into the cell for CCR-5-tropic HIV_1 strains. Thus, it prevents the virus from entering the host cell and has uses similar to raltegravir. It is given orally. Both the drugs are under further evaluatıon.

The current trend in anti-HIV therapy is to begin HAART *(Highly Active Anti Retroviral Therapy)* with two NRTI plus an NNRTI or triple NRTI regimen; and to modify the therapy by adding booster PI regimen in case of treatment failure, adverse reactions, drug interactions, poor patient compliance, pregnanacy or co-morbidity. Combination therapy aims to delay the development of drug resistance and to reduce the viral load to the minimum possible.

The toxicity of combination therapy, the need for adherence to it, the inconvenience of some regimens and the high cost of lifelong therapy necessitate restrictive treatment to severely symptomatic patients and asymtomatic patients with low CD_4 counts (<200 cells/cu mm) and/or very high viral loads.

To improve adherence to ART, single tablet, fixed dose combinations (e.g. Trioimmune, Duovir-N) are now available. They improve long term compliance, and help to reduce the viral load and emergence of resistant strains.

AIDS and pregnancy: To prevent transmission of HIV to the fetus, chemotherapy of the pregnant woman in full doses, started as early in pregnancy as possible, is recommended. Further, the newborn is also treated in the early weeks of life. Even AZT alone, taken orally for just 3-4 weeks before delivery and during labour, is reported to reduce the risk of transmission by 50%. The use of AZT during pregnancy has not been associated with fetal malformations, but mitochondrial dysfunction has been reported.

Many physicians, however, prefer to use a combination of AZT + an NRTI + a protease inhibitor during pregnancy. For women who are already in labour, a combination of AZT + lamivudine, given at the onset of labour and to the infant for one week, or a single dose of nevirapine to the mother and to the infant within 72 hours of birth, can also decrease the risk of perinatal transmission.

STD – Prophylaxis

Avoidance of promiscuous sexual contact is the best method of preventing STD. Failing this, physical methods such as the use of a condom and thorough washing of the genitals and the surrounding areas with soap and water after an intercourse can help to prevent infection.

Chemoprophylaxis of STD: Procaine penicillin, IM 2.4 mega units into each buttock (a total of 4.8 mega units), preceded by 1 g. of probenecid, helps to prevent both gonorrhoea and syphilis. It is more effective in preventing gonorrhoea than syphilis. Hence, a patient so treated should be kept under observation for the possible development of clinical manifestations and positive serology of syphilis.

In patients allergic to penicillin, doxycycline may be used in the dose of 100 mg bid for 15 days. This regimen has the advantage of being effective in preventing chancroid, granuloma inguinale and lymphogranuloma venereum. But, it is less effective than penicillin in preventing syphilis.

The general principles of prevention of STD also apply to AIDS. In addition, sterilization of needles and syringes (preferably the use of disposable material), good blood banking practices and avoidance of pregnancy by women known or suspected to harbour the virus are important measures to check its spread. HIV is killed by sterilization with pressurized steam (in an autoclave or pressure cooker) at 121° C for at least 20 minutes and with boiling water (100° C) for at least 20 minutes.

Table 51.6: Antiretroviral drug regimens for PEP

Exposure status	Drugs
Mild or moderate risk	Lamivudine 150 mg bid and AZT 300 mg bid (Basic regimen)
High risk	Above drugs *plus* Indinavir 800 mg tid or Nelfinavir 750 mg tid (Expanded regimen)

Table 51.7: Points to remember about the management of STDs

- STDs often occur concurrently.
- Compliance with treatment and followup are often dismal.
- It may be better to treat even when an STD is suspected, preferably with single dose therapy (see Table 51.3).
- Serious complications including infertility may occur from lack of adequate treatment.
- Perform serological test for syphilis on patients with other STDs.
- Perform pregnancy test on all females with STD.
- Counsel patients about STD prevention and about HIV testing.
- Advise all patients that the sexual partner must be treated to prevent re-infection.

Post-exposure prophylaxis (PEP): Universal precautions against HIV infection are the best prophylaxis against the disease. However, treatment with antiretroviral drugs may be appropriate following occupational exposure (in health professionals) to HIV contaminated material such as blood or bloody fluids, infected needles, or contact of abraded skin or mucosa with the above material. The regimens for PEP are outlined in Table 51.6.

(a) **No treatment except local cleansing** is required in persons with contamination of intact skin.

(b) **Basic therapy** (for 4 weeks) in persons with non-intact skin or mucosa contaminated with small or large volumes of infected material (mild or moderate risk).

(c) **Expanded regimen** (for 4 weeks) in persons with deep puncture wounds with hollow needles (high risk).

Important points to remember about STDs are outlined in Table 51.7.

Chemotherapy of Tuberculosis 52

Tuberculosis (TB) is an infectious disease, caused by several species of mycobacteria. The important human pathogens of this class are *M. tuberculosis* and *M. bovis*. Tuberculosis has been described as 'King of Diseases' in the Vedas and was mentioned by Charaka and Sushruta, about 600 B.C. With the discovery of tubercle bacillus, the causative organism, by Robert Koch in 1882, the disease became known as tuberculosis.

Tuberculosis is a systemic disease, the commonest form in man being the chronic pulmonary variety.

It is world's second commonest cause of death from infectious disease, after HIV/AIDS. India accounts for nearly 1/3rd of global tuberculosis burden. HIV and multidrug resistant TB threaten to make the situation even worse. Infection with *M. bovis* is less common than in the past but infection with atypical mycobacteria now accounts for 1-4% of cases considered to have TB. The atypical mycobacteria are, in general, of low virulence but the disease caused is usually resistant to therapy.

The disease spreads by droplet infection. These are delivered by the infected pulmonary or laryngeal TB patients during sneezing, coughing, singing and even simply talking. Because of their small size, they remain air-bone for a few hours.

Unlike other bacterial infections, tuberculosis is a difficult disease to treat. The reasons are:

- ***Tubercle bacilli grow slowly, dividing only once in 1-2 days, even in the most favourable circumstances*** such as in an open cavitary, pulmonary lesion. In less favourable circumstances, such as a closed, caseous lesion, the bacteria become metabolically dormant and may 'persist' (persisters) for many years although they are drug sensitive. Only rifampicin acts against such persisters. In an open cavity, there may be many bacilli resistant to one drug even before drug therapy is commenced.
- ***The caseation and fibrosis tend to block the blood vessels supplying the necrotic area,*** making penetration by drugs difficult. The caseated material itself is impenetrable to many anti-TB drugs.
- ***Tubercle bacilli remain viable and multiply even when ingested by macrophages.*** The chemotherapeutic agents (except INH, rifampicin, and pyrazinamide) penetrate poorly into the macrophages.
- ***CMI develops 2-8 weeks after the infection*** in most infected patients. This gives some protection from its spread. Deficient CMI as in AIDS accelerates the spread.
- ***The organisms tend to develop resistance to the chemotherapeutic agents,*** and multi-drug resistant (MDR) bacilli are now on the rise.

Drug therapy for TB forms the most important aspect of its management. The drugs used are:

I **First line drugs :**

- ***Bactericidal:*** Isonicotinic acid hydrazide (H), Rifampicin (R), Streptomycin (S) and Pyrazinamide (Z).
- ***Bacteriostatic***: Ethambutol (E) and Thiacetazone (T).

II **Second line drugs :**

- ***Bactericidal***: Amikacin, Capreomycin (A) and Kanamycin (K); Fluoroquinolones (Q); Linezolid.
- ***Bacteriostatic***: Ethionamide (Et), Cycloserine (C) and Clofazimine.

A single drug should never be used in tuberculosis, as this leads to the rapid development of drug resistant tubercle bacilli. This is preventable by the employment of drug combinations.

Standard Chemotherapeutic Agents

ISONICOTINIC ACID HYDRAZIDE (H): This is the cheapest and one of the most effective antituberculous drugs. Its bactericidal potency is equalled only by rifampicin. It 'decimates' the population of tubercle bacilli within a few days of starting the treatment. It acts on the bacilli multiplying in the walls of the cavities, as well as those inside the macrophages. Further, it is more effective than other drugs in preventing drug resistance to other drugs. *However, unlike rifampicin, it does not eliminate the persisters.*

Fig. 52.1: Isonicotinic acid hydrazide

Mechanism of action: INH is a prodrug. It is activated by the mycobacterial catalase-peroxidase to an active compound which inhibits the synthesis of mycolic acid, an important constituent of the mycobacterial cell wall. In addition, the drug inhibits the same catalase-peroxidase and makes the organisms susceptible to oxidative mechanisms.

INH resistance: When INH is used alone, the mycobacteria can develop *in vitro* resistance to it very rapidly by mutation. The importance of *in vitro* INH resistance, however, is doubtful as it does not correlate with the drug response in patients, where the drug can still continue to remain effective. INH, therefore, should not be discontinued because of apparent failure to achieve the therapeutic objectives or because of *in vitro* evidence of resistance, but the other drug administered along with INH should be changed. Primary INH resistance is rare.

Absorption, fate and excretion: INH is rapidly and completely absorbed on oral administration. Peak plasma levels are reached within an hour and effective blood levels may persist for as long as 24 hours. *The absorption of the drug from the GI tract is so complete that oral and parenteral doses produce comparable plasma and tissue levels.* Antacids interfere with its GI absorption. After absorption it is distributed throughout the body. It penetrates well into the saliva, milk, pleural fluid and CSF. Its concentration in CSF in normal human volunteers is about 20% of the plasma levels but in the presence of tubercular meningitis, higher (50%) concentrations are achieved. It can cross the placental barrier freely. Its concentration in the breast milk is similar to that in the plasma.

INH penetrates and acts intracellularly, and diffuses into macrophages and the necrotic centres, and even after its disappearance from tissues like brain and muscles, tissues like liver, skin, lungs and caseous material still retain an appreciable amount of the drug. Tuberculostatic concentrations of INH may persist for as long as 4 days in caseous masses, after a single oral dose, but these are not enough to destroy the persisters.

INH is mainly metabolized in the liver by acetylation. Individuals may differ in their ability to metabolize it. Thus,

- ***Rapid inactivator*** is one whose 6 hour serum level of active INH following a single test dose of 4 mg. per kg. is 0.2 mcg per ml. or less.

• ***Slow inactivator*** is one, whose 6 hour level is 0.8 mcg per ml. or more after an equivalent dose. Acetylation status is a genetically determined character. Rapid inactivation is found commonly in Japanese and Eskimos and has also been reported in Indians. Rapid acetylation is of no therapeutic importance when doses are administered daily; but subtherapeutic levels may result when once weekly dose is given.

Approximately 75 to 95 per cent of orally administered INH is excreted in the urine within first 24 hours, mainly as acetyl isoniazid and isonicotinic acid. In addition, small quantities are excreted after conjugation with glycine and as isonicotinoyl hydrazone.

INH is safe in chronic renal failure and 300 mg./day can be administered when plasma creatinine is less than 12 mg.%. Dose adjustment (1/3 rd to ½) is necessary in the presence of liver damage.

Adverse reactions: In general, INH is a remarkably safe drug. The important adverse effects encountered clinically involve mainly the peripheral and the central nervous systems. The manifestations are:

• ***Allergy***: These include fever, malaise, skin eruptions, sometimes with lymphadenopathy and jaundice. Infectious mononucleosis, blood dyscrasias and diffuse vasculitis have been reported rarely.

• ***Peripheral nervous system***: The drug causes peripheral neuritis leading to anaesthesia, paraesthesiae, burning and pain along the distribution of sensory nerves in extremities. Isoniazid promotes increased excretion of pyridoxine. Pyridoxine deficiency causes peripheral neuritis, sometimes accompanied by anemia and skin changes. Neuropathy is dose related and is more frequent in undernourished, chronic alcoholics and diabetic patients. It is rare with the 200-300 mg./day regimen. *In the dose of 10-15 mg. per day, pyridoxine prevents such neuropathy.* Optic neuritis leading to atrophy may rarely develop. Hence, INH should be discontinued if visual disturbances develop.

• ***Central nervous system***: INH stimulates the CNS. Psychotic behaviour may be seen rarely with a normal dose but such episodes are commoner in patients with a history of epilepsy or psychosis. The psychic disturbances consist of euphoria, transient loss of memory, separation of ideas and reality, loss of self control and personality changes. Large doses of the drug may cause ataxia, muscle twitching, paraesthesiae and toxic encephalopathy.

• ***Liver damage***: The drug can sometimes cause hepatitis. The liver shows bridging and multilobular necrosis. The incidence is highest in individuals older than 50 years of age. Acetylhydrazine may have some role to play. Patients receiving INH should be monitored for possible hepatotoxicity and the drug should be stopped if the SGPT increases to more than 3 times the upper limit of normal.

• ***Miscellaneous*** : These include dryness of mouth and GI discomfort. INH depresses the hepatic biotransformation of diphenylhydantoin and the latter drug often proves toxic when used concurrently with INH. INH also interacts with disulfiram. Toxic doses (40 mg. per kg. or higher) may cause severe metabolic acidosis, hyperglycemia, glycosuria, seizures and coma. Convulsions may respond to pyridoxine.

Preparations and dosage :

(i) Isoniazid tablet 100 and 300 mg. Usual dose, 200 to 300 mg. (3-5mg/kg) daily given in a single dose. In twice weekly regime, 15 mg/kg twice a week. In miliary and meningeal tuberculosis, 10-15 mg/kg daily. In chemoprophylaxis 5 mg/kg daily.

(ii) Isoniazid syrup 50-100 mg. per 5 ml.

(iii) Isoniazid injection 100 mg. per ml.

RIFAMPICIN or R (R-cin, Rimactane) : It is a semisynthetic derivative of rifamycin B, isolated from *Streptomyces mediteranei.* Its important property is its effectiveness against *Mycobacterium tuberculosis* and *Mycobacterium leprae.* The former organism is inhibited by doses of the same magnitude as with INH but the sterilizing action is faster than that of INH. It is also active against *Staph. aureus* and *albus* and *Cl. welchii.* It is as effective as erythromycin or lincomycin against *Streptococcus viridans* and *beta hemolyticus, Pneumococci, Bacillus anthracis, C. diphtheriae, N. gonorrhoeae* and meningococci. It is only moderately active against *H. influenzae* and *Streptococcus faecalis.* It is also active *in vitro* against many Gram-negative bacilli like *E. coli,* Proteus, Salmonella, Shigella, *Pseudomonas aeruginosa* and Brucella. However, unlike with penicillin, many organisms develop early resistance to rifampicin.

Mechanism of action : Rifampicin acts by inhibiting bacterial DNA-dependent RNA polymerase, thus stopping the expression of bacterial genes. Human RNA polymerase is not inhibited. The drug is :

- ***Bactericidal and acts against both intra- and extra-cellular organisms.***
- ***Effective against tubercle bacilli resistant to other standard drugs and against some of the atypical mycobacteria***; and
- ***The only drug which acts on the persisters.***

Absorption, fate and excretion: Rifampicin is well absorbed from the gut. After a dose of 600 mg. orally, given at least ½ hour before breakfast, the peak level is achieved within 2-3 hours and therapeutically useful concentration persists for more than 12 hours.

Food interferes with its absorption. Almost 85% of the drug gets bound to serum proteins. It is widely distributed throughout the body and is present in effective concentrations in many organs and body fluids including the CSF. It crosses the placenta. The drug is largely metabolized in the liver to desacetyl rifampicin which undergoes entero-hepatic circulation and is active against *M. tuberculosis*. High concentrations of the drug occur in the bile and the saliva. It is largely (60%) excreted in feces as desacetylated form. Small amount is excreted in the urine unchanged.

Since rifampicin is largely metabolized by the liver, the serum concentration is raised in liver disease while renal failure has little effect. Hence, dosage adjustment is not necessary in the presence of renal damage.

Adverse reactions: These occur in less than 5% of patients with the usual doses. They include skin rashes, diarrhoea, ataxia, dizziness, hepatitis, jaundice, proteinuria, leucopenia and thrombocytopenia. It is advisable to check hepatic function before starting the drug. Patients on rifampicin therapy should be told that their urine, faeces, saliva, sputum, tears, sweat and even contact lenses may turn harmless orange red.

Acute hepatic and renal failure, allergic reactions including shock and a flu-like syndrome have been reported in patients taking large doses of rifampicin (>900 mg.) intermittently. Some of these may have immune mechanisms. However, intermittent therapy with smaller doses (450-600 mg.) appears to be safe. It causes teratogenic effects in animals, and it is better avoided during pregnancy.

The drug induces hepatic microsomal enzymes and thus could cause *increased metabolism of several drugs, e.g., hydrocortisone, oral contraceptives, phenytoin, sulfonylureas, warfarin, digoxin, dapsone, verapamil, zolpidem, simvastatin, methadone, theophylline, nonnucleotide reverse transcriptase inhibitors and most protease inhibitors.* This action is of less clinical importance when the drug is administered once a month as in leprosy.

Preparations :

(i) Rifampicin caps 150, 300, 450 and 600 mg.

(ii) Rifampicin syrup for children.

Therapeutic uses:

- ***Tuberculosis*: ** Because of the likelihood of the emergence of resistant bacteria and availability of other potent antibiotics for the Gram-positive and negative organisms, rifampicin is mainly reserved for the treatment of tuberculosis. (See later).

When re-starting rifampicin after it has been discontinued for any reason, it is advisable to start with a smaller dose (150 mg/day) in order to prevent allergic reactions.

- ***Brucellosis*** (Chapter 46)
- ***Leprosy*** (Chapter 52).
- ***Serious staphylococcal** septicaemia* resistant to the conventional drugs
- ***Legionnaire's disease***
- ***Prophylaxis of meningococcal infection and infection with H.influenzae (type B) because of high concentration of rifampicin in the saliva.***

RIFAPENTINE: This semisynthetic rifamycin antibiotic has a spectrum similar to that of rifampicin but it is longer-acting. Given orally, it is readily absorbed and is metabolized in the liver to the active metabolite 25-desacetyl rifapentine. The t½ of both rifapentine and its active metabolite is 13 hours. It is highly protein bound and is mostly (70%) cleared by the liver. It can induce hepatic CYP450 enzymes. Its toxicity is similar to that of rifampicin. It is administered in the dose of 600 mg once or twice weekly. It is not recommended for initial phase treatment in HIV patients because of increased risk of acquired rifampicin resistance. It can be given during the continuous phase.

STREPTOMYCIN or S: This aminoglycoside is considered in detail in Chapter 46.

- ***It is not absorbed orally and must be administered IM. The injection is painful.***
- ***It is bactericidal*** to the tubercle bacilli rapidly multiplying at neutral pH in the walls of the tuberculous cavities,
- ***It does not penetrate into the macrophages nor into caseous material.*** It is less potent than INH.
- ***Its concentration in the CSF is poor.***
- ***It is much more toxic than INH and rifampicin .***

Streptomycin should be used with caution in the elderly; 0.75 g. daily is considered the preferred regime in such patients. It is better avoided in those with known renal insufficiency.

PYRAZINAMIDE or Z (Pyzina, Unipyranamide): This drug, related chemically to thiosemicarbazones and nicotinamide, is effective orally against *M. tuberculosis* of human type resistant to streptomycin and INH but is ineffective against the bovine and atypical forms of tubercle bacilli. It is bactericidal. It shows anti-tubercular activity *in vitro* at an acidic pH and is effective only against tubercle bacilli within macrophages. It has good meningeal penetration. In combination with streptomycin, INH and rifampicin, pyrazinamide exerts a potent sterilizing effect on the tuberculous lesions during the first two months of therapy.

The **mechanism of action** of pyrazinamide is not definitely known. It is a prodrug and is converted to the active compound pyrazinoic acid. Like INH, it inhibits the bacterial synthesis of mycolic acid.

Absorption, fate and excretion: Pyrazinamide is rapidly absorbed from the GI tract. The peak plasma levels are reached within 1 to 3 hours and the drug can be detected in the plasma upto 15 hours. It is widely distributed in the body and *achieves a concentration in the CSF almost equal to the plasma levels.* The drug is deaminated in the liver. The degradation products and the free drug are excreted in urine.

Adverse reactions: Most patients complain of a metallic taste and sulfurous eructations. Apart from arthralgia, anorexia, nausea, vomiting, malaise, mild skin rashes and rarely photosensitivity resulting in bright red-brown discolouration of the exposed parts of the body, the serious toxic effects involve the liver. Toxic hepatitis may occur at any time during the course of treatment. It does not appear to be dose-related. Death may occur due to hepatic necrosis. The drug, therefore, is contraindicated in the presence of hepatic insufficiency.

Rise in serum uric acid level due to increased tubular reabsorption of urates and precipitation of gouty arthritis have been reported.

Preparations and dosage: It is available as 500, 750 and 1000 mg. tablets, Dose 25 mg/kg/day (not exceeding 1.5 g/day) in one or 2 divided doses. For children: 15-30 mg. per kg daily.

Morphazinamide (Dynazide): This drug, related structurally to pyrazinamide, is claimed to be more potent than the parent compound. The adverse effects are similar to those of pyrazinamide.

$$H-\underset{C_2H_5}{\overset{CH_2OH}{C}}-NH-CH_2-CH_2-HN-\underset{CH_2OH}{\overset{C_2H_5}{C}}-H$$

Fig. 52.2: Ethambutol

ETHAMBUTOL or E (Themibutol, Combutol): Ethambutol is the dextrorotatory isomer of 2,2' (ethylenediamine)-di-1-butanol. The levorotatory form is inactive against the mycobacteria but is equally toxic.

- ***It is effective orally against mycobacteria resistant to INH, streptomycin and ethionamide as well as against many atypical mycobacteria.***
- ***It is bacteriostatic.***
- ***Primary resistance to this drug has not been reported.***
- ***When it is used along with other drugs, resistance to ethambutol develops slowly,*** and the development of resistance to the other drugs is greatly delayed.

Mechanism of action: It acts mainly against rapidly multiplying organisms in the walls of the cavities. It inhibits the synthesis of bacterial cell wall arabinosyl transferase.

Absorption, fate and excretion: Nearly 70 per cent of the drug is absorbed after oral administration. It penetrates into erythrocytes which serve as the depot from which the drug is released into circulation. It, however, does not persist in other tissues and body fluids, the CSF level being only 50% of the plasma level.

Approximately 50 per cent of the oral dose is eliminated unchanged in urine within 24 hours; 15 per cent of the drug is excreted in the form of two metabolites. It accumulates in the presence of renal damage.

Adverse reactions: The main adverse effect is retrobulbar optic neuritis on prolonged therapy. The early symptoms are blurring and haziness, followed by progressive decrease in visual acuity, contraction of the visual fields, central scotomas and poor colour discrimination, particularly, loss of ability to see green colour. The symptoms may disappear when the drug is discontinued. Optic neuritis is likely to occur in 2% of patients treated with 25 mg/kg/day but is rare in patients receiving 15 mg/kg/day. Peripheral neuritis has also reported. The drug should be avoided in children below 8 years because of the difficulty in identifying early reduction in visual acuity in them. Other adverse reactions include nausea, anorexia, confusion, headache and allergic reactions.

Tests for visual acuity should be done before, during and after the treatment.

Preparations and dosage: Ethambutol is available as 200, 400 and 800 mg tab. For doses, see later.

THIACETAZONE or T: Thiacetazone, a thiosemicarbazone derivative, is used as a companion drug to INH. Initial resistance to thiacetazone is uncommon. It is bacteriostatic. The drug is satisfactorily absorbed from the gut. Peak plasma levels are reached within 4 hours. It rapidly diffuses into the various body tissues and also crosses the placental barrier. About 40 per cent of the drug is excreted in urine within 48 hours. It is also secreted in milk.

Adverse reactions : These usually manifest itself within first 3 months of therapy. Anorexia, nausea and vomiting are the commonest symptoms. Drug fever, skin rashes and Stevens-Johnson syndrome (erythema multiforme) appear occasionally. The serious toxic manifestations include progressive anemia, granulocytopenia and even agranulocytosis; it also causes kidney and liver damage.

It should never be used in HIV patients as it can cause severe and fatal skin reaction.

The usual recommended dose of the drug is 150 mg. (2 mg/kg) daily in a single dose given with INH. Thiacetazone and INH tablet contains 50 mg. of thiacetazone and 100 mg. of isoniazid. Dose : 3 tablets daily in an adult.

Table 52.1 summarises properties of the standard antituberculosis drugs.

Table 52.1: Properties of standard antituberculosis drugs

Drug	Oral absorption	Distribution	Disposal	Action	Action on persisters	CSF level	Serious toxicity
H	90%	Wide (IC)	Hepatic	Cidal	None	Good	Neuro, Hepato
R	90%	Wide (IC)	Hepatic	Cidal	Yes	Good	Hepato, Immuno
S	Negligible	Mainly EC	Renal	Cidal	None	Poor	Neuro, Nephro
Z	Good (70%)	Wide (IC)	Hepatic	Cidal (IC)	None	Excellent	Hepato
E	Good (77%)	All tissues except CSF	Renal	Static	None	Fair	Ocular

IC = Intracellular; EC = Extracellular; Neuro = Neurotoxicity; Hepato = Hepato toxicity; Nephro= Nephrotoxicity; Immuno = Immunological toxicity; Cidal = Bactericidal; Static = Bacteriostatic. For full forms of drug names, see earlier.

Reserve Chemotherapeutic Agents

Majority of the reserve antitubercular drugs are less effective and more toxic than the standard drugs. Further, they need to be given daily. Hence, they are used mainly in cases either resistant to or intolerant of standard drugs.

ETHIONAMIDE or Et (Rigenicid, Trescatyl): Ethionamide is structurally related to INH and acts by inhibiting the mycolic acid synthesis. It is effective against tubercle bacilli resistant to other drugs and has proved effective in infections due to atypical mycobacteria. It is effective against intracellular as well as extracellular organisms. Resistance can develop both *in vivo* and *in vitro*. Such organisms show cross resistance to thiosemicarbazones.

Absorption, fate and excretion: Ethionamide is absorbed fairly rapidly from the gut. It is GI irritant. The drug is widely and rapidly distributed in the body tissues and achieves a significant concentration in the CSF. It is metabolized in the liver to several metabolites. Less than 1 per cent of the drug is excreted in the active form in urine.

Adverse reactions: The toxicity of ethionamide is considerable and makes drug withdrawal mandatory in about 30 per cent of cases. Mild allergic manifestations include skin rashes and alopecia, but occasionally, serious manifestations like purpura and anaphylactoid shock may develop. GI disturbances occur in majority of the patients and include anorexia, nausea, vomiting and diarrhoea. To minimize this, it is given in a single dose after the evening meal or at bed time.

The nervous system disturbances are similar to those observed following INH but occur more frequently. The drug also causes toxic hepatitis.

The miscellaneous adverse effects include

endocrinological disturbances like gynecomastia, menorrhagia and impotence. Pellagra-like symptoms including stomatitis and diarrhoea occur in a few cases.

Preparations and dosage: Ethionamide 125 and 250 mg. tablets. The optimum dose of the drug is 1 g. daily; because of gastrointestinal intolerance, it is administered initially in the dose of 250 mg. twice daily and then increased gradually by 250 mg. every fortnight.

CAPREOMYCIN (Capastat) : This antibiotic, obtained from *Streptomyces carpreolus,* is a polypeptide, highly soluble in water. Its *in vitro* activity against mycobacteria is about half that of streptomycin but it is effective against mycobacteria resistant to the standard agents. It is bactericidal. Resistance to it occurs slowly. Its mechanism of action, pharmacokinetics and adverse reactions are similar to those of streptomycin.

Capreomycin should be administered with caution in the presence of renal impairment.

Preparations and dosage: The recommended dosage for adults is 15 to 20 mg. per kg. (approximately 1 gm.) daily, IM for 60 days and then twice weekly for 18 months. Suggested dosage in children is 15 mg. per kg. given according to the similar dosage schedule.

Kanamycin and Amikacin, aminoglycoside antibiotics, have been discussed in detail in Chapter 46. They are bactericidal and are active against mycobacteria resistant to streptomycin, INH and cycloserine.

CYCLOSERINE (Themiserine): It is an antibiotic useful in the treatment of tuberculous as well as Gram-negative infections. It is given orally and is mainly tuberculostatic. It is effective against tubercle bacilli resistant to INH or streptomycin and against atypical mycobacteria, although its antitubercular activity is less than that of these two drugs. Cycloserine acts by inhibiting the synthesis of the bacterial cell wall.

Absorption, fate and excretion: Cycloserine is rapidly absorbed from the gut; peak plasma levels are reached within 4 hours and decline by 12 hours. Repeated administration leads to accumulation of the drug in the plasma. It is distributed throughout the body and achieves the same concentration in the CSF as in the plasma, particularly when the meninges are inflamed.

Approximately 50 per cent of the orally administered drug appears in the urine unchanged within 12 hours, and 65 per cent is excreted by the kidney within 72 hours. Renal impairment leads to high plasma concentrations.

Adverse reactions: The use of cycloserine is limited by its toxicity. The neurological effects include peripheral neuropathy, ataxia, slurred speech and seizures. The psychic effects include nervousness, insomnia, anxiety, psychotic reactions, delusions and hallucinations. Some patiens become suspicious while others become paranoid and develop suicidal tendencies. Alcoholics, patients receiving isoniazid and persons with chronic convulsive disorders are more prone to have seizures. Pyridoxine 150 mg/day may help to reduce neurotoxicity In view of its serious neurotoxicity, the drug should be avoided in patients with a history of epilepsy or psychosis and in those with renal impairment.

Preparations and dosage: Cycloserine tartrate 250 mg. The recommended dose of the drug is 0.5 to 1g. daily, administered in two divided doses. A satisfactory regime is to start with 250 mg. every 12 hourly, and to add 250 mg. every ten days until the patient is receiving 1-2 g. daily in about 2 months. In children, a dose of 10-15 mg. per kg. per day is used.

FLUOROQUINOLONES (Q) : See Chapter 44. Experimentally, ciprofloxacin, ofloxacin, levofloxacin, and moxifloxacin are active against *M.tuberculosis*, even those resistant to the other drugs. They are given orally or IV. These drugs readily penetrate into macrophages. Levofloxacin, in addition, has a relatively long elimination half life and is given once daily. They are useful for treating infections with *M.tuberculosis* and *M.avium* complex (see later) resistant to standard drugs and in cases with relapse.

MACROLIDES: Newer macrolides, **azithromycin** and **clarithromycin** also have action against acid-fast bacilli. They are used to treat atypical mycobacterial infection (see later) and cases with relapse.

Management of Pulmonary Tuberculosis

The presence of active pulmonary tuberculosis can be suspected from clinical features and routine laboratory investigations like the ESR; nevertheless, it should be confirmed by a skiagram and repeated sputum examinations. However, 15-20% of subjects with active pulmonary lesions have negative smears. Ideally, culture is required for definite diagnosis. Culture is also useful for drug sensitivity studies. Polymerase chain reaction (PCR) for mycobacterial antigen has been claimed to be highly sensitive and specific for identification of active TB, including TB meningitis. *It is important to remember that an active disease can exist even in the absence of significant symptomatology.* In difficult cases, a strong positive Mantoux test (induration more than 15 mm diameter) is helpful in diagnosis.

The aims of chemotherapy are:

- ***To kill the dividing bacilli in the lung lesions*** so as to render the sputum negative and the patient non-infectious.
- ***To kill the 'persisters'*** so as to avoid relapse and to ensure total cure; and
- ***To prevent emergence of drug resistance.***

Chemotherapy is the mainstay of the treatment of tuberculosis (Table 52.1) and all other forms of treatment like diet, climate and bed rest are only of secondary importance.

Activity, moderate exercise and work are not harmful in asymptomatic patients. But rest is necessary in very ill patients. *In drug resistant cases, bed rest and continued use of INH may sometimes salvage the apparently hopeless case.* The type of climate is not so important. Patients with diminished pulmonary ventilatory reserve should, however, avoid high altitudes. There is no special diet for tuberculosis; the patient should take a well balanced and adequate diet according to his or her purse and liking.

Necessity for hospitalisation will depend upon:

- ***The severity and extent of the lesion.***
- ***The general condition of the patient***; and
- ***The presence of complications such as pneumothorax and hemoptysis.***

Majority of the patients can now be treated successfully as out-patients. However, patients in the communicable stage of the disease should be strictly isolated from infants for a few weeks. It is reassuring to know that adequate chemotherapy makes sputum-positive patients 'non-infectious' in 3-6 weeks.

Upto 90-95% of drug-resposive new cases of pulmonary TB can be cured by standard DOT therapy. *The major difficulty is how to persuade patients to take drugs regularly for adequate periods of time.* Majority of treatment failures are due to either failure to take prescribed therapy or infection with resistant bacilli.

When instituting chemotherapy, it is vital to launch a vigorous attack on the mycobacteria by using an adequate, uninterrupted and prolonged drug regimen. It is likely that a second opportunity to cure the disease may not present itself because of the development of drug resistance. Reactivation obviously indicates the failure of the drugs to sterilize the lesion in the first instance; they are even less likely to accomplish this the second time.

Selection of chemotherapeutic regimen:

INH, rifampicin, streptomycin and pyrazinamide are the four bactericidal anti-tuberculous drugs. Drugs are always administered in combinations in order to:

- ***Delay the development of acquired resistance and prolong the effective therapy.***
- ***Eliminate persisters.***
- ***Shorten the course of therapy;*** and
- ***Reduce ADR.***

There are many ways of combining the standard antituberculous drugs. These combinations vary in their effectiveness and the choice of the regimen depends upon:

- ***Administrative facilities for giving injections.***
- ***Drug tolerability.***
- ***Possibility of drug resistance.***
- ***Associated diseases such as DM.***
- ***Patient acceptability;*** and
- ***Cost.***

In countries like India, the conditions of treatment vary from ideal to barely minimum and the optimal regimen may not always be practicable. Tuberculosis is one of the diseases where the use of *fixed dose drug combinations* is justified. Its advantages are :

- ***Reduction in the number of pills to be swallowed.***
- ***Improvement in drug compliance;*** and
- ***Convenience in mass-treatment of populations.***

On the large populations of bacilli actively multiplying at neutral pH in the walls of pulmonary cavities, INH, rifampicin and streptomycin are bactericidal; ethambutol is bacteriostatic; pyrazinamide is inactive. The most active drug against the small bacterial population that multiplies inside macrophages in an acid medium is pyrazinamide, followed by INH and rifampicin. Streptomycin is inactive in acid medium. Only rifampicin is active against intermittently multiplying persisters in solid caseous lesions; therefore, it is particularly effective in preventing a relapse.

Thus, from the bacteriological standpoint, INH + rifampicin is the most effective antituberculous combination. To enhance the effectiveness of this combination and avert the consequences of drug resistance, it is desirable to add one or two supplementary drugs (Z; or Z+E; or Z+S) in the **initial intensive phase of treatment.**

The greater the bacterial population at the start of the treatment, as in patients with a cavity, the greater is the chance of developing drug resistance. Hence, **the initial intensive**

Table 52.2: Dosage of commonly used drugs

Drug	Daily dosage		
	Adults		Children
	< 50 Kg	> 50 Kg	
Rifampicin (R)	450 mg.	600 mg. Max. 600 mg.	10 mg/kg;
Isoniazid (H)	300 mg.	300 mg.	5-10 mg/kg; Max. 300 mg
Pyrazinamide (Z)	1000 mg.	1500 mg.	15-30 mg/kg.
Streptomycin (S)	0.75 g.	1.0 g.	20-30 mg/kg; Max. 0.75 g.
Ethambutol (E)	25 mg/kg (see text)	-	Not recommended
Thiacetazone (T)	150 mg.	150 mg.	4 mg/kg.

1. All drugs are given in a single dose.
2. Use pyridoxine 10 mg. daily as supplement when high doses of INH are used, as in miliary tuberculosis and meningitis.
3. Before starting streptomycin, check kidney function, particularly in patients over 60 years of age; reduce the dose accordingly, if necessary.

phase *treatment should always be with three or four drugs, all bactericidal.* The drugs are administered daily (if unsupervised) or thrice weekly (supervised). For short course chemotherapy (6-9 months), a minimum of three drugs must be given for the first 2 months, *The duration of treatment must never be shorter than 6 months.*

The various regimens used are:

(1) **Daily, combination drug therapy :** A six month course consisting of daily H+R+Z+E for two months, followed by H+R daily (self administered) or twice weekly (supervised) for 4 months is the preferred therapy for patients with fully susceptible organisms (*usually newly diagnosed cases*). Drugs may also be given three times a week throughout under supervision. During the initial intensive phase, most of the actively growing tubercle bacilli are killed and the patient becomes non-infectious. The **continuation or sterilizing phase** is necessary to eliminate the persisters and reduce the failure.

In patients who are unable to take Z, a nine month regimen consisting of H+R with or without E/S is given initially daily for 8 weeks, followed by H+R daily or 3 times a week (supervised) for further 24-28 weeks.

(2) **Directly Observed Treatment, Short Course (DOTS)** chemotherapy has proved to be highly cost effective. Instead of supplying the drugs to the patient for self administration at home, the drugs are administered under supervision. This ensures that the drugs are actually consumed. Because of the difficulties in organizing such 'supervised treatment' every day, intermittent, thrice weekly regimens were tested and found effective (Table 52.3). DOTS regimen:

(a) Ensures high rate of treatment completion.

(b) Decreases the possibility of acquired drug resistance; and

(c) Prevents relapse.

DOTS is mandatory when drugs are prescribed less often than daily; when drugs are prescribed to be taken daily, the regimen is on self-administration basis.

The initial DOTS-based National Tuberculosis Programme of India (NTP, 1962) was converted into the Revised National Tuberculosis Control Programme (RNTCP, 1993). The basic principles of RNTCP are :

(a) Good quality diagnosis primarily by sputum microscopy in patients complaining of cough.

(b) Regular and uninterrupted good quality drug supply, including the use of a patientwise carry-home box for dispensing drugs to patients.

(c) Direct observation of consumption of every dose of treatment in the initial *intensive* phase of therapy and at least of the first dose of the week in the *continuation* phase of treatment; and

(d) Systematic monitoring and supervision by the health-care giver and accountability for every patient diagnosed.

In the intensive phase of DOTS, all the drugs are administered thrice weekly,on alternate days, under direct observation. **Medications for the continuation phase** are packed into weekly blister packs, and the consumption of the first dose from each blister pack is directly observed. Evidence that the patient has taken the medicines is available by checking the empty blister packs.The programme is made domiciliary by appointing health workers or trained volunteers for supervision.

E or S may be unnecessary in areas where primary INH resistance is less than 4% and resistance to R is rare. Patients who are unable to take HR during the continuation phase for some reason can be given HE daily for 6 months. However, this regimen has high failure and relapse rates.

In any regimen which contains R, all the drugs are best administered together as single dose, half an hour before breakfast.

In patients with bone or joint tuberculosis, tubercular meningitis, miliary tuberculosis and those with HIV infection, it is advisable to extend the treatment for at least 12-18 months, preferably for 24 months (see later).

Routinely, one should consider managing all patients with DOTS which is highly cost effective. However, it has been reported that in

Table 52.3 : DOTS regimens* of RNTCP

Category	Patient type	Regimen (Duration in months) Intensive	Maintenance
Category I	**Serious, sputum positive **Serious, sputum negative **Serious, extrapulmonary	HRZE (2)	HR (4)
Category II	Sputum positive, relapse Sputum positive, failure Sputum positive, default	HRZES (2)+ HRZE (1)	HRE (5)
Category III	Not serious, sputum negative Not serious, extra-pulmonary	HRZ (2)	HR (4)

***All drugs are administered thrice weekly.** Higher doses are used : H-600 mg, R-450 mg, Z-1500 mg, E-1200 mg and S-750 mg. Patients who weigh more than 60 kg receive additional R-150 mg per dose. Patients older than 50 years and/or those weighing less than 30 kg receive S-500 mg. Patients in category I and II, whose sputum remains positive after the initial intensive phase treatment receive an additional month of intensive phase treatment.

** Meningitis, disseminated TB, pericarditis, spinal TB, intestinal and genitourinary TB, bilateral or extensive pleurisy and smear positive or negative pulmonary TB with extensive parenchymal involvement are considered serious forms of TB.

a population with high degree of drug resistance, a DOTS programme with first line drugs resulted in overall cure rate of 54% despite excellent compliance. Under such conditions DOTS therapy may simply be eliminating the drug sensitive strains of the mycobacterium leaving the more resistant strains to thrive.

Treatment regimens, except for dosage, are generally the same for children as for adults, except that *ethambutol is avoided in young children below 8 years.*

As a rule, reserve drugs are rarely required in the initial treatment. They may, however, be needed because of primary resistance to the basic drugs, or because of intolerance or toxicity. When using reserve drugs, care should be taken to avoid drug combinations with similar toxic effects such as liver or kidney damage.

The response to chemotherapy depends on the duration of the lesion rather than the extent of the lesion. Lesions of recent origin, even though extensive, may be completely reversible. The response can be gauged by :

- ***Clinical improvement*** (usually within 2-3 weeks) as shown by improvement in appetite, weight gain and a feeling of well-being.
- ***Bacteriological improvement***: Negative sputum cultures on two occasions, one of which is at the end of 3 months of therapy, is considered as cure. Bacteriological monitoring of patients with extra-pulmonary tuberculosis is difficult.
- ***Radiological improvement***: With adequate chemotherapy, cavity closure or its disappearance without surgical intervention has been reported in 75 to 90 per cent of patients within 3-6 months.
- ***Periodic determination of ESR.***

Ideally, *in vitro* susceptibility tests to determine the sensitivity of the organisms to chemotherapeutic agents should be carried out before and during the drug therapy. This, however, is many times impracticable.

Apart from doing audit for efficacy of treatment, patients should be monitored for possible serious toxicity of drugs. H, R, and Z all can cause liver damage while H may cause neuropsychiatric syndromes. Pyrazinamide should not be used in patients with known chronic liver disease. In decompensated liver disease, R should be avoided. However, *S, E and Q can be used in subjects with fulminating liver disease.* Induction of autoimmune thrombocytopenia by R, impaired vision by E or H and gouty arthritis by Z mandate their withdrawal. *The usual doses of H, R, Z can be given in renal failure* as they are eliminated in bile or metabolized to nontoxic products.

Adjuvant therapy: If the tuberculosis is very extensive or is complicated by marked pulmonary insufficiency secondary to emphysema, chronic bronchitis or pulmonary fibrosis, oxygen or ventilatory assistance or both may be required. Cleansing of bronchopulmonary secretions, and a tracheostomy if necessary, may be life saving. Patients should avoid smoking and respiratory irritants. Secondary respiratory infection must be promptly treated with appropriate antibiotics; so also associated diseases like diabetes mellitus.

Dry, hacking, spasmodic cough can be controlled by codeine phosphate 15 mg. bid.

Pulmonary haemorrhage leading to hemoptysis needs prompt evacuation of the bronchopulmonary secretions to prevent aspiration and bronchial spread of the disease. The bleeding lung should be kept in a dependent position to avoid such a spread. The commonly used positions are the semi-reclining or the lateral. Light sedation is advisable but over-suppression of the cough reflex favours atelectasis. If bleeding continues beyond 24 hours, blood transfusion may be necessary.

Failure to obtain reversal of infectiousness (sputum or tracheobronchial secretions free of tubercle bacilli after smear and culture) after 3 months of therapy, or closure of cavities after 4 or 6 months demands revision in chemotherapy. Failure of drug therapy is likely to be due to several causes (Table 52.4) of which non-compliance is the most important.

Table 52.4: Causes of failure of drug treatment of tuberculosis

- Failure of the patient to take the drugs (Non-compliance).
- Incorrect prescribing of drugs.
- Primary drug resistance.
- Secondary drug resistance.
- Persisters which are dormant and therefore have not been affected by the drugs.
- Poor general health due to malnutrition, diabetes or chronic alcoholism; and
- Associated disease such as diabetes mellitus or AIDS.

The reasons for non-compliance can be

- ***Quick symptomatic relief giving a false sense of security.***
- ***Adverse reactions to the drugs.***
- ***Having to attend the TB clinic repeatedly*** with loss of wages and the inconvenience of travel.
- ***Staff attitude towards the patients.***
- ***Lack of social support and poverty;*** and
- ***Failure to educate the patient.***

Failure rate after DOTS is around 2% and 6% in categories I and II, respectively. In patients who have failed to respond to or shown relapse after first course of chemotherapy, drug resistance to R or H may be suspected. This could be due to:

- ***Inadequate/irregular drug therapy.***
- ***Patients coming from an area with high prevalence of drug resistance;*** or
- ***Known exposure to a patient with drug resistant disease.***

In these patients, the proportion of bacilli still susceptible to standard anti-tuberculous drugs may be usually high. Bacteriological relapse after completion of a regimen containing H + R is due to late replication of persisters, which have escaped the effect of the drugs by remaining dormant. Therefore, re-treatment regimen (i.e. of Category II) should be given for 8 months under direct observation. This can cure the majority of patients, having either still-susceptible bacilli or exhibiting resistance to INH and/or streptomycin, but still susceptible to rifampicin.

In patients who have failed to be cured after second course (supervised category II) of chemotherapy, the proportion of resistant bacilli is up to 80% and that of MDR bacilli about 50%. **MDR is defined** as resistance to INH *and* rifampicin along with/without resistance to other drugs. *Treatment of MDR tuberculosis is complex, needs elaborate evaluation and drug sensitivity testing, and is best left to experts.*

The sputum samples of all these patients need drug susceptibility studies to the standard drugs. Until the results of susceptibility tests are available, the patient should be put on a 3-4 drug regimen consisting of antimicrobial agents which the patient has never received before. **Fluoroquinolones and newer macrolides** are now used as additional reserve drugs to treat the infection due to resistant organisms. *The addition of only one new drug at a time to an ineffective regimen must be avoided as resistance to that drug is bound to develop.* After sputum negativity (seen after 3-4 months of treatment), the continuation phase should be started with 2 best tolerated and more active drugs (ethionamide and ofloxacin) for 18 months.

When results of susceptibility tests are available, treatment is selected depending on resistance pattern (Table 52.5). The initial regimen is with at least 3 drugs to which bacteria are sensitive *in vitro* and which preferably have not been used earlier. Of these, one is injectable and others oral. After 3-6 months of initial regimen (required to achive sputum negativity), 3 effective oral drugs are used to complete the continuation phase of 15-18 months.

Reserve drugs used to treat the resistant cases are less effective and more toxic; they need daily administration. Although most of the drug toxicity with these agents takes place in the early months of therapy, the hepatic toxicity of pyrazinamide and the psychoses caused by cycloserine may occur at any time during the treatment. Cases for re-treatment with these drugs, therefore, should be hospitalised. Organisms rapidly develop resistance to the reserve drugs. Sputum is examined every month. In most patients, sputum conversion occurs by 5 months. Persistent cavitation in the presence of positive sputum after 6 months of secondary chemotherapy or relapse calls for surgical intervention.

Treatment programme for MDR-TB thus uses individualized treatment regimens (ITRs)

Table 52.5: Treatment of resistant tuberculous infection

Resistance to	Treatment till sputum negativity	Treatment after sputum negativity
H ± S but not R	Re-treatment regimen (Category II)	R + E (9 months)
H + E ± S	Z + R+ K/ Amikacin + Q/Et	R + Q/Et (9 months)
H + R ± S	Z + E + Q + AG	Q + Et + Cycloserine (15-18 months)
H + R + E ± S	Z + Et + Q + Cycloserine + AG	Q + Et + Cycloserine (15-18 months)

If resistance to H + S, capreomycin can be used. If resistance to Z, include Cycloserine.
AG = Aminoglycoside

based on drug sensitivity test (DST) results in each patient. However, countries like India do not have adequate resources to manage MDR-TB in this manner. Hence the alternative strategy of treating all MDR-TB patients with standardized treatment regimen, based on common DST profile of the prevalent MDR-TB strains, has been proposed under DOTS-Plus programme of RNTCP. DOTS-Plus includes diagnosis and management of MDR-TB. Sputum samples of Category II patients who remained smear positive at the end of 4 month of therapy or later are processed at RNTCP accredited laboratory for culture and DST. After confirmation of MDR TB, the patient is switched to Category IV regimen, which is a standardized treatment. It involves 6-9 mths of intensive threapy with 6 drugs (K + Ofloxacin + Et + Z + E + cycloserine), followed by 18 mths of continuation phase with 4 drugs (Ofloxacin + Et + E + cycloserine). PAS is indluded if any of the drugs is not tolerated. All the drugs are given as single daily dose with 100 mg pyridoxine.

Extensively drug resistant TB (XDR-TB) is defined as resistance to at least INH and rifampicin (i.e MDR-TB) plus resistance to any of the fluoroquinolones and any one of the second-line injectable drugs (amikacin, kanamycin, or capreomycin). When such DST results are available from an accredited laboratory, an individualized regimen may be used in such patients after obtaining a detailed history of previous anti-TB treatment.

Other Forms of Tuberculosis

Drug regimens proven effective in pulmonary tuberculosis are effective in extrapulmonary tuberculosis as well. Some authorities, however, advocate that *short courses should not be used to treat severe extra-pulmonary forms of tuberculosis*. Severe forms of tuberculosis like tuberculous meningitis, tuberculous pneumonia, tuberculous pericarditis and acute miliary tuberculosis are treated with the three or four drugs for 18-24 months. Glucocorticoids may be required to overcome severe toxemia.

Tuberculous meningitis: H + S + R + Z is the preferred initial combination in this disease. INH is used in the dose of 10-15 mg/kg/day. Intensive chemotherapy is administered for 4-6 months or till CSF returns to normal, followed by maintenance therapy. Total duration of chemotherapy should be 2 years. Pyridoxine is prescribed e.g. to prevent INH toxicity.

Steroids should be used in all severely ill patients, in those with a suggestion of cerebrospinal block and probably also in children under 1 year of age. The initial adult dose of prednisolone is 80 mg. per day (1 mg. per kg. in children) in 4 equally divided doses. The dose should then be gradually reduced till a maintenance level of 25 to 30 mg. daily is reached within 2 to 3 weeks. For withdrawal of glucocorticoids see Chapter 64.

The same regime including steroids is also applicable to miliary tuberculosis, tuberculous pericarditis and tuberculous pneumonia.

Tuberculous lymphadenitis: This condition which is often due to atypical mycobacteria usually responds unsatisfactorily to chemotherapy. If no progress is apparent within 6 to 8 weeks, the glands may be removed surgically. Sometimes surgical evacuation of pus deep to the fascia is necessary.

Miscellaneous tuberculous infections: Tuberculosis of the genitourinary tract, bones, joints, skin, larynx and intestine responds well to routine chemotherapy. INH and rifampicin are the safest drugs in the presence of renal failure. Streptomycin and ethambutol are retained in patients with renal failure and must be used with caution. For ocular tuberculosis, topical and systemic glucocorticoid therapy may be required in addition to systemic chemotherapy.

Tuberculosis during pregnancy : This should be treated with H + R + Z + E together with pyridoxine for 9 months. Streptomycin should be avoided.

Glucocorticoids in Tuberculosis

Glucocorticoids are known to impair host defence mechanism and promote dissemination of infection. However, their anti-inflammatory action may sometimes be helpful. They are useful when the excessive inflammatory reaction of the body is likely to threaten life or is likely to lead to extensive fibrosis on healing. *They must never be used without cover of effective antitubercular chemotherapy.* The indications are:

- ***To relieve toxic symptoms and hypoxemia in fulminating, rapidly progressive infection in pulmonary tuberculosis, tuberculous pneumonia or miliary tuberculosis.*** As they do not affect the final outcome of the treatment, they should not be used in the average case of pulmonary tuberculosis.
- ***To prevent bronchial stenosis in endobronchial tuberculosis.***
- ***To reduce toxemia, hasten the absorption of the exudate and prevent the formation of adhesions, arachnoiditis and hydrocephalus in tuberculous meningitis***
- ***To hasten the reabsorption of fluid in tuberculosis of the serous membranes like the pleura and the pericardium.*** Use of glucocorticoids in abdominal tuberculosis, however, is dangerous as it may lead to intestinal perforation.
- ***As an adrenal cortical hormone replacement***, e.g. in Addison's disease, when it occurs with tuberculosis elsewhere in the body.
- ***To counter the hypersensitivity reactions to antituberculous drugs***, particularly when the patient's condition is serious and the drugs are still effective.
- ***To arrest the dire consequences in rapidly enlarging mediastinal tuberculous lymph nodes.***
- ***To prevent the serious consequences of fibrosis in ocular and genito-urinary tuberculosis.***

The detailed pharmacology of steroids is discussed in Chapter 64.

Treatment of tuberculosis is essentially medical. Moreover, it must be emphasized that surgical removal of the lesion does not mean that the disease is completely eradicated. The patient must, therefore, be treated with adequate chemotherapy before, during and after such procedures.

Chemoprophylaxis of Tuberculosis

Chemoprophylaxis of tuberculosis means the use of anti-tuberculous drugs for its prevention. INH is the ideal drug for this purpose as it is cheap, effective orally and has minimum toxic effects. Chemoprophylaxis can be:

Primary chemoprophylaxis: In this case, drugs are given to tuberculin negative, uninfected persons, particularly infants and children below the age of 3 years, who have had close contact with an infectious case of pulmonary TB (especially the mother). It prevents the implantation of tubercle bacilli and hence reduces the risk of serious clinical tuberculosis in 60-90% of subjects. No immunity develops. INH is given in doses of 5 mg. per kg. daily usually for 3 months and at the end of this period, if the child is tuberculin negative, it receives BCG vaccine to provide active immunity. *BCG vaccination should not be carried out during INH prophylaxis.* INH resistant BCG vaccine, if available, may be used.

Secondary chemoprophylaxis: INH is given to high risk patients with the intention of preventing the development of disease after infection has already taken place and the tuberculin test has already become positive within preceding 2 years, or with the intention of preventing a breakdown of apparently inactive disease e.g. following an attack of measles or whooping cough. For this purpose, INH is administered in the dose of 5 mg. per kg. for a period of 1 year. This is particularly important in tuberculin positive children under the age of 5 years in whom the disease and its complications can be severe. Secondary chemoprophylaxis is also justified (a) in individuals showing recent tuberculin conversion from negative to positive, and (b) in ex-tuberculous patients, in whom the disease appears inactive at present, during treatment with glucocorticoids or immunosuppressants, and times of stress such as pregnancy, puerperium, surgery and serious intercurrent illness.

BCG VACCINE: This is prepared from *Bacille Calmette Guerin,* a strain of bovine tubercle bacillus with greatly attenuated virulence, developed in France by Calmette and Guerin. The aim of the vaccination is to increase the patient's resistance by producing artificial primary tuberculous infection with an organism which causes only a local lesion and some swelling of the adjacent lymph nodes.

Before vaccination, a tuberculin test is carried out where 0.0001 mg. or 5 test units of purified protein derivative (PPD) obtained from the mycobacterium is injected intradermally on the ventral surface of the forearm. If the test is negative, it is repeated after 6 weeks. If the tuberculin test still remains negative, 0.1 ml. of the vaccine is injected intradermally in the deltoid region. This leads to the formation of a papule followed by an ulcer within 4 to 6 weeks. The regional glands are slightly enlarged. Healing occurs gradually thereafter, but the papule may be detectable upto a period of 12 months. After vaccination, the tuberculin test becomes positive within 6 to 12 weeks indicating the development of immunity.

A rare complication of BCG vaccination is a glandular cold abscess. This should be treated with chemotherapy in the usual way. Just an enlargement of lymph nodes needs no treatment. Still rarer is the occurrence of fatal disseminated tuberculosis mainly in children with hypogammaglobulinemia. Hence, those with hypogammaglobulinemia or eczema should not be vaccinated.

BCG vaccination has been shown to be useful

- ***In tuberculin negative school children.***
- ***In contacts of cases with active tuberculosis; and***
- ***In persons living in areas with high incidence of tuberculosis.***

Ideally, it is given within first six months of life. Pretesting with PPD is not needed if BCG is given immediately after birth. Preliminary tuberculin testing can also be dispensed with during mass vaccination programme as administration of BCG to tuberculin positive children is not hazardous.

BCG has contributed to the control of tuberculosis. But, the efficacy of different BCG vaccines ranges from 0% to 80% in different populations. Its efficacy is about 70% against serious form of disease in children (meningitis and miliary TB) but variable against pulmonary tuberculosis in adults. *It must not be given to anyone with symptomatic HIV infection.* BCG is probably the safest among vaccines in use today. However, it gives relative degree of resistance to clinical tuberculosis. The protection, is "not complete, nor permanent, nor predictable, nor measureable". Further, the presence of widespread infection with mycobacteria other than tubercle bacilli can interfere with the protection given by BCG.

BCG and host defence: BCG enhances the host defence mechanisms. It has been observed to stimulate the reticuloendothelial system and confer upon mice resistance to bacterial and viral infections. Its administration can prevent the growth and cause regression of transplanted tumours in animals. In man, local intra-lesional injection of BCG or PPD has been observed to produce beneficial effects in skin neoplasms such as malignant melanoma, carcinoma, reticulum cell sarcoma and superficial bladder cancer.

The mechanism of antimalignancy action of BCG is not well understood. It probably has an immunological basis. The agent activates the natural killer cells and the production of hemopoietic stem cells. Macrophages affected by BCG become more active killer cells and more effectively clear antigens and immune complexes, and recruit other cells. Finally, BCG has been reported to cross react with cells of certain malignancies such as melanoma, leukemia and hepatoma. BCG has also been shown to be useful in leprosy prophylaxis.

Nontuberculous Mycobacterial Infections

These infections are caused by organisms such *as M.kansasii, M.avium, M. murinum,* and *M.scrofulaceum*; they are grouped under the term ***M. avium* complex (MAC)**. Of these, *M. scrofulaceum* causes cervical lymphadenitis especially in children; and *M. marinum* causes skin disease. They are frequently resistant to many of the commonly used drugs. Whenever possible, surgical removal of the infected tissue is recommended, followed by chemotherapy with clarithromycin/azithromycin and ethambutol. In some situation, rifabutine, amicacin, clofazimine and/or fluoroquinolone are added.

Fluoroquinolones such as ciprofloxacin, ofloxacin, moxifloxacin and gatifloxacin have inhibitory activity against MAC. Ciprofloxacin is used in the dose of 750 mg bid and ofloxacin in the dose of 400 mg/day.

RIFABUTIN (Mycobutin): is a semisynthetic antibiotic derived from rifamycin S. Its action is similar to that of rifampicin. It is more active than rifampicin against MAC and even against MAC stranis resistant to rifampicin. It is readily absorbed and tissue levels are 5-10 times higher than plasma concentration. CSF concentration is 30-70 % that of the plasma. Its plasma t½ is 45 hours, compared to 3-5 hours of rifampicin. It is mainly eliminated in bile and no dose adjustment is needed in kidney damage. Adverse effects include GI disturbances, neutropenia, myalgia and impairment of taste. Other adverse effects are similar to those of rifampicin. It too induces hepatic microsomal enzymes.

Rifabutin is given in a dose of 300-600 mg/day along with other drugs in pulmonary MAC infection for upto six months. Smaller doses are used for treating pulmonary TB. It is used as a single agent for prophylaxis against MAC. It is recommended in place of rifampicin in the treatment of HIV positive individuals,who are also taking protease inhibitors as it does not cause changes in serum level of these drugs.

CLARITHROMYCIN: This macrolide is used for the treatment of disseminated MAC in a dose of 500 mg bid, in combination with ethambutol and rifampin (Chapter 46). It is more potent than azithromycin but the latter has better intracellular penetration.

Tuberculosis and HIV Infection

HIV infection causes a specific and progressive destruction of the helper T lymphocytes (CD4 cells) and impairs the function of the B lymphocytes and macrophages. This makes an HIV infected person :

- ***More liable to undergo reactivation of old, healed tuberculosis***
- ***To get a fresh infection***; and
- ***To progress rapidly to active clinical tuberculosis.***

Further, the severity of tuberculosis increases as the destruction of the immune system by HIV progresses. Both *M.tuberculosis* and the MAC can infect these patients. The infection appears in the early stages of HIV infection, much before the other opportunistic infections do. Treatment is with the standard four drug regimen (INH, rifabutin, S/E and Z) for 9-12 months, pyrazinamide being dropped after the first two months. However, treatment is more difficult and relapses are frequent.

Other drugs used in the treatment of MAC associated with AIDS are clofazimine and clarithromycin. Therapy needs to be continued for life if clinical and radiological improvement is observed.

Chemotherapy of Leprosy 53

Leprosy is caused by ***Mycobacterium leprae*** which produces characteristic lesions in the skin and the peripheral nerves. ***M.leprae*** is an obligate intracellular organism and its ability to survive within the macrophages and Schwann cells is a key feature of its pathogenicity. The disease is common in South-East-Asia, Africa and other tropical and subtropical countries. Although the leprosy bacillus was discovered by Hansen in 1873, almost 12 years before the discovery of tubercle bacillus, the progress in the chemotherapy of leprosy has been much slower than in that of tuberculosis. This is because, until recently, it was not possible to culture the leprosy bacillus. Further, unlike tuberculosis, human leprosy cannot be transmitted to animals so easily.

Human leprosy bacillus from nasal washings and skin biopsies has now been cultivated successfully in the foot pads of mice; and the disease has been successfully transmitted to some species of armadillo. The infected armadillo tissues contain a large number of leprosy bacilli, thus, providing a good experimental model of human leprosy.

Types of leprosy: Clinically, there are four main types of leprosy:

- *Lepromatous* (LL).
- *Tuberculoid* (TL).
- *Indeterminate* (IL); *and*
- *Dimorphic* (borderline, BL).

They are determined by the degree of CMI (Cell mediated immunity) in the host against the lepra bacilli.

In **LL**, the **CMI** is low (negative lepromin test), the lesions abound in lepra bacilli and the disease progresses rapidly. The disease affects mainly the face, nose, ears, eyes and lymph glands. The typical lesion of LL is a macule, a hypopigmented, circular, erythematous patch not associated with itching or hypoalgesia. Macules are usually small, smooth and symmetrically distributed. Eventually, the skin becomes furrowed and nodulated, giving a pecular 'leonine facies'. Eyelashes fall off. Later, ulceration occurs with marked tissue destruction involving eyes, nose and larynx. *The nerves are affected late in the disease.* Inspite of marked destruction, leprosy, *per se,* is rarely the cause of death. Histologically, the lesion of LL is essentially a granuloma consisting of many macrophages, called lepra cells, containing numerous bacilli.

In **TL**, the **CMI** is intact (strongly positive lepromin test), the organisms are few, *nerves are predominantly affected first*, and the progress of the disease is slow. The typical tuberculoid lesion is a large, flat, atrophic, hairless, hypopigmented skin area, with red, raised margin showing marked impairment of sensation. The peripheral nerves are thickened. Although 70% of leprosy skin lesion have diminished sensation, the nonanaesthia 30% of lesion occur in patients with multi-bacillary disease (see later). The prognosis is better than in LL and gross mutilation occurs only secondary to nerve destruction and anaesthesia. Histologically, the lesion consists of focal masses of epitheloid cells and giant cells with lymphocytic infiltration. Since this picture resembles that seen in tuberculosis, it is called tuberculoid leprosy.

IL or the confusing form is an early stage where the lesions are slight and do not give a clue about the type of disease.

BL is an unstable condition, where immunity is low and which becomes lepromatous if left untreated.

LL and BL forms have plenty of bacilli in the lesions and are called **multibacillary leprosy**, whereas TL and IL lesions show fewer bacilli and are called **paucibacillary leprosy**. In the field classification, the presence of more than 5 skin patches is treated as multibacillary.

The diagnosis of leprosy is essentially clinical, supported by bacteriological evidence from smears from the lesions, nodules, earlobes, or from scrapings of the nasal mucosa. The lepromin test is of no diagnostic value because persons who have never been in contact with leprosy but are Mantoux positive may have a positive lepromin test. It is always negative in lepromatous leprosy and weakly to strongly positive in tuberculoid leprosy.

All patients with active leprosy should be treated with chemotherapy. *It is, however, unjustifiable and even dangerous to treat this disease on mere suspicion.* This not only exposes the patient to prolonged therapy with potentially toxic drugs but can also cause severe psychological trauma. In case of doubtful diagnosis, it is better to wait for definite diagnosis because little harm can be done by waiting. The important aims of therapy are :

- ***To achieve clinical cure.***
- ***To achieve bacteriological cure;*** and
- ***To treat physical deformities resulting from nerve and tissue damage.***

The psychosocial aspect of the patient and his environment also need attention.

Drugs Used in Leprosy

Table 53.1 lists the drugs used in the treatment of leprosy.

SULFONES: Sulfones are derivatives of 4-4' diaminodiphenyl sulfone (DDS, **Dapsone**) (Fig. 53.1). It is interesting to note that DDS was first synthesized in 1908 but its antibacterial property remained unknown until 1937 and its value as an antileprotic drug was discovered only in 1941!

Table 53.1: Drugs used in leprosy

- Sulfones : Dapsone
- Rifampicin
- Clofazimine
- Ethionamide/Prothionamide
- Fluoroquinolones : Ofloxacin; Pefloxacin
- Other antibiotics Minocycline; Clarithromycin

$NH_2-C_6H_4-SO_2-C_6H_4-NH_2$

Fig. 53.1 : Diamino-diphenylsulfone (DDS)

Sulfones are chemically related to sulfonamides and although they are highly effective in experimental streptococcal infection, they are too toxic for use for this purpose in man. They are, however, very useful in the treatment of leprosy because the doses needed are very small. Among the various sulfones, dapsone still remains the drug of choice.

Mechanism of action: Sulfones are essentially bacteriostatic and probably act by inhibiting the de-novo synthesis of folic acid by *M. leprae*. The action of DDS is antagonised by para-amino-benzoic acid.

Sulfones have bacteriostatic action also

against other bacteria susceptible to sulfonamides and against the tubercle bacilli. They are, however, not used in the treatment of infection with these organisms because of their toxicity.

Absorption, fate and excretion : DDS is slowly but completely absorbed from the GI tract. The peak plasma level is reached within 1-3 hours after oral administration and the drug remains detectable in the plasma for 8-12 days (t ½ 27 hours). Sulfones are cumulative drugs. They are distributed throughout the body fluids and tissues and can be detected in the tissues upto 3 weeks after stoppage of therapy. Sulfones get concentrated more in the leprosy-affected skin than in the normal skin. These compounds are metabolized in the liver and excreted in urine as glucuronic acid conjugates. They are also excreted in large quantities in bile; this portion however, is reabsorbed. Excretion also occurs in human milk.

Dapsone resistance: Both primary and secondary resistance of *M. leprae* to dapsone is well established, and is associated with gene mutation. However, primay resistance to dapsone is rare. Low dose monotherapy and irregular treatment are mainly responsible to development of secondary resistance.

Adverse reactions : These are similar to those due to sulfonamides. They commonly cause anorexia, nausea and vomiting. They can give rise to allergic reactions like dermatitis and drug fever. Skin sensitization can occur in about 3 per cent of dark skinned patients. Fatal exfoliative dermatitis (Stevens-Johnson syndrome) associated with drug fever, hepatitis and psychosis can rarely occur.

Sulfones are powerful oxidant drugs and can cause hemolytic anemia. Patients with G6-PD deficiency are more susceptible. They can also cause anemia, methemoglobinemia and agranulocytosis. Other toxic effects include hematuria, liver damage and goitrogenesis.

Although the list of toxicity is formidable, sulfones are remarkably well tolerated by most of the leprosy patients in the dosage recommended.

Preparations and dosage:

(i) Dapsone (DDS): 50-100 mg. tablets. It is given in the dose of 100 mg. daily. Such dosage results in peak plasma levels that exceed the MIC of dapsone against *M. leprae* by a factor of about 500. Such high levels inhibit the multiplication of mutants of *M. leprae* with low or moderate degrees of dapsone resistance.

(ii) Dapsone injection is a 20 per cent w/v suspension in arachis oil. Dose : 0.2 ml. IM, weekly, gradually increased to a maximum of 0.8 ml. weekly.

Other uses of sulfones: Dermatitis herpetiformis is a chronic disease characterised by intensely itching papules, urticaria-like lesions, vesicles and bullae on the extensor surfaces of the body. A gluten-sensitive enteropathy is observed in many patients with this disease. Dapsone, in the dose of 50 mg. orally, daily, increased by 25 mg. (daily dose) once in 10-15 days to 25 mg. three to four times daily, rapidly controls the skin lesions. If the patient adheres strictly to the gluten-free diet, the dose of dapsone can be reduced or the drug may even be stopped.

Dapsone has also been used to treat *Pneumocystitis carinii* infection, and in combination with pyrmethamine, MDR falciparum malaria. (Chapter 54).

RIFAMPICIN: This antibiotic has been discussed in Chapter 52. Its introduction has revolutionised the management of leprosy. It is bactericidal and given orally, it is highly effective in leprosy. Few toxic effects have been reported so far in the case of monthly administration. Supervised administration of 600 mg. of rifampicin *single dose once a month* is as effective as daily administration of 600 mg. in leprosy. Bacterial resistance to rifampicin has been reported.

ETHIONAMIDE: This drug is described in detail in Chapter 52. It is expensive and more toxic than dapsone but perhaps has faster bactericidal action against *M. leprae* than full dosage dapsone. It is administered orally, daily. **Prothionamide** has similar properties as ethionamide.

CLOFAZIMINE (Lamprene, Hansepran): This red-purple phenazine dye is well absorbed after oral administration. It is principally retained in tissues of the reticuloendothelial system and concentrated by macrophages of the skin. It acts by inhibition of mycobacterial DNA synthesis. It is bactericidal and has action against dapsone resistant organisms. It also possesses anti-inflammatory properties. Bacterial resistance to clofazimine is rare. It is excreted in the urine slowly for several weeks.

It imparts a reddish black hue to the skin of patients, which persists for several months. Clofazimine is also deposited in the intestine where it may cause segmental thickening leading to crampy pain and diarrhoea. Otherwise, it is remarkably free of toxicity.

In the dose of 100 mg. three times a day, it is of great value in lepra reactions because of its simultaneous bactericidal and anti-inflammatory actions. It can effectively relieve the agonizing pain in lepra reactions in tuberculoid leprosy. It is also claimed that the drug enhances the ability of human macrophages to kill listeria.

New drug regimens: The currently available drugs for the treatment of leprosy can be arranged in decreasing order of *in vitro* bactericidal activity as: rifampicin, **ofloxacin/pefloxacin** (400 mg/day), **minocycline** (100 mg/day), **clarithromycin,** ethionamide/protheonamide, clofazimine and DDS. Studies indicate that 100 mg. of minocycline with 500 mg. of clarithromycin given daily produces beneficial effects. Such regimens are particularly useful in patients allergic to sulfones and those with resistant infection.

Chaulmoogra and Hydnoarpus oils, used previously, are now of historical interest.

Management of Leprosy

Leprosy, which was once considered to be an incurable disease can now be cured completely. As in the case of tuberculosis, the main difficulty in the treatment of leprosy is in persuading the patient to continue the drug therapy regularly for a prolonged period. In many countries adequate facilities are still not available for detecting, treating and following such cases in various villages. The medical treatment of leprosy can be wholly undertaken by practitioners or by trained medical auxilliaries in the majority of patients. Some knowledge about the natural history of the disease, details about the drug therapy and a sympathetic outlook towards the patient are all that is necessary for managing the patients.

The disease is transmitted by prolonged and intimate contact with untreated, open lepromatous patients whose cutaneous lesions and mucosal discharges teem with leprosy bacilli. The multiplication time of *M. tuberculosis* is 18 hours whereas that of *M. leprae* is 12 days. Therefore, rifampicin has to be given twice a week in tuberculosis whereas in leprosy even once a month administration is effective. *A single dose of 600 mg rifampicin kills over 95% of lepra bacilli within 4 days and hence there is no public health problem after 4 days in such patients.*

Majority of the patients can be treated as outdoor patients, in mobile clinics or in primary health centres. Only a few may need hospitalization. Segregation must not be advocated very loosely as this would cause social disruption and considerable psychological trauma, particularly in a society ridden with prejudices and traditions where a patient may be outcast for life and made miserable. Usually, the patients developing reactions during drug therapy and those with impending eye or nerve damage need hospitalization. Isolation is indicated in patients with LL who are untreated or in whom treatment has lapsed; these are the patients whose skin lesions and mucosal discharges teem with leprosy bacilli. Such patients can be rapidly rendered non-infectious by using rifampicin. There is no danger in admitting other forms of leprosy patients to general hospital wards if simple principles of barrier nursing are observed and routine hygienic precautions are strictly followed.

Choice and duration of therapy: Although approximately 99.9% of leprosy bacilli are killed in about 3-4 months by dapsone or clofazimine given daily and within 3-7 days by rifampicin adminstered in a single dose of 600-1000 mg., it is known that some bacilli may still persist for a long time, despite the bactericidal concentrations of an anti-leprosy drug. This is probably so because, though drug sensitive, the bacilli are not metabolically active.These **persisters** may cause relapse over 3-30 years. So far, no drug given alone can eliminate all "persisting" *M. leprae.* Hence, as in TB, combinations of drugs are recommended in order to:

- ***Prevent drug resistance to monotherapy.***
- ***Eliminate persisting organisms***; and
- ***Reduce the required duration of effective therapy.***

Rifampicin, dapsone and clofazimine are the first line drugs in leprosy. All patients should receive a multidrug combination **(MDT)** *as recommended by WHO (Table 53.2). Tuberculosis must be excluded before starting monthly rifampicin.*

For low body weight (less than 35 kg) **multibacillary** patient rifampicin is given 450 mg. single dose monthly and dapsone in the dose of 50 mg. daily. Similar doses are used for adolescents. It is recommended that MDT be given for 1 year and be continued, when possible, upto smear negativity in LL cases. In case clofazimine is not acceptable because of its skin pigmentation, ethionamide in the dose of 250 mg. daily plus INH 300 mg. daily (self-administered) may be given. Alternatively, minocycline 100 mg daily or ofloxacin 400 mg daily may be substituted for clofazimine.

Table 53.2 : WHO recommended regimen for leprosy

Leprosy type	Drugs	Duration
Tuberculoid (pauci-bacillary)	Dapsone 100 mg/d, unsupervised + Rifampicin 600 mg monthly (supervised)	6 months
Lepromatous (multi-bacillary)	Dapsone 100 mg/d + clofazimine 50 mg/d (unsupervised) and + rifampicin 600 mg clofazimine 300 mg monthly (supervised)	12 months

In case of **paucibacillary** leprosy (tuberculoid and indeterminate), WHO recommends rifampicin 600 mg. once a month (supervised) and dapsone 100 mg. daily (self administered), for six months. Indian experience, however, suggests that for the best results, the duration of dapsone therapy should be extended to 12 months. In all cases, the maximum dosage of dapsone should be used from the start and need not be reduced during lepra reaction.

Doses recommended in children are given in Table 53.3.

Table 53.3 : Suggested doses for leprosy in children

Drug	Age: 10-14 yrs	Age: < 10 yrs
Dapsone	50 mg/day	25 mg/day
Rifampicin	450 mg/monthly (supervised)	300 mg/monthly (supervised)
Clofazimine	150 mg/monthly supervised and 50 mg on alternate days (unsupervised)	100 mg/monthly supervised; and 50 mg twice a week unsupervised

WHO recommends one time dose for treating a single skin lesion of paucibacillary leprosy, using rifampicin 600 mg + ofloxacin 400 mg + minocycline 100 mg, all taken together (ROM therapy). Smaller doses are used in children. *Other experts do not recommend such a single dose regimen* but advocate more intensive and prolonged regimens (daily dapsone and daily R) in all patients with leprosy.

Since leprosy is exacerbated during pregnancy it is important to continue the treatment with dapsone, rifampicin and clofazimine.

It must be pointed out that the above mentioned MDT may be beyond the reach of many of patients in developing countries. Hence, DDS in the dose of 100 mg. daily may be the only drug available **for mass use**. *Prolonged dapsone monotherapy for 1-2 years is claimed to be curative in almost 80% of TL cases.* Dapsone, if used alone, should be continued for 2-3 years after the disease becomes inactive. In LL (which takes 2-6 years to become inactive) dapsone should be continued for 10 years after the disease becomes inactive. If, at this stage, the lepromin test is positive (indicating the presence of normal CMI), dapsone may be discontinued. If it is negative, dapsone must be continued lifelong.

The disease is considered inactive when during a 12 month period:

- ***The disease is clinically inactive.***
- ***No acid fast bacilli are demonstrated by the slit-and-scrape samplings from the skin sites;*** and
- ***Skin biopsies are negative for acid-fast bacilli.***

Clinical activity in **tuberculoid leprosy** is denoted by:

(a) Increase in the size of previous lesions or the appearance of new ones.

(b) Persistence of erythema or infiltration in the lesions.

(c) Progressive sensory impairment and motor loss; and

(d) Continuation or worsening of local tenderness of peripheral nerves.

In **lepromatous leprosy,** clinical activity is indicated by (a) continued presence of hypopigmented macules or nodules; and (b) tenderness on peripheral nerves.

All patients should be periodically tested for sensory and motor nerve involvement in all four limbs. Prednisolone (20-40 mg/day) should be added to the specific chemotherapy promptly on suspicion of sensory or motor involvement. Prednisolone should be tapered over a period of 8-12 months.

Following drug therapy, early lesions disappear completely. Late cutaneous lesions in LL show atrophy, tissue paper like wrinkling and scarring. In TL, nerves already damaged may remain permanently thickened. Local treatment may be necessary for neuropathic ulcerations of the extremities, caused by repeated trauma to insensitive tissues.

Minocycline and a fluoroquinolone can be substituted in dapsone-resistant cases.

Prognosis with early drug therapy is excellent and recovery is almost complete without any residual damage. Mild anemia is not a contraindication to dapsone therapy. Dapsone may be used (along with hematinics) to treat a patient with hemoglobin less than 50 per cent.

Patients who show allergy to DDS may be desensitized. The drug should, however, be withdrawn completely if the rash recurs, and desensitization with lower doses be resumed.

Following adequate MDT, the tuberculoid or indeterminate leprosy rarely recurs and usually no treatment is necessary after the clinical cure. In case of lepromatous leprosy, patients should be followed up at regular intervals for detecting a possible recurrence. Impairment of nerve function can occur even during or after MDT, and needs to be monitored for 2-3 years.

Lepra reactions: The acute exacerbation that occurs during the course of leprosy is called lepra reaction, but they are usually precipitated by anxiety, malaria, acute infections and during treatment with sulfones.

Lepra reactions are of two types:

- ***Type I reaction***; and
- ***Type II reaction.***

In **type I reaction,** (Reversal Reaction) the existing lesions show increased erythema and swelling and tender peripheral nerves. Loss of nerve function may occur. The constitutional symptoms are not marked and often it leads to a decrease in the number of bacilli in the lesions. This type of reaction usually occurs in tuberculoid leprosy. The mechanism of type I reactions is thought to be delayed type of hypersensitivity; it occurs in patients with good CMI towards *M. leprae*. The treatment is mainly directed at controlling acute inflammation, reversing the eye and nerve damage.

Type II reaction occurs usually in about 20% of lepromatous leprosy and is characterised by **erythema nodosum leprosum** (ENL). The basic lesion is a vasculitis following deposition of (antigen + antibody) immune complexes. Suddenly, many crops of bright erythematous nodules and raised patches appear and the existing lesions become worse. These may be associated with fever, iritis, neuritis, arthritis orchitis and lymphadenitis. This is a more severe reaction than the first one. It is difficult to treat and can relapse.

Clofamizine and **prednisolone** are administered in both types of reactions: clofamizine is given in the dose of 100 mg tid for several days; and **prednisolone** in the dose of 40 mg/day x 2 weeks, 30mg/day x 2 weeks, 20 mg/day x 2 weeks, 10 mg/day x 2 weeks and then 5 mg/day. The treatment is continued for 3-12 months, depending on the severity of the reaction. The severe pain in lepra reaction in tuberculoid leprosy, arising from swollen nerves, responds well to clofazimine and prednisolone. The earlier the introduction of prednisolone, the more likely is it to prevent permanent nerve damage.

DPT is continued in full doses throughout both types of lepra reactions.

Thalidomide, a selective TNF alpha inhibitor (Chapter 76), in the dose of 400 mg daily, is very useful and even better than steroids for managing acute severe and chronic ENL. It causes dryness of mouth, constipation and diarrhoea. It is highly teratogenic and is *absolutely contraindicated in pregnancy.* In chronic ENL, thalidomide may have to be given for many years. *Severe type II reactions need prolonged treatment with prednisolone and thalidomide.*

Leprosy prophylaxis: It is advisable to avoid skin to skin contact with patients with LL with open lesions. Pus from ulcers is highly infectious. Airborne droplet infection is a distinct possibility and mechanical transmission by biting insects cannot be ruled out.

Antitubercular **BCG vaccine** has been shown to endow some protection against leprosy. Similarly, prophylactic dapsone at half the therapeutic dose is sometimes recommended in close contacts, particularly in children of leprotic mothers.

Chemotherapy of Malaria 54

The term 'Malaria' is coined from the Italian phrase 'mal aria', meaning 'bad air' The disease was very active in Rome for centuries, and at least four Popes are believed to have died from malaria. It is caused by parasitic protozoa of the genus *Plasmodium* and is characterised by fever with rigor, anemia and splenomegaly. The morbidity due to malaria in Asia and Africa has been greatly underestimated. Currently, it is estimated that nearly half a billion people in the world suffer from malaria, and more than a million die from malaria every year, most of them from the developing countries. Nearly 50% of the cases the world over are caused by *P. falciparum.* The widespread resistance of the anopheles mosquitoes to the economical insecticides such as DDT, and the increasing prevalence of drug resistance in *P.falciparum* makes the situation worse.

Life cycle of plasmodium : There are four major types of plasmodia which infect man :

- ***P. vivax.***
- ***P. falciparum.***
- ***P. ovale;*** and
- ***P. malariae.***

P. vivax causes benign tertian malaria which, though mild, has a tendency to relapse. *P. falciparum* infection results in malignant tertian malaria, a fulminating infection, which, if not treated promptly, may result in death; but the disease, once cured, has no tendency to relapse. In both these infections, the infected individual develops pyrexia with rigors every 3rd day, and hence the term 'tertian'. *P. ovale* and *P. malariae* infections are usually mild; the infected individual develops pyrexia every 4th day and hence, it is described as 'benign quartan'.

An individual is infected by malarial parasites through the bite of a female Anopheles mosquito. The disease can also be transmitted by transfusion of infected blood and from mother to the foetus by the passage of organisms across the placenta. The salivary glands of the infected female anopheles mosquito contain a large number of *sporozoites* and these are introduced into the blood stream of the host, namely man, during mosquito bite (Fig 54.1).

After the entry, the sporozoites develop further through various stages:

(1) Pre-erythrocytic Stage

(2) Erythrocytic Stage;

(3) Development of sexual forms.

In the **pre-erythrocytic stage,** sporozoites disappear rapidly from the circulation and invade the hepatic cells **(Hepatic cycle - Site I)**. The duration of the pre-eryhrocytic stage varies with the species of plasmodium. It is 5 to 7 days for *P. falciparum* and 8 days to several months for *P. vivax.* The host does not develop any symptoms during this phase. At the completion

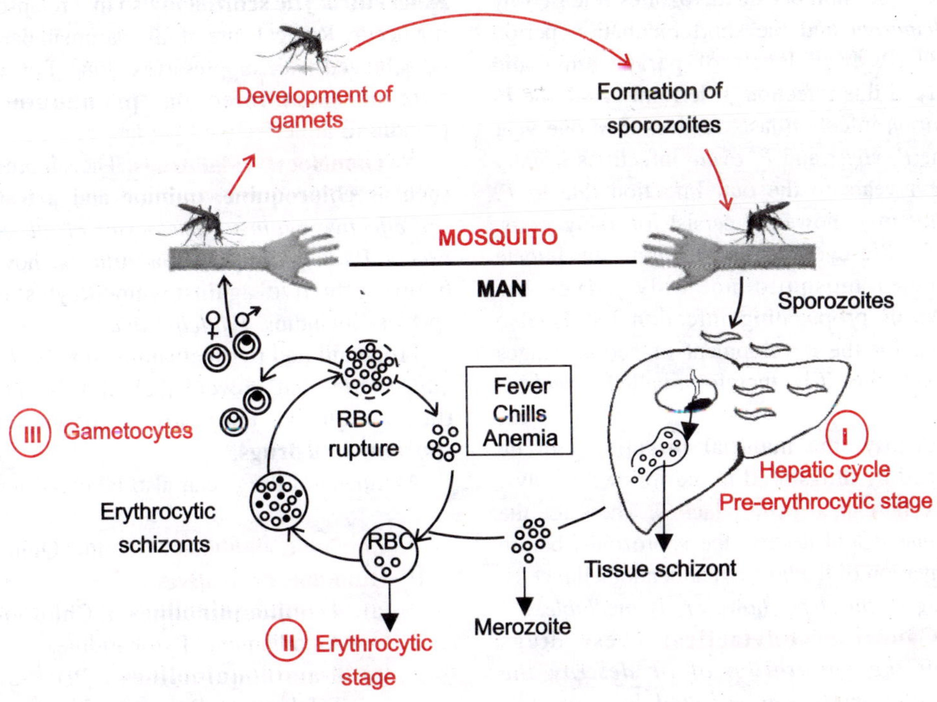

Fig. 54.1 : Life cycle of malarial parasite (*P.falciparum*)

of this phase, the infected reticuloendothelial cell, termed **tissue schizont** (*primary exo-erythrocyte form*) releases several thousand *merozoites* into the blood stream.

In the **erythrocytic stage (Site II),** merozoites invade the erythrocytes and undergo further development and multiplication, giving rise to **erythrocytic schizonts** (*asexual erythrocyte forms*). The infected RBCs eventually rupture, and release thousands of merozoites into the blood. This periodic release of merozoites from the infected erythrocytes is associated with paroxysms of fever with rigor. The merozoites thus released invade fresh erythrocytes, and the cycle of erythrocytic schizogony repeats.

Development of **sexual forms** starts with the differentiation of some of the released merozoites into **male (macro) and female (micro) gametocytes (Site III).** During a mosquito bite, these forms are sucked in from the peripheral blood and undergo further development into gametes in the mosquito gut. The female gamete is eventually fertilized by the motile male gamete to form a **zygote**. The zygote invades the gut wall of the mosquito to form an **oocyst.** The mature oocyst contains several thousands of sporozoites. After about 1 to 4 weeks, depending upon the species of plasmodium, the oocyst ruptures releasing **free sporozoites** which eventually reach the salivary glands of the mosquito and are ready to be injected in the man.

The above cycle in case of *P. falciparum*, terminates at this point. However *P vivax* and *P. ovale* differ from *P. falciparum* in that they have **persistent hepatic cycle** due to presence of **hypnozoites**, also known as latent tissue phase or **exo-eryhrocytic phase.** The delayed formation of tissue schizonts from such latent hypnozoites explains the relapses of *P. vivax* and *P. ovale* malaria. In case of *P. malariae*, the relapse may originate from erythrocytic forms remaining in the body for upto 30 years, there being no exoerythrocytic schizogony.

The larger number of merozoites released by *P. falciparum* and the short incubation period explain the high levels of parasitaemia and severity of this infection. If left untreated, the *P. falciparum* infection lasts for less than one year and the *P. vivax* and *P. ovale* infections usually take 3-4 years to die out. Infection due to *P. malariae* may, however, persist for many years.

In the life cycle of plasmodium, the female Anopheles mosquito not only serves the purpose of propagating infection but is also essential for the development of certain stages of the parasite. It is, therefore, called a **vector**.

Clinically, the malarial infection can be controlled by drugs used in the following ways:

I **True causal prophylactics:** These are the drugs that would destroy the sporozoites before their invasion of the host reticuloendothelial cells. *No drug of this type, however, is available.*

II **Causal prophylactics:** These drugs *prevent the maturation of or destroy the sporozoites within the infected hepatic cells (Site I) and prevent erythrocytic invasion.* They are also known as *primary tissue schizonticides*. **Primaquine, pyrimethamine and proguanil** act as causal prophylactics against *P. falciparum* but their efficacy against *P. vivax* is doubtful.

III **Suppressives:** These drugs (*schizonticides*) *inhibit erythrocytic schizogony (Site II) and prevent the rupture of the infected erythrocytes.* This leads to freedom from rigors and pyrexia (clinical cure). However, they do not necessarily eradicate the infection. The suppressive agents include **quinine, 4-aminoquinolines, mefloquine, artemisinin, proguanil, pyrimethamine and tetracycline.** Treatment with *suppressives can cure P. falciparum infection* as the parasite does not undergo secondary exoerythrocytic schizogony. Since these drugs do not affect the persistent tissue phase of *P. vivax* (**hypnozoites**) relapses can occur with the stoppage of suppressive therapy.

IV **Radical curatives:** This term refers to **eradication of both erythrocytic and secondary exoerythrocytic schizogony** so that relapse does not occur. Radical cure of falciparum malaria can be achieved with suppressives alone. For radical cure of vivax infection, **primaquine** and **proguanil** are effective (See later).

V **Gametocytocidal drugs:** The suppressives such as **chloroquine, quinine** and **artesunate** *are effective against gametocytes of all species except P.falciparum.* **Primaquine** is, however, highly effective against gametocytes of all species, including *P.falciparum.*

Proguanil and pyrimethamine *do not destroy gametocytes* but prevent their development in the mosquito. They are also known as **sporonticidal drugs.**

Antimalarial drugs can also be classified as :

I **Cinchona alkaloids :** Quinine, Quinidine

II **Quinoline derivatives :**

(a) **4-aminoquinolines :** Chloroquine, Amodiaquine, Pyronaridine.

(b) **8-aminoquinolines :** Primaquine, Tafeloquine, Bulaquine.

(c) **Quinoline methanol :** Mefloquine, Halofantrine, Lumefantrine.

III **Antifolates :**

(a) **Biguanides:** Proguanil.

(b) **Diaminopyrimidines :** Pyrimethamine.

(c) **Sulfonamides :** Sulfadoxine.

IV **Artemisinin compounds :** Artesunate, Artether, Artemether.

V **Antimicrobials:** Doxycycline, Clindamycin, Atovaquone.

Table 54.1 summarises the actions of the commonly used antimalarials.

Cinchona Alkaloids

QUININE is an alkaloid isolated from the bark of the cinchona tree, originally a native of Peru, South America, and known for many years as 'Jesuit's bark'. Quinine, the oldest of all the therapeutic agents used to treat malaria is still useful in the treatment of cerebral malaria and chloroquine-resistant *P. falciparum* infection.

Table 54.1: Actions of commonly used drugs on the life cycle of the malarial parasites

Drug	Hepatic phase	Erythrocytic phase		Latent tissue phase (responsible for relapse)	Development of gametocytes in the mosquito (sporonticidal action)
		Asexual parasites	Sexual forms (gametocytes)		
Quinine	No action	Fast action	Active against *P. vivax* and *P. malariae.* No direct action on *P. falciparum*	No action	No action
Chloroquine Amodiaquine	No action	Fast action	As quinine	No action	No action
Primaquine	Active and can be used for prophylaxis	Weakly active	Direct and fast action on all species but particularly *P. falciparum*	Highly active	Highly active
Proguanil	Active particularly on *P. falciparum*	Active but relatively *slow*	No direct action	No action	Highly active
Pyrimethamine	As proguanil	As proguanil	No evidence of direct action	Some action on *P. vivax*	Little evidence
Sulfones and Sulfonamides	Possible action	Action slow	As pyrimethamine	Little evidence	——
Mefloquine	No action	Marked but slow	As quinine	No action	No action
Artesunate	No action	Fastest acting	Acting against *P.vivax*	No action	No action
Atovaquone	No	More active than chloroquine	No	No	No

Pharmacological actions :

• ***Antimalarial action*** : Quinine is schizonticidal and, therefore, useful only as a suppressive. *It is also gametocidal against all species except P.falciparian.* It has no effect on the sporozoites, the pre-erythrocytic stage and the persistent tissue forms.

Mechanism of action of quinine is like that of chloroquine (see later) but as the drug is not extensively concentrated in the parasites, other mechanisms may also be involved.

• ***Local irritant action*:** Quinine has been termed as a 'general protoplasmic poison'. It depresses a variety of enzymatic processes, reduces ciliary activity, and inhibits phagocytosis and the growth of fibroblasts. Quinine also causes pain, edema, and reactive fibrosis. Sterile injection abscesses and venous thrombosis may occur after its IM and IV use respectively.

• ***GI tract*:** Quinine has an intensely bitter taste and can cause nausea, vomiting and epigastric pain.

• ***Cardiovascular actions*:** Like quinidine, another cinchona alkaloid, quinine directly depresses the myocardium, reduces its excitability and conductivity and lengthens the refractory period. Quinine IV can produce profound hypotension due to depression of the myocardium and dilatation of the arterioles.

• ***Miscellaneous actions*:** It has a mild analgesic and antipyretic activity. It stimulates the uterine smooth muscle. However, in the doses in which it is used in malaria, it causes hardly any adverse effects on the pregnant uterus. It has a curarimimetic action on the skeletal muscles.

Absorption, fate and excretion: Administered orally, it is almost completely and rapidly absorbed from the small intestine; and the peak plasma levels are reached within 1 to 3 hours after a single dose. It readily crosses the placental barrier.

Quinine is mainly metabolized in the liver. Its plasma $t^1/_2$ is about 10 hours but it is usually prolonged in the acute stage of falciparum infection because of hepatic impairment. Approximately 5 per cent of the total dose appears in urine unchanged.

Adverse reactions: The major reason for the decline in popularity of quinine is its toxicity. The salient toxic manifestations are:

• ***Cinchonism*:** This syndrome, which occurs when quinine is administered in full doses for a long time, resembles salicylism. When mild, the symptoms consist of ringing in the ears, nausea, headache and visual impairment. With large doses, tinnitus, deafness, vertigo, blurred vision, disturbances of colour vision and photophobia appear. Toxic amblyopia occasionally leading to total blindness has been rarely reported. With severe intoxication, skin rashes, headache, fever, vomiting, confusion and delirium are seen. As the poisoning progresses, the skin becomes cold and cyanotic, the respiration is depressed, BP falls, and eventually death occurs due to respiratory arrest. Even if the patient recovers, visual and auditory impairment may not be entirely corrected.

The treatment of quinine poisoning is essentially symptomatic.

• ***Idiosyncrasy*:** The idiosyncratic manifestations are similar to those seen with cinchonism but occur with a therapeutic dose of the drug. The commonest manifestation is intense flushing accompanied by generalized pruritus. Quinine may precipitate angioneurotic edema or asthmatic attacks in sensitive individuals. Rarely, it causes thrombocytopenic purpura, hemolytic anemia and agranulocytosis.

• ***Cardiovascular toxicity*:** Like quinidine, quinine is a myocardial depressant and can cause cardiac arrest when given IV.

• ***Black water fever*:** This condition, characterised by acute intravascular hemolysis, hemoglobinuria and fever and sometimes progressing to acute renal failure, is encountered with chronic *P. falciparum* malaria. Focal hepatic necrosis may develop in severe cases. Blackwater fever may occur during the natural course of malaria, and is often triggered by quinine treatment. It is probable that the reaction has immunological basis and is caused by a state of hypersensitivity attributable to the presence of incompletely suppressed falciparum infection. It is important to continue appropriate antimalarial therapy in such a patient. Fresh blood transfusion to maintain hematocrit above 20% may be necessary. The fluid and electrolyte imbalance, should be corrected along with treatment of hypotension and shock. *Alkalinization of urine and use of glucocorticoids are controversial.* Further management is that of oliguria or established renal failure, when present. Later, the patient should be evaluated for his G6PD status.

- ***Hypoglycemia*:** Quinine can cause hypoglycemia by releasing insulin from the pancreatic beta cells.
- ***Miscellaneous*:** Quinine IV may cause convulsions.

Preparations and dosage:

(i) Quinine sulfate (Quinarsol, Quininga) tablet 300 mg. Dose : 300 to 600 mg.

(ii) Quinine hydrochloride tablet 300 mg. Dose: 300 to 600 mg.

(iii) Quinine sulfate injection (Quininga, Rubiquin) contains 300 mg. of the salt per ml. It can be administered by IV infusion or by deep IM route. Dose: 300 to 600 mg.

Therapeutic uses:

- ***Malaria*:** It is an important drug for treating severe falciparum infection (see later).
- ***Myotonia congenita*:** This hereditary myopathy, characterised by tonic spasm of skeletal muscles, is often benefited by 300 to 600 mg. of quinine hydrochloride given twice or thrice daily by mouth. Other myopathies characterised by wasting and weakness of skeletal muscles do not respond to quinine.
- ***Cramps*:** The drug has been used in the dose of 200 to 300 mg. before retiring to prevent nocturnal muscle cramps.

4-Aminoquinolines

The 4-aminoquinolines constitute the mainstay of suppressive therapy of malaria. In addition, they are useful in a variety of other conditions. The therapeutically useful compounds of this class are **chloroquine, hydroxychloroquine** and **amodiaquine.**

CHLOROQUINE (Resochin, Lariago): This is the most frequently used compound and is used as the diphosphate salt.

Fig. 54.2: Chloroquine

Mechanism of action: Malarial parasites digest haemoglobin in their lysosomes to utilize amino acids. The released heme is highly toxic but is converted by the parasitic polymerase to nontoxic hemozoin. Chloroquine, being a basic drug, concentrates in the acidic lysosomes and binds to liberated heme. The heme-quinoline complexes get incorporated into the growing polymer chain interrupting the heme polymerization. Whether raised heme levels, heme-quinoline complexes or both exert cidal effects is yet unknown. But there is an oxidative damage to membranes, digestive proteases and other bio-molecules of parasites.

Pharmacological actions:

- ***Antimalarial activity*:** Chloroquine kills the erythrocytic forms of *P. vivax* and ”*P. falciparum*. It is also effective against the gametocytes of *P. vivax, P. ovale* and ”*P. malariae*. It, however, has no effect on the sporozoites, the pre-erythrocytic stage and the persistent tissue forms. As a suppressive, chloroquine is superior to quinine.

Resistance to chloroquine by *P. falciparum* develops in endemic areas. It is due to an efflux mechanism by which the parasite pumps the drug out of the cell. Such organisms exhibit cross-resistance to other 4-aminoquinolines.

Chloroquine and amodiaquine are considered safe antimalarials during pregnancy.

- ***Other antiparasitic actions***: In addition to its activity against plasmodia, the drug is effective in giardiasis, taeniasis and extraintestinal amoebiasis.

- ***CVS***: Like quinine, chloroquine also has a depressant effect on the myocardium and may exert a direct relaxant effect on vascular smooth muscles when given in sufficiently large doses.

- ***Miscellaneous actions***: It has some anti-inflammatory, antithistaminic and local anaesthetic activities.

Absorption, fate and excretion: Chloroquine is rapidly and almost completely absorbed from the intestinal tract. Effective plasma concentration is attained within 2-3 hours of oral dose and within 15 minutes of IM administration. Approximately 55 per cent of the drug in plasma is protein bound. It is highly concentrated in the liver, spleen, kidney, lung and leucocytes. The brain and the spinal cord levels, however, are only 10 to 30 times the plasma levels. Because of its high volume of distribution, a loading dose is necessary to initiate therapy. Because of its affinity for the tissue proteins, the drug persists in the body for a considerable time after discontinuation of medication.

Chloroquine is metabolized in the liver to the active metabolite 4-hydroxychloroquine. Acidification of urine hastens its renal excretion.

Adverse reactions: Chloroquine used as an antimalarial is a relatively safe drug. Commonly it causes nausea and vomiting. The drug, however, may produce serious toxicity when used in large doses for prolonged periods. The important toxic manifestations are:

- ***Intolerance***: Skin rashes with or without pruritus, angioneurotic edema, photosensitivity, pigmentation and even exfoliative dermatitis have been reported. Long term treatment may lead to bleaching of the scalp hair, eyebrows and eyelashes. Rarely, thrombocytopenia, and pancytopenia may occur.

- ***Eye***: Ocular complications have become commoner with the high dosage, prolonged chloroquine therapy of rheumatoid arthritis, discoid lupus and lupus erythematosus. *They are very rare during the treatment of malaria.* Temporary loss of accommodation with blurring of vision or diplopia may develop during therapy. Difficulties in focussing eyes have been reported in pilots taking chloroquine prophylactically. This phenomenon is reversible on discontinuation of the treatment. Lenticular opacities and posterior subcapsular cataracts have been reported. The retinal changes (*retinopathy),* consist of constriction of the retinal arteries, edema and abnormal blue-black pigmentation of the retina and depigmentation of the macula accompanied by macular degeneration. The field of vision is constricted and scotomata may appear. These changes are not reversible and need immediate discontinuation of the treatment. Because of its prolonged sojourn in the body, the ocular changes may appear even a few years after discontinuation of chloroquine. *It is recommended, therefore, that any patient on long term chloroquine therapy (as in RA) should undergo periodic ophthalmoscopic examination.*

- ***Central Nervous System***: Insomnia and transient depression are common. Acute psychotic episodes, seizures and, rarely, neuromyopathy may occur. Ototoxicity has also been reported.

- ***Cardiovascular System***: Abnormalities of ST segment and T waves may be seen during chloroquine therapy. *Chloroquine IV can cause abrupt fall in blood pressure and cardiac arrest especially in children, and also convulsions.*

Preparations and dosasge:

(i) Chloroquine phosphate tablet 250 mg. (150 mg. of the base). Dose: as a suppressive in acute attack : initial dose : 1 g. followed by 0.5 g. after 6 hours and 0.5 g. daily thereafter for 2 days followed by 0.5g once a week for 3 months: For prophylaxis in an individual who is going into an endemic area, 0.5 g. weekly.

(ii)* Chloroquine sulfate tablet contains 150 mg. of chloroquine base. Dosage: same as above.

(iii) Chloroquine injection contains

chloroquine phosphate or sulfate equivalent to 40 mg. of the base per ml. Dose: 200 to 300 mg. of the base IM, divided between two injection sites, or IV, slowly, diluted with 100 ml. of glucose saline. The total parenteral dose within 24 hours should not exceed 900 mg. of the base.

Therapeutic uses:

- ***Malaria***: It is still the first line of treatment for *P.vivax* malaria and uncomplicated falciparum malaria due to sensitive strains. (See later).
- ***Hepatic amoebiasis***: Chapter 55.
- ***Giardiasis***: Although chloroquinc phosphate, mepacrine and amodiaquine are effective in this condition, metronidazole is preferred (Chapter 56).
- ***Clonorchis sinensis (Chinese liver fluke) infestation***: Chloroquine phosphate, 250 mg. daily, is given for 6 weeks.
- ***Rheumatoid arthritis***: Chapter 71.
- ***Discoid lupus and disseminated lupus erythematosus***: Chloroquine is useful only in the milder forms of this disease and as a supplementary therapy to glucocorticoids in severely ill patients in whom the dose of adrenocortical steroids cannot be safely increased further. The arthritic and the cutaneous lesions improve markedly with chloroquine therapy. Chloroquine phosphate is given in the dose of 250 to 500 mg. daily for 1 to 4 weeks or until a clear response is obtained. The dose is then reduced to a maximum of 250 mg. and maintained subsequently.
- ***Miscellaneous***: In lepra reaction (Chapter 53).

HYDROXYCHLOROQUINE: This drug is less toxic than chloroquine, and has similar properties and uses as chloroquine.

AMODIAQUINE (Camoquin): This drug is as effective as chloroquine, in a single oral dose. Its pharmacological actions are similar to those of chloroquine. It is rapidly absorbed and is highly concentrated in the liver and the spleen. It is largely (95%) metabolized in the body. The adverse effects reported include GI disturbances, headache, photosensitivity reactions and rarely, agranulocytosis.

Amodiaquine tablet contains 250 mg. of the salt. Dose : as a suppressive in an acute attack of malaria : 0.5 to 0.75 g. (0.4 to 0.6 g. of the base) on the first day and then 2 tablets daily for two days. *P. falciparum* strains resistant to chloroquine may still be sensitive to amodiaquine. However, *it is not recommended for prophylactic (chronic suppressive) therapy* because of possible hepatitis and agranulocytosis.

Amopyroquine has similar properties as amodiaquine but can also be given parenterally.

Pyronaridine, structurally related to amodiaquine, is a promising new anti-malarial developed in China and can be given orally as well as parenterally. It has good schizontocidal activity against *P. falciparum* and *P. vivax* and is effective against chloroquine-resistant malaria. The drug needs further evaluation.

8-Aminoquinolines

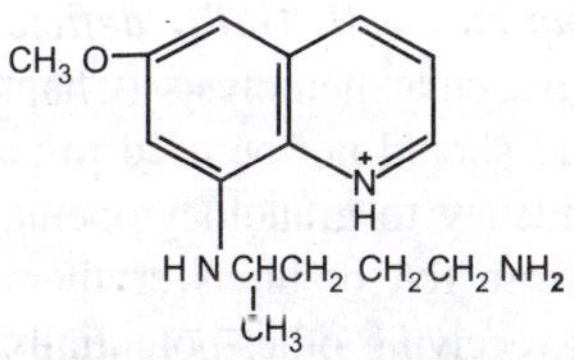

CH_3O — $\overset{+}{N}H$ — $HN\,\underset{CH_3}{CH}CH_2\,CH_2CH_2\,NH_2$

Fig. 54.3 : Primaquine

PRIMAQUINE : This drug is effective against:

- ***The persistent tissue forms of P. vivax;*** and
- ***The pre-erythrocytic (hepatic) and sexual forms (gametocytes) of all species of human malarial parasites.***

Primaquine probably acts by generating toxic, reactive species and/or by interfering with electron transport in the parasite.

Following the administration of primaquine, only a proportion of gametocytes in the blood are destroyed, while the rest are rendered incapable of undergoing further maturation in the mosquito. The drug has a weak schizonticidal activity against *P. vivax* but exerts no effect on the schizonts of *P. falciparum.* It is, therefore, not effective as a suppressive but given along with a 4-aminoquinoline, it can produce radical cure in *P. vivax* infection. Significant *in vivo* resistance to primaquine has not been reported.

Absorption, fate and excretion: Given orally, it is rapidly and completely absorbed. It is concentrated in the liver; large amounts are also present in the lung, brain, heart and the skeletal muscle. It is rapidly metabolized in the liver, and the products excreted in the urine; only 1% of the drug is excreted unchanged.

Adverse reactions: At the recommended dosage, toxicity is not common. The adverse reactions are :

- ***Gastrointestinal*:** Epigastric distress and abdominal cramps can be minimised by taking the drug with or after food and by antacids.
- ***Hemopoietic*:** *Moderate doses* cause mild anemia and leucopenia; and *large doses* may cause methemoglobinemia, cyanosis and agranulocytosis.
- ***In patients with G6PD deficiency,*** it can cause intravascular hemolysis (Chapter 35).

The drug should not be used in patients who have a tendency to granulocytopenia e.g. those suffering from RA or lupus erythematosus and in patients receiving other potentially hemolytic drugs. Proguanil potentiates its toxicity.

Although it has not been established that primaquine is teratogenic in humans, its use should be postponed till after delivery. It can cause hemolysis in G6PD-deficient fetuses.

Preparations and dosage: Primaquine tablet contains 7.5 mg. of primaquine base. The dose for radical cure of vivax malaria is 15 mg. daily for 14 days given along with chloroquine 1 g. on the first day and 500 mg. daily for 2 days.

Bulaquine (Aablaquine) an analogue of primaquine, is claimed to be as effective as primaquine. The drug is under evaluation.

Tafenoquine is a new, long acting, potent, primaquine-like drug which achieves radical cure in 3 days. It is under evaluation.

Quinoline Methanol

MEFLOQUINE (Lariam) is a quinoline methanol derivative. It probably acts like chloroquine. It:

- ***Acts on the erythrocytic stage.***
- ***Is highly effective in a single dose against P. falciparum including chloroquine resistant and MDR strains.***
- ***Can be given 12 hours after the last dose of quinine. However, because of long half life of mefloquine, quinine should not be administered after it as both are cardiotoxic.***
- ***Has no action on the persistant tissue forms.***

Given orally, mefloquine is rapidly and completely absorbed, is highly protein bound and is extensively distributed in the tissues. It is eliminated slowly in feces with a plasma t½ of about twenty days. The parasites can develop resistance to it.

Adverse reactions:

- ***GI tract:*** Mefloquine commonly causes dizziness, nausea, vomiting, diarrhoea or abdominal pain; these generally resolve without specific treatment.
- ***Neuropsychiatric disturbances:*** The most common of these are affective disorders, anxiety disorders, hallucinations and sleep disturbances. A single dose may cause lightheadedness and loss of concentration. Transient depressive feeling occurs more commonly with mefloquine than with chloroquine. Rarely, psychosis, toxic encephalopathy and convulsions have been reported. Patients treated a second time within a month after the first dose are at seven fold risk of adverse effects.
- ***CVS*:** Like chloroquine and halofantrine, mefloquine causes bradycardia and sinus arrhythmia. Patients who have recently received mefloquine should not receive halofantrine

which exaggerates the lengthening of QT interval.

● ***Teratogenicity*:** Mefloquine is teratogenic and should be avoided in the first trimester of pregnancy. However it may be used in the second and third trimesters. *If it is used in non-pregnant women of childbearing age, the patients should be advised to avoid pregnancy for three months after the treatment.* Women who are treated with mefloquine may continue breast-feeding.

● ***Miscellaneous*:** Allergic skin reactions, hepatitis and blood dyscrasias can occur.

Preparations and dosage: Mefloquine is available as 250 mg tablets. A single dose of 750 mg (15 mg/kg) orally is sufficient in most areas to treat uncomplicated malaria. However, in certain areas, the same dose may have to be repeated in 6 hours to ensure a cure. In the single dose of 1.5 gm, mefloquine is uniformly effective in curing multidrug resistant (MDR) malaria in almost 100% of patients. However, such a dose invariably causes severe nausea and vomiting. A second dose of 1 gm may have to be given to patients living in areas of mefloquine resistance.

Due to fear of the development of drug resistance, mefloquine is not used as a single drug for prophylaxis in endemic areas.

HALOFANTRINE (Halofan): This blood schizonticide is a phenanthrene methanol compound, discovered in the forties, but restudied nearly 40 years later. It is as effective as chloroquine against chloroquine sensitive strains of *P. falciparum.* It is also effective against strains resistant to chloroquine, pyrimethamine and quinine. The mechanism of action is like that of other quinolines.

Given orally, it is slowly and variably absorbed, peak concentration being reached 4-6 hours after ingestion. The drug should not be taken along with fatty foods. The plasma half-life of the parent compound is about 1-2 days, although the major N-desbutyl metabolite, with therapeutic activity, has a longer half-life of about 3-5 days. Unlike most antimalarials, the drug is palatable. It is administered in three doses of 500 mg. 6 hours apart, repeated after 1 week, if necessary. This regimen has a cure rate of greater than 90% in case of *P. falciparum* and *P. vivax.* It is also available for parenteral use.

Adverse reactions: These include nausea, vomiting, abdominal pain, diarrhoea and rise in liver enzymes. It's major disadvantge is that it causes prolongation of QT interval and even ventricular arrhythmias leading to death; *it should not be used in patients receiving quinine, chloroquine or quinidine, antidepressants and antipsychotics. It is not suitable for prophylaxis.*

Lumefantrine is structurally similar to quinine. Used in combination with artemether, it is well tolerated and efficacious in uncomplicated falciparum malaria, and is used where resistance to monotherapies is being experienced. It can be combined with mefloquine.

Acridine Derivatives

MEPACRINE : This suppressive drug, once used extensively in malaria, is now rarely recommended. Although not a drug of choice, it is sometimes used in giardiasis and in discoid lupus erythematosis.

Biguanides

PROGUANIL (Chloroguanide, Paludrine): The commonly used salt of this drug is proguanil hydrochloride.

Proguanil has negligible antiplasmodial action *in vitro.* Its antimalarial action *in vivo* is attributed to its conversion into a cyclic ring triazine metabolite (**cycloguanil**) in the human body. This compound binds to an enzyme dihydrofolate reductase, which converts folic acid to folinic acid, more strongly in the malarial parasite than in the human tissues. Deficiency of folinic acid prevents the completion of schizogony. As the sulfonamides prevent the conversion of PABA into folic acid, they synergize with the antimalarial effect of proguanil. It :

- ***Is an effective schizonticide against both P.vivax and P.falciparum;*** but its action is slower than that of 4-aminoquinolines.
- ***Is effective against the primary pre-erythrocytic forms of P.falciparum,*** and is useful in causal prophylaxis of falciparum malaria.
- ***Prevents the development of gametes encysted in the gut wall of the mosquito.*** It is, thus, valuable in sporonticidal prophylaxis; however
- ***Has no action against the persistent tissue forms of P.vivax.***

Although it is a biguanide derivative, proguanil has no hypoglycemic action.

West African strains of *P. falciparum* are usually *genetically resistant* to proguanil while all the varieties of plasmodia have been demonstrated to develop an *acquired resistance* to this agent. This is due to mutation in the parasite that leads to decreased drug binding at the active site.

Absorption, fate and excretion: Given orally, it is rapidly and adequately absorbed, mostly from the small intestine. Approximately 75 per cent is bound to proteins. The drug achieves a higher concentration within erythrocytes than in plasma. Its elimination is slow, mainly in the urine, with plasma t½ of 12-21 hours.

Adverse reactions: Proguanil is free from significant toxic effects when used in therapeutic doses. Gastrointestinal disturbances, stomatitis, and mouth ulcers may develop occasionally. A reduction in the leucocyte count and megaloblastic anemia may occur rarely.

Preparations and dosage : Proguanil hydrochloride tablets 100 mg. The base content of the salt is approximately 87 per cent.

Therapeutic uses:

It is not a drug of choice for controlling an acute attack. For causal prophylaxis, a dose of 100 to 200 mg. daily is used depending upon the sensitivity of the strain prevalent in the particular area.

Proguanil 100 mg in combination with atovaquone 250 mg **(Malarone)** is used to treat MDR falciparum malaria. The combination is generally well tolerated. For doses, see later. *The drug is considered safe during pregnancy.* It can be combined with folic acid 5 mg daily, which does not affect its efficacy.

Diaminopyrimidines

PYRIMETHAMINE (Daraprim): Like proguanil, it is selectively toxic to the malarial parasite by binding to its dihydrofolate reductase. It is more potent than proguanil.

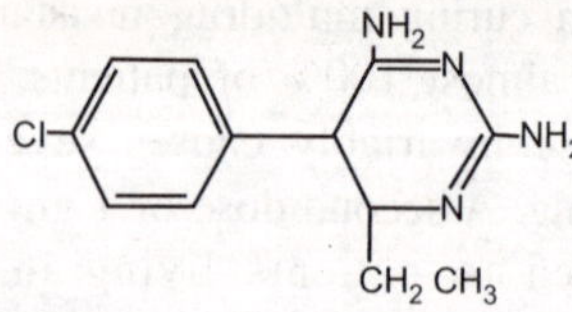

Fig. 54.4 : Pyrimethamine

Development of resistance to the drug *in vivo* has been reported and some degree of cross-resistance between pyrimethamine and proguanil can also occur. The antimalarial activity of the drug is enhanced by combination with sulfonamides. Chloroquine resistant strains of *P. falciparum* are frequently resistant to proguanil and pyrimethamine.

Unlike other antimalarials, it is tasteless and, therefore, suitable for children.

Absorption, fate and excretion: Pyrimethamine is completely but relatively slowly absorbed from the small intestine. It is extensively metabolized and slowly excreted by the kidney. Thus, following the administration of a single dose of 25 mg., pyrimethamine persists in the plasma and continues to be excreted in the urine for more than 14 days.

Adverse reactions: The drug is relatively safe. It can cause GI disturbances, ataxia and megaloblastic anemia, which responds to oral folic acid. Folic acid does not block its antimalarial activity. The drug appears to be safe in antimalarial doses during pregnancy.

Preparations and dosage : Pyrimethamine is dispensed as a 25 mg. tablet. For relief of an acute attack of *P. vivax* 50 mg. on the first day followed by 25 mg. daily for 2 days. However, given alone it is not the drug of choice for acute attacks. It is generally used in combination.

Pyrimethamine 25 mg. is available in combination with sulfadoxine (**Fansidar**, **Rimodar**) (dose 3 tablets once), and with sulfadimethopyrazine (500 mg) as **Metakelfin.** Combination of pyrimethamine 12.5 mg. with dapsone 100 mg. (**Maloprim**) is also available.

Therapeutic uses:

- ***Malaria***: See later.
- ***Toxoplasmosis***: It is used in the dose of 25 mg. twice a day, followed by 25 mg. once daily for one month, along with sulfadiazine 4 gm daily. A loading dose of 50-100 mg. of pyrimethamine may be used in the event of ocular complications (Chapter 56).
- ***Polycythemia vera.***

Trimethoprim has similar anti-malarial actions (anti-folate) as pyrimethamine but is much less potent. (Chapter 44).

SULFONAMIDES: Sulfonamides and sulfones have antimalarial activity similar to pyrimethamine, but their mechanism of action is different (see Chapter 44). They are effective against the asexual blood forms; their action, however, is too slow. When administered with pyrimethamine or proguanil (DHF-reductase inhibitors), these compounds potentiate the action of the former drugs. Hence, these combinations have been used against *P. falciparum* infection resistant to chloroquine or pyrimethamine.

A long acting sulfonamide such as **sulfadoxine** (half life 200 hours), is usually preferred.

Sulfonamide-containing combinations such as Fansidar are not recommended for prophylaxis because of Stevens-Johnson syndrome it is known to cause.

The sulfone, DDS, has been used in the dose of 25 mg. daily for 4 weeks from the 7th day of illness onwards, in combination with quinine/chloroquine/pyrimethamine, to prevent recrudescence in chloroquine-resistant falciparum malaria.

Artemisinin Compounds

ARTEMISININ: This is obtained from the Chinese plant *Artemisia annuta* (Qinghaosu, sweet worm wood) which has been used in China for the treatment of fever for almost 2000 years. Chemically, it is a sesquiterpene lactone endoperoxide. The drug is lipophilic and poorly soluble in water. Derivatives of artemisinin include **artesunate** (water soluble), **artether** and **artemether** (both lipid soluble).

Mechanism of action: Artemisinin and related compounds covalently bind to and damage the parasitic proteins by free radicals. The latter are generated by clevage of endoperoxide bridge in artemisinin by intraparasitic heme iron.

These act mainly as schizonticides against all malarial parasites, including those resistant to chloroquine and quinine. They have no effect on the hepatic stage. Recrudesence may occur.

They reduce parasitemia and gametocytemia rapidly and dramatically. They are also useful in cerebral malaria. So far, there is no evidence of high level resistance to this drug.

Orally, they are well absorbed and are metabolized to the active form, dihydro-artemisinin. The t½ of artesunate is about 23 minutes, while that of artemether is about 45 minutes. This is a disadvantage.

Adverse reactions: No serious adverse reactions have been reported. ADR include nausea, vomiting, abdominal pain, loss of appetite and leucopenia. Higher doses may produce bradycardia, prolongation PR and QT intervals and transient increase in SGOT/SGPT values. They are contraindicated during the first trimester of pregnancy, lactation, and in immunocompromised patients.

Preparations and dosage:

(i) Artesunate (Falcigo) is available as 50 mg tablets. For chloroquine resistant malaria and cerebral malaria, two doses of 100 mg are administered on the 1st day followed by 50 mg twice daily for 5 to 7 days.

Artesunate injection for IV/IM use contains 60 mg. It is administered in a dose of 120 mg on day one, followed by 60 mg 12 hours later; and 60 mg once daily for the next 4 days.

(ii) Artether (E-male) is a synthetic ethyl derivative of artemisinin. It is available for IM injection 150 mg. given once daily for 3 consecutive days. Children are given 3mg/kg. for three days.

(iii) Artemether (Paluther) is available as an injection containing 80 mg/ml in arachis oil. It is administered in a dose of 80 mg IM on first day followed by 80 mg daily for the next 5 days.

(iv) They are available as suppository.

Artemisinin and its derivatives are safe and effective alternative to quinine in the treatment of falciparum malaria. However, its use should be restricted to the treatment of MDR malaria. *It is now recommended that artemisinin derivatives should never be used alone but in combination with other drugs so as to prevent or slow down the development of drug resistance.* For use of artemether in schistosomiasias, see Chapter 58.

Antimicrobials

DOXYCYCLINE: This drug exerts a slow but potent action against the blood schizonts and the primary exo-erythrocytic forms of *P. falciparum,* including those resistant to chloroquine and proguanil. It is used in combination in resistant cases as resistance to tetracyclines is rare.

CLINDAMYCIN has also been found useful in combination with other drugs (see later).

ATOVAQUONE: This is a highly lipophilic, hydroxynaphthoquinone compound which has potent activity (in animal models) against *P.carini*, *Plasmodia* and *T.gondii.* It acts by selectively interfering with mitochondrial electron transport in susceptible parasites.

Its absorption after oral administration is slow and incomplete but is increased threefold by fatty foods. Its plasma t½ is 2-3 days and it is excreted, mostly unchanged, in feces.

Proguanil potentiates the antimalarial activity of atovaquone. Atovaquone + proguanil is useful as a prophylactic against. *P. falciparum* and in treating MDR malaria. The combination is active against the circulating parasites but not the hepatic stage of plasmodium. It is claimed to be more effective than mefloquine. Atovaquone is available as **Malarone**, containing atovaquone 250 mg + Proguanil 100 mg for adult use and atovaquone 62.5 mg + Proguanil 25 mg for pediatric use. For prophylaxis, the dose is one tablet daily taken with food. For treatment of MDR malaria, it is 4 tablets as a single dose for 3 consecutive doses. Tetracycline, rifampicin and metoclopramide decrease the efficacy of atovaquone.

When it is used as monotherapy, the parasites develop resistance to it rapidly, by genetic mutation.

Adverse reactions : These include fever, vomiting, anorexia, headache, diarrhea, dose related maculopapular rash, anemia and neutropenia.

Other Uses: In the oral dose of 750 mg. three times a day for 21 days, it is helpful in treating mild to moderate *P.carini* pneumonia in AIDS patients. In the treated AIDS patients, its adverse effects have been difficult to distinguish from the manifestations of the underlying disease. Its use in toxoplasmosis is considered experimental.

Table 54.2 shows the plasma t½ of the commonly used antimalarial drugs.

Table 54.2: Half-life of the commonly used antimalarial drugs

Drug	Half-life
Chloroquine and amodiaquine	3 weeks
Quinine	10-12 hours
Mefloquine	15-33 days
Pyrimethamine	80-100 hours
Primaquine	8.5 hours
Proguanil	12-21 hours
Sulfadoxine	100-200 days
Atovaquone	2-3 days
Tetracycline	5-10 hours

Management of Malaria

Prophylaxis: *When residents of a non-endemic area wish to travel to an endemic area,* anti-malarial drug(s) are recommended to prevent or suppress symptoms caused by malarial parasites. The choice depends on the likely strain of malarial parasites in the region and its known sensitivity pattern (Table 54.3). The therapy should be started before the start of the travel, continued during the travel in endemic area and even after departure from the area. Presumptive anti-relapse terminal prophylaxis to eliminate hepatic forms of *P. vivax/P. ovale* is generally indicated only for persons who have had prolonged exposure in malaria-endemic areas.

All infants and children travelling to endemic areas need antimalarial prophylaxis. Chloroquine is the drug of choice. For areas with resistant strains, mefloquine is an option. To use doxycycline, the age of the child should be above 8 years and for atovaqone/proguanil, weight should be at least 5kg.

Ideally, pregnant women should be advised to avoid travel to endemic area. If it is not possible, chemoprophylaxis is given, which reduces the incidence of severe maternal anaemia and other adverse outcomes like abortion, still birth, prematurity, and low birth weight. Chloroquine remains the drug of choice for sensitive organisms, while mefloquine is currently the only medication recommended for chloroquine resistant organisms. Doxycycline is contraindicated and atovaquone/proguanil is not used because of insufficient safety data.

Very small amounts of chloroquine and mefloquine are excreted in the breast milk and hence can be given for prophylaxis in lactating women. Atovaquone/proguanil is not recommended. Limited data are available for doxycycline. Primaquine is given only after testing the infant for G6PD deficiency.

The traveler should also be urged to avoid contact with the night biting anopheles in the endemic area; the methods include covering exposed parts, netting over the bed, fitting window-screens, using insecticides and mosquito repellents.

Such chemoprophylaxis is not 100% effective; hence the diagnosis of malaria should be considered in a patient who has visited an endemic area and gets fever after returning home though he has received chemoprophylaxis.

Treatment of an acute attack: The diagnosis of malaria is confirmed by microscopy of stained thick and thin blood films. The intracytoplasmic parasites should be identified (if the species is uncertain, it should be considered to be *P.falciparum*) and counted. In severe malaria, the developmental stage of the parasite should be noted. The prognosis worsens with *P.falciparum* infection, higher parasitic counts and more mature parasites. Smear examination should be repeated every 12 hours in serious cases, for monitoring the efficacy of therapy. The initial treatment of acute malaria is the same irrespective of the species of parasite, unless the infection is severe and due to *P. falciparum,* particularly in children and in non-immune subjects. It is the follow up therapy of relapsing malaria that differs.

The drug regimens used in an acute clinical

Table 54.3: Drug regimens for malarial prophylaxis

Drug, dose, frequency	When to start before entering ende-mic area	How long to continue after leaving the area	Remarks
Chloroquine sensitive *P. falciparum and *P.vivax/P.ovale***			
Chloroquine (base) 300 mg OW	1 week	4 weeks	Choice for infants/ children/pregnant & lactating mothers
Proguanil 200 mg OD	2 days	4 weeks	
Chloroquine – resistant *P falciparum* and MDR strains**			
Mefloquine 250 mg OD	1 week	4 weeks	Same as above
Doxycycline 100 mg OD	1-2 days	4 weeks	Not in children< 8 yrs/ pregnant women.
Atovaquone 250 mg + proguanil 100 mg; one tablet OW***	1-2 days	7 days	Not in children < 5kg/ pregnant & lactating women.
Terminal prophylaxis to prevent relapse of *P. vivax/P. ovale*			
Primaquine 30 mg OD		14 days along with post-expo-sure prophy-lactics (or after its completion).	Not in pregnancy In infants & children, including those of lactating mothers, after ruling out G6PD deficiency

OD = once daily OW = once weekly

* If not tolerated in the recommended doses, mefloquine, doxycycline or atovaquone + proguanil can be given

** If the traveler cannot tolerate any of these regimens, Primaquine 30 mg 1-2 days before, throughout the stay and 7 days after leaving

*** Choice for mefloquin resistant malaria in Southeast Asia(Burma, China, Combodia, Vietnam)

attack of malaria with *P.vivax*, *P.ovale*, *P. malariae* and chloroquine susceptible *P.falciparum*, in adults, are shown in Table 54.4.

Quinine still remains a potent and reliable antimalarial drug. Further, children tolerate it well. However, it takes longer to exert the full effects and hence, chloroquine is generally preferred. It can be given orally as well as parenterally.

In case of severe *P. falciparum* infection, particularly in a non-immune individual, treatment must be immediate and IV quinine may be life-saving. Artemisinine suppositories can be used immediately at home before transferring the patient to the hospital.

Postural hypotension is common in uncomplicated malaria and is exacerbated by quinine and chloroquine. Febrile patients, both adults and children, should therefore be kept in the horizontal position. *Mothers should be advised that febrile babies should not be carried vertically, especially after any of the above drugs is given parenterally.*

In non-endemic areas, freedom from

Table 54.4: Treatment of chloroquine sensitive acute malaria

- ***In patients who can take orally*:**
  Chloroquine (base) 600 mg. followed 6 hours later by 300 mg. on day one; 300 mg. once daily on days two and three.
  OR
  Amodiaquine (base) 600 mg. followed by 200 mg. (base) on day one; 400 mg. once a day on days two and three.
  OR
  Quinine (salt) 300 mg. tablets, 6 tablets daily for three days, followed by 4 tablets daily for the next 5-10 days.
- ***In patients who cannot take orally*:**
  Chloroquine IM 2.5 mg./kg every 4 hours or 3.5 mg./kg. every 6 hours (total dose not to exceed 25 mg/kg. base).
  OR
  Chloroquine IV 10 mg./kg. base over 4 hours, followed by 5 mg./kg. base (given in a 2 hour infusion) every 12 hours (total dose not to exceed 25/mg./kg base).

NB: For *P.falciparum* infection, primaquine (gamatocytocidal) 0.75 mg/kg, given as a single dose on first day of treatment, is a must to prevent spread.

recrudescences of falciparum infection can be ensured by follow up treatment with 300 mg. (one tablet) of chloroquine, taken once a week for three months.

Most of these anti-malarial drugs are very bitter and hence, they may be given along with milk or fruit juice. Care must be taken to ensure that the patient swallows the tablets and does not vomit later. This can be helped by prior administration of prochlorperazine (Stemetil) or a similar antiemetic drug, if necessary. If vomiting occurs within 1 hour of drug ingestion, repeat the full dose of the drug; in the case of mefloquine repeat half the initial dose. If vomiting occurs after one hour, it is not necessary to repeat the drug.

Since latent exoerythrocytic forms persist in the liver in infections with *P. vivax* and *P. ovale,* **delayed true relapses** occur in the majority of patients. In such cases, radical cure can be obtained by primaquine in the dose of 7.5.-15 mg. daily for 14 days, started after treating the acute attack. In this dosage, the drug is generally well tolerated and hemolysis, if it occurs, is mild and self-limiting. In some cases, higher doses of primaquine (30 mg. daily for 14 days) may be needed; such regimen, however, needs supervision for possible adverse effects. *Primaquine used in a single dose of 45 mg. is also sufficient to destroy falciparum gametocytes which are not affected by chloroquine or quinine.* In pregnant women and infants, *chloroquine is given weekly for 3 months* to prevent relapse of *P. vivax or P. ovale infection.*

Cerebral malaria with pronounced CNS symptoms occurs as a complication of *P. falciparum* infection and carries high mortality. It needs emergency treatment including excellent nursing care and repeated monitoring. Quinine is administered in high dilution and by very slow IV infusion (see later). If there are no facilities for IV infusion, quinine can be given in the dose of 0.25-0.5 g. in 20 ml. glucose saline IV, over not less than 10 minutes by the clock. *More rapid injection may cause a fall in BP, cardiac arrhythmias and cardiac arrest* Alternatively, quinine can be given IM provided the solution is sterile and nearly neutral in reaction. Alternatives to quinine are parenteral artemether and arteether.

Severe and even fatal **hypoglycemia** has been reported in patients with cerebral malaria; this complication does not respond well to glucose by IV bolus and to glucagon. A somatostatin analogue octreotide which inhibits the stimulatory effect of quinine on the beta cells of the pancreas may be used.

Chloroquine is as good as quinine for susceptible *P. falciparum* infection and in severe cases it can be given IV or IM in similar way as quinine. The single average adult IV dose is 200-300 mg. of the base in a 5% solution.

Table 54.5: Dosage schedule for oral treatment of moderate and severe malaria in children

Drug	Dose, mg Upto 1 yr	1-3 yr	4-6 yr	7-11 yr	12-14 yr	Regimen
Quinine	100-200	200-300	300-500	500-1000	1000-2000	Daily dose to be divided into 3 parts and continued for 7 days
Chloroquine	75	150	300	300	400-600	i) Loading dose
(base) in mg	75	150	150	150	225-300	ii) Second-one follow 6 hours after first
	37	75	150	150	150-300	iii) One dose daily on day 2 & 3
Amodiaquine	50	100	150	200-300	400-600	i) Dose for first day
	50	50	300	50-200	250-400	ii) Daily dose for day 2 & 3
Sulfadoxine 500 + pyrimethamine 25 mg per tablet	½ tab	½ tab	1 tab	1 tab	2 tab	Single dose

Modified from: The Clinical Management of Acute Malaria, WHO Reg. Pub., South East Asia Series No. 9, New Delhi.

Intramuscular route, however, is safer and is preferred. It can be repeated upto a total of 900 mg. in 24 hours. In all these cases, oral therapy should be started as soon as possible.

Quinidine is as effective as quinine in the treatment of malaria. If quinine is not available, quinidine is an acceptable substitute for the emergency treatment. Doses and precautions are the same as with quinine.

Glucocorticoids, urea and mannitol which were used in the past to treat the cerebral edema of falciparum malaria, are of doubtful value and infact may have deleterious effects in these cases; they are better avoided.

Treatment of malaria in children is essentially similar to that in adults. Quinine is better tolerated by children but its parenteral use is associated with high toxicity. Chloroquine injection may cause convulsions in infants and small children, and should be avoided whenever possible. Relapsing vivax attacks in small children may be treated with pyrimethamine 12.5 mg. base once a week, between the attacks. Primaquine should be avoided in the neonates for fear of hemolysis. Mefloquine should not be used in children under 15 kg of weight. For details of dosages see Table 54.5.

Acute malaria in pregnant women can be treated with chloroquine or quinine in the usual doses. For chloroquine-resistant malaria, chloroquine + clindamycin combination is safe. Mefloquine is probably safe in the second and third trimesters and may be used when benefits outweigh the risk. Artemisinin has no deleterious effect on the fetus and can be considered, if the situation demands. However the data about its safety are inadequate. Associated anemia needs the administration of folic acid and iron. *Primaquine and tetracycline should be avoided.*

Malaria in G6PD deficient persons: Such patients should be treated with the usual doses of either chloroquine or quinine. If indicated, primaquine in the dose of 30-45 mg once a week for 4-8 weeks is an acceptable treatment in areas of milder variants of G6PD deficiency.

Chloroquine resistant malaria: Chloroquine resistant *P. falciparim* malaria is now widespread in many areas, including India.

Table 54.6: Treatment of chloroquine resistant malaria

- ***In patients who can take orally***

Quinine 600 mg tid + doxycycline 100 mg bid / clindamycin 10 mg/kg bid for 7 days.

OR

Sodium artesunate : 100 mg. orally 12 hourly on day one, then 50 mg. 12 hourly for 4 days.

OR

Mefloquine 750 mg orally, repeated after 6 hours.

OR

Atovaquone 250 mg + proguanil 100 mg combination, 4 tablets (single dose) daily for 3 days.

OR

Pyrimethamine-sulfadoxine 3 tablets (single dose), followed by quinine 600 mg orally tid for 2 days.

- ***In patients who cannot take orally***

Quinine hydrochloride by IV infusion: 20 mg/kg in 500 ml. of 5% dextrose-saline in 4 hours; followed by 10 mg./kg. infused over 2 hours, every 8 hours, until the patient is able to swallow and parasite density is <1%. Complete the therapy with oral quinine 600 mg tid till total therapy is of 7 days AND tetracycline 250 mg IM 6 hourly until patients start taking orally, followed by doxycycline 100 mg bid till total of 7 days.

OR

Artemether or arteether IM (see text).

Chloroquine resistance should be suspected.

- ***In all patients with a complication of malaria*** such as cerebral malaria, severe anemia, jaundice or renal failure.
- ***In any patient who has already received a full course of chloroquine within the last one month*** as that suggests the possibility of recrudescence from a resistance strain; and
- ***When hemoglobin continues to fall in the absence of bleeding, and asexual forms of the malarial parasite persist, along with symptoms, after 48 hours of treatment.*** The gametocytes may persist for several weeks after treatment and that does not represent failure of treatment.

Widespread development of parasitic resistance to chloroquine and fansidar in falciparum malaria in many countries necessitates the use of combination therapy as the first line treatment in this condition. Artemisinine-based combination therapy (ACT) is to be preferred. The major drawback of ACT is the cost. Table 54.6 shows the drug regimens used in the treatment of chloroquine resistant malaria.

Multidrug resistant (MDR) malaria is always to be treated with drug combinations (Table 54.7).

Table 54.7 : Currrently used antimalarial drug combinations for MDR falciparium malaria

Artesunate + SP/ mefloquine/amodiaquine*
Artemether + lumefantrin*
SP + chloroquine /amodiaquine/quinine/ mefloquine
Quinine + tetracycline/clindamycin
Atovaquone + proguanil
Chlorproguanil + dapsone
Sulfadoxine + pyrimethamine (SP)

*The combinations to which resistance has not been reported.

SP is always given as a single dose. All other drugs are given for 3 days, except quinine + tetracycline combination, which is given for 7 days.

Radical cure: Radical cure should be aimed at only in infections occurring in a nonendemic area. Such a patient should receive primaquine in the dose of 15 mg. of the base daily for 2 weeks. Simultaneously, he should continue to receive 300 mg. of the chloroquine base weekly for suppression of an overt attack. Such primaquine therapy is essential mainly in vivax malaria.

Recrudescence: Early recrudescence of malaria (within 28 days of mefloquine treatment) should not be treated by either mefloquine or halofantrine because of their enhanced cardiac toxicity. It should be treated with artemisinin.

Adjuvant therapy in malaria: Cerebral malaria sometimes causes coma and shock. Blood pressure should be maintained by IV fluids and dopamine. Management of coma is similar to that of coma due to other causes. However, in some cases, lumbar puncture to reduce intra-cranial tension may cause dramatic recovery. Convulsions are treated with parenteral diazepam.

Severe malaria can sometimes cause renal failure leading to oliguria, anuria and death due to uremia. In the initial stages, the osmotic diuretic mannitol may be useful. However, later hemodialysis or peritoneal dialysis can be life. It is also important to remember the possibility of such a complication, since administration of excess parenteral fluids during the period of unrecognized renal impairment can precipitate fatal pulmonary edema. Falciparum malaria can cause severe hypoglycemia; this should be remembered while treating such patients.

Chronic malaria is usually associated with iron deficiency anemia, which responds to oral iron therapy. In severe anemia, parenteral iron and even blood transfusion may be necessary.

Immunity in malaria: Development of partial immunity is recognized in *P. falciparum* infection. The immunity is basically humoral. Immune antibodies cross the placental barrier and confer passive immunity on the foetus, who is protected for some months after birth. The immunity operates against the erythrocytic stage, but is ineffective against other stages of the parasite. Immunity in malaria is not only species-specific, but to some extent also strain-specific. Thus, a person who has developed immunity to a *P. falciparum* strain in a particular area may get infected with a different strain when in another area. It is not absolute and diminishes when an immune adult moves for a year to a nonendemic area. The development of anti-malarial vaccine is still experimental.

Malaria eradication: This concept is based on the idea of completely eliminating the disease from a particular area so as to halt its transmission completely, at the same time, preventing the reintroduction of the disease from outside. Malaria eradication, therefore, envisages a vigorous attack on the parasites in human patients with the suppressive, causal prophylactic and radical curative drugs, along with eradication of the vector mosquitoes. The latter includes improving environmental hygiene, the use of various insecticides and larvicides such as synthetic pyrethroids, DDT and organo-phosphorous compounds.

Unfortunately, mosquitoes have developed resistance to the first highly effective, reasonably safe and cheap insecticide DDT.

Mosquito repellents: Highly effective, dependable and totally safe mosquito repellent is not yet available. It is extremely difficult to ensure 100 per cent protection from the hungry Anopheles mosquitoes. A simple remedy which acts as mosquito repellent by its smell has the following composition:

Cedar wood oil ..	18 ml.
Citronella oil ..	42 ml.
Spirit of camphor to ..	100 ml.

Citronella oil can also be applied in the form of vanishing cream. It is nonirritant, non-toxic, cheap and not so unpleasant. Probably more effective is a 35 per cent emulsion of dimethyl phthalate which acts as an irritant to insect's feet. It must be rubbed into every part, avoiding eyelids, lips and scrotum. Other agents used are ethohexadiol, butopyronoxyl, diethyl-toluamide (DEET), n-butyl acetanilide, picaridin and pyrethroid. These are also irritants and have an intensely bitter taste. Allergic reactions and bronchial spasm may occasionally develop with their use. Insecticide-(permethrin)-treated bed nets are also available for this purpose.

For antimosquito tablets and coils containing synthetic pyrethyroids, see Chapter 60.

Chemotherapy of Amoebiasis 55

Amoebiasis is an infectious disease caused by the protozoon, *Entamoeba histolytica*. The disease, though labelled as 'tropical', is not uncommon in temperate zones. It primarily affects the colon, but other organs like liver, lung and brain may get secondarily involved. The disease is characterised by gastrointestinal and constitutional symptoms and has a tendency to chronicity. Acute amoebic dysentery is associated with bloody, mucoid stools, abdominal pain and tenesmus. Chronic amoebiasis usually presents with vague symptoms like anorexia, abdominal pain and intermittent diarrhoea or constipation. There may be tenderness over the caecal region. Many infected persons, who pass the cystic forms of the protozoan in feces, however, may remain completely symptomless and act as 'carriers'.

E. histolytica usually lives as a harmless commensal in the lumen of human bowel, a state which might be termed **asymptomatic amoebiasis**. The parasite subsists on debris and bacteria and not on the tissues of its host. When it becomes a pathogen, the trophozoites become larger and hematophagous, having many erythrocytes in the endoplasm, and cause **invasive amoebiasis**. Invasion is mediated by the destruction of epithelial cells and killing of neutrophils and lymphocytes.

Intestinal amoebiasis results in ulceration of the colon. The regions involved in descending order of frequency are the caecum, the ascending colon and the rectosigmoidal area. In fatal cases, the entire colon and even the terminal portion of the ileum may be involved leading to acute necrotizing colitis and sometimes toxic megacolon. Amoebic involvement of the caecum and appendix may cause a clinical attack of appendicitis. A granulomatous lesion of the caecum giving rise to a lump in that region, known as **amoeboma**, may cause obstructive symptoms.

Life cycle of E. histolytica: *E. histolytica* exists in two forms :

- ***The trophozoites,*** present in the intestinal lumen and in infected tissues; and
- ***The cysts,*** which develop from the trophozoites within intestinal lumen.

The trophozoites with amoeboid movements are the active form. However, they die rapidly after elimination in the stool. The cysts represent a dormant stage and are resistant to freezing and partial drying and transmit infection from person to person.

Cysts are usually ingested following fecal contamination of water or food. Bad hygiene and insects like flies assist in the propagation of infection. In the intestine of the host, the cyst wall is weakened by the intestinal enzymes and the trophozoites released invade the wall of the colon and enteroportal circulation. The organism may then find its way to the liver and other tissues, giving rise to **extra-intestinal amoebiasis**.

The drugs used in chemotherapy of amoebiasis are :

I **Drugs used only in intestinal amoebiasis** (**Luminal amoebicides**): Halogenated oxyquinolines, Diloxanide furoate, Antibiotics and Kurchi.

II **Drugs used in both intestinal and extraintestinal amoebiasis** (**Tissue/mixed amoebicides**): Emetine, Dehydroemetine, Metronidazole, Tinidazole, Secnidazole.

III **Drugs used only in extraintestinal amoebiasis:** Chloroquine.

An alternative chemical classification is:

I **Emetine group** e.g. Emetine, Dehydroemetine and its resinate.

II **Imidazole derivatives :** Metronidazole, Tinidazole, Secnidazole.

III **Quinoline derivatives :**

- ***Halogenated hydroxyquinolines***: Diiodohydroxyquinoline, Iodochlorohydroxyquinoline.
- ***4-aminoquinolines***: Chloroquine.

IV **Antibiotics:** Tetracyclines, Paromomycin.

V **Miscellaneous:** Diloxanide furoate, Nitazoxanide and Kurchi.

Emetine Group

EMETINE: Emetine is an alkaloid obtained from ipecac, the root of the plant *Cephalis ipecacuanha*. The other alkaloid, cephaline, though amoebicidal, is too toxic for use.

Antiamoebic action: *In vitro,* emetine has a direct lethal effect on the trophozoites of *E. histolytica* in concentrations that can be achieved in the blood but probably not in the lumen of the bowel after parenteral therapeutic doses. It has, however, little effect on the cystic forms. The drug inhibits protein synthesis. Trophozoites affected by emetine show degeneration of the nucleus and reticulation of the cytoplasm. This arrests their multiplication and leads to their phagocytosis.

Absorption, fate and excretion: Emetine has a bitter taste and is absorbed from the gut but because of its irritant nature, it is administered by deep IM injection. The drug gets concentrated in the liver. Significant amounts are also present in the lung, kidney and spleen. Since the drug is slowly eliminated in urine, repeated injections can lead to cumulation.

Adverse reactions: The major drawback of emetine is its toxicity. The adverse reactions are:

- ***Local reaction***: These often appear when it is administered SC but are uncommon when the drug is given deep IM. It may cause local pain, tenderness, stiffness and weakness of the muscles, and rarely, an abscess.
- ***G I system***: Occurrence of nausea, vomiting, diarrhoea, headache, dizziness and prostration are common. Vomiting (hence the word "emetine") occurs both as a result of gastric irritation and stimulation of the CTZ.
- ***Cardiovascular system***: The important cardiotoxic effects of emetine are tachycardia, precordial pain, hypotension, myocarditis and pericarditis. The ECG offers an early index of cardiotoxicity. The changes include lowering and inversion of T-wave, deformation of ST segment and QRS complex, prolongation of PR and QT intervals, atrial tachycardia and premature beats.

It is advisable to confine the patient to bed during emetine therapy and to avoid undue exertion for three weeks thereafter. It is necessary to observe the pulse rate and BP during the therapy; ideally, an ECG should be taken before starting the therapy, repeated after the 5th dose and again after a week.

- ***Miscellaneous***: It may cause weakness, aching and tenderness of the muscles, especially those of neck and limbs. The weakness is probably because of its blocking action on the neuromuscular junction.

Emetine should be avoided in patients with cardiac or renal damage, in pregnant women, in old people and in young children.

Preparations and dosage:

(i) Emetine hydrochloride injection, 60 mg. of the salt per ml. Dose : 30 to 60 mg. daily by SC or deep IM injection.

(ii) Syrup of ipecac is the preferred agent for inducing emesis but *never the liquid extract of ipecac which is too potent.* Dose 30 ml. in adults.

Therapeutic uses:

(1) As a tissue amoebicide (see later).

(2) For the treatment of *Paragonimus westermanii* (lung fluke) and *Fasciola hepatica* infestations, (Chapter 58)

(3) Ipecacuanha syrup as an emetic (Chapter 40).

DEHYDROEMETINE: This semisynthetic drug, claimed to be less toxic than emetine, is preferred to emetine. Dehydroemetine injection contains 60 mg. of the drug per ml. Dose: 1 mg. per kg. IM daily for 5-7 days. Dehydroemetine resinate is a slow release preparation given orally. Dose : 50 mg. daily for 10 days.

Imidazole Derivatives

H—C—N
‖ C—CH_3
O_2N—C—N
|
CH2 CH2 OH

Fig. 55.1: Metronidazole

METRONIDAZOLE (Flagyl, Unimezol, Metrogyl) : Metronidazole, a nitroimidazole derivative, is the drug of choice in most forms of amoebiasis except in asymptomatic cyst passers. It is

- ***A potent amoebicide.***
- ***Effective in both intestinal and extra-intestinal amoebiasis;*** and
- ***Relatively less toxic and cost effective***

It is also highly effective against (1) anaerobic protozoa *(T. vaginalis, G. lamblia and Balantidium coli);* and (2) non-sporing, anaerobic, Gram positive and negative bacilli such as bacterioides, including the *B. fragiles* group, *Clostridium difficile* and *H. pylori.*

Metronidazole also has a radiosensitizing effect on hypoxic tumour cells.

Mechanism of action: The susceptible organisms carry electron transport components (ferredoxins) that donate electrons to metronidazole, which reduces the 5'-nitro group of metronidazole; the short lived intermediates of that reaction interact with the bacterial DNA with a lethal effect. It is not activated by the aerobes and therefore does not affect them. Resistance to metronidazole has been reported in *T. vaginalis* and *G. lamblia* but not in *E. histolytica* infection.

Absorption, fate and excretion: Metronidazole is rapidly and almost completely (80%) absorbed from the small bowel and very little reaches the colon. *It is, therefore, relatively ineffective in the asymptomatic cyst-passers and in chronic intestinal amoebiasis.* Food does not affect its bioavailability. Protein binding is 20% and except for placenta, the drug diffuses into all tissues. It also achieves concentrations lethal to the sensitive organisms in CSF, bile, bone and abscesses. It is metabolized mainly in the liver, into a relatively inactive acid metabolite; and a hydroxy metabolite active against anaerobes. Its t½ is 8 hours. The metabolites are excreted by the kidneys, imparting a red colour to urine. Renal insufficiency does not significantly alter its kinetics, but hepatic insufficiency prolongs its plasma t½. The drug is present in the milk.

Adverse reactions : These, as a rule, are mild and seldom necessitate discontinuation of therapy. They include :

- ***Common***: Marked nausea, anorexia, abdominal pain and metallic taste in the mouth.
- ***Less common***: Vomiting, diarrhoea, headache, stomatitis, cystitis, dizziness, vertigo, ataxia, urticaria, pruritus and flushing.
- ***Rare***: Peripheral neuropathy, seizures, ataxia and incoordination.
- ***Mild blood dyscrasia*** in the form of neutropenia, associated with the nitro group in the drug. It is reversible.
- ***Antabuse-like reactions*** on alcohol consumption (Chapter 6), during and for upto 3 days of metronidazole therapy.

Possible tumorigenic and mutagenic effects occur in experimental animals but are not observed in clinical practice.

Preparations and dosage:

(i) Tablets 200 and 400 mg for oral use.
(ii) Pediatric suspension 200 mg/5 ml.
(iii) Vaginal tablets containing 500 mg.
(iv) Rectal supposatories 1.0 and 1.5 g.
(v) Solution for IV use (Unimezol, Metrogyl) For doses, see text.

Therepeutic uses:

• ***Intestinal and hepatic amoebasis :*** It is a drug of choice (See later).

• ***Anaerobic infections***: Metronidazole is effective in chemoprophylaxis and treatment of infections due to nonsporing, Gram negative anaerobes (bacteroides) and has been used in combination with other antimicrobials in gynecological and colorectal surgery to reduce postoperative morbidity. Initially, it is given rectally as suppositories in the dose of 1 g. eight hourly until oral feeding begins. It is then administered orally in the dose 800 mg. initially, followed by 400 mg. 8 hourly for 7-10 days. If necessary, it can also be administered in the dose of 15 mg/kg followed by 7.5mg/kg by IV infusion 6-8 hourly. Each dose is infused over a period of 1 hour. In severe abdominal and pelvic sepsis. The combination of gentamicin with either metronidazole or clindamycin has been shown to be synergistic. It can also be used for surgical prophylaxis in the dose of 400 mg, 24 hours and 8 hours before surgery.

For use in pseudomembraneous colitus see Chapter 48.

It may be noted that anaerobes are implicated in a multitude of infections including those of gut, soft tissues, skin ulcers, abscesses of the lung and brain and in septicemia. Metronidazole is as effective as neomycin in hepatic encephalopathy.

• ***Ulcerative gingivitis*** (Vincent's stomatitis): The causative organisms are a spirochaete, *Treponema vincenti,* and Gram-negative bacilli, *Leptotrichia buccalis*. The preferred treatment is with penicillin G. Metronidazole orally in the dose of 200 mg thrice daily for 3-4 days is also useful. Tetracycline and clindamycin are other drugs used.

• ***H. pylori Infection*** ((Chapter 42)

• ***Trichomoniasis and other protozoal infections*** (Chapter 56).

• ***Dracunculosis***: (Chapter 58)

TINIDAZOLE (Tini): This analogue of metronidazole has a longer t½ (13 hours) and is probably better tolerated than metronidazole. In acute amoebic dysentery, it is given in the dose of 600-800 mg orally tid for 5 days or in the dose of 2g (50mg/kg in children) once daily for 3 days. In anaerobic infections, it is used orally in the dose of 2 g. initially, followed by 1 g daily (single dose) for 5-6 days. For surgical prophylaxis, it is administered in the dose of 2 g. once 12 hours before surgery.

SECNIDAZOLE (Secnil): This analogue of metronidazole has a longer t½ and similar uses. In acute amoebic dysentery, it is administered orally in a single dose of 2 gm. In children a single dose of 30 mg/kg is given orally. In hepatic amoebiasis, the dose of secnidazole is 1.5 g per day for five days. In giardiasis, the single oral doses are: 2 g in adults; 500 mg in children weighing 10-15 kg; 750 mg in children weighing 16-26 kg and 1g in those weighing over 26 kg.

ORNIDAZOLE (Ornizen) is a newer imidazole with similar properties as secnidazole. It is available as 500 mg tablets.

Quinoline Derivatives

Amongst these, **diiodohydroxyquinoline**, **iodochlorohydroxyquinoline** and **broxyquinoline** are halogenated hydroxyquinolines while **chloroquine** is a 4-aminoquinoline derivative. They act by direct contact with the trophozoites of *E. histolytica*. All the halogenated oxyquinolines also have some antibacterial and antifungal properties. The mechanism of action of halogenated oxyquinolines is unknown.

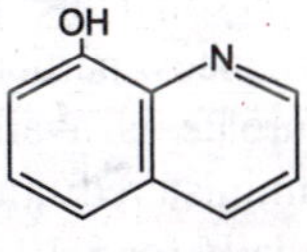

Fig. 55.2: Hydroxyquinoline nucleus

DIIODOHYDROXYQUINOLINE (Iodoquinol, Diodoquin): This halogenated quinoline (Fig. 55.2 and 55.3) is an effective luminal amoebicide, against both motile and cystic forms of the protozoan, more so against the former. Clearance of cysts is partially due to elimination of trophozoites. It is, however, not effective in extraintestinal amoebiasis.

Absorption, fate and excretion: Diiodohydroxyquinoline is insignificantly absorbed from the intestinal tract and 90% of it is excreted in feces.

Adverse reactions: These are mild and uncommon. The drug may occasionally cause headache, nausea, vomiting and diarrhoea. Chills, fever, skin eruptions and iodine dermatitis have been reported. It is contraindicated in patients with iodine intolerance.

Preparations and dosage: Di-iodohydroxyquinoline tablet 300 mg. Dose : 600 mg. thrice daily for 15 days. Another course may be given after 2 to 3 weeks. In infants, the drug is given in the daily dose of 50 to 100 mg. thrice daily; in children between 1 to 5 years, 150 to 300 mg. 2 or 3 times daily and in those between 6 to 12 years, 300 mg. thrice daily. Because of its relative insolubility in water, the drug cannot be given as a retention enema.

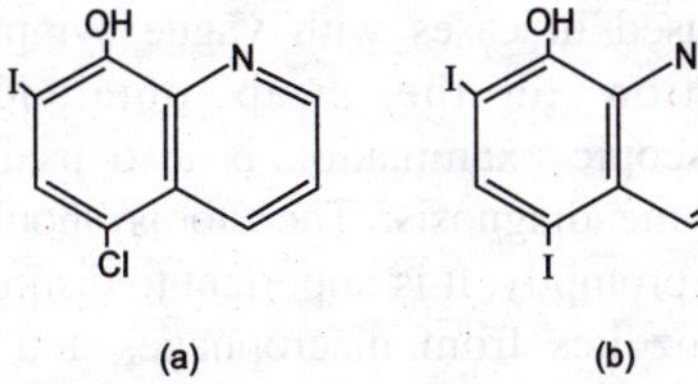

Fig. 55.3 : (a) Iodochlorohydroxyquinoline (b) Di-iodohydroxyquinoline

IODOCHLOROHYDROXYQUINOLINE (Quiniodochlor, Enteroquinol): This drug resembles di-iodohydroxyquinoline in anti-amoebic action. It is probably more useful in cyst carriers. It is not much absorbed from the GI tract and owes its antiamoebic action to a local effect. It also has antibacterial, antifungal and antitrichomonal actions.

Adverse reactions: These are usually mild and include diarrhoea or constipation, abdominal pain, anal pruritus and mild iodism. A neurological syndrome consisting of myelitis, peripheral neuritis and sometimes optic nerve involvement (Subacute Myelo-Optic Neuropathy-SMON) has been reported in patients receiving this drug over prolonged periods. These cases were mostly reported from Japan. *They are very rarely reported from other areas.* Early symptoms can improve following the stoppage of the drug. Usually, oral daily doses of upto 750 mg. for 10-12 days are considered relatively safe in adults. *Larger doses should be avoided.*

Preparations and dosage:

(i) Iodochlorohydroxyquinoline tablets 250 mg. Dose: 750 mg. daily in 3 divided doses for 10 days. The course may be repeated once after a week. It may be used along with emetine or alternated with other drugs.

(ii) Retention enema: It is prepared by suspending 2 g. of the drug in 200 ml of water. It is instilled on alternate nights 5 times.

(iii) Iodochlorohydroxyquinoline 3% cream for topical dermal use.

Therapeutic uses: Besides its use in luminal amoebiasis, it is also used topically in fungal infections of the skin. The major disadvantage of topical application is yellow staining of clothes and linen.

CHLOROQUINE: The pharmacology of chloroquine is discussed in Chapter 54. Given orally, it is completely absorbed and concentrated in the liver. It has a minimal effect in intestinal amoebiasis because of poor concentration in colonic lumen and wall. Its use in hepatic amoebiasis has declined following the availability of metronidazole.

Antiamoebic Antibiotics

TETRACYCLINE: The intestinal bacteria are essential for the production of intestinal amoebic lesions. They probably act by creating an environment congenial to the growth of amoebae, by manufacturing certain metabolites and vitamins on which the protozoa thrive, and by producing secondary infection. Tetracycline, though exhibiting an antiamoebic action *in vitro* in large doses, probably acts *in vivo* by altering the intestinal bacterial flora and creating a medium unfavourable for the growth of amoebae. It may be administered in the dose of 0.25 g. 6 hourly for 10-15 days, in combination with metronidazole to treat amoebic liver abscess particularly when bacterial co-infection is suspected.

PAROMOMYCIN (Aminocidin, Humatin): This aminoglycoside antibiotic (Chapter 46) given orally in the dose of 500mg tid for 10 days is effective as luminal amoebicide. It is also used in the treatment of leishmaniasis (Chapter 56).

Miscellaneous Agents

DILOXANIDE FUROATE (Furamide): This potent direct amoebicidal drug is mainly effective in chronic intestinal amoebiasis, in cyst passers and partially useful in mild acute cases. It is of no value in extra-intestinal amoebiasis.

Fig. 55.4 : Diloxanide Furoate

Given orally it is hydrolysed to diloxanide which is partly absorbed. Nonabsorbable portion acts as a luminal amoebicide. The drug is well tolerated, safe and almost non-toxic. The adverse effects reported are mild and include mainly GI disturbances, particularly flatulence.

Diloxanide furoate is available as 500 mg. tablets and is administered orally in the dose of 500 mg. 3 times daily for 5-10 days. As the drug is non-cumulative, a second course may be given immediately following the first course.

Nitazoxanide is a prodrug. After absorption, it gets converted to an active metabolite, tizoxanide, which is active against *E. histolytica.* Adverse effects are mild GI disturbances. It is given to children in the dose of 100-200 mg bid for 3 days. It also acts against, *Cryptosporidium parvum* and *G lamblia* (Chapter 56).

KURCHI: Kurchi consists of the dried stem bark of *Holarrhena antidysenterica.* Kurchi has mild antiamoebic activity and is useful only in mild intestinal amoebiasis. It may produce nausea and vomiting but is otherwise well tolerated. Powdered roots of this plant are used as a household remedy in India for ages for abdominal pain and diarrhoea.

Management of Amoebiasis

Amoebiasis, in general, is a difficult disease to treat because of its tendency to chronicity and the inability of various drugs to eradicate the cystic forms of the parasite completely.

The diagnosis of acute intestinal amoebiasis without demonstration of trophozoites in stools is rarely justified. This form is most readily found in diarrhoeal stools and a saline purgative may be used in cases with vague symptoms. Examination of the swab obtained on sigmoidoscopic examination is also useful in clinching the diagnosis. The stools should be examined promptly. It is important to distinguish the trophozoites from macrophages and even experts may find it difficult to identify an active amoeba as *E. histolytica* when it is seen without engulfed red blood cells.

Cysts are found in formed stools. However, the period of their formation varies in different individuals. A casual failure to identify cysts does not, therefore, exclude the presence of amoebiasis and repeated stool examination is necessary. *ELISA assays that detect specific stool antigen can distinguish between pathogenic E. histolytica from non-pathogenic E. dispar ; the latter needs no treatment.*

Definitive diagnosis of amoebiasis can also be made by antigen detection by PCR and by detection of anti-amoebic antibodies in the serum. But, these tests have limitations.

The administration of antimicrobial agents like sulfonamides and tetracyclines greatly increases the difficulty of detecting *E. histolytica.*

In the presence of symptoms of hepatitis, demonstration of *E. histolytica* in stools aids the diagnosis. This is often not possible, particularly if the patient has received antimicrobial therapy empirically for fever. If the patient with hepatitis is acutely ill, it is justifiable to carry out a therapeutic test with metronidazole purely on clinical grounds.

Table 55.1 summarises the suggested treatment of amoebiasis.

Table 55.1: Summary of suggested treatment of amoebiasis

Cyst passers:	Diloxanide furoate 500 mg tid for 10 days.
	or
	Diiodohydroxyquinoline 650 mg tid for 15 to 20 days.
	or
	Iodochlorhydroxyquinoline 250 mg tid for 10 days
Invasive:	Metronidazole 400 to 800 mg tid for 5 days.
	or
	Tinidazole 2 gm daily for 2 to 3 days.
	or
	Secnidazole 2 gm single dose followed by a luminal amoebicide for 10 to 20 days.
Severe cases and hepatic abscess :	Metronidazole IV or Dehydroemetine (DHE) IM for 5 days. (See text).

Acute intestinal amoebiasis: Metronidazole in the dose of 600-800 mg. (15 mg./kg. in children) three times a day for five to seven days is the treatment of choice. It is much less toxic than emetine and is effective orally. Almost 90% of patients with moderate amoebic dysentery respond clinically to oral metronidazole therapy. The symptoms are relieved within 24 hours. Severe cases may need IV metronidazole or IM emetine. An equally effective regimen is to give 2.4 g (30 mg/kg) of metronidazole in a single daily dose for two successive days. Additional advantage of this drug is its effectiveness in hepatic amoebiasis which can never be entirely excluded in any case of amoebic dysentery.

Parasites persist in the intestine in almost 30-40% of the patients who receive only metronidazole. Therefore, metronidazole therapy should be followed by a course of a luminal amoebicide to ensure a cure.

Emetine, is valuable for rapidly controlling the symptoms of severe infection, but its usefulness is limited by its cardiotoxicity. It is used in the dose of 1 mg. per kg. (60 mg. in an adult) by deep IM injection with the precautions mentioned previously. The drug should be given in two divided doses on the first day so as to detect any idiosyncratic manifestations. Treatment should not be continued beyond 5 days. It should be followed by diloxanide furoate 500 mg tid for 10 days or by di-iodohydroxyquinoline 600 mg bid or 500 mg tid for 15 days. In patients presenting with fulminating amoebic colitis with toxic symptom, it is advisble to use oral tetracycline in addition, to eliminate the intestinal bacteria.

Adjuvant therapy includes the use of antispasmodics for relief of colicky pain and correction of dehydration in severe cases. A cardiac lesion should be excluded before starting emetine and strict bed rest should be enforced during its use. None of the regimens gives entirely satisfactory results, and relapse may occur even a month after apparent cure.

Asymptomatic cyst passers and chronic intestinal amoebiasis: The drug regimens recommended in such cases are:

(a) Diloxanide furoate 500 mg. 3 times daily for 10 days.

(b) A combination of di-iodohydroxyquinoline 1.8 g. daily and tetracycline 1 g. daily, in divided doses for 10 days.

Chronic amoebic colitis is sometimes difficult to treat and usually more than one drug, given in rotation, is needed to achieve success. It must be remembered that some of the symptoms of colitis may be due to 'irritable colon' or certain pathological changes which may not regress rapidly, even though the colon is cleared of organisms. Hence, other supportive and symptomatic therapy such as a high fibre diet and antispasmodics may be more useful.

Hepatic amoebiasis : Metronidazole is the drug of choice. Emetine hydrochloride and chloroquine diphosphate are also effective.

Metronidazole (800 mg. three times a day for 10 days) rapidly controls hepatic amoebiasis in majority of cases. An alternative regime is 2.4 g. (30 mg/kg) in a single daily dose for two successive days. In this dose nausea is likely to be severe and should be prevented by administration of metoclopramide. Metronidazole may also be administered IV in the dose of 15 mg./kg. (0.75-1g. for an adult) as a loading dose, followed by 7.5 mg./kg. every six hours for 7-10 days. Each dose is infused slowly over one hour. Neutralized solutions should not be refrigerated, lest precipitation occurs.

Aspiration is usually necessary in addition to chemotherapy whenever an abscess is present. Simultaneous administration of tetracycline therapy may be beneficial.

Chloroquine diphosphate is given in the dose of 500 mg. thrice daily for 2 days followed by 250 mg. twice daily for 2 to 3 weeks; however, the relapse rate is high.

Emetine hydrochloride or dehydroemetine is given deep IM in the dose of 1 mg. per kg. of body weight for a period of 10 days. The above treatment should be followed by a course of a luminal amoebicide.

In patients in whom the diagnosis between amoebic and pyogenic liver abscess is not certain, metronidazole alone should be avoided because a pyogenic liver abscess may temporarily respond to metronidazole.

Other forms of extra-intestinal amoebiasis: These respond well to metronidazole.

Criteria for cure of amoebiasis: Failure to detect *E. histolytica* in stool specimens obtained at regular intervals for next 2 years is taken as the criterion for cure of amoebic infection. Clinical cure does not signify cure of the disease and relapses can occur.

Prevention: The cysts responsible for propagation of the disease are resistant to the agents routinely used to purify water. Chlorine, in the concentration employed to purify water, fails to kill them. It is, therefore, necessary to avoid fecal contamination of water by sanitary disposal of feces. Fly control and detection and treatment of carriers is equally important. *The surest way to eliminate cysts from water is to boil it*. There is no effective prophylactic therapy. Prophylactic use of small doses of luminal amoebicides has been tried. Although they have been claimed to be useful, such a procedure will have very limited application, particularly in those areas where possibility of frequent reinfection is always present.

Chemotherapy of Other Protozoal Infections

56

Leishmaniasis is a vector-borne infection caused by intracellular protozoa of the genus *Leishmania.* It exists in three main forms, (a) visceral leishmaniasis or kala-azar, (b) cutaneous leishmaniasis or oriental sore and (c) mucocutaneous leishmaniasis localized largely in South America and hence termed American leishmaniasis.

Visceral Leishmaniasis or Kala-azar

This form of the disease, produced by *Leishmania donovani* and *L. infuntum* (India, Nepal, Bangladesh and Sudan) and *L. chagasi* (Latin America) is transmitted by Phlebotomus sandflies. It is characterized by hepato-splenomegaly, irregular fever, anemia, leukopenia and hyperglobulinemia. In India, it is mostly confined to Assam, Bihar, Orissa and Bengal.

Life cycle : During its life cycle, the protozoan exists in two forms : (1) the **Leishmania forms**, (amastigotes) found within the reticuloendothelial cells of the liver, spleen and lymph nodes, and within the macrophages of the infected person; and (2) the flagellated **leptomonad forms** (promastigotes) which develop from the leishmania forms within the digestive tract of the sandfly, after it has fed on the blood of an infected individual; this form exhibits motility. The development of the leptomonad forms within the sandfly takes about 10 days; they are injected by the sandfly into man during its bite. In man, they attack the reticuloendothelial cells, are phagocystosed by macrophages and get transformed into the leishmania forms.

Diagnosis of kala-azar depends upon the demonstration of the leishmania forms in the peripheral blood or in the aspirate obtained by sternal, splenic, liver or lymph node puncture. Blood culture is a more certain but time-consuming method of diagnosis.

The treatment of leishmaniasis is still disappointing. The drugs available are :

I **Pentavalent antimony compounds:** Sodium stibogluconate and Meglumine antimonate.

II **Diamidine derivatives:** Dihydroxy-stibamidine isethionate and Pentamidine isethionate.

III **Miscellaneous:** Amphotericin B, Aminocidin, Miltefosine.

They are also summarized in Table 56.1.

I **Pentavalent antimony compounds:** The pentavalent antimony compounds exhibit little activity against the leptomonad forms of Leishmania *in vitro.* Their efficacy *in vivo* suggests their reduction into trivalent antimony compounds in the body.

Table 56.1 : Drugs for leishmaniasis

Drug	Dose (adults and children)
Sodium stibogluconate	20 mg of Sb/kg/day, IV or IM for 28-30 days
Meglumine antimonate	Same as above
Amphotericin B	0.5 to 1.0 mg/kg IV, every second day for 15 infusions
Liposomal amphotericin B	3 mg/kg/day on days 1-5, 14 and 21 (Tatal 21 mg/kg)
Pentamidine	2-4 mg/kg daily or every second day IV or IM upto 15 doses.
Miltefosin	2.5 mg/kg/day for 4 weeks.

SODIUM STIBOGLUCONATE (Pentostam, Solustibosan) : Currently, this is the drug most preferred for the treatment of leishmaniasis. It acts by suppressing both glycolysis and fatty acid metabolism and by diminishing the net generation of ATP and GTP in the amastigotes. Given IV/IM, it is excreted in two phases : a short phase with t½ of two hours and long phase with t½ of more than 24 hours. Leishmania can develop resistance to antimonials; high degree of resistance has been reported from Bihar in India.

Adverse reactions to antimony compounds: The common adverse effects include a metallic taste in mouth, nausea, vomiting, diarrhoea and giddiness. Myalgias, authralgia, hepatitis, panereatitis and arrythmias may occur. ECG may show flattening or inversion of T waves, and prolongation of QT interval. A few cases of anaphylactoid shock and renal failure have been reported.

II **Diamidine derivatives:** These drugs are more potent but more toxic than the pentavalent antimony compounds. However, they are not so effective in Indian Kala-azar. They are usually reserved for cases resistant to antimonial chemotherapy. They are also useful for prophylaxis against *T. gambiense* and in the treatment of early Gambian and Rhodesian trypanosomiasis.

PENTAMIDINE : Two pentamidine salts are available, isethionate (Pentamidine) and mesylate (Lomidine). They are administered IM.

It is concentrated in the liver; very little gets into the brain tissue. The drug can be detected in the urine for 6-8 weeks. The mechanism of action is not known. It interferes with amino acid transport, disrupts the mitochondria and inhibits the transformation of amastigotes to promastigotes.

Adverse reactions : Following the IM injection, it may cause local irritation, breathlessness, nausea, vomiting, facial flushing, pruritus, tachycardia, arrthythmia and hypotension. The systemic toxicity includes hepatotoxicity, leukopenia, thrombocytopenia, acute renal failure and hypocalemia. About 5% of patients may develop insulin dependent diabetes mellitus. It appears to have a direct action on the pancreatic beta cells, resulting in initial insulin release followed by impaired insulin secretion.

Therapeutic uses

- ***Visceral leishmaniasis and mucocutaneous leishmaniasis*** resistant to pentavalent antimony therapy are treated with a course of pentamidine or amphotericin B.
- ***Pneumocystis carinii pneumonia*** : Although cotrimoxazole is highly effective in *P. carinii* pneumonia, its increased toxicity in patients with AIDS makes some physicians prefer pentamidine. It is also used for prophylaxis. A dose of 300 mg aerosolised, given once every 4 weeks, appears to be 60-70% effective in preventing the first episode of pneumonia in patients with AIDS. The other drugs used for the same purpose are daily co-trimoxazole and weekly Fansidar. (Chapter 54)
- ***Trypanosomiasis:*** See later.

DIHYDROXYSTILBAMIDINE SETHIONATE: This is given IV in the dose of 250 mg. daily for 10 days. The course may be repeated after an interval of 2 weeks and a total dose of 7.5 g., should be given over a period of 4 to 5 weeks. Its toxicity is similar to that of pentamidine.

III **Miscellaneous :**

AMPHOTERICIN B: This antifungal antibiotic, (Chapter 48) is useful in patients not responding to antimony compounds. However, it is expensive, toxic and not easily available. Liposomal preparations are less toxic as they are targeted specifically toward macrophages, and may be preferred.

Amphotericin damages an ergosterol-like membrane steroid of leishmania. It is considered the drug of choice for Indian Kala-azar. The disease can relapse but responds to repeat therapy. Freedom from relapse for 6 month indicates cure.

MILTEFOSINE: This phosphocholine derivative has been reported to be highly effective orally particularly in Indian visceral and cutaneous leishmaniasis. It acts by interfering with cell signaling pathways. Given orally in the dose of 100 mg (2.5 mg/kg) per day for 4 weeks, it is reported to produce high cure rates in visceral leishmaniasis. It has a long t½ (154 hours). Adverse effects reported are vomiting, diarrhoea and transient, hepatic and renal damage. *It is teratogenic and should be avoided in pregnancy.*

AMINOCIDIN (Paromomycin): This aminoglycoside antibiotic has been reported useful in the treatment of visceral leishmaniasis. Given in the dose of 15-20 mg/kg/day, in 3 divided doses IM, for 21 days, it is claimed to be superior to sodium stibogluconate. It needs further evaluation. (Chapter 46).

Oriental Sore

This condition is caused commonly by *Leishmania tropica (L. major).* The parasite is transmitted by another species of sandfly. It is characterised by nodular skin lesion that later ulcerates. Mild lesions may be left to heal by themselves. More severe cases require local as well as systemic antimonial therapy. Ketoconazole in the dose of 200-400 mg/day for 4-6 weeks may be useful.

Sores on the face and hands often get secondarily infected and tend to become chronic. This would need additional antibiotic therapy.

American Mucocutaneous Leishmaniasis

It is caused by *Leishmania brasiliensis and L. mexicana.* It is characterised by skin granulomas and ulcerative lesions of the nose, mouth and pharynx. The treatment is similar to that of visceral leishmaniasis. However, the disease is relatively resistant to antimonials; and amphotericin B is perhaps the best alternative.

Trypanosomiasis

This disease, caused by parasites of the genus *Trypanosoma,* is characterised by chronic irregular fever, skin eruptions, lymphadenitis, and physical and mental lethargy. It can be divided into :

(1) **African typanosomiasis** or sleeping sickness caused by *Trypanosoma gambiense* and *Trypanosoma rhodesiense* transmitted by tse-tse and open woodland flies respectively.

(2) **South American trypanosomiasis** caused by *Trypanosoma cruzi* transmitted by blood sucking Reduviid bugs.

African trypanosomiasis: Therapeutic response is better if the treatment of sleeping sickness is undertaken in its earlier stage when the parasite has not invaded the CNS. The drugs used are:

SURAMIN SODIUM: This drug, a complex organic urea compound, is particularly useful in treating the more acute rhodesian form of African trypanosomiasis and early infections with *T.gambiense*. It is also a useful prophylactic agent but has now been replaced by pentamidine for this purpose.

The mechanism of action is not clear. Parasites treated with the drug lose their infectivity but still survive *in vitro* for over 24 hours after exposure. In addition to trypanocidal activity, the drug is effective against the adult forms of *Onchocerca volvulus.*

Absorption, Fate and Excretion: Suramin is administered IV as the drug is not adequately absorbed from the gut; IM administration is painful. It gets extensively bound to plasma proteins and persists in the plasma for as long as 3 months after a single dose. *It does not cross the blood brain barrier and is, therefore, useless in the encephalitic stage of the disease.* In such cases, the arsenical, melarsoprol, is used. The drug is excreted in urine.

Adverse reactions: These include nausea, vomiting, dermatitis, chills, fever, pruritus, paraesthesias, photophobia, and sometimes loss of consciousness and shock. Blood dyscrasias may develop occasionally. The drug is nephrotoxic and may give rise to cylindruria, albuminuria and hematuria.

Preparations and dosage: A freshly prepared 10 per cent solution in distilled water is given IV at intervals of 5 to 7 days for 5-6 injections. The initial dose is 0.5 gm. followed by 1 gm. in subsequent injections. A child under 3 years is usually given 0.25 g., from 3 to 10 years 0.5 gm. and those above ten years 1 gm. As the drug is nephrotoxic, urine should be examined before each injection. For use of suramin in onchocerciasis (Chapter 58).

PENTAMIDINE ISETHIONATE: This drug may serve as a substitute for suramin. It is administered in the dose of 3 to 4 mg. of the base per kg. of body weight, on every alternate day for 10 doses IV. A single IM dose (300-400 mg.) once every 6 months has been shown to protect against the Gambian but not the Rhodesian disease. Hypotension and hypoglycemia are common adverse effects. The drug doses not cross the BBB.

The organic arsenical compounds used in African trypanosomiasis are **Mel B and Mel W**. These compounds are toxic and are mainly used to treat meningo-encephalitic stage of the disease.

MEL B (Melarsoprol): This trivalent organic arsenical, effective in the early and the late meningoencephalitic stages of trypanosomiasis, is administered IV, slowly, in increasing doses of 0.36-3.6 mg. per kg. (upto a maximum of 200 mg.) dissolved in propylene glycol. The injection is given on alternate days for 3 days. The course may be repeated after an intermission of 3 weeks in cases with involvement of the CNS. Nearly 95% of the patients can be cured without serious complication, whereas 1-5% die during treatment. The toxic manifestations include vomiting, abdominal colic, proteinuria, neuritis, blood dyscrasias and arsenical encephalopathy.

Mel B is contraindicated in severely debilitated patients and in those with hepatic and/or renal damage.

MELARSONYL POTASSIUM (Mel W, Trimelarson): This water soluble derivative of Mel B is given as a 5 per cent solution, by IM injection. The first dose is 2 mg. per kg.; then 4 mg. per kg. given daily for 3 days. In severe cases, another course of 4 mg. per kg. daily for 4 days may be given after a week. The preparation is probably less toxic but also less effective than the parent compound in advanced *T. rhodesiense* infection, but may be equally effective in *T. gambiense* infection. The drug is also useful in onchocerciasis.

NITROFURAZONE (Furacin): The drug has been employed for trypanosomiasis in patients who have relapsed after other forms of treatment. It is given orally in doses of 500 mg.

3 times daily for 7 to 10 days. For children, a dose of 30 mg. per kg. is recommended. The adverse manifestations include GI disturbances, peripheral neuritis, seizures and hemolysis in G6PD deficient patients.

EFLORNITHINE HYDROCHLORIDE (Difluoromethylornithine, DFMO) has been shown to give high cure rates in late stages of gambian trypanosomiasis. It is an irreversible inhibitor of synthesis of polyamines required for cell division and differentiation. The drug can cause alopecia, diarrhoea, anemia, leucopenia and thrombocytopenia. Headache, hallucina-tions, convulsions and hearing loss may occur. It is teratogenic. It is administered by IV infusion in the dose of 400 mg/kg/day in four divided doses for 14 days. It is expensive and should be considered as an alternative in patients who relapse after melosoprol.

Eflorinthine cream has been found useful in reducing the rate of growth of facial hair in women; however it needs to be used for prolonged periods of time (Chapter 67).

South American Trypanosomiasis (Chagas' disease) : There is no effective and safe agent available for the treatment of this condition. A variety of drugs, including pyrimethamine, nitrofurans, amphotericin B and puromycin have been given a trial. None of these gives complete cure. They only cause a transient disappearance of parasitemia.

Two drugs **nifurtimox** and **benznidazole**, effective orally, appear to kill circulating trypanosomes. Nifurtimox is given orally in a dose of 8 to 10 mg/kg per day in 4 divided doses, for 90 to 120 days. The drug may cause GI disturbances, weight loss, insomnia, arthralgia, neuropathy, leucopenia and seizures. Benznidazole is administered in a dose of 5-10 mg/kg day in two divided doses for 60 days. It can cause GI disturbances, polyneuropathy and bone marrow suppression. They are not useful in chronic disease.

Toxoplasmosis

Toxoplasmosis is a common disease of birds and mammals, caused by infection with the obligate intracellular protozoon *Toxoplasma gondii*. The organisms are arc shaped (toxon=arc; gondii=the name of a North American rodent). Infection in the animal world occurs by ingestion of cysts that contain sporulated oocytes (**bradyzoites**) by an intermediate host such as the rat or the sheep. The bradyzoites released in the gut enter the epithelium of the small intestine and transform into rapidly dividing **tachyzoites**, which can infect all mammalian cells except the RBCs. Seven to 10 days after the tachyzoite infection, tissue cysts containing many tachyzoites are formed. The parasites' sexual phase (feline phase) takes place in the definitive host like the cat which ingests the infected rats. The infected cats may excrete millions of sporozoites containing oocytes which may remain viable for many years in the soil. Human infection occurs following ingestion of either soil contaminated with sporulated oocytes or undercooked meat containing tachyzoites. Cysts are commonly found in tissues such as the brain, and skeletal muscles.

Toxoplasmosis is largely asymptomatic and self limiting, but a small percentage of patients get lymphadenopathy, fever and malaise. Retino-choroiditis forms an important manifestation (25-35%) in children but is rare in adults. Encephalitis, myocarditis and pneumonitis can occur. *Repeated abortions can occur in infected women*. There is no drug which will kill the trophozoites or eradicate the cysts. Spontaneous cure is known to occur. A combination of pyrimethamine and sulfadiazine is effective in inhibiting the trophozoites. No treatment is recommended for asymptomatic infection in immunocompetent subjects.

Pyrimethamine, a DHF reductase inhibitor, is given orally in the initial dose of 75 mg. daily, followed by 25-50 mg. daily. **Sulfadiazine** is used in the dose of 2 gm followed by 0.5-1.0 g orally every six hours. The combination treatment is given for 4-6 weeks. The other drugs used are **co-trimoxazole, clindamycin** and **atovaquone spiramycin, azithromycin** and **clarithromycin.** Pyrimethamine is combined with clindamycin or azithromycin.

The regimen recommended in affected, pregnant women is **spiramycin**, a macrolide, in the dose of 1g tid orally continued throughout pregnancy. In all cases, folic acid supplement should be given. Monthly ultrasonography is suggested to detect any fetal abnormality. The presence of hydrocephalus is an indication to terminate pregnancy.

Congenitally infected neonates are treated aggressively with oral pyrimethamine (0.5 to 1.0 mg/kg/day) and sulfadiazine (100 mg/kg/day) along with folic acid for one year. Spiramycin (100 mg/kg/day) may also be useful. However, a macrolide alone may not be beneficial unless combined with pyrimethamine. Clindamycin can be substituted for sulfadiazine in all patients allergic to sulfonamide.

Trichomoniasis

Vaginal discharge is a common complaint in general practice. It must be emphasized that *many discharges are non-infective* and hence it is wrong and may even be harmful to use systemic or local antimicrobial drugs unless proper diagnosis is made.

In women of the child-bearing age excessive vaginal discharge (**leucorrhoea**) may simply be due to pelvic congestion or increased secretion of the cervical glands as in cervical erosion or during oral contraceptive medication. In such cases bacteriological examination is negative and no drugs are indicated. What is needed is reassurance and advice on simple hygiene and cauterization of the cervical erosion.

Vaginal discharge due to infection should be treated according to the causative organism. *Trichomonas vaginalis* is by far the commonest one, followed by *C. albicans.* Typically, trichomoniasis presents as an intense vaginitis with a purulent, greenish yellow profuse, frothy, offensive discharge. Other symptoms include pruritus, burning, edema, dyspareunia and urinary frequency. Candidial vaginitis is less intense with thin and curd like or 'cheesy' discharge and adherent plaques on the vaginal wall. Sometimes, accurate clinical differentiation between these lesions is difficult.

Trichomonas vaginalis is the infectious protozoan most commonly associated with vulvovaginitis during reproductive years. Infection in males is often symptomless. The condition is diagnosed by microscopic examination of fresh material from the vagina, of semen, of prostatic fluid obtained by massage and of urinary sediment. The flagella of the protozoan can be identified in a wet smear.

Drugs for local treatment : They are useful when extravaginal sources of reinfection are not present. They include:

1. Halogenated hydroxyquinolines like Iodochlorohydroxyquinoline, Diiodohydroxy-quinoline;
2. Agents like Furazolidone, surfactants like Sodium lauryl sulfate, Dioctyl sodium sulfosuccinate, Triclobisonium and Povidone iodine.

These drugs are discussed elsewhere. They are often combined with deodorizers like thymol, menthol, or eucalyptol. Other local agents like vinegar,boric acid and lactic acid are used to lower the vaginal pH to its usual acidity (3.5 to 4.5). This facilitates the growth of the normal vaginal flora and results in suppression of the trichomonal infection.

Drug for systemic therapy: *Oral metronidazole is the drug of choice for trichomtoniasis.* It is discussed in detail in Chapter 55.

Trichomoniasis responds well to oral metronidazole 400 mg. twice daily for 7-10 days. A second course may be instituted after 4-6 weeks. A single dose of 2 g. has also been reported to give equally good results. *Since trichomoniasis is a urogenital infection, simply using local pessaries without systemic therapy is unsatisfactory. However, addition of topical treatment to systemic therapy increases local concentration, which may be beneficial in refractory carcinoma.*

Trichomoniasis is sexually transmissible and it is advisable to administer a course of metronidazole to the sexual consorts of the infected persons. It is advisable to avoid sexual intercourse until cure has been confirmed. Infections due to *C. albicans* and gonococcal and puerperal infections need appropriate antibiotic therapy (Chapter 51).

Metronidazole, given in the dose of 400 mg. twice daily for 7 days, is also useful in the treatment of mixed vaginitis (**non-specific vaginitis**) due to an aerobe *(Gardnerella vaginalis)* and anaerobes. The infection causes a malodorous, off-white, vaginal discharge of high pH, giving a positive amine test. There is no inflammation of the vaginal wall.

TINIDAZOLE (Tini, Tiniba) : It is effective in a single oral dose of 2 g. in the treatment of vaginal trichomoniasis and giardiasis (See Chapter 55).

Secnidazole:. Dose 2gm. as a single dose.

Giardiasis

Giardia lamblia is a flagellate protozoan parasite of the small intestine. Like *E. histolytica,* it has no animal host and is transmitted from man to man by fecal contamination of food and water. It can cause diarrhoea, anorexia, nausea, vomiting, abdominal pain and weight loss. Both the cysts and trophozoites may be found in the stools. *Giardiasis is quite common and often exists in association with E. histolytica infection.*

Metronidazole is the drug of choice in giardiasis. It is given in the dose of 200 mg tid for 5 days in adults and 15 mg/kg/day in 3 divided doses for 5 days in children.

Nitazoxanide is effective against metronidazole resistant G. lamblia. **Other drugs used** are tinidazole, 2 g single dose, furazolidone (100 mg qid for 7 days), mepacrine and paramomycin. These drugs have been discussed earlier.

Chemotherapy of Viral Infections 57

Unlike with bacterial infections, satisfactory treatment of viral infections still remains difficult. A virus is made up of a nucleic acid core enclosed in a protein coat called **capsid** which consists of repeating, identical subunits called **capsomeres.** Certain other constituents protect the nucleic acid moiety from the action of various body fluid enzymes. Viruses, unlike bacteria, have no cell wall and the enzyme systems associated with it.

Viruses are of two types (Table 57.1):

- ***Deoxyribonucleic acid (DNA) viruses;*** and
- ***Ribonucleic acid (RNA) viruses.***

Table 57.1: DNA and RNA viruses

- ***DNA viruses:*** Herpes simplex; varicella-zoster; smallpox; hepatitis B; human cytomegalovirus (CMV).
- ***RNA viruses:*** Rabies; rubella; measles; dengue; yellow fever; poliomyelitis; HIV; influenza.

Most viruses survive outside the host cell only for a short time. After penetration into the target cell, viral replication occurs in following steps:

(a) Uncoating of viral nucleic acid strands
(b) Early, regulatory protein synthesis
(c) Replication of viral DNA/ RNA
(d) Late structural protein synthesis
(e) Coating and maturation of viral particles; and
(f) Their release from the target cell.

Antiviral drugs can act at any of these steps.

The major difficulties involved in the chemotherapy of viral infections are:

- Viruses, unlike bacteria are intimately parasitic on host cells. They are obligatory intracellular agents. Hence, a drug that is expected to destroy the virus is likely to be toxic to normal host cells.
- Certain viruses multiply in the cytoplasm while others do so in the nucleus of the infected cell. A drug which acts on a virus in the cytoplasm may not necessarily act on a virus that multiplies in the nucleus and vice versa.
- The severity of infection produced by a virus and its response to a given chemotherapeutic drug differ considerably in different species of animals.
- Precise diagnosis of many virus infections is difficult. The laboratory screening tests for antiviral compounds are also difficult. Further, *in vitro* efficacy of a new drug may not predict its therapeutic efficacy.
- In many viral infections, the greater part of the viral multiplication takes place before the clinical diagnosis can be made. The antiviral compounds are likely to be most effective during the stage of replication of the virus, which is difficult to detect clinically.

- Antiviral drugs inhibit viral replication. However, viruses start replicating after stopping the drug. This is a common problem in immunocompromised patients. Moreover, antiviral drugs may not eliminate nonreplicating or latent viruses.
- Viruses undergo structural changes and develop drug resistance.

At the onset of infection, the viruses are usually adsorbed on to the surface of a host cell. In a few cases, they react with the cell membrane receptor sites specific for the virus. Viruses cause cell injury by :

- ***Direct lysis resulting from viral replication;***
- ***Lysis induced by antiviral antibody and the complement***; and
- ***Cell mediated immune mechanisms.***

In addition, viral infection may transform cells so that they may proliferate and produce tumours. Since the multiplication of a virus is heavily dependent on host cell mechanisms, an effective antiviral agent must act intracellularly and selectively.

Antiviral compounds – Classification :

I **Compounds interfering with the nucleic acid synthesis,** e.g., Idoxuridine, Adenine arabinoside, Acyclovir, Ribavirin, Trifluridine, and Azidothymidine (AZT).

II **Inhibitors of attachment/penetration,** e.g., Amantadine, Zanamivir.

III **Inhibitors of reverse transcriptase** e.g. Lamivudine.

IV **Acting through immune mechanism** e.g. Interferon, Gamma globulin and Monoclonal antibodies.

IDOXURIDINE (5-Iodo-2'-Deoxyuridine, Ridinox): This compound is chemically related to thymidine and acts by competing with it in the synthesis of DNA, thereby preventing the utilisation of thymidine. The drug interferes with the synthesis of normal cellular DNA and, hence, is too toxic for systemic use. It has been employed locally as 0.5% drops or ointment in the treatment of herpetic keratitis. It is now superseded by drugs such as acyclovir.

TRIFLURIDINE: This nucleoside analogue has been used as 0.5% ophthalmic ointment to treat ocular herpes. It is less specific and not used systemically.

ADENINE ARABINOSIDE (Vidarabine): This purine nucleoside analogue inhibits a variety of DNA viruses *in vitro*. Topically (as 3% ointment) it has been used to treat ocular herpes simplex. It has also been used to treat herpes encephalitis. The drug causes CNS, hematological and GI toxicity and has now been replaced by acyclovir and related compounds.

ACYCLOVIR: (Cyclovir, Zovirax): This guanosine analogue is a potent antiviral drug of low toxicity.

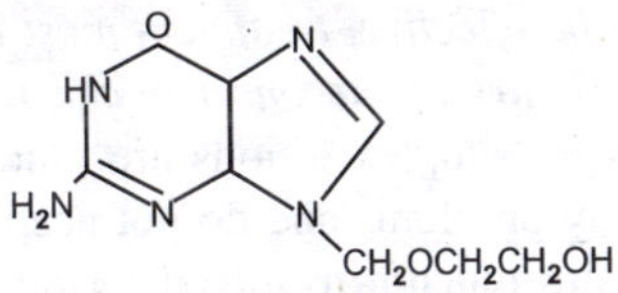

O, HN, N, H_2N, N, N, $CH_2OCH_2CH_2OH$

Fig. 57.1: Acyclovir

Mechanism of action: The drug is phosphorylated by viral-specific thymidine kinase to monophosphate derivative, which is further phosphorylated by host cell kinase to form acyclovir triphosphate. The latter inhibits viral DNA synthesis.

The antiviral spectrum includes Herpes simplex virus (HSV) 1 and 2, Varicella zoster virus (VZV) and Epstein barr virus (EBV). HSV and VZV can develop resistance to acyclovir, particularly in HIV positive patients.

Absorption, fate and excretion: Given orally, it has a bioavailability of 15-30%; the CSF level of the drug is only 50% that of plasma. Hence, for viral encephalitis it is given IV. Its t½ is 3 hours. It is mostly excreted unchanged in the urine; 15% is metabolized in the liver.

Applied locally, it is effective in corneal lesions. (Ocular keratitis).

Adverse reactions: Locally it may cause stinging and reversible superficial keratopathy. Orally, the drug is generally well tolerated. Given IV, it may cause headache, thrombophlebitis and elevation of blood urea and creatinine (crystalline nephropathy). CNS toxicity includes delirium tremors, abnormal EEG and hallucinations. (Neuropsychiatric reaction).

Preparations and dosage

(i) Tablets 200 mg. Dose 200-400 mg 4-5 times a day.

(ii) IV infusion 250 mg/ml. Dose 5-10 mg/kg over 1 hour at 8 hour interval.

(iii) Eye ointment 3%.

(iv) Cream 5% for skin application.

Therapeutic uses : Both, HSV and VZV produce their effects by destroying the epithelial cells by replicating in them. Once the damage is done, the healing time in an **immunocompetent** individual is largely unrelated to the virus. *Hence, to be effective, treatment must be started within 24 hours of the onset of the rash.* Most of the herpes simplex lesions are mild and heal without any problems and do not need the drug.

In an **immunocompromised** person, however, failure to curtail viral replication may lead to prolongation of the local lesions and dissemination of infection; hence, in such patients, treatment with acyclovir should be begun at any stage of the infection. In these patients acyclovir reduces visceral complications but has no effect on healing of skin lesions or pain. The indications for use of acyclovir are :

- ***Herpes simplex* virus infection**

(a) **Primary and recurrent genital infections:** It is highly effective in an oral dose of 200 mg 5 times a day for 7 days. It can be administered IV in severe cases.

(b) **Gingivostomatitis and pharyngitis :** also responds to above-mentioned regime.

(c) **Keratoconjunctivitis :** Topical administration is used.

(d) **Meningitis and encephalitis:** IV acyclovir is the treatment of choice.

- ***Varicella zoster* virus infection** VZV causes varicella (chickenpox) as primary infection. Reactivation of the virus, which remains latent in dorsal root ganglia, results in herpes zoster.

(a) **Varicella :** Acyclovir is not routinely used if VZV infection is uncomplicated in children. In adults, 800 mg orally 5 times a day for 7 days decreases time to crusting, its erruption and duration of fever. But treatment should be started within 24 hours of rash. Intravenous therapy is needed for severe varicella pneumonia and encephalitis.

(b) **Localized herpes zoster :** Oral treatment with acyclovir in *immunocompetent individuals* should probably be reserved for those who have very early lesions and for those in whom the attack threatens to be widespread or in a critical area such as the face.

If given within 72 hours of rash, 800 mg acyclovir 5 times a day for 7-10 days decreases pain and healing time but does not reduce the intensity of post-herpetic neuralgia. It also decreases ocular complications of keratitis or uveitis. It may be life saving in patients with encephalitis. It can also be given, by IV infusion.

Both varicella and herpes zoster in the immunocompromized patient should always be treated with IV acyclovir.

- ***Prophylaxis with acyclovir*:** Prophylactic treatment with acyclovir is given to immunocompromized patients undergoing bone marrow transplant or chemotherapy.

Valacyclovir and **famciclovir** are prodrugs for acyclovir and **penciclovir** respectively and have similar applications.

The use of glucocorticoids in herpes zoster is best left to the specialists.

GANCICLOVIR: It is an acyclic nucleoside analogue of guanine with action similar to that of acyclovir. It is given orally or by IV infusion. Its concentration in infected cells is high and remains so for more than 24 hours.

The adverse reactions include GI disturbances, myclosuppression and aspermatogenesis. CNS symptoms like headache, behavioural changes and convulsions are also observed. It may also cause liver and renal dysfunction. It is carcinogenic, teratogenic and mutagenic in animals. Because of its toxicity, its use is presently limited to immunocompromised host with serious cytomegalovirus (CMV) infection of the retina and colon.

Valganciclovir is a prodrug for ganciclovir.

FOSCARNET SODIUM: This drug, an inorganic pyrophosphate compound, is given by IV infusion to treat CMV retinitis in patients with AIDS, as an alternative to ganciclovir. It has potent activity against HSV as well. It inhibits DNA polymerase. It does not require activation by viral thymidine kinase. It is effective against acyclovir-resistant and ganciclovir-resistant strains. The drug can cause GI toxicity, nephrotoxicity, anemia and CNS disturbances like headache. Hypocalcemia, hypokalemia and hypomagnesimia have also been reported.

SORIVUDINE is a pyrimidine nucleoside analogue which can be used in both immunocompromised and immunocompetent patients with herpes zoster infection.

RIBAVIRIN (Virazol): This purine nucleoside analogue has a broad spectrum antiviral activity against DNA and RNA viruses. It has been shown to be of some use against influenza A and B infections, respiratory syncytial virus (RSV) infection, Lassa fever and hepatitis C. It is administered in aerosolised form or by nebulization.

Adverse reactions : Ribavirin has been shown to be teratogenic, mutagenic, embryotoxic and gonadotoxic in small animals, and is contraindicated in pregnancy. A woman must avoid conception for 6 months after cessation of ribavirin. Further, passive exposure to aerosolized ribavirin should be avoided by pregnant women. It causes dose dependent anemia, bone marrow suppression, cardiac and neurological toxicity. Aerosolization is generally well tolerated and produces no evidence of systemic toxicity except allergic reactions.

INTERFERONS (Inf) : Interferons are species specific cellular glycoproteins, produced naturally by virus-infected cells, and have antiviral protective action. They are not virus specific and can interfere with a wide variety of DNA and RNA viruses. They are, therefore, considered as potent, broad spectrum, antiviral compounds with a high therapeutic ratio. There are many interferons which vary from species to species. Each species produces at least three types of interferons;

- ***Alpha*** and ***Beta*** from nearly all cell types induced by viruses, double stranded RNA and cytokines like Il-1, Il-2 and TNF
- ***Gamma*** from immunologically stimulated T lymphocytes and NK cells.

Each of these can now be produced by recombinant DNA technology. Virus-induced human interferon differs from the interferon produced by lymphocytes during immune response in several respects. Alpha and beta interferons have 166 amino-acids and molecular weight ranging from 16,000- 26,000. Gamma interferon has 146 amino-acids with molecular weight 20,000 to 25,000. It is less antiviral and more immunoregulator.

Mechanism of action : Certain agents like the live attenuated measles virus, microbial extracts and anionic polysaccharides can stimulate the production of endogenous interferon.

Interferons act by binding to specific, cell-surface receptors and inducing the production of new cellular RNA and proteins, which in turn inhibit protein synthesis of viruses. They inhibit several steps of viral reproduction including viral penetration, uncoating, synthesis of mRNA, translation of viral proteins and/or viral assembly and release. Interferon may also act as an immune modulator, thus increasing cytotoxic T lymphocyte activity, enhancing NK cell activity and activating macrophages. Hence, patients with an intact immune system are more likely to benefit from exogenous interferon. Interferon has no effect on extracellular virus.

Little is known about the metabolism of interferons in man. They do not penetrate CSF readily. IFN-α predominantly undergoes proteolytic degradation in the renal tubules.

Adverse reactions: These include hypersensitivity reactions, fever, flu-like syndrome, lethargy, myalgia, arthralgia and ocular symptoms. Dose-related myelosuppression, nephrotoxicity and hepatotoxicity have also been reported. Larger doses cause alopecia, neurotoxicity, personality changes, depression, reversible hearing loss, retinopathy, thyroid dysfunction, azotemia and impaired fertility. Antibodies to interferon can decrease its therapeutic effect.

Table 57.2: Therapeutic uses of the commonly used antiviral (non HIV) drugs

Drug	Route	Indications
Idoxuridine	T	HSV keratitis
Trifluridine	T	HSV keratitis dermatitis
Acyclovir	T, O	Herpes genitalis; mucocutaneous HSV; local herpes zoster.
	IV	Herpes simplex encephalitis; Severe herpes genitalis; herpes zoster in the immunocompromised
Ganciclovir		CMV infections.
Foscarnet	IV	CMV retinitis; acyclovir resistant HSV infection.
Amantadine	O	Influenza A
Rimantadine	O	Influenza A
Zanamivir	Inhalation	Influenza A and B
Oseltamivir	O	Influenza A and B
Adefovir	O	HBV infection
Lamivudine	O	HBV infection
Ribavirin	Aerosol	Respiratory syncytial virus infection
Interferon alpha 2a/2b	SC IV	Chronic hepatitis B C and D; condyloma acuminata

T = Topical; O = Oral; SC = Subcutaneous; IV = Intravenous; CMV = Cytomegalovirus; HIV = Human immunodeficiency virus; HSV = Herpes simplex virus;

Preparations and dosage:

(i) Interferon alpha 2b (Intron A): 10 million units / ml IM/SC injection.

(ii) Interferon alpha 2a (Raferon A): 3-9 million units.ml injection.

(iii) Pegylated interferon alpha 2a and 2b: These are polyethylene glycol attached to interferons. They have sustained absorption and reduced clearance resulting into increased $t^1/_2$

(iv) Interferon beta 1a (Avanex): It is a glycosylated recombinant product from mammalian cells, 6 million units / ml injection.

(v) Interferon beta 1b (Betaferon): It is a nonglycosylated recombinant product from mammalian cells. 6 million units / ml injection.

Therapeutic uses: Recombinant alpha interferon 2b has been used successfully in the treatment of :

- ***Chronic hepatitis B,*** where it provents progressive liver damage, along with histological improvement.
- ***Chronic hepatitis C and D*** : All forms of interferon are useful in this condition. Combination with ribavirin has been claimed to give better results.
- ***Condyloma acuminata.***
- ***Hairy cell leukemia.***
- ***Chronic myelogenous leukemia where it may induce remission.***
- ***Multiple sclerosis*** where interferons beta la and lb have been shown to reduce both frequency and severity of exacerbations. They are currently recommended for relapsing/ remitting multiple sclerosis.
- ***All severe viral infections,*** where it may be of some use.

Experimentally, interferons restrain the growth of various tumours in mice. Partially purified interferons have been shown to produce antitumour effects in osteogenic sarcoma, multiple myeloma, lymphoma and breast cancer nodules in human beings.

AMANTADINE (1-Admantanamine hydrochloride) : This drug acts by inhibiting uncoating of viral RNA of influenza A virus within infected cells, thus inhibiting viral replication. Clinically, it is useful in the prophylaxis and treatment of influenza A, but not influenza B. Its therapeutic usefulness, however, appears to be limited.

Adverse effects are not a major problem though the drug can cause confusion, high headedness, slurred speech, insomnia, anxiety, difficulty in thinking, hallucinations, urinary retention and skin rash. It is also used in parkinsonism (Chapter 14).

The drug is administered orally in the dose of 100 mg. once or twice daily for 5-7 days. To be effective, it must be administered within the first 24-48 hours after the onset of symptoms.

RIMANTADINE: This drug has actions similar to those of amantadine but is 4-10 times more active. However, the CNS toxicity occurs less often than with amantadine and no dosage adjustment is necessary in patients with renal impairment except in those with end stage renal failure. It has a longer t½ of 24-36 hours than amantadine. Both are teratogenic in animals.

ZANAMIVIR: This drug is a potent inhibitor of the viral neuraminidase. It prevents the entry of influenza A and B viruses into the target cell. It has been shown to be useful against both type A and type B influenza viruses. It is given as 5 mg powder bid for 5 days by inhalation. It can be used prophylactically once daily by inhalation for the prevention of influenza. The drug can cause nausea, vomiting and bronchospasm.

OSELTAMIVIR (Tamiflu) has similar actions as zanamivir. Given orally within 36 hours of onset of symptoms, it can also decrease the severity of influenza A and B and swine flu. It can also be used prophylactically.

DOCOSANOL is a new antiviral agent, an OTC product, available as 10% cream. It is used for recurrent orolabial herpes simplex. It blocks the fusion between cellular and viral envelope membranes and thus inhibits viral replication.

FOMIVIRSEN, an oligonucleotide agent, is used IV for the treatment of difficult cases of CMV retinitis. It can cause vitritis, cataract and increase in intraocular pressure.

GAMMA GLOBULIN: It prevents viral adsorption to and their penetration into the target cell. (See Chapter 76 for details).

Antiviral drugs used to treat AIDS (HIV-infection) are discussed in Chapter 51. Lamivudine, an anti-HIV drug, has also been used for treating chronic HBV infection.

For **antiviral monoclonal antibody palivizumab,** see Chapter 76.

Chemotherapy of Helminthiases 58

Worm infestation (helminthiasis) is one of the major global public health problems, more so in tropical countries. Besides the environmental conditions peculiar to tropics, poverty, illiteracy, lack of adequate sanitary facilities and of pure water supply make total eradication of this problem very difficult. The number of people suffering from worm infestation in developing countries runs into several millions. The commonest parasites observed are roundworms, hookworms, threadworms, tapeworms, filarial worms and schistosomes.

Worms can cause various GI and general symptoms. In addition, some of them can cause blood loss, nutritional deficiencies, urticaria and other allergic manifestations, intestinal obstruction and hepatosplenomegaly. Roundworms have been implicated in the pathogenesis of bronchial asthma in endemic areas. Peripheral blood eosinophilia occurs in all nematode infestations (except enterobiasis), but not in platyhelminth or protozoal infestations. A careful examination of stool may often spare the unnecessary removal of teeth and tonsils, usually blamed for 'septic foci', in cases with 'resistant urticaria'.

The helminths are multicellular organisms possessing three germ layers and exhibiting a bilateral symmetry. They are classified into two major phyla (1) phyllum nemathelminthes (roundworms : nematodes) and (2) phyllum platyhelminthes (flat worms : cestodes and trematodes). **Anthelmintics** are drugs used in the treatment of helminthiasis.

For a clinical trial of a potential anthelmintic agent, a well established anthelmintic drug with a similar spectrum should always be incorporated in the experimental design so as to ensure an effective comparison. The efficacy of the new drug can be gauged by counting the ova or eggs present in the stools. Efficacy of a drug against taeniasis, however, can only be judged by the appearance of the scolex in the stools. Patients suffering from multiple parasitic infestations are ideal for investigating a new anthelmintic drug claimed to have a broad spectrum of action.

In endemic areas, the main aim of anthelmintic treatment should be to reduce the load of infection below the level of clinical significance. Complete parasitological cure is often not possible. In achieving this, safety and economic considerations must determine the choice of the drug in mass therapy.

An anthelmintic drug which kills the worm is called **vermicidal**, while that which affects the worm in such a way that it is easily expelled is known as a **vermifuge**.

Many anthelmintics with either selective or broad spectrum actions and low toxicity, relatively safe even in the undernourished individuals, are now available. They are convenient to administer as no prior preparation is necessary and no follow up purgation is required unless constipation is present.

Table 58.1: Common forms of helminthiasis and the drugs used in their treatment

Helminth	Common name	Drug of choice	Alternative drugs
Nematodes (intestinal)			
Ascaris lumbricoides	Roundworm	Albendazole Mebendazole	Pyrantel, Piperazine
Ancylostoma duodenale	Hookworm	Albendazole Mebendazole	Pyrantel, Thiabendazole
Enterobius vermicularis	Pinworm	Albendazole Mebendazole	Pyrantel, Piperazine
Trichuris trichura	Whipworm	Mebendazole	Albendazole, Thiabendazole
Strongyloides stercoralis	Threadworm	Ivermectin	Thiabendazole, Albendazole
Trichinella spiralis	Pork roundworm	Albendazole	Thiabendazole, Mebendazole
Nematodes (somatic)			
Wuchereria bancrofti	Lymphatic filarial worm	Diethylcarba-mazine	Ivermectin
Oncocerca volvulus	Oculodermal filarial worm	Ivermectin	Diethylcarbamazine
Onchcerca loa loa	Oculodermal filarial worm	Ivermectin	Diethylcarbamazine
Dracuncula medinensis	Guineaworm	Metronidazole	Mebendazole
Cestodes			
Tenia saginata	Beef tapeworm	Praziquantel	Niclosamide
Tenia solium	Pork tapeworm	Praziquantel	Niclosamide
*Cysticerca cellulosae**	Larva of T. solium	Albendazole	Praziquantel
Diphyllobothrium latum	Fish tapeworm	Praziquantel	Niclosamide
Hymenolepsis nana	Dwarf tapeworm	Praziquantel	Niclosamide
Echinococcus granulosus	Hydatid larva	Albendazole	Mebendazole
Trematodes			
Schistosoma hematobium	Blood flukes	Praziquantel	Metrifonate
S.mansoni	Blood flukes	Praziquantel	Oxamniquin
S.japonicum	Blood flukes	Praziquantel	
Flukes			
Fasciola hepatica	Liver fluke	Praziquantel	Niclosamide
Clonorchis sinensis	Chinese liver fluke	Praziquantel	Niclosamide
F. busci	Giant intestinal fluke	Praziquantel	Niclosamide
Paragonimus westermani	Lung fluke	Praziquantel	Niclosamide

* Glucocorticoids are administered concurrently to reduce edema.

Table 58.2 : Mechanisms of action of common antihelmintics

Site	Drug(s)	Mechanism
Neuromuscular transmission		
(a) Ganglionic nicotinic ACh receptors at neuromuscular junction*	Levamisole, Pyrantel palmoate	Stimulation produces persistent depolarization resulting in muscular contracture/paralysis
(b) GABA receptors at neuromuscular junction.	Piperazine	GABA agonist causing hyper Polarization and flaccid paralysis
(c) Glutamate-gated, chloride channel at neuromuscular junction in invertebrates	Ivermectin	Causes tonic paralysis of microfilariae which are then immobilized and phagocytosed by RE cells
Acetyl cholinesterase	Metrifonate	Inhibition, causing muscular contracture
Cell membrane	Praziquantel	Increases Ca^{++} influx leading to muscular contracture
Microtubules in cytoskeleton	Benzimidazole: Mebendazole, Albendazole; Thiabendazole	Bind to beta-tubuline and inhibit polymerization of microtubules
Mitochondria	Niclosamide	Inhibition of anaerobic phosphorylation of ADP leading to death

* The ACh receptors at the neuromuscular junction of the nematodes are of the ganglionic nicotinic types. The agonists cause contractions of the worm. Experimentally, it can be reversed by the ganglionic blocker mecamylamine.

The anthelmintic drugs used commonly for therapy are listed in Table 58.1.

Mechanism of actions : Various mechanisms by which the anthelmintics act are summarised in Table 58.2.

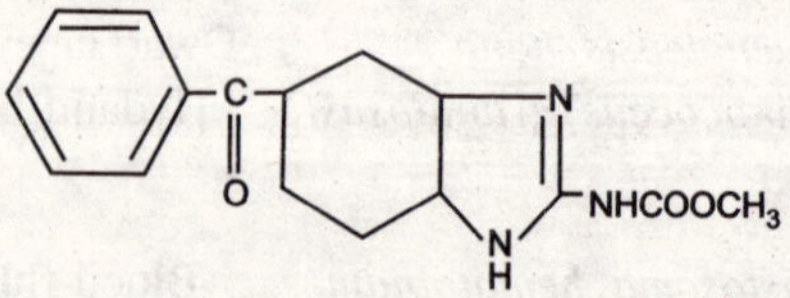

Fig. 58.1: Mebendazole

Drug Therapy of Roundworms

MEBENDAZOLE (Pantelmin, Mebex, Wormin): This broad spectrum anthelmintic is a benzimidazole derviative. Given orally it is poorly (less than 10%) absorbed. It inhibits microtubule polymerization by binding to beta-tubulin.

It is effective in ascariasis, enterobiasis, trichuriasis and in hookworm infestation. It is the drug of choice in enterobiasis and in trichuriasis. It also has some action against *S. stercoralis*. The drug is slow-acting and it may take 2-3 days for parasitic clearance from the gut. It also adversely affects the ova of the trichuris and the hookworm. It is effective *in vivo* against the larvae of

Trichinella spiralis and exerts a lethal effect on the germinal membrane of the larvae of *Echinococcus granulosus* (Hydatid Worm).

Adverse reactions: These are usually mild and consist of abdominal pain, nausea and diarrhoea. Very large oral doses, may cause vertigo, dizziness, headache and arthralgia. Benzimidazoles are embryotoxic and teratogenic in animals, and should be avoided in pregnancy.

Preparation and Dosage: It is available as tablets and liquid suspension. A single dose of 100 mg. repeated after one week is effective in enterobiasis. It is administered in the dose of 100 mg. twicc daily for 3 days for hookworm and round worm infestations. For taenia infestations, doses upto 300 mg. three times a day for three days have produced 100% cure rates. Used orally in the dose of 400-600 mg. tid for 21-30 days, it has been claimed to be effective in causing regression of hydatid cysts of the liver. Such treatment may, however, rarely cause bone marrow aplasia. Hence, albendazole is preferred for treatment of hydatid disease.

ALBENDAZOLE (Zentel): This broad spectrum benzimidazole has actions similar to those of mebendazole. It also has larvicidal actions in hydatid disease, ascariasis and ankylostomiasis and ovicidal properties in ascariasis, ankylostomias and trichuriasis.

Given orally, it is rapidly absorbed and has better bioavailability than mebendazole. After absorption, it undergoes first pass metabolism in the liver to its active metabolite, albendazole sulfoxide. It is well distributed in tissues, bile, CSF and hydatid cyst. It has plasma t½ 8-12 hours. *Its major advantage is that it is effective against many common intestinal worms in a single dose and is cost effective.*

The drug is well tolerated and adverse reactions are mild, mainly GI disturbances. When used in hydatid disease for long term therapy, it may cause alopecia, liver damage and bone marrow depression.

Therapeutic uses

- ***Ascariasis, ankylostomiasis and trichuriasis :*** Usually 400 mg single dose. Hookworm and trichuriasis may need a repeat dose.
- ***Enterobiasis:*** 400 mg single dose, repeated after 4 weeks.
- ***Hydatid disease:*** 400 mg bid for one months, repeated if necessary.
- ***Strongyloidiasis:*** 400 mg twice daily for 3 days, repeated after 3 weeks if necessary.
- ***Trichinella spiralis :*** 400 mg bid for 8-14 days.
- ***Cysticercosis:*** It is considered the drug of choice because of short course, less toxicity than praziquantel, better penetration into CSF and cost. It is given 400 mg bid for 21 days. A glucocorticoid is started prior to albendazole to reduce the intensity of the inflammatory reaction to the dead parasites.

PYRANTEL PAMOATE (Combantrin, Nemocid): This drug, a tetrahydropyrimidine derivative, is highly effective against round worms and *E. vermicularis* and a little less effective against hookworms. In contrast to piperazine, it has a depolarizing, neuromuscular blocking action and causes spastic paralysis of the worms. It is not much absorbed from the gut. In ascariasis and enterobiasis, it is usually given in a single dose (10 mg./kg.upto a maximum of 1 gm.); for hookworm infestation, the same dose is repeated on three successive days. Cure rates over 90% are reported with this drug. The dose can be repeated after 2 weeks, if needed. *It can be used during pregnancy.*

Adverse reactions: These are usually mild and include GI disturbances, abdominal pain, headache, drowsiness, skin rashes, and raised plasma SGOT levels.

Oxantel pamoate, an analogue of pyrantel, is also claimed to be useful in trichuriasis. It is given in a single dose.

PIPERAZINE: This drug is useful in the therapy of ascariasis and enterobiasis. Apart from the anthelmintic action, the drug does not show any significant pharmacological activity in the human host.

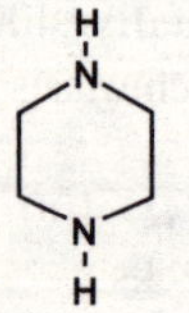

Fig. 58.2: Piperazine

Mechanism of action: The drug acts as a GABA agonist and causes hyperpolirization of ascaris muscle resulting in faccid paralysis of the worms which are then easily expelled by peristaltic movements. This eliminates the danger of worm migration.

Absorption, fate and excretion: Piperazine is absorbed from the gut, to the extent of about 30%. The drug is partly metabolized in the body and partly excreted unchanged in the urine.

Adverse reactions: Piperazine has a wide margin of safety. Adverse effects are rare, and usually due to cumulation after large doses. They include nausea, vomiting, diarrhoea and urticaria. Neurotoxic effects, observed rarely; include vertigo, muscular incoordination, hypotonia, ataxia of cerebellar type (*'worm-wobble'*), paraesthesiae, blurring of vision and very rarely, seizures. The adverse effects disappear rapidly after discontinuation of the treatment. *The drug appears to be safe during pregnancy.*

Preparations and dosage: A variety of piperazine salts are available for therapy. They are equally effective.

(i) Piperazine citrate is available as 300 mg. tablets (equivalent to about 250 mg. of piperazine hydrate), as an elixir containing 18 g. of the salt in 100 ml. of water and as a mixture for infants containing 720 mg. of the drug per 5 ml.

For ascariasis in adults, a single dose of 5 g. is administered. The equivalent dose of the elixir is upto 30 ml. For children, it is given in the dose of 75 mg. per kg. (5 to 7 ml. of the mixture for infants per year of age to a maximum of 30 ml.) in a single dose. Preliminary fasting is not necessary. The drug is preferably administered in the evening and a saline purge may be given on the next morning to facilitate the expulsion of parasites. A purge, however, is not obligatory.

(ii) Piperazine hydrate. Dose: Adults, 4 g as a single dose.Children,120 mg/kg, upto a total dose of 4 g.

The doses of other piperazine salts are expressed in terms of hydrate equivalents. As piperazine paralyses the adult worm, it may be preferred in subjects with intestinal/biliary obstruction due to worms.

For use of piperazine in enterobiasis, see later.

LEVAMISOLE (Decaris): Levamisole is l-tetramisole and accounts for most of the antehelmintic activity of the racemic mixture, tetramisole. Like pyrantel, it causes sustained contracture of somatic muscles of the worm by an irreversible, non-competitive, depolarization type of neuromuscular block. It is rapidly and considerably absorbed and about 60% is excreted in the urine, mostly as metabolites, within 24 hours.

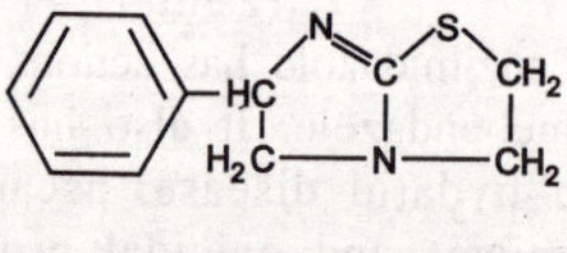

Fig. 58.3: Levamisole

Levamisole also has **immunostimulant** properties (Chapter 76).

Levamisole is available as a single dose tablet containing 150 mg. for adults and 50 mg. for children.

In ascariasis, it is effective in the dose of 2.5-5.0 mg./kg. given as a single oral dose. It is also effective against hookworms though to a smaller extent. In tricho-strongyliasis, a single dose is effective in over 95% of the cases.

Adverse reactions reported are usually mild and include nausea, vomiting, abdominal pain, diarrhoea, giddiness and drowsiness.

These drugs are not active against larvae and hence follow-up re-evaluation of treated patients is necessary.

Drug Therapy of Hookworms

A. duodenale infestation is extremely common in tropical countries and represents an important cause of iron deficiency anemia due to intestinal blood loss. Acute clinical manifestations can be due to larval migration through various tissues and skin. The infestation often exists along with ascariasis. In such a situation, it is preferable to treat ascariasis first, as drugs used solely against ancylostomiasis may irritate the roundworms causing their migration or their aggregation into ball-like masses. The former may lead to invasion of the bile duct and the liver, while the latter may precipitate acute appendicular or intestinal obstruction and rarely, perforation. Hence, drugs effective against both roundworms and hookworms are to be preferred.

It should be noted that no single drug is able to eradicate all the hookworms in 100 per cent cases, and it is necessary to repeat the same drug or give another drug after an appropriate interval. **Albendazole** (400 mg single dose), **Mebendazole** and **Pyrantel** are the preferred drugs in ancylostomiasis. (see above). Multiple doses are often needed to ensure complete cure.

Bephenium hydroxynaphthoate (Alcopar): This drug, given in a single dose, is effective in removing roundworms and hookworms of the species *Ancylostoma doudenale*. It is less effective against *Necator americans*. This drug is not commonly used now because of availability of better drugs.

Adjuvant treatment: This includes administration of iron salts for the correction of anemia. Regular, oral administration of iron daily can prevent the anemia and maintain the hemoglobin levels to 12 g/dl even without immediate treatment of worms. Provision of footwear to avoid larval penetration should be encouraged in endemic areas.

Drugs Therapy of Pinworms

E. vermicularis is a common parasite found in the caecum and the vermiform appendix. The infestation is more common in children. The majority of cases are asymptomatic.The gravid female worm deposits eggs on the perianal and perineal skin leading to intense itching. Scratching of this region may lead to autoinfection by ingestion of ova carried under the nails. To prevent this, patients should be advised to trim the nails and wash the hands thoroughly before the meals. Symptomatically, an antihistaminic cream applied around the anus relieves itching. Infection can also occur through underclothing, bed linen, lavatory contamination and water contamination.

Gravid female worms sometimes migrate into the female genital tract, causing pelvic pain, valvo-vaginitis, pruritus and even granuloms.

Besides the drug therapy, additional measures are desirable in resistant cases. At night, the patient should wear pants under the pyjamas, and gloves which can be boiled. Hands should be washed repeatedly and it may be useful to treat the whole family simultaneously. Infection can also be disseminated by inhalation or ingestion of dust.

Mebendazole 100 mg, or **albendazole** 400 mg. single dose, repeated after 2 weeks, and **pyrante palmoate** are the drugs of choice in pinworm infestation. Single doses of mebendazole produce 90-100% cure rates. The other drug used is piperazine; though effective, it is now rarely used.

Drug Therapy of Strongyloidiasis

The adult female of *Strongyloides stercoralis* lives in the mucosal epithelium of the duodenum and the jejunum. There is no parasitic male; the reproduction is parthenogenic. Ova passed by the adult worm develop into rhabditidiform larvae in the intestine; they metamorphose into the infective filariform larvae in the soil. The infective larvae invade the human host by penetrating the skin and travel through the venous circulation to the lungs. They migrate through the alveolar capillary walls, ascend the respiratory tract to the epiglottis, and are swallowed to reach the small intestine where they mature. Alternatively, the rhabditidiform larvae develop into infective larvae in the intestine; the latter penetrate the intestinal wall to reach the circulation *(internal auto-infection).* Internal autoinfection leads to persistence of the infection for upto 20 years. In immunosuppressed or malnourished patients internal autoinfection may assume massive proportions with ectopic migration of larvae, resulting in *hyper-infection syndrome*. The intestinal parasites cause epigastric pain and diarrhoea; heavy infections may produce malabsorption. Hyperinfection syndrome is a serious complication with acute onset of fever, abdominal pain and distension, often accompanied by shock and pneumonitis. As *strongyloides* ova do not appear in stools, diagnosis depends upon identification of larvae; repeated stool examination or examination of the duodenal contents may be necessary for identifying the larvae.

Ivermectin in the dose of 100-200 mcg/kg daily for 2 days is considered the therapy of choice (see later).

THIABENDAZOLE (Mintezol): This drug, a benzimidazole derivative, has a broad spectrum of activity and is effective against roundworms, hookworms, pinworms and strongyloid worms. It acts in the same way as other benzimidazoles.

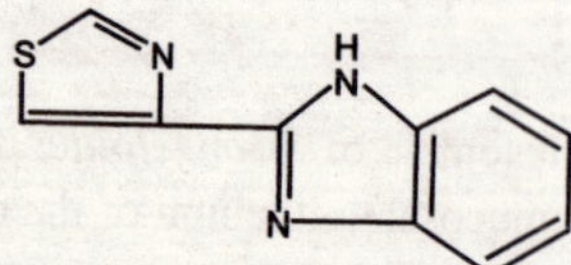

Fig. 58.4: Thiabendazole

Thiabendazole is partly absorbed after oral administration and largely metabolized in the liver and excreted by the kidney as the hydroxylated derivative.

Adverse reactions: These occur in 15 to 30 per cent of patients and include skin reactions, anorexia, nausea, vomiting, epigastric distress, dizziness and fever. Other adverse effects are hypoglycemia and disturbances of colour vision. Blood pressure may fall; liver damage and crystalluria have also been reported.

In majority of cases with strongyloid infestation, 25 mg. per kg. in adults and 30 mg. per kg. in children in 2 divided doses at 12 hourly intervals for 3 days are highly effective. It is now rarely used because of toxicity.

Drug Therapy of Trichuriasis (Whipworm)

Trichuriasis caused by *Trichuris trichura* (whipworm) is frequently encountered along with roundworms and hookworms. Trichuriasis is acquired after consumption of food contaminated with parasite eggs. Children are unusually susceptible and develop anemia.

Rarely, the worms may lodge in the appendix or may penetrate the bowel wall and cause peritonitis.

Mebendazole is highly effective. It is given orally in the dose of 100 mg twice daily for 3 days or as a single 500 mg dose. A second course may be given after 3 weeks with a cure rate of almost 90%.

Albendazole is less effective and has to be given in a single daile dose of 800mg. for 4 days.

Drug Therapy of Filariasis

Filarial infections are caused by parasitic tissue-dwelling filarial nematodes, which are transmitted by biting insects (Table 58.3).

Table 58.3: Types of filariasis

Type	Species	Vector
• ***Lymphatic***	*W.bancrofti* *B. malayi*	Mosquitoes
• ***Subcutaneous and ocular***	*O.volvulus*	Blackfly (simulium)
• ***Dermal***	*Loa loa*	Biting flies (chrysops)

Different varieties of this worm infect over 250 million people in the world, causing elephantiasis and blindness in severe cases. The drugs available for cure and prevention of this condition are **diethylcarbamazine** and **ivermectin.**

DIETHYLCARBAMAZINE (DEC, Hetrazan, Banocide, Unicarbazine): This drug, a piperazine derivative, inactive *in vitro,* leads to a rapid disappearance of microfilariae of *W. bancrofti, B. malayi* and *Loa loa* from the human peripheral blood. The drug probably acts by sensitizing the microfilariae so that they become susceptible to phagocytosis and are trapped by the fixed reticuloendothelial cells in the liver sinusoids. DEC also enhances cell mediated immunity of the human host and thus his resistance to the infestation. The microfilariae of *W. bancrofti* in a hydrocoele, however, are not affected. The drug kills the adult worms of *B. malayi* and *Loa loa* and possibly those of *W. bancrofti.* However, this action is slower than the effect on microfilariae and needs longer/repeated course. The drug has no action against the adult worm of *O. volvulus.* It has some action in ascariasis.

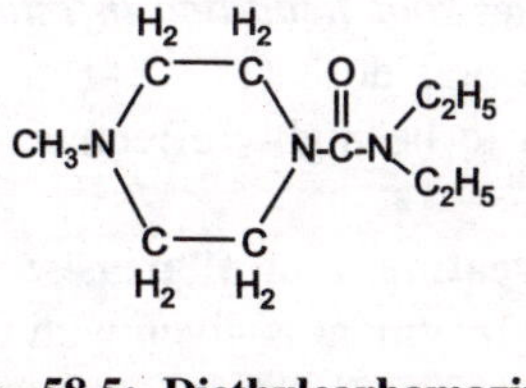

$$CH_3\text{-}N\langle(CH_2CH_2)_2\rangle N\text{-}C(=O)\text{-}N(C_2H_5)_2$$

Fig. 58.5: Diethylcarbamazine

Absorption, fate and excretion: Diethylcarbamazine is rapidly absorbed from the GI tract. Peak plasma levels are achieved within 3 hours. It is uniformly distributed in the body with the exception of fat. It is metabolized in the liver and eliminated in urine within 30 hours.

Adverse reactions: The drug is usually well tolerated. The common ADR include anorexia, nausea, vomiting, headache and drowsiness. These are rarely troublesome. Allergic reactions, due to release of foreign proteins in the tissues by the death of larvae or adult worms, include fever, tachycardia, bronchospasm, lymphadenopathy, muscular pains, arthralgias and urticaria. The allergic reactions are sometimes severe and may involve the eyes, particularly in onchocerciasis (**Mazzoti reaction**). They may start within a few hours of first oral dose and persist for 3-7 days. It is recommended, therefore, to start the therapy with a small dose (50 mg, single dose) and then increase it gradually. Severe ocular reactions can be controlled by instillation of 5 per cent hydrocortisone drops. Administration of antihistaminics or glucocorticoids can minimise systemic allergic effects. Very large doses may cause muscle tremors and convulsions.

Preparations: Diethylcarbamazine tablet usually contains 50 mg or 100 mg of diethylcarbamazine citrate. The syrup contains 10 mg of the drug per ml.

Therapeutic uses:

- ***Filariasis*:** For active lymphatic filariasis *(W. bancrofti* and *Loa loa* infestation), the recommended dose is 6 mg. per kg. body weight in single or divided doses daily for 12 days. The course may be repeated after one month. It has both anti-micro and anti-macro-filarial properties. However evidence indicates that a single dose of 6 mg./kg may be equally useful. Combination of a single dose with a single dose of DEC with invermectin or albendazole is synergestic.
- ***Filarial prophylaxis*:** (See later).
- ***Tropical eosinophilia*:** Pulmonary eosinophilia resulting from parasitic infestation may take the form of a mild illness with fever and cough that last for only a few days (Loeffler's syndrome). This is due to transient allergic

pneumonitis in response to parasitic antigens during the invasive stage of larval migration of roundworm and hookworm. This responds to appropriate anthelmintic treatment.

Classical **tropical eosinophilia** with typical mottling in the lung, fever, anorexia, weight loss and attacks of dyspnoea resembling bronchial asthma is an inflammatory response to microfilaria. It is associated with leucocytosis and marked eosinophilia (more than 3000/cmm). DEC in doses of 6 mg per kg. body weight daily orally for 7 to 10 days is highly effective and is the drug of choice. Resistant cases may be treated with double the dose.

- ***Larva migrans*** (creeping eruption): In this condition, a dose of 3 mg. per kg. is given daily for 10 to 15 days. Thiabendazole is less effective and more toxic. **Albendazole** 400 mg daily for 3 days or **Ivermectin,** 200 mcg/kg/as a single dose, is considered the drug of choice.

Although DEC does have microfilaricidal effect in onchocerciasis caused by *O. volvulus* it gives rise to various adverse effects, including worsening of the ocular condition. Ivermectin is now preferred.

IVERMECTIN (Mectizan): Ivermectin was originally obtained from *Streptomyces avermitilis* found in the soil sample of a Japanese golf course. This macrocyclic lactone has been found to be highly effective against a broad range of parasites and arthropods, and is extensively used in veterinary medicine. It is the drug of choice in onchocerciasis. It probably acts on glutamate gated chloride channel and causes tonic paralysis of microfilariae, which are then immobilized and phagocytosed by reticuloendothelial system. However, the drug has no lethal effect against adult worms. Its efficacy to eliminate the microfilarie from the skin and ocular tissues is as good as that of DEC but perhaps more sustained. In addition, it has the advantage of being effective in a single dose.

Absorption, fate excretion : It is well absorbed and is highly protein-bound in the plasma. More than 97% is metabolized in the liver and is mostly eliminated in the feces. Its elimination t½ is 12-56 hour.

Adverse reactions: As compared to DEC, it causes less severe and fewer systemic and ocular adverse reactions. These are mostly due to the death of microfilariae (Mazzoti reaction), which causes ocular inflammation that may lead to blindness. Commonly, it may cause itching, skin edema, arthralgia, headache and fever. Ivermectin has GABA agonistic activity, and hence the drug should not be used in meningitis and along with CNS depressants.

Therapeutic uses:

- ***Onchocerciasis:*** Given orally in a single dose of 150 mcg/kg, it is highly effective in the treatment of onchocerciasis. It needs to be given in a dose of 150 mcg/kg once in 6-12 months for upto 10 years or until the patient is asymptomatic. If symptoms recur, then the same dose is given every 3 months instead of once a year, for the rest of the period. It appears that a single dose of ivermectin once every 6-12 months may be useful in preventing this disease. When onchocerciasis and loiasis coexist, a single annual dose of 400 mcg/kg can be used.

As a curative treatment of severe onchocerciasis, suramin is sometimes used. It kills the worm but is highly toxic.

- ***Lymphatic filariasis:*** Ivermectin is also effective against the microfilairae of *W.bancrofti*. Single annual doses of 400 mcg/kg are effective and safe in lymphatic filariasis.
- ***Intestinal nematode infection:*** Ivermectin as a single dose of 100 mcg/kg is used for strongyloidiasis. A higher dose of 150-200 mcg/kg is used when ascariasis, trichuriasis and enterobiasis coexist.
- ***Scabies and head-lice infestation:*** Given as a single oral dose (150-200 mcg/kg) it has been found to be highly effective.

Mass treatment of filariasis: In endemic areas, mass treatment is given with the objective of reducing microfilariae to subinfective levels. DEC incorporated in table salt (0.2-0.4% of the base by weight) has been found to reduce the prevalence. Either (DEC 6 mg/kg +albendazole

400 mg) or (ivermectin 200 mcg/kg +albendazole 400mg) in single doses every 6-12 months has shown to be more effective than either drug used alone in controlling the transmission of filariasis, including lymphatic filariasis. The combination of DEC 6 mg/kg and ivermectin 400 mcg/kg, given as a single dose, once a year, is also highly effective.

Recent Egyptian studies suggest that yearly rounds of DEC + albendazole for 5 consecutive years can possibly eliminate filariasis from an endemic area.

Drug Therapy of Guinea Worm

Dracunculus medinensis infestation is transmitted by drinking of water containing infected cyclops (water flea). The adult female usually remains in subcutaneous tissue and may come out through a small ulcer, usually on the foot. The treatment mainly consists of mechanical removal of the worm. **Metronidazole** has been shown to be helpful in this process. **Mebendazole** in the dose of 200 mg t.i.d. orally for 7-10 days is also claimed to be effective in helping easy expulsion.

The important treatment of dracontiasis, as in any other worm infestation, is preventive. This is very simple as the intermediate host, cyclops, can easily be filtered out from the drinking water by using a piece of cloth.

Drug Therapy of Tapeworms

This infestation is transmitted by ingestion of infected beef or pork and can be prevented by avoiding the ingestion of suspected meat or by its thorough cooking.

PRAZIQUANTEL: *It is the drug of choice in taeniasis.* In a single dose of 10 mg/kg it is highly effective against intestinal taeniasis, *T.saginatum, T.solium* and *D. latum* infections in humans, as well as in cysticercosis of the brain. A single dose of 25mg/kg. is used to treat *H. nana* infection. For details, see later.

MEBENDAZOLE/ALBENDAZOLE : These drugs are used to treat hydatid disease of the liver (see earlier).

NICLOSAMIDE (Chlorsalicylamid, Yomesan, Niclosan): This drug is effective in *T. saginata, T. solium, D. latum* and *H. nana* infestations. Given orally, it is not absorbed. It acts by inhibiting anaerobic phosphorylation of ADP by the mitochondria of the parasite.

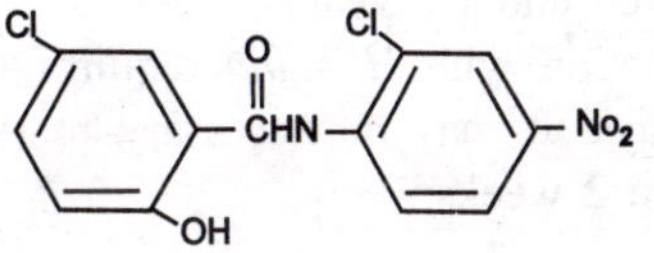

Fig. 58.6 : Niclosamide

Niclosamide is a vermicidal drug. The segments of the worm which are voided after its administration are partially digested by the action of the intestinal proteolytic enzymes; this makes indentification of the scolex impossible. The criterion for cure with this drug, therefore, is absence of eggs and proglottids in the stools for 3 to 4 months after therapy. This is the period required for *T. saginata* to mature and shed mature proglottids from the scolex.

Identification of scolex is important when treating *T. solium* infestation, as cysticercosis, i.e., harbouring of the larval forms (cysticerci) in the tissues of the host may develop if the infestation is not completely eradicated. This makes it mandatory to use a purge within 1-2 hours after the drug is given, in order to prevent digestion of the segments. As the lethal action of niclosamide does not extend to the ova, regurgitation of viable ova into the duodenum in case of *Taenia solium* exposes the patient to the risk of digestion of the ova, autoinfection with larvae and thus cysticercosis. *Niclosamide is not effective against cysticercosis. Hence, in the treatment of infection with T. solium praziquantel is preferred.*

The major advantage of niclosamide is its lack of toxicity except mild GI disturbances. After keeping the patient on a low residue diet on the day before and fasting overnight, 2 tablets of the drug (1 g.) are given in the morning on an empty stomach. The tablets should be chewed, and not swallowed, in order to ensure a thorough mixing of the drug with the intestinal contents. Another 1 g. is given after 1 hour. A saline purge may be given 1 to 2 hours after the second dose but is not essential except in *T. solium* infestation. The dosage in children is 1 g. for those between 2 to 8 years and 0.5 g. in children under 2 years.

Infestation with *H. nana* requires treatment for 5 days. It may be necessary to repeat the course in 2 weeks.

Drug Therapy of Schistosomiasis

Schistosomiasis (bilharziasis) is caused by blood flukes (Schistosomes) that parasitize the venous channels of the definitive hosts. The three common species are *S. hematobium, S. mansoni* and *S. japonicum.* Unlike the other infestations, schistosomal infestations can be considered as systemic, as the parasites are localised in organs other than the gut. Man and domestic animals act as hosts for schistosomes, the ova of which contaminate water. Hatched miracidia invade the water snail (intermediate host). Free living cercariae, emerging from the snail, penetrate the human skin and mature into the adult worms. The infection causes:

- ***Cercarial dermatitis (Swimmer's itch)*** due to repeated exposure to larvae.
- ***Acute schistosomiasis or Katayama's fever***, a serum sickness-like illness more common with *S. japonicum;* and
- ***Chronic illness associated with the formation of egg granulomas*** in various tissues such as urinary bladder and intestines, leading to obstructive and inflammatory lesions. *S. mansoni* causes intestinal and hepatic schistosomiasis whereas *S. hematobium* causes urinary disease.

PRAZIQUANTEL (Biltricide, Cysticide): This pyrazino-iso-quinoline compound is highly effective against all species of schistosomes found in man, at all ages and in all areas. Further, it is effective against liver, lung and intestinal flukes as well as against cestodes causing taeniasis and cysticercosis. The drug increases the permeability of cell membrane to calcium ions, leading to strong muscular contractions and tegumental damage causing the schistosomes to detach from the wall of the vein. It has negligible effect on eggs.

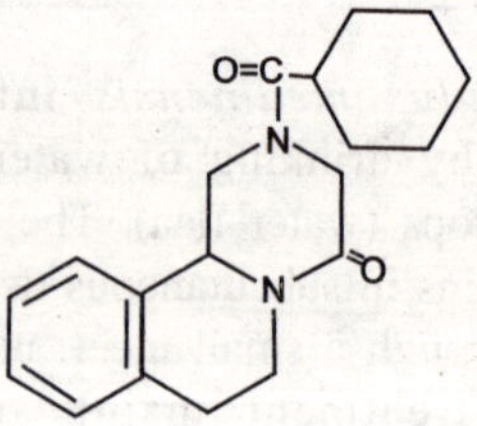

Fig. 58.7 : Praziquantel

Absorption, fate and excretion: Given orally, praziquantel is rapidly absorbed, but significant proportion of the drug is metabolized during the first pass. Its absorption is increased by a high carbohydrate meal. It acts within 1 hour of ingestion. Approximately 70 - 80% of a dose is excreted in urine within 24 hours. Its plasma t½ is 1-1.5 hours.

Adverse reactions: These are dose dependent and are usually mild such as headache, anorexia, drowsiness, lassitude, colic and allergic reactions. Rarely, it may cause hallucinations, excitement or psychotic symptoms, particularly in the Japanese. Experimental evidence indicates that it has no mutagenic, carcinogenic, embryotoxic or teratogenic effect. It is considered safe in children and pregnant women.

Therapeutic uses:

- ***Schistosomiasis*** : It is the drug of choice and is given orally in the dose of 40 mg/kg for

S. hematobium infection and 60 mg/kg for *S. mansoni* and *S. japonicum* infections. The total dose may also be divided into two doses given four hours apart. It is very bitter and the tablet should be swallowed and not chewed. A cure rate of 80-90% has been claimed in *S. hematobium* infection and more than 60% in infection with the other species, at one year follow-up. Even in those in whom the disease is not cured, the egg count drops by more than 90%. The dose may be repeated after 6-8 weeks, if required. Because of its short t½, it is not used for prophylaxis.

The drug, however, cannot kill the schistosomules (migrating larvae) that are 3-21 days old. **Artemether** does kill them during the first 21 days in the body, and may be given in the dose of 6 mg/kg every 2 weeks. A combination of artemether and praziquantel is synergistic in killing the adult worm. Katayama fever which is a hypersensitivity reaction is mainly treated with a glucocorticoid, along with praziquantel.

- In ***taeniasis***, a single dose of 10 mg/kg produces high cure rates. Praziquantel does not kill the ova and hence a post-treatment purge is advised in *T. solium* infection. A single dose of 20 mg/kg is highly effective in *H. nana* infection. Although it is effective in the treatment of cerebral cysticercosis in the dose of 50 mg/kg/day in three divided doses for 14 days, albendozole is preferred in the dose of 15 mg/kg/day for 8 days. Treatment may be continued upto 30 days, if necessary.
- In ***fluke infestations***: See later.
- ***Hydatid disease :*** It may be used as an adjunct to albendazole.

OXAMNIQUINE (Vansil): This is a tetrahydroquinoline derivative. Given orally, it is well absorbed. It is effective only against *S. mansoni* (African) infestation. Generally, it is well tolerated. Adverse reactions include dizziness, somnolence, abdominal pain, headache and diarrhoea. It is better tolerated after meals. Rarely, it causes hallucinations and seizures. The urine may be coloured red. It should be avoided during pregnancy.

The dose varies according to the geographical region. In South America and the Caribbean islands, it is given as a single dose, 15 mg/kg in adults and 20 mg/kg in children under 14 years of age. The dose can also be split into 2 doses given 3-8 hours apart. In the Arabian peninsula and in East and Central Africa, a total dose of 30 mg/kg is given, divided into 2 equal doses, administered on two consecutive days. Higher doses such as 40-60 mg/kg are needed in countries such as Egypt, Sudan, Zaire, Zimbabwe and Uganda; in these places, it is administered in 20 mg/kg single doses on 2-3 consecutive days. The cure rate is 60-90%.

METRIFONATE (Bilarsil): This organophosphorus insectcide is a prodrug and its therapeutic effects are due to its metabolite dichlorovas, which is a cholinesterase inhibitor (Chapter 18). It is effective only in *S.hematobium* infestation with a cure rate of 40-80%. The adverse effects are usually mild and transient; they consist of GI disturbances, weakness, dizziness and vertigo.

Recently, **artemisinin derivatives,** artemether and artesunate, have been shown to possess activity against schistosomes and may be combined with praziaquantel.

Drug Therapy of Flukes

PRAZIQUANTEL: This drug has revolutionized the treatment of infestation with these parasites (paragonimiasis). It is highly effective against lung and intestinal flukes. The recommended dose is 75 mg/kg, divided into three doses given on the same day. The dose may be repeated (see above).

Thiabendazole given in a single dose of 10 mg/kg for liver and lung flukes infestation, is also useful.

Bithionol 30 mg/kg daily for 5 days is also effective but more toxic.

Chemotherapy of Malignancy 59

In the genesis of malignancy (cancer), multiple factors are implicated, the environmental carcinogen being the major culprit. Only in a few cases (10%), it is genetically inherited. Chemotherapy of malignanacy differs in some respects from that of infections in that:

(a) In infections, the invading microbe is biologically 'foreign' to the host and its metabolic reactions are so different from those of the host tissue cells that a chemotherapeutic agent can attack it selectively without affecting the host tissue cells. No such clear cut differences in metabolic reactions have been demonstrated between malignant and normal cells; drugs probably destroy the cancerous tissue preferentially because it is a rapidly growing tissue. Thus, many anticancer drugs lack the selectivity of the antimicrobial drugs.

(b) In infections, the body helps the antimicrobial drug with its own defence system in the form of antibodies, phagocytosis etc. Although antibodies have been demonstrated against certain cancer cells, such host defence is usually lacking or ineffective. It is necessary, therefore, to use the drugs in such doses so as to destroy all the malignant cells. In most instances, this is impracticable because of non-specificity and high tissue toxicity of these compounds.

(c) Malignant cells can develop resistance to drugs.

Cancer of the epithelial tissues is called **carcinoma** and that of the non-epithelial (mesenchymal) tissues is known as **sarcoma.**

The characteristics which distinguish the cancer cells from normal cells are:

- ***Uncontrolled (autonomous) proliferation.***
- ***Dedifferentiation and loss of function.***
- ***Invasiveness;*** and
- ***Metastasis.***

The normal cell proliferates through a definite **cell cycle**, that causes programmed DNA replication. The mechanism of cell division is essentially the same in all dividing cells and is divided into five phases (Fig. 59.1). Thus, the cell successively goes through:

(1) **G_0 (gap 0 or resting) non-proliferative phase.**

(2) **G_1 (gap 1 i.e. presynthetic) phase,** during which the cell determines its readiness to commit to DNA synthesis.

(3) **S (synthetic) phase,** involving DNA synthesis.

(4) **G_2 (gap 2 i.e. post-synthetic) phase,** during which the accuracy of DNA replication is determined, and errors are corrected; and

(5) **M (mitotic) phase,** during which the replicated chromosomes are separated into two nuclei for the two daughter G_1 cells. These cells may re-enter the cycle or pass into the resting G_0 phase.

Topoisomerases 1 and 2 play an important role during DNA replication. The cell-cycle transition between G_1 and S and that between G_2 and M are so well regulated that the cell divides properly with a minimum of errors. Check points in G1 and G2 determine whether the cell will enter S and M, respectively. These check points are regulated by protein kinases (cyclin-dependent kinases CDK) and kinase-associated proteins called cyclins.

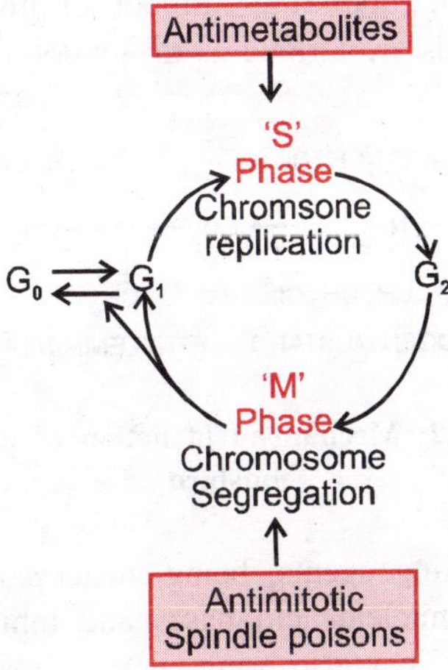

Fig. 59.1: Cell cycle and sites of action of drugs

Progress through the cell cycle depends on the balance between positive and negative regulatory forces. The positive forces include growth factors and a series of cyclins and cyclin-dependent kinases (**cDKs**). The negative forces are the proteins which are induced by genes such as tumour suppressor gene p53. When there is damage to the DNA, these inhibitors normally halt the cycle, allowing repair. If repair fails, the cell undergoes degradation of nuclear DNA leading to death called **apoptosis** (programmed cell death). Apoptosis helps to eliminate abnormal cells that have become redundant during development and differentiation. It thus acts as the first line of defence against mutations and renewal of cells with abnormal DNA that could become malignant.

In the cancer cell, the cell cycle control is disrupted by:

- ***Abnormal growth factor function.***
- ***Abnormal cdk function.***
- ***Abnormal DNA synthesis;*** and
- ***Abnormal decreases in negative regulatory forces due to mutation in the tumour suppressor gene.***

Anticancer drugs, classification :

I **Phase-specific, cell-cycle active** e.g. Antimetabolites, Bleomycin, Taxane, Epipodophylotoxin and Vinca alkaloids.

II **Phase non-specific** which can injure DNA at any phase of the cell cycle but appear to block the check points before the cell division e.g. Alkylating agents, Antitumour antibiotics Camptothecins and Platinum analogues.

III **Hormones** and **antihormone;** or

IV **Miscellaneous** eg Monoclonal antibodies (mAb).

Since the cytotoxic drugs act by affecting the cell division, they also affect all rapidly dividing cells leading to common toxicity such as:

- ***Bone marrow suppression.***
- ***Loss of hair (Alopecia).***
- ***Damage to GI mucosa and ulceration, nausea and vomiting.***
- ***Damage to gonads.***
- ***Impaired wound healing.***
- ***Growth inhibition in children;*** and
- ***Teratogenicity.***

The anticancer drugs currently employed can also be classified as :

I **Alkylating agents:**

- ***Nitrogen mustards,*** e.g., Mechlorethamine, Cyclophosphamide, Melphalan, Uracil mustard and Chlorambucil.
- ***Ethylenimines,*** e.g., Triethylene thiophosphoramide (Thio-TEPA).
- ***Alkyl sulfonates,*** e.g., Busulfan.

II **Antimetabolites:**

- ***Folic acid antagonists,*** e.g., Methotrexate.
- ***Purine antagonists,*** e.g., 6-Mercaptopurine, Azathioprine.
- ***Pyrimidine antagonists,*** e.g., Fluorouracil, Fluorodeoxyuridine, Cytosine arabinoside.

III **Radioactive isotopes,** e.g., Radioiodine, Radiogold, Radiophosphorus.

IV **Cytotoxic antibiotics,** e.g., Actinomycin-D, Mitomycin-C, Rubidomycin, Doxorubicin, Bleomycin, and Mithramycin.

V **Antimitotic plant products** – Vinblastine, Vincristine, Vindesin, Taxane, Etoposide, Camptotheptin analogues.

VI **Hormones and Anti-hormones :**

- ***Glucocorticoids*** eg, Prednisolone.
- ***Estrogens*** and ***Progestius.***
- ***Antiestrogens*** eg, Flutamide.
- ***Aromatase inhibitors*** eg, Letrozole.
- ***GnRH agonists*** eg, Luprolide, Goserelin
- ***GnRH antagonist*** eg, Abarelix
- ***Somatostatin analogues*** eg, Octreotide.

VII **Miscellaneous:** Hydroxyurea, Procarbazine, Mitotane, 1-Asparaginase, Cisplatin, Tretinoin, Arsenic trioxide.

VIII **Monoclonal antibodies and tyrosine kinase inhibitors:** Trastuzumab, Rituximab and Imatinib.

IX **Biological response modifiers:** Interferons (Chapter 57), BCG, Levamisole (Chapter 76).

Chemotherapy of cancer is a specialized field, to be handled only by an oncologist. Precise adherence to treatment protocols is mandatory because of the low therapeutic index of many drugs. Its detailed discussion is beyond the scope of this book. Only the guidelines and some important drugs used are described below.

Alkylating Agents

The compound sulfur mustard was first used in 1917 in chemical warfare. It caused severe vesication of the skin and the mucous membranes, GI ulcerations and myelosupression. The pharmacological properties of nitrogen mustards became known only after the end of World War II.

Mechanism of action: Nitrogen mustards are called alkylating agents because these compounds can transfer an alkyl radical to a suitable receptor site. Alkylating agents, in neutral or alkaline solution, form highly reactive quaternary ammonium derivatives, ethyleniminium cations (Fig. 59.2). These cations react with (alkylate) groupings like amino, sulfhydryl, hydroxy or phosphate in the physiologically important molecules in the cells and render them unavailable for the normal metabolic reactions. Depending upon the number of groups, the compounds are termed as di- or polyfunctional.

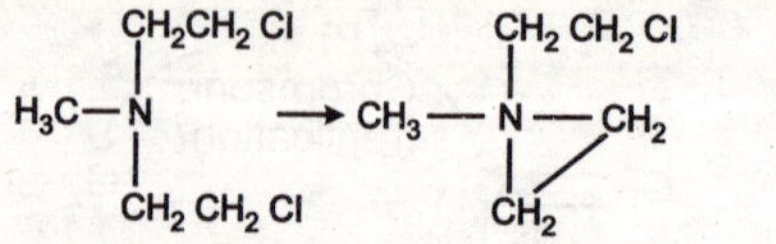

$$H_3C-N(CH_2CH_2Cl)_2 \rightarrow CH_3-\overset{+}{N}(CH_2CH_2Cl)\begin{matrix}CH_2\\|\\CH_2\end{matrix}$$

NITROGEN MUSTARD — ETHYLENIMINIUM ION

Fig. 59.2: Mechanism of action of nitrogen mustard

Alkylating agents, being nucleophilic, react with the nucleic acid bases and inhibit DNA synthesis. They also bring about a cross-linkage of DNA strands in resting as well as in dividing cells and thus interfere with cell replication.

Pharmacological actions common to various alkylating agents are described below; individual differences are mentioned under each drug.

- ***Cytotoxic action:*** In general, these drugs damage the nuclei of growing and multiplying cells. The hemopoietic system is highly susceptible to this action. Thus, they cause leucopenia, anemia, thrombocytopenia and, in toxic doses, aplasia of the bone marrow. Although the net result is similar, the mode of action of individual drugs may differ. Thus, chlorambucil is more effective against the cells of lymphoid series while busulfan has predominant action against myeloid tissue.

These drugs also affect epithelial tissues such as those of cornea and the intestinal mucosa causing nuclear fragmentation and desquamation, leading to the formation of ulcers. Hair follicles are also damaged causing alopecia. They impair spermatogenesis irreversibly in males and may cause amenorrhoea and fetotoxicity in females.

- ***Immunosuppressant action :*** Alkylating

agents suppress antibody production and hence act as immunosuppressants.

- ***Miscellaneous actions:*** All the alkylating agents produce severe nausea and vomiting.

Nitrogen mustards are also called **Radiomimetic drugs** as their actions resemble to some extent the biological effects of ionizing radiation. All alkylating agents, however, are not radiomimetic to the same extent.

MECHLORETHAMINE (Mustine): This is the first nitrogen mustard introduced in cancer therapeutics. Locally, it is a vesicant, the most susceptible tissues being those of the skin, the eyes and the respiratory tract.

When dissolved in water, the drug undergoes very rapid intramolecular chemical transformation to the active form within a few minutes and hence, is given IV immediately. It is largely metabolized in the body. Extravasation of the drug into the tissues causes severe irritation and sloughing.

It is supplied as hydrochloride, 10 mg. of which are triturated with 90 mg. of anhydrous sodium chloride to increase the bulk. The usual total dose is 0.4 mg./kg. of body weight given either singly or in 2 to 4 divided portions.

Adverse reactions: Mechlorethamine is a very toxic drug. Commonly, it produces anorexia, severe nausea and vomiting. Hence it is usually administered at bed time along with a prophylactic antiemetic like chlorpromazine. Delayed toxicity involves anemia, severe bone marrow depression, aplasia and death. It can cause menstrual irregularities in females.

Therapeutic uses: Mechlorethamine and other alkylating agents are used in combination with other drugs to treat various hematologic and solid cancers and lymphomas.

Because of its serious toxicity, mechlorethamine has been replaced by less toxic drugs such as **lomustine** (given orally) and **carmustine** (given IV). They are lipid soluble and penetrate the blood brain barrier. Hence, they are preferred for the treatment of brain tumours. **Estramustine** is a stable combination of an estrogen and mustine, designed to deliver mustine to the estrogen receptor site of a tumour such as prostate cancer. It has both local cytostatic effect and a hormonal effect due to its estrogen component.

CYCLOPHOSPHAMIDE (Endoxan): The pharmacological actions of this compound are mostly similar to those of mechlorethamine hydrochloride. It is a pro-drug and is converted in the body to its active form. In contrast to nitrogen mustard, it is not a local irritant and it can be given orally as well as parenterally. It is less likely to cause thrombocytopenia.

Absorption, fate and excretion : Cyclophosphamide is well absorbed from the GI tract. It is converted in the liver to active metabolites, hydroxyphosphamide and aldophosphamide. They are metabolized further to inactive compounds. About 14 per cent of the drug appears in the urine unchanged.

Adverse reactions: Toxicity of cyclophosphamide is similar to that of mechlorethamine. Sometimes, it causes chemical cystitis and hepatic damage. The toxicity to the urinary tract epithelium is due to the metabolite acrolein. **Mesna,** a synthetic sulfhydryl compound, given simultaneously with cyclophosphamide and again 4 and 8 hours later, reacts with the toxic metabolite in the urinary tract, thus preventing hemorragic cystitis.

Preparations and dosage: Cyclophosphamide is supplied as 50 mg. tablets and in vials containing 100-200 mg. of powder. Solution for injection is prepared by adding 5 ml. of sterile water to 100 mg. of the drug. The solution remains stable for 3 hours. The drug can be given IV, intrapleurally, intraperitoneally, intra-arterially and directly into the tumour. The usual daily dose is 3.5-5 mg. per kg., orally or IV for 8 days, followed by the daily oral maintenance dose of 100 mg. for 30-40 days. It can be repeated after 6-8 weeks.

Therapeutic uses: Commonly, cyclophosphamide is used as a part of a multiple-drug regimen to treat various malignancies. It is used to treat chronic lymphatic leukemia, lymphoma and solid tumours. Because of the possibility of hemorrhagic cystitis, the patient is advised to take plenty of fluids.

Its use as an immunosuppressing agent is discussed in Chapter 76.

MELPHALAN (Alkeran, 1-Sarcolysin): This is a phenylalanine nitrogen mustard and has properties similar to the other alkylating agents. It is effective orally. It is less irritant locally and alopecia is rare following its use. Other systemic toxic effects are similar to those of mechlorethamine.

Melphalan is administered orally in 2 mg. tablets; the dose recommended is 0.25 mg./kg daily for 4 days every 4-6 wk. The drug is used in the treatment of multiple myeloma.

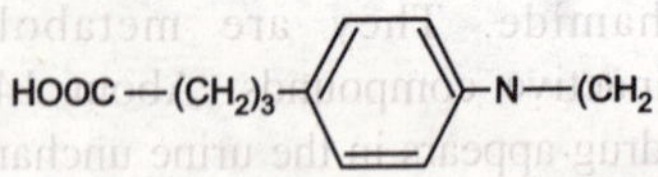

$HOOC-(CH_2)_3-C_6H_4-N-(CH_2CH_2Cl)_2$

Fig. 59.3: Chlorambucil

CHLORAMBUCIL (Leukeran): This compound, chemically related to mechlorethamine, has similar pharmacological and toxicological properties.

Chlorambucil, however, is the shortest acting nitrogen mustard. It is effective orally, predominantly against malignant cells of lymphoid series. It is not a local irritant and is less likely to cause alopecia even after prolonged use. Its myelosuppressive effect is dose dependent and usually reversible.

Chlorambucil is supplied as 2 mg. tablets. It is given orally, usually in the dose of 0.1-0.2 mg. per kg. of body weight daily for 3 to 6 weeks.

Therapeutic uses: The drug can be used for similar purposes as cyclophosphamide but is the drug of choice in the treatment of chronic lymphocytic leukemia.

THIOTEPA: This compound has similar actions as mechlorethamine but is not a local irritant. It is not well absorbed orally and is given IV. It is also used by bladder instillation for superficial bladder tumours.

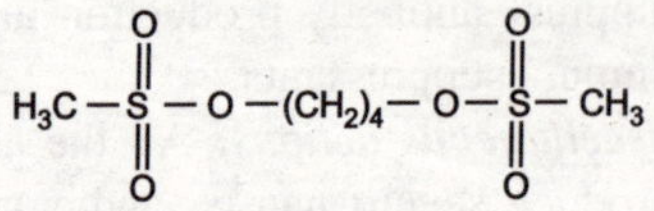

$H_3C-SO_2-O-(CH_2)_4-O-SO_2-CH_3$

Fig. 59.4: Busulfan

BUSULFAN (Myleran): This drug differs from nitrogen mustards in its mechanism of action. It is more effective against cells of the myeloid series. The drug gets selectively bound to nuclei and causes a selective depression of granulocyte and platelet production; it does not have a significant action on the intestinal epithelium or the lymphoid tissue. In combination with chlorambucil, it can produce actions similar to radiation.

Absorption, fate and excretion: Given orally it is well absorbed. Given IV, it disappears from the blood within 2 to 3 minutes. It is excreted in the urine as methanesulfonic acid.

Adverse reactions: These are similar to those of other alkylating agents. It causes much less nausea. Because of its selective action, the incidence of thrombocytopenia is higher. Prolonged administration may cause amenorrhoea, wasting, pigmentation, gynecomastia, anhydrosis and pulmonary fibrosis.

Therapeutic uses: It is the drug of choice in the treatment of chronic myeloid leukemia. The treatment is initiated with 2-8 mg. daily orally and then, depending upon the leucocytic count, the dose is tapered to a daily maintenance dose of 0.5-2 mg.

Antimetabolites

Chemical substances which take part in cellular metabolic reactions are called as metabolites. An antimetabolite is a chemical agent which, by virtue of its close structural similarity to the metabolite, blocks its actions. It can achieve this either by preventing the combination of the metabolite with its specific enzyme or by itself combining with the specific enzyme and thus getting transformed into a compound which is either metabolically inactive or harmful to the cell. The latter process is sometimes called as lethal synthesis.

Clinically useful growth inhibiting anti-metabolites are structural analogues of :

- ***Substances essential for the synthesis of the nucleic acid bases,*** e.g., folic acid antagonist methotrexate; and
- ***Substances which get incorporated into the nucleic acid chains,*** e.g., purine and pyrimidine antagonists; they act as pseudometabolites.

METHOTREXATE (Amethopterin): This is a 4-amino substituted folic acid analogue which acts as a **folic acid antagonist**.

Mechanism of action: Folic acid is essential for the production of the coenzyme, tetrahydrofolic acid (THF). The conversion of folate to THF is carried out by an enzyme, folate reductase (Chapter 34). Methotrexate competes with folic acid for this enzyme and succeeds in binding the folate reductase irreversibly, thus restricting the production of THF. Lack of the coenzyme THF leads to inhibition of DNA synthesis and consequently of cell replication. Methotrexate is, therefore, more toxic to tissues with a high proportion of rapidly dividing cells, such as the bone marrow.

Pharmacological actions:

- ***Cytotoxic actions:*** Methotrexate has a predominant action on the bone marrow. It inhibits erythropoiesis, myelopoiesis and finally may cause aplasia of the bone. This causes marked peripheral granulocytopenia, reticulocytopenia and moderate lymphopenia. The drug also causes ulceration of the intestinal mucosa leading to severe hemorrhagic, desquamating enteritis. It can cross the placental barrier and interfere with embryogenesis causing foetal abnormalities and death.
- ***Immunosuppressive action:*** Methotrexate is a potent immunosuppressant and acts by preventing the clonal expansion of both B and T lymphocytes.
- ***Anti-inflammatory action:*** Used in small doses, it reduces lymphocyte proliferation, rheumatoid factor production, and interferes with the release of inflammatory cytokines like IL-2, IL-6, IL-8 and TNF-α. Thus it acts as an anti-inflammatory agent. It is used as a disease modifying drug in rheumatoid arthritis (Chapter 71).

Absorption, fate and excretion: Methotrexate is well absorbed from the intestines. The metabolism of methotrexate differs in some respects from that of folate. Thus, it disappears from the blood rapidly and remains in the tissue longer than folate. It thus causes a prolonged inhibitory effect. Its concentration in the CSF is poor. About 50-90 per cent of the dose is rapidly excreted in the urine, in free form. Renal impairment is a contraindication to it use.

Adverse reactions: These are due to deficiency of THF and include megaloblastic anemia, thrombocytopenia, leucopenia, aplasia, oral and intestinal ulceration, nausea, vomiting and diarrhoea, alopecia, dermatitis, ulcerative stomatitis and liver damage. These cannot be reversed by giving folic acid as its conversion to THF is blocked. Hence, ideally THF should be administered to antagonise its toxicity. Since THF is too unstable for therapeutic use, a related compound folinic acid (N5-formyl THF, citrovorum factor) is used in the form of calcium folinate or calcium levofolinate. Folinic acid is administered IM or IV, beginning 8-24 hours after the initiation of methotrexate therapy. It is given in the dose of 120 mg (in divided doses) in the first 24 hours, followed by 15 mg. orally or by IM injection 6 hourly for the next 48 hours.

Simultaneous administration of ketoprofen and methotrexate may cause prolonged and striking elevation of plasma methotrexate level. It is possible that similar drug interactions may occur with other NSAID.

Preparations and dosage: Methotrexate is supplied as 2.5 mg. tablets and as powder for injection. Daily recommended dose is 2.5 to 5.0 mg. In case of choriocarcinoma, larger doses of 10-30 mg. daily for five days are usually given. Methotrexate can be given intrathecally, to treat meningeal infiltration in acute leukemia, in a single dose of 0.1-0.5 mg. per kg. body weight.

Therapeutic uses:

- ***Acute lymphatic leukemia*** in children.
- ***Choriocarcinoma:*** It is extremely useful in this condition where it has almost produced 'cure' in certain cases.
- ***Soft tissue sarcoma, breast cancer and acute myeloid leukemia:*** It has some place in the treatment of these conditions.
- ***Rheumatoid arthritis*** (Chapter 71).
- ***Psoriasis*** (Chapter 69).
- ***As an immunosuppressant*** in steroid resistant asthma, Crohn's disease and transplant rejection; and
- ***For medical termination of pregnancy*** (Chapter 66).

6-MERCAPTOPURINE (Purimethol): This purine analogue acts by interfering with the synthesis and interconversion of purines. It is converted in the cells to ribonucleotide of 6-mercaptopurine, which then suppresses the de novo biosynthesis of purines and hence of DNA. The drug is mainly toxic to the bone marrow and intestinal epithelium. Its pharmacological actions are similar to those of methotrexate.

Fig. 59.5 : 6-Mercaptopurine

Absorption, fate and excretion: The drug is well absorbed orally. It is metabolized rapidly by xanthine oxidase, which is also required to synthesize uric acid. Use of the xanthine oxidase inhibitor allopurinol decreases the inactivation of 6-mercaptopurine (Chapter 71). Mercaptopurine and its metabolites are rapidly excreted by the kidneys. Its penetration into the CSF is poor.

Adverse reactions: These are similar to those of methotrexate and are mainly related to bone marrow and GI tract. Sometimes, it causes hepatic necrosis. It may also cause hyperuricemia with hyperuricosuria due to massive destruction of the cells of lymphoid tissues. Hence, urine should be maintained alkaline and its volume adequate.

Therapeutic uses: Mercaptopurine is useful in the treatment of acute leukemia, particularly in children. It is supplied as 50 mg. tablets. The usual daily oral dose is 2.5 mg. per kg. given as a single dose. It is regulated by noting the hematological and clinical improvement. Mercaptopurine is also effective in choriocarcinoma and chronic myelogenous leukemia. The drug acts more slowly than methotrexate. Repeated use may lead to the development of resistance.

Other purine analogues like **6-thioguanine** and **azathioprine** also possess cytotoxic actions. However, they do not seem to have any distinct advantages over mercaptopurine as antileukemic agents. Azathioprine (Imuran) is usually favoured as an immunosuppressive agent in organ transplantation and in certain autoimmune diseases like hemolytic anemias, glomerulonephritis and rheumatoid arthritis.

Drugs like **azaserine** and **duazomycin** (N--acetyl DON), though not purine analogues, interfere with purine synthesis by acting as glutamine antagonists. However, clinically they are not so useful.

5-FLUOROURACIL: This fluorinated analogue of pyrimidine acts by binding the enzyme thymidylate synthetase, thus preventing the production of thymine, the basic component of DNA. It also gets incorporated into RNA in place of uracil. It is toxic to the bone marrow alimentary epithelium and CNS. It is usually administered by slow IV infusion to prevent its first-pass degradation in the liver. Fluorouracil and its derivative, fluorodeoxyuridine have been used in the treatment of carcinoma of stomach, colon, rectum, breast and ovaries. The dose recommended is 15 mg./kg. body weight daily for 3-5 days, followed by 7.5 mg./kg. every second or third day till toxicity is seen. It is relatively a less toxic drug. It is available as solution 50 mg./ml.

CYTOSINE ARABINOSIDE (Cytarabine): This pyrimidine analogue is considered to be the drug of choice in inducing remission in acute myeloid leukemia, especially in adults. It is an 'S' phase specific antimetabolite and acts by interfering with pyrimidine synthesis. The toxic effects include nausea, vomiting, bone marrow depression and cerebellar ataxia.

Gemcitabine, a related compound, is phase nonspecific and is used in pancreatic carcinoma.

Radioactive Isotopes

These are the isotopes of various elements which act because of their physical property of emitting beta and gamma radiation. The radiations given out produce ionization in the cells, thereby disrupting the cellular metabolism, and cell destruction. The therapeutically useful radio-isotopes are radioiodine ^{131}I, radiogold ^{198}Au, and radio-phosphorus ^{32}P.

RADIOIODINE (Na ^{131}I): The drug is given as Na ^{131}I orally. It is concentrated by the thyroid gland and causes acinar destruction. It acts by emitting beta radiation. It is useful in certain cases of thyroid carcinoma. Usually, in thyroid carcinoma, surgery is preferred with or without radiation. Only those tumours which can concentrate enough radioiodine e.g. follicular carcinoma, can be destroyed by this therapy.

Combined therapy with surgery followed by radioiodine can achieve excellent results in selected cases. Usually, the patient is allowed to develop myxedema before the administration of radioiodine. This ensures the maximum uptake by the left-over "thyroid tissue". Generally, 2-3 doses of 150 mCi. each at the interval of 2-3 months are considered adequate and the total dose should not exceed 500 mCi. During radioiodine therapy, the patient must be isolated and special arrangements made for the disposal of urine in order to reduce the possible radiation hazard to other people (Chapter 62).

RADIOACTIVE PHOSPHORUS (Sodium phosphate ^{32}P): Radioactive phosphorus is a beta emitting isotope. It is metabolized by the body like stable phosphorus and is distributed in different tissues in proportion to their total phosphorus content. It is taken up rapidly by those cells where the metabolic turnover of phosphorus is high e.g. multiplying cells, bone marrow, spleen and lymph nodes. It is deposited in bones and is incorporated in nucleoproteins of growing cells. Because of its wide distribution, it causes generalized body irradiation including that including that of lungs, GI tracts and gonads. Excessive irradiation of bone marrow may cause leucopenia, thrombocytopenia and anemia.

It is administered in the form of sodium phosphate ^{32}P, either orally or intravenously.

Therapeutic uses: Its most important use is in the treatment of polycythemia vera, where it is used alone or with phlebotomy. The drug is given orally in doses of 5-6 mCi. About 25 per cent of the dose is not absorbed and appears in feces. It suppresses the production of RBCs, platelets and leucocytes; it does not destroy the already formed mature RBC. Therapeutic effect is seen after an interval of 6-8 weeks. It can be given IV. The drug may be repeated, if necessary, after 3-4 months. Repeated doses of ^{32}P in a case of polycythemia vera may sometimes cause acute leukemia in a few patients and hence, some authorities prefer to avoid this therapy. The other drug used is hydroxyurea (see later).

RADIOACTIVE GOLD (1yAu): This radioisotope gives out low energy beta and gamma radiations. Because of its beta radiations, it was used to produce localized tissue destruction in the treatment of malignant pleural and peritoneal effusions.

Cytotoxic Antibiotics

This group of antibiotics derived from the

Streptomyces species act by inhibiting DNA and/or RNA synthesis. Their cytotoxic property and ADR are similar to those of the polyfunctional alkylating agents.

ACTINOMYCIN D (Dactinomycin): This antibiotic has toxicity similar to that of mechlorethamine. It can damage the skin, particularly that exposed previously to x-ray irradiation. It is mostly used as an experimental tool to block the production of ribosomal ribonucleic acid in cell metabolism studies.

RUBIDOMYCIN (Dunomycin, Daunorubicin): This antibiotic, obtained from a strain of *Streptomyces coeruleorubidus* is also cytotoxic. When used along with vincristine and prednisolone, it is reported to produce remission in many cases of acute leukemia in children. It is also useful in acute myeloblastic leukemia in adults. It causes profound bone marrow suppression and toxic cardiomyopathy.

DOXORUBICIN (Adriamycin): This antibiotic is obtained from *Streptomyces pneuceticus.* It acts as an inhibitor of topoisomerase I and II, thus interfering with DNA replication. It produces a complete remission in acute lymphoblastic leukemia and lymphoblastic lymphosarcoma in patients who failed to respond to or had relapsed after stopping standard chemotherapy. Its toxicity is similar to that of rubidomycin. It has also been used in other malignancies. It is used IV and can also be given by instillation into the bladder.

Epirubicin and **Idarubicin** are newer analogues of doxorubicin.

BLEOMYCIN: This drug, derived from *Streptomyces verticillus*, is useful in epidermoid carcinomas of the skin, the upper respiratory passages, the oral cavity and the genito-urinary tract and in lymphomas resistant to other drugs. Radiation can be given after bleomycin which is a radiosensitizer but prior radiation impairs its effectiveness. Its main toxicity is nausea, vomiting, dermographia, scleroderma like changes in the skin, pneumonitis, and occasionally pulmonary fibrosis. It is rarely a myelosuppessant. It is used IV, IM or SC.

MITOMYCIN C: This antibiotic is obtained from *Streptomyces caespitosus*. It has been employed by IV or intra-arterial injection, in the treatment of chronic myeloid leukemia and Hodgkin's disease. Like alkylating agents the drug may cause local tissue necrosis on extravasation, severe bone marrow depression, bleeding, toxic hepatitis and hemolytic uremic syndrome. The usual dose is 6-10 mg/m^2 IV bolus every 6 weeks.

MITHRAMYCIN (Plicamycin): This drug derived from *Streptomyces plicatus*. It has been found to be useful in embryonal cell carcinoma of the testis, in hypercalcemia due to malignant disease and in Paget's disease. It has high toxicity and causes myelosuppression, thrombocytopenia, liver and kidney damage and bleeding due to suppression of clotting factors.

Ixabepilone is derived from apothiline, a cytotoxic macrolide. It has actions similiar to those of taxane but can be used in taxane resistant cases. It is used in combination to treat advanced metastatic breast cancer. It is a CYP3A4 substate. It causes peripheral sensory neuropathy.

Antimitotic Plant Products

VINCA ALKALOIDS: From the various alkaloids isolated from periwinkle plant (Vinca rosea; Catharanthus rosens), three compounds, **vinblastine, vincristine** and **vindesine**, have been shown to be useful in the chemotherapy of malignancy. Vinorelbine is a semisynthetic derivative.

Mechanism of action: They cause cell-cycle arrest in mitosis. They bind to tubulin and prevent the formation of the mitotic spindle (**antimitotic spindle poison**).

Pharmacological actions: These alkaloids have similar spectrum of cytotoxic activity. Interestingly, there is no cross resistance between these two agents, in spite of the close similarity in their chemical structure.

In addition, vinca alkaloids produce certain neurological effects. They affect neuromuscular transmission and cause peripheral neuropathy. They may also cause mental depression, ataxia and tremors. It should be noted that the molecules of these alkaloids contain indole and dihydroindole groups, similar to other psychotropic drugs like LSD.

Because of their large molecular size, vinca alkaloids are not well absorbed by oral route. These drugs, being highly irritant, are administered through a freely running IV infusion. They are excreted primarily by the liver into the biliary tract. They are not used intrathecally because of severe neurotoxicity.

Adverse reactions: Although these drugs are chemically related, their toxicity is relatively different. Vinblastine is more toxic to the bone marrow while vincristine causes more neurotoxicity and alopecia. Common toxic effects include nausea, anorexia and vomiting, mental depression, constipation and alopecia. Neurotoxicity includes cranial nerve palsies and peripheral neuropathy. Signs of intestinal obstruction due to severe constipation with paralytic ileus may occur. They are teratogenic.

Therapeutic uses: The commonly employed drug is vinblastine sulfate (Velbe). The drug should not be used unless the total WBC count is at least 4000 per cmm.

Vinblastine is mainly useful in Hodgkin's disease and other lymphomas, where it produces remission in 50-60 per cent of cases. It can also be used in methotrexate resistant choriocarcinoma and lymphosarcoma.

Vincristine (Oncovin) is useful in the treatment of acute lymphatic leukemia in children to initiate remission.

PACLITAXEL (Taxol): This drug has been isolated from the bark of the Western yew tree. It binds to the beta subunit of tubulin and results in the formation of a stable non-functioning microtubule bundle, thus interfering with mitosis. This action differs from that of vinca alkaloids which inhibit microtubules. It also induces apoptosis and has anti-angiogenic property. It is metabolised in the liver. The drug is used to treat cancer of the ovary, breast, lung, esophagus, head and neck. It is administered by infusion.

Adverse reactions : The primary toxic effect of paclitaxel is on the bone marrow. Neutropenia occurs 8-11 days after a dose but reverses rapidly after 2-3 weeks. Several patients complain of myalgias for a few days after receiving paclitaxel. Other adverse reactions are asymptomatic bradycardia or episodes of silent ventricular tachycardia. Paclitaxel can cause alopecia, skin rashes, neuropathy and hypersensitivity reactions.

Docetaxel, an analogue of paclitaxel with similar properties but a longer half-life, is used for similar indications.

Camptothecin analogues: These have been isolated from the Chinese tree *Camptotheca acuminata* and include **irinotecan** and **topotecan.** They inhibit nuclear topoisomerase1 and thereby inhibit DNA replication.These drugs have been tried in advanced colorectal and ovarian cancer. Their main adverse effects are neutropenia and diarrhoea.

ETOPOSIDE : It is a semisynthetic compound prepared from podophyllotoxin obtained from Podophyllum peltatum. It acts by inhibiting topoisomerase II, leading to DNA damage. It is given orally or IV. The adverse reactions are similar to those of radiomimetic agents. It has been used in a wide variety of cancers.

Hormones and Anti-Hormonal Drugs

Hormones act differently from the cytotoxic drugs and hence can be usefully combined with them in certain malignancies. They may act in one of the several ways:

- ***Inhibition of cell growth and differentiation,*** e.g., androgens in breast cancer and estrogens in prostatic cancer.
- ***Stimulation of differentiation of cells which then regain their ability to respond to the body's controlling and inhibitory influence,*** e.g., estrogens in breast cancer in postmenopausal women.
- ***Selective lysis of leukemic lymphocytes:*** they are effective in acute lymphatic leukemia. They stimulate the granuloblasts and are therefore ineffective in acute myeloid leukemia.
- ***Inhibition of the circulating concentration of a substance which stimulates the malignant cells,*** e.g., thyroxine is believed to suppress certain thyroid cancers by inhibiting TSH secretion.

Hormones do not directly kill the susceptible malignant cells, do not cause hyperuricemia and are slower in their effect. Pharmacology of these hormones is discussed elsewhere. Their application in the treatment of malignancies is discussed below:

ESTROGENS: Carcinoma of the prostate is androgen dependent; bilateral orchidectomy, in patients with prostatic carcinoma can produce marked improvement. Similar beneficial effects are obtained by the administration of estrogens. The best results are obtained by combining estrogens with orchidectomy. Synthetic estrogens which are as effective as the natural ones but much cheaper are preferred. **Diethylstilbestrol** is given in the dose of 5 mg. thrice daily for several days and then reduced to 1 mg. thrice daily. Adverse effects due to estrogen therapy are described in Chapter 65. In males, these mainly include sexual impotence and gynecomastia;

Aromatase inhibitors: These nonsteroidal drugs inhibit the enzyme aromatase responsible for the conversion of the adrenal androgen androstenedione to estrone (Chapter 65). They markedly reduce the circulating estrogen levels. The aromatization occurs in the body fat. Such estrogen synthesis may be important in the pathogenesis of breast cancer growth in postmenopausal women. They are selective in action and do not inhibit synthesis of adrenal glucocorticoids. They are given orally and are generally well tolerated. Adverse reactions are mild and include nausea, headache, fatigue, hot flushes and arthralgia.

They are now increasingly used as first line drugs in postmenopausal women to treat ER +ve breast cancer, including that which has progressed inspite of tamoxifen therapy. They can be combined with other drugs.

The currently used non-steroidal aromatase inhibitors are **anastrozole** and **letrozole**.

Exemestane is a steroidal hormonal compound. It acts by irreversibly inactivation of aromatase and has similar uses as other aromatase inhibitors.

TAMOXIFEN (Nolvadex): This nonsteroidal antiestrogen is structurally related to diethylstilbestrol. Given orally, it competes with the circulating estrogens for binding to the cytoplasmic estrogen receptors (ER). The metabolites of tamoxifen have a much stronger affinity for the receptors and are not easily displaced by circulating estradiol. At low concentrations, they have a cytostatic effect on ER positive cells. Higher concentrations cause cytotoxic effects characterized by cell death of ER positive and receptor negative cells.

Absorption, fate and excretion: Given orally, it is well absorbed and has a long half-life. It is extensively metabolized in liver to active metabolites and undergoes enterohepatic circulation. With a standard dose of 10 mg twice a day, a steady state serum concentration is achieved by 4 weeks of treatment. The approximate biological half-life of tamoxifen and its metabolite N-desmethyltamoxifen are 7 and 14 days, respectively. Hence, the drug can be detected in the serum for 4 weeks after treatment is discontinued. Approximately 30% of the dose is excreted in faeces.

Adverse reactions: The drug is well tolerated and adverse effects are minimal. The most frequent side effect has been hot flushes. About 10% of the patients may experience mild nausea and vomiting. Rarely, it causes bone pain associated with hypercalcemia, particularly in patients with bone metastasis. It may also give rise to vaginal bleeding and ocular toxicity. Higher incidence of deep vein thrombosis and endometrial cancer has been reported in a few women on prolonged tamoxifen therapy.

Therapeutic uses: Tamoxifen is well tolerated, reasonably safe and of proven efficacy in patients with breast cancer. It is the adjuvant treatment of choice in the postoperative patients, irrespective of their age, pre- or post-menopausal status, the ER status of the excised tumour and whether the axillary lymph nodes are positive or negative. Understandably, the results are better in patients with ER positivity. It can be combined with chemotherapy.

The dose is 10 mg. orally twice daily. The optimum duration of treatment is uncertain; but the drug should be given for at least 2 years, and probably for 5 years or even lifelong. Larger doses are not more beneficial.

The observation that there is less osteoporosis in women treated with tamoxifen lead to the development of a new series of its anlogues called **Selective Estrogen Receptor Modulators** (SERM) such as raloxifene, which are used for prevention and treatment of osteoporosis (Chapter 68).

PROGESTINS: The endometrial carcinoma in humans is believed to be due to prolonged unopposed stimulation by estrogens. **Hydroxyprogesterone caproate and megestrol acetate** have been used with success in metastatic endometrial carcinoma. The former is usually given IM in the dose of 1-3 g. at weekly intervals, and the latter orally in the dose of 40 mg. four times a day. Medroxyprogesterone has also been used for this purpose in the dose of 100-500 mg. per day orally (Chapter 65). Both agents have also been used to treat cachexia associated with cancer and AIDS.

FLUTAMIDE (Cytomid): This is a non-steroidal anti-androgen compound which binds to androgen receptor and blocks the effects of androgens. It exerts substantial anti-tumor activity in patients with metastatic cancer of prostate. The drug does not inhibit either the production of gonadotropins or adrenocortical steroidogenesis.

Given orally, it is rapidly and completely absorbed. Its adverse effects are nausea, vomiting, loss of libido, sexual impotence and hot flushes. Serious hepatotoxicity is rare.

It has been used in conjunction with a GnRH analogue in the treatment of prostatic cancer. In this combination it blocks the effects of testosterone. The combination is as effective as but less toxic than stilbestrol. As flutamide blocks the inhibitory feedback of testosterone on LH secretion, the levels of plasma testosterone rise, and this partly offsets the direct beneficial effect of flutamide on prostatic cancer. However, flutamide, used as a single drug in the dose of 250 mg tid is effective in the management of early prostatic cancer; it can also be used as the sole drug in orchidectomised patients, in whom it blocks the effects of the adrenal androgens. **Nilutamide** and **bicalutamide** are other antiandrogen with similar properties (Chapter 67).

LH-RH AGONISTS: **Leuprolide** and **goserelin** have been used to treat metastatic cancer of the prostate. (Chapter 65).

ABARELIX : This GnRH antagonist causes supression of LH and FSH and lowers the testosterone levels. It is used for treating advanced prostatic cancer.

SOMATOSTATIN ANALOGUES such as **octreotide** and **lanreotide** are sometimes used in the treatment of carcinoid tumours.

GLUCOCORTICOIDS: Hydrocortisone, and related glucocorticoids like prednisolone have been shown to be useful in following conditions:

(a) In acute lymphatic leukemia in children and in malignant lymphoma. This is due to their direct lympholytic effect. They suppress mitoses in lymphocytes. Steroids are not useful in the myeloid and monocytic types of acute leukemias.

(b) These steroids are also useful to prevent the accelerated erythrocytic destruction and thus prevent anemia in disseminated cancer patients; further, they effectively counter the hemolytic and hemorhagic complications (due to thrombocytopenia) accompanying chronic lymphocytic and myeloid leukemias, and malignant lymphomas.

(c) They are useful in treating cerebral edema due to intracranial tumour metastases.

(d) They are also useful to control the hypercalcemia caused by certain tumours or following cancer chemotherapy.

(e) They can be used in critically ill patients along with cytotoxic drugs to produce symptomatic relief and a sense of well being.

(f) Dexamethasone is useful as an adjunctive antiemetic with chemotherapy.

Prednisolone is generally started in doses of 60-100 mg. daily in divided doses, and then, depending upon the response, reduced to a maintenance dose of 20-40 mg. daily.

l-THYROXINE SODIUM: Follicular and papillary types of thyroid carcinomas are probably dependent on thyroid stimulating hormone (TSH). The primary treatment of these conditions is surgical. Papillary carcinoma is very slow growing and metastasizes largely to cervical lymph nodes; post-operatively it has been treated lifelong with thyroxine. Follicular carcinoma metastasizes early and widely; post operatively it is best treated with radioactive iodine, thyroxine being used only to treat the resultant hypothyroidism.

Miscellaneous Agents

PROCARBAZINE HYDROCHLORIDE (Matulane, Natulan): This drug, a methylhydrazine, has been found to be effective orally in the treatment of Hodgkin's disease. It inhibits DNA, RNA and protein synthesis. The toxic effects reported are restlessness, drowsiness, disorientation, leucopenia, thrombocytopenia and anemia. It also has some MAO inhibiting property and may cause disulfiram – like reaction following alcohol ingestion. It is leukemogenic and mutagenic.

MITOTANE : This drug, structurally related to the insecticide DDT, gets selectively concentrated in the adrenal cortex and acts as adrenolytic. It has been used in the treatment of Cushing's syndrome due to adrenocortical carcinoma. The adverse effects include anorexia, nausea, diarrhoea, somnolence and lethargy. Most patients who receive the drug for more than a week require maintenance therapy with a synthetic glucocorticoid to prevent the development of clinical adrenal insufficiency.

L-ASPARAGINASE (Erwinase, Elspar): This enzyme, which deaminates asparagine to aspartic acid is prepared from E. coli. Asparagine is a non-essential amino acid normally synthesized by the mammalian tissue cells. Certain malignant tumours, however, are unable to synthesize asparagine and consequently, are dependent on supplies from the host. Asparaginase acts by depleting asparagine from the host, hydrolysing circulating l-aspargine to aspartic acid, thus denying the malignant cells the essential metabolite. It is relatively nontoxic to normal cells. Given IV, it has produced relief in cases of lymphoblastic leukemia and reticulum cell sarcoma. It may cause hypersensitivity, pyrogenic reactions and skin rashes.

Cis-PLATIN (Neoplatin, Cisplastine): This platinum complex is given IV. Upon entering a cell it gets converted into active form, a potential mustard-like alkylating agent. It inhibits DNA biosynthesis and kills cells at any stage of cell-cycle. Used in combination with other drugs such as vinblastine and bleomycin, it produces prolonged remissions in a high percentage of patients, even in those with metastatic testicular tumours. It is also useful in many solid tumours. The drug is, however, toxic. It commonly causes marked nausea, vomiting and anemia and prophylactic administration of an antiemetic is mandatory. Anaphylactoid reactions are sometimes observed. Dose-related renal damage, autotoxicity, neuropathy and myclosuppression can occur. Aminoglycosides can aggravate its renal toxicity. Aggressive hydration with saline plus mannitol/furosemide is recommended to reduce the nephrotoxicity.

Carboplatin and **oxaliplatin** are newer analogue.

HYDROXYUREA is mainly used in the management of myeloproliferative disorders. It acts by inhibiting the enzyme ribonucleoside diphosphate reductase which is responsible for the conversion of ribonucleotides to deoxyribonucleotides, a rate limiting step in the biosynthesis of DNA. Hydroxyurea is almost 100% absorbed from the gut.

Adverse reactions include leukopenia, megaloblastic anaemia, thrombocytopenia, GI disturbances, skin reactions, stomatitis, alopecia, and neurological manifestations.

It is used in chronic granulocytic leukemia, polycythemia vera, thrombocytosis and sickle cell anaemia.

Tyrosine Kinase Inhibitors and Monoclonal Antibodies (mAb)

Identification of the molecular and genetic changes that cause malignant transformation has proved useful in developing new anticancer drugs.The family of **Epidermal Growth Factor Receptor** (EGFR) tyrosine kinases has attracted considerable interest because many epithelial tumours, particularly breast cancer, express excess amounts of HER2 which is a member of the epidermal growth factor receptor family and is associated with clinical resistance to cytotoxic and hormonal therapy. The intracellular domain of HER2 encodes tyrosine kinase which inhibits apoptosis and promotes metastases.

TRASTUZUMAB (Herceptin): This is a humanized, cDNA derived antibody against HER2. Blocking these receptor prevents the tumour growth. It can cause nausea, vomiting, fever, delayed bone marrow suppression and cardiomyopathy. It is used in patients with breast cancer.

BEVACIZUMAB (Avastin): This is a recombinant, humanized, monoclonal anti- VEGF (**Vascular Endothelial Growth Factor**) antibody, which prevents the latter's binding to endothelial receptors. VEGF binding initiates angiogenesis (endothelial proliferation and the formation of new blood vessels). Bevacizumab inhibits angiogenesis and thus retards further growth of all tissues including the metastases. Approved for the treatment of metastatic colorectal cancer, it has also been used for treating other cancers such as breast cancer, malignant mesothelioma and prostate cancer (off-label use); it is administered by IV infusion. It is administered by intraocular injection to prevent angiogenesis and macular degeneration in AMD. The adverse reactions are those to an injected foreign protein.

Panitumumab is a humanized monoclonal antibody targetting EGFR and used in the treatment of metastatic colorectal cancer.

Other humanized monoclonal antibodies used are **rituximab** for non-Hodgkin lymphoma and **alemtuzumab** for chronic B cell lymphatic leukemia. The latter depletes the leukemic and the normal lymphocytes by direct antibody-dependent lysis (see also Chapter 76)

^{131}Iodine-Tositumonab is a monoclonal antibody labelled with radioiodine. Given IV, it is taken up more specifically by the tumour cells than by normal tissues. A single course of treatment can produce a clinical response in about 60% of patients" with refractory non-Hodgkin lymphoma.

IMATINIB (Gleeve) is the first tyrosine kinase inhibitor which is highly effective, orally, in the treatment of chronic myeloid leukemia (CML). Most of the patients with CML have a translocated, shortened chromosome 22, termed the Philadelphia chromosome.This translocation creates a tyrosine kinase fusion gene called BCR-ABL gene which phosphorylates effector proteins and drives cell proliferation. Imatinib acts specifically by binding to the BCR-ABL gene and blocks the phosphorylation of the effector proteins.

Imatinib mesylate is well absorbed orally and is highly protein bound. Its plasma t½ is 18 hours and that of its active metabolite is about 40 hours. It is metabolized in the liver and the metabolites eliminated in the feces.

In patients with CML in the chronic phase who have failed to respond to interferon, imatinib induces a complete hematological remission in almost 88% and a complete cytogenic remission in 30%. It is also useful in CML in the acute phase, and to a smaller extent in CML in blast crisis.

Adverse Reactions: These are usually mild and include nausea, vomiting, edema, muscle cramps and diarrhoea. Neutropenia, thrombocytopenia, and increased hepatic aminotransferases may be observed. Since imatinib is a competitive inhibitor of hepatic microsomal enzymes, it may increase the serum concentration of warfarin, whereas the administration of itraconazole or erythromycin may increase the plasma concentration of imatinib.

Nilotinib, a tyrosine kinase inhibitor, is claimed to be effective in CML patients intolerant of or resitant to imatinib. **Dasatinib**, a multiple tyrosine kinase inhibitor has activity against all phases of CML and Philadelphia chromosome positive acute lymphoblastic leukemia. **Lapatinib** is an oral inhibitor of HER2 and EFGR1. It is used to treat metastatic breast cancer.

Gefitinib is a quinazoline derivative and is a specific inhibitor of EGFR tyrosine kinase. It has been approved for the treatment of patients with non-small cell carcinoma of the lung who are resistant to standard chemotherapy.

Sunitinib and **sorafinib** are other oral, multiple tyrosine kinase inhibitors, which are used in renal cell carcinoma.

Biological Response Modifiers

For immunostimulants and other biological modifiers such as BCG, levamisole and interferon alpha, see Chapter 76.

Drug Therapy of Malignant Diseases

Chemotherapy has definitely improved the outlook in this otherwise hopeless malady, and in a few conditions, long term remissions (almost cure) can be obtained by chemotherapy. These are acute lymphatic leukemia in children, Hodgkin's lymphoma, choriocarcinoma in females, Wilm's tumour in children, disseminated testicular cancer and histiocytic lymphoma. In majority of the conditions, however, chemotherapy, being purely suppressive, is recommended to help the patient to return to his near-normal mode of life. It is not usually recommended simply for prolonging the act of dying, in an otherwise terminally ill patient.

The diagnosis must be firmly established before using these drugs. A detailed discussion of drug therapy in individual diseases is beyond the scope of this book. Certain principles, however, are outlined below:

- Traditional cytotoxic therapy has been based on the broad histologic categories of cancer such as lung, breast or colon cancer. Single-agent response rarely exceeds 30% of these tumours. Hence, it is liable to undergo continual change. In general, irradiation is recommended in a localised malignant growth, after palliative surgery, wherever possible. This, if carried out early, may prevent the spread and also will cause less damage to healthy tissues. Generally, chemotherapy should not be given simultaneously with local irradiation.

Newer methods of selecting the cancer chemotherapeutic agent e.g. gefitinib (see above) which acts on a specific molecular target (in addition to the traditional histologic category of the tumour) may make future anticancer therapy dedicated and more effective.

● The drugs are usually given in combination and the treatment is administered in 'cycles'. This allows the normal body tissues (especially the bone marrow) to recover from the adverse effects of the drug.

● Nearly all cytotoxic drugs act by interfering with cell replication. It is possible to devise a combination of drugs acting by different mechanisms and providing greater benefit than single agents do individually. Thus, in many conditions such as acute leukemia, Hodgkin's lymphoma and testicular tumours combinations of drugs have been found to be highly effective.

By the time a tumour is clinically detectable, only about 10% of the cells are actively proliferating and therefore susceptible to the action of anti-cancer drugs. The remaining 90% are in the resting phase but are known to re-start proliferating if the total tumour mass is reduced (by surgery or by radiotherapy) and become susceptible to the action of drugs.

● A single dose of a cytotoxic drug kills not a fixed number of cancer cells but a constant proportion of those present. Hence, chemotherapy has the maximum chances of being curative when few tumour cells are present. Once a clinical remission is obtained, continuation of chemotherapy (perhaps with a different drug) in the presence of inapparent, residual disease is highly effective.

● Conditions like acute leukemia, certain sarcomas and Hodgkin's lymphoma which show rapid progression need prompt attention, while a condition like chronic lymphatic leukemia, particularly in old people, may progress so slowly that patients may enjoy good health and can survive almost a normal span of life without any chemotherapy.

Table 59.1: Palliative symptom control in the terminally ill cancer patient

- Frequent re-evaluation is important as symptoms change often.
- Enquiring daily about frequency of bowel movements is more important than monitoring pulse, temperature and BP.
- **Never say "Nothing can be done"**. Consult or refer if the patient is uncomfortable.
- ***Pain***: See Chapter 9.
- ***Anorexia***: Prednisolone 15-30 mg. or dexamethasone 2-4 mg. per day may be helpful.
- ***Nausea and vomiting***: See Chapter 38. They may be morphine-induced.
- ***Dyspnoea***: It may respond to morphine, diazepam or a glucocorticoid.
- ***Headache***: If severe, it may be due to raised intracranial tension and may respond to dexamethasone 16 mg/day for a few days, followed by 4-6 mg/day.
- ***Noisy upper respiratory secretions*** ('death rattle') are troubling to the family but not generally to the patient. They can be reduced by SC injection of atropine 200-400 mcg. every 2-4 hours, as needed.
- ***Convulsions***: These are especially liable to occur in patients with cerebral tumours and should be treated with phenytoin or carbamazepine; when oral medication is no longer possible, rectal diazepam may be employed. In very restless patients, midazolam may be used by SC infusion in the dose of 20-40 mg. per 24 hours.
- ***The treatment of other symptoms*** (constipation, cough, restlessness-confusion and pruritus) has been described elsewhere in the book.
- ***Use of bone marrow growth factors*** can reduce the degree of neutropenia and protect against infection (Chapter 34).

● In most cases, drugs have to be given in such doses that toxic effects are inevitable. Patients should have regular hematological supervision and with drugs like methotrexate, evidence of damage to the alimentary epithelium should be looked for.

- All anticancer drugs have adverse effects. The most frequent adverse reactions are severe nausea, vomiting, infections and hemorrhage due to bone marrow suppression. Hyperuricemia following the breakdown of large number of tumour cells can be prevented by using allopurinol which interferes with uric acid synthesis.
- Use of bone marrow growth factors eg., G-CSF and GM-CSF may reduce the frequency and severity of anemia, neutropenia and thrombocytopeme (Chapter 34).
- Cytotoxic drugs are contraindicated during pregnancy as they cause abortions or foetal abnormalities.
- In choosing a drug regime one must always keep in mind its "cost effectiveness" as chemotherapy in general is very expensive. These drugs should not be used simply to prolong the 'act of dying' in otherwise hopeless terminal cases.

Response to therapy may be judged by:

(1) Improvement of the sense of well-being of the patient.

(2) Decrease in tumour markers.

(3) Normalisation of organ function; and

(4) Shrinkage of the tumour mass.

The best results are generally obtained in patients in good nutritional state and without severe metabolic disturbances or other complications. Ideally, the patient should have adequate hepatic, renal and bone marrow function, uncompromised by tumour invasion, previous chemotherapy or irradiation.

Chemotherapy is only a part of the overall approach to the care of terminally ill cancer patient. When one can neither cure an illness nor prolong life, one must strive to *improve the quality of life of the patient.* Towards this end, the following contribute significantly:

- ***Maintenance of nutrition.***
- ***Treatment of anemia and neutropenia*** (Chapters 33, 34) and ***cachexia.***
- ***Protection from infection*** as the chemotherapeutic agents, acting as immunosuppressants, reduce the body's resistance to infection.
- ***Control of symptoms*** particularly pain on a day to day basis (see Table 59.1).
- ***Occupational therapy,*** and
- ***Adequate emotional and spiritual support*** to the patient and the family. This is very important particularly in a condition like incurable cancer where the physician can hardly do anything specific but watch helplessly.

Antiseptics, Disinfectants and Insecticides

60

Sterilization can be defined as freeing an article, a surface or a medium, by *removing or killing all micro-organisms including vegetative bacteria, spores, fungi* and *viruses.*

Disinfection (high level disinfection) is the term used for *destruction of all pathogenic organisms* such as vegetative forms of bacteria, mycobacteria, fungi and viruses but not spores. If spores are killed during the process, only then it is equivalent to **sterilization**. Sterilization and disinfection can be achieved by physical and chemical methods. A **disinfectant** or *germicide* is a chemical which *causes disinfection.* It may be bactericidal or bacteriostatic. *They are generally used to disinfect inanimate objects.* They are classified into

- ***Bactericides.***
- ***Viricides;*** and
- ***Fungicides.***

Drugs toxic to the external parasites are called ***ectoparasiticides***.

An **antiseptic** *is a chemical disinfectant (usually bacteriostatic in the concentration used) that can be diluted sufficiently to be safe for application to living tissues (intact skin, mucus membranes or wounds) while still retaining its antimicrobial property.* Antiseptics and disinfectants are used not only in the original form but are often added to easily available every day utilities like soaps, toothpastes, mouth wash and after-shave lotions. They are also used to disinfect excreta, fumigate rooms and bedding, and sterilize instruments (endoscopes) and complicated apparatus (heart lung machines and respirators) that cannot be sterilized by heat.

Classification:

(A) **Physical agents** e.g. heat, filtration and radiation.

(B) **Chemical agents:** They are classified as:

I **Acids:**

- ***Inorganic acids***: Boric acid;
- ***Organic acids***: Benzoic acid, Salicylic acid.

II **Alkalis:** Sodium and Potassium hydroxide.

III **Alcohols:** Ethanol and Isopropyl alcohol.

IV **Aldehydes:** Formaldehyde, Gluteraldehyde.

V **Surfactants:**

- ***Anionic***: Soaps, Sodium lauryl sulfate, Sodium cetostearyl sulfate.
- ***Ampholytic*** Surfactants.
- ***Cationic***: Benzalkonium, Cetylpyridinium, Dequalinium and Triclobisonium.
- ***Nonionic***: Polysorbates.

VI **Phenols and related compounds :** Phenol, Cresol, Chlorocresol, Hexylresorcinol, Bithionol, Thymol, Hexachlorophane, Chlorhexidine.

VII **Halogens and halogen containing compounds:** Chlorine and Chloramines; Iodine and Iodophors.

VIII **Oxidizing agents:** Hydrogen peroxide and

other Peroxides, Potassium and Zinc permanganates.

IX **Dyes:** Crystal violet, Brilliant green, Methylene blue, Acriflavine, Proflavine.

X **Heavy metals:** Silver nitrate, Zinc compounds.

XI **Gases:** Ethylene oxide.

Mechanism of action: They may act by one or more of the mechanisms listed in Table 60.1.

Table 60.1: Mechanisms of action of disinfectants and antiseptics

- Coagulation of the bacterial proteins.
- An alteration in the properties of the bacterial cell wall.
- Binding of free sulfhydryl (--SH) groups essential for enzyme action; and
- Competition with essential substrates for the important enzymes in the bacterial cell.

Factors which determine the therapeutic efficacy of these agents are:

- ***Drug concentration and its therapeutic index***: In general, antiseptic effect increases with a rise in concentration. Alcohol, however, is an exception and shows maximum antiseptic activity in a 70 per cent concentration. The potency of a particular concentration is meaningful only in relation to the tissue toxicity *(Therapeutic Index)*. Presence of necrotic tissue reduces their penetration and lowers their effective concentration. Anionic surfactants like soaps reduce the effective concentration of cationic surfactants by chemical neutralization.
- ***Species susceptibility***: Some forms, particularly spores and some species of bacteria, are resistant to many antiseptics. *Viruses are susceptible to alkalis but resistant to phenol.*
- ***Temperature and duration of contact***: A limited rise in environmental temperature and prolonged contact can enhance Soporicidal activity. A rise of temperature by 10° C generally doubles the antibacterial activity of chemical agents whereas it increases that of moist heat a hundredfold.

Physical Agents

(1) **Heat** applied at the right temperature and for optimum length of time is the best and most effective sterilizing agent available. It may be applied either in the form of moist heat or dry heat.

Moist heat: Moist heat kills micro-organisms by coagulating the proteins. It can be applied in several ways:

- ***Pasteurization***: This is commonly used to kill the pathogenic micro-organisms (not all sporulating bacteria) in milk.
- ***Boiling***: Boiling in water for 20 minutes is an efficient method of *high level disinfection;* spores are often resistant to boiling.
- ***Steam***: Steam is a very efficient means of *sterilization* because of its high penetrating capacity and because it gives up a large amount of heat (latent heat). Steam may be used at atmospheric pressure (temperature 100°C) to sterilize culture media that decompose at higher temperatures. More commonly, steam is used at higher pressures (2 atmospheres) which raise its temperature to between 108° and 147°C for at least 20 minutes. By selecting the correct temperature and time cycle, a wide variety of materials can be sterilized.

Dry heat: Dry heat kills the organisms by oxidizing their cell constituents. It can be used in several ways.

- ***Hot air*** in an oven is commonly used to dry *sterilize* glass syringes, instruments, and glassware. Dry sterilization must be carried at 160° C - 180° C for 60-120 minutes.
- ***Flaming***: i.e., direct heating in a bunsen flame, is commonly used in a bacteriology laboratory to *sterilize* inoculating wires, etc.
- ***Incineration***: This is suitable for soiled dressings, pathological material, animal carcasses and heavily soiled bedding.

(2) **Filtration** through different types of filters including the modern Millipore membrane filters is an efficient way of removing larger particles and bacteria from liquids that cannot be treated by other means, e.g., human serum albumin. It is also used to remove heat-resistant, pyrogenic cell-wall endotoxins from other solutions prior to autoclaving them. However, viruses, especially the smaller ones, may pass through filters.

(3) **Radiation** used for *sterilization* is of two types: non-ionizing and ionizing.

(a) **Non-ionizing radiation:** Two types of non-ionizing radiation, infrared and ultra-violet, are used for sterilization.

- ***Infrared*** radiation is another form of dry heat sterilization.
- ***Ultra-violet*** radiation is absorbed by the proteins and nucleic acids and kills microorganisms by the chemical reactions it sets up in the bacterial cell. It has low penetrating capacity and its main application is to reduce the bacteria in air, water and on contaminated surfaces. All forms of bacteria and viruses are vulnerable to ultraviolet rays below 3000A°. Excessive exposure of skin can produce serious burns. Care must be taken to protect the eyes while using UV radiation.

(b) **Ionizing radiation:** The lethal action of ionizing radiation is due to its effect on the nuclear DNA and on the other vital cell components. There is no appreciable rise in temperature. High energy **gamma rays** from cobalt-60 are used to sterilize articles such as foods, syringes, swabs, culture plates, catheters and plastic material including disposable plastic heart-lung machines.

Acids and Alkalis

BORIC ACID: Boric acid and sodium borate (Borax), are weak bacteriostatic and fungistatic agents. It is soluble in water upto 5 per cent. This concentration, however, inhibits phagocytosis. Locally, boric acid is not an irritant. Aqueous solutions of boric acid (2-4%) are used as mouth washes, eye and skin lotions. Mixed with starch, talc or zinc oxide, it is used as a dusting powder.

Preparations:

(i) Boric talc dusting powder contains 2.3 g. of boric acid, 5 g. of starch and 50 g. of sterilized, purified talc.

(ii) Boric acid eye lotion contains 3.4 g. of boric acid dissolved in 100 ml. of freshly boiled and cooled purified water.

(iii) Borax glycerin: This contains 12 per cent w/v of borax with glycerin and is used for painting throat and tongue.

BENZOIC ACID: This organic acid has antibacterial and antifungal properties; in a concentration of 0.1 per cent, it is used as a preservative. The antimicrobial activity of the drug is decreased if the pH of the medium exceeds 5. Taken orally, benzoic acid is conjugated with glycine in the liver to form hippuric acid which is excreted in the urine. Compound benzoic acid-salicylic acid ointment (Whitfield's ointment) has been used to treat ringworm infection (see Chapter 69).

SALICYLIC ACID: This drug has bacteriostatic, fungicidal and keratolytic properties. It is applied externally for the treatment of seborrhoeic dermatitis, acne, and fungal diseases. Further, it produces a slow and painless destruction of the epithelium; and it is applied in the form of a paint in a collodion base, or as a plaster, for the destruction of warts and corns. Its keratolytic property makes it useful in psoriasis (Chapter 69).

Preparations:

(i) Salicylic acid ointment 2 per cent.

(ii) Whitfield's ointment : See Chapter 69.

(iii) Salicylic acid compound dusting powder contains 1.5 g. of salicylic acid and 2.5 g. of boric acid, made up to 50 g. with sterilised, purified talc.

(iv) Salicylic acid ear drops contain 0.12 g. of salicylic acid with 8 ml. of glycerin and 15 ml. of specially denatured spirit.

(v) Salicylic acid collodion contains 12 g. of salicylic acid in 100 ml. of flexible collodion.

Alkalis like sodium hydroxide and potassium hydroxide are used for disinfecting excreta from patients with poliomyelitis. In addition, both these alkalis are caustic and may be used for removal of warts.

Alcohols

ETHANOL: Ethyl alcohol in the concentration of 70 per cent is a skin antiseptic. It, however, exhibits poor activity against bacterial spores and hydrophilic viruses. It acts by denaturation of cellular protein. As it evaporates quickly, it lacks residual activity. It should not be allowed to come in contact with cornea.

ISOPROPYL ALCOHOL: This is an inflammable secondary alcohol with an unpleasant burning taste. It is about twice as toxic as ethyl alcohol. As a germicide, it is slightly more potent than ethyl alcohol and has a marked degreasing action. It is used in the concentration of 68 to 72 per cent v/v, for disinfection of skin.

Aldehydes

FORMALDEHYDE: Formaldehyde, a gas at room temperature, is used as a fumigant or as a 40% w/v aqueous solution containing methanol (Formalin). The solution, in the concentration of 1:200, is a highly effective disinfectant against several bacteria, viruses and fungi; a higher concentration and prolonged exposure are necessary to eliminate spores. It acts by alkylation of proteins and nucleic acids.

Formaldehyde solution has a pungent odour and is extremely irritant to the mucous membranes. It precipitates tissue proteins in high concentration. When applied to the unbroken skin, it hardens the epidermis.

Uses: A 10 per cent solution is used for disinfection of excreta, sputa and brush bristles. It is sometimes used in dentistry as a mummifying agent for residual pulp tissue. A 3 per cent solution is available for removal of warts on the palms and soles, and a 20 to 30 per cent solution is employed to treat hyperhidrosis. A 4 per cent solution in saline is a common preservative for pathological specimens.

Gaseous formaldehyde is used for sterilization of those articles which cannot be wetted with solutions or subjected to high temperatures. Formaldehyde gas is obtained by heating formaldehyde solution or formalin tablets. It does not damage metal, plastics or fabrics.

GLUTARALDEHYDE (Cidex): Glutaraldehyde is a saturated aldehyde which produces a slightly acid solution in water. It is a potent bactericide, sporicide, viricide and fungicide. The solution must be alkalinised to pH 7.4-8.5 for activation. The shelf life of activated solution is 14 days. A rise of pH above 8.5 causes polymerization of glutaraldehyde with loss of activity. It is less irritant than formaldehyde to the eyes and the skin. Unlike formaldehyde, it does not damage lenses and cementing material in endoscopes and is superior to it for sterilizing rubber, plastic and metal appliances. It can also be used to sterilize complicated apparatus like respirators. It is available as a 2% solution which is buffered to a pH of 7.5-8.5 with sodium bicarbonate before use. As 2% aqueous solution, it is used as a local application to treat idiopathic hyperhidrosis of palms and soles.

Surfactants

Surfactants are chemical compounds which lower the surface tension of solutions, usually aqueous ones. They are also termed as *detergents.* They can be classified into:

ANIONIC SURFACTANTS: Soaps belong to this category. Anionic surfactants dissociate in aqueous solution to form a relatively large and complex anion, which is responsible for the surface tension lowering activity. Soaps are mainly effective against Gram-positive and acid-fast organisms. It is likely, however, that their cleansing action is secondary to emulsification of the lipoidal secretions in which the bacteria are embedded; the micro-organisms are subsequently enmeshed in the lather and washed away with rinsing. In general, **soft soaps** derived by combination of unsaturated fatty acids with potassium hydroxide or sodium hydroxide are more efficient germicidal agents than **hard soaps** formed by the treatment of saturated fatty acids with sodium or potassium hydroxide. The disadvantages of soaps are their:

- ***Narrow antimicrobial spectrum.***
- ***Incompatibility with cationic surfactants.***
- ***Tendency to precipitation by hard water;*** *and*
- ***Ability to cause drying and cracking of the skin.***

Preparations:

(i) One part of soft soap in 20 parts of warm water is used as an enema to soften impacted feces. Soap liniment which is an alcoholic solution of soft soap, camphor and lemon grass oil, is a mild counterirritant, and is used in the treatment of sprains and bruises.

(ii) Sodium lauryl sulfate : This anionic surfactant is effective in hard water. It is active in both acidic and alkaline media. It is used in medicated shampoos and as a preoperative skin cleanser, usually along with another antiseptic.

(iii) Sodium cetostearyl sulfate is used like sodium lauryl sulfate.

Other anionic surfactants include dioctyl sodium sulfosuccinate used as a fecal softening agent, and sodium tetradecyl sulfate used as a sclerosing agent for varicose veins. These are discussed elsewhere.

CATIONIC SURFACTANTS : Cationic surfactants dissociate into a large and relatively complex cation, which is responsible for the activity and a smaller inactive anion. The cation usually contains pentavalent nitrogen atom, which is often present as a quaternary ammonium, pyridinium or piperidinium group. In addition to emulsifying and detergent actions, the cationic surfactants have a marked bactericidal activity against both Gram-positive and Gram-negative organisms. They are, however, less effective against spores, viruses and fungi.

The mechanism of their antibacterial activity is not clear. It is postulated that by lowering surface tension, they damage the cell membrane. They may also inactivate certain enzymes.

Cationic surfactants are most effective in neutral solution. They are incompatible with anionic surfactants like soaps. A significant quantity of these agents is absorbed by cotton, rubber and porous material resulting in a reduction in their effective concentration. As these agents combine readily with proteins, their activity is greatly reduced in the presence of serum, pus and other organic matter. When applied to skin, they tend to form a film under which bacteria, particularly *Pseudomonas aeruginosa* and *Mycobacterium tuberculosis,* may remain viable.

The solutions of cationic surfactants are generally colourless, odourless, non-irritating and non-toxic in bactericidal concentrations. They remain stable for a long time and do not deteriorate on boiling or autoclaving. This group is the most favoured of the antiseptics at present.

Preparations:

(i) Benzalkonium chloride: This occurs as a white or yellowish white amorphous powder or as gelatinous pieces. It has an aromatic odour, markedly bitter taste and is water soluble.

A 1:1,000 solution may be used for the pre-operative disinfection of intact, unbroken skin.

A 1:1000 to 1:4,000 solution has been used for storing sterilised surgical instruments, usually along with 0.5 per cent sodium nitrite to retard rusting. A 1:8,000 solution is used for soaking baby napkins to prevent napkin rash.

Instruments and polythene tubes, treated with the drug must be thoroughly washed before use as the cationic surfactants have a deleterious effect on nerve tissue.

It is not recommended as an antiseptic because resistant pseudomonas and other Gram negative bacteria can grow in the antiseptic solution. It is used only as a disinfectant.

(ii) Cetrimide (Cetavlon) : A concentration of 0.1 to 1 per cent in water is used for similar purposes as benzalkonium chloride. A 1:20,000 concentration is used as a preservative for eye drops. Cetrimide cream contains 5.0 g. of cetrimide, 50.0 g. of cetostearyl alcohol and 500 g. of liquid paraffin made upto 1000 g. with water. Certrimide lotion contains 1 per cent centrimide in water.

(iii) Miscellaneous : Other cationic surfactants available include cetylpyridinium chloride, dequalinium acetate and triclobisonium chloride.

AMPHOLYTIC SURFACTANTS: Ampholytic surfactants are derivatives of long chain N-substituted amino acids and can have anionic, non-ionic or cationic properties depending on the pH. They are anionic at a pH above their isoelectric point and cationic at a pH below it. They have the detergent properties of anionic surfactants and the antiseptic properties of cationic surfactants. They, however, are incompatible with both anionic and cationic agents. The compounds available for use include sodium N-dodecyl alanate, and dodecyldi-(aminoethyl)-glycine hydrochloride.

POLYSORBATES: The elimination of one molecule of water from the hexahydric alcohol sorbitol results in the formation of compounds termed sorbitans, while elimination of another water molecule results in the formation of sorbides. By esterification of these with fatty acids, non-ionic surfactants are produced. These are termed polysorbates. These substances are active water in oil emulsifying agents, while their polyoxyethylene derivatives are non-ionic, oil in water emulsifying agents.

The polysorbates and their polyoxyethylene derivatives such as Tween 80 are used in pharmacy in the preparation of cream, ointment and suppository bases and for emulsification of oils. They may be employed internally to improve the absorption of fat and fat soluble vitamins. They are also used as surface active agents in insecticides and fruit spraying solutions, as industrial detergents and in the manufacture of cosmetic creams. They are devoid of antiseptic activity.

Phenols and Related Compounds

PHENOL (Carbolic acid): Phenol, one of the oldest antiseptics, was introduced into medicine in 1867 by Lord Lister. It occurs as pinkish, needle-shaped, deliquescent crystals, sparingly soluble in water but freely soluble in alcohol. It is a potent bactericidal and fungicidal agent. It acts by denaturing the bacterial proteins and disrupting the cell wall. It is mainly effective against nonsporulating pathogens. *All spores and most viruses are resistant.* It rapidly penetrates the skin, the mucous membranes and other tissues and acts as a corrosive. It is extremely irritating to exposed tissues and may cause necrosis. The antiseptic and corrosive properties are greatly reduced if it is dissolved in alcohol, glycerine or a fixed oil. It is carcinogenic.

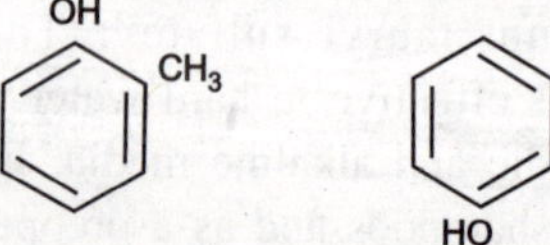

Fig. 60.1 : Ortho-cresol Phenol

Phenol is rapidly absorbed on oral administration. It can also penetrate intact skin. The degradation products, upon oxidation, impart a greenish tinge to the urine.

Ingestion of phenol results in severe GI corrosion, pain, vomiting and shock. Collapse occurs within a few minutes, body temperature falls and even convulsions may occur; death is usually due to respiratory failure. Treatment is essentially symptomatic.

Uses: Phenol is no longer used even as a disinfectant because of its corrosive properties. It may, however be used as an *in vitro* deodorant. A 0.5 per cent solution is occasionally used as antipruritic on the skin.

It has been occasionally used as a 5 per cent oily solution in almond oil for sclerosing unprolapsed haemorrhoids.

CRESOL: Cresol is a mixture of the ortho, meta and para methyl derivatives of phenol. In the commercially available product, the meta isomer is the major constituent. Cresol is 10 times as active as phenol and has a wider margin of safety. It is an almost colourless to pale brownish yellow liquid, becoming darker on keeping or on exposure to light, and with a characteristic phenolic odour. It is sparingly soluble in water and is used as 2 per cent solution.

LYSOL (Cresol with soap solution): This is prepared by saponification of a mixture of cresol with a vegetable oil or the mixed fatty acids derived therefrom. It contains 50 per cent v/v of cresol. The bactericidal value of lysol varies according to the soap used in its preparation. Lysol is a useful disinfectant for hospital and domestic use. However, because of its highly irritant nature, it has largely been replaced by safer preparations like iodophors.

CHLOROXYLENOL (Dettol): It is a less toxic chlorinated phenol. It is supplied as a 4.9% solution in water. It is effective against Gram-positive and Gram-negative organisms. Surgical dettol used for pre-operative preparation of skin contains 1.44 per cent of chloroxylenol; dettol used for disinfection of surgical instruments contains 6.25 per cent of the agent while a 1-3 per cent concentration is employed in the antiseptic cream.

BITHIONOL: This is a non-irritant bactericide, particularly effective against Gram-positive cocci, usually employed in soaps and soap solution in a concentration varying from 0.5 to 5 per cent.

THYMOL: Thymol and chlorothymol possess both antiseptic and antifungal properties. Both these, however, are irritating to wounds, have a poor water solubility and lose their bactericidal power considerably in the presence of proteins. They are used in mouth washes and antiseptic solutions.

HEXACHLOROPHANE (G-11): This chlorinated phenol exhibits bacteriostatic activity against a wide variety of organisms mainly Gram+ve organisms. It retains its activity in the presence of soaps but not so much in the presence of serum or pus.

It can get absorbed from burnt or denuded skin and from mucous membrane and even from the unbroken skin in premature infants. Severe neurotoxicity in the form of a myelopathy and cerebral edema has been reported in infants washed regularly with a 3% solution. Accidental ingestion or the application of high concentration (6%) to children has caused cardiovascular disturbances, convulsions and respiratory arrest.

Phenolic disinfectants are not to be used in the nursery.

CHLORHEXIDINE (Hibitane) : It is a cationic biguanide with low water solubility. Chlorhexidine digluconate is water soluble. This compound acts against a wide range of Gram-positive and Gram-negative organisms and against fungi at pH 5.5 to 7.0. Bacterial spores are prevented from germinating but are not killed. It is effective even in the presence of blood or pus. It is rapid acting, non-irritating and has residual activity. It has low potential for producing contact dermatitis and photosensitivity. It is absorbed poorly. It is available as 5% aqueous concentrate or 1% water miscible cream. Its activity is reduced in the presence of neutral soap, surfactants and anionic agents. Oral toxicity is low because it is poorly absorbed. Commercial preparation **Savlon** contains hibitane and cetrimide.

Halogens and Halogen Containing Compounds

CHLORINE AND CHLORAMINES: Chlorine is the most commonly used halogen, largely for purification of water. Chloramines, which release chlorine slowly, are used for disinfection. Chlorine exerts a bactericidal action against a variety of Gram-positive and Gram-negative organisms in a concentration as low as 0.0002 per cent. The acid-fast organisms, however, require a much higher concentration. The agent also kills protozoa and viruses including HIV. The bactericidal action is significantly reduced in the presence of blood, serum, feces and other organic matter.

It is a strong oxidizing agent and its antibacterial activity is due to the formation of hypochlorous acid (HOCl). *Interestingly, the killing of bacteria ingested by neutrophils in the animal body involves synthesis of HOCl by the intracellular action of the enzyme myeloperoxidase on H_2O_2 and halide.* Sodium hypochlorite 5.25% made up in tap water (pH 7.5) retains activity for months. An alkaline medium greatly reduces the antiseptic activity of hypochlorous acid by causing dissociation of the acid molecule.

Chlorine poisoning is characterised by severe irritation of the respiratory passage leading to pulmonary edema, and by metabolic acidosis. Treatment is symptomatic.

Solutions of hypochlorous acid are corrosive to aluminium, stainless steel and silver.

Preparations:

(i) Chlorinated lime and boric acid solution (Eusol) is prepared by dissolving 1.25 g. of calcium hypochlorite and an equivalent quantity of boric acid and calcium hydroxide powder in 100 ml. of water. The solution is irritating and should, therefore, be diluted with saline before using on denuded surfaces.

(ii) Chloramine: This is an organic chloride. A 2 per cent solution of the agent is used for irrigation of wounds, while a 0.2 to 0.5 per cent solution is recommended for mouth wash and for irrigation of bladder and urethra. The solution has to be freshly prepared for use.

(iii) Chlorinated lime (Bleaching powder) is extensively used for purification of water.

IODINE: Iodine is probably the oldest and the most widely used of the antiseptics. It is the most potent bactericidal agent and in addition, also possesses high sporicidal, fungicidal, amoebicidal and a moderate viricidal activity. The germicidal activity of iodine is less influenced than that of chlorine by pH, temperature and the time of contact. However, like chlorine, its activity is inhibited by reducing agents and organic material, whereas it is enhanced by alcohol.

Iodine, though employed routinely for treatment of wounds and abrasions, stains the skin, is irritating, painful and may delay the healing. In rare cases, it causes severe reactions, such as fever and skin eruptions. Elemental iodine, if ingested, can cause severe GI irritation and shock. Treatment consists of gastric lavage with a solution of soluble starch or 5 per cent sodium thiosulfate, and correction of dehydration.

Iodism, may occur following prolonged systemic use of iodides (Chapter 62).

Preparations:

(i) Strong iodine tincture contains 10 per cent w/v of iodine, 6 per cent w/v of potassium iodide, and 1 per cent w/v of water in 90 per cent alcohol.

(ii) Weak iodine tincture contains 2 per cent w/v of iodine and 2.5 per cent w/v of potassium iodide in 50 per cent alcohol.

(iii) Iodine compound paint contains 0.31 g. of iodine and 0.62 g. of potassium iodide with mentha oil, water and 90 per cent alcohol in glycerin base. A slightly different composition, containing peppermint oil instead of mentha oil and termed *Mandl's paint* is also available.

(iv) Non-staining iodine ointment contains 5 per cent iodine with arachis oil and yellow soft paraffin.

(v) Aqueous iodine solution (Lugol's solution) is used in thyrotoxicosis. (Chapter 59).

Uses: Iodine tincture may be employed for disinfection of skin prior to surgery. Iodine crystals have been used to sterilise water for drinking during hiking expeditions and water for soaking fresh vegetables to disinfect them before consumption. *Iodine 1:20,000 solution is bactericidal in one minute and kills spores in 15 minutes.*

Iodine glycerin preparation (Mandl's paint) is applied to the mucous membranes in the treatment of follicular tonsillitis and pharyngitis. Iodine ointments are used as counterirritants and have also been used externally as fungicides in the treatment of ringworm. Iodinated hydroxyquinolines are used in amoebiasis and as topical antifungal agents.

The use of iodides as expectorants and in the treatment of thyrotoxicosis is discussed elsewhere.

Unlike iodine, iodides have no antibacterial action.

IODOPHORS: Iodophors are developed by complexing iodine with surfactants like non-ionic detergents, quaternaries and macromolecules. The detergents act as solubilizers and carriers, combining detergent property with antibacterial activity. Iodophors are non-irritating, non-staining and water-miscible in all dilutions. They owe their germicidal activity to the slowly released elemental iodine. As compared to aqueous or tincture iodine, they are less irritating, less toxic and non-sensitizing to the skin, though somewhat less effective. They are sporicidal on prolonged contact.

The iodophors available are:

(i) **Povidone-iodine** 5% (Betadine): A complex of iodine with polyvinyl pyrrolidone, available as solution, ointment and eye-drops.

(ii) Undecoylium chloride iodine: A complex of iodine with the cationic surfactant undecoylium chloride.

Iodophors are commonly used as mouth and hand washes, for preoperative skin preparation, as local antiseptics, in ringworm and in oral and vaginal moniliasis.

Povidone eye drops (5%) are sometimes used for dry eye conditions. Iodophors may also be used for disinfection of operation rooms, wards, nurseries, etc.

Oxidizing Agents

HYDROGEN PEROXIDE: This colourless, odourless liquid is used mainly as a disinfectant and an antiseptic. It is a potent oxidizer and owes its action to its ready release of nascent oxygen, when applied to tissues. It has a broad spectrum of activity. Concentrations of 10-25% are sporicidal. Vapour phase H_2O_2 is a cold gaseous sterilant and can be used as a substitute for formaldehyde.

Its application causes an effervescence which mechanically removes the tissue debris from otherwise inaccessible regions. The action, however, is of short duration. Solutions of hydrogen peroxide have poor power of penetration. It has the advantage that it does not combine with tissue proteins and its degradation product is non-toxic.

Hydrogen peroxide solution contains not less than 6.0 per cent w/v of H_2O_2, corresponding to about 20 times its volume of available oxygen and hence, is described as '20 volume'.

Peracetic acid prepared from H_2O_2 is a more potent bactericidal and sporicidal agent used in food processing industry.

Uses: It is used for cleansing wounds, abscesses, for the removal of adhering dressings and for irrigation.

In dentistry, hydrogen peroxide solution is used to clean septic sockets and root canals; diluted with 3 to 8 parts of water, it is a useful deodorant gargle and mouth wash. It is also used as ear drops for the removal of ear wax.

Other peroxides: These include magnesium peroxide and zinc peroxide. The last one is used most commonly. It releases nascent oxygen, leaving behind zinc oxide, which has a mild astringent action. It is applied locally as a 40 per cent suspension for disinfecting, deodorising, and promoting healing of burns and other wounds contaminated with anaerobic bacteria. A 25 per cent suspension in water is used as a mouth wash to treat anaerobic infections.

POTASSIUM AND ZINC PERMANGANATES: These compounds possess oxidising and astringent properties. Zinc permanganate is more astringent than the potassium salt. The permanganates are caustic as crystals and concentrated solutions.

Their ingestion may provoke severe gastriontestinal irritation; potassium permanganate, in addition, causes cardiovascular depression and kidney damage.

Preparations:

(i) Potassium permanganate occurs as dark purple crystals, having a metallic lustre. It is moderately soluble in water.

(ii) Potassium permanganate gargle contains 25 mg. of potassium permanganate in 100 ml. of water (1 in 4000). It should be freshly prepared.

(iii) Zinc permanganate occurs as brownish-black iridescent deliquescent crystals soluble 1 in 3 parts of water.

Uses: The value of potassium permanganate is limited owing to its rapid reduction in the presence of body fluids. It is used as a gargle, mouth wash or for vaginal irrigation; 1 in 10,000 to 1 in 5,000 for urethral irrigation and as wet dressings and in baths for acute dermatoses with a secondary infection. A 1 per cent solution has been used in mycotic infections such as athlete's foot and in poison ivy dermatitis. A 5 per cent solution has a powerful styptic action.

Because of its oxidising property, potassium permanganate as a crystalline insufflation has been employed topically to oxidise venom in case of snake and scorpion bite. A 0.02 per cent solution in water is used for stomach wash in the treatment of alkaloidal poisoning.

Potassium permanganate is commonly employed to purify well water and to disinfect vegetables and fruits.

Zinc permanganate, because of its greater astringent activity, is preferred to the potassium salt for urethral irrigation.

Dyes

Dyes have been used since ancient times in foods, medicines and cosmetics. The natural dyes have been replaced by the more stable synthetic dyes. These are used as antiseptics, chemotherapeutic, diagnostic and colouring agents. They are non-irritant. They are sometimes used as aqueous solutions or ointments applied topically in the treatment of burns, impetigo and chronic ulcers of the skin and mucous membranes. They are claimed to promote healthy granulation and thus help in healing of ulcers. They cause local staining. The commonly used dyes are: **gentian violet** 0.1 %, **brilliant green** 0.5-1.0 % and **acriflavine** 2 %.

METHYLENE BLUE: Methylene blue occurs as a dark greenish, crystalline powder with a metallic lustre. It is hygroscopic and soluble in water. Used in small doses, it facilitates the conversion of methemoglobin to haemoglobin and has been used as an antidote in the treatment of cyanide poisoning and drug induced methemoglobinemia. For this purpose, it is given IV as a 1 per cent solution in doses of 1 to 4 mg. per kg. bodyweight. It is also used in the treatment of idiopathic methemoglobinemia in the dosage of 300 mg. orally daily along with large amounts of ascorbic acid.

Heavy Metals

The pharmacology of heavy metals is discussed in Chapter 72. Heavy metal salts used exclusively as antiseptics destroy the micro-organisms in very low concentrations, an action referred to as the *oligodynamic action*. The antiseptic activity is due to precipitation of the bacterial proteins.

SILVER COMPOUNDS:

(i) **Silver nitrate:** This occurs as colourless or white crystals, extremely soluble in water. Silver nitrate has antiseptic, astringent and caustic properties. If ingested, it produces severe GI irritation, vertigo, coma and convulsions. Applied to the skin, it stains the area.

The prophylactic use of aqueous solution containing 1 per cent of silver nitrate as eye drops (two drops) for conjunctivitis and ophthalmia neonatorum is still used. Aqueous solution of 0.5% is sometimes applied on second and third degree burns as prophylaxis against infection.

Silver nitrate stick has been used to remove warts and other small skin growths and for cauterization of wounds and trachoma follicles. The stick should be moistened before use.

(ii) **Silver sulfadiazine** (Chapter 44).

ZINC SALTS: Zinc salts possess astringent, corrosive and weak antiseptic properties. The commonly used salts are:

(i) **Zinc sulfate:** Zinc sulfate occurs as odourless, colourless, efflorescent crystals or as a white crystalline powder. It has an astringent metallic taste and is soluble in water.

Externally, zinc sulfate is used as an astringent lotion for indolent ulcers and to assist granulation. Eye drops in the concentration of 0.1 to 1 per cent are sometimes used in angular conjunctivitis and in chronic inflammation of the cornea. The salt is the major ingredient of many commercially available deodorant anhidrotics.

(ii) **Calamine** is a pink powder, almost odourless and tasteless, practically insoluble in water. Chemically, it is basic zinc carbonate (98%) with a small amount of ferric oxide which imparts the pink colour. It has mild astringent and antiseptic actions and is used as a lotion and a dusting powder in skin conditions like sunburns, eczema and urticaria, where it also acts as a soothing and protective agent.

Calamine lotion contains 15 per cent of calamine, 5 per cent each of zinc oxide and glycerine, 3 per cent of bentonite, 0.5 per cent each of liquified phenol and sodium citrate, with rose water as the vehicle. It can also be used as oily lotion or cream (Chapter 69).

(iii) Zinc phosphate is **toxic** and is used as **rat poison**.

Gases

Ethylene oxide, formaldehyde and betapropiolactone in the gaseous form are powerful agents used for sterilization. Beta-propiolactone has been reported to have carcinogenic properties.

ETHYLENE OXIDE: This is colourless liquid with a boiling point of 10.7° C. At normal room temperatures, it is a *highly inflammable and highly explosive* gas with a sweet ethereal smell. The explosive tendency can be limited by mixing it with an inert gas such as nitrogen or carbon dioxide and keeping down the concentration of ethylene oxide to 10%.

A relative humidity of about 30% is necessary for satisfactory sterilization. It has powerful bactericidal, sporicidal and viricidal properties and a high penetrating capacity. The presence of protein impairs its effectiveness. Its safe use necessitates special equipment which is not commonly available; this is its main drawback. Otherwise, its properties make it an excellent agent for sterilizing complicated equipment like heart-lung machines and respirators as well as suture material. It is mutagenic and carcinogenic.

Choice of Method of Sterilization and Disinfection

All instruments and apparatus to be sterilized

should be first thoroughly cleaned by washing and scrubbing. The same applies to areas for fumigation as the presence of organic matter reduces the efficacy of chemical disinfectants.

Autoclaving is the method of choice for sterilizing all theatre appliances that will withstand it. Those which cannot withstand autoclaving are sterilized by chemical methods: lysol, chloroxylenol or iodophor for surgical blades and scissors; formaldehyde or gluteraldehyde for endoscopes and specialized rubber equipment; and ethylene oxide for heart-lung machines. Syringes are sterilized by autoclaving, hot air sterilization or gamma radiation. Diabetics are commonly advised to keep their syringe and needle permanently immersed in spirit and to boil them once a week. Gamma radiation is now increasingly used to sterilize many types of disposable articles on a massive scale so that they are available ready-to-use. Autogenous and some types of synthetic grafts used in cardiovascular surgery are sterilized with antibiotics.

It is customary to sterilize the air in operation threatres with ultra-violet radiation or with iodophor spray. Ultra-violet radiation is also used to sterilize the air inside sterile dispensing cabinets. Solutions of biological materials such as sera and antibiotics which cannot be sterilized by heat are often 'sterilized' by filtration, though a few vaccines will withstand sterilization by steam at 100°C. Laboratory glassware is ordinarily sterilized in a hot air oven after thorough, preliminary cleansing.

Wards, theatres and sick rooms and the contaminated furniture can be swabbed with formalin or iodophor solution, fumigated with gaseous formaldehyde or sprayed with iodophor solution or with a commercial mixture containing glutaraldehyde, chemically bound formaldehyde and benzalkonium chloride (Bacillocid). Books and bedding can be fumigated with gaseous formaldehyde or ethylene oxide. Cotton clothing and rubber mattresses can be autoclaved. Cotton mattresses, however, cannot be autoclaved and have to be exposed to sunlight and fresh air. Incineration is the method of choice for soiled dressings, pathological materials and animal carcasses. If facilities for incineration are not available they are best disinfected with lysol or iodophor. Lysol and iodophor can also be used for disinfecting the excreta of patients with infectious diseases before disposal.

The skin, especially its deeper layers, cannot be sterilized. The best method for reducing the bacterial count on the skin is thorough scrubbing and washing followed by the application of a suitable antiseptic. For preoperative preparation of the skin, the preferred antiseptics are tincture of iodine (mitis), aqueous iodophor (2%) solution and a 2% solution of hibitane in alcohol. Acriflavine and chloroxylenol are the popular wound antiseptics though heavily infected wounds are best treated with systemic antibiotics. Although Condy's lotion (a 0.1% aqueous solution of potassium permanganate) is still the favourite for bladder washes, 1% aqueous solutions of acetic acid and silver nitrate are far more effective for this purpose.

Chloroxylenol is a popular and effective disinfectant for hand-washing by attendants and for sick-room swabbing. Feeding utensils of patients with communicable disceases are best kept separate, washed and finally scalded with boiling water. Soiled bed linen and clothes of patients treated at home should be soaked in a disinfectant such as chloroxylenol and then washed. After recovery of the patient, bed linen and clothes are best laundered and heavy articles such as mattresses exposed to sunlight.

Swimming pools and water supplies are generally disinfected by chlorination whereas potassium permanganate is a convenient domestic disinfectant for water, fruits and vegetables.

Table 60.2 summarises the chemical methods of high level disinfection. Boiling is used to disinfect, whereas steam, dry heat and radiation are used for sterilization (see earlier).

It is worth remembering the following points about disinfectants:

Table 60.2: Some chemical methods of high level disinfection

Chemical	Concentration	Uses and comments
Sodium hypochlorite	0.1 to 1.0 %	Efficient for disinfecting linen, clothing, spills, stainless steel instruments; syringes and needles before autoclaving/disposal. Solution must be freshly prepared as it is unstable. Cheapest disinfectant.
Chloramine T	4%	Similar to above. More stable.
Ethanol	70%	Useful for hand washing, spills, instruments, equipment.
Cetrimide	Stock solution diluted 1:100	Useful for furniture, spills, fittings, equipment.
Povidone iodine	One part of 10% solution added to 3 parts of boiled water	Similar to ethanol. Immerse for 15 minutes
Formaldehyde	35-40% solution diluted 1:10	Disinfection after 30 minutes immersion; sterilisation after several hours. Toxic.
	Tablets releasing vapour	Requires special apparatus.
Glutaraldehyde	2%	30 minutes immersion for disinfection, 10 hours for sterilisation. Needs activation before use.
Hydrogen peroxide	6%	Disinfection after 30 minutes of immersion.

- Most are highly active against Gram positive bacteria.
- Acid fast bacilli are less susceptible to these agents and need higher concentrations. They are resistant to chlorhexidine, oxidizing agents and cresol.
- Aldehydes, sodium hypochlorite and povidone iodine have action against fungi too.
- Spores are usually resistant to all except aldehydes, sodium hypochlorite and high concentrations of povidone iodine.
- Hydrophilic viruses are usually resistant except to aldehydes and high concentrations of sodium hypochlorite.
- Prions are resistant to most agents except high concentrations of sodium hypochlorite.
- *Hand washing is the important method for preventing transmission of infection from person to person and is best done with soap and warm water, with or without a disinfectant,* as a disinfectant can cause irritation, dryness and sensitization of the skin.

Insecticides

These drugs, primarily used to destroy insects, are important because of their toxicological properties.

Classification :

I **Organochlorines :**

(a) Chlorophenothane (DDT) and related compounds

(b) Cyclodienes e.g. Aldrin, Endrin, Diledrin, Heptachlor, Chlorolane, Endosulfan, Chlordecone

(c) Gammabenzene hexachloride (Gammexane); and

(d) Toxaphene and related compounds.

All these compounds persisting in the environment can accumulate in the body tissues.

II **Carbamate insecticides :** Carbaryl, Dimetan, Pyrolan, Zectran and Carbofuran.

III **Organophosphorus compounds:** Malathion, Parathion, TEPP, and Diazinon.

IV **Botanical compounds:** Pyrethrum, Limonoids and Rotenone.

I Organochlorines :

CHLOROPHENOTHANE (DDT, Dicophane), chemically dichloro-diphenyl-trichloroethane, occurs as a white powder, practically insoluble in water but slightly soluble in alcohol and kerosene. It was the first highly effective and relatively safe insecticide discovered by Muller who was later awarded the Nobel prize in Medicine in 1948.

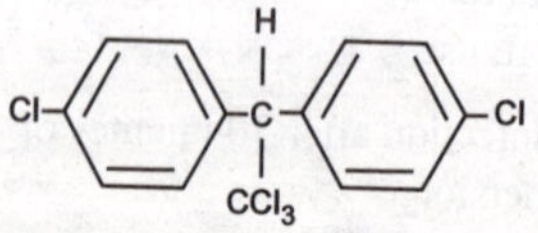

Fig. 60.2 : Dicophane (DDT)

DDT is lethal to many arthropods including fleas, body lice, houseflies and mosquitoes. It is a stomach and contact poison i.e. it is absorbed through both the chitinous exoskeleton and the GI tract of the insect. It paralyses the CNS.

DDT, because of its low volatility, retains its insecticidal action for a long time. The agent does not have an immediate lethal effect like pyrethrum and rotenone, but these may be combined to advantage with DDT. Its value as an insecticide has, however, diminished considerably due to the development of resistance in many strains of insect species.

Absorption, fate and excretion: DDT is slowly and incompletely absorbed from the GI tract of man and other large animals. Although it does not penetrate the intact skin in powder form, when dissolved in the various organic solvents, appreciable percutaneous absorption can occur. Absorption may also occur through accidental inhalation in workers engaged in spraying the insecticide and in animals consuming the fodder dusted with DDT.

Following absorption, large amounts of DDT are stored in body fat depots and in the liver. The drug is excreted unchanged in milk to some extent but most of it is slowly degraded in the tissues and the products eliminated in urine.. DDT stimulates the hepatic microsomal enzyme systems and this may enhance the biotransformation of drugs like barbiturates. Slow poisoning can occur due to consumption of animal milk/meat containing DDT.

Adverse reactions:

- ***Acute poisoning***: This is characterised by vomiting, diarrhoea, paraesthesiae, giddiness and fatigue followed by tremors, convulsions and coma; associated solvents like kerosene can cause pulmonary edema. Death occurs from respiratory arrest or from ventricular fibrillation as DDT sensitises the myocardium to adrenaline. The human lethal dose of the insecticide is estimated to be between 10 and 20 g.

Treatment of acute poisoning is symptomatic and includes gastric lavage, saline purgation, diazepam for the treatment of convulsions, artificial respiration and oxygen. Treatment has to be continued for many days in view of the possible drug storage. Milk, oily substances and sympathomimetic amines should be avoided. Workers engaged in spraying the insecticide should wear protective clothing and face masks.

- ***Chronic poisoning***: Early symptoms of chronic poisoning are loss of appetite, muscular weakness, fine tremors and mental apprehension. Rarely, it may cause motor neurone disease. Occasionally, anemia, leucocytosis, liver and kidney damage may develop. It has been shown to produce cancer of the bladder in animals.

Uses: DDT is useful for eliminating fleas, bugs, mosquitoes, cockroaches and body lice. For this purpose, a 10 per cent mixture of DDT with a suitable inert diluent like talc is employed. However, bugs and headlice have become resistant in many countries. Further, it is not ovicidal. The walls and furniture can be sprayed with a solution of DDT in kerosene; about 100 mg. per square feet usually ensure effective control for about 6 weeks.

DDT was a widely used pesticide in agriculture and in horticulture (0.1 to 1 per cent aqueous suspension or a 5 to 10 per cent dust). *Its storage in human body, its possible long term neurotoxicity and its carcinogenicity are a matter of great concern which has lead to a decrease in its use.*

ENDRIN AND DIELDRIN: These compounds are more toxic than DDT particularly to fish and birds. Endrin is 2 to 3 times more toxic than dieldrin. These agents are employed for residual spraying, usually as 0.6 to 1.2 per cent suspension for similar purpose as DDT.

GAMMA BENZENE HEXACHLORIDE (Gammaxane): Chapter 69.

All **organochlorine insecticides are CNS stimulants** and can cause convulsions. As they are lipid soluble, they tend to concentrate in the tissues and have prolonged t½. They may also undergo enterohepatic circulation. **Endosulfan** ingestion causes prolonged convulsions, disseminated intravenous coagulation and myoglobinuria. Its treatment is mainly symptomatic : gastric lavage, activated charcoal and anticonvulsants like benzodiazepines. The patient may return after discharge for repeat convulsions a few days later, due to release of the compound from deposits in the fat.

II **Carbamate insecticides :** These agents act as acetylcholinesterase inhibitors and cause actions similar to the organophosphorus compounds (see below). However, they have shorter duration of action and larger margin of safety. They are considered as nonpersistent insecticides. (Chapter 18).

III **Organophosphorus insecticides:** The organophosphorus compounds such as malathion, chlorpyrifos and fenitrothion are effective against a variety of arthropods like lice, flies and mosquitoes. They act against both the larvae and the adult insects and are widely used as agricultural and horticultural pesticides (For toxicity and treatment, see Chapter 18).

IV **Botanical compounds:**

PYRETHRUM FLOWERS: These are the dried flower heads of *Chrysanthemum cineratiaefolium*. They owe their insecticidal activity to the two esters, pyrethrin 1 and pyrethrin ll. Pyrethrum flowers are mainly used in the form of an extract and are superior to DDT in being rapidly lethal to the insects.

Pyrethrum acts mainly by contact and has no appreciable effect on ingestion. It mainly affects the central nervous system of the insect.

Pyrethrum has relatively low human toxicity. Excessive ingestion, however, may cause initial stimulation of the CNS followed by paralysis. The agent also produces contact dermatitis.

Pyrethrum is usually sprayed as solutions containing 0.4 to 0.6 per cent of total pyrethrins. Its applications are similar to those of DDT.

PYRETHROIDS: Synthetic pyrethroids are chemically related to natural pyrethrins and are esters of certain acids (e.g., chrysanthenic acid) and alcohols (e.g., allethrolone). They act as neuropoisons by virtue of their action on sodium channels in the axons in the peripheral and CNS. A single dose produces toxic signs, such as tremors, hyperexcitability, choreoathetosis and convulsions, tetanic paralysis in mammals. In small doses, the action is reversible but at near–lethal doses, they cause structural changes in the nervous system, such as axonal swelling and/or breaks and myelin degeneration. Such neurotoxicity is especially liable to occur in children. Pyrethrum is absorbed following ingestion or inhalation but not significantly from the skin. Hence, when they are being heated they should be kept away from infants and children. Further, mats/coils cotaining pyrethroids, when heated, cause irritation of the eyes and nose, and suffocation.

Synthetic pyrethroids include **allethrin, resmethrin, tetramethrin** and **permethrin.** They are generally metabolised through ester hydrolysis, oxidation and conjugation and there is no tendency to accumulate in tissues. In the environment, synthetic pyrethroids are fairly rapidly degraded in soil and in plants. They are adsorbed on soil and sediments and hardly eluted with water. There is little tendency for bioaccumulation in organisms. Because of low application rates and rapid degradation in the environment, residue in food is generally low. For similar reasons, in the dose levels used as insecticides, no serious adverse effects have been noticed in fish, aquatic arthropods and honey beas. Because of their excellent activity against a wide range of insect pests and their non-persistence in the environment, they are now extensively used as agricultural insecticides and for control of household insects.

They have high ovicidal and pediculocidal property, a 1% cream-rinse permethrin preparation, applied and kept for 10 minutes, eleminates head-lice infestation after a single application. Similarly, a 5% permethrin dermal cream is highly effective against scabies (Chapter 69).

LIMONOIDS : Limonoids are derived from the ancient Indian plant, neem (*Azadirachta indica*). Several biological active compounds have been isolated from the oil, seeds, bark and leaves of neem. Neem oil or neem leaves have been used for centuries by households and farmers in India to protect the foodgrains.

The limonoid azadirachtin and other similar compounds are highly effective in minute quantities against a variety of insects. Since neem is a collection of active ingredients the development of resistance by insects is probably difficult. They appear to be harmless to humans and to useful insects such as honey-bees. Unlike the modern chemical insecticides, azadirachtin is not an instant killer but is a growth inhibitor, anti-feedant and repellant. Its biodegradability is an additional advantage. Neem oil is also claimed to possess spermicidal and antibacterial properties. A number of neem based pesticides are now available.

ROTENONE: Rotenone is the principal active insecticidal constituent of *Derris* or *Tuba root.* Rotenone is a stomach and contact insecticide. Its action is more rapid but less persistent than that of DDT and less rapid but more persistent than that of the pyrethrum.

Rotenone may cause GI irritation, conjunctivitis, pharyngitis and rarely, respiratory stimulation and convulsions. It is used either as a dusting powder diluted with talc or as an insecticidal wash.

Section XIII
Drugs Used in Endocrine Disorders

Anterior Pituitary Hormones 61

The important functions of growth, sclf preservation (homeostasis) and species preservation (reproduction) in a multicellular organism demand the highest degree of integration of the various body systems and adaptation to external environment. This integration is brought about by the 'neuroendocrine complex' consisting of the CNS, the ANS and the endocrine glands. The endocrine glands and the ANS serve to carry messages from the highest integrating authority, the CNS, to the body organs and cells. In turn, the ANS and the endocrine glands influence the functioning of the CNS. Finally, there is 'cross talk' between the endocrine system and the cells of the immune system. Thus, the glucocorticoids are potent immunosuppressants, whereas cytokines and interleukins exert profound effects on the functions of the various endocrine glands.

The introduction of the radioimmunoassay technique for measuring hormones in biological fluids by Berson and Yallow in 1960 revolutionised the diagnosis of endocrine disorders.

Endocrine Physiology-Introduction

The word **hormone** is derived from the Greek word *Hormao* which means 'to impel'. It is defined as a substance secreted by specialized cells and transported to a distant site to exert its action upon specific tissues.

The endocrine glands consist of groups of highly specialized cells located at various sites in the body. They synthesize and discharge their specialized secretions (hormones) directly into the circulation without the intervention of a duct (hence the name 'ductless' glands).

Hormones are secreted by well organized endocrine glands such as the thyroid and the adrenals, and by not so well organized endocrine cells in the GI tract which secrete gastrin, secretin, pancreozymin and cholecystokinin (gut hormones). Kidneys secrete renin and erythropoietin. 1,25 Dihydroxy- cholecalciferol, the active metabolite of vitamin D synthesized by the kidney, also qualifies as a hormone. The heart is the major source of atrial natriuretic peptide (ANP).

Generally, a hormone is stored in the same gland which synthesizes it. The hormones of the neurohypophysis, vasopressin and oxytocin, are, however, synthesized in the hypothalamus but are stored in the neurohypophysis. The hypothalamic regulatory hormones are synthesized in various areas of the hypothalamus but are stored in the median eminence.

The hormones of the endocrine glands can be grouped into five major classes:

- ***Amino acid derivatives*** e.g. Catecholamines, Dopamine and Thyroid hormones.

- ***Peptides*** e.g. Hypothalamic regulatory hormones (TRH, GnRH, CRH and others), Somatostatin and Vasopressin.
- ***Proteins*** e.g. Insulin,GH and PTH.
- ***Steroids*** e.g. Adrenocortical and Gonadal steroids.
- ***Vitamin derived*** e.g. Vitamin D derivatives and Retinoids.

A hormone may act

(a) On other endocrine glands e.g. hypothalamic regulatory (releasing and release inhibiting) hormones and trophic hormones of the anterior pituitary; or

(b) Directly on the tissues e.g. insulin, growth hormone (GH), prolactin (PRL), parathyroid hormone (PTH), and hormones of the adrenals and gonads.

Regulation and release of a hormone: A hormone is directly released into venous blood, generally in discrete pulses, at a slow basal rate, which in the case of many hormones, shows a natural diurnal rhythm. There are many factors which either increase or decrease the hormonal synthesis and secretion:

(a) Various **releasing and release- inhibiting hormones** of the hypothalamus act on the anterior pituitary to modify the synthesis and release of its trophic hormones. They have an intrinsic diurnal rhythm set on them by the brain.

(b) Hormones of the anterior putuitary stimulate synthesis and release of hormones of the target glands, (thyroid, adrenal cortex and gonads). In the absence of these hormones, the target glands not only cease functioning but also undergo atrophy. Hence, these hormones are called **trophic hormones**. In turn, elevated plasma concentrations of hormones produced by the target glands act on the hypothalamus to alter the rate of release of regulatory hormones and on the pituitary to reduce its responsiveness to the latter, and thus reduce the secretion of the respective trophic hormones of the anterior pituitary (TSH, ACTH, FSH, LH). On the other hand, a fall in the plasma concentration of a target gland hormone leads to a greater release of the corresponding trophic hormone. Thus, in health, any change in the plasma concentration of a target gland hormone tends to correct itself by altering the anterior pituitary function. This mechanism of mutual regulation of hormone activity is called **feed-back system** (Fig 61.1). It helps to maintain the plasma concentration of the target gland hormones within a delicately balanced narrow range.

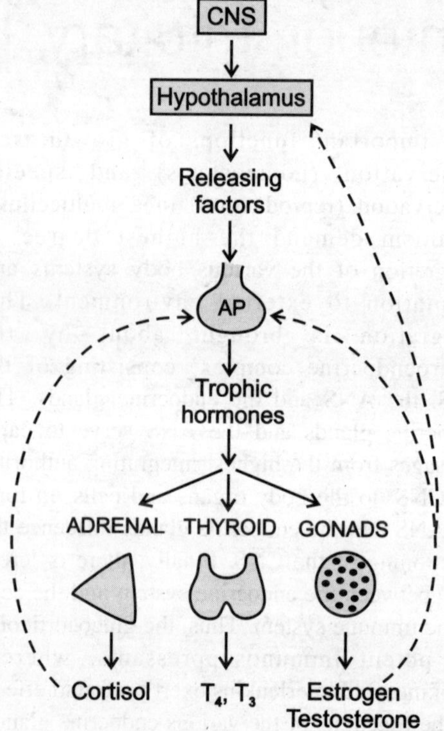

Fig. 61.1 : Hormone release and feedback mechanisms AP = Anterior Pituitary

(c) The rate of release of a hormone may also be influenced by changes in the concentration of non-hormonal chemical substances in the plasma. For example, hyperglycemia stimulates the release of insulin from the pancreas but supresses the release of GH from the anterior pituitary; hypoglycemia has the opposite effects. A decrease in the level of plasma calcium stimulates the release of PTH but supresses that of calcitonin; an increase in the level of plasma calcium has the opposite effect.

This is another type of *feed-back mechanism* which is also homeostatic in nature.

(d) In addition to the classical feedback, local regulatory systems exist which control hormonal secretion. *Paracrine regulation* involves the release of a hormone by one type of cells that acts on adjacent cells in the same tissue e.g. somatostatin from the pancreatic islet D cells inhibits insulin secretion by the beta cells. *Autocrine regulation* involves the action of a hormone on the same cells that produce it e.g. insulin-like growth factor 1 (IGF 1) acts on many cells that produce it, including chondrocytes, gonadal cells and breast epithelial cells.

(e) Psychoneurogenic factors can alter the rate of secretion of hormones e.g. depression may inhibit gonadotropin secretion; acute stress increases the release of catecholamines from the adrenal medulla and glucocorticoids from the adrenal cortex.

(f) Increased plasma level of GH is to be found in patients with malnutrition, anorexia nervosa and dwarfism due to end organ resistance to GH. This increase is thought to be due to diminished feedback by IGF-1, the levels of which are low in these conditions. In acromegaly, it is due to the activity of the pituitary tumour cells.

Role of hypothalamus: The hypothalamus synthesizes and releases several chemical substances which reach the pituitary either along neurons (vasopressin and pitocin) or via the portal circulation. Those which are of known chemical structure and are available as synthetic substances are called 'hormones'; others are called 'factors'. As a group, they are called *hypothalamic regulatory hormones* (Table 61.1). They are synthesized in the cell bodies of the neurons in different parts of the hypothalamus, and are stored in the median eminence. In response to appropriate stimuli, they are released into the portal circulation and travel to the anterior pituitary to exert their releasing or release-inhibiting actions on the trophic hormone producing cells of the latter. The hypothalamic releasing hormones and factors are released in nanogram or smaller quantities. They cause the synthesis and release of much larger, microgram quantities of pituitary trophic hormones. In turn, the trophic hormones cause synthesis and release of still larger, milligram quantitites of target gland hormones. This can then be considered as a 'cascading amplifier' system of greatly multiplying the original hypothalamic signals. Some of the hypothalamic regulatory hormones act not only on the corresponding pituitary cells but also on others to stimulate or inhibit the release of their hormones. For vasopressin and pitocin see Chapters 38 and 43, respectively.

Table 61.1: Hypothalamic regulatory hormones

Releasing hormone (RH) or factor (RF) for:
Thyrotrophin (TRH)
Luteinizing hormone and follicular stimulating hormone (LH/FSH—RH or Gn—RH)
Growth hormone (GH—RH)
Corticotrophin (CRH)
Melanocyte stimulating hormone (MSH-RF)
Release inhibiting hormone (RIH) or factor (RIF) for:
Growth hormone (GH-RIH, Somatostatin)
Melanocyte stimulating hormone (MSH-RIF) Prolactin (PIF)

The hypothalamic neurons which secrete the regulatory hormones are themselves under the control of specialized monoaminergic, neurotransmitter neurons in the midbrain. Thus,

- ***Dopamine*** is concerned in the release of GH and inhibition of release of PRL.
- ***Noradrenaline*** is concerned in the release of GH, TSH, and gonadotrophins.
- ***Serotonin*** (5-HT) is concerned in the release of GH and PRL and inhibition of TSH release.

In turn, these midbrain nuclei are under the control of the 'visceral brain' and are responsive to stress and emotional disturbances. The pituitary secretion of some hormones (GH, ACTH and PRL) is primarily regulated (via hypothalamus) by intrinsic brain rhythms related to sleep-wake cycle or to change to lighting conditions rather than by any specific homeostatic requirements.

The release of one pituitary hormone may be governed by different bioaminergic mechanisms under different circumstances e.g. it appears that sleep induced GH release is 5-HT mediated whereas hypoglycemia-mediated GH release is mediated by noradrenaline. Growth hormone and prolactin secretion appears to be controlled by the CNS itself. That of ACTH, TSH and gonadotrophins is regulated by complex feedback mechanisms.

Many drugs (reserpine, chlorpromazine, 1-dopa, amphetamine, imipramine, bromergocriptine etc.) act on the hypothalamus and influence the local monoamine concentration and thus, bring about alterations in the secretion of anterior pituitary hormones particularly prolactin. *Thus, the hypothalamus can be regarded as the highest relay centre which integrates the endocrine and the ANS and ensures their smooth coordination by the cerebral cortex.*

TRH, somatostatin and gut hormone containing neurons are widely distributed in the CNS outside the hypothalamus.

Transport and metabolism of hormones: The hormones are carried in the plasma partly protein bound and partly free. The free form is the active form. The bound form, though inactive, has a reservoir function, releasing more free hormone as it is degraded.

The metabolic degradation of free hormones occurs in the liver, in the target endocrine glands and in the tissues on which they act. Conjugation of steroid hormones to sulfates and glucuronides occurs in the liver. Generally, metabolic degradation renders the hormone less active or inactive. With some hormones, however, metabolic transformation (e.g. thyroxine to tri-iodothyronine) renders the hormone biologically active. The kidney excretes conjugated steroid hormone and a trace of the free original hormone.

Knowledge of the t½ of the circulating hormones helps to establish effective, physiological, hormonal replacement therapy as the time required to achieve a steady state plasma level is generally related to the t½ of the hormone(s). Most protein hormones such as insulin, ACTH and GH have short t½ (minutes), whereas the steroids and the thyroid hormones have longer t½ (hours to days).

The responses of body cells to hormones are considerably influenced by genetic as well as environmental factors. Important among these are species, race, age, sex, time of the day, season, temperature, nutrition, presence of disease and prior effect of other hormones.

The important differences between the peptide hormones and the steroid hormones are shown in Table 61.2. In general, catecholamines behave like the peptide hormones and the iodothyronines (with important differences) behave like the steroid hormones.

Mechanism of action of hormones: Hormones act through specific receptors which may be divided into two major classes:

(1) **Cell membrane receptors;** and
(2) **Nuclear receptors.**

Generally, amino acid derivatives and peptide hormones interact with cell-surface-membrane receptors; whereas steroidal and thyroidal hormones, vitamin D and its derivatives, and retinoids, which are lipid soluble, interact with nuclear receptors (Table 61.3).

The glycoprotein hormones TSH, FSH, LH and hCG consist of two subunits alpha and beta.The alpha subunit is common to all of them whereas the beta subunit of each one of them is distinctive and is responsible for its specific biological action. Structural similarities also exist between insulin and insulin-like growth factors, IGF I and IGF II. Such similarities among the

Table 61.2: Important differences between peptide and steroid hormones

Parameter	Steroids	Peptides
Biosynthesis	Multiple enzymes	Single protein, prohormone
Storage in the gland	Minimal	Often substantial
Half life	Long (hours)	Short (minutes)
Binding proteins	Present	Less common
Peripheral transformations	Common	Do not occur
Initial binding site	Cytoplasmic receptor	Plasma membrane receptor
Principal site of action	Nucleus	Plasma membrane
Principal mechanism of action	Activation of genome	Activation of second messenger
Degradation products	Sometimes retain activity	Inactive
Administration	Oral, parenteral	Parenteral
Allergy	No	Yes

hormones explain the overlapping actions of related hormones.

A persistent increase in the concentration of a hormone brings about a reduction in the concentration of its specific receptors **(down regulation)**. A hormone may bind to more than one class of receptors e.g. insulin at high concentrations binds to somatomedin receptors and can have growth stimulating actions. Several clinical syndromes are due to mutational abnormalities in the receptors, e.g., GH resistance, resistance to thyroid hormones etc.

Hormones as drugs: Hormones for clinical use may be obtained from natural sources such as animal glands or may be prepared synthetically; these as well as their synthetic analogues are widely used as drugs. In many instances e.g. with steroid and thyroid hormones which are available as chemically pure substances, their biological actions in humans are independent of their source. In other instances e.g.with insulin, the pharmacokinetics in humans may differ with the source of the drug though the biological actions are identical. In contrast, GH activity is species specific and only human GH is therapeutically effective in humans.

Synthetic analogues may have the advantage(s) of abundant and cheap supply e.g. prednisolone, improved bioavailability because of resistance to metabolic degradation; longer or shorter duration of action as desired e.g. rDNA analogues of human insulin;or greater specificity because of elimination of trace contaminants e.g. rDNA-FSH.

Hormones are used:

- ***For diagnostic purposes*** e.g. ACTH is used to diagnose Addison's disease, and dexamethasone to diagnose Cushing's disease. *Rarely*, they may be used for a *therapeutic trial* to confirm or refute a diagnosis when the laboratory tests are equiuvocal e.g. hypothyroidism.
- ***For therapeutic purposes***, either (a) as *replacement therapy* to supplement or replace a deficient natural hormone e.g. insulin in diabetes mellitus; or (b) as *pharmacotherapy* e.g. glucocorticoids in asthma.

Table 61.3: Different types of hormone receptors

Receptor type	Hormones
Membrane receptors	
(a) GPCR	Catecholamines, LH, FSH, TSH, ACTH, hypothalamic releasing factors, somatostatin
(b) Tyrosine kinases	Insulin, insulin-like growth factors, epidermal growth factor
(c) Cytokine regulated kinases	GH, PRL
(d) Serine kinases	Activin, transforming growth factor
Nuclear receptors *	
(a) Type I-in cytoplasm**	Steroids e.g., glucocorticoids, estrogens, progesterone
(b) Type II-in nucleus	Thyroid hormones, vitamin D, retinoids

*All nuclear receptors ultimately act to increase or decrease gene transcription.
**After ligand binding, the ligand-cytoplasmic-receptor complex translocates to the nucleus.

The Pituitary Gland

The pituitary gland, together with the hypothalamus, forms a neuroendocrine relay station for messages from the brain to the rest of the body.

Pituitary gland weighs 0.4 to 1.1 g. in adults and is larger in females than in males. It consists of **adenohypophysis** developed from the oropharynx and **neurohypophysis** developed from the floor of the third ventricle. The former consists of the *anterior lobe*, the *pars tuberalis* and the *pars intermedia.* The neurohypophysis consists of the posterior lobe of the pituitary and the infundibular stalk which connects it to the hypothalamus.

The pituitary gland has a rich arterial blood supply and also has a 'portal system' which connects it with the median eminence of the hypothalamus. The latter transmits the hypothalamic regulatory hormones to the pituitary via the portal system. The blood flow in the pituitary portal circulation is bi-directional; this would permit the pituitary hormones to have a regulating effect on the secretory neurons in the hypothalamus.

The anterior lobe of the pituitary contains three types of cells :

- ***Chromophobe,***
- ***Eosinophil***; and
- ***Basophil***.

Electron microscopy and immuno-fluorescence microscopy have permitted the identification of specific-hormone-producing cells (Table 61.4).

Six adenohypophysical hormones have been definitely identified. These are GH and PRL (eosinophil cells); and ACTH, TSH, FSH, LH (basophil cells). Of these ACTH, prolactin and GH are peptides and TSH, LH and FSH are glycoproteins. The melanocyte stimulating hormone (MSH) exists in the pars intermedia of the anterior pituitary. Vasopressin and oxytocin are present in the neurohypophysis.

The various tropic hormones are described in detail along with the respective target gland hormones elsewhere. For posterior pituitary hormones see Chapter 38 and 43.

Effects of hypopituitarism: Manifestations of hypopituitarism depend upon the age of the subject.

- ***In children***: Retardation of linear growth

Table 61.4: Hormones of the anterior pituitary

Pituitary cell	Hormone produced	Stimulators	Inhibitors	Target gland	Biologic effects
Somatotrope	GH	GHRH	Somatostatin, IGF1	Liver, bone, other tissues	Growth promotion, IGF1 production, insulin antagonism
Corticotrope	ACTH	CRF, AVP	Glucocorticoids	Adrenal cortex	Glucocorticoid production
Thyrotrope	TSH*	TRH	T_4, T_3, Dopamine, Glucocorticoids	Thyroid	T_4, T_3 synthesis and release
Gonadotrope	FSH*, LH*	GnRH,	Sex steroids, Inhibin	Testes, ovaries	Sex steroid production, follicular growth, germ cell maturation
Lactotrope	PRL	Estrogen, TRH	Dopamine	Breast, other tissues	Milk production, metabolic effects

AVP = Arginine vasopressin. * = Glycoproteins

and of bone age are the two important effects of GH deficiency (GHD) in children. They are due to IGF1 deficiency secondary to GH deficiency. These children appear normal at birth. As they grow, the deviation from normal height becomes more and more marked. They are small but intelligent, delicate and graceful.

A selective growth hormone deficiency may occur, in which case the diagnosis is made by the radioimmunoassay of plasma GH. When GHD occurs as a part of panhypopituitarism, the associated deficiencies of ACTH and TSH make the clinical diagnosis easier. Panhypopituitarism may be idiopathic or may be due to destruction of the anterior pituitary by a granuloma or a tumour. Isolated GHD is generally idiopathic and often genetic in origin. In some cases, manifestations of GHD are due to GH resistance in the peripheral target tissues.

- ***In adults***: Panhypopituitarism may be produced in adults by destruction of the pituitary by a pituitary tumour, therapeutic hypophysectomy (as in the treatment of a pituitary tumour) or postpartum pituitary necrosis (Sheehan's syndrome). It may also be due to continuation of childhood panhypopituitarism into adult life.

The clinical manifestations are due to deficiency of:

- ***Gonadotropins***, such as infertility, impotence, amenorrhoea and total loss of sexual hair.
- ***TSH***, giving rise to hypothyroidism.
- ***ACTH***, such as hypotension and fasting hypoglycemia. Pigmentation of Addison's disease is not seen, and aldosterone production is relatively unaffected; and
- ***GH***. These can be subtle and comprise fatigue, lethargy, and impaired physical performance, accompanied by reduction in muscle and bone mass, increased adiposity and increased cardiovascular mortality, emotional lability and feelings of social isolation. Treatment with human growth hormone (hGH) reverses many of these in manifestations and has beneficial effects in adult GHD.

The patients become moderately plump but not obese; cachexia is absent.

Effects of hyperpituitarism: Excessive production of anterior pituitary hormones may occur in the presence of demonstrable pituitary disease or in its absence. Such excessive production is associated with gigantism, acromegaly, one form of Cushing's syndrome, the galactorrhoea-amenorrhoea syndrome and rarely, hyperthyroidism. Excessive production of the anterior pituitary hormones (TSH, ACTH and Gonadotropins) also occurs in response to failure of function of the respective target glands.

High levels of plasma GH are seen in acromegaly, GH resistance, uncontrolled diabetes mellitus, anorexia nervosa and protein calorie malnutrition. In some cases, such excess of pituitary hormone may give rise to important clinical features e.g. pigmentation of Addison's disease, probably due to excess of ACTH.

GROWTH HORMONE (GH) : A growth hormone is found in all vertebrates. In addition to its growth promoting properties, it possesses several important metabolic effects which are essential for health but do not appear to be absolutely necessary for survival.

Source and chemistry: It is synthesized and stored by the (eosinophil) somatotrophic cells of the adenohypophysis. It is present in the pituitary gland at all ages. GH secreting cells constitute upto 50% of the total anterior pituitary cell population. Human growth hormone (hGH) is a polypeptide consisting of a series of 191 amino acids and has been synthesized. About 5-15 mg. of hGH can be obtained from one anterior pituitary gland. hGH for clinical use is now obtained by recombinant DNA technique.

The growth promoting effect of GH appears to be species specific in that a species responds to GH of homologous origin and to that from higher but not from lower species. The human being responds only to human GH.

Plasma levels and regulation of GH secretion: Plasma level of hGH as measured by an immunoassay is undetectable between GH pulses in an adult. It rises (as high as 25 ng per ml or higher) several times in spikes during the day, mostly during exercise, deep sleep (especially in children), and several hours after a meal. These spikes are higher in women than in men and can be distinguished from pathological increases in plasma GH levels by their suppression after glucose administration. Stimulated by the sex steroids,especially estrogen, GH levels rise during puberty.

Hypoglycemia is the most consistent stimulus to GH secretion and insulin-induced hypoglycemia is the gold standard for diagnosis of GHD. GH responsiveness to insulin hypoglycemia is depressed in obesity, hypopituitarism, hypothyroidism, chronic alcoholism and in individuals on glucocorticoid therapy. Clonidine, levodopa and arginine are the other stimuli to GH release in normal persons.

The rate of release of GH by the pituitary is regulated by GH-RH and somatostatin (GH-RIH). It is stimulated by ghrelin, a polypeptide, synthesized by the stomach. Ghrelin also causes increase in appetite and obesity. GH secretion is profoundly influenced by nutritional factors and is stimulated by high protein diet.

The amount of GH secretion is estimated to be about 200-2000 mcg/24 hours, depending on the age, sex and obesity. A substantial part of this occurs during the early hours of sleep. The latter is probably important in the anabolic and repair processes of the body.

Pharmacological actions: Endogenous GH circulates in the blood with a plasma t½ of about 20 minutes, though its metabolic effects last much longer. It exerts:

(I) **Metabolic effects**, directly, by acting on the tissue GH receptors which are widely distributed in the body; and

(II) **Growth related effects,** predominantly indirectly, through IGF-1; and directly to a smaller extent.

Both these categories of effects are more easily demonstrable in GHD patients than in normals.

I **Metabolic effects:**

- ***Carbohydrate metabolism***: Effects on carbohydrate metabolism are complex and difficult to explain in terms of a single basic action of GH.

Plasma levels of glucose and insulin do not change during the diurnal peaks of hGH but after such peaks, the individual becomes resistant to insulin, and glucose tolerance is slightly and transiently impaired.

Acute administration of hGH to normal humans and to non-diabetic, hypophysectomised individuals causes transient hypoglycemia. On the other hand, during chronic administration, it impairs glucose tolerance. Hypophysectomy ameliorates diabetic retinopathy; individuals so treated are prone to hypoglycemia.

- ***Protein metabolism***: GH has a strong anabolic action which can be demonstrated in animals with intact pancreas. Retention of nitrogen, phosphate and potassium occurs. Blood urea falls and urinary excretion of hydroxyproline rises indicating increase in muscle mass and collagen synthesis. GH stimulates the transport of amino acids into the cells and accelerates intracellular protein synthesis.

- ***Fat metabolism***: The fasting plasma free fatty acid (FFA) level rises on administration of GH, due to the lipolytic action of GH on acute administration. Intracellular accumulation of FFA also occurs. In addition, during chronic administration, it inhibits lipogenesis from glucose and acetate. The FFA thus released are utilised by the tissues and inhibit the utilization of glucose (Chapter 63). Under physiological conditions in which GH is secreted without concomitant release of catecholamines, as during sleep, there is little change in plasma fatty acids. GH may, therefore, be of minor importance in lipolysis in man.

- ***Mineral metabolism***: As mentioned earlier, retention of potassium, sodium and phosphorus occurs during administration of GH. Calcium absorption is increased. The hypercalciuric action of GH is not seen in the absence of endogenous parathyroid hormone activity.

II **Growth-related effects:** Growth is brought about by the indirect (through IGF-1) and direct actions of GH (see above), the former being the main mediator. Seventyfive per cent of the circulating IGF-1 is synthesized by the liver in response to GH; it produces widespread effects by binding to specific IGF-1 receptors in the tissues; the rest comes from the spill-over of that produced for paracrine action by numerous tissues (bone, cartilage, erythroid precursors, myocytes and kidneys). IGF-1, unlike most other protein hormones, circulates in the blood bound to IGF binding proteins (IGFBPs 1-5). These proteins serve a carrier function.

The basic actions of IGF-1 are:

- ***Positive nitrogen and mineral balance; and synthesis and accretion of protein in most tissues;*** *and*
- ***Cellular proliferation.***

They are responsible for generalized, coordinated and balanced linear growth in childhood; and unbalanced, local growth (wound healing at all ages and growth of the contralateral kidney after unilateral nephrectomy in childhood)

The other actions of IGF-1 are:

- ***Rise in GFR*** (25%)
- ***Hypoglycemia*** if sufficient amount is given.
- ***Marked increase in insulin sensitivity*** in type 2 diabetics.
- ***Inhibition of GH secretion***; and
- ***Partial reversal of the catabolic effect of nutrient deprivation and glucocorticoids***.

The growth due to GH affects every tissue and organ in the body with the possible exception of the brain and the eye. In children whose epiphyses have not yet closed, it promotes linear bone growth without accelerating skeletal or sexual maturation. It acts on the epiphyseal growth plate but does not advance epiphyseal fusion. The increase in body mass produced by GH mainly affects the lean body mass and is due to retention of water, nitrogen and minerals but not of fat. The growth promoting effect is dramatic in children with GH deficiency (GHD). In most of such children, the effect continues during many (8-10) years of hGH therapy, although a few become refractory after some months. It is noteworthy that hGH injected at intervals of 2-3 days will promote growth, although the metabolic effects produced by it are of short duration. The growth stimulating effect of hGH in GHD is more dramatic in younger than in older children.

- ***Miscellaneous***: GH induces visceromegaly as seen in patients with acromegaly. Rats receiving GH develop a variety of tumours.

Absorption, fate and excretion : GH is administered by SC or IM route. The peak level after SC administration occurs after 2-4 hours, and the active blood level persists for 36 hours. It is metabolized in the liver.

Adverse reactions: Recombinant hGH is well tolerated and safe, and causes few adverse reactions in children. During treatment of GH deficient children, it causes hypothyroidism which must, therefore, be looked for regularly. It may cause glucose intolerance, especially in adults. The other adverse reactions in adults, not seen in children are edema, myalgia and arthralgia. In diabetics, it may aggravate hyperglycemia and cause ketosis. Rarely, it may cause headache, seizures and benign intracranial hypertension, particularly after surgery in patients with craniopharyngiomas. Antibodies to GH appear in about 30% patients on GH but they are present in low titre and rarely intefere with growth stimulation.

Preparations and dosage: The currently available hGH is produced by recombinant DNA technology. *One mg of hGH equal three units.* The preparations are:

(i) Somatrem (methionyl hGH) is available as (1) Protropin; and (2) Somatonorm; and

(ii) Somatropin (non-methionyl hGH) is available as (1) Humatrope; (2) Genotropin; and (3) Norditropin;

A long acting, encapsulated form of somatropin (Nutropin depot) for injection once or twice a month is also available.

Somatrem and somatropin are therapeutically equivalent. The dose in children with GHD is 20-40 mcg/kg/day, IM or SC, given daily. The therapy is started with the lower dose. If growth acceleration is considered inadequate at the end of the first year, larger doses may be used. As SC injections are as effective as and less painful than IM injections, the former route is preferred. In adults, the dose is 3-4 mcg/kg/day, administered daily.

Therapeutic uses:

- ***GHD with short stature in children*** **:** GH administration stimulates rapid linear growth and 5-10 cm. of height may be added during the first year. This rate of growth slows down from the second year onwards. Most patients continue to respond for several years. A few, however, become refractory after some months; in some of these, the refractoriness can be explained on the basis of development of antibodies. Unlike with anabolic steroids, the advancement of bone age is not greater than the increase in linear growth with GH. Hypothyroidism is known to occur during hGH therapy.
- ***GH deficiency in adults.***
- ***Turner syndrome;*** and
- ***Chronic renal failure with short stature***.

Since GH is prohibitively expensive, its use in short stature on suspicion of GHD is not recommended.

The utility of GH in the following conditions is not proven : old age; osteoporosis; athletes; idiopathic short stature; and cachexia and other catabolic states.

GH therapy is contraindicated in : (a) Acute critical illness; and (b) Patients with neoplasms.

MECASERMIN (IGF-1): This is rDNA human IGF-1, given SC. It is metabolized in the liver and the kidney. Its actions are similar to those of GH. The common ADR is hypoglycemia, occurring in over 40% of subjects. Overgrowth of fat, facial bones and kidney can occur after prolonged treatment. Other ADR are similar to those of GH.

It is used to treat severe IGF-1 deficiency, growth failure and patients resistant to GH because of antibodies. It is not recommended for GH responsive GHD subjects. It is contraindicated in patients with closed epiphyses. It is very expensive.

SOMATOSTATIN (GH-RIH): Somatostatin, a peptide containing 14 amino acids, is secreted by the hypothalamus and the delta cell of the islet of Langerhans, and is also found in the gut wall. It is widely distributed in the brain.

Apart from inhibition of the release of growth hormone (GH), somatostatin inhibits release of insulin and glucagon from pancreas, and of gastrointestinal peptides. Hence, it has been nicknamed 'Omnistatin'. It also often inhibits the target tissues. It inhibits secretion of gastric acid independently of its action on the release of gastrin. It decreases the splanchnic blood flow. It has a very short plasma half-life.

OCTREOTIDE (Sandostatin, Octride): This synthetic, longer acting analogue of somatostatin is used to control severe diarrhoea caused by carcinoid syndrome and by metastatic vasoactive intestinal polypeptide tumors (VIPomas), and to treat glucagonomas, malignant insulinomas and pituitary tumour causing acromegaly. Its adverse effects are nausea, flatulence, abdominal discomfort and asymptomatic gallstones. Its other uses are dumping syndrome, acute pancreatitis and esophageal variceal bleeding. A long acting preparation with action for 30 days is also available.

Lanreotide (Somatulin LA) is a long acting analogue of octeotride, effective for 7-14 days. Its properties and uses are similar to those of octeotride.

Pegvisomant, a genetically altered GH antagonist, has been found to be useful in the treatment of acromegaly. It blocks the binding of GH to its tissue receptor.

SOMATORELIN, (GH-RH) : This polypeptide with 40 amino acids acts on the somatotrophs. It is used to test the ability of the anterior pituitary to synthesize and release hGH (hGH reserve).

rDNA synthetic analogues of GH-RH, unlike similar analogues of GnRH (Chapter 65), do not cause a down regulation of their own receptors in the pituitary somatotropes. Their use in children with short stature due to idiopathic (hypothalamic), GH deficiency is under active investigation.

SERMORELIN (Geref[50]) is a GH-RH analogue with 29 aminoacids, that has been introduced for diagnostic test for GH secretion.

Thyroid Hormones and Antithyroid Drugs

62

The thyroid gland was discovered by Wharton in 1656 but its function was not known. In 1874, Gull described thyroid hypofunction in man. In 1895, Magnus Levy reported increased basal metabolic rate (BMR) in patients with hyperthyroidism. The isolation and crystallization of the thyroxine (T_4) was achieved by Kendall in 1915 and its chemical structure was determined by Harrington and Barger in 1926. Tri-iodothyronine (T_3) was detected, isolated and synthesized by Gross and Pitt-Rivers in 1952.

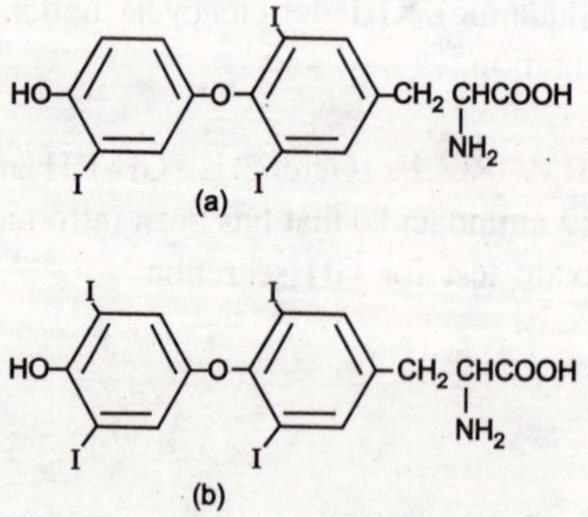

Fig. 62.1 : Thyroid hormones

The thyroid gland acini synthesize :

- ***Thyroxine*** and
- ***Tri-iodothyronine.***

The third hormone, thyrocalcitonin, secreted by the interstitial cells, is discussed in Chapter 68. Chemically, thyroxine (T_4) is 3, 5, 3', 5'tetra-iodothyronine, and tri-iodothyronine (T_3) is 3, 5, 3' tri-iodothyronine (Fig.62.1).

Synthesis of thyroid hormones: Sea fish is a good dietary sources of iodide. Dietary iodide is absorbed from the upper GI tract and is carried in the plasma as inorganic iodide. The thyroid hormones are synthesized as follows:

- ***Iodide trapping:*** The thyroid traps the plasma iodide circulating through it, against a concentration gradient between the thyroid follicular cells and the plasma. This active process is stimulated by thyroid stimulating hormone (TSH, Thyrotropin). It is competitively inhibited by thiocyanate and perchlorate ions. The other organs which compete with thyroid for iodide are the kidneys which excrete it in urine, and to a smaller extent the salivary glands, the gastric and intestinal mucosa, the liver, the placenta and the mammary glands.
- ***Organic binding of iodine:*** The iodide is first oxidized by H_2O_2 and thyroid peroxidase to hypoiodate. Hypoiodate iodinates the tyrosine residues in the thyroglobulin (TG) to form mono- and di-iodotyrosine (MIT and DIT) successively. These two reactions are extremely rapid but may be defective in certain disease states and are inhibited by thiourea drugs. Both reactions are stimulated by TSH.
- ***Coupling:*** Thyroxine (T_4) is formed by coupling of two molecules of DIT, and tri-iodothyronine (T_3) by coupling of one molecule

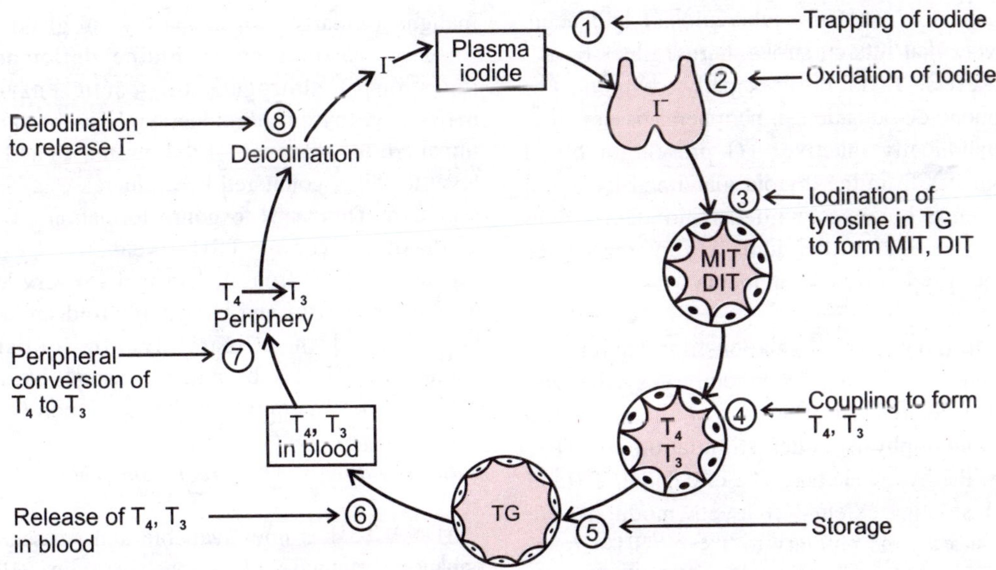

Fig. 62. 2 : Synthesis of thyroid hormone

of MIT and DIT each. The coupling reactions occur while MIT and DIT are bound by peptide bonds within the thyroglobulin molecule. They are oxidative reactions and need the same peroxidase involved in oxidation of iodide to hypoiodide. They are inhibited by thioamides.

- ***Hormonal release:*** TG which contains T_4 and T_3, is stored within the thyroidal follicular lumen. It is taken up by the thyroid follicular cells by endocytosis. Under the influence of TSH, a protease acts on the intracellular thyroglobulin to release T_4, T_3, MIT and DIT. MIT and DIT are deiodinated and the iodine is reutilized for iodinating globulin while T_4 and T_3 directly enter the circulation.

About 90% of the body iodine is in the thyroid gland, mainly as organic iodine. This large thyroidal pool of iodine (5-7 mg.) turns over very slowly at the rate of 1% per day.

Plasma iodine: The plasma in health contains about 0.2 to 0.4 μg. of inorganic iodide and 4 to 15 μg. of hormonal iodine per 100 ml. The hormonal iodine is made up mostly of T_4 (4-13 μg./dl.) and a small quantity of T_3 (80-200 ng./dl.). T_4 and T_3 circulate in the plasma partly protein bound and partly as free hormones. The major binding protein is **thyroxine binding globulin** (TBG) which accounts for 60% of the binding capacity of the plasma. The level of TBG is influenced by estrogens and rises during pregnancy and oral contraceptive use. The *mean* concentration of circulating *free* T_4 is 1.5 ng/100 ml. (about 0.03% of the total plasma T_4) and of *free* T_3 0.3 ng% (about 0.3% of the plasma total T_3). The free hormones are physiologically active. In states of iodine deficiency, the thyroid synthesizes T_3 in preference to T_4. A similar situation exists in case of T_3 thyrotoxicosis in which plasma T_3 alone is elevated.

About 80% of the thyroid hormones (T_4 and T_3) are disposed of in the body by deiodination; the remaining 20% are excreted in stools. About 40% of T_4 released by the thyroid is converted peripherally to T_3; this accounts for almost 80% of the total T_3 formed in the body. Thus, T_4 acts not only as a hormone but also as a prohormone. Although the thyroid normally forms more T_4 than T_3, the latter is the physiologically active hormone, at least as far as most tissues are concerned. The peripheral conversion of T_4 to T_3 is inhibited by drugs such as propylthiouracil, glucocorticoids and propranolol; as well as during chronic (rheumatoid arthritis, tuberculosis) and acute (myocardial infarct, stroke, burns) illnesses.

Reverse T_3 (rT_3) is principally a byproduct of T_4 mono-deiodination in peripheral tissues. It is metabolically inactive. TG present in blood originates from the thyroid gland and its serum concentration rises with thyroid damage, in thyrotoxicosis, in thyroiditis and in some cases of metastatic thyroid carcinoma.

Pituitary thyroid relationship: Thyrotropic hormone (TSH), a glycoprotein, is synthesized and released by the thyrotropes in the adenohypophysis under stimulation by TRH from the hypothalamus. The circulating T_3 (and to a smaller extent T_4) levels modulate the response of the pituitary to TRH. TSH acts on the TSH receptors in the thyroid follicular cell membrane to accelerate all the reactions in the synthesis and release of thyroidal hormones. Its action on the thyroid is modulated by the thyroidal organic iodine content (see thyroid auto-regulation) and is mediated by adenylyl cyclase-cyclic AMP mechanism. Repeated administration of TSH in animals:

- ***Increases the weight and vascularity of the thyroid gland.***
- ***Reduces its colloid and iodine content;*** and
- ***Increases the height of its acinar epithelium histologically.***

In the absence of adenohypophysis, the thyroid gland undergoes atrophy which is reversible on administration of TSH. The plasma t½ of TSH is about 1 hour and the estimated daily secretory rate between 50 and 200 mcg.

TSH secretion rises in the presence of low and falls in the presence of increased circulating T_4 and T_3 levels, respectively. The mutual regulation of secretory activity by the adenohypophysis and the thyroid is called the **feed-back system.** The negative feed back is believed to occur at the level of the pituitary rather than the hypothalamus. It has been implicated in the pathogenesis of some cases of simple goitre, a non-inflammatory, non-malignant enlargement of the thyroid gland. If, for any reason such as iodine deficiency, ingestion of goitrogens or genetic enzyme deficiency, thyroid hormone synthesis becomes impaired, the tendency of the plasma T_4 and T_3 level to fall is countered by an increase in TSH secretion. This leads to goitre formation.

Plasma level of TSH (measured by an immunoassay) is from undetectable to very low in hypopituitarism and in hyperthyroidism, and is elevated in primary hypothyroidism. Although TSH may be initially responsible for the development of some forms of non-toxic goitre, *plasma TSH levels are elevated only in goitrous patients who are hypothyroid.*

rDNA TSH is now available and is used to enhance the uptake of radioactive iodine (^{131}I) by the metastases of well differentiated thyroid cancer in patients who are being treated with radioiodine.This helps to ablate the metastases. It is very expensive.

TRH (Protirelin): This synthetic substance is a tripeptide, (pyro) Glu-His-Pro (NH_2). Human, ovine, bovine and porcine TRH have the same chemical structure. Intravenous TRH results in a rapid rise in plasma TSH level. This test was used in the past in the diagnosis of subclinical thyrotoxicosis; it has now been replaced by highly sensitive plasma TSH assay.

Synthetic TRH also stimulates the release of prolactin, FSH (in men), LH (in women at luteal peak) and GH (in acromegaly).

Thyroid autoregulation: This term is used to indicate the maintenance of the thyroidal organic iodine stores constant by the thyroid itself, without the mediation of the negative feedback mechanism. An acute increase in the supply of iodide to the thyroid tends to increase its organic iodine content. This is resisted by immediate local inhibition of the iodide trapping mechanism (Wolff Chaikoff effect). Further, the thyroid responsiveness to a constant circulating TSH level diminishes in these circumstances. This autoregulation is the first, homeostatic,

Table 62.1: Differences between T_4 and T_3

	Thyroxine (T_4)	Triiodothyronine (T_3)
Equipotent doses	100 mcg	25 mcg
Free hormone (% of total) in plasma	0.03	0.3
Onset of action	7-10 days	6-8 hours
Elimination t/2	7 days	1 day
Wearing out of effect after cessation of therapy	Long	Short

defence mechanism of the thyroid against acute changes in the supply of iodine.

Mechanism of action of thyroid hormones: Thyroid hormones are thought to interact with the cells at three receptor sites:

(1) **The nucleus** where they cause transcription of mRNA necessary for the synthesis of cellular proteins which are responsible for the increase in the oxygen consumption and calorigenesis. Their anabolic effects are also due to their nuclear interaction.

The non-genomic actions of T_4 are at the plasma membrane and mitochondria.

(2) **The plasma membrane of the cells:** This occurs early in the course of the exposure of cells to thyroid hormones and requires energy. It facilitates the entry of substrates such as amino acids, calcium and of the thyroid hormones themselves. It also stimulates adenylate cyclase activity in the cell membrane.

(3) **The mitochondrial inner membrane** which is the site for oxidative metabolism. This is also an early action and stimulates the generation of ATP.

Uncoupling of oxidative phosphorylation is not a physiological effect of thyroid hormones but plays a role in their calorigenic action in patients with thyrotoxicosis.

Difference between T_3 and T_4: The overall effects of T_4 and T_3 are qualitatively similar. Table 62.1 shows the important differences.

Physiological and pharmacological actions of thyroid hormones:

- ***Calorigenic action***: The thyroid hormones stimulate oxygen consumption and heat production in all tissues except the brain, gonads, lymph nodes, spleen, thymus and dermis.Thus, they regulate the basal metabolic rate (BMR). The calorigenic response to externally administered thyroid hormones is most marked in the hypothyroid individual. However, there is a latent period of several hours or even days between the administration of the hormone and the response.

- ***Growth***: The thyroid hormones are essential for intra-uterine tissue differentiation and as well as extra-uterine growth. Intra-uterine thyroid deficiency causes defective brain development leading to cretinism with mental retardation. Deficiency of thyroid hormones appearing after birth leads to retardation of physical growth, characterised by a marked delay in the bone maturation (retarded bone age). A characteristic epiphyseal dysgenesis, where calcification appears as multiple, small irregular foci causing stippled, porous, fluffy or fragmented appearance in x-rays, is seen. It is associated with significant decrease in the serum alkaline phosphatase level.

Thyrotoxicosis occurring during childhood leads to a temporary acceleration of linear growth.

- ***Metabolic actions***: In physiological doses, the thyroid hormones promote growth and protein synthesis and are, therefore, anabolic in their effects. In excessive amounts, as in thyrotoxicosis, their effect is catabolic.

The thyroid hormones increase the rate of absorption of glucose from the gut. Peripherally, they increase the rates of cellular entry and intracellular utilization of glucose. Larger doses may cause glucose intolerance.

The thyroid hormones enhance the rate of cholesterol synthesis by the liver, its rate of biliary excretion, its conversion to bile acids and its faecal loss. The preponderance of increased synthesis over metabolic degradation accounts for the elevated levels of serum cholesterol in hypothyroidism. In hyperthyroidism, serum cholesterol is normal unless the individual is malnourished. The thyroid hormones also enhance the lipolytic action of catecholamines on the fat cells, though they do not exert a lipolytic action themselves.

They also affect the water and electrolyte metabolism. Thus, the hypothyroid subject retains water and sodium and cannot excrete an added load of water. Diuresis and natriuresis occur soon after starting thyroid medication.

• ***Cardiovascular system***: Thyroxine stimulates the rate as well as the force of contraction of the myocardium. It also increases the cardiac output, probably secondarily to peripheral vasodilatation. It acts on the myocardium partly by a direct genomic action and partly by sensitizing it to the effects of catecholamines. Only the latter action is inhibited by beta adrenergic blocking drugs.

• ***Central nervous system***: Thyroxine is essential for myelination of the CNS. Hence, its deficiency during foetal life leads to irreversible CNS damage. A variety of neurological changes such as mental retardation and slow tendon reflexes are seen in hypothyroidism, while increased irritability, tremors and hyperkinesia are characteristic of hyperthyroidism. Psychosis may also be seen in hypothyroidism.

• ***Gastrointestinal tract***: Diarrhoea and constipation are common in hyper and hypothyroidism, respectively. Achlorhydria is frequent in both these conditions. The liver may be depleted of glycogen in hyperthyroidism.

• ***Reproductive tract and the breast***: Gonadal function is disturbed in males as well as in females in hypothyroidism; menorrhagia is seen in women and infertility in both the sexes. No specific changes are observed in hyperthyroidism. In dairy animals, *but not in humans*, thyroxine is a potent galactopoietic.

• ***Hemopoietic system***: Anemia, correctible only by thyroid medication, as well as megaloblastic anemia, are seen in hypothyroidism.

• ***Skin***: Thyroxine deficiency causes deposition of a complex mucopolysaccharide material in the connective tissue of the skin which causes the pallor and roughness of the skin.

• ***Miscellaneous actions***: Excess of thyroxine impairs the conversion of creatine to creatinine and also the formation of phosphocreatine, leading to wasteful creatinuria. Various types of myopathies and periodic paralysis are seen in hyperthyroidism. Plasma level of creatine kinase (CPK), lactic dehydrogenase (LDH) and creatinine are increased in hypothyroidism. Conversion of carotene to vitamin A is defective in thyroid deficiency, while requirement of both water and fat soluble vitamins is enhanced in thyrotoxicosis.

In some species, these hormones have special functions such as stimulation of oxygen consumption in fish, metamorphosis in amphibia and plumage growth in birds.

Absorption, fate and excretion: Both thyroxine (40-75%) and triiodothyronine are well absorbed when given orally. *The absorption is more complete when they are taken on an empty stomach but can be variable and incomplete when taken with food.* Injected labelled thyroxine is concentrated mainly by the liver and the kidney, while T_3 gets distributed to a variety of organs and tissues. These hormones are progressively de-iodinated in the peripheral tissues and iodine thus liberated is returned to the extrathyroidal iodide pool for re-utilization. Plasma t½ of thyroxine in health is 6-7 days and that of T_3 is 1-2 days. These are shortened in hyperthyroidism and prolonged in hypothyroidism. The hormones are conjugated with sulfuric acid in the liver and are excreted in the bile. Oxidative deamination and decarboxylation also occur. Sulfates are partly hydrolysed and reabsorbed in the intestines. About 20-40 per cent of the amount present in the bile is excreted in feces.

Adverse reactions: These are similar to the symptomatology of thyrotoxicosis and include diarrhoea, weight loss, palpitation, tremor, hyperkinesia, irritability and occasionally anginal pain. Administration of large doses for

Table 62.2 : Thyroid function tests (plasma levels) in health and disease.

	Normal	Hypothyroidism, primary	Hypothyroidism, secondary	Thyrotoxicosis	Enthyroid, sick syndrome*	Pregnancy, OC pill use
Total T_4 (mcg/dl)	4-13	↓	↓	↑/N	N	↑
Free T_4 (ng/dl)	0.8-2.0	↓	↓	↑/N	N	N
Total T_3 (ng/dl)	80-200	N/↓	N/↓	↑	↓	N/↑
Free T_3 (pg/ml)	2.5-5	N/↓	N/↓	↑	↓	N
TSH (microunit/ml)	0.5-5.0	↑	N (inappropriately low)	↓	N/↓	N

* Seen in chronic/severe acute, medical and surgical illness

prolonged periods can cause osteoporosis especially in menopausal women; left ventricular hypertrophy; and pseudotumour cerebri. *If a patient with combined hypothyroidism and hypocortisolism is not pre-treated with a glucocorticoid, thyroxine can precipitate hypoadrenal crisis.* Occasionally, agitation and even psychosis may occur. The additive tartrazine in thyroxine tablets is occasionally associated with cutaneous allergic reactions.

Preparations and dosage:

(i) Thyroxine sodium (Eltroxin, Thyrox, Thyronorm) 25 mcg, 50 mcg, 100 mcg and 200 mcg tablets. Dose: 0.05 to 0.2 mg. once daily, on an empty stomach in the morning.

(ii) Levothyroxine sodium injection 200, 500 mcg. Dose in myxedema coma: 200-500 mcg IV on first day; 100-200 mcg on second day.

(iii) Liothyronine sodium (l-triiodothyronine sodium, Tetroxin) 20 mcg. tablets. Dose: 20 mcg 1-3 times a day.

(iv) Liothyronine sodium injection, 10 mcg/ml. Dose in myxedema coma : 25-50 mcg IV.

T_3 is not used routinely as its rapid onset of action may precipitate angina or congestive cardiac failure, especially in the elderly patients. Further, the longer half-life of T_4 maintains a substantial peripheral pool of T_4 from which T_3 is slowly formed. This provides a buffer against lapses in treatment. Because of its shorter half-life, T_3 lacks this buffering effect. Thyroid extract and thyroglobulin are no more used in therapy.

Although combinations of T_4 and T_3 are available for replacement therapy, claims for their superiority over thyroxine remain unsubstantiated.

Table 62.2 summarises the thyroid function tests in health and disease.

Therapeutic uses of thyroid hormones:

● ***As substitution therapy***: In **cretinism,** therapy must be started as soon after birth as possible, preferably within 4 weeks. With proper treatment, normal physical development and linear growth can be achieved. Some degree of mental retardation can, however, occur especially in the athyrotic cretins. In cretins with goitres, the thyroid deficiency is milder.

Therapy is started with a small dose (25 mcg) and is increased by 25 mcg only at fortnightly intervals. The entire daily dose is given once a day (see Table 62.3). *Once started, thyroid medication must be continued lifelong.* This must be impressed upon the parents.

The dose of thyroxine is adjusted to maintain plasma T_4 between 9 and 12 mcg %. When such facilities are not available, the dose is adjusted clinically. In the infant, the mental milestones are the crucial guide to adequacy of treatment. In older children, it can be monitored by the rate of linear growth and bone age.

Table 62.3: Thyroxine substitution therapy in hypothyroid infants and children

Age	Dose mcg/kg	Total mcg/day
Birth-6 months	10-15	25-50
6-12 months	6-10	50
1-5 years	5-6	75
6-18 years	3-5	100

Overtreatment can result in symptoms and signs of hyperthyroidism; worse, it can lead to premature craniosynostosis of the skull.

In **adult hypothyroidism,** a complete reversal of the physical and metabolic abnormalities can generally be achieved by adequate replacement therapy, unless the patient proves intolerant of such therapy. This is likely to happen in patients with coronary heart disease in whom angina may be precipitated or aggravated by thyroxine. In the younger patients with no concomitant disease, therapy is started with 50-100 mcg. of thyroxine per day. The daily dose is increased by 50 mcg. once in three months until the plasma TSH becomes normal (1-5 microunits/ml). In most patients, the maintenance dose is 0.1 to 0.2 mg. (about 1.5-2 mcg./kg.) of T_4 per day. After the maintenance dose is determined, therapy can be monitored clinically and by plasma TSH.

The lethargic, obese patients may need slightly larger doses than the anxious thin ones. The dose must be smaller in older patients. It is also about 0.05 mg. smaller in the hot summer months than during the cold winter months, in regions where the variations in ambient temperatures are marked. *Thyroxine must be continued in slightly larger doses throughout pregnancy*. In patients with ischemic heart disease, therapy is initiated with doses as small as 0.01 or 0.015 mg. per day; use of larger doses is known to precipitate angina and acute MI.

Therapy must be continued lifelong in most patients. In some situations, hypothyroidism is transient and thyroid replacement therapy may be omitted after a few months. In patients with secondary hypothyroidism, associated cortisol deficiency, if any, should be corrected.

- ***Non-toxic goitres***: Normal plasma TSH levels are seen in most patients with non-endemic, simple goitres. Such goitre is thought to be due to locally generated growth factors. Hence, the mechanism of action of T_4 in these patients remains obscure; formerly, it was thought to encourage regression of the goitre by suppressing the plasma TSH level. It also corrects any associated mild hormonal deficiency. It is used in the dose of 100-200 mcg. per day. The goitre regresses in about 60 per cent of the patients. Whether a given patient will respond or not cannot be predicted. The best responses are, however, seen (a) in the large, diffuse, soft, enzyme-deficiency goitres and (b) in the diffuse puberty goitres in patients who have not recently received iodine. In the former group, lifelong treatment is desirable. In the latter group, therapy is continued for 2-3 years but may occasionally have to be given lifelong. Similar dosage is used in the treatment of auto-immune thyroiditis (Hashimoto's disease) with hypothyroidism.

- ***Hyperthyroidism***: Thyroxine (100-200 mcg. per day) given concurrently prevents / reverses the enlargement and the increased vascularity brought about by thioamides in the diffuse toxic goitre of Grave's disease.

- ***Thyroid carcinoma***: Surgery is the treatment of choice in all cases of thyroid carcinoma. It is followed by radioiodine therapy in patients with papillary and follicular carcinoma. Thyroxine has been used instead of ^{131}I after surgery in patients with small, well differentiated carcinomas as they are TSH dependent. The dose of T_4 here must be larger than that customarily used in hypothyroidism and the plasma TSH must be maintained at unmeasurable level.

- ***Therapeutic trial***: Thyroxine may occasionally be used as a therapeutic test for hypothyroidism when laboratory investigations are not possible or fail to establish the diagnosis in clinically strongly suspected cases.

Table 62.4: Principles of treatment of myxedema coma

- Hospitalize, preferably in an ICU.
- Glucocorticoids.
- Levothyroxine in large dose IV /orally.
- Triiodothyronine IV, if available.
- Antimicrobials
- Slow warming; and
- Management of hypoventilation, hyponatremia and other electrolyte disturbances.

- ***Antithyroid drug treatment during pregnancy*:** Thyroxine may be added to the antithyroid drug during pregnancy to avoid hypothyroidism in the mother. However, thyroid hormones do not cross the placenta whereas the antithyroid drugs do. Hence, it is necessary to keep the dose of the antithyroid drug to a minimum during pregnancy.

Thyroid hormone treatment does not appear to alter the course of the exophthalmos in Grave's disease.

Treatment of Myxedema Coma

Myxedema coma is a serious complication of long standing, untreated hypothyroidism. It is characterised by coma, hypothermia, marked bradycardia and hypotension. It is most likely to occur in elderly people and during cold season. Inadequate treatment, exposure to cold, infection and trauma act as precipitating factors. Alveolar hypoventilation with carbon dioxide narcosis, hypoglycemia, lactic acidosis and dilutional hyponatremia are important associated abnormalities. The diagnosis is essentially clinical but may be confirmed by plasma hormone estimation. *Therapy should be started without waiting for the result of the tests.* The principles of treatment are given in Table 62.4.

Because of a 5% to 10% incidence of co-existing, decreased adrenal reserve, IV administration of glucocorticoid should precede that of thyroid hormones. If available, thyroxine sodium is given IV in a loading dose of 150-300 mcg, followed by 100 mcg IV every 24 hours. If IV thyroxine preparation is not available, 500 mcg can be given through a nasogastric tube as a loading dose. Some physicians prefer to add tri-iodothyronine in the dose of 10 mcg IV, every 8 hours, for a few days, because the peripheral conversion of thyroxine to tri-iodothyronine is diminished in severely hypothyroid patients. Over-aggressive treatment with thyroxine (>500 mcg/day) or tri-iodothyronine (> 75 mcg/day) is associated with increased mortality rate. Prophylactic antibiotics are recommended in these patients. Warming should be slow, with blankets. Hypoventilation, if present, should be treated by placing the patient on a respirator; and hyponatremia with fluid restriction rather than with hypertonic saline. Fluid and electrolyte balance should be carefully monitored to avoid overhydration. Therapy of myxedema coma remains unsatisfactory and mortality is high.

Iodine and the Endemic Goitre

Endemic goitre is a manifestation of iodine deficiency. The daily iodine requirement is 1-2 mcg. per kg. body weight and can be met with by ingestion of 200 g of sea fish 2-3 times a week. Sea-fish and unpurified common salt obtained from sea water are important dietary sources of iodine. As the common salt obtained by evaporation of sea water contains very little iodide, endemic goitre can be prevented by iodization of the common salt by adding 50-80 mg of *sodium iodate* to 1 kg of common salt. This provides 30-50 ppm (parts per million) of *iodine* at the source of production. Considering the loss of iodine during storage to be about 50%, 10 g of salt, the usual daily consumption, provides about 150-250 mcg of iodine, which is the intended daily supplement. An alternative method is the administration of Lipiodol which is poppy seed oil with 38% by weight of iodine. It is administered IM in the dose of 1 ml every 2-5 years or orally in the same dose once a year; the latter is preferable. Treatment of an existing simple goitre with iodine is generally unsuccessful. Instead, therapy with thyroxine is more effective.

Excess of iodine can cause goitre ± either hypothyroidism or hyperthyroidism (see later).

Antithyroid Drugs

The clinical manifestations of hyperthyroidism are due to an excess of circulating thyroid hormones. They can be ameliorated by using **Antithyroid Drugs,** which *interfere* with the synthesis, release or action of thyroid hormones.

Classification of antithyroid drugs :

I **Those which interfere with hormonal synthesis-**

(1) **Ion inhibitors** which inhibit iodine trapping and binding e.g. Potassium perchlorate and thiocyanate.

(2) **Thioamides** which inhibit thyroid peroxidase and block the synthesis of MIT, DIT; and prevent the coupling reaction e.g. Propylthiouracil, Carbimazole.

II **Those that interfere with the hormonal release and promote its storage** e.g. Iodides, Lugol's iodine; and

III **Radioiodine** that destroys the acinii.

Antithyroid drugs such as iodide and propylthiouracil may act by more than one mechanism.

Drugs interfering with hormonal synthesis (Class I) reduce the plasma T_4 and T_3 levels. This in turn stimulates TSH synthesis by the pituitary, stimulates the thyroid, which undergoes hypertrophy and hyperplasia; thyroid vascularity increases. The height of the acinar epithelium increases'. Since this causes enlargement of the thyroid gland, these drugs are called **goitrogens.**

In addition, there are several other compounds which have antithyroid actions as a side effect; they are not used clinically as antithyoid drugs. When used for other, clinical purposes, they may interfere with the interpretation of the thyroid function tests. Thus, sulfonamides, PAS, lithium and resorcinol interfere with thyroidal synthesis, while amiodarone prevents the conversion of T_4 to T_3. Hepatic enzyme inducers such as rifampicin, phenytoin and carbamazepine promote rapid inactivation of the thyroid hormones. Further, the iodine-containing contrast media used in radiology can also interfere with thyroid function. All such agents thus, can cause ' Drug-\induced thyroid disorders' (Hypo- or Hyper-thyroidism).

ION INHIBITORS : **Potassium thiocyanate and perchlorate** competitively inhibit the iodide trapping by the thyroid gland. This action is countered by an excess of iodide ions. Thiocyanate is not used in practice because of its potential toxicity but may be responsible for the goitrogenic action of certain staple foods (e.g. cassava).

Potassium perchlorate has been used in the treatment of hyperthyroidism, initially in the dose of 600-800 mg. daily in divided doses. The maintenance dose is 200-400 mg. daily. It is effective in controlling the symptoms of hyperthyroidism. Its ADR includes gastric irritation, fever, skin rashes, lymphadenopathy, agranulocytosis and rarely aplastic anemia. Most patients tolerate the drug well; it is cheap but is not available easily. It is a useful alternative in patients allergic to the thioamides.

Perchlorate is also used to demonstrate defective organic binding of iodine in the thyroid gland in congenital goitrous cretinism and in Hashimoto's thyroiditis.

THIOAMIDES: The important drugs belonging to this group are methyl- and propyl-thiouracil, methimazole and carbimazole (Fig. 62.3). They have similar modes of action but differ in pharmacokinetics, dosage and the incidence of adverse reactions.

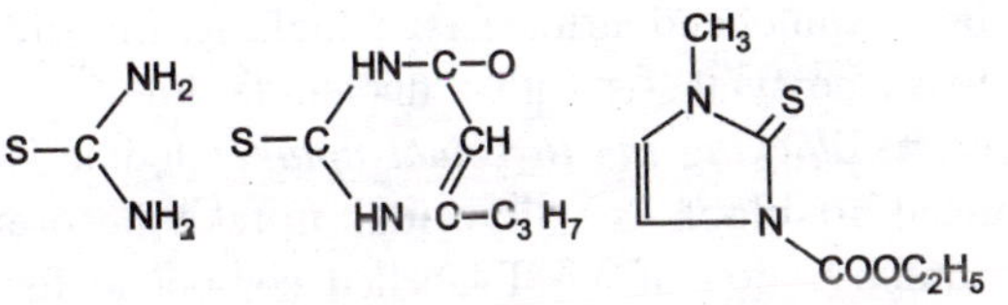

Thiourea Propylthiouracil Carbimazole

Fig. 62.3 : Thioamides

Mechanism of action: These drugs bind to and inhibit the thyroid peroxidase; they thus block thyroid hormone synthesis by inhibiting:

- ***Coupling of iodotyrosines.***
- ***Conversion of MIT to DIT; and***
- ***Formation of MIT.***

Propylthiouracil (but not carbimazole) in addition inhibits the peripheral conversion of T_4 to T_3. Carbimazole has also been claimed to encourage a remission in Grave's disease by suppressing the autoimmune process in the thyroid. The plasma t½ of PTU is about 75 minutes while that of carbimazole is 4-6 hours.

Absorption, fate and excretion: These drugs are rapidly absorbed (20-30 minutes) after oral administration. They are concentrated by the thyroid gland. The duration of action of a single oral dose is less than 8 hours. Hence, they are administered every six to eight hours. Some physicians prescribe the entire daily dose of thioamides on a once a day basis.

They are partly metabolized in the liver and the thyroid and partly excreted in the urine unchanged. Carbimazole is metabolized to the active metabolite methimazole. They cross the placental barrier and are secreted in milk.

Adverse reactions: The incidence of the adverse effects is reasonably small and does not probably exceed 5 per cent. The milder ADR include drug fever, pruritus, urticaria, edema of the feet, arthralgia, lymphadenopathy and hair loss. The more serious effects are leucopenia, agranulocytosis, thrombocytopenia and liver damage. Hypothyroidism is an extension of the pharmacological action of these drugs and is reversible after stopping the therapy.

Preparations and dosage:

(i) Propylthiouracil : 50 mg. tablets. Dose: 300-600 mg. daily in divided doses.

(ii) Methimazole 5 and 10 mg. tablets. Dose: 5 to 20 mg.

(iii) Carbimazole (Neomercazole, Antithyrox) 5, 10 and 20 mg. tablets; dose: for control 30 to 60 mg. daily; for maintenance, 5 to 20 mg. daily.

Therapeutic uses: Hyperthyroidism (see later).

II IODIDE: Iodide is the oldest remedy for thyroid disorders including hyperthyroidism. *It is the quickest acting drug in hyperthyroidism and its action becomes apparent within 24 hours.* The BMR falls at a rate comparable to that seen after subtotal thyroidectomy. The gland becomes less vascular and firm. The acinar cells become smaller in size and the colloid content increases. The maximum clinical benefit is seen within 10-14 days. The hyperthyroid state is, however, only partially controlled by iodide and after a variable period of time, the beneficial effects seem to wear off. With continued treatment, hyperthyroidism may return in its initial intensity.

Mechanism of action : Iodide rapidly shuts off the release of the preformed thyroid hormones and promotes their storage. This effect (thyroid constipation) is availed of while using iodine in the management of thyrotoxic crises (see later). When given along with a thiourea compound, it prevents the increase in the size of the goitre which may occur following antithyroid drugs given alone. This is probably related to the decreased responsiveness of an iodine-rich gland to the circulating TSH.

Adverse reactions : Chronic iodine intoxication (iodism) may occasionally occur in a susceptible individual, giving rise to skin rash, rhinorrhea, lacrimation and increased salivation. Iodide causes an escape of thyrotoxicosis if used in a patient on potassium perchlorate. Prolonged use of iodides (as in cough mixtures) has been reported to occasionally produce goitre and even myxedema. Iodides cross the placenta and may cause goitre/cretinism in the foetus. *They must, therefore, be avoided during pregnancy.*

They may precipitate thyrotoxicosis (Jod-Basedow effect) in an occasional patient with a non-toxic goitre, especially in iodine-deficient areas. This effect has been occasionally reported also after the use of an iodine-containing organic dye as for IVP or coronary angiography, as well as after the antiarrhythmic drug amiodarone.

Preparations and dosage : Preparations used are *Lugol's iodine* and saturated solution of potassium iodide (SSKI). The former is prepared by dissolving 5 g of iodine in 100 ml of 10 % solution of potassium iodide and it *provides 150 mg of iodine per ml; the dose is 0.1 - 0.3 ml three times a day.* SSKI is prepared by dissolving 30 g of KI in 21 ml of water to give 30 ml of *SSKI* and *it provides 1 g of KI per ml.* The dose of iodine needed to control hyperthyroidism is about 6 mg per day; however, much larger doses are used in thyrotoxic crisis.

Therapeutic uses:

- ***Prevention of endemic goitre*** (See earlier)
- ***Preoperative preparation*:** They are used in the preoperative preparation of a hyperthyroid patient to reduce the vascularity of the gland. This is the most important use of iodides. It is given for 10-14 days preoperatively *in addition to a thiourea drug,* but *must be carefully avoided in patients on potassium perchlorate.* Thyroxine given concurrently with antithyroid drugs can obviate the need for the pre-operative addition of iodide to therapy.
- ***Rapid control of hyperthyroidism*:** Iodides along with a thioamide are used when it is imperative to control hyperthyroidism very rapidly as in a patient with thyrotoxic crisis or with CHF.

Patients with hyperthyroidism tend to have little hormonal iodine stored in their glands. Iodide administration can increase the hormonal content of the gland. If such a patient is then given a thioamide drug, it fails to act quickly because thioamide blocks synthesis but not release of thyroid hormones. Hence, iodide administration to a hyperthyroid patient should be commenced after first blocking thyroid hormone synthesis with a thioamide drug.

- ***Blocking the thyroidal uptake*:** Iodide is used to block the thyroidal uptake before administration of a ^{131}I labelled compound for the localization of a pheochromocytoma and in cases of a nuclear accident with possible release of ^{131}I into the environment.

IPODATE (Oragrafin): This is an organic-iodine contrast dye, used in oral cholecystography. It suppresses thyroid function in normals and in hyperthyroid patients. Five hundred mg. once a day inhibits thyroid hormone secretion, inhibits peripheral conversion of T_4 to T_3 and thus lowers T_4 and T_3 concentrations in the plasma. The secretion of thyroid hormones is often stimulated by the slow release of iodide resulting from the metabolism of ipodate, leading to a high rate of relapse. **Recurrent hyperthyroidism** after the use of ipodate is resistant to treatment with thioamides.

Lithium (Chapter 13) interferes with iodination of tyrosine but it is too toxic for therapeutic use.

III RADIOACTIVE IODINE: Radioactive iodine, (radiocodine) ^{131}I, is concentrated selectively by the thyroid gland. It emits gamma and beta radiations. Gamma radiation is useful for external counting in thyroid scan. Beta radiation are particles that penetrate only upto 3-5 mm. in the soft tissues. Within this compass, they dissipate their energy to the tissues and act as ionizing radiation. They destroy the thyroidal follicles, produce fibrosis and impair the ability of the remaining follicles to replicate.

Preparation and dosage: Radioiodine iodine ^{131}I is available as a solution of Na ^{131}I. It is administered orally in the dose of 3-10 mCi. on an empty stomach or after a light breakfast. Patients can be treated on an out-patient basis but are instructed to dispose of their urine carefully into latrine and to avoid close contact with children for 2 weeks. The effect of a dose becomes apparent within 3 to 4 weeks and maximum effect is seen within 3-6 months. About 50 per cent of the patients become euthyroid after a single dose. Others may need a second or even a third dose. Decision about the need for a second dose is generally taken at the end of 4-6 months.

Adverse reactions:

- ***Focal soreness in the neck*** due to irradiation and an ***aggravation of the hyperthyroid state*** are rare.
- ***Hypothyroidism*:** This occurs in 40-60% of the patients in the long run. Hence, treated patients must be followed up for long periods. The incidence of hypothyroidism is lower when smaller and more conservative doses are used than with larger doses, but then so is the cure rate of hyperthyroidism.
- ***Damage to the foetal thyroid*:** The foetal thyroid picks up iodine (and hence radioiodine) from the 16th week onwards. *The foetal thyroid is extremely susceptible to radiation and may be quickly destroyed.*
- ***Thyroid carcinoma*:** Radiation is known to be carcinogenic and the possibility of development of thyroid cancer following radioiodine cannot be totally ruled out, especially if it is used to treat hyperthyroidism in children. Therefore, many physicians reserve radioiodine treatment for adult patients.
- ***Genetic damage*:** So far, this has not been demonstrated.

Pharmacotherapy of Hyperthyroidism

T_4 and T_3 assays are helpful in confirming the diagnosis of **thyrotoxicosis**, which is defined as the clinical state caused by persistent elevation of plasma T_4 and T_3. Thyrotoxicosis may be due to an excessive, ongoing production of thyroid hormones **(hyperthyroidism, with elevated ^{131}I uptake)** as in Grave's disease or the nodular toxic goitre, or may occur in its absence (low ^{131}I uptake). Only the patients with hyperthyroidism benefit from treatment with antithyroid drugs and they alone should be treated with modalities (surgery or radioactive iodine) which destroy the thyroid gland.

Thyrotoxicosis without hyperthyroidism occurs in thyroiditis and during administration of excessive doses of thyroid hormones as treatment. These patients need withdrawal of thyroid hormone treatment, supportive treatment (propranolol and a benzodiazepine), and in case of de Quervain's thyroiditis, an anti-inflammatory drug (NSAID or a glucocorticoid). As the thyroiditis is self- limiting, destructive forms of treatment (surgery and radioactive iodine) should not be employed in these patients.

As the pathogenesis of hyperthyroidism is not known with certainty, the treatment is empirical and is aimed at reducing the production of the thyroid hormones. Plasma TSH levels are markedly suppressed in this condition. LATS, or long acting thyroid stimulator, is demonstrable in the plasma of some patients with Graves' disease. It is an antibody which binds to the TSH receptor on the thyroid cells (TSHRAb) and stimulates the synthesis and release of thyroid hormones.

Grave's disease often undergoes spontaneous remissions and exacerbations. In some cases, the exacerbations are related to entry of large amounts of iodine into the body. Response to drug therapy is variable.

Table 62.5: Indications for antithyroid drugs

- ***Children.***
- ***Pregnant women*:** Propylthiouracil is preferred to carbimazole because it is more protein bound and crosses the placenta to a smaller extent.
- ***Young adults with small goitres and mild thyrotoxicosis of recent onset.***
- ***Before thyroidectomy*** in all cases; and
- ***After radioiodine therapy***, for a few weeks, starting 7-10 days after ^{131}I dose.

There are three forms of treatment available for therapy of hyperthyroidism. They are :

- ***Antithyroid drugs.***
- ***Radioactive iodine***; and
- ***Surgery.***

Advantages of thioamide drugs:

- They are well tolerated by most patients and are fairly rapidly effective; clinical benefits being apparent in about 2 weeks. The patient is rendered euthyroid in about 2-3 months. This euthyroid state can be maintained as long as it is desired by the maintenance doses. If therapy is continued for 2 years, permanent remission is achieved in about 40-50 per cent of the cases.
- If hypothyroidism occurs, it is reversible.
- They do not generally aggravate the endocrine exophthalmos.
- They can be used safely in children in whom radioiodine is contraindicated and thyroidectomy is technically difficult.
- *They can also be used during pregnancy.* However, the dose used must be smaller.
- They can be used to perform a therapeutic test in patients with doubtful diagnosis.

Disadvantages of drug therapy:

- Prolonged treatment and follow up are essential. This is difficult in the case of uneducated or uncooperative patients.
- In spite of adequate treatment, recurrence occurs in 40-60 per cent of the cases. Such patients are liable to have recurrence after further courses of therapy and hence, need more definitive treatment with radioiodine or surgery.
- In patients with severe CHF, their action is too slow. In such cases, iodide may be used along with a thiourea drug.
- *They rarely cause serious toxicity such as agranulocytosis.*

Advantages of radioiodine:

- The treatment is convenient, effective and can be carried out on an out-patient basis. It can be used with certainty of effects even in unintelligent or undependable patients.
- It is pleasant to take without any discomfort or fear and very acceptable to the patient. It avoids surgery and its attendant complications.
- There is no fear of recurrence once the patient becomes euthyroid.
- It is relatively inexpensive as it saves hospitalization required for surgery. In many cases control can be achieved with a single dose.
- It can be offered to patients in whom surgery is not possible and to those who refuse surgery, and can be used routinely in all patients past the age of 35-40 years.

Disadvantages of radioiodine:

- Because of high incidence of hypothyroidism, it cannot be recommended for children.
- *It cannot be given to a woman of the child bearing age without ascertaining that she is not pregnant.*
- It is slow acting. However, the administration of radioiodine may be followed by a period of antithyroid drugs to achieve early clinical control.
- There is a rare possibility of late development of thyroid carcinoma. Thyroid neoplasms, some of them malignant, have been reported in children following radioiodine treatment.
- Since the effects are irreversible, it cannot be used as a therapeutic trial.
- Prolonged observation for several years is necessary in order to detect late onset "hypothyroidism.
- Special facilities for handling the radioactive material are necessary.

Choice of therapy: Indications for various forms of therapy are outlined in Tables 62.5, 62.6 and 62.7. The treatment of thyrotoxicosis is essentially medical. In most instances, the choice rests between an antithyroid drug and radioiodine. However, surgery may be the treatment of choice in selected cases.

Table 62.6: Indications for radioiodine

- ***All patients above the age of 35 years***; in severe cases, the patient is first made euthyroid with a thioamide, before radioiodine administration.
- ***Recurrent hyperthyroidism after an adequate course of thioamide drugs or after surgery.***
- ***Allergy to thioamides***; and
- ***In young patients in whom a severe, associated systemic disease contra-indicates surgery and predicts shortening of the life expectuncy.***

Table 62.7: Indications for surgery

- ***Multinodular toxic goitre.***
- ***Solitary toxic nodule.***
- ***A large diffuse, toxic goitre***, especially when it fails to regress and disappear on thioamide treatment.
- ***Recurrence*** after adequate treatment with a thioamide; and
- ***When malignancy cannot be ruled out.***

Pregnancy is an absolute contraindication to radioiodine. It should also be avoided in children.

Women who receive radioiodine treatment should be advised to avoid pregnancy for one year, because they may need retreatment during that period.

Supportive measures: These comprise

(a) A sedative/tranquilizer to allay anxiety.

(b) Administration of calcium orally (1000 mg/day) may be helpful in avoiding possible osteoporosis.

(c) **Propranolol** (30-120 mg/day) to control, palpitation, tachycardia and tremor. It does nor correct the hyperthyroid metabolic state. Hence, propranolol alone should not be used for preoperative preparation of the patient.

(d) Treatment of CHF and AF; propranolol is the preferred drug.

(e) Vitamin supplememnts.

Treatment is generally ambulatory; rest at home is rarely required.

Thyrotoxic Crisis – Treatment

This is a manifestation of extreme hyper-metabolism in a thyrotoxic patient and may occur:

(a) After thyroidectomy in an inadequately prepared patient (surgical storm); and

(b) In the presence of an infection, injury or any surgical procedure other than thyroidectomy (medical storm).

The manifestations are hyperpyrexia, marked tachycardia, extreme irritability and delirium. Nausea, vomiting and diarrhoea may add to the dehydration caused by hyperpyrexia. It is a medical emergency and the treatment must be immediate (see Table 62.8).

In spite of all this hectic treatment, mortality is still high; hence, it is best prevented by adequate therapy of every thyrotoxic patient.

Drug-induced thyroid disease: See earlier.

Amidodarone, containing 37% by weight of iodine, can cause either hypothyroidism or *hyperthyroidism* due to iodine released (3 mg/100 mg) during its metabolic degradation. The drug can also cause chemical thyroiditis with resultant *thyrotoxicosis* without hyperthyroidism; this does not respond to a thioamide. Amiodarone should be stopped, if permissible. Hypothyroidism is treated with thyroxine replacement. As iodine-induced hyperthyroidism and thyrotoxicosis due to thyroiditis are difficult to distinguish, such patients should be treated with prednisolone 30-40 mg/day for about 3 months, and a thioamide.

Glucocorticoids in thyroid disorders : Glucocorticoids are valuable in treating

- ***Myxedema coma.***

Table 62.8: Principles of treatment of thyrotoxic crisis

- ***Hospitalization***, preferably into an I.C.U.
- ***Treatment of the precipitating cause.***
- ***Large doses of an antithyroid drug*** (propylthiouracil is preferred because it inhibits peripheral convertion of T_4 to T_3. 200 mg. or carbimazole 20 mg. every 4 hours).
- ***Iodide***, started a couple of hours *after* the thioamide drug. It may be given intravenously (sodium iodide 1 g. by infusion) or through a nasogastric tube (0.3 ml of SSKI every 8 hours). These doses are in excess of that which controls hyperthyroidism.
- ***Propranolol*** (IV) 2-10 mg. repeated every 4 hours, or reserpine 2.5 mg. (IM) every 4-6 hours.
- ***Supportive measures*** including dexamethasone 0.5-1.00 mg. IM 8 hourly. oxygen, adequate intravenous fluids and glucose, B complex vitamins, antimicrobials, and treatment of hyperpyrexia with aspirin, wet packs or ice packs. Congestive heart failure, if present, needs to be treated with digoxin.

- ***Thyrotoxic crisis.***
- ***Schmidt syndrome:*** Concurrent Graves disease and hypoadrenalism, both due to autoimmune disease.
- ***de Quervain's subacute thyroiditis with low-uptake thyrotoxicosis***
- ***Amidodarone-induced thyrotoxicosis but not hypothyroidism.***
- ***Graves' opthalmopathy.***

There is no evidence that the use of glucocorticoids benefits the average case of Graves' disease or Hashimoto's disease.

Iodine-Containing Contrast Media

Several iodine-containing, organic compounds are used for delineating the vascular tree in various parts of the body. Iodine forms about 50% by weight of the contrast molecule.

The older ionizable contrast media iothalamate (Conray) and diatrizoate (Urografin) are liable to cause hyperosmolality-based, anaphylactoid reactions (see below). With the newer non-ionizable media metrizamide (Amipaque) and iopamidol (Niopam), such reactions are rare; the newer contrast media are expensive but safer.

Although these contrast media are safer than most other drugs injected intravascularly, adverse reactions do occur occasionally. Rarely, even a test dose of 1 ml is known to cause a severe reaction and death.

They may be either local or systemic :

- ***Local reactions*** comprise pain at the site of injection which may spread proximally in case of thrombophlebitis, and edema of the limb involved.
- ***Mild systemic reaction*** may consist of a sense of warmth due to vasodilatation, itching and urticaria.
- ***Severe anaphylactoid reactions*** (Chapter 2) comprising collapse, bradycardia, bronchospasm and hemolysis. The major pathogenic factor is the high osmolality of the contradst medium, causing endothelial damage.
- ***Precipitation of hyperthyroidism (Jod Basedow phenomenon)*** has been reported especially in iodine-deficient persons.
- ***Acute renal failure,***especially in patients with longstanding diabetes mellitus.

Insulin, Oral Antidiabetic Drugs and Pharmacotherapy of Diabetes Mellitus

63

Though diabetes mellitus (Madhumeha) as a disease is known for ages; its pharmacotherapy, is just over 80 years old. The presence of sugar in the urine of diabetics was demonstrated by Dobson in 1755. In 1889, von Mering and Minkowski discovered that pancreatectomized dogs become diabetic in addition to developing digestive disturbances. The non-digestive part of the pancreas, islet cells, was thought to be responsible for the substance which prevented diabetes and it was christened 'insulin' by de Mayer (1909), long before its extraction by Banting and Best in 1921. The Latin word insula means islands. There are few episodes in medical research as dramatic as the discovery of insulin, a life saving agent.

Insulin is ineffective orally. Hence, the search was continued for an orally effective agent. Synthalin A, a biguanide, was the earliest oral hypoglycemic agent (OHA), to be used in therapy but was found to be too toxic. A chance observation by Janbon (1942) led to the discovery of hypoglycemic action of sulfonamides. This was confirmed by Frank and Fuchs in 1955, who observed the blood sugar lowering action of carbutamide, a sulfonamide, during its trial in infectious diseases. Since then, many sulfonylurea compounds have been introduced as OHA. In 1957, Unger reintroduced phenformin, a biguanide, as an oral antidiabetic drug.

Physiology of energy metabolism: The main carbohydrates consumed by humans are starch, a polysaccharide, and sugar, a disaccharide. The ingested polysaccharides are split to a small extent by the salivary amylase but largely by the pancreatic amylase into oligosaccharides in the duodenum and upper jejunum. The oligosaccharides and disaccharides are cleaved by alpha-glucosidases in the brush border of the jejunal enterocytes into monosaccharides (glucose, fructose and galactose) which are promptly absorbed in the upper jejunum.

Tissues differ in their dependence on glucose and free fatty acids (FFA) for energy. The brain utilizes only glucose most of the time while most other tissues can utilize glucose as well as FFAs. In fact, in the fasting state, the skeletal and cardiac muscle can derive 90 per cent of their energy from FFA.

By facilitating the entry of glucose into the cells, insulin makes possible its utilization by tissues at lower blood glucose levels than would be possible without insulin. Deficiency of insulin causes diabetes mellitus.

Immediately on entry into the cell, glucose is phosphorylated by *hexokinase* to glucose-6-phosphate (G-6-PO_4) (Fig. 63.1) which is further metabolized by:

(1) ***Glycolysis*** (Triose phosphate pathway) which is an intracytoplasmic anerobic process by which G-6-PO_4 is converted to pyruvate. When pyruvate production exceeds the cell's oxidative capacity, it is reduced to lactate. When oxygen

is available, lactate is converted back to pyruvate. Glycolysis is a relatively inefficient method of energy production. However, it is quantitatively a major route in (a) the brain, (b) the red blood cells, (c) the exercising skeletal muscle and (d) the ischemic cardiac muscle.

(2) ***Pentose-phosphate shunt*** which is an aerobic multicyclic process that converts a part of G-6-PO_4 to 3-phospho-glyceraldehyde by a different pathway. This pathway is an important source of NADPH (reduced nicotinamide adenine dinucleotide phosphate).

(3) ***Glucuronic acid pathway*** which converts G-6-PO_4 to uridine diphospho-glucose (UDPG) via G-1-phosphate. UDPG is utilized for synthesis of glycogen and mucopolysaccharides and contributes glucuronic acid required for hepatic conjugation of many substances such as bile pigments and steroids.

(4) ***Glycogenesis*** whereby glycogen is derived from UDPG by the action of *glycogen synthetase*.

(5) ***Conversion to glucose*:** Liver and kidney are the only two organs which contain the enzyme *glucose-6-phosphatase* which converts G-6-PO_4 to glucose. The reaction is irreversible. Muscle cannot convert glycogen to glucose but converts it by glycolysis to lactate which is either utilized locally for energy or is transported to the liver where, it is utilized for neoglucogenesis.

The key enzymes in the liver are glucokinase, (an isoform of hexokinase), phosphorylase, glycogen synthetase, glucose-6-phosphatase and the enzymes concerned with neoglucogenesis.

More than 90 per cent of the energy from glucose is derived from the aerobic oxidation of pyruvate by the tricarboxylic acid cycle (Kreb's cycle, Fig. 63.1). The citric acid formed in this cycle is further metabolized:

(a) To produce CO_2, NADH (reduced nicotinamide adenine dinucleotide) and $FADH_2$ (reduced flavine adenine dinucleotide); the last two are concerned in the generation of ATP (adenosine triphosphate).

(b) To produce oxaloacetate which carries further acetate (acetylcoenzyme A) into the cycle.

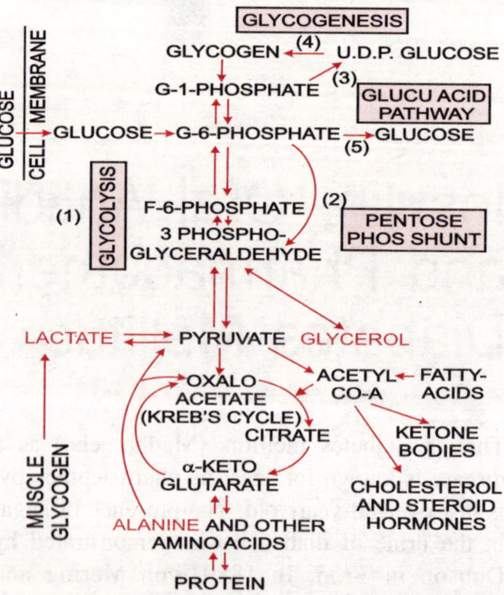

Fig. 63.1 : Glucose metabolism
G = Glucose; F = Fructose

NADH produced is required for neoglucogenesis in the liver. NADPH is important for lipogenesis; its deficiency causes impaired lipogenesis; and consequently contributes to ketoacidosis in DM.

Acetylcoenzyme A is also derived by successive beta oxidation of long chain fatty acids. Further metabolism of acetylcoenzyme A can occur in various ways:

(a) It enters Kreb's cycle.

(b) It is re-synthesized to long chain fatty acids.

(c) It is converted by liver (but not by other tissues) to ketone bodies (acetoacetate, beta hydroxybutyrate and acetone) which are utilized by peripheral tissues, and during prolonged fasting by the brain, for energy production; and

(d) It is utilized for the synthesis of cholesterol and its derivatives such as bile salts, and adrenocortical and sex steroids.

Thus, pyruvate metabolism (Kreb's cycle) is the meeting ground for the metabolism of carbohydrates, fats and proteins.

During absorption of glucose after a meal, it is utilized preferentially by all tissues for energy production and/or storage. Between meals, the liver converts the stored glycogen to glucose **(Glycogenolysis)** for release into circulation; it also converts non-carbohydrate sources (lactate; glucogenic amino acids alanine and glutamine; and glycerol) to glucose **(Neoglucogenesis or Gluconeogenesis)**. Neoglucogenesis occurs to a smaller extent also in the renal cortex. As insulin inhibits hepatic glycogenolysis and neoglucogenesis, its deficiency in diabetics leads to exaggerated neoglucogenesis. The liver also converts other sugars such as fructose, galactose and sorbitol to glucose.

In health, out of the glucose derived from the daily ingested foodstuffs, about 3 per cent is stored in the liver and muscle as glycogen; about 30 per cent is converted to fatty acids; the rest enters Kreb's cycle and is utilized partly for energy production and partly for synthesis of amino acids.

INSULIN: Insulin is secreted by the beta cells of the islets of Langerhans. It was extracted from the pancreas by Banting and Best in 1921 and was isolated in crystalline form by Abel in 1930.

It is a polypeptide with a molecular weight of about 6000, consisting of two amino acid chains, A and B, linked by two disulfide bridges. The chains contain 21 and 30 amino acids respectively (Fig. 63.2). The disulfide bridges are essential for its biological activity. Insulin was traditionally obtained from bovine and porcine pancreas. 'Human' insulin biosynthesized by cultures of bacteria *(E. coli)* and yeasts (recombinant DNA or rDNA insulin) is now commonly used in clinical practice. Its primary structure (amino acid sequence), but not the secondary and tertiary structures, is identical with that of insulin derived from human pancreas. Bovine and porcine insulin are structurally similar to human insulin in all except 3 and 1 amino acid residues, respectively. This explains their relatively low antigenicity in humans. Between the two, porcine insulin is less antigenic. rDNA synthetic, modified, human insulin analogues (lispro, aspart, glargine, etc) have different pharmacokinetic but the same pharmacodynamic properties as native human insulin.

Insulin is soluble in water but undergoes molecular aggregation to hexameric form at extremes of pH (3.2 and 10). Such aggregation is further enhanced by zinc which brings about its crystallization. Insulin is relatively insoluble at the pH range of 4 to 7. It also combines with protamine with prolongation of its action.

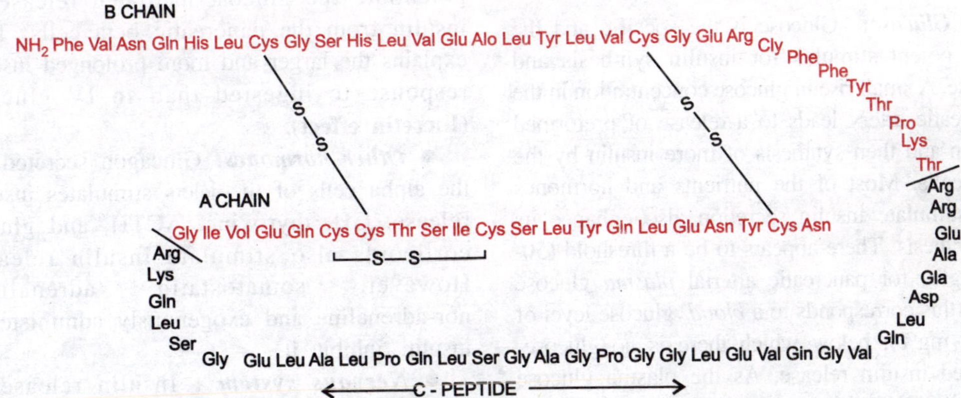

Fig. 63. 2 : Human proinsulin, a precursor of insulin

Synthesis and storage: The islets constitute 1 per cent by weight of the pancreas. The islets contain:

- ***Alpha or A cells which secrete glucagon.***
- ***Beta or B cells which secrete insulin.***
- ***Delta or D cells which secrete somatostatin; and***
- ***PP or F cells which secrete pancreatic polypeptide (PP)***

Insulin is synthesized within the beta cells as a single chain polypeptide precursor called *preproinsulin* which is converted to *proinsulin.* Proinsulin is biologically only 1/8th as active as insulin and forms only 3-6% of the total insulin within the pancreas. It is not stored within the beta cells but is soon cleaved by proteolytic enzymes to form the single chain C peptide and double chain insulin, (Fig. 63.2). It is stored in the granules of beta cells.

The pancreas of a normal human adult contains about 200 units (8 mg) of insulin. It secretes about 50 units of insulin in 24 hours, of which about 50% is degraded by the liver in the first pass. About half of the total daily insulin output is released at a slow rate, in repeated pulses, to provide a basal plasma insulin level while the other half is secreted after meals. The plasma level of insulin fluctuates throughout the day with peaks after meals.

Factors determining insulin release:

- ***Glucose*:** Glucose is the specific and the most potent stimulus for insulin synthesis and release. A small rise in glucose concentration in the pancreatic artery leads to a release of preformed insulin and then synthesis of more insulin by the beta cells. Most of the nutrients and hormones that stimulate insulin secretion also enhance its biosynthesis. There appears to be a threshold (50-90 mg%) for pancreatic arterial *plasma* glucose level (this corresponds to a *blood* glucose level of 45-80 mg%), below which there is no glucose-induced insulin release. As the plasma glucose level rises, there is a progressive increase in insulin release which reaches its maximum at glucose level of 300-350 mg%.

Glucose enters the beta cells via the 'glucose transporters'. It is metabolized in the beta cells, raising the ATP/ADP ratio. As a result, the ATP dependent K channels in the cell membrane close, causing its depolarisation. When the depolarisation reaches a threshold value, the Ca^{++} channels open, causing an influx of calcium into the cell. The elevated cytoplasmic calcium brings about exocytosis of the insulin granules. The sensitivity of this insulin-releasing mechanism to glucose is dependent upon the prior carbohydrate intake. It is markedly depressed by restriction of dietary carbohydrate and by even short periods (48 hours) of fasting. Further, chronic hyperglycemia may cause selective unresponsiveness of beta cell to glucose (**glucotoxicity**).

- ***Other substrates*:** Amino acids, especially arginine, fatty acids of all chain lengths, ketones and non-glucose sugars (fructose, mannose and ribose) also stimulate insulin synthesis and release.
- ***Hypokalemia*** inhibits insulin release.
- ***Gut hormones*:** Ingestion of glucose or a meal causes the release into the portal circulation of (a) gut hormones gastrin, secretin, pancreozymin, glucose-dependent insulinotropic polypeptide (GIP) and glucagon-like peptide-1 (GLP-1); and (b) pancreatic hormones insulin and glucagon. They modulate the plasma glucose level postprandially. GIP and GLP-1 potentiate the glucose-mediated release of insulin from the pancreatic beta cells. This explains the larger and more prolonged insulin response to ingested than to IV glucose (**Incretin effect**).
- ***Other hormones*:** Glucagon secreted by the alpha cells of the islets stimulates insulin release. GH, thyroxine, ACTH, and glucocorticoids also stimulate insulin release. However, somatostatin, adrenaline, nor-adrenaline and exogenously administered insulin inhibit it.
- ***Nervous system* :** Insulin release is enhanced by parasympathetic (vagal) stimulation and by selective beta-adrenergic stimulation. It is under tonic inhibition by pancreatic $alpha_2$

adrenoreceptors; this is seen in conditions associated with increased sympatho-adrenal discharge such as hypoxia, severe burns, surgery and MI with shock.

- ***Drugs***: Glucose-induced insulin release is enhanced by xanthines which inhibit phosphodiesterase. Sulfonylureas stimulate insulin release (see later). It is inhibited by the thiazides, diazoxide and phenytoin.

Transport, fate and excretion: Insulin circulates in the plasma in a free form. It disappears rapidly from the plasma with a t½ of 5-6 minutes. It is degraded by the liver, kidneys and skeletal muscles. Sixty percent of *exogenous insulin* is degraded by the kidney while the hepatic clearance accounts for 30-40% of the drug used. The reverse is true in the case of *endogenous insulin.* Only traces of free insulin appear in the urine. *Insulin degradation is retarded in chronic renal disease which can alter insulin dosage in such patients.*

Mechanism of action: There is no single action of insulin which accounts for its diverse effects. Insulin affects all aspects of energy metabolism. Many of its actions on protein and fat metabolism are independent of those on glucose metabolism.

Insulin binds to specific insulin receptors in the cell membrane of most tissues. The main target sites are the adipose tissue, the liver, and the skeletal muscles. The insulin receptor comprises two subunits :

(1) **The extracellular alpha subunit** which serves as the recognition site; and

(2) **The transmembrane beta subunit** which contains the **tyrosine kinase**.

Binding of insulin to the alpha subunit causes autophosphorylation and activation of the enzyme tyrosine kinase in the beta subunit; the latter brings about the subsequent physiological effects of insulin, mediated via:

- ***The insulin receptor substrate (IRS) proteins*** which regulate the intermediary metabolism viz. carbohydrate, lipid and protein metabolism (**immediate effects**); and
- ***Mitogen-activated protein kinase (MAPK) pathway*** that stimulates growth and mitogenic processes (**long term effects**).

The phosphorylated receptor phosphorylates insulin receptor substrate 1 (IRSI). The IRS1 then phosphorylates other protein substrates in the cell, thus initiating a cascade effect. This network of phosphorylations within the target cell probably acts as the second messenger. Such phosphorylation activates some enzymes while it inactivates others. The cascade is responsible for multiple (**pleotropic**) effects of insulin on intermediary metabolism.

Insulin stimulates carrier-mediated transport of glucose by recruiting **glucose transporters** (GLUT) from the cytoplasm to the cell membrane. The liver cells are freely permeable to glucose which enters them via 'glucose transporters'; insulin stimulates such glucose uptake. The rise of intracellular glucose to very high levels can stimulate, by mass action, many of the chemical reactions concerned in glucose utilization. In addition, insulin directly stimulates certain aspects of glucose utilization within the cell. It increases the cellular uptake of amino acids and potassium independently of the increased glucose uptake.

Further, insulin action causes a reduction in the concentration of *cyclic AMP* in the hepatocytes and the adipocytes, and inhibition of the cAMP dependent processes.

The **long term effects of insulin** include stimulation of DNA transcription, cell proliferation and differentiation. These actions are mediated by IGF-1 and local growth factors. Examples of this action are stimulation of synthesis of GLUT and the hexokinases; the hepatotrophic effect of insulin; and the fetal growth for which insulin is largely responsible.

Insulin also stimulates lipoprotein-lipase on the surface of the vascular endothelium. The latter hydrolyses the triglyceride core of the chylomicrons and VLDL in circulation. The FFA thus released are taken up by the adipose tissue and reconverted to triglycerides.

Pharmacological actions : Insulin modifies various metabolic processes in a dose-dependent manner. Thus, it inhibits lipolysis at plasma concentrations of 1-20 microunits per ml; levels of 10-50 microunits/ml are needed to suppress hepatic glucose production; while levels of 30-500 microunits/ml are needed to stimulate peripheral glucose uptake by muscle and adipose tissue. Increased transport of potassium into cells requires even higher levels of plasma insulin, such as are achieved during IV glucose-insulin drip in the treatment of hyperkalemia.

Most of the major biological effects of insulin on intermediary metabolism are mediated by its actions on the adipose tissue, liver and skeletal muscle. They are summarised in Table 63.1.

Effects on carbohydrate metabolism and regulation of blood glucose level: The blood glucose is measured by the specific glucose oxidase method. *The capillary blood glucose level is similar to venous plasma glucose level in the fasting state; after ingestion of glucose or food, the former exceeds the latter by 10-60 mg/dl.*

- ***In the fasting state,*** in a healthy individual, the plasma glucose fluctuates between 60 and 100 mg/dl. After a meal, it rises to a maximum of 140-150 mg/dl and returns to the fasting level within 2-3 hours. The arterial blood glucose is maintained so as to supply glucose to brain which ordinarily utilizes only glucose as its fuel. Some other tissues (renal medulla, RBCs. and bone marrow) also utilize only glucose.

The main determinants of the variations in the blood glucose are ingestion of food and the plasma levels of various hormones especially insulin. The central theme of these processes is:

(a) To promote storage of glucose and other metabolic fuels (fatty acids and amino acids), as well as their peripheral utilization after a meal; and,

(b) To make glucose available to the brain by glycogenolysis and neoglucogenesis, and FFA to the other tissues, in the post-absorptive state.

- ***Ingestion of a mixed meal*** **:** Absorption of food during the ***postprandial*** period results in elevation of blood glucose, amino acids and FFA. All of them induce insulin release. Glucagon release is enhanced by amino acids but is inhibited by hyperglycemia and FFA.

Table 63.1: Actions of insulin on the major target organs

Metabolism	Adipose tissue	Liver	Skeletal muscle
Carbohydrate	Increased glucose uptake.	Increased glycogen synthesis and storage. Decreased glycogenolysis and neoglucogenesis.	Increased glucose uptake and utilisation. Increased glycogen synthesis and deposition.
Fat	Decreased lipolysis (antilipolytic action). Increased formation of triglycerides (lipogenesis)	Increased lipogenesis Decreased ketogenesis	Decreased lipolysis.
Protein		Decreased protein breakdown. Increased protein synthesis	Increased amino acid transport into the cell and protein synthesis. Decreased protein breakdown.

Both insulin and glucagon are released into portal circulation and reach the liver in high concentrations. *The overall effect of food ingestion and absorption is to increase the insulin/glucagon ratio. The reverse occurs during the post-absorptive period, during starvation and in severe diabetes.*

The liver plays a central role in regulation of the blood glucose level. The enhanced insulin/glucagon portal vein ratio during food absorption stimulates glucose uptake and inhibits glucose output by the liver. This curbs the rising blood glucose level. The reversal of insulin/glucagon release ratio in favour of glucagon in the *post-absorptive state* increases the hepatic glucose output. *In the fasting state*, this enhances the other counter-regulatory anti-insulin hormones leading to stimulation of gluconeogenesis by GH, corticosteroids, catecholamines and thyroid hormones whereas glycogenolysis is stimulated by catecholamines.

The peripheral utilization of glucose results in the production of CO_2, water, heat and substances such as pyruvate, NADPH, NADH and ATP. *Many of the biochemical consequences of insulin deficiency can be explained by deficiency of these substances.* Insulin is not necessary for glucose uptake by brain, leucocytes and RBCs, for its GI absorption nor for its renal tubular reabsorption. The most easily demonstrable effect of insulin deficiency is hyperglycemia although its other metabolic effects are equally important.

- ***In the post-absorptive state***, (a) The anti-insulin hormones (see above) stimulate lipolysis with release of FFA into circulation. The tissues (except the brain, RBCs, renal medulla and bone marrow) utilize FFA as the main metabolic fuel and thus conserve glucose (b) Conservation of glucose is aided by the inhibitory action of catecholamines and FFA on tissue uptake of glucose, and (c) Glucocorticoids by their anti-anabolic action make amino acids available for neoglucogenesis by the liver. This hormonal profile is further exaggerated during prolonged fasting as well as in severe insulin deficiency.
- ***During pregnancy***, the dominant theme is to make glucose available to the fetus. This is achieved by an excess of anti-insulin influences from mother's own adrenal cortex as well as by insulin degradation. Pregnancy is, therefore, a potentially diabetogenic state.
- ***During lactation***, extraction of glucose by the breast for milk production further affects blood glucose level.

Effects on lipid metabolism: The net effect of antilipolytic, lipogenic and glycerogenic actions of insulin is to enhance fat storage. The weight gain during insulin therapy is largely due to obesity. One of the earliest defects in diabetes (before the abnormality of carbohydrate tolerance) is elevated plasma FFA in the overnight fasting state and after exercise. The oxidation of these FFA in the liver to acetyl CoA provides the energy necessary for neoglucogenesis. Acetyl CoA is converted by the liver to ketone bodies. *Ketogenesis is a necessary accompaniment of neoglucogenesis.*

In the decompensated diabetic state, the greater availability of FFA (from enhanced lipolysis in adipose tissue and muscle) leads to *excess synthesis of ketone bodies by the liver.* This causes **ketoacidosis** and possibly **insulin resistance**. Thus, in a diabetic who is overeating, hyperglycemia is unlikely to be accompanied by ketosis; on the other hand, in a diabetic who is unable to eat due to an acute illness, hyperglycemia due to neoglucogenesis from oversecretion of the counter-regulatory hormones particularly glucagon is likely to be accompanied by ketonuria.

Effects on protein metabolism: Insulin is a protein anabolic hormone. Its deficiency leads to negative nitrogen balance by reducing the peripheral protein synthesis and by diverting the amino acids for neoglucogenesis. This is wasteful as only 56 g of glucose can be produced from each 100 g of protein broken down. Insulin is also necessary for the anabolic action of GH.

Other actions of insulin:

- ***Vascular actions*** : Insulin has vasodilatory properties, probably exerted via activation of endothelial NO production. NO-mediated vasodilatation is impaired in diabetes, thus promoting atherosclerosis. Hyperglycemia also may impair endothelium-dependent vasodilatation. Hyper-insulinemia of Type 2 DM, via the MAPK pathway, may stimulate the proliferation of vascular smooth muscle cells.

• ***Anti-inflammatory action:*** Insulin quenches the inflammatory process, especially in the vasculature.

• ***Fibrinolysis*:** Decreased fibrinolysis, associated with hyperinsulinemia and hypertriglyceridemia in uncontrolled T2DM, has been implicated in atherogenesis.

• ***Growth and cancer*** : Insulin plays an important role in intra- and extra-uterine growth.

• ***Steroidogenesis*** : Hyperinsulinemia may be responsible for the ovarian and adrenal hyperandrogenism in women with polycystic ovary syndrome.

Factors modifying the actions of insulin:

• ***Muscular Exercise*:** Exercise training increases the sensitivity of muscles to insulin and lowers the blood glucose.

• ***Other hormones*:** Counter-regulatory hormones (glucagon, catecholamines, cortisol and growth hormone) oppose the metabolic actions of insulin and elevate blood glucose.

• ***Anti-insulin antibodies*:** These are present in the plasma of all individuals who have received insulin. Their presence in high concentrations can cause 'insulin resistance'.

Plasma insulin: Plasma insulin can be measured by radioimmunoassay (IRI or immunoreactive insulin) and by bioassay (ILA or insulin like activity).

Immunoreactive insulin (IRI): The commercial kits measure both insulin and pro-insulin. In healthy individuals, the fasting level of IRI is 5-30 microunits per ml of plasma. It rises sharply on IV glucose and less sharply but to higher levels on ingestion of glucose. In patients with mild T2DM, the rise of plasma IRI following glucose is sluggish initially but it reaches supranormal levels later **(hyperinsulin response)**. *This sluggish, initial response of plasma IRI is the primary defect in genetic diabetes* and the subsequent hyperinsulin response is due to the excessive rise of plasma glucose due to the inadequate initial rise of IRI. A greater hyperinsulin response is seen in some non-diabetic obese individuals.

A **hypoinsulin response** is, on the other hand, seen in patients with T1DM, those with diabetes due to pancreatectomy or chronic pancreatic disease, and those with severe T2DM of long duration.

ILA: The term 'Insulin-like activity' indicates what is measured by the bioassay because the effect is the sum total of insulin itself, its potentiators and inhibitors. The adipose tissue methods give higher ILA values than the rat diaphragm method.

Absorption, fate and excretion: Oral insulin is ineffective. It must be given parenterally. Addition of zinc and/or protein slows down its absorption and prolongs its duration of action. Insulin released from the pancreas and circulating in the plasma is in the *monomeric* form, which is highly diffusible and biologically active. Therapeutically used **conventional** and **Standard Recombinant (SR) human** insulin preparations (see later) contain insulin in *tetrameric or hexameric* form and are minimally diffusible; hence monomeric insulin must first be released from the injected insulin, thus delaying its onset of action. When insulin is injected in a concentrated solution, its release and absorption from the site of injection are slow. Absorption of subcutaneous conventional (Table 63.2) and SR insulins (Table 63.3) is fastest from the abdominal wall, less rapid from the arm and slowest from the thigh.

The time-course of action of SR insulins and insulin analogues are shown in Table 63.4. VRA insulin analogues lispro and aspart exist as hexamers in the commercial preparations, but dissociate instantly on SC injection; hence they are absorbed very rapidly, and require no lag time, defined as the time interval between the injection and the meal. Further, the rate of their

Table 63.2: Conventional insulin preparations of bovine origin

Preparation	pH and appearance	Added protein	Activity in hours		
			Onset	Peak	Duration
		SHORT ACTING			
Regular	3.2 clear	None	½	4	5-8
Insulin zinc suspension, amorphous (semi lente)*	7.2 cloudy	None	1	8	12-14
		INTERMEDIATE ACTING			
Isophane (NPH)**	7.2 cloudy	Protamine	2	12	18-24
Insulin zinc suspension, (lente)*	7.2 cloudy	None	2	6-8	18-24
		LONG ACTING			
P.Z.I., *	7.2 cloudy	Protamine	7	16	24-36
Insulin zinc suspension, crystalline (ultra lente)*	7.2 cloudy	None	7	16	20-36

* Although PZI and lente insulins are no longer available commercially, they are listed in this table because of their historical importance** This does not contain excess of protamine or zinc. Regular insulin can be added to it, as needed. **Highly purified bovine insulin** is available as regular (Fastact), isophane (Interact) and 30:70 mixture of regular and isophane (Mixact).

absorption is independent of the site of injection. Inhaled insulin is also absorbed rapidly.

Human insulins are faster acting and have a shorter duration of action than the conventional bovine preparations. Excercising the limb into which regular insulin is injected speeds up its absorption and may even cause hypoglycemia. Finally, repeated injections at the same site can cause local fibrosis and delay absorption. Varying rates of absorption probably contribute as much to the variations in the degree of control of hyperglycemia as the variations in the insulin requirement in a given patient.

Preparations : See Tables 63.2 and 63.3. Regular insulin is commonly injected SC about ½ hour before a meal. The intermediate and long acting preparations are injected once a day (at bedtime) or twice a day, before the breakfast and either before dinner or at bed time.

Insulin mixtures: The action of short acting insulins is so short that several injections a day

Table 63.3: Currently available insulins

Animal insulins (bovine and porcine): Most manufacturers have discontinued their production.

Human insulins

(1) ***Human insulin converted biochemically from porcine insulin***

(2) ***Standard Recombinant (S R) insulins:***

(a) Rapid acting: Regular (Zinc insulin amorphous; Actrapid)

(b) Intermediate acting: NPH (Insulatard);

(3) ***Human Insulin analogues, recombinant***:

(a) Very rapid acting (VRA): Lispro; Aspart; Glulisine; and

(b) Long acting :Glargine; Detemir

Table 63.4: Time course of action of SR insulins and human insulin analogues

Insulin	Onset of action	Peak action	Duration of action
SR human insulins			
Regular (Actrapid, Huminsulin R)	30-60 min	2-3 hrs	8-10 hrs
NPH (Insulatard, Huminsulin N)	2-4 hrs	4-10 hrs	18-24 hrs
Analogues			
Lispro and aspart	5-15 min	30-90 min	4-6 hrs
Glulisine	5-15 min	30-90 min	1-2.5 hrs
Glargine	2-4 hrs	None	20-24 hrs
Detemir	2 hrs	None	6-24 hrs

are required to control diabetes adequately. The action of long acting insulin starts too late to cover the first meal of the day (breakfast) when an injection is taken in the morning. Hence, appropriate mixtures of the two are commonly used in practice. Such mixtures have a fairly rapid onset and act for about 12-16 hours. They are given before breakfast and dinner.

I **Mixtures of conventional and highly purified animal insulins :**

(a) That which is *commercially available*, ready to use, and stable during proper storage: Mixact (Table 63.2 footnote).

(b) Those which are *prepared by the patient* by mixing regular and NPH insulins in the syringe immediately before use (not to be stored). Their advantage is that they can be tailor-made to suit the requirements of an individual patient.

II **Mixtures of monocomponent human insulin:** These are all neutral in pH. *NPH insulin does not contain an excess of either zinc or protamine; hence it can be mixed with regular insulin in any proportion immediately before use.*

Readymade mixtures (Mixtard) of actrapid and monocomponent NPH insulin are convenient and effective in T2DM but may not be adequate in T1DM; in the latter, the prescribed quantities of regular and NPH insulins are mixed in a syringe immediately before injection.

Monocomponent human Insulins: Their advantages are that they are

- ***Purer than the conventional insulin.***
- ***More stable.***
- ***Neutral in PH and less likely to cause subcutaneous fat atrophy.***
- ***Less antigenic and can be used effectively in patients allergic to beef insulin and in those with circulating antibodies to beef insulin.*** In the last case, when changing from an older insulin preparation to a purified insulin, the dose should be reduced in order to avoid hypoglycemic episodes.

However, they are all expensive.

Insulin analogues : (Designer insulins): Insulin analogues are molecules that differ from human insulin in amino acid sequence but that bind to insulin receptors and act like native insulin. They are

(1) **Lispro** (Humalog) : This preparation exists as an insulin hexamer which, on injection, dissociates instantly into monomers. For its properties, see Tables 63.4 and 63.5. It can be injected immediately before or within 5 minutes of commencing a meal. Its advantages are : (a) It is more effective in reducing the postprandial rise in blood glucose. (b) The incidence of hypoglycemic reactions is lower. (c) Variation in

Tables 63.5: Properties of and comparison among available insulins

	SR regular insulin	**SR NPH**	**VRA analogues, Lispro & Aspart**	**Long acting analogue Glargine**
Physical properties	Clear and neutral	Turbid and neutral	Clear and neutral	Clear and acidic
Administation	SC;IM;IV	SC	SC;IM	SC
Can be mixed with	SR NPH	SR regular, Lispro, and Aspart	SR NPH	None
Premixed prep.	Regular+NPH	Regular+NPH	Lispro+ Lispro protamine Aspart+ Aspart protamine	None
Lag period*	30-60 minutes	2-4 hrs	5-15 min	2-4 hrs
Peak plasma level**	2-3 hrs	4-10 hrs	30-90 min; Twice as high as with SR regular	No peak
Duration of action***	8-10 hrs	18-24	4-6 hrs	20-24 hrs
Hypoglycemia	Late during action	4-10 hrs	Early during action	Uncommon
Weight gain	Yes	Yes	Yes	Uncommon
Use during pregnancy	Yes	Yes	Lispro and aspart may be used	No

With **glulisine**, * and ** are similar to lispro and aspart; & *** is 1.2-5 hrs. With **detemir insulin** * is 2 hrs; there is no peak; and *** is 6-24 hrs. Control of HbA_{1c} is similar with SR insulins and insulin analogues. SR insulins are expensive; analogues are more expensive.

the injection site has less effect on its absorption. It may be particularly useful in intensive insulin regimens; it is very effective for use in continuous SC insulin infusion (CSII).

(2) **Aspart insulin** (NovoRapid) is short acting and has properties,uses and limitations similar to those of lispro, but with somewhat longer duration of action. Aspart insulin has also been protaminated to produce a long-acting insulin. A premixed preparation (NovoMix 30) containing the rapid-acting and the long-acting aspart insulins (30:70) is available. It is equivalent to the human mixtard insulin preparation. It is claimed to cause fewer between-meals hypoglycemic reactions in spite of maintaining lower postprandial blood sugars than human mixtard insulin. It is injected SC twice a day within +/- five minutes of commencing the meals.

(3) **Glulisine insulin**: See Table 63.4.

(4) **Glargine insulin** (Lantus) is a long acting analogue (Tables 63.4 and 63.5). It provides a prolonged, continuous, low, plasma insulin concentration (plateau). It does not cause hunger due to hypoglycemia between meals, and there is less/no weight gain. *Because of its acid pH (pH 4.1), it cannot be mixed with any of the SR insulins.* It is given SC once a day, and

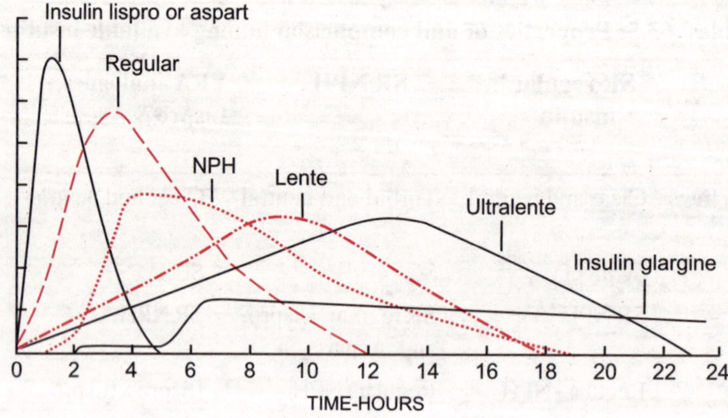

Fig. 63.3. Extent and duration of action of various types of insulin

a very short acting insulin is injected additionally before each major meal (basal-bolus regimen). This mimics the delivery of endogenous insulin in non-diabetics except that it is into systemic and not portal circulation.

(5) **Detemir insulin** has a fatty acid side chain that allows albumin binding, resulting in prolongation of its action. Its duration of action increases as the amount injected as a single dose increases. However, for most purposes it is shorter than that of insulin glargine, requiring twice daily injections in T1DM. Its efficacy is similar to that of NPH insulin (Table 63.4).

Figure 63.3 shows the time-action curves of various insulins.

Inhaled insulin (Exubera): This rapid acting preparation of human regular insulin is administered as aerosolized dry powder and is absorbed in the pulmonary capillaries. Of the administered dose, about 40% reaches the pulmonary alveoli, with a bioavailability of about 10%. Clinically, it appears to be as effective as regular insulin. Adverse reactions include mild cough and some decrease in pulmonary function on prolonged use. The elimination of the need for injections is its main advantage. However, the cost, the special bulky inhaler required, poor bioavailability and the need for multiple inhalations make it less acceptable. Because of poor demand, it has been withdrawn from the market.

Adverse reactions:

- ***Hypoglycemia*:** Hypoglycemia is a common adverse effect of insulin. The common causes of hypoglycemia during insulin therapy are : too large a dose; failure to eat; vigorous physical exercise; and ingestion of alcohol. It is also frequent during 'intensive insulin regimens'. It is especially frequent in T1DM, aged diabetics and diabetics with diabetic nephropathy.

Table 63.6: Symptoms of hypoglycemia

- ***Sympathetic*** (Adrenergic) due to adrenaline liberation: hunger, anxiety, cold limbs due to vasoconstriction, tachycardia, palpitation, tremulousness, pallor, sweating, piloerection and subjective feeling of impending disaster. The body temperature tends to be lowered in hypoglycemic coma and this is of diagnostic importance.
- ***Cerebral*** (Neuroglycopenia) due to the brain being starved of glucose: confusion, bizarre behaviour, depression, coma, convulsions and focal lesions such as hemiplegia or visual disturbances. Cerebral edema or organic damage may cause these symptoms to persist after correction of the low blood sugar level.
- ***Non-specific:*** Nausea, headache.

Table 63.7: Differences in hypoglycemic episodes on different types of insulin

Preparation	Hypoglycemia, onset	Important features
Short acting Before a meal	After 3 hours; rapid in onset	Adrenergic symptoms predominate
Intermediate acting Before breakfast	Late afternoon and evening; gradual in onset.	Cerebral symptoms predominate and may not be recognized as due to hypoglycemia
Before dinner or at bedtikme	Early morning the next day	Cerebral symptoms predominate. Morning headaches.

Prior ingestion of a non-selective ß- blocker like propranolol can delay the recovery from hypoglycaemia (*hypoglycemia unresponsiveness*). *Selective* β_1 *- blocking agents like atenolol or metaprolol are less liable to do so.*

Table 63.6 gives the important symptoms of hypoglycemia. Table 63.7 lists the important differences among hypoglycemic episodes on different types of insulin.

Patients with T1DM of long duration may fail to recognize the symptoms of hypoglycemia (*hypoglycemia unawareness*). Table 63.8 lists the causes of hypoglycemia unawareness. The principles of management of hypoglycemia unawareness are listed in Table 63.9.

Attacks of hypoglycemia must be prevented because:

- ***An unrecognized attack during night is followed by rebound hyperglycemia with glycosuria next morning (Somogyi effect)***: This is likely to lead to an increase in the dose of insulin with repetition of hypoglycemia.
- ***Hypoglycemia can be followed by hypoglycemia unawareness.***
- ***They are harmful in patients with cardiovascular disease;*** and
- ***Frequent attacks may cause permanent neurological damage*; *and worsening of retinopathy.***

Table 63.8: Causes of hypoglycemia unawareness

- Ignorance of symptoms of hypoglycemia.
- T1DM
- Increasing duration of diabetes.
- Repeated severe hypoglycemia.
- Impaired glucose counter-regulation (but *not* autonomic neuropathy); and
- Strict glycemic control.

Patients on insulin therapy should be explained the symptoms of hypoglycemia. They should be warned about the dangers of missed meals, unplanned vigorous exercise and alcohol. They should carry sugar with them at all times and swallow it at the first symptom of hypoglycemia. Finally, a patient started on insulin therapy should be forbidden to swim, to work near machines and to drive till the dose is stabilized.

Oral glucose/sucrose, a sugar-containing food, can relieve hypoglycemic symptoms if it is administered early. In a comatose patient, IV glucose or IM glucagon (1 mg.) rapidly awakens the patient. If coma persists after correction of hypoglycemia, mannitol and large doses of glucocorticoids may be administered IV to relieve the cerebral edema.

Coma in a diabetic that is not diagnosable with certainty should be first treated with IV

Table 63.9: Principles of management of hypoglycemia unawareness

Prevention:
- Educating the patient about symptoms of hypoglycemia.
- Strict avoidance of hypoglycemia (blood glucose less than 70 mg/dl in this context) as even moderate hypoglycemia causes transient impairment of glucose counter-regulation for as long as 24 hours.
- Between-meals and bedtime snacks.
- Reduction in insulin dose before vigorous exercise.
- Avoidance of glycated hemoglobin concentrations in the non-diabetic range.
- Night-time insulin dose reduction after vigorous exercise; and
- Regular blood glucose monitoring.

Treatment:
- Hospitalization.
- Blood glucose monitoring especially at 3 AM, as hypoglycemia at that hour often goes unrecognized; and
- At least three weeks of scrupulous avoidance of hypoglycemia can restore hypoglycemia awareness.

glucose (50 ml. of 50 per cent). A rapid arousal during the injection confirms the diagnosis of hypoglycemia.

• ***Insulin allergy***: Allergy to insulin is IgE-mediated. It may consist of local itching, redness, swelling and pain. Generalized urticaria and lymphadenopathy are uncommon. Anaphylactic reactions are rare. Allergic reactions are uncommon with non-protein containing insulins but can occur with any insulin preparation.

• ***Insulin lipodystrophy***: This occurs at the site of injection and is of two types.

(1) **Lipohypertrophy** which is a spongy lump and is due to the lipogenic property of insulin injected repeatedly into a given area. The skin around the growth becomes anaesthetized, and this may encourage further injections in the same area. It is advisable to rotate the injection site. Switching to human insulin has no effect.

(2) **Lipoatrophy,** in which there is a loss of fat tissue, is probably of immunological origin. It is more common in females, in those who use conventional insulin preparations and in those who are allergic to insulin. The treatment consists of injection of human insulin at the borders of the lipoatrophic area. Resolution may take as much as 4-6 months.

• ***Insulin presbyopia***: When hyperglycemia is rapidly controlled with insulin, the patient often develops loss of visual accommodation due to alterations in the physical properties of the lens. It usually settles down within a few weeks.

• ***Insulin neuropathy***: In an occasional patient, rapid control of hyperglycemia with insulin either precipitates peripheral neuropathy or worsens a pre-existing one.

• ***Obesity***: Insulin therapy without dietary restriction and exercise may increase the body weight. This increases the insulin requirement and sets up a vicious cycle.

• ***Edema*** may be seen in some patients on initiating insulin therapy.

• ***Hepatomegaly*** due to glycogen deposition occurs in an occasional patient.

Therapeutic uses of insulin:

• ***Idiopathic diabetes mellitus***: discussed below in detail.

• ***Secondary diabetes mellitus***: Diabetes due to pancreatic diseases such as pancreatitis or hemochromatosis generally needs to be treated with insulin.

• ***Glucose—insulin IV drip*** is used to treat hyperkalemia.

• ***Glucose—insulin—potassium (GIP)*** drip has been used to treat patients with MI complicated by arrhythmias due to hypokalemia. The drip drives potassium into the cells.

• ***Insulin tolerance test*** with determination of plasma hGH has been used to test pituitary reserve and to diagnose hypopituitarism.

Pharmacotherapy of Diabetes Mellitus

Diabetes mellitus (DM) is a chronic metabolic disease caused by a variable combination of insulin deficiency and insulin resistance. The result is disordered utilization and storage of the proximate nutrients (carbohydrates, proteins and fats) and reduced production of ATP. Hyperglycemia is its most easily measured laboratory marker and the liability to chronic degenerative disease in almost all body tissues is its hallmark.

The etiology of DM is still obscure although it has a strong genetic basis. However, with proper management with diet, drugs and exercise a diabetic can enjoy an almost normal life.

Diabetes Mellitus is currently classified as shown in Table 63.10.

(1) **Type 1 DM (T1DM):** This is insulin dependent (IDDM) and the patient's survival depends upon uninterrupted insulin therapy.

(2) **Type 2 DM (T2DM):** This is not insulin dependent (NIDDM) and the patient's survival (except in emergencies) does not depend upon insulin therapy.

(3) **Type 3 DM** which is due to other hormonal disorders such as acromegaly, and drugs such as glucocorticoids; it may often respond to oral antidiabetic agents; and

(4) **Type 4 DM (Gestational DM; GDM);** this must be treated with diet with or without insulin.

Clinically, T2DM occurs in obese and normal weight adults, is stable and less likely to cause ketoacidosis. It also occurs in adolescents and even pre-adolescents. T1DM, on the other hand, occurs mostly in younger, underweight persons, in whom it often starts during puberty, is labile and is often complicated by ketoacidosis. In T1DM, there is an absolute deficiency of insulin and hence, it tends to be more severe. In T2DM, on the other hand, the insulin deficiency is less severe, and insulin resistance is the major contributory cause. Other varieties usually lie in between these two extremes.

Symptoms such as polyuria, polydipsia and polyphagia along with a random plasma glucose of 200 mg make the diagnosis of T2DM. In the absence of symptoms, criteria listed in Table 63.10 may be used.

In the early stages, T2DM subjects, especially the obese ones, have a relative excess of insulin in their plasma in response to a glucose load. This is the consequence of peripheral insulin resistance in the adipore tissue and muscles.

Overeating leads to excessive insulin secretion which reduces the concentration and affinity of insulin receptors in peripheral tissues; the insulin sensitivity normalises after weight reduction. In T2DM, a progressive age-dependent diminution of the beta cell function/ regeneration is responsible for the development and worsening of diabetes and its long term complications. By the time diabetes is diagnosed (FBS 126 mg/dl), 75% of the beta cells have been destroyed.

Table 63.10: ADA diagnostic venous plasma glucose values in T2DM

Plasma venous glucose (PVG) mg/dl	Fasting	2 hr. post glucose	Random
Normal	Less than 100	Less than140	
Impaired fasting glucose (IFG)	100-125	Less than140	
Impaired glucose tolerance (IGT)	Less than 100	140-199	
Diabetes mellitus (DM)	126 or more	200 or more	200 or more*

IFG/IGT may occur independently of each other. *= Plus symptoms of DM

On the contrary, the plasma of patients with T1DM lacks measurable insulin. The destruction of the pancreatic islets is due to autoimmune 'insulitis'. Islet cell antibodies are present in the plasma of some of these patients. Certain HLA phenotypes are found to be present frequently in T1DM.

Pathogenesis of T1DM: Genes on chromosome 6 determine the susceptibility to T1DM. In predisposed persons, immunological insulitis with beta cell damage and antibody formation start and progress insidiously; there is progressive diminution in insulin secretion during this preclinical stage which may last for years. The disease manifest acutely, commonly following a virus infection. By that time, serious damage to the insulin synthesizing/secreting capacity has occurred.

Pathogenesis of T2DM: T2DM has multifactorial pathogenesis (polygenic). The two basic mechanisms involved are: (1) Insulin resistance; and (2) Impaired insulin secretion.

- ***Insulin resistance (IR)*** **:**. The term insulin resistance indicates inadequate response to a given dose/level of insulin. Obesity is a major antecedent of IR. In obesity, increased intra-adipocyte triglyceride stores, especially in the visceral fat promote the growth of large, intrinsically insulin-resistant, intra-abdominal adipocytes. The adipocytes release FFA and inflammatory cytokines (IL6 and TNFα) which interfere with the insulin signaling cascade in the tissues and contribute to IR. This inhibits insulin induced suppression of lipolysis. *Endogenous glucose production is accelerated in spite of hyperinsulinemia.* TNFα enhances lipolysis in the peripheral adipose tissue. Circulating FFA and glycerol aggravate IR in the skeletal muscle and the liver. The current evidence indicates that hepatic insulin resistance is the key event in the pathogenesis of T2DM.

The concentration of the adipose-specific **adiponectin**, which increases insulin sensitivity, diminishes in T2DM, adding to IR. Adiponectin acts via AMP kinase, an enzyme involved in various metabolic responses such as suppression of hepatic neoglucogenesis, glucose uptake in the exercising skeletal muscles, fatty acid oxidation and inhibition of lipolysis.

A decrease in the mitochondrial oxidation of FFA in the liver and the muscle, leading to triglyceride accumulation, has also been suggested.

Further, it has been suggested that a genetic variant of the normal PPARγ (see later) results in/contributes to IR, primarily in the adipose tissue and secondarily in the liver. In predisposed individuals, an insulin secretory defect, present possibly on a genetic basis, obesity, acute illness or simply ageing. might further expose or aggravate the underlying defect, leading to the onset of T2DM.

- ***Insulin deficiency*****:** The normal pancreatic beta cells respond to IR by secreting more insulin (**hyperinsulinemia**) and maintaining the plasma glucose at or just above the upper limit of normal. Over a period of time, the beta cells develop insulin secretory defect as a result of progressive elevation of plasma glucose (**glucotoxicity**) and elevated FFA levels (**lipotoxicity**). Hyperglycemia may be toxic to the beta cells by inhibiting fatty acid oxidation (substrate competition) and local accumulation of FFA. The subject may then progress through the stages of IFG/IGT (see above) to diabetes mellitus.

In addition to IR, genetic predisposition, age, severe stress, multiple pregnancies and treatment with certain drugs, especially glucocorticoids, diminish the capacity of the beta cells to secrete insulin. Unless treated aggressively, the insulin secretory capacity of the beta cells continues to deteriorate after the diabetic state is established; and that is responsible for the progressive worsening of diabetes in most patients.

Insulin deficiency results in:

- ***Decreased peripheral utilization of glucose.***
- ***Decreased production of ATP.***
- ***Decreased synthesis of glycogen in liver and muscle.***
- ***Increased protein catabolism and neoglucogenesis.***

Table 63.11: Aims of therapy of diabetes mellitus

- To control symptoms with diet, exercise and drugs.
- To maintain the optimum body weight.
- To correct the metabolic disturbances; and
- To prevent or delay the degenerative vascular complications.
- To maintain normal growth in children.

- ***Increased lipolysis with increased plasma levels of FFA; and decreased lipogenesis.***
- ***Increased neoglucogenesis with increased hepatic glucose output.***
- ***Increased ketogenesis***; and
- ***Depressed cell mediated immunity (CMI).***

Diabetes, if left untreated, can cause impairment of general health, increased susceptibilty to infections, retinal, renal, cardiovascular and neurological complications, diabetic coma and premature death. The aims of therapy are given in Table 63.11.

An ideally controlled diabetic should :

(a) Be free from classical diabetic symptoms of polyuria, polyphagia and polydipsia.

(b) Have steady, ideal body weight.

(c) Have venous plasma glucose levels as near normal (fasting less than 110 mg% and post-prandial less than 140 mg%) as is possible without getting frequent/severe hypoglycemia. *However, in old people and in patients with severe liver and kidney disease, cardiac disease and cerebrovascular disease, one often has to be satisfied with higher levels of blood glucose.* A similar compromise is generally necessary in IDDM (especially long standing IDDM) in order to avoid repeated hypoglycemia.

(d) Have **less than 7% glycosylated hemoglobin** (HbA_1c) level: HbA_1c level is an index of the 'time averaged' blood sugar level over the previous 8-12 weeks **(Blood Sugar Memory)**. In non-diabetics, HbA_1c level is less than 6% of the total hemoglobin.

(e) Not develop ketoacidosis without severe provocation and

(f) Have normal plasma lipid levels.

Diabetic children should have normal growth; and diabetic women should have normal pregnancies and deliveries, and normal babies

Table 63.12 summarises the *venous plasma glucose* and HbA_1c criteria for judging the level of metabolic control. *Capillary blood glucose* values are higher than venous plasma glucose values.

Education of the patient is important and must include an understanding of his own disease, diet control urine examination, insulin administration, adjustment of the insulin dosage, the danger of neglecting the disease and the rewards of adherence to the prescribed regimen. Home blood glucose monitoring (HMBG) helps to improve the control.

Table 63.12: Venous plasma glucose and HbA_{1c} criteria for the degree of metabolic control

	Good	Acceptable	Fair	Poor
Venous plasma glucose :				
Fasting	< 110	120-140	140-180	Above 180
Postprandial	< 140	140-180	180-235	Above 235
Hemoglobin A_{1c}%	< 6 *	6-7.5 *	7.5-9	> 9

* Not to be attempted in T1DM. Good/excellent control mandatory during pregnancy.

The diet should be adjusted to bring the weight down to optimum and to maintain it there. Weight reduction in obese diabetics is accompanied by considerable improvement in hyperglycemia. In growing children, one must consider their continually changing caloric requirements. The total calories are generally divided as follows: protein calories 10-20%, fat calories 10-20% and carbohydrate calories 60-80%. Sugar consumption must be limited to less than 5% of the total daily calories consumed; and most of the carbohydrates be derived from starchy foods (complex carbohydrates).

The total daily intake should be divided into three meals and two snacks. The distribution of calories among the meals should be constant from day to day; this is desirable in all diabetics but is of critical importance in those on insulin. Overeating and fasting must be avoided. **Guar gum** (Carbotard) in the dose of 5 g in 200 ml of water before each meal or sprinkled on food is used to slow the absorption of glucose derived from the meal.

Daily, physical exercise reduces insulin requirement. Sudden, unaccustomed, vigorous exercise, however, may precipitate hypoglycemia especially in patients on insulin; if it is unavoidable, extra food (15 g of carbohydrate for each hour of anticipated exercise) should be eaten prophylactically. In the juvenile diabetic who has omitted insulin, vigorous exercise can precipitate ketoacidosis.

Along with lifestyle modification, prophylactic aspirin, unless contraindicated, is recommended in all patients with T2DM . A statin may be added, regardless of the baseline lipid levels, in those who are at higher risk for CVD or have CVD.

Not all diabetics need insulin all the time. The choice of therapy depends on whether it is T1DM or T2DM. The distinction between the two may sometimes not be clear. Further, what appears T2DM at the onset may sometimes be the earliest stage of late onset T1DM. And, adolescents may have T2DM rather than T1DM. T2DM patients can be controlled with diet, exercise and OHA for variable lengths of time, after which they may need insulin. In addition, T2DM patients may need insulin temporarily in the presence of a complication (Insulin Requiring DM, IRDM). T1DM patients need insulin lifelong for survival. *Hence, phenotyping the patients into IDDM, NIDDM or IRDM can help the clinician in the choice of therapy, "insulin" or "no insulin."* The indications for insulin are listed in Table 63.13.

Table 63.13: Indications for insulin therapy

- IDDM.
- NIDDM patients who are under-weight, those who have a history of onset before 30-35 years and those whose diabetes is of long standing.
- All diabetics with complications such as ketosis, infection, intractable pruritus, gangrene, congestive cardiac failure or progressive retinopathy.
- During surgical procedures.
- Diabetic pre-coma and coma.
- Primary or secondary failure following OHA therapy; and
- Pregnant diabetics.

Choice of insulin preparation: For routine control of NIDDM, the intermediate acting preparation NPH (Table 63.2), given before breakfast, can control some diabetics with a single daily injection. If this does not help, regular insulin may be added to NPH insulin.

The main merits of *regular* (i.e. plain or soluble) insulin are its rapidity and short duration of action. This makes it convenient in diabetic coma; *in intensive insulin treatment* (see later); in unstable diabetes and postoperatively. For the same reason, it must be used when an illness such as infection, vomiting or diarrhoea prevents regular intake of meals and the patient is likely to get hypoglycemia with longer acting insulins. When it is decided to change over from short to intermediate acting insulin, it is desirable to commence therapy with a dose of the latter only 2/3rds of the total daily dose of the former.

The rDNA synthetic, human insulin analogues (lispro, aspart, glargine) have much to offer in terms of flexibility of the daily routine;but they are expensive. They are, however, not necessarily more effective in terms of lowering HbA_1c than the conventional and the SR insulins in all patients.

Animal insulins have been claimed to be at least as good as human insulins. This claim has been supported by a Cochrane review. Diabetics who are well controlled on conventional insulins need not be shifted to newer insulins routinely. However, animal insulins, which are cheaper, are difficult to obtain now, as their production has been discontinued by most manufacturers.

Insulin therapy : Every diabetic may require insulin at some time in his life and it is life-saving in some situations. Although no insulin preparation available can mimic the need-oriented release of insulin by the patient's own pancreas, majority of diabetics can be managed by a judicious use of the available preparations. With the modern insulin syringes (1 ml divided into 40 or 100 parts), insulin dose can be adjusted in multiples of 1 unit.

• ***Management of an adult with T2DM without any complication***: *In most such patients, diabetes is stable and relatively mild. It can be controlled with diet and exercise with or without oral antidiabetic drugs (OHA; see later).* If insulin is acceptable to the patient, the intermediate acting NPH insulin is started with 5-10 units dose SC half an hour before breakfast. Blood sugar is determined while fasting, before lunch, before dinner and at bed time (*day-profiling*). The dose of insulin is increased by 2-5 units once in 3-4 days till pre-dinner blood sugar is normal. If the pre-lunch blood sugar is still high, a small dose (5-10 units) of short acting regular insulin is added to the pre-breakfast dose of NPH. Persistence of hyperglycemia at bedtime is treated by giving an additional dose of regular insulin before dinner. If the dose of NPH given before breakfast does not control next morning's fasting hyperglycemia while normalizing the blood sugar at other times, a small dose of NPH should be added before dinner or at bed time. A few patients may ultimately need a mixture of regular and NPH before breakfast and before dinner with or without regular insulin before lunch. In some of these, addition of an OHA may improve the diabetic control.

Some physicians initiate therapy with a small (5-10 units) dose of NPH at bedtime, to normalise the fasting blood glucose. Some patients may be controlled by BIDS (Bedtime Insulin and Daytime Sulfonylurea) regimen.

Persistent elevations of post-prandial blood sugars contribute in a major way to the occurrence of chronic degenerative complications of diabetes. As stated earlier, very short-acting insulin analogues, **lispro** and **aspart**, are effective in controlling postprandial hyperglycemia even when injected immediately before or within 5 minutes of commencing a meal. This makes them easier to use than SR insulin preparations.

Currently, it is felt advisable to start insulin therapy immediately on diagnosis of T2DM rather than wait till other forms of therapy have failed. This is so because although tablets are easier to take, early initiation of insulin therapy may result in lower HbA_1c levels and better long term preservation of endogenous insulin secretion as compared with a sulfonylurea.

• ***Management of an adult with T2DM on insulin and a complication such as acute infection*** : Under these conditions, insulin requirements go up and ketoacidosis may develop. If the patient can continue to take his normal meals, the insulin regimen need not be changed. If the patient cannot take his normal meals, he must be given a liquid diet containing plenty of salt and about 200 g. of carbohydrates per day (Sick Day Dietary Regimen). He is encouraged to take portions of this every 3-4 hours and regular insulin (10-50 units) is given SC every 6 hours after appropriate blood sugar determination. Salted buttermilk, vegetable soup, milk, fruit juice, with added sugar, are suitable items of food for these patients. As soon as the patient can take solid food, he can resume his original insulin regimen.

• ***T1DM*** : In these patients, diabetes tends to be severe and unstable. Attacks of diabetic coma and hypoglycemia are liable to occur because these patients tend to be unpredictable in their eating habits, sporadic in their exercise and prone to emotional outbursts, all of which interfere with the smooth control. Added to this are the over-anxious parents of a diabetic child.

Most patients need (a) an injection of regular insulin before each major meal with or without an additional dose of NPH before dinner or at bed time; (b) a mixture of regular with NPH insulin (50:50 rather than 30:70) before breakfast and before dinner; or (c) an injection of glargine insulin at bed time + an injection of lispro, aspart or SR regular insulin before each major meal, which can offer the patient the maximum flexibility. This, however, is an expensive regimen.

In some unstable, poorly controlled patients, regular insulin has to be injected SC several times a day (**intensified insulin treatment**) under guidance from blood sugar determination (by patient) on capillary blood, using finger prick and a portable reflectance meter, several times a day (**home blood glucose monitoring**, HMBG). Besides its therapeutic value, such therapy is also educative for the patient; he can see the blood sugar values instantly, correlate them with his symptoms and can learn to take corrective measures by increasing or decreasing the dose of insulin. *Not multiple daily doses of insulin but such immediate corrective action after each blood glucose determination is the essence of the intensive treatment.* The treatment is effective in improving the glycemic control but difficult to follow for long periods. The **UKPDS and the Diabetes Control and Complications Trial (DCCT),** studies have demonstrated that aggressive treatment of T1DM and probably T2DM to achieve tight control of hyperglycemia reduces the microvascular complications of DM but not IHD. Rigorous control of BP is more effective for the latter purpose. However, such regimens demand intelligent, highly motivated and disciplined patients, which makes it difficult in practice. Further, the patients need a 24 hour access to the health care provider.

Although battery operated, computerized, portable, insulin pumps have been used to deliver insulin under the skin, at a constant, predetermined rate, their use is tedious, inconvenient, and needs very careful supervision.

A needle-free system (Jet injection) for SC delivery of insulin is available.

Resistance to insulin is defined as the requirement of more than 2 units/kg/day. It may be acute or chronic.

Acute insulin resistance is associated with surgical or other trauma, emotional disturbance or infection; its treatment is the elimination of the cause and administration of as much insulin as is required to attain normal blood sugar levels.

Chronic insulin resistance may be due to:

• ***Noncompliance*** by the patient.

• ***Associated medical/endocrine disorders*** such as acromegaly or hypercortisolism.

• ***Genetic, insulin-receptor abnormality*:** This is associated with hyper-insulinemia, hypertriglyceridemia, hypertension and IHD (Reaven Syndrome), a precursor of T2DM.

• ***Insulin antibodies***; Insulin antibodies develop in all persons who receive the available preparations of insulin. *They are likely to develop in high titre in patients who have received insulin intermittently rather than continuously. Such resistance responds to prednisolone (60-100 mg. daily)*

• ***Lipoatrophic type of diabetes***.

Management of Emergencies in the Diabetic

Keto-acidotic diabetic coma :

In ketosis prone T1DM patients, diabetic coma can be precipitated by merely omitting insulin. In T2DM, it is likely to be precipitated by a severe infection or acute MI.

Pathophysiology: The deficiency of effective insulin action under these cirumstances brings about:

• ***Failure of peripheral glucose utilization,***

increased mobilization of muscle protein and increased neoglucogenesis, leading to hyperglycemia.

- ***Impaired oxidation of glucose leading to non-availability of pyruvate.***
- ***Excessive mobilization of FFAs from the adipose tissue, leading to excessive production of ketone bodies*** acetoacetic and beta-hydroxy butyric acids. These organic acids contribute to metabolic acidosis and by being excreted as salts of sodium and potassium in the urine, deplete the body sodium, potassium and water. Metabolic acidosis causes a shift of potassium and phosphorus out of the cells, their loss in the urine, severe potassium and phosphate depletion and moderate insulin resistance; and
- ***Increased hepatic glycogenolysis resulting in depletion of liver glycogen.***

Hyperglycemia and glycosuria promote a solute diuresis leading to dehydration and hypovolemia which aggravate the acidosis.

The urine is loaded with sugar and ketone bodies and the breath smells of acetone. The blood sugar is commonly in the range of 600-800 mg%. Plasma bicarbonate is markedly reduced and the blood pH is lowered.

Management: The diagnosis must be confirmed before starting treatment. If hypoglycemic coma cannot be ruled out, IV glucose (50 per cent, 50 ml) should be tried first.

On admission, blood is withdrawn for the following estimations, which must be repeated every 2 hours: glucose, bicarbonate, serum potassium, sodium, creatinine and hematocrit.

The following clinical data are recorded on admission and one hourly after that : pulse rate, blood pressure, temperature, fluid intake and output, glycosuria, ketonuria and ketonemia.

The principles of management of keto-acidotic diabetic coma are outlined in Table 63.14.

Table 63.14: Principles of management of diabetic coma

- Rapid correction of dehydration.
- Regular insulin, early and enough.
- Correction of acidosis.
- Treatment of precipitating cause, if found.
- Correction of hypokalemia and hypophosphatemia.
- Nursing management.

- ***Correction of dehydration*:** Normal saline is infused as follows: 1.5 litre in the first hour; one litre per hour for the next 3-4 hours; and 1 litre every 4 hours, thereafter. Half strength (0.45%) saline is used only if the initial plasma sodium is more than 150 mEq/litre. In elderly patients and in those with cardiovascular disease, titrate the rate of infusion according to the CVP. Plasma expanders may be used to treat severe hypotension. When blood glucose reaches 250 mg%, glucose and potassium should be added to the saline infusion.
- ***Insulin: Continuous, low dose, insulin infusion (CLDII)*** is effective, physiological and safe. Administration of 5-10 units (generally 0.1 unit/kg) of regular insulin per hour by continuous infusion maintains the plasma insulin at about 100-200 microu/ml, which is effective in correcting the diabetic ketoacidosis. In general, patients with infection show less response to and need larger doses of insulin. Acidosis does contribute to insulin resistance but the greater part of resistance is due to infection. Advantages of CLDII are listed in Table 63.15.

With minor modifications, the same regimen can be used to treat hyperglycemic, hyperosmolar, nonketotic diabetic coma.

Possible adsorption of insulin to the glass bottle and the tubing can be overcome by addition of albumin to the infusate. In actual practice, isotonic saline serves the purpose equally well. About 20-50 ml of insulin in saline should be run through the infusion set before connecting it to the patient.

Operationally, an insulin infusion may be set up as follows : add 100 units of regular insulin to 1000 ml of isotonic saline solution. Start a drip through a pediatric scalp vein set, the needle being inserted into a forearm vein. Infuse at the rate of 40-50 ml/hour (10 drops/minute). This works out to 5-6 units/hour. Taking into account

Table 63.15: Advantages of CLDII

- It provides a predictable fall of blood glucose, 60-100 mg% per hour. In the presence of infection, the rate of fall is lower.
- It is safe and rarely causes hypoglycemia, hypokalemia or cerebral edema. Stopping the insulin drip quickly corrects the hypoglycemia, should it develop.
- Previous insulin therapy does not affect the response to it.
- It has sound pharmacokinetic basis; and
- It is simple to use and can be administered by trained nursing staff.

the adsorption of insulin to the glass and the tubing, the effective rate of delivery may be 3-4 units per hour. If blood glucose shows no response at the end of 2 hours, double the rate of insulin administration.

When blood glucose comes down to 250 mg%, (a) decrease insulin to 3 units per hour; and (b) add 50 g of glucose and 20 mEq of potassium to each litre of infusion fluid. *Continue the infusion till the patient starts eating normally. Then, start SC insulin 30 minutes before discontinuing the infusion. Nothing else should be added to the insulin saline drip.* It is advisable to run this drip as a side drip into the tubing of the main fluid drip.

If IV infusion of insulin is not possible, regular insulin may be injected IM (Not SC) in the dose of 20 units initially, followed by 5 units once every hour. When IM route is used, rehydration becomes critical, Usually, one litre of isotonic saline is given rapidly followed by another litre in one hour.

Subcutaneous insulin as used in the past often failed to be absorbed in the presence of dehydration and shock, thus creating an apparent initial picture of 'insulin resistance'. Further, after correction of shock, large quantities of insulin were absorbed rapidly, causing hypoglycemia. On the other hand, because of short half life of insulin, intermittent, large, IV doses of insulin produce markedly fluctuating plasma insulin levels. Hence, the rate of reduction of blood glucose could not be controlled. An excessively rapid reduction in blood glucose can cause:

(a) **Severe hypoglycemia.**

(b) **Hypokalemia,** as the extracellular potassium accompanies glucose into the cell; and

(c) **Cerebral edema** as the plasma osmolality diminishes rapidly. This last complication is abetted by rapid correction of acidosis as well.

- ***Correction of acidosis*** **:** Acidosis, if severe (arterial blood pH less than 7.0), is corrected by IV sodium bicarbonate (Chapter 36).
- ***Treatment of the precipitating cause*****:** Infection is treated with antibiotics. Routine administration of antibiotics prophylactically is, however, not recommended.
- ***Potassium and phosphorus*****:** As soon as urine output is satisfactory, 20 mEq of potassium per hour through the drip is started. It is generally given as potassium chloride (2 g. = 26 mEq of K). If available, K_2HPO_4 (equivalent to 20 m Eq of potassium) may be added to the drip instead of KCl. It gives not only potassium but also phosphorus which is depleted in these cases. As soon as the patient can take orally, milk can be given as a rich source of phosphorus, and fruit juice and soups can provide potassium.
- ***Nursing care*****:** *Excellent nursing care is essential in the management of a patient in diabetic coma. Attention to skin, mouth, position and bladder are a must.* Catheterization of bladder should be avoided. After second day of the recovery, the patient should return to his normal food and insulin regimen.

Hyperglycemic, Hyperosmolar, Nonketotic coma: This is a less common form of metabolic coma which occurs in aged diabetics who have just enough (exogenous or endogenous) insulin to prevent ketosis but not hyperglycemia. The blood sugar level may be in excess of 1000 mg. per cent and may be as high as 2700 mg.%. Dehydration is severe. The treatment is similar to that of diabetic coma except that 0.45% sodium chloride solution is required in very large quantities. Insulin should be omitted when the blood sugar reaches about 250 mg%.

Surgery in a diabetic: Patients detected to be diabetic just before an emergency operation, T1DM patients, and patients with T2DM on insulin and on OHA should be managed with low dose continuous insulin infusion during and after major surgery. Those on tablets and undergoing minor surgical procedures such as cataract surgery (after which the meal pattern will not change) can be managed with tablets alone. Those on diet alone should receive insulin as and when necessary after surgery.

Hyperglycemic Agents

GLUCAGON : Glucagon is a single-chain polypeptide made of 29 amino acids, with a molecular weight of 3485. It is synthesized, stored and secreted by the alpha cells of the islets of Langerhans in response to a fall in blood glucose and a rise of plasma amino acids.

Pharmacological actions: Glucagon is the most potent glycogenolytic hormone known and produces a rapid rise in blood glucose by activating the hepatic phosphorylase via cyclic AMP. It is the body's second defence against hypoglycemia in healthy people, the first being reduction in plasma insulin level in response to diminishing blood glucose concentration; the latter is not operative in patients receiving either insulin or an OHA. Glucagon stimulates neoglucogenesis only in the presence of glucocorticoids and stimulates lipolysis in the peripheral tissues, which, in turn stimulates ketogenesis.

Paradoxically, glucagon stimulates secretion of insulin from the beta cells in man and it has been proposed that it is involved in the secretion of insulin after ingestion of glucose.

Glucagon also has a significant positive inotropic and chronotropic action on the heart.

Absorption, fate and excretion: Given orally, it is destroyed by proteolytic enzymes. After parenteral administration, it is absorbed rapidly but has a short plasma half life (3-6 minutes). It is degraded mainly in the liver, kidneys and plasma.

Preparations and dosage: Injection glucagon hydrochloride, 1 mg. Dose: 0.5-1 mg. S.C., IM or IV.

Therapeutic uses:

- ***For treating insulin hypoglycemia.*** Glucose IV is the treatment of choice. If this is not available, glucagon may be administered. If an IM injection of 1 mg. does not restore consciousness, inject 1 mg IV.
- ***To diagnose the hepatic form of glycogen storage disease*** in which it fails to raise the blood sugar level on IV injection.
- ***In beta-blocker toxicity with shock*** (Chapter 30).
- ***In radiology of the bowel as it relaxes the intestinal muscle.***

DIAZOXIDE: This benzothiadiazine analogue is a potent oral hyperglycemic agent. Its effects are reversible.

- ***It inhibits the insulin release from the beta cells of the pancreas by an alpha-adrenergic mechanism.***
- ***It stimulates release of catecholamines from the adrenal medulla.*** The latter also inhibit insulin release by beta cells.
- ***It increases the hepatic glucose output,*** through a beta-adrenergic mechanism; and
- ***It is a direct vasodilator*** when administered IV (Chapter 29).

The important adverse effects are water retention with edema, hirsutism and with high doses nausea, vomiting and hypotension.

The oral dose is 3-5 mg/kg/day in 2-3 divided doses. A thiazide diuretic is commonly given along with it to prevent edema.

Therapeutic uses:

- ***In the treatment of resistant hypoglycemias*** such as those due to insulinoma, glycogen storage disease and leucine-sensitive hypoglycemia.

- ***In hypertensive emergencies*** (Chapter 29).

Oral Anti-Diabetic Agents

Oral anti-diabetics must be distinguished from the hypoglycemic drugs such as salicylates which are too toxic for clinical use in doses that effectively lower the blood sugar. An ideal antidiabetic drug should : (a) be effective orally; (b) be nontoxic; and (c) correct the other metabolic defects in a diabetic, in addition to lowering the blood sugar. Although the drugs available at present do not meet these requirements fully, they are useful as monotherapy or in combination for controlling T2DM.

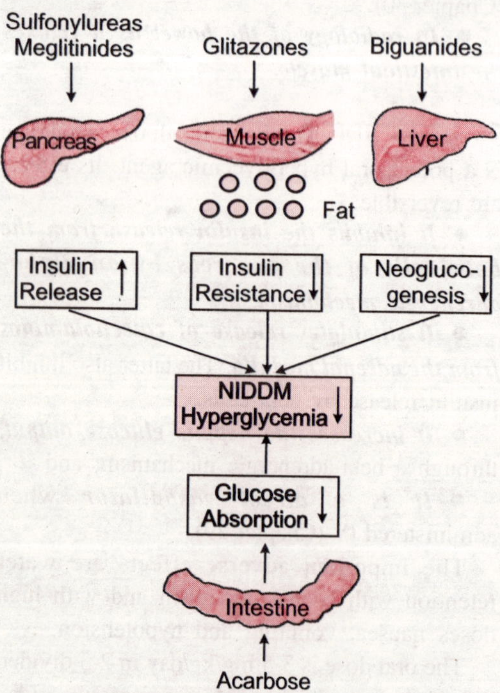

Fig. 63.4: Mechanism of action of oral antidiabetic drugs

The oral antidiabetic agents can be classified according to their predominant mechanism of action (Fig. 63.4)

I **Stimulators of insulin release by beta cells,** e.g., Sulfonylureas, Meglitinides

II **Inhibitors of hepatic gluconeogenesis,** e.g., Biguanides.

III **Inhibitors of intestinal α–glucosidases,** e.g., Acarbose, Miglitol.

IV **Drugs which reduce insulin resistance,** e.g., Glitazones; and

V. **Inhibitors of dipeptidyl dipeptidase-4 (DDP-4)** eg. Sitagliptin

SULFONYLUREAS: These compounds are chemically related to sulfonamides and have a basic structure as follows:

$$R-C_6H_4-SO_2NH\overset{O}{\overset{\|}{C}}NH-R_2$$

Fig. 63.5: General structure of sulfonylureas

Mechanism of action:

- ***Pancreas***: Sulfonylureas stimulate the release of insulin by the pancreas beta cells by increasing their sensitivity to glucose. hence they are effective only in the presence of a functioning pancreas.

They act on **sulphonylurea receptors** linked to the ATP-dependent K channels in the cell membrane of the islet beta cells. Activation of the receptors causes the K channels to close and the cell membrane to depolarise. There then occurs a calcium influx into the cell, with release of stored insulin from the granules.

Sulfonylureas release insulin slowly and for prolonged periods into the portal circulation where its primary action is on the liver, in contrast to the injected insulin which directly enters the systemic circulation.

- ***Liver muscle and adipose tissue***: Sulfonylureas inhibit hepatic neoglucogenesis and glycogenolysis. Hepatic glucose output decreases while the glucose uptake by the muscle increases. The hepatic glycogen stores are increased.

The basic action of all the sulfonylureas is identical. They differ in their pharmacokinetic properties, potency and hypoglycemic activity

Table 63.16 : Commonly used sulfonylurea compounds*

	Tolbuta-mide	Chlor-propa-mide	Glipi-zide**	Gliben-clamide (Glybu-ride)	Glicla-zide	Glime-piride ***
	Rasti-non	Diabenese Copamide	Gly-nase	Daonil Euglucon	Diami-cron	Amaryl
Tablets	0.5 and 1.0 g	0.1 and 0.25 g	5 mg	5 mg	80mg	1, 2, 4 mg
Plasma half life (hrs)	4 – 5	35	4	12	8 – 12	3 – 4
Duration of action (hrs)	6 – 10	24 – 72	12 – 24	12 – 24	12 – 24	16 – 24
Doses per day	2 – 3	1	1 – 2	1 – 2	1 – 2	1
Relative frequency of severe hypoglycemia	< 1	4 – 6	2 – 4	10-15	–	< 1%
Daily dose (g/day)						
Average	1.5	0.25	0.005	0.005	0.080	0.002
Max.	2.0	0.50	0.020	0.020	0.320	0.008

* Sulfonylureas are best taken 15-30 minutes before meals; food may interfere with their absorption.

** Also available as a sustained release preparation Glytop SR (5 and 10 mg). The tablets are swallowed intact.

***Rapid onset of action.

of their metabolites, all of which decide their biological t½. However, the plasma t½ of sulfonylureas bears little relationship to the duration of their hypoglycemic effect.

Pharmacological actions: These drugs:

(a) Lower the blood sugar in non-diabetics and selected diabetics.

(b) Lower the elevated FFA levels even before they lower the blood sugar.

(c) Normalise the metabolic state of the diabetic; and

(d) Promote weight gain.

The beneficial effects of sulfonylureas on serum on the serum lipids and lipoproteins are due to improved control of diabetes.

Absorption, fate and excretion: Sulfonylureas are rapidly absorbed from the GI tract when taken on empty stomach. They appear in the blood within 1-2 hours of their ingestion and peak levels are achieved in 4-6 hours. Food and hyperglycemia can reduce their absorption. They are all extensively (>90%) protein bound and are mainly metabolized in the liver (Table 63.16).

Chlorpropamide is extensively metabolized by the liver. As 20% is excreted unchanged in the urine, renal impairment enhances its hypoglycemic effect. Because of its long half-life, 7-10 days are required for it to achieve plateau plasma levels. Hence, its dose should not be increased more often than once in 10 days. Further, the drug should be avoided in patients with chronic renal disease.

Adverse reactions: Considering the number of diabetics taking sulfonylureas, their toxicity is remarkably low. The important adverse reactions are :

- ***Weight gain:*** This is moderate.
- ***Hypoglycemia*** can be precipitated by an excessive dose, decreased food intake, vomiting or by associated liver/kidney disease. Drugs like oral anticoagulants and salicylates, potentiate their hypoglycemic effect by displacing them from protein binding. MAO inhibitors and propranolol produce a state of **hypoglycemia unresponsiveness** and their combination with sulfonylureas or insulin can be dangerous. Alcohol can produce dangerous hypoglycemia in patients on a sulfonylurea.
- ***Allergic reactions*:** Sulfonylureas which are closely related to sulfonamides sometimes give rise to allergic skin rashes and very rarely bone marrow suppression.
- ***Liver*:** Chlorpropamide can cause cholestatic jaundice and occasionally pulmonary eosinophilia.
- **CVS:** See later.

Drug interactions: They sometimes potentiate and prolong the CNS effects of barbiturates and other sedative-hypnotics. By potentiating the action of circulating ADH on the renal tubules, chlorpropamide causes water retention and hyponatremia. Alcohol induced flushing is seen in some patients on sulfonylureas, especially chlorpropamide.

Preparations and dosage: Table 63.16.

Therapeutic uses :

- ***T2DM*** (fresh cases) : Sulfonylureas are useful in treating symptomatic patients with T2DM, including those who develop it during adolescence, and patients with **Maturity Onset Diabetes of the Young** (MODY), most of whom cannot be controlled for long periods of time by diet and exercise only. Patients most eligible for sulfonylurea therapy have the profile shown in Table 63.17. Out of those selected on the basis of these criteria, about 70 per cent show satisfactory response whereas the remaining are termed **primary failures**.

Usually, it takes 1-2 weeks to achieve the maximum effect of a given dose; hence the dose should not be increased more often than once in 1-2 weeks. In patients older than 60, with declining renal function, who are also liable to be forgetful about eating, a short acting sulfonylurea (tolbutamide/glipizide) is preffered.

Table 63.17: Profile of sulfonylurea-responsive patients

- Over 40 years of age and obese (or at least not underweight) at the time of diagnosis.
- Diabetes of recent onset.
- No significant ketonuria.
- Fasting blood sugar is less than 300 mg/dl.
- If on insulin, the daily requirement is less than 40 units.
- No acute complication likely to lead to ketoacidosis.
- No serious cardiac, kidneys or liver disease.
- Not candidates for surgery.

Of the patients who are initially well controlled with sulfonylureas, 5-10% escape from control every year (**secondary failure**). The important causes of secondary failure are dietary excess, intercurrent disease, inadequate dose, poor compliance and progressive deterioration of pancreatic function. This can be treated by (a) improving patient compliance; (b) changing over to another sulfonylurea; (c) addition of a biguanide or acarbose; or (d) addition of/change over to insulin.

If a patient with T2DM well controlled by less than 20 units of insulin wishes to change over to oral therapy, insulin can be stopped abruptly and a sulfonylurea introduced. However, if the insulin requirement is between 20 and 40 units daily, the dose of insulin is progressively reduced while that of a sulfonylurea is progressively increased, till the latter completely takes over. *Such changeover from insulin to oral drugs, if done repeatedly, can lead to the development of antibodies to insulin and insulin resistance because of intermittent insulin therapy.*

- Some patients with T2DM may show a better response to **sulfonylurea-insulin combination** than to either drug alone.

● *Diabetes insipidus*: Chlorpropamide has been used in diabetes insipidus (Chapter 38).

Limitations of sulfonylureas: These are outlined in Table 63.18.

Table 63.18: Limitations of sulfonylureas

Sulfonylureas are ineffective in:
- IDDM.
- Very long standing T2DM
- Diabetic coma.
- Diabetes due to pancreatectomy or destruction of pancreas by disease.
- Surgical diabetics; and
- The presence of infection and / or heavy ketonuria.
- Further, they cannot be used in pregnant women and in patients with severe liver or kidney disease.

Choice of the sulfonylurea preparation: **Tolbutamide** is well tolerated and is relatively safe. But it has to be taken 2-3 times a day. **Chlorpropamide** controls hyperglycemia in a single daily dose. Although doses larger than 500 mg. per day are pharmacologically more effective, they may cause a disproportionate increase in adverse effects. Chlorpropamide is generally effective in 'primary and secondary failures' on tolbutamide therapy. **Glipizide** is intermediate between tolbutamide and chlorpropamide. **Glibenclamide** is effective in a single daily dose and may be effective in patients who are not controlled by maximum doses of chlorpropamide. However, its tolerated dose varies from 2.5 to 20 mg. per day and it can cause a higher incidence of hypoglycemia than chlorpropamide, glipizide and glimepiride. It is, therefore, used in divided doses when more than 5 mg/day is being used. In patients with renal impairment, tolbutamide or **gliclazide** is the preferred drug. *If good glycemic control is not achieved with maximum doses of sulfonylureas, one should use combination oral drug therapy or change to insulin.*

Meglitinides : These drugs, unrelated chemically to sulfonylureas, have the same mechanism of action. They do not stimulate further release of insulin in patients on maximum dose of a sulfonylurea, cause hypoglycemia, and can be used in patients with decreased renal function. Their usefulness is similar to that of sulfonylureas. They are:

REPAGLINIDE (Novonorm, Eurepa) : It is administered shortly before each major meal in the dose of 0.5 to 4.0 mg. It has a rapid onset and a short duration of action (4 hours) and controls postprandial hyperglycemia effectively. Because of its short duration of action, it is less likely than sulfonylureas to cause repeated hunger, frequent eating, and weight gain. It is cleared primarily by the liver. It is useful in the treatment of NIDDM, as a monotherapy or along with metformin.

Nateglinide is unrelated chemically to repaglinide. Its onset of action and duration of action (2-3 hours) are shorter.

BIGUANIDES: The general chemical structure of biguanides is shown in Fig. 63.6. A free guanidine radicle is thought to be essential for the hypoglycemic effect of biguanides.

$$(R_1)(R_2)N-C(=NH)-NH-C(=NH)-NH_2$$

Fig. 63.6: General Structure of Biguanides

Mechanism of action: The exact mechanism of action of biguanides is not clear. They do not stimulate insulin release from the pancreas; and the presence of either exogenous or endogenous insulin is necessary for their action.

Several mechanisms may be involved in the antidiabetic effect of biguanides. They:

● ***Inhibit hepatic neoglucogenesis*** and decrease hepatic and renal glucose output. This is probably their major action.

● ***Increase the peripheral glucose utilization*** by enhancing anaerobic glycolysis.

● ***Act as insulin sensitizers in the muscle and adipose tissue, and reduce hyperinsulinemia.*** But, they have less robust effect on insulin resistance, inflammatory markers and vascular function than the glitazones (see later).

- ***Delay glucose absorption;*** and
- ***Reduce the appetite,*** which may be helpful in obese subjects.

Pharmacological actions: These agents do not lower the blood sugar in normal subjects but they do so in diabetics. By themselves they do not produce hypoglycemia in diabetics. They potentiate the hypoglycemic action of insulin and sulfonylureas.

They do not inhibit ketogenesis in the liver. Hence, diabetics on these drugs may develop ketoacidosis with minimum hyperglycemia and glycosuria. Further, biguanides decrease the glycogen content of the liver.

They reduce plasma total and LDL cholesterol and triglyceride levels, and increase plasma fibrinolytic activity. Lipolysis, FFA production and lipid oxidation are reduced by biguanides.

Protein break down and aminoacid turnover are not affected; and weight loss is mainly due to reduction in appetite. Their main benefit is prevention of weight gain in contrast to sulfonylureas where it is common.

Absorption, fate and excretion: Metformin is absorbed rapidly from the GI tract and gives adequate plasma levels. Its t½ is 1.5-4 hours. It is largely excreted unchanged in urine.

Adverse reactions: Metformin is generally well tolerated. In 20% of the patients, it produces an unpleasant, bitter or metallic taste, anorexia, nausea, and abdominal discomfort. This can be minimized by starting with a small dose and giving it with, rather than before, meals. The time disintegrating tablet is tolerated better. They also produce lethargy, muscular weakness and an excessive weight loss in some patients. The drug may produce vitamin B_{12} deficiency during long term use. Severe allergic reactions are rare.

Lactic acidosis has been reported rarely during metformin therapy, but it could be lethal during an acute illness such as a severe infection. *Before prescribing a biguanide to an elderly patient, serum creatinine should be measured to assess the renal function.* Patients undergoing a radiocontrast study (CT scan or coronary angiography) should be advised to omit metformin one day before and for 48 hours after the procedure. Metformin should be omitted and insulin substituted the day before major surgery. In both instances, metformin administration may be resumed after normal renal function is demonstrated. Its use is contraindicated in patients with liver disease, chronic kidney disease, COPD, CHF and chronic alcoholism.

Preparations and dosage:

(i) Metformin 500 and 850 mg. tablets. It is generally started in the dose of 250 mg 2-3 times a day with major meals, and the dose increased gradually upto 2000 mg per day. *Fixed dose combinations with a sulfonylurea do not allow individualization of the doses of the two drugs and should generally be avoided.*

(ii) Metformin SR 500 mg tablet once a day.

Therapeutic uses:

- ***Obese patients with T2DM,*** who could be controlled with diet alone but find this therapy unacceptable. In such patients, the anorectic action of metformin is of additional help in making the patients lose weight.
- ***Secondary sulfonylurea failure:*** Metformin may be added to a sulfonylurea in cases of secondary failure (see above).
- ***Polycystic ovaries syndrome (PCO) :*** In obese patients with PCO and oligo-ovulation, regular ovulation may be restored, leading to conception. (Chapter 66).
- ***Non-alcoholic steato-hepatitis (NASH).***

UGDP and UKPDS studies: The UGDP study showed that morbidity and mortality from vascular disease were higher in patients treated with tolbutamide or phenformin than in those treated with diet alone or with diet plus insulin. This conclusion was not universally accepted, nor was it substantiated by the subsequent UKPDS study. *Both studies, however, focussed attention on the importance of diet and exercice, with or without insulin, in controlling* *hyperglycemia to prevent long term degenerative complications.*

ACARBOSE (Glucobay, Acar): This is an oligosaccharide of microbial origin.

Mechanism of action : It binds competitively to carbohydrate binding regions of alpha glucosidases enzymes in the brush border of the enterocytes in the jejunum. It thus inhibits the intestinal absorption of carbohydrates but not of glucose because it does not interact with the sodium dependent glucose transporter in the small intestine.

Pharmacological actions : Given orally, acarbose reduces postprandial hyperglycemia which is known to activate coagulation cascade; acarbose reduces this phenomenon.

It is administered in the dose of 25-50 mg, chewed and swallowed after eating the first few morsels during each meal. As acarbose interferes with the digestion of sucrose, *patients receiving insulin or a sulfonylureas as well as acarbose should carry glucose not sucrose.*

Adverse reactions: These include flatulence, abdominal discomfort and loose stools. Occasionally, liver enzymes may be elevated.

Therapeutic uses: The drug is useful in patients on high carbohydrate diet and is generally used in combination with other drugs.

Miglitol is similar to acarbose but is claimed to be less hepatotoxic.

Both the drugs are contraindicated in patients with chronic intestinal disease, including inflammatory bowel disease, and in intestinal obstruction.

THIAZOLIDINEDIONES (Glitazones) : The introduction of glitazones in the treatment of T2DM was a major breakthrough since the introduction of sulfonylureas in 1950s. **Rosiglitazone** and **pioglitazone** are the two glitazones available currently.

Mechanism of actions: These drugs are potent agonists of the Peroxisome Proliferator-Activated Receptors gamma (PPARγ) which are nuclear receptors abundantly present in the adipose tissue but are also present in the liver, heart and skeletal muscle. After binding to the receptor PPARγ, glitazones modulate gene expression involved in glucose and lipid metabolism, insulin signal transduction, and adipocyte differentiation and proliferation. *Their primary action is to increase the insulin sensitivity of the adipose tissue, liver and muscle* **(insulin sensitizers).**

They also help to preserve the pancreatic beta-cell function by reducing the FFA and cytokine-induced islet cell damage.

In addition, they also have action on the vascular endothelium, immune system, ovaries and tumour cells.

Pharmacological actions: These drugs;

- ***Increase the insulin sensitivity of the adipose tissue and lower the plasma FFA levels.*** As a result, insulin sensitivity in liver and the muscle increases as well. They ameliorate hyperinsulinemia and thereby may protect the body from *the damaging effects of chronic endogenous hyperinsulinemia. Exogenous insulin therapy has no such long term ill effects.*
- ***Reduce the production of the proinflammatory cytokines by the visceral adipocytes and increase the adipose tissue production of adiponectin.*** This further increases the insulin sensitivity of other insulin responsive tissues such as liver and muscle.
- ***Increase the subcutaneous, small-adipocyte mass***, and divert the triglyceride storage from the visceral adipocytes to the subcutaneous adipose tissue.
- ***Lower the hepatic fat content*** and ameliorate dyslipidemia.
- ***Lower the hepatic glucose production and increase glucose uptake by skeletal muscle*** via glucose transporters; thus they reduce hyperglycemia.
- ***Preserve and enhance beta cell and vascular function by*** reducing the inflammatory milieu in the body.

Overall, they enhance insulin action (directly) and beta cell function (indirectly). They are classified as **insulin sensitizers,** and, by definition, require the presence of endogenous insulin. *Hence, they can be used only in T2DM but not in T1DM.* As insulin sensitizers, they are more potent than metformin.

They have multiple beneficial effects on the laboratory indices of the diabetic state. They:

- ***Ameliorate hyperglycemia and lower the levels of glycosylated hemoglobin.*** *By themselves, they do not cause hypoglycemia.*
- ***Lower plasma levels of FFA and triglycerides.***
- ***Increase plasma HDL levels.***

However, they (especially rosiglitazone) increase the plasma LDL level. Further, their beneficial effects on microvascular complications of diabetes have not yet been convincingly demonstrated. Finally, a meta-analysis has concluded that "rosiglitazone was associated with a significant increase in the risk of death from myocardial infarction and with an increase in the risk of death from cardiovascular causes". Pioglitazone has been claimed to be free from these disadvantages. It must be remembered that there is more to the treatment of DM than the control of hyperglycemia.

Since their action is genetic regulation, their maximum effect is seen after weeks or months. They synergise with sulfonylureas and metformin, as well as insulin in their antidiabetic effects.

Before prescribing a glitazone it is necessary to check for edema and its cause; and for cardiac, renal and hepatic status. Its use together with insulin should be avoided.

Absorption, fate and excretion: They are generally prescribed for use once daily. They are completely absorbed and are metabolized extensively by the liver. The metabolites of rosiglitazone are weakly active and are excreted by the kidney; whereas those of pioglitazone are more active and are excreted in the bile.

Adverse reactions: These are

(a) **Liver:** These drugs cause elevation of hepatic enzymes, which mandates periodic monitoring. Fatal hepatotoxicity was reported with troglitazone, which was, therefore, withdrawn from the market. It is rare with rosiglitazone and pioglitazone. Pioglitazone induces hepatic drug metabolizing enzymes and can decrease the effctiveness of the drugs which are substrates of these enzymes e.g. oral contraceptives.

(b) **Weight gain:** All glitazones cause weight gain (2-4 kg) in dose dependent manner. It is caused by proliferation of new adipocytes and redistribution of fat stores, plus fluid retention.

(c) **Fluid retention/CHF:** Fluid retention and increase in plasma volume can occur, and this may precipitate or worsen CHF. It is more common with concomitant insulin therapy.

(d) **Miscellaneous:** Anovulatory women may resume ovulation. These drugs may cause very unpleasant hunger sensation, especially when they are used in combination with other antidiabetic drugs. Retarded fetal development has been noted in animals; hence *they are not recommended during pregnancy.*

Preparations and dosage :

(i) Rosiglitazone (Avandia, Result, Enselin): 4-8 mg /day in single or divided doses.

(ii) Pioglitazone (Actos, Pioz, Pioglit): 15-45 mg/day in single or divided doses.

Therapeutic Uses :

- ***T2DM*:** They are used as monotherapy, or in combination with other OHA in resistant cases. They should be used cautiously, if at all, in combination with insulin.

In spite of all the claims in favour of the glitazones, it should be remembered that sulfonylureas and metformin have been in use for over four decades and their efficacy and safety profiles are fairly well known. The glitazones were introduced only recently and long term studies are needed to establish their correct status in the treatment of T2DM. Moreover, the glitazones are expensive compared to sulfonylureas and metformin, and their routine use may not be affordable by many.

- ***Other insulin resistant states*** such as polycystic ovary syndrome.
- ***Non-alcoholic steatohepatitis*** (NASH)

Table 63.19 outlines a suggested plan for the management of uncomplicated NIDDM.

Table 63.19: Management of uncomplicated NIDDM

- ***Initial treatment:*** *
  Diet and exercise

If poor response

- ***Initial drug treatment***

FPG (mg/dl)	Bodily habitus	Drug
< 140	Normal weight or obese	Metformin
< 140	Underweight	Insulin or sulfonylurea
> 140	Moderately or severely obese	Metformin
> 140	Underweight	Insulin or sulfonylurea

If poor response

● ***Underweight***	Add insulin/glitazone
● ***Normal weight or obese***	Add sulfonylurea or metformin

If poor response

● ***Underweight***	Change to insulin
● ***If normal weight or mildly obese***	Pre-breakfast and bedtime NPH or lente insulin
● ***If moderately or severely obese***	Add pre-dinner mixture (30:70) of plain and NPH insulin

FPG = Fasting plasma glucose
OHA = Oral hypoglycemic agents. For use of acarbose and glitazones, see text. Some authorities use a glitazone as the first line drug in T2DM.
* *Use of insulin from the diagnosis is now favoured by many authorities* (see text).

Table 63. 20 summarises the important drugs used in T2DM.

Use of OHA Combinations: This has advantages such as

(1) Additive effect because of different mechanisms of actions.

(2) Lower incidence of ADR of individual drugs; and

(3) Effectiveness in patients showing resistance to monotherapy.

Although fixed-dose combinations of metformin with a sulfonylurea, a glitazone or sitagliptin are available, they lack the flexibility of dose adjustment of the individual drugs.

Newer antidiabetic agents :

(A) PRAMLINTIDE (Symlin): The polypeptide, **amylin**, which is co-secreted with insulin is markedly reduced in diabetics. It helps to control postprandial hyperglycemia by (a) suppressing endogenous glucagon production, especially postprandially; (b) reducing the gastric emptying rate; and (c) inducing centrally mediated satiety, by opposing the action of ghrelin. Amylin has a short t ½. A long acting synthetic amylin analogue **pramlintide** has been used successfully in treating T1DM and T2DM patients in whom the PP hyperglycemia is difficult to control. It is injected SC, tid, along with insulin (by a separate injection) just before each meal. It helps to reduce weight. The frequency of hypoglycemia increases. The other adverse reactions are nausea, anorexia, early satiety and vomiting. It needs further, long term evaluation.

(B) GLP-1 BASED DRUGS: The intestinal L-cells-derived Glucagon – Like Peptide-1 (GLP-1) is the main mediator of the **Incretin Effect**, already described. The other, clinical effects of GLP-1 are (a) suppression of inappropriate postprandial hyperglucagonemia, gastric emptying, and appetite; and (b) weight loss. Stimulation of islet growth, differentiation and regeneration has been described in animals. It is degraded by the enzyme dipeptidyl dipeptidase-4 (DDP-4), and has a t ½ of 2-5 minutes.

Table 63.20 Important drugs used in T2DM

Drug	Site of action	Blood glucose Fasting	Blood glucose PP	ADR	Weight gain	Dose and schedule
Insulin	Multiple	Excellent	Excellent	Hypo.	Marked	See text
Sulfonyl ureas	Beta cells	Good	Good	Hypo.	Moderate	OD/BID
Metformin	Liver	Good	Good	Anorexia, nausea	Less gain or loss	OD/BID
Glitazones	Muscle/ adipocytes	Good	Good	Hepato toxicity	Moderate	OD/BID
Glucosidase inhibitors	Intestine	Fair	Excellent	Bloating	Less gain	With each meal
Repaglinide	Beta cells	Fair	Good	Hypo.	Moderate	Just before each meal
Nateglinide	Beta cells	Poor	Excellent	Less hypo.	Moderate /less	Just before each meal

Hypo = Hypoglycemia

EXENATIDE (Byetta), is a longer acting (t ½ 2.4 hours), synthetic analogue of GLP-1. It has been used by pre-meal SC injection, bid, in the treatment of T2DM with resistant postprandial hyperglycemia. It lowers the blood sugar and HbA_{1C} modestly. Its main merit is the weight loss it causes. Nausea, vomiting, diarrhea and upper respiratory symptoms are the most common ADR. However, post-marketing reports of acute pancreatitis have appeared.

It is generally used as an add-on drug with metformin or a sulfonylurea.; but not with insulin. By itself, it does not cause hypoglycemia though it may cause it when used along with a sulfonylurea. It needs further, long-term toxicity evaluation.

Liraglutide is an exenatide analogue with similar properties, uses and limitations. It can be used once a day.

DDP-4 INHIBITORS: **Sitagliptin** and **vildagliptin** are orally administered DDP-4 inhibitors which prolong the t ½ of endogenous GLP-1, and therby increase insulin levels. This may improve the glycemic control. They have been used orally in combination with an OHA (metformin, a sulfonylurea or a glitazone) They are primarily excreted in the urine. They are less effective than the established OHAs; and they have no extra- hypoglycemic benefits. The drugs are generally well tolerated except for mild GI upset. Rarely, they may cause allergic skin reactions, sometimes severe.

They are not recommended as monotherapy. Their long term safety is not known.

The newer antidiabetic agents described above are therapeutically weaker than the older agents. The older OHA drugs have been in use for many years, and their efficacy and safety profiles are fairly well known. The newer drugs have been in use for much shorter periods, and long term studies are needed to define their correct place in therapeutics. They cannot be recommended for monotherapy. Further, some of them must be injected; and all are expensive.

Insulin substitutes : From time to time, claims are made about the indigenous preparations derived from plants or metals, found to possess hypoglycemic action in experimental diabetes. As hyperglycemia and glycosuria are prominent manifestations of DM, a new potential antidiabetic agent is usually tested for its ability to correct these abnormalities. It must be emphasized, however, that DM is not synonymous with hyperglycemia and glycosuria. It is a disease due to deranged total energy metabolism and the new drug must help to correct the fundamental defects in metabolism. While accepting such an agent, therefore, one should know the mechanism of its hypoglycemic action and also the possible long term effects. Otherwise, it is difficult to justify its use in place of established remedies which have been shown to prevent the complications which is the major problem of DM. Using a drug simply to lower the blood sugar is like applying a dye to the hair "which though it helps one to look younger, does not reverse the fundamental process of senescence".

Table 63.21 lists the drugs which affect the blood glucose level.

Table 63.21: Drug induced hyperglycemia and hypoglycemia

- ***Drugs which cause hyperglycemia:***
  Hormones: Glucagon, GH Glucocorticoids; Thyroid hormones; Estrogens; Progestogens; Adrenaline and Noradrenaline.
  Other drugs: Beta adrenergic receptor agonists; Diazoxide; Phenytoin; Thiazides; Nicotinic acid in large doses.
- ***Drugs which cause hypoglycemia*:** MAO inhibitors; Beta adrenergic receptor blockers; Disopyramide; Alcohol; ACE inhibitors; Quinine; Lithium; large doses of Salicylates; Pentamidine;
- ***Drugs which cause hypoglycemia unawareness*:** Nonselective beta adrenergic blockers, e.g., Propranolol.

Sweetening Agents

These are non-carbohydrate substances devoid of food value, useful as sugar substitutes in diet and beverages. Used in small amounts, they are considered harmless including in pregnancy. They do not contribute to dental caries. They are:

(1) **Saccharin** : It is commonly employed as the sodium salt which is comparatively free from the unpleasant after-taste of saccharin. Saccharin tablet contains 12 mg. of saccharin. One tablet is approximately equivalent to 1 teaspoonful of sugar (7.5 g. sucrose).

(2) **Aspartame** (Equal): Aspartame is a dipeptide formed by a synthetic combination of two natural amino acids, L-aspartic acid and the methyl ester of phenylalanine. It is 200 times sweeter than sucrose. It decomposes if exposed to high temperatures as in cooking and then loses its sweet taste.

(3) **Neotame:** This new analogue of aspartame is water soluble and more heat stable at neutral pH. It is, therefore, suitable for use in cooked food. It is about 30-60 times sweeter than aspartame, and is claimed to have 'flavour enhancing' property. It increases the perception of flavours such as fruit flavours.

(4) **Sucralose** (Splenda) : This zero calorie trichlorinated sucrose is 600 times as sweet as the native sucrose. The body does not recognize it as either carbohydrate or fat. It is not absorbed, nor metabolized, and is excreted unchanged in the faeces.

Adrenal Cortical Steroids 64

Publication by Thomas Addison's in 1855 on the clinical picture of adrenal destruction attracted the attention of physiologists to the importance of the adrenal cortex. Subsequent experiments established that the adrenal gland was necessary for survival and that the cortex and not the medulla was essential for survival. Of the steroids isolated from the cortex, hydrocortisone, cortisone, corticosterone, desoxycorticosterone, dehydrocortisol and aldosterone were shown to be biologically active. In the meanwhile, adrenocorticotropin (ACTH) or corticotropin, isolated from the adenohypophysis (1943), was shown to be responsible for the structural and functional integrity of the adrenal cortex. The work by Hans Selye, who postulated the relationship between the adrenal cortex and stress, stimulated extensive work in adrenal physiology. Observation of the relief of symptoms of rheumatoid arthritis during pregnancy led to the use of cortisone in its treatment by Hench, who was awarded the Nobel prize in medicine, jointly with Kendall and Reichstein.

The adrenals consist of an outer cortex and an inner medulla, which are structurally and functionally different from each other. The adrenal cortex consists of three zones; from without inwards, they are **zona glomerulosa, zona fasciculata and zona reticularis**.

Pituitary-adrenal relationship: The hypothalamus, pituitary and the adrenal cortex form the HPA axis. ACTH is the specific adenohypophyseal hormone which maintains the structure and regulates the function of the adrenal cortex. It is secreted by the basophil cells (corticotrophs) and is a polypeptide with 39 aminoacids. The first 24 aminoacids which determine its biological activity are common to the hormone obtained from cattle, pig, sheep and man. The arrangement of the remaining 15 amino acids shows species variation and is responsible for its antigenicity. Melanocyte stimulating hormone (MSH) from the anterior pituitary has a sequence of amino acids identical with that of the first 13 of ACTH.

Adrenocorticotropin

Regulation of ACTH release: A corticotropin releasing hormone (CRH) is formed by hypothalamus is stored in the medial eminence, and from there reaches the anterior pituitary via the portal circulation. It stimulates the synthesis and release of ACTH. ACTH, together with beta lipotropin, is derived from a larger parent polypeptide called pro-opio-melanocortin (POMC). 5-HT probably plays an important role in the release of ACTH.

Cyproheptadine, a 5-HT antagonist, inhibits the normal rise of plasma cortisol following insulin-induced hypoglycemia. Further, oral administration of this drug causes a significant depression in the plasma cortisol (hydrocortisone) level. *The term cortisol refers to the native hormone of the adrenal cortex present in the biological fluids; whereas the term hydrocortisone is used to refer to the synthetic substance used therapeutically.*

Diurnal fluctuations in the rate of release of ACTH regulate the rates of secretion of cortisol and corticosterone. The plasma level of cortisol modulates the rate of release of CRH and in turn that of ACTH by negative feedback mechanism. Thus, increased plasma level of cortisol inhibits ACTH release and reduces the ACTH store of the adenohypophysis. The synthetic glucocorticoids have a similar but more prolonged inhibitory action. Decreased plasma level of cortisol, as in Addison's disease, stimulate ACTH secretion, via the hypothalamus. This delicately balanced mechanism thus adjusts the plasma level of cortisol to within normal limits.

Under stressful situations, neuronal impulses from higher centres stimulate release of CRH which ultimately elevates the output of cortisol to meet the increased demands of the body. This important homeostatic mechanism which overrides the diurnal variations in ACTH secretion as well as its regulation by plasma cortisol level is deranged in various disease states and in the functional suppression of the HPA complex by glucocorticoid administration.

The rate of secretion of cortisol is maximum in the early hours of the morning, declines during the day and reaches a minimum at about midnight, the plasma level being highest at about 6 AM. The 24 hours rhythmic secretion of ACTH and cortisol appears to be related to the sleep pattern.

Synthetic CRH is a 41 amino acid polypeptide that can be used to evaluate ACTH reserve of the anterior pituitary.

In addition to CRH, arginine vasopressin (Chapter 38) also stimulates the release of ACTH from the corticotropes. It likely plays an important role in the full magnitude of the stress response.

Pharmacological action of ACTH:

- ***On the adrenal cortex*** : ACTH stimulates the adrenal cortex to synthesize and secrete cortisol and corticosterone, and weak androgens. In hypophysectomised animals, the adrenal cortex undergoes atrophy and secretion of cortisol is markedly depressed and does not rise in a normal fashion in response to 'stressful' stimuli. Such atrophy can be prevented by administration of ACTH. The rate of secretion of aldosterone is, however, relatively unaffected after hypophysectomy.

The adrenal cortex uses cholesterol from two sources for steroidal synthesis: uptake of circulating LDL and local intracellular synthesis of cholesterol; both are enhanced by ACTH, acting on the cell membrane receptors, activating the adenylyl cyclase system and increasing intracellular cyclic AMP content. Further, ACTH accelerates the intracellular conversion of cholesterol to pregnenolone, the rate limiting step in the synthesis of adrenocortical steroids.

Prolonged elevation of ACTH level causes hyperplasia and hypertrophy of the adrenal cortex with increased secretion of cortisol, corticosterone and weak androgens. *The pharmacological actions of ACTH are in fact the pharmacological actions of these hormones, mainly cortisol.* (See later).

- ***Extra-adrenal effects***: These are of less clinical importance and include cutaneous pigmentation, lipolysis in adipose tissue, ketosis and insulin resistance.

Absorption, fate and excretion: ACTH is administered IM/IV. It is well absorbed after IM injection with plasma t½ is about 15 minutes. It is rapidly metabolized and only a negligible amount appears in the urine. The quantitative response to a given dose of ACTH is greater when it is given:

- ***In the morning than in the evening;*** and
- ***By slow IV infusion than as an IV bolus.***

The maximum adrenocortical stimulation is obtained in adults with 20 IU of corticotropin infused over 8 hours, 40 IU of depot corticotropin given IM every 12 hours and by 1 mg. of depot Synacthen given once a day.

Assay of ACTH : Plasma ACTH is measured by chemiluminescence assay.

Adverse reactions: Apart from the rare allergy, all other adverse actions of ACTH are due to increased secretion of adrenocorticosteroids. Further, *ACTH obtained from the animal pituitaries* contains significant amounts of vasopressin, which can lead to hyponatremia; *it is no more recommended.*

Preparations and dosage :

Synthetic ACTH (Cosyntropin, Synacthen, Cortrosyn) : This contains the first 24 of the 39 amino acids of natural ACTH, and shows similar pharmacological actions. The biological activity of 1 mg. is equal to 10 units of the natural preparation. The preparations are:

(i) Cosyntropin solution, 250 mcg for IM or IV injection (Synacthen).

(ii) Cosyntropin zinc-phosphate suspension, 1.0 mg (Synacthen Depot) IM.

Cosyntropin solution is used to perform the Short ACTH Stimulation Test (see below). Cosyntropin-zinc-phosphate suspension is used to prime the adrenal cortex by 1.0 mg IM daily for 3 days before the short ACTH stimulation test, in order to distinguish between primary and secondary adrenocortical failure.

Uses of ACTH:

- ***Diagnostic*:** Short ACTH stimulation test is performed by injecting 250 mcg of cosyntropin IM or as an IV bolus and measuring plasma cortisol at 60 minutes; a level of 18 mcg/dl or higher indicates normal functioning of the HPA axis.

It has no therapeutic uses.

Hormones of the Adrenal Cortex

The adrenal cortex is divided into three zones which elaborate *corticosteroids* (mineralocorticoids and glucocorticoids) and weak *androgens*. The zones are:

- ***Zona glomerulosa*** which elaborates aldosterone and desoxycorticosterone (mineralocorticoids).
- ***Zona fasciculata*** which secretes cortisol (glucocorticoid); it synthesizes but does not secrete cortisone; and
- ***Zona reticularis*** which forms dehydroepiandrosterone (DHEA) and androstenedione (androgens) and traces of estrogens.

Chemistry and synthesis: The adrenal cortical hormones are steroids (Fig. 64.1) consisting of cyclopentanophenanthrene ring with various functional groups (-H, -CH3, -OH, = O) attached to different carbon atoms. All steroid hormones have similar basic structure, with relatively minor differences which, however, cause striking alteration in their biological activity. They are sparingly soluble in water and circulate in association with binding proteins.

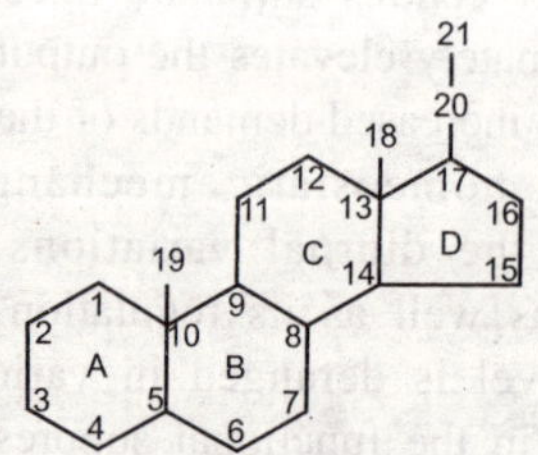

Fig. 64.1: Cyclopentanophenanthrene ring

All the steroids can be synthesized basically from 2-carbon acetate chains via cholesterol. Cholesterol is converted through pregnenolone to progesterone. Progesterone is an intermediary in the synthesis of other steroids and is not secreted by the adrenal cortex. After progesterone, the synthetic pathways for the three groups of hormones separate out. (Fig. 64.2). These steroids are secreted into the blood as they are formed, and are not stored in the adrenal cortex in any significant quantities. Administered cortisone is converted in the body to the active compound cortisol.

Table 64.1 shows secretory rates of the

Table 64.1: Secretory rates of adrenocortical hormones in humans

Hormone	Secretory rate (mg./day)
Cortisol	10
Aldosterone	0.05-0.2
Corticosterone	2-4
DHEAS	7-15
D^4 Androstenedione	1-1.5

physiologically important adrenocortical hormones.

The various steps in the synthesis of these steroids are governed by specific enzymes. These enzymes, especially those concerned in synthesis of cortisol, are sometimes congenitally deficient, leading to a deficiency of cortisol and an excess of ACTH and the adrenal androgens.

Steroidal synthesis can be reduced by :

- ***Metyrapone*** which selectively inhibits synthesis of cortisol and corticosterone. It was used for testing adrenal function.
- ***Aminoglutethimide*** which acts by blocking the conversion of cholesterol to pregnenolone. It reduces the synthesis of all steroid hormones.
- ***Ketoconazole***, an antifungal agent, which is a nonselective inhibitor of adrenal and gonadal steroid synthesis. It is sometimes used in Cushing syndrome; and
- ***Mitotane,*** an anticancer drug, which causes necrosis of the adrenal cortex (see "Chapter 59).

Mifepristone, an antiprogestin, (Chapter 66) which in large doses blocks the glucocorticoid receptors. It has been used in Cushing syndrome due to adrenal carcinoma.

Regulation of the secretion of adrenal cortical hormones: The rate of secretion of the glucocorticoids is regulated by the variations in the blood levels of ACTH. Although exogenously administered ACTH increases the secretion of aldosterone, physiologically aldosterone output is independent of ACTH. Aldosterone secretion is mainly regulated by Angiotensin II, and serum potassium levels. A reduction in salt intake and a contraction of circulating blood volume are potent stimuli, via the *rennin-angiotensin I -angiotensin II pathway*, to aldosterone secretion (Chapters 24 and 30). Increase in the intake of potassium stimulates aldosterone synthesis and release.

Metabolism and excretion of adrenal corticoids: The adrenal corticoids circulate in the plasma partly free and mostly bound to cortisol binding protein. The former is the biologically active form, the latter, a reserve form. These steroids are metabolized in the liver and the metabolites are excreted in the urine as conjugates of sulfuric and glucuronic acids. The corticosteroids being water insoluble, are excreted in the urine only in traces. The urinary metabolites can be estimated as neutral 17-ketosteroids and 17-ketogenic steroids. (Fig. 64.2). Aldosterone is excreted in urine partly as free aldosterone and partly as conjugates of tetrahydroaldosterone.

Glucocorticoids and Mineralocorticoids

Adrenocorticoids exert a wide variety of physiological effects and pharmacological actions. They enable the organism to withstand various noxious stimuli and environmental changes termed as 'stress'. In the absence of the adrenal cortex, survival is possible only under rigidly controlled and protected conditions wherein food and salt are available in plenty at all times and the environmental temperature is regulated. When exposed to 'stress', the adrenalectomized animal dies quickly unless pre-treated with a glucocorticoid. Under optimum conditions, a small dose of hydrocortisone is sufficient to maintain such animal in a state of well being, while under conditions of 'stress' larger doses of steroids

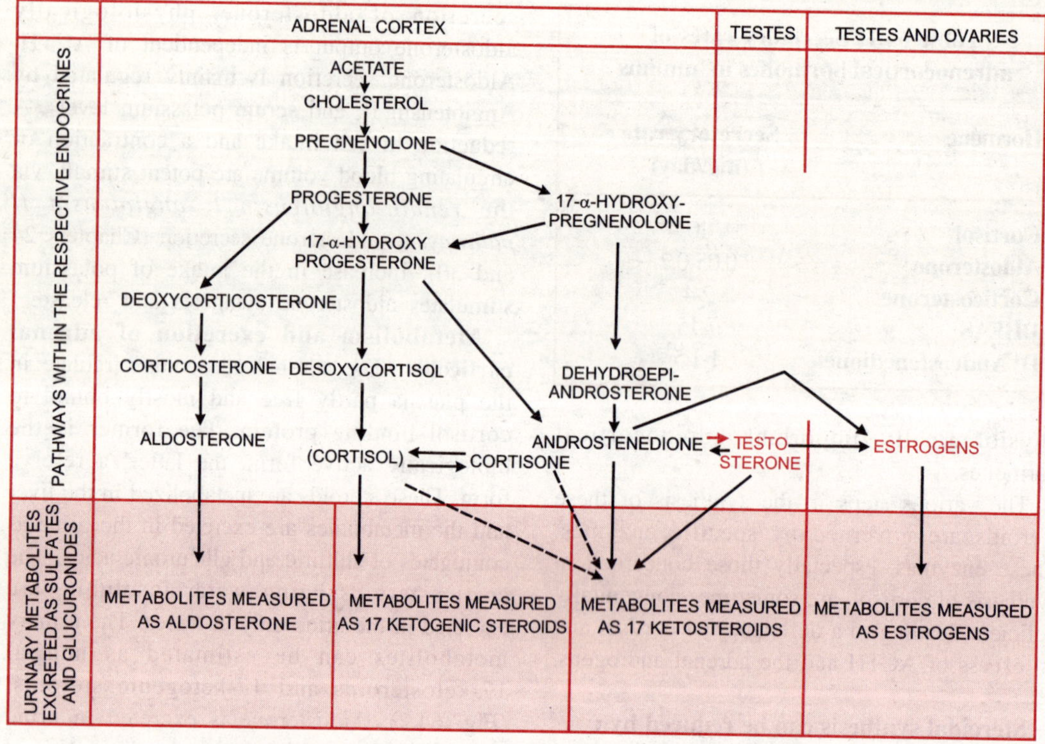

Fig. 64.2: Synthesis and metabolism of steroid hormones

are needed for survival; if given to healthy animals, they produce 'hypercortisolism'.

Experimental evaluation of synthetic steroids: The easily quantifiable actions of adrenocorticoids are :

- ***Sodium retention in adrenalectomized animals.***
- ***Liver glycogen deposition.***
- ***Suppression of H-P-A axis***; and
- ***Anti-inflammatory action.***

The ability of a corticosteroid to maintain life in an adrenalectomized animal parallels its sodium retaining potency. On the other hand, the potencies based on suppression of HPA axis, liver glycogen deposition, anti-inflammatory action, work capacity of the skeletal muscles and involution of the lymphoid tissue parallel one another. There can be, however, in the case of synthetic steroids, a dissociation between sodium retaining potency and liver glycogen deposition potency.

A corticosteroid with predominantly sodium retaining effects is called a **mineralocorticoid** e.g. aldosterone and desoxycorticosterone. A corticosteroid with predominantly liver glycogen depositing and neoglucogenetic action is called a **glucocorticoid** e.g. hydrocortisone, cortisone and most of the newer synthetic steroids. Corticosterone, a natural corticosteroid and 9-alpha-fluorohydrocortisone, a synthetic steroid, have marked mineralocorticoid as well as some glucocorticoid activities.

Structure-activity relationship : The natural glucocorticoids like cortisone and cortisol are pregnane derivatives with ketone groups at 3 and 20, a hydroxyl group at 21 and are unsaturated between carbon atoms 4 and 5 (Fig. 64.1). Introduction of an aldehyde group in the 18th position increases the mineralocorticoid potential markedly, e.g. aldosterone. The anti-inflammatory and glucocorticoid potency is markedly increased by introduction of a double bond between 1 and 2 carbon atoms as in prednisone or prednisolone, by alpha-methylation in the 6 position as in 6 alpha methyl prednisolone and by 9 alpha fluorination and substitution at 16 position as in triamcinolone, dexamethasone and betamethasone.

GLUCOCORTICOIDS: The important glucocorticoid secreted in man is cortisol. It has some mineralocorticoid activity too. Since the pharmacological actions of hydrocortisone (cortisol) are, in fact, its physiological actions, they are discussed together.

Mechanism of action : Glucocorticoids enter the cell as free molecules and bind to cytosolic steroid receptors; the complex translocates to the nucleus and the steroid binds to the glucocorticoid responsive element (GRE) in the regulatory region of the concerned gene. This leads to transcription of mRNA which is exported to the cytoplasm. In the cytoplasm., the mRNA causes translation of proteins responsible for the hormonal synthesis.

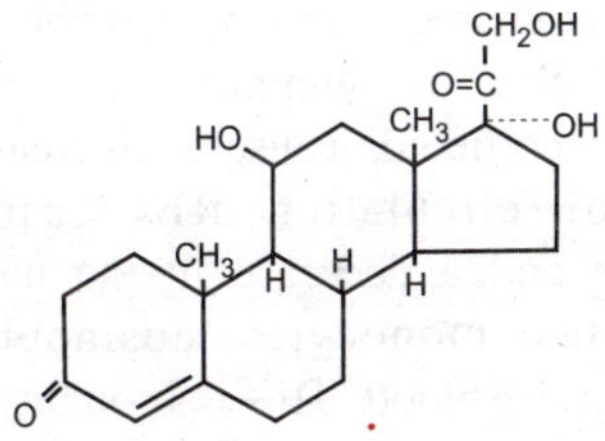

Fig. 64.3: Hydrocortisone

Pharmacological actions: Glucocorticoids exert a variety of physiological effects and pharmacological actions. Those effects of corticosteroids that involve concerted actions with other regulatary hormones are termed *permissive.* They probably reflect the steroid-induced changes in synthesis of proteins that modify the tissue response to the other hormones.

Metabolic effects: The glucocorticoids affect the metabolism of carbohydrates, proteins, fats, electrolytes, water and calcium.

• ***Carbohydrate and protein metabolism*:** Glucocorticoids inhibit the peripheral utilization of glucose by skeletal muscle and adipose tissue. Further, they inhibit the incorporation of amino acids into protein in the peripheral tissues (*antianabolic action*) and stimulate their conversion into glucose (*neoglucogenesis*) in the liver. The plasma amino acid level rises significantly due to muscle catabolism. Simultaneously, the plasma glucagon level also rises markedly during chronic but not acute administration. All this helps to maintain an adequate glucose supply to the brain.

The adrenalectomized animal cannot maintain normal blood sugar level while fasting; while chronic administration of glucocorticoids causes hyperglycemia and glycosuria.

In physiological doses, glucocorticoids stimulate protein and RNA synthesis in the liver; large supraphysiological doses cause catabolic and antianabolic effects in the skin, muscles, lymphoid and connecting tissues. This leads to wasting of muscle, thinning of the skin and osteoporosis.

• ***Fat metabolism*:** Glucocorticoids play a 'permissive' role in the mobilization of fat from the peripheral fat depots by adrenaline and GH. Prolonged administration of excessive glucocorticoid causes a re-distribution of body fat, with a loss from the extremities and a deposition in the neck (**buffalo hump**), supraclavicular area and face (**moon face**). The mechanism of this re-distribution is not known. Plasma lipids are not changed consistently in either hypocorticism or hypercorticism.

• ***Electrolyte and water metabolism*:** Hydrocortisone has a relatively weak salt retaining and potassium wasting effect. However, when large doses (300 mg./24 hours) are used, sufficient salt retention occurs to make the concurrent use of a mineralocorticoid unnecessary. Twenty-five mg of hydrocortisone has the same mineralocorticoid activity as 0.1 mg of fludrocortisone. The potent synthetic steroids, dexamethasone, betamethasone and triamcinolone, produce marked sodium loss in the urine.

Cortisol is essential for excreting a water load. Adrenalectomized animals cannot excrete a water load and tend to develop water intoxication. This defect is corrected by a glucocorticoid.

• ***Calcium metabolism and bone***: In pharmacological doses, glucocorticoids antagonize the action of vitamin D on the gut and reduce absorption of calcium. Large doses for prolonged periods may interfere with the development of cartilage and inhibit linear growth in children. As a result of the protein catabolic action, glucocorticoids inhibit formation of new bony tissue. Hence, the continuous resorption which occurs as a part of bone remodelling leads to severe osteoporosis in chronic states of hypercorticism.

Cardiovascular system: The important cardiovascular changes which occur in adrenal insufficiency are partly due to mineralocorticoid deficiency which acts through its effects on electrolyte and water metabolism, and partly due to glucocorticoid deficiency. Usually, the blood volume and blood pressure diminish and blood viscosity increases. These defects are only partially corrected by administration of sodium chloride and/or a mineralocorticoid. Addition of a glucocorticoid completely restores the circulation to normal.

The absence of glucocorticoids leads to increase in capillary permeability, inadequate vasomotor responses of smaller blood vessels and reduction in the cardiac output. Glucocorticoids potentiate the pressor response of blood vessels to adrenaline and NA by upregulating the adrenergic receptors in the vessel wall. In pharmacological doses, they have a positive inotropic action on the heart.

Hypertension is seen during chronic administration of glucocorticoids and in the patients with Cushing's syndrome. In the latter condition, it is an important cause of death.

Muscles: Permissive concentration of cortisol is necessary for the normal functioning of the skeletal muscle. Muscular weakness is a feature of Addison's disease. It is largely due to inability of the circulatory system to respond to the stress of exercise. It is specifically corrected by a glucocorticoid. On the other hand, the muscle weakness of hypercortisolism is due to hypokalemia and to muscle wasting (**steroid myopathy**) (see later).

Central nervous system: Patients with Addison's disease show apathy, depression, irritability and sometimes psychosis. All these are corrected by a glucocorticoid.

Patients on large doses of glucocorticoids may show mood elevation, euphoria, nervousness, restlessness, depression and even psychosis. These are all reversible.

Hematological action: Hyperplasia of the lymphoid tissue and peripheral lymphocytosis are seen in Addison's disease while Cushing's syndrome is characterized by lymphocytopenia and dissolution of lymphatic masses in the body. Glucocorticoids cause an increase in the number of circulating RBCs, platelets, neutrophils and a decrease in the number of lymphocytes, monocytes, eosinophils and basophils in the blood. This is brought about by a redistribution of the cells between the blood and other compartments; there is no lysis of lymphocytes in normal persons. However, in patients with acute lymphoblastic leukemia, the lymphocytes are rapidly destroyed by the corticosteroids. A mild secondary polycythemia is common in Cushing's syndrome.

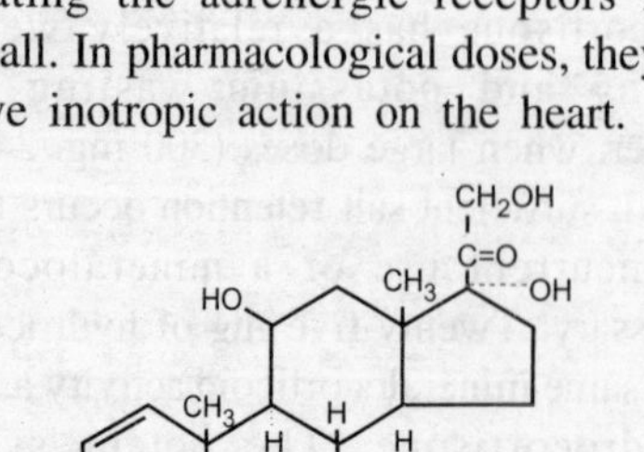

CH_2OH, C=O, CH_3, OH, HO, CH_3, H, H, H, O

Fig. 64.4 : Prednisolone

CH_2OH, C=O, CH_3, OH, OH, CH_3, CH_3, H, H, F, O

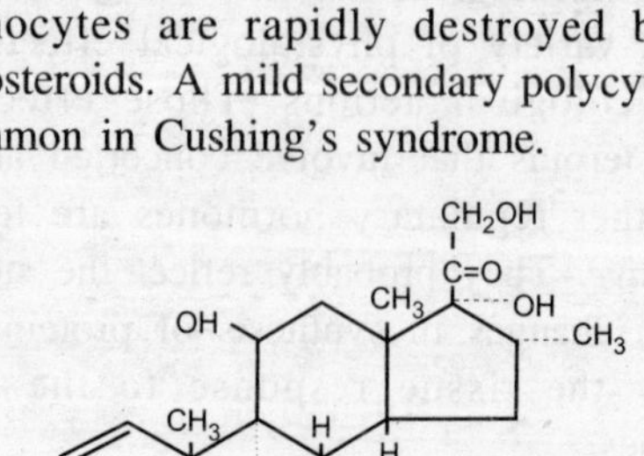

Fig. 64.5 : Dexamethasone

GI tract: Glucocorticoids increase both basal and nocturnal gastric acid secretion; and inhibit the secretion of prostacyclin.

Antiinflammatory action: Glucocorticoids prevent or suppress the symptoms and signs of inflammation such as local heat, redness, swelling and tenderness. At the tissue level, they suppress the *early phenomena* (edema, fibrin deposition, capillary dilatation, and migration of phagocytes into the inflamed area) as well as the *late manifestations* (capillary proliferation, fibroblastic proliferation, deposition of collagen and cicatrization). They interfere with wound healing. Fibrous tissue, once formed, is not affected.

The mechanisms which possibly contribute to their **anti-inflammatory action** are :

(a) The inflammatory process involves migration of leucocytes into the affected tissue. This is inhibited by glucocorticoids, leading to suppression of the proinflammatory cytokines and chemokines.

(b) Glucocorticoids diminish the neutrophil and monocyte functions viz. chemotaxis and lysosomal enzyme synthesis. This decreases the recruitment of neutrophils and macrophages into the affected area.

(c) They inhibit the release of arachidonic acid from phospholipids by inhibiting the enzyme phospholipase-A_2, (see Figure in Chapter 24) and hence diminish the production of PGs, LTs, PAF and related compounds which play an important role in inflammation. They also decrease capillary permeability by reducing the amount of histamine released by the basophils and mast cells.

(d) At high concentrations, they stabilize lysosomal membranes, thus preventing the spillage of hydrolytic enzymes.

This anti-inflammatory effect of glucocorticoids forms the basis for their clinical use in many different conditions.

Immunosuppressive and anti-allergic actions: Glucocorticoids in large therapeutic doses (40-60 mg. of prednisolone per day):

- ***Inhibit the function of macrophages*** and reduce their ability to respond to antigens. This affects phagocytosis and bactericidal action. Further, production of TNFα, some interleukins and interferons is reduced.
- ***Inhibit the activation of cytotoxic T lymphocytes and their proliferation***; they cause transient peripheral lymphopenia.
- ***Cause lysis of the T lymphocytes.***
- ***In humans, the complement is not affected but its effects are inhibited.***
- ***Suppress cell-mediated hypersensitivity reaction. The glucocorticoid doses that modify CMI usually do not suppress the antibody production. (Humoral immunity)***; and
- ***Prevent homograft rejection;***

Large doses (100-200 mg. of prednisolone/ day) diminish the effective concentration of specific IgG antibodies.

Although glucocorticoids do not, in moderate doses, interfere with antibody production or with antigen-antibody union nor with the liberation of histamine from the tissues damaged by such union, they suppress the inflammatory response to it. This last action is important in the suppression of such allergic phenomena as urticaria, allergic rhinitis and bronchial asthma.

Clinically, glucocorticoids modify the course of many diseases involving the immune responses. Although they do not modify the basic disease process, they suppress the inflammatory response to injury and thus, protect the tissues. However, *they increase the susceptibility to a variety of bacterial, fungal, viral and parasitic superinfections.*

It was thought in the past that the antiinflammatory and immunosuppressive actions of glucocorticoids were limited to pharmacological doses. It is now realized that glucocorticoids produced normally, as a part of the response to stress, exert a beneficial antiinflammatory-immunosuppressive effect and help to limit the damage caused by such reactions. Further, they may prevent possible cardiovascular collapse due to the depressant action of released immune mediators on the vascular tone (physiological action).

Miscellaneous actions: Glucocorticoids have uricosuric and non-specific antipyretic effects. Their analgesic effect depends upon their anti-inflammatory action. Glucocorticoids markedly increase the activity of phenylethanolamine-N-methyltransferase, an enzyme located almost exclusively in the adrenal medulla and which catalyses the conversion of NA to adrenaline. They play an important role in the structural and functional maturation of the fetal lung.

Inhibition of HPA axis: *Glucocorticoids given in supraphysiological doses for longer than 1 week suppress the HPA axis and cause adrenocortical atrophy.* Such patients, during therapy, and for long periods (as long as 12 months) thereafter, are unable to increase the endogenous cortisol output in response to stress. During this period the pituitary function recovers first; plasma ACTH progressively reaches supranormal levels in 4-5 months. Only then the atrophic adrenal cortex starts recovering its function. But it can take the HPA axis as long as 8-12 months to be able to respond normally to stress. *This recovery of the HPA axis is not accelerated by administration of exogenous ACTH.* However, physiological doses of a glucocorticoid (20 mg. of hydrocortisone or 5 mg. of prednisolone, per day) may be used for prolonged periods after cessation of prolonged, large dose glucocorticoid therapy, without interfering with the recovery of HPA axis.

Patients who are on small doses of any glucocorticoid (20 mg. of hydrocortisone or equivalent doses of other glucocorticoids per day) and those who are on high doses of intermediate acting glucocorticoids (see Table 64.2) **on alternate days** show little or no suppression of the HPA axis. When large doses are used daily and for prolonged periods, the suppression is most marked when the entire daily dose is given at bed time and is least when it is given on rising in the morning. The other advantage of the alternate day therapy is the minimization of the nitrogen and calcium imbalance. It, therefore, permits safer administration of much larger total dosage of glucocorticoids. Hence, whenever possible, in patients requiring high-dose, prolonged glucocorticoid therapy, *the* **alternate day regimen** should be attempted. *Because of their very prolonged action, the long acting glucocorticoids are not suitable for alternate day administration.*

The long acting compounds, however, are eminently suited for uniform and continuous suppression of ACTH secretion in the syndrome of congenital, virilizing, adrenocortical hyperplasia. As the peak secretion of ACTH occurs at night (in this condition as in normal persons), the entire daily dose of the long acting glucocorticoid should be given at bedtime.

Patients on long term glucocorticoid treatment should be considered to be suffering from adrenal insufficiency and during stress the dose of the glucocorticoid should be increased.

- ***During minor stress***, such as a febrile illness, severe exercise, bouts of gastroenteritis with vomiting and diarrhoea, and minor surgery, the normal adrenals respond by secreting about 100 mg. of hydrocortisone per day; this then is the requirement of hydrocortisone (or an equivalent dose of another glucocorticoid) during such situations. The dose can be abruptly reduced to the maintenance dose as soon as the stressful event is over.
- ***During major stress***, such as major surgery, severe burns and MI, the daily requirement of 300-400 mg. of cortisol can be met with by giving 100 mg. by IV infusion every six to eight hours on the first day. From the next day onwards, the dose is halved every day till the physiological maintenance dose is reached, if the recovery is uneventful. In case of doubt about the grading of the stress as minor or major, it is safer to use the larger dose.

While withdrawing long term glucocorticoid therapy, the reduction upto the physiological maintenance dose may be as rapid as the disease will permit. Too rapid a reduction can cause (a) a flare up of the disease under treatment; and (b) nonspecific 'withdrawal symptoms' comprising fever, malaise, myalgia and arthralgia.

After reaching the physiological maintenance dose, it should be continued upto 1 year in order to allow the HPA axis to recover its function fully; during this period, any stressful situation is covered by larger doses of a glucocorticoid as detailed above; failure to do so may precipitate an acute adrenal crisis. *Patients undergoing surgery should always be asked for history of glucocorticoid therapy during the past 1 year.*

The placenta metabolizes hydrocortisone and prednisolone to the inactive cortisone and prednisone. Unlike the mother, the fetus cannot convert cortisone and prednisone to hydrocortisone and prednisolone. By contrast, dexamethasone and betamethasone cross the placenta to achieve high concentrations in the fetal circulation and can suppress the fetal HPA axis. *Therefore, if a pregnant woman needs treatment with a glucocorticoid, prednisolone should be used in preference to dexamethasone and betamethasone.*

Absorption, fate and excretion of hydrocortisone and the synthetic glucocorticoids: The oral bioavailability of hydrocortisone is about 50% and variable (30-90%) on administration as an enema. The absorption from aqueous suspension of acetate given IM is slower than that of orally administered hydrocortisone and hence the effect lasts longer. Absorption of prednisolone is almost complete (80 - 100%) after both oral and rectal administration. It is worth noting that as much as 50% of intraarticular prednisolone, administered in patients with rheumatoid arthritis, is absorbed into systemic circulation. Dexamethasone is well absorbed (80%) on oral administration. The bioavailability of oral methylprednisolone is variable (50 - 80%).

Cortisone acts in the body after conversion to hydrocortisone, and prednisone to prednisolone, in the liver.

Hydrocortisone is highly protein bound in the plasma and so is prednisolone. Dexamethasone is less protein bound than hydrocortisone.

Table 64.2: Comparison of various glucocorticoids

Drug	Biological half-life (hours)	Glucocorticoid activity	Mineralocorticoid activity	Pituitary suppression	Comparative doses*(mg.)	Affinity**
Short acting						
Cortisone	8-12	0.8	1	1	25	1
Hydrocortisone	8-12	1	1.25	2.5	20	100
Intermediate acting						
Prednisolone	18-36	4	0.5	5	5	220
Methylprednisolone	18-36	5	0	8	4	1350
Triamcinolone	18-36	5	0	—	4	—
Long acting						
Dexamethasone	36-54	25	0	100-200	0.75	540
Betamethasone	36-54	25	0	100-200	0.75	400

* These dose relationships apply to oral and intravenous administration of these compounds but not to intramuscular or intra-articular administration of these compounds or their derivatives.

** Affinity for human, intracellular, glucocorticoid receptor.

Therapeutic efficacy in inflammatory disorders is proportional to the glucocorticoid activity.

Hydrocortisone is largely metabolized by conversion to tetrahydrocortisone and conjugation; prednisolone by hydroxylation and conjugation. The pharmacokinetic parameters of methylprednisolone are similar to those of prednisolone.

The concentration of prednisolone in breast milk is about 10% that of plasma concentration, and no restriction on breast feeding is considered necessary when the mother is receiving upto 20 mg. of prednisolone per day.

The biological t½ of the glucocorticoids and their relative affinity for human, intracellular, glucocorticoid receptor are given in Table 64.2.

Adverse reactions: These are related to individual susceptibility, dosage and duration of therapy.

Single large doses, prednisolone 1-2 mg/kg or equivalent doses of other glucocorticoids, are harmless and may, therefore, be used without hesitation in situations where life is threatened by adrenocortical or pituitary insufficiency or by cerebral edema. **Short term therapy** *(generally 1-2 weeks)* with small or moderate doses is unlikely to produce any harmful effects.

Prolonged therapy with glucocorticoids in doses higher than 20-30 mg. of hydrocortisone or equivalent doses of other steroids per day is liable to cause adverse effects. Hence, this is the generally recommended maximum maintenance dose in prolonged glucocorticoid therapy. *The only exception is life threatening conditions* where doses large enough to suppress the clinical manifestations of the disease are needed, and then one accepts adverse effects as the price one has to pay for keeping the patient alive.

The ADR, other than sodium retention, are shared by all glucocorticoids. However, certain adverse effects seem to be unique to triamcinolone; these are : anorexia; muscle wasting; weight loss; sedation and depression. *It should be avoided in renal diseases.*

The important adverse effects of glucocorticoid therapy are :

- ***Gastrointestinal tract*:** Acute erosive gastritis with hemorrhage may occur during intensive therapy, and peptic ulceration may be troublesome during prolonged therapy. Intestinal perforation and pancreatitis are the other reported GI complications.
- ***Endocrine system*:** These are an extension of their pharmacological actions and comprise hypercortisolism.
- ***Metabolic effects*:** Clinical manifestations (including, ketoacidosis and non-ketotic, hyperglycemic, hyperosmolar coma) of idiopathic diabetes mellitus can be precipitated. *Pre-existing diabetes, however, is not an absolute contraindication to glucocorticoid therapy and development of hyperglycemia during therapy in itself does not warrant cessation of treatment.* Some patients develop hyperlipidemia and hypophosphatemia.

Prolonged therapy causes central obesity with moon face and buffalo hump. Pink florid striae appear on the abdomen, hips and pectoral regions and the skin may become friable. The patient may get spontaneous ecchymosis and bruise easily (**Cushingoidism**).

- ***Suppression of inflammation and immune responses*:** Glucocorticoids may mask the clinical features of a serious illness e.g. fever and abdominal rigidity may be absent when a patient on these drugs develops acute peritonitis, which may, therefore, be missed. Further, preexisting infections like tuberculosis can spread and superinfection with other organisms can occur.
- ***Retardation of linear growth*** occurs in children who receive high doses. In equivalent therapeutic doses prednisolone is twice and dexa-and beta-methasone are thrice as growth inhibiting as hydrocortisone. Mean estimated doses of glucocorticoids (mg/M^2/24 hours), optimal for growth in children with congenital adrenal hyperplasia are: cortisone acetate 22 (oral), 14 (IM); hydrocortisone 18.4; prednisone 3.7; methylprednisolone 2.4 and dexamethasone 0.23.
- ***Cardio-vascular and renal system*:** Hypertension, salt and water retention and

rarely hypokalemic alkalosis can occur. They are uncommon with dexamethasone, betamethasone and triamcinolone.

● *CNS :* Glucocorticoids readily enter the brain and can influence mood, sleep patterns and EEG activity; patients may complain of insomnia. Acute psychotic reactions may occur especially during intensive therapy. Benign intracranial hypertension and aggravation of epilepsy particularly in children can occur.

● ***Musculoskeletal effects***: Proximal myopathy and osteoporosis with compression fractures of the vertebrae are serious complications. Biphosphonates are reported to prevent the osteoporosis. Rarely, acute avascular necrosis of bone may occur.

● ***Eyes***: Glaucoma occurs in some patients during local glucocorticoid therapy, and posterior subcapsular cataract has been reported during their long term systemic use.

● ***Miscellaneous changes***: These include hypercoagulability of blood with thromboembolic complications, acne, hirsutism, loss of scalp hair, subcutaneous atrophy and delayed wound healing.

Rapid IV injection of large pulse doses (see later) can cause flushing of the face and chest, vasoactive reaction, cardiac arrest and seizures.

The **Cushingoidism** produced by glucocorticoid therapy differs in certain respects from Cushing's syndrome produced by endogenous hypercortisolism. Pseudotumour cerebri, glaucoma, cataract, pancreatitis, aseptic necrosis of bone, panniculitis and vasculitis are almost unique to the iatrogenic form of Cushing's syndrome.

There are certain differences between the adverse effects of ACTH and glucocorticoids. With oral glucocorticoid therapy dyspepsia, gastric complications, bruising, striae formation, loss of muscle mass and osteoporosis are more common. With ACTH, on the other hand, there is a higher incidence of hypertension, pigmentation, hirsutism and acne.

Table 64.3 shows the important *adverse reactions to topical use of glucocorticoids* on the skin. They are especially likely to occur :

Table 64.3: Adverse skin reactions to topical glucocorticoids

- Epidermal and dermal atrophy (thinning of the skin, striae, telangiectases superficial fissures and purpura).
- Acne, folliculitis, miliaria.
- Hypertrichosis.
- Hypopigmentation.
- Allergic contact dermatitis (uncommon).
- Rebound of the lesion under treatment, on abrupt withdrawal especially of the potent steroids.
- Masking or aggravation of dermatophytoses, impetigo or scabies.

(a) In infants, children and the elderly.

(b) With the use of potent steroids, especially when used in large doses for prolonged periods.

(c) With the use of occlusive dressings; and

(d) When used in areas such as the face with thin skin.

Drug interactions : See Table 64.4.

Synthetic glucocorticoids: The synthetic glucocorticoids include prednisone, prednisolone, triamcinolone, paramethasone, dexamethasone, betamethasone and 6-methylprednisolone (Table 64.2). Prednisone is converted in the body to the active compound prednisolone. The last four synthetic steroids show negligible or almost absent mineralocorticoid activity. However, none is superior to prednisone and prednisolone with respect to the peptic ulceration, osteoporosis and hyperglycemia. All of them are potent pituitary inhibitors. In addition, triamcinolone has a greater propensity to cause myopathy while the incidence of increased capillary fragility and echymosis is more with triamcinolone, dexamethasone and betamethasone.

The synthetic glucocorticoids are rapidly absorbed orally. Their long-acting esters used topically and intra-articular injection are poorly absorbed. Like hydrocortisone, they are metabolized by the liver but more slowly.

Table 64.4: Drug interactions of glucocorticoids

- ***Glucocorticoid dosage is decreased:*** Antibiotics (erythromycin, trioleandomycin), cyclosporin, isoniazid and ketoconazole reduce the metabolic clearance of glucocorticoids. Estrogens increase the levels of corticosteroid binding protein and thus reduce the free fraction; they also reduce the clearance.
- ***Glucocorticoid dosage is increased*:** Cholestyramine decreases the intestinal absorption. Antiepileptic drugs (barbiturates, phenytoin, carbamazemine), rifampicin, aminoglutethimide increase the metabolism by inducing hepatic microsomal enzymes.
- ***Glucocorticoid dosage needs adjustment*:** Antianxiety and antipsychotic drugs: Recurrent or poor control of CNS symptoms due to inherent glucocorticoid effects.
- ***Anticholinesterases:*** May precipitate myasthenic crisis.
- ***Anticoagulants*:** Effectiveness of anticoagulants decreases.
- ***Antihypertensives*:** Their effectiveness decreases.
- ***Oral hypoglycemics*:** Their effectiveness decreases.
- ***Sympathomimetics*:** Their effectiveness increases.
- ***Salicylates*:** Their clearance is increased.

The synthetic steroids have pharmacological actions and adverse effects identical with those of hydrocortisone except the mineralocorticoid actions. They are less extensively protein bound than hydrocortisone and hence diffuse more completely into the tissues. They are effective in smaller doses. Such smaller doses, however, should not be construed to give them any superiority over the older preparations as in equivalent therapeutic doses their adverse effects are similar. Another advantage of the newer steroids is that it has been possible to prepare a variety of their esters suitable for topical application and local injection into tissues.

Preparations and dosage of glucocorticoids:

- ***For systemic use:***

(i) Cortisone acetate (Corlin) tablets, 25 mg. Dose : 25-37.5 mg (replacement therapy).

(ii) Cortisone injection, a suspension of cortisone acetate (25 mg. per ml.). Dose: 50 to 200 mg. daily IM in single or divided doses.

(iii) Hydrocortisone tablet 10 mg. and 20 mg.

(iv) Hydrocortisone hemisuccinate (Efcorlin) being readily water soluble is administered IM, by IV infusion or as a retention enema. Approximately 133 mg. of the salt contains 100 mg. of hydrocortisone. Hydrocortisone 100 mg by IV bolus lasts for 4 hours only. A continuous infusion 4 mg/hour provides adequate plasma levels (30-40 mcg/dl) for surgical cover. For retention enema, a dose equivalent to 100 mg. of hydrocortisone, dissolved in 120 ml. of normal saline is given each night.

(v) Prednisone tablet 5 mg. or as an equivalent amount of prednisone acetate. Dose: 10 to 100 mg. daily in divided doses.

(vi) Prednisolone tablet 5 mg. or an equivalent amount of prednisolone acetate. Dose: 10 to 100 mg. daily in divided doses.

(vii) Prednisolone acetate suspension 25 mg. per ml. It is administered by IM, intra-articular or peri-articular injection.

(viii) Prednisolone or prednisone pediatric drops 5 mg. of prednisolone or prednisone per ml. Dose : new-born, 0.3 to 0.4 mg. per kg. per dose; infants, 0.2 to 0.3 mg. per kg. per dose; older children, 0.15 to 0.2 mg. per kg. per dose.

(ix) Prednisolone sodium phosphate., in contrast to prednisolone or its acetate, is soluble in water. Approximately 27 mg. of the salt are equivalent to 20 mg. of prednisolone. Dose : equivalent to 20-100 mg. of prednisolone IV and 20 mg. by retention enema.

(x) Methylprednisolone 4 mg. tablets. Dose : 2-40 mg. daily in divided doses.

(xi) Methylprednisolone sodium succinate (Inj. Medrol). Dose : equivalent to 40-120 mg. of methyl-prednisolone base IM or IV, 40 to 120 mg. as a retention enema; pulse dose 500-1000 mg. by slow IV infusion.

(xii) Methylprednisolone acetate injection (Depot Medrol) for IM use.

(xiii) Triamcinolone tablet (Kenacort) 4 mg. Dose : 2-24 mg. daily in divided doses.

(xiv) Triamcinolone diacetate injection for IM or intra-articular use. Dose : 5 to 40 mg.

(xv) Betamethasone tablet (Betnelan) 0.5 mg. Dose : 0.5 to 5 mg. daily.

(xvi) Betamethasone sodium phosphate, a water soluble salt is available as tablets and for injection (Betnesol); nearly 1.3 mg. of the salt is equivalent to 1 mg. of betamethasone. Dose: equivalent to 0.5 to 5 mg. of betamethasone by mouth; for acute adrenal insufficiency, 10 to 20 mg. by IV or IM injection daily in divided doses.

(xvii) Dexamethasone tablet (Decadron) 0.5 mg. Doses similar to betamethasone tablets.

(xviii) Dexamethasone 21-phosphate injection (Decadron injection) contains 4 mg. of the salt per ml. Roughly 1.3 mg. of the salt is equivalent to 1 mg. of the base. Dose : 4 to 20 mg. of the base by IM or IV injection.

• ***For topical use***: Numerous preparations containing either the glucocorticoids alone or in combination with antibiotics are available for topical therapy. The *topical skin preparations* can be divided into four groups in increasing order of potency (Table 64.5). The potency of the topical preparations is proportional to their ability to cause vasoconstriction and cutaneous blanching on local application.

Table 64.5: Topical glucocorticoid preparations

Mild: Hydrocortisone 1% (Wycort)

Moderately potent: Clobetasone butyrate 0.05% (Eumosone); Hydrocortisone 2.5% (Wycort).

Potent: Betamethasone valerate 0.1% (Betnovate); Hydrocortisone butyrate 0.1% (Lococid); Fluocinolone acetonide 0.025% (Flucort); Triamcinolone acetonide 0.2% (Ledercort).

Very potent: Clobetasol propionate 0.05% (Tenovate).

The skin preparations as creams or ointments and topical preparations for nasal, conjunctival and intra-articular use are available.

Beclomethasone dipropionate, budesonide and fluticasone as inhaled steroids in bronchial asthma are discussed in Chapter 26.

Hydrocortisone oral paste 0.5% (Orabase HCA) may be useful in treating painful, nonherpetic, oral ulcers.

Therapeutic uses of glucocorticoids: These can be divided into:

I **Substitution therapy: This is used in the management of adrenocortical (AC) insufficiency** arising from adrenal disease (**Addison's disease**; primary AC insufficiency) or hypopituitarism (secondary AC insufficiency). Either may be chronic or acute.

• ***Chronic adrenal insufficiency*** due to Addison's disease is treated with replacement doses of a glucocorticoid. They are given in a dose that reduces hyperpigmentation and abolishes postural hypotension which is the hallmark of adrenocortical insufficiency. Hydrocortisone with its moderate salt retaining property is preferred; however, as it is difficult to obtain, prednisolone in equivalent doses is used. Hydrocortisone is generally given in the dose of 30 mg. daily, divided into two doses, 20 mg. in the morning and 10 mg. in the evening. However, the replacement dose of hydrocortisone in Addison's disease may vary from 10 to 50 mg/day, because of its very short half life.

Once the patient is regulated on hydrocortisone, addition of 9-alpha-flurohydrocortisone (0.1 to 0.2 mg. daily) helps to complete the replacement therapy. Alternatively, the same purpose may be achieved by prescribing additional intake of salt (2-4 g. per day). *Additional quantities of salt must not be prescribed to patients taking mineralocorticoids.*

In patients with adrenocortical insufficiency secondary to hypopituitarism, smaller maintenance doses are sufficient; and a mineralocorticoid is not required.

It is essential to explain to the patient that treatment of this condition is lifelong and that it is dangerous to stop it abruptly. In times of stress, the dose must be rapidly increased 3 to 4 fold.

● ***Acute adrenal insufficiency*** may arise (a) as a result of an acute infection, injury or surgery in a previously known Addisonian patient; (b) as a result of abrupt withdrawal of glucocorticoids from a patient who is on large doses; or (c) in a fulminating meningococcal infection. It is a medical emergency requiring energetic and immediate treatment. The principles of therapy are shown in Table 64.6.

Table 64.6: Principles of treatment of acute adrenal insufficiency

- Hydrocortisone hemisuccinate by IV infusion, 100 mg every 4-6 hours.
- Dextrose in normal saline in adequate amounts.
- Vasopressor drugs to maintain blood pressure; and
- Antibiotics.

As the large doses of hydrocortisone cause sufficient salt retention, mineralocorticoids are not needed at this stage. Following recovery, 4th-5th day onwards, hydrocortisone is given orally in maintainance doses, together with 9-alpha-fluorohydro-cortisone.

● ***Septic shock :*** Chapter 31.

II **Pharmacological therapy :**

● ***Pulse therapy*:** Methylprednisolone IV, in dose of 150-300 mg., injected over ½ hour, once daily, for three consecutive days, is useful in threatened acute rejection of a renal graft, vision-threatening Graves' exophthalmos and similar dire emergencies. Methylprednisolone in similar IV doses for 3-5 days can shorten the duration of relapse, and accelerate recovery from an acute exacerbation of multiple sclerosis. Long term course of the disease is not altered. *Rapid IV administration of such large doses can cause cardiac arrhythmias.* High dose oral prednisolone is probably equally effective. The drug is combined with immunosuppressive and immunomodulatory drugs for reducing the frequency and severity of relapses in multiple sclerosis (Chapters 14 and 76).

● ***Intensive short term therapy*** can save life and reduce morbidity in certain potentially lethal conditions in which the inflammatory or the metabolic response of the body itself threatens life. These conditions include: allergic emergencies such as anaphylactic shock; status asthmaticus; circulatory collapse unresponsive to pressor amines; acute necrotizing vasculitis; water intoxication; central hyperthermia; and acute hypercalcemia accompanying vitamin D intoxication or hormone therapy of metastatic breast cancer. In status asthmaticus, the glucocorticoids take several hours to act and their use supplements that of the bronchodilators. In circulatory failure a single massive dose (preferably of a long acting compound) sometimes restores the blood pressure to normal. In hypercalcemic crisis, glucocorticoids take several days to reduce the plasma calcium and must be used along with other quicker acting measures. Glucocorticoids used as adjuncts have been shown to be effective in preventing or minimizing the long term sequelae (such as deafness) of acute bacterial meningitis.

In all these conditions, *large doses* such as 100-200 mg. (1-2 mg/kg/day) of prednisolone per day may have to be used but therapy with such doses seldom lasts longer than 48-72 hours. In such cases, the adverse effects mainly consist of burning and itching at the mucocutaneous junctions, and rarely of multifocal ventricular premature beats, precipitation of ketoacidotic coma in idiopathic diabetes, and acute erosive gastritis with hemorrhage.

● ***Cerebral edema:*** Glucocorticoids are life saving in cerebral edema due to neoplasms, either primary or metastatic. *Their value in treating cerebral edema due to head injury, stroke and cerebral malaria is unproven; in fact they may be harmful.* Also see Chapter 38.

• ***Prolonged, high-dose, suppressive therapy*** is indicated in severe acute rheumatic fever, severe ulcerative colitis, coeliac disease not responding to gluten-free diet, subacute hepatic necrosis, chronic active hepatitis, alcoholic hepatitis, autoimmune hemolytic anemia, idiopathic thrombocytopenic purpura, acute lymphatic leukemia, disseminated Hodgkin's disease, nephrotic syndrome, acute homograft rejection, pemphigus and collagen diseases. In these diseases, the initial dose may be as high as 100-200 mg. of prednisolone per day, the therapy continues longer than 7-10 days and the maintenance dose may be 15 mg. of prednisolone or more per day. The fear of adverse reactions is utmost in this group and the patients need close supervision. A rapid reduction in the dose can cause an acute exacerbation of the disease being treated. On the other hand, abrupt cessation is dangerous and can precipitate acute adrenocortical insufficiency; the patients must be warned about this possibility. In order to minimise the suppression of the HPA axis during such prolonged, high-dose therapy, the alternate day regime should be tried once the clinical improvement has stabilized; if it is unable to maintain the clinical remission, the entire daily dose may be given in the morning with the same objective in mind.

• ***Low-dose, chronic, palliative therapy*** consists of the use of small doses of a glucocorticoid (2-10 mg. of prednisolone per day) as an adjunct to some other drug e.g. salicylates in rheumatoid arthritis. Here, total relief of symptoms is not aimed at, in order to avoid the adverse effects of the glucocorticoid. *Such low-dose therapy should not be tried on alternate days as it is ineffective in controlling the disease adequately.* As the therapy is generally very prolonged, sometimes lifelong, the patients need close supervision. The dose of the glucocorticoid should be raised 2-4 times during such stress as surgery or a severe infection.

• ***Chronic, suppression of ACTH secretion*** is indicated in congenital, virilizing, adrenocortical hyperplasia. This is achieved with the use of a long acting compound such as dexamethasone or betamethasone in the dose of 0.5 mg. at bedtime daily. Such therapy adequately suppresses the plasma level of 17(OH) progesterone and rarely causes any adverse effects. It must be impressed upon the parents of such a child that the therapy must continue lifelong.

• ***Neonatal respiratory distress syndrome (prevention)***: Lung maturation in the fetus is influenced by fetal cortisol secretion. This may be affected by prematurity. Betamethasone is administered to pregnant women in the dose of 12 mg, to be repeated after 18-24 hours (Chapter 43), to prevent neonatal respiratory distress syndrome when delivery is anticipated before the 34th week of gestation (preterm).

• ***Topical application*** is valuable in many dermatological, ocular and external ear conditions. Ocular conditions benefited by local therapy are interstitial keratitis, phlyctenular conjunctivitis, spring catarrh, iritis and iridocyclitis, whereas, posterior uveitis and sympathetic ophthalmia need systemic medication.

Local steroid therapy is valuable in inflammatory dermatoses and for controlling exacerbations of pruritic eczema and psoriasis. *It is not recommended for urticaria.* Unfortunately, steroid ointments are misused as a dermatological panacea because they give dramatic relief in inflammatory and pruritic skin conditions. Their indiscriminate use, is not only wasteful but also harmful. *Application of a steroid ointment for such conditions as herpes simplex, herpes zoster, fungal infections and impetigo may lead to their exacerbation.*

Glucocorticoids accelerate the fungal growth, and cause local skin atrophy with resultant telangiectasia, purpura and striae. Systemic toxicity including adrenal suppression can occur following local therapy, more so in infants; and hence, potent preparations like betamethasone valerate, triamcinolone acetonide, fluocinolone acetonide and clobetasol propionate should not be prescribed for treating infantile eczema.

Similarly, potent steroids should not be applied to facial skin as atrophy and telangiectasia occur more quickly on the face.

The practice of adding a glucocorticoid to antibiotics and antifungal agents is difficult to justify. The same is true of use of glucocorticoids in ointments for hemorrhoids.

- ***Intra-articular and intratendinous use***: Long acting esters of glucocorticoids have been used successfully to treat painful osteoarthritis and painful tender fascial nodules by local infiltration. Such therapy has the added advantage of minimum systemic absorption and consequent reduction in toxicity. Such injections should not be given more than 3 times a year.
- ***Miscellaneous***: Glucocorticoids have been used empirically in a wide variety of conditions such as Bell's palsy, acute infective polyneuritis, encephalitis, infective hepatitis, complete heart block, hypsarrhythmia and so on. Their usefulness in these conditions is doubtful.

Table 64.7: Precautions during glucocorticoid therapy

Before starting therapy

- Enquire about and check for : peptic ulcer, diabetes mellitus, tuberculosis, any other infection (especially one not amenable to chemotherapy).

During therapy

- Prescribe the drug with food.
- Diet low in calories and sodium, and high in potassium.
- Check periodically for: weight gain, edema, hyperglycemia, hypertension, infection, GI bleeding, hypokalemia, ocular changes.
- Monitor growth in children.
- Instruct the patient not to stop the drug abruptly.
- Increase the dose in case of any stress (severe infection, major surgery).
- Prescribe oral calcium and vitamin D supplements; alendronate; (Chapter 68); antacids; H_2 receptor blockers

While stopping therapy

- Taper therapy slowly (see text).

Precautions during corticosteroid therapy: These apply especially to the prolonged, high dose, suppressive therapy and are listed in Table 64.7. There are no absolute contraindications to glucocorticoid therapy other than Cushing's syndrome and ocular herpes zoster. Proper precautions have to be taken in using them in diabetes mellitus, peptic ulcer, hypertension, CHF, osteoporosis; in debilitated or old patients; and in the presence of infection.

Choice of the glucocorticoid : *For routine systemic use, prednisolone is the drug of choice as it is effective orally and cheap.* When a potent glucocorticoid is indicated, dexa-/beta-methasone is preferred; they do not cause sodium retention.

MINERALOCORTICOIDS: The important natural mineralocorticoids are **aldosterone** and **desoxycorticosterone.** They have identical effects on electrolyte and water metabolism and on cardiovascular system except that aldosterone is thirty times more potent than desoxycorticosterone.

Physiological and pharmacological actions of aldosterone:

- ***Electrolyte and water metabolism***: Physiologically, the major stimulators of aldosterone production are angiotensin II and potassium. Aldosterone secretion rises after consumption of foods rich in potassium and after vigorous exercise that causes release of potassium from the exercising muscle.

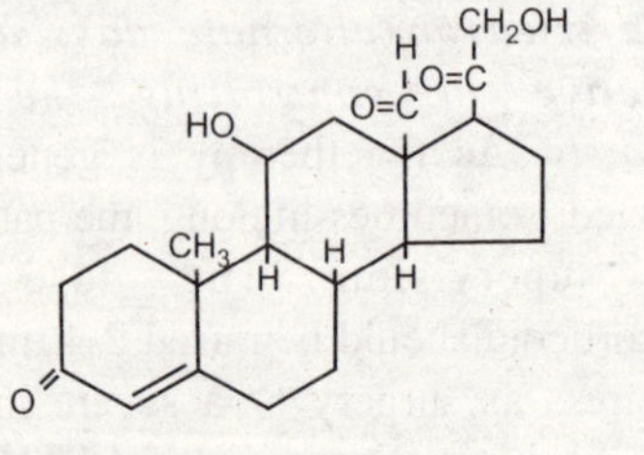

Fig. 64.6 : Aldosterone

Single doses of aldosterone promote sodium resorption and increased excretion of potassium by the kidney, intestine and sweat and salivary glands. On repeated administration of aldosterone, and in patients suffering from an aldosterone producing adenoma (primary hyperaldosteronism) however, the subject escapes from the sodium retaining effect; potassium loss, however, continues. Neither aldosterone nor desoxycorticosterone has an effect on GFR and unlike hydrocortisone, neither hormone can restore the ability to excrete a water load in an adrenalectomized animal.

The results of **aldosterone deficiency** are clearly seen in Addison's disease. In hypopituitarism, aldosterone secretion is relatively unimpaired. In aldosterone deficiency, the distal renal tubule is unable to conserve sodium, causing marked sodium loss with associated osmotic diuresis and a fall in plasma sodium. The extracellular fluid space becomes contracted and at the same time hypo-osmolar. As a result, water moves into the cells which become over-hydrated. Contraction of the blood volume may lead to collapse and death. Azotemia is likely to occur as a result of contracted blood volume. Potassium excretion by the kidneys is impaired. Hyperkalemia and acidosis add to the burden of metabolic disturbances. Increased intake of salt or administration of a mineralocorticoid corrects all the above abnormalities, but the muscular weakness still remains and the patient is unable to withstand stress. Addition of a glucocorticoid is necessary for complete correction of circulatory instability and muscular weakness in Addison's disease.

Aldosterone exerts similar effects on cellular sodium transport at other sites such as the intestines. Further, although aldosterone is primarily produced by the adrenal gland, its local production by the endothelial cells and the vascular smooth muscle cells of the heart and the blood vessels has been demonstrated. The production of aldosterone by the heart is regulated by angiotensin II. (Fig. 64.7).

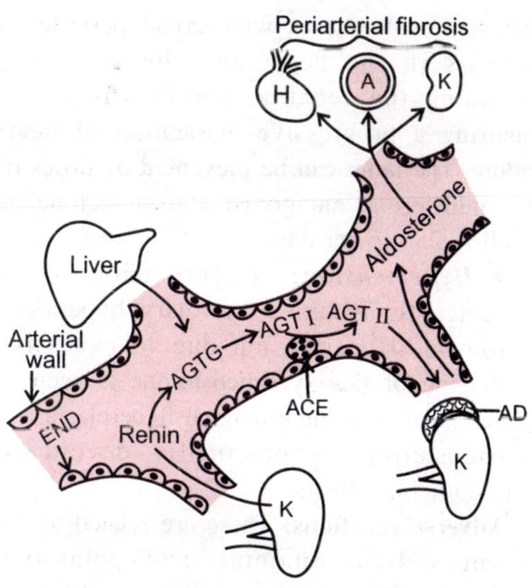

Fig.64.7 : Pathogenesis and deleterious effects of secondary hyperaldosteronism in CHF

Endo = Vascular endothelium. K = Kidney.
AGTG = Angiotensinogen. AD = Adrenal gland.
AGT I = Angiotensin I. AGT II = Angiotensin II.
ACE = Angiotensin converting enzyme.
H = Heart. A = Small arteries and arterioles.

- ***Cardiovascular effects :*** Along with angiotensin II, aldosterone also plays a role in blood coagulation, in contraction of systemic arterioles and in stimulating thirst. They are also involved in regulating inflammatory and reparative processes that follow tissue injury.

The excess of aldosterone in congestive heart failure (**secondary hyperaldosteronism**) can cause widespread damage. In the initial stages of LV dysfunction, the patients have *compensated* heart failure, with natriuresis due to the natriuretic peptide secreted by the cardiac atria. When moderate or severe reduction in renal perfusion occurs because of worsening (*decompensated*) heart failure, the kidneys secrete an excess of renin with resulting excess of circulating angiotensin II and consequent hyperaldosteronism. This overrides the beneficial effects of the atrial natriuretic peptide. With angiotensin II causing sodium reabsorption in the proximal renal tubule and aldosterone in the distal tubule, salt retention is almost complete. The combination of hyperaldosteronism and an excess of salt causes widespread periarterial fibrosis in the heart and the arterioles including the renal arterioles (fig 64.7), ensuring a progressive worsening of heart failure. The latter can be prevented by doses of the aldosterone antagonist spironolactone as small as 25 mg per day.

• ***Hypertension***: Hypertension is a characteristic feature of primary hyperaldosteronism. Hypertension due to excessive production of desoxycorticosterone is seen in one form of congenital adrenal hyperplasia.

Aldosterone is practically devoid of glucocorticoid effects.

Adverse reactions: These are related to the potent sodium retaining and potassium depleting actions and consist of weight gain, edema, hypertension and hypokalemia. Patients with Addison's disease are extremely sensitive to these effects and hence, the dose of a mineralocorticoid has to be adjusted carefully in such patients.

Preparations and dosage: Aldosterone, because of very transient action is not therapeutically useful. 9 α-Fluoro-hydrocortisone (Fludrocortisone, Florinef) is available as 0.1 mg. tablets. It is used when a mineralocorticoid is needed. Dose: in adults: 0.05 - 0.30 mg daily; in children upto 12 years, 5 mcg/kg/day. The dose in patients with Addison's disease is best adjusted to maintain plasma potassium (± plasma renin activity) within normal limits.

Therapeutic uses: Fludrocortisone is used in the treatment of:

• ***Addison's disease.***

• ***Salt losing congenital adrenal hyperplasia.***

• ***Hyporeninemic hypoaldosteronism*** as in chronic kidney disease due to diabetes mellitus and other causes; and

• ***Severe postural hypotension from autonomic neuropathy of any etiology.***

Hyperaldosteronism: Aldosterone output may be raised in two entirely different groups of conditions:

• ***Primary hyperaldosteronism***: This is generally due to an adenoma of the adrenal cortex. The patient suffers from hypertension, hypokalemia, polyuria, alkalosis, periodic paralysis and occasionally abnormal glucose tolerance. Edema is very rarely seen. Serum sodium and total body sodium may remain within normal limits as the kidneys escape from the sodium retaining effects of aldosterone after the first few days. The treatment is essentially surgical. Spironolactone is used for preparing the patient for surgery.

• ***Secondary hyperaldosteronism***: This refers to an increased production of aldosterone in response to activation of the renin angiotensin system or because of decreased metabolism of aldosterone by the damaged liver. It occurs in edematous patients with hepatic cirrhosis, CHF and nephrotic syndrome. It is likely to occur after sodium depletion in response to vigorous diuretic therapy. Spironolactone is used to treat these patients (Chapter 38).

Adrenal Function Tests

The plasma levels of cortisol, 17 alphahydroxyprogesterone, aldosterone, and the adrenal androgens are measured by immunoassays, under basal conditions and during dynamic tests. Examples of such tests are:

Short, ACTH stimulation test: This has already been described earlier.

Overnight dexamethasone suppression test: Plasma cortisol level is measured the morning after administration of 1 mg of dexamethasone orally at 10 p.m. A level of less than 5 mcg% indicates normal suppression.

Gonadotropins, Estrogens and Progestins

65

Harvey Cushing, in his studies (1911) on hypophysectomised dogs, established the role of the pituitary in regulating the gonadal function. The first substance with gonadotropic activity was isolated from the urine of pregnant women by Zondek and independently by Fluhmann in 1929.

The anterior pituitary secretes two distinct gonadotropic hormones They are:

(1) **Follicle stimulating hormone** (FSH)

(2) **Luteinizing hormone** (LH), also known as interstitial cell stimulating hormone (ICSH).

The molecular weights of human FSH and LH are estimated to be about 33,000 and 28000, respectively. However, these hormones can exist in monomer, dimer or tetramer forms. Secretion of FSH and LH is regulated by a hypothalamic releasing hormone (GnRH).

Physiology of pituitary gonadotropins: Complex interactions between the hypothalamus, the anterior pituitary and the gonadal sex steroids regulate the ovulation in women and spermatogenesis in men. This system is controlled by three feed-back mechanisms :

- ***Long feed-back mechanism*:** Gonadal sex hormones act on the hypothalamus by way of negative feed-back mechanism (estrogen, progesterone, testosterone) or a positive feed-back mechanism (estrogen).
- ***Short feed-back mechanism*:** This involves a direct action of the sex hormones on the anterior pituitary, regulating the secretion of FSH and LH, and
- ***Ultra-short negative feed-back mechanism*:** This comprises regulation of the hypothalamic GnRH by the pituitary FSH and LH.

Dopamine found at the nerve endings in the hypothalamus is involved in the release of GnRH, which in turn affects both FSH- and LH-secretory cells of the anterior pituitary. Secretory activities are modulated differently by estrogen, progesterone and testosterone. The mode of action of GnRH is believed to be similar in both sexes except for its cyclicity in women.

The regulatory mechanisms in the hypothalamus reside in two centres : (a) **the tonic centre** in the ventromedial nucleus and the arcuate nucleus and (b) **the cyclic centre** in the pre-optic suprachiasmatic area. In males the tonic centre is dominant and causes activation of the pituitary and thereby a stimulation of the testes, producing spermatogenesis and testosterone synthesis. In females, it is probably the lack of the androgenic influence, which allows the development of the 'hypothalamic clock', essential for the cyclic release of the gonadotropins. Thus, the cyclic centre is dominant in the female. This centre is sensitive to external and internal stimuli. In the presence of female sex hormones, it is activated (or suppressed) and indirectly activates the tonic centre producing an increased release mostly of

LH from the anterior pituitary and consequently ovulation.

The natural GnRH isolated from the human, porcine, ovine and bovine hypothalami is a decapeptide. They are identical in structure and have been synthesized. Since it predominantly causes release of LH and less of FSH, it is also known as LH-RH. The evidence for the existence of a separate FSH-RH as distinct from the LH-RH is still insufficient.

The sequence of various hormonal changes that occur during a normal 28 days menstrual cycle in women is shown in Figure 65.1. Day one is defined as the first day of menstrual flow, while the day preceding the first day of the next menstrual flow is designated as the last day of the cycle. Generally, cycles between 21 and 35 days are accepted as normal, the duration of menstrual flow being 2-7 days.

Ovarian follicular growth, once initiated by FSH, proceeds independently to the preovulatory phase. A rise of FSH early in the cylces is followed by a rise in blood estradiol. Under the influence of FSH alone, the follicle cells do not secrete estrogens unless a small amount of LH is also present. Most FSH-stimulated follicles undergo atresia whereas one follicle (the dominant follicle) per menstrual cycle becomes the graffian follicle and ovulates. The ovulatory peaks of FSH and LH occur betwen days 11-23 of the menstrual cylce (Fig. 65.1). Its timing has no relationship to the length of the cycle. Following this large quantity of LH (LH surge), the follicle size increases resulting in follicular rupture and release of an ovum. The peaks of plasma estradiol and 17-alpha hydroxy-progesterone precede the mid-cycle LH peak. This indicates that theca interna cells which predominantly synthesise estradiol produce 17-alpha hydroxy-progresterone as an intermediate product. Estimation of these hormones, therefore, gives some idea about the follicular function.

Following rupture, the follicle undergoes reorganization to form a **corpus luteum**, which secretes mainly progesterone, and also 17-alpha hydroxy-progesterone, estradiol and some other steroids.

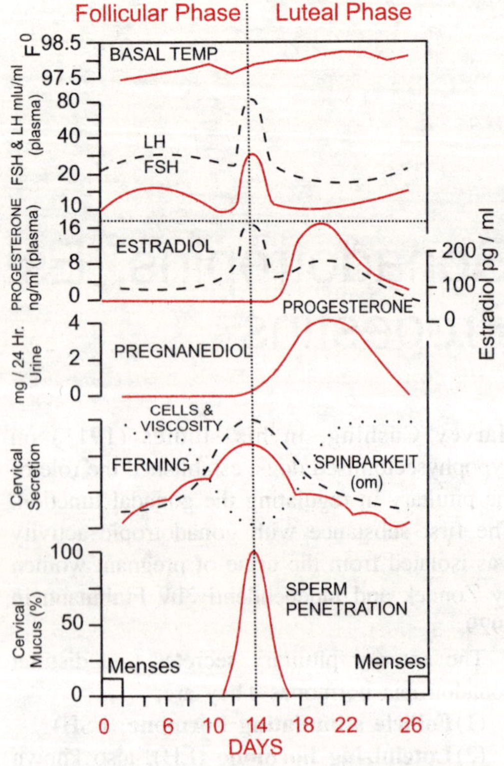

Fig. 65.1 : Hormonal changes in blood and urine during the menstrual cycle in human female. Dotted line denotes the day of LH surge.

Corpus luteum (CL) is an independent endocrine organ. In rodents, CL has a limited life span of 3-4 days unless prolactin is secreted by the pituitary. In this species, prolactin acts as luteotropic hormone (LTH), necessary for initiation and maintenance of CL. Such role of prolactin, however, has not been demonstrated in human females in whom LH itself is luteotropic. The life span of CL during a non-pregnant cycle in humans averages about 11 days, while the functional life span of the CL of pregnancy is 9-10 weeks. Since 17-alpha hydroxy-progesterone is synthesized mainly by the CL (not by human placenta) its blood level reflects the function of CL during pregnancy.

It appears that the preovulatory LH surge is partly initiated by an increase in the pituitary sensitivity to GnRH. This increase in sensitivity is the result of the high estradiol levels present at this time of the cycle. In addition, an increased discharge of GnRH has been demonstrated at this stage. Thus, in response to the 'ovarian signal' (in the form of estradiol) a large quantity of LH is released abruptly (LH surge) leading to ovulation and the subsequent formation of CL. Unlike that of most other mammals, the human CL secretes estradiol as well as progesterone, the latter in larger quantities. The increased estrogen and progesterone following ovulation suppress the sensitivity of the hypophysis to GnRH, in addition to suppressing the hypothalamus. In the absence of conception, the progesterone and estrogen levels remain high for eight days and then fall abruptly leading to menstruation. These hormonal changes before and after ovulation are associated with the characteristic **proliferative** and **secretory** changes, respectively, in the endometrium.

Although it is difficult to predict the day of ovulation in a given cycle in a human female, the reproductive cycle shows a remarkable regularity and in the majority, it is repeated every 26-30 days. What keeps the system cycling so regularly is not well understood. The usual way of judging ovulation clinically by noting the rise in basal body temperature (BBT) is not accurate.

Gonadotropic hormones stimulate the biosynthesis of sex steroids in the gonads. LH increases the accumulation of adenosine 3', 5'-monophosphate (cyclic AMP) as one of its early effects. Cyclic AMP triggers synthesis of various sex hormones starting from the C27 compound cholesterol leading to the formation of various C21, C19 and C18 sex steroids (Fig. 65.2). As seen in this figure progesterone is necessary for the synthesis of androgens, and androgens are obligatory precursors of estrogens.

The non-pregnant human female synthesizes two biologically active estrogens estradiol (E_2) and estrone (E_1) and much larger amounts of prohormone estrone sulfate. The last is converted to estrone in the peripheral tissues. The third, weakly active estrogen, estriol, is synthesized by the placenta.

Apart from estrogens and progesterone, the ovarian extract also contains 17-alpha-hydroxyprogesterone, and androstenedione, a precursor of testosterone.

Although the ovaries normally cease their gametogenic and hormonal function in the fifth decade of life, leading to menopause, postmenopausal women have some circulating estrogen. This is due to conversion of the adrenal androgens into estrogens in the peripheral adipose tissue.

Hypothalamo-pituitary-ovarian relation-ship: In addition to the **cyclical** release in relation to the menstrual cycle in women, LH release is characterized by **pulsatility**. Thus, it is released in discreet bursts (pulses) every 1-2 hours, separated by periods of little or no release. Similar pulsatile release is also seen in men. This is probably based on a similar, pulsatile release of GnRH from the hypothalamus. This intermittent release of a hormone permits the regeneration of its receptors in the end organ and maintenance of sensitivity of the latter to the concerned hormone.

The secretion of LH and FSH from the anterior pituitary is regulated by the interaction between the sex steroids and hypothalamic GnRH. Both progesterone and testosterone suppress the discharge of LH and FSH stimulated by GnRH. In contrast, estrogen appears to exert a biphasic effect on the pituitary response to hypothalamic GnRH. As the follicular phase in women progresses, the rising plasma FSH levels cause the plasma estradiol level to rise. The sharp rise in the estradiol level at the end of follicular phase exerts a *positive feedback* on the pituitary and is responsible for the midcycle LH surge. The decline in the levels of estradiol and progesterone in the late luteal phase are responsible for the commencing rise in the plasma FSH level even before the menstrual bleeding commences, an example of *negative feedback*. The increased levels of gonadotropins after the menopause are due to the loss of the estrogen's inhibitory influence.

Pharmacological doses of an estrogen exert only a negative feedback on the pituitary,

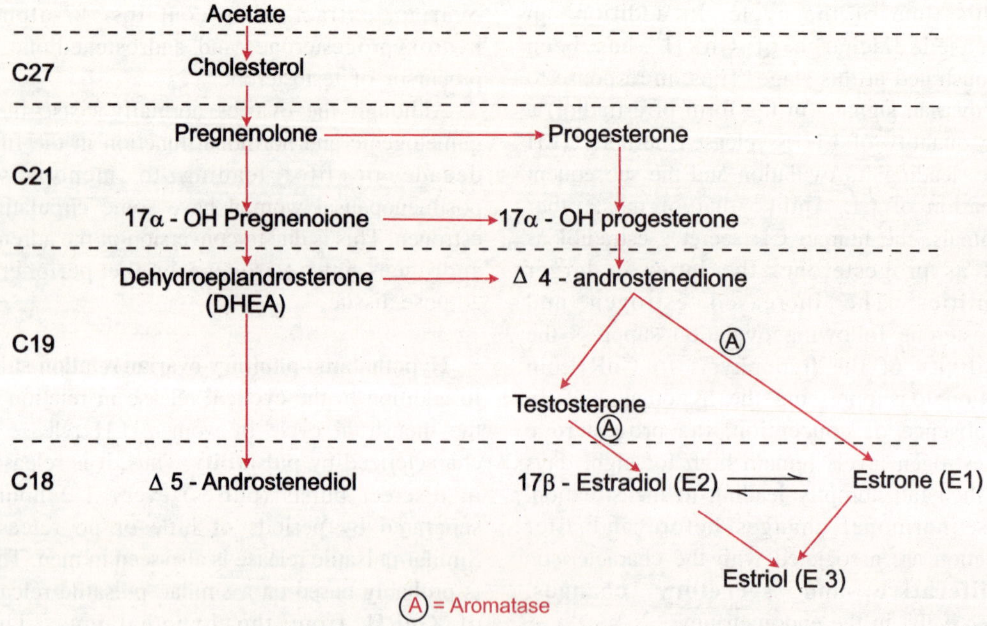

Fig. 65.2: Biosynthesis of sex steroids in the gonads.

causing inhibition of gonadotropin release in a dose dependent manner.

GnRH: The first lot of GnRH (then called LH-RH) was isolated by Schally in 1971 by extracting and processing one million pig hypothalami! The GnRHs of sheep, pigs, cows and human origin are identical in structure. GnRH is a decapeptide. It is synthesized in the hypothalamus and is secreted in a pulsatile fashion. It is also found in human placenta. Placental GnRH may be involved in the synthesis and release of human CG (hCG). GnRH also appears in high concentration in the breast milk. Its plasma t½ is 2-8 minutes.

The main function of GnRH is the promotion of synthesis and release of LH and FSH from the anterior piuitary. The relative amounts of FSH and LH released after administration of GnRH are related to the puberal status of the individual. Prior to the onset of puberty, FSH is the predominantly released gonadotropin, whereas after puberty it is LH which is predominantly released. Given in an intermittent, *pulsatile* manner, GnRH increases the responsiveness of the pituitary gonadotropes to GnRH itself. This self-priming effect is not observed following a *continuous* GnRH infusion, which results in an initial increase for a short time, followed by a sustained and progressive decline, in LH secretion. This is due to a 'down regulation' of the GnRH receptors.

Clinically, **pulsatile GnRH** administration with appropriate frequency and amplitude of pulses appears to be a requirement for the restoration of normal gonadotropin release pattern in patients with hypothalamic hypogonadism. The pituitary's response to Gn-RH varies throughout the menstrual cycle, being maximum at mid-cycle.

Preparations and dosage: Synthetic GnRH (Gonadorelin, Fertiral) is available as 500 mcg/ml in 2 ml ampoules. It is administered by *pulsatile subcutaneous infusion,* 10-20 mcg over 1 minute, to be repeated every 90 minutes, for the treatment of amenorrhoea and infertility due to abnormal release of endogenous LH-RH. It is also available as 100 mcg ampoules (Relefact) for assessment of pituitary function.

Therapeutic uses :

● ***Assessment of the function of the pituitary gonadotropes*** to distinguish between delayed puberty and hypogonadotropic hypogonadism; the results of this test are often inconclusive.

● ***Induction of ovulation*** in patients with polycystic ovary syndrome not responding to clomiphene.

● ***Treatment of males and females with idiopathic, hypothalamic, hypogonado-"trophic hypogonadism (Kallman syndrome).***

GnRH ANALOGUES: The analogues are of two types:

(1) **Agonists;** and

(2) **Antagonists.**

The **agonists** bind to the GnRH receptors on the pituitary gonadotropes, and following prolonged receptor occupation they cause their *down-regulation.* Unlike the GnRH antagonists, the agonists enhance the release of gonadotropins initially; this is a disadvantage in the treatment of the hormone dependent cancers treated with GnRH agonists. Exogenous estrogens, progestins and androgens inhibit the GnRH release, but only progestin exert this effect at doses that do not have marked hormonal effect.

GnRH analogues are administered SC/IM and by nasal spray. They have higher affinity for the GnRH receptors and are metabolized more slowly than the native GnRH.

Adverse reactions : These include hot flushes, sweating, vaginal dryness, headache and occasionally diminished libido and depression. Prolonged treatment causes osteoporosis.

The **GnRH agonists** (Table 65.1) are used in the treatment of:

● ***Certain hormone dependent cancers*** e.g. cancer of the prostate and the breast.

● ***Central precocious puberty.***

● ***Endometriosis.***

● ***Large uterine fibroids;*** and in

● ***IVF regimens, as an adjunct to GnRH,*** in order to inhibit untimely release of LH from the pituitary.

As GnRH is not easily available, leuprolide may be used for gonadotropin stimulation test.

The **GnRH antagonists** act by competitive inhibition of the binding of endogenous GnRH to the GnRH receptors and suppress the release of LH and FSH from the onset of administration. They are more expensive; further, they often act as releasers of histamine.

Ganirelix, a GnRH antagonist, causes less histamine release than the other antagonists. Unlike GnRH agonists, it does not cause initial stimulation phase but blocks the release of FSH

Table 65.1: Some clinically used GnRH agonists

Name	Potency	Half life (minutes)	Dose and mode of administration
GnRH (Gonadorelin, Fertiral)	1	5	See text
Leuprolide acetate (Lupron)	15	180-220	1 mg SC daily
Leuprolide acetate polymer			3.75 mg SC monthly
Buserelin acetate (Suprefact)	20	75-85	40 mcg/kg/day, in divided doses, intranasally; or 1 mg SC daily
Nafarelin (Nasarel)	150	120-160	200-400 mcg intranasally, twice daily
Triptorelin microspheres (Decapeptyl)	144	--	4 mg IM monthly
Goserelin acetate polymer (Zoladex)	100	--	3.6 mg SC monthly

without down regulation of the receptor. It is usually given SC. Currently, it is used during IVF regimen as a means of preventing LH surges during ovarian stimulation.

Gonadotropins

All the gonadotropins are glycoproteins. They have varying plasma half lives and undergo metabolic degradation by plasma proteases. The gonadotropins available for human therapy are:

- ***Human chorionic gonadotropin (hCG)***, and
- ***Human menopausal urinary gonadotropin (hMG).***

The other two, pituitary FSH and LH, are not used in therapy.

The gonadotropins used in therapeutics are capable of eliciting antibody formation.

Bioassay: These are usually conducted on hypophysectomised immature rats and mice and are based on the measurement of increase in ovarian or uterine weight (for FSH), increase in weight of the ventral prostate (for LH), or histological changes in the ovary, uterus and vagina. In the past, biological tests based on the detection of hCG in the urine were used in the diagnosis of pregnancy. These tests are based on observation of (a) ovulation in the rabbit (Friedman test), or in the mouse (Ascheim Zondek test); (b) ovarian hyperemia in immature rats; or (c) presence of spermatozoa in the cloaca of the male frog (Frog test), a few hours after the injection of the urine sample in these animals. These have now been replaced for clinical purpose by immunological tests.

HUMAN CHORIONIC GONADOTROPIN (hCG): This glycoprotein hormone of human pregnancy is secreted by the foetal placenta. It can be detected in the maternal plasma several days before the first missed period. Sufficient amounts of it is absorbed into the blood and sustains luteal function until the placenta starts secreting estrogen and progesterone by the 3rd month of pregnancy. Its physiological role after that time is unknown.

The amino acid sequences of the alpha subunits of the human glycoprotein hormones are identical but those of the beta subunits differ. *LH and hCG have biologic activities in common,* reflecting the 80 per cent structural homology between their beta subunits. hCG, however, differs chemically from LH mainly in that it has additional 32 amino acids.

Besides the placenta, certain tumours secrete hCG. Gestational trophoblastic tumours, derived from the placenta, are invariably associated with abnormally high hCG blood levels and its serial estimation is valuable for monitoring therapy and detecting tumour recurrence. Similarly, it has been used as a tumour marker to diagnose recurrence and to monitor therapy in men with nonseminomatous germinal cell tumours.

Pharmacological actions: Like pituitary LH, small doses of hCG can preserve the CL and prolong the secretory phase of the menstrual cycle. This is associated with an increased urinary excretion of pregnanediol. The hCG can induce a decidual reaction in the endometrium even in the absence of conception (pseudopregnancy). It does not promote follicle maturation in humans; however, in immature animals, it can evoke follicular growth and induce ovulation.

Injected into the males, hCG stimulates the interstitial cells of the testes to secrete androgen.

Adverse reactions : These include headache, edema, gynaecomastia, precocious puberty and occasionally depression.

Preparation and dosage: hCG (Pregnyl, Choragon, Life) 2000 IU, 5,000 IU, 10,000 I.U. and 20,000 I.U. with 10 ml of diluent.

Therapeutic uses:

- ***Ovulation induction***: hCG therapy can induce ovulation in an adequately developed follicle following endogenous FSH or exogenous hMG, leading to conception.
- ***Cryptorchism***: Cryptorchism denotes failure of the testes to descend into the scrotum. hCG is used to promote this descent. It is given

in doses of 3000-5000 IU every 3-4 days for 4 injections. If descent does not occur, orchidopexy is indicated. Evidence indicates that non-descent of the testes into the scrotum can damage them from very early age, and hence treatment should be initiated as early as 2-3 years of age. The hormone should not be used if mechanical obstruction is present.

- ***Delayed puberty in boys*:** This is treated with 500-1000 I.U. of hCG 3 times a week for 4 weeks, repeated, if necessary, after several months. Once initiated, the puberty progresses without further treatment. If such progression fails to occur, hypogonadotrophic hypogonadism is diagnosed.
- ***Testing the responsiveness of the immature testes to gonadotropins*:** For this purpose, serum testosterone is measured before and 3-4 days after an injection of 5000 I.U. of hCG. A post-injection level of 2 ng/ml is considered a normal response. It also confirms the presence of testicular tissue in a patient in whom the testes are not palpable and not demonstrable by imaging techniques.
- ***Treatment of hypogonadotropic hypogonadism:*** For this purpose, 2000 I.U. are injected 2-3 times a week for prolonged periods. Enlargement of the testes and development of secondary sex characters are stimulated. Addition of hMG may be necessary for inducing spermatogenesis.
- ***Treatment of luteal phase defect*:** hCG may be used to support the production of adequate amounts of progesterone in the luteal phase of the menstrual cycle in patients with luteal phase defect. Alternatively, progesterone has been used to supply the deficient hormone.

HUMAN MENOPAUSAL URINARY GONADOTROPIN (hMG, Menotropins, Pergonal) : This is prepared from the urine of menopausal women and is available in ampoules containing 75 IU of FSH and LH each. It is used, together with hCG, to induce ovulation in women with anovulation due to pituitary-hypothalamic disorders but with normal ovaries, and those with polycystic ovaries. Various regimens have been used. In one such regimen the initial dose used is 75 I.U. (one ampoule) injected IM daily for 7 days, while monitoring the follicular growth by ultasonography and plasma estradiol levels. If on day 8, plasma estradiol is > 200 pg/ml and follicular size > 10 mm, the dose is maintained. When the follicle is increased to 16-18 mm. size, 5000-10,000 IU of hCG is injected IM to induce ovulation. If ovulation fails to occur with the lower dose of hMG, the dose is increased in the subsequent cycles; a dose of 75-300 IU of FSH and LH each daily is usually sufficient for this purpose. Ovulation can be successfully induced in 90% of selected cases, and pregnancy occurs in about 50%; of these, 20% end in abortion and multiple births may occur in 20-30%. The above regimen can also be used in IVF technique. The growth and development of children so born have been normal.

hMG has also been used with variable success in men with idiopathic oligospermia.

Because menotropins is an *unpurified* preparation, it is injected IM and not SC, in order to reduce the occurrence of allergic reactions. The *highly purified* FSH preparation (Metrodin HP, devoid of LH activity), prepared by immuno-concentration with monoclonal antibodies, as well as follitropin (Puregon), an *rDNA monocomponent FSH preparation*, may be injected either IM or SC.

Adverse reactions: The main complication of this therapy is **hyperstimulation syndrome** after hCG injection. The ovaries become very large and friable due to maturation of many follicles. This causes abdominal pain and nausea. If the friable ovary ruptures into the abdomen, the patient may develop ascites and shock. The management is conservative. Prevention implies (a) keeping the dose of hMG low; and (b) not injecting hCG if the plasma estradiol level exceeds 2000 pg/ml.

PROLACTIN: The human pituitary gland secretes prolactin (hPRL, M.W. 21500). Unlike with the other pituitary hormones, the secretion of prolactin is under control of a hypothalamic **prolactin-inhibiting factor** (PIF), now identified as **dopamine** in the median eminence. In the pituitary, D_2 receptors are predominant and mediate the PRL inhibition.The normal adult serum PRL levels are about 10-25 ng/ ml in women and about 10-20 ng/ml in men.

Serum hPRL concentration increases during pregnancy and postpartum. Breast feeding and stimulation of the nipple can cause a marked rise in serum hPRL levels. Increased levels are also observed following exercise, psychological and surgical stress.

- ***Endocrine actions:*** PRL acts on a receptor belonging to type I cytokine receptor family. The main actions of prolactin are the preparation of the breasts for lactation, and the initiation and maintenance of lactation. Following prolactin, the lobuloalveolar epithelium of the breast proliferates. The mechanism that converts the developed and potentially secretory mammary gland into an active secretory organ at delivery is not well understood; but other hormones such as estrogens, corticosteroids, insulin and thyroid are also necessary for galactopoiesis.

Excess of circulating prolactin inhibits reproductive function and suppresses sex drive. By inhibiting GnRH and consequently gonadotropin secretion, it impairs gonadal steroid production and blocks the development of the ovarian follicles, causing anovulation. Its direct luteolytic effect leads to inadequate luteal phase. In males, it causes low plasma testosterone and decreased spermatogenesis.

- ***Metabolic actions:*** PRL increases calcium absorption and mobilizes calcium from the bone. Hyperprolactinemia is associated with increased bone loss and osteoporosis. PRL receptors are present in the osteoblasts of developing bone. Hypoestrogenimia present in hyper prolactenemic women probably causes increased bone loss. PRL also induces pancreatic beta cell growth. By acting centrally, it increases appetite and is probably involved in parenting behaviour.

Hyperprolactinemia is observed in prolactin secreting pituitary adenomas. It can also be drug induced, which is reversible (Table 65.2). It causes galactorrhoea, amenorrhoea and infertility in women, and sexual impotence in men. Its rational therapy involves the use of drugs that decrease the hPRL secretion. The drugs used are **bromoergocriptine, lisuride, pergolide, cabergoline and quinagolide.**

Table 65.2: Drugs causing hyperprolactinemia

- ***Blockers of dopamine (D_2) receptors***: Antipsychotic phenothiazines; haloperidol; metoclopramide; domperidone.
- ***Dopamine synthesis inhibitors:*** α methyldopa.
- ***Central dopamine depletors***: Reserpine.
- ***Antidepressants:*** Imipramine, amitryptiline, fluoxetine.
- ***Hormones:*** TRH; oral contraceptives; antiandrogens.
- ***Miscellaneous:*** Cimetidine; verapamil; opiates.

BROMOERGOCRIPTINE (Bromocriptine, Parlodel, Proctinal): This semisynthetic ergot alkaloid is a selective D_2 receptor agonist. Since dopamine is a neurotransmitter or local hormone at various sites in the brain, bromocriptine can produce various motor, behavioural and endocrine effects. Its oxytocic and cardiovascular actions, however, are negligible.

Pharmacological actions:

- ***Hormonal actions***: Dopamine (PIF), released by the hypothalamus, inhibits prolactin release from pituitary lactotrophes. Bromocriptine acts as a D_2 agonist on the pituitary lactotrophic cells to inhibit synthesis and release of prolactin and to decrease the replication of the tumorous lactotrophs. Given to patients with hyperprolactinemia, it causes a marked fall in serum prolactin levels, accompanied by restoration of the normal cyclic release of gonadotropins.

Bromocriptine causes a **brief rise** in plasma GH levels in normal subjects but a **sustained fall** in plasma GH in patients with acromegaly. The exact mechanism of this paradoxical effect is not known.

• ***Motor effects***: Bromocriptine causes a reduction in dopamine turnover with a decrease in concentration of the dopamine metabolites and an increase in dopamine content of the brain. It thus produces beneficial effects in Parkinson's disease. But the doses required are almost 10 times higher than those which suppress prolactin.

• ***Behavioural effects***: Prolonged treatment, particularly with larger doses, can cause altered behaviour and awareness, sometimes accompanied by hallucinations. This probably results from hydrolysis of the LSD fragment of the bromocriptine molecule.

• ***CVS:*** These drugs cause vasodilatation (see adverse reactions below).

Absorption, fate and excretion: The drug is rapidly and almost completely absorbed from the gut and readily crosses the BBB. Following a single dose, plasma level remains high for several hours and low levels can be detected for upto four days. The drug is extensively metabolized and only 6 to 7% is excreted in the urine. The rest appears in the bile and feces.

Adverse reactions : These include postural syncope, gastric upset, nausea and drowsiness. Continuous high doses may cause constipation, nasal congestion, cramps in legs, hallucinations, dystonic reactions, arrhythmias and postural hypotension. The drug should be avoided in patients with a history of mental illness, ischaemic heart disease and peripheral vascular disease. Long term use may rarely produce retroperitoneal fibrosis.

Preparations and dosage:

(i) Bromocriptine mesylate tablets 2.5 mg.

(ii) Bromocriptine mesylate inj. 40 mg/ml. This is used IM in cases of prolactinomas compressing the optic chiasma. Tumour shrinkage can occur and vision saved, while the patient awaits surgery.

(iii) Vaginal preparation may be useful in patients intolerant of oral bromocriptine.

Therapeutic uses:

• ***Hyperprolactinemia-galactorrhea syndrome***: Given in the dose of 2.5-10 mg daily in divided doses, it restores serum prolactin levels to normal and stops galactorrhea in patients with prolactinomas and those with functional hyperprolactinemia. Further, amenorrhea is corrected and fertility is restored in women, within 4-12 weeks of therapy. It is, however, not effective in amenorrhea due to gonadotropin deficiency or ovarian failure.

In patients with prolactinomas, bromocriptine in the dose 2.5 to 10 mg. daily produces tumor regression and resolution of visual field defects. It is considered a specific and safe primary treatment for prolactin-secreting adenomas. However, bromocriptine is not a cure for all such tumours; recurrence can occur after stopping even prolonged drug treatment.

• ***Prolactinoma with impotence in males***: It lowers serum prolactin levels and restores potency in these patients. Further, the tumour size may regress in prolonged treatment.

• ***Acromegaly***: Bromocriptine in the dose of 15-20 mg daily causes a sustained, dose-related decrease in plasma GH levels and the hormonal, metabolic and clinical responses have been maintained for upto five years in individual cases. However, it is not advocated as a substitute for surgical or radiation therapy of this condition as complete clinical remission occurs in only a minority of patients. Further, following its stoppage, the plasma GH and the disability return to previous status.

• ***Parkinson's disease*** : Though it has a more prolonged action than levodopa, it cause higher incidence of neuropsychiatric adverse reactions (Chapter 14).

Its use to suppress puerperal lactation has caused hypertension, seizures, stroke and psychosis. The use of bromocreptine and other D_2 agonists for that purpose should also be avoided.

LISURIDE (Dopergin): This drug has properties and uses similar to those of bromocriptine. It is available as 0.2 mg tablets.

CABERGOLINE (Dostinex, Caberlin): This is a long acting analogue of bromocriptine and can be administered once a week. The dose is 500 mcg once a week, increased by 500 mcg increments, upto a maximum of 2 mg/week. The adverse reactions to this drug are different from those to bromocriptine : palpitation, epigastric and abdominal pain, epistaxis, hemianopia, syncope and hot flushes. Patients resistant to bromocriptine may respond to this drug.

QUINAGOLIDE (Norprolac): This drug has properties, adverse reactions and therapeutic uses similar to bromocriptine. It is used in the daily dose of 25 mcg at bedtime, increased weekly to a maximum daily dose of 75-150 mcg at bedtime.

Pergolide (Permax): This is a long-acting dopamine agonist as effective as bromcriptine. However it has been withdrawn from the market in USA because of cardiotoxicity.

As 5-HT_{2B} receptor agonists, pergolide and cabergoline can cause fibrosis of the cardiac valves during long term therapy of parkinsonism but not hyperprolactinemia. Other dopamine receptor agonists do not have this adverse effect (Chapter 23).

Placental Hormones

The placenta serves the important function of sustaining the growth and nutrition of the developing embryo. In addition, it is an endocrine organ secreting hormones. One of these, the chorionic gonadotropin (hCG), has already been discussed. hCG appears in the urine very early after implantation of the fertilized ovum and disappears from the urine within a few days after delivery. Factors that control the production of hCG are not known. It helps to maintain the functioning corpus luteum during early pregnancy.

Another placental peptide related to human pituitary growth hormone has been isolated. The substance has lactogenic, luteotropic and growth promoting activities. It is present in human serum, urine and amniotic fluid during pregnancy and disappears immediately after delivery. The hormone is named *'placental growth hormone or placental lactogen (hPL)'*. It is believed to act as a anabolic hormone in the mother and the fetus.

During pregnancy (probably from the 3rd month), the placenta produces large amounts of estrogen and progesterone. The placental progesterone, besides having a physiological effect on maternal organs, also acts as an important precursor for foetal corticosteroids and androgens.

During pregnancy, the urinary excretion of estrogen shows a great preponderance of estriol over that of estrone and estradiol. Since the fetus plays a specific role in the synthesis of estriol, assay of the level of estriol in maternal urine provides useful information about the well-being of the foetus. A fall in urinary estriol level may denote foetal distress or retarded foetal growth.

Although the placenta contains large amounts of corticosteroids there is no conclusive evidence to suggest that these are synthesized in the placenta.

Estrogens

In humans, the estrogens are produced mainly by the ovary and the placenta; small amounts may be produced by the adrenals and testes. The synthesis of estrogens from acetate and cholesterol is shown in Fig. 63.2. In certain animals like the horse, large quantities of estrogens are produced by the testes. Estrogens are also present in various plants and seeds. The natural estrogens are steroids. However, typical estrogenic activity is also shown by chemicals which are not steroids. Hence, the term 'estrogen' is used as a generic term to describe all the compounds having an estrogenic activity.

The pituitary gonadotropins regulate the production of the ovarian steroids. LH stimulates the production of the *androgens, androstenedione and testosterone* by the theca cells of the ovarian follicles. These two androgens are taken up by the adjacent granulosa cells of the ovarian follicles. The granulosa cells proliferate and express aromatase under the influence of FSH. *Aromatase converts the androgens into estrogens, estrone and estradiol, respectively (two cell theory).* The liver and the adipose tissue also contain aromatase and convert the circulating androgens into estrogens. Unlike in the gonads, estrogen production in other sites is unregulated.

During childhood, small amounts of the pituitary gonadotropins keep up a limited ouput of estrogenic and androgenic hormones which bring about the normal, gradual development of the genitalia. At puberty, increased output of gonadotropins leads to an increased production of the ovarian estrogens.

Physiological functions of estrogens: These are:

- ***Development of female reproductive tract*** (uterus, fallopian tubes and vagina).
- ***Development of female secondary sex characters***, such as breasts (ductal growth), body contours, hair, skin and voice. They are also responsible for the psychological and emotional get up typical of feminity.
- ***Stimulation of the proliferative or preovulatory phase of endometrium.*** The cyclical changes in estrogen secretion during the normal menstrual cycle and inhibitory role of excessive estrogens on pituitary FSH have already been discussed earlier.
- ***Vasodilatation of capillaries*** in general and those of the endometrium in particular.
- ***Metabolic effects*** such as retention of nitrogen, sodium and fluid in tissues.
- ***Cardioprotection*** in women of the reproductive age; this is mediated by maintenance of the LDL levels at a lower level than in males, as well as probably by other mechanisms. Menopausal women lose this protective influence of estrogen, leading to increased incidence of ischemic heart disease.
- ***Maintenance of the integrity of the skeleton in women of reproductive age;*** following menopause women suffer from osteoporosis as a result of estrogen deficiency.
- ***Promotion of the union of the epiphyses with the metaphyses*** thus controlling the height in females. Because of this action, the epiphyseal fusion is accelerated following the onset of menarche in females and once the epiphyses are fused, no further increase in height can occur.

Classification of Estrogens: These drugs can be classified into three groups:

I **Natural estrogens** estradiol, estrone and estriol and their esters.

II **Semisynthetic estrogens** e.g. ethinyl-estradiol and mestranol.

III **Synthetic estrogens :** (a) Those which are steroids e.g. mestranol; and (b) those which are not steroids but derivatives of diphenylethylene (stilbene) e.g. stilbestrol, and triphenyl-ethylene e.g. chlorotrianisene (TACE) (Fig. 66.1). Stilbestrol and chlorotrianisene are now used only to treat patients with carcinoma of the prostate and the breast (Chapter 59).

All the estrogenic compounds produce similar pharmacological actions and hence, are discussed together.

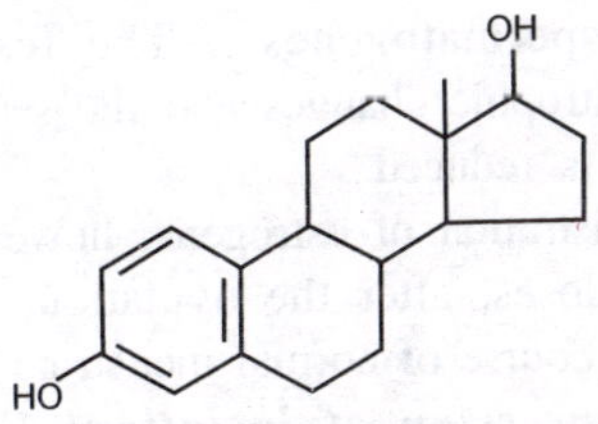

OH

HO

Fig. 65.3: Estradiol

Mechanism of action: Estrogens bind to the nuclear estrogen receptors in estrogen responsive tissues. The steroid-receptor complex undergoes conformational change and binds to the estrogen responsive element (ERE) located on the target gene, where it brings about changes in transcription.There are two types of estrogen receptors:

(1) ERα, present in the female genital tract, breasts, hypothalamus, endotheial cells and vascular smooth muscle and

(2) ERβ, present in bone, brain, prostate and ovaries.

The vascular actions of estrogen do not require gene activation and are mediated by the membrane receptors.

Pharmacological actions: These drugs, when used as substitution therapy, produce actions similar to the physiological actions of natural estrogens.

• ***Estrogen and menstruation***: In women with deficient ovarian function, estrogens in appropriate doses produce proliferative changes in the endometrium. Following these changes, withdrawal of estrogens causes menstrual flow known as *withdrawal bleeding*. This obviously cannot be compared with the natural menstruation where progesterone withdrawal plays an important role. The response depends upon the size of the dose and the duration of treatment. With very small doses irregular bleeding can occur even without the interruption of the drug (*break-through bleeding*).

• ***Gonadotropin inhibition***: Continuous administration of estrogens suppresses the secretion of FSH and also of midcycle LH surge resulting in inhibition of ovulation. In males, it inhibits spermatogenesis. The testes may undergo atrophic changes and the secretion of androgen is reduced.

Administration of estrogens, however, even in large doses, after the ovulation, does not affect the course of normal menstrual cycle.

• ***Suppression of lactation***: Estrogens suppress lactation without affecting prolactin levels.

• ***Metabolic actions***: They have a weak anabolic action. Given over a long period, they may cause sodium and water retention. Estrogens reduce the level of plasma cholesterol but increase that of triglycerides. They promote urate reabsorption by the proximal renal tubule. This accounts for the lower mean 24 hours urinary urate excretion in women than in men.

Large doses of estrogens given over a long period inhibit the growth of epiphyseal cartilage.

• **Bones**: Estrogens have a positive effect on the bone mass which is mediated by complex actions. Osteoblasts and osteoclasts express both ERα and ERβ. The former play a major role.

(a) Estrogen directly regulates the osteoblasts and brings about their differentiation.

(b) It increases the osteoblast and osteocyte survival by inhibiting their apoptosis.

(c) The major effect is to decrease the number and activity of the osteoclasts via altering the cytokine signals from the osteoblasts. Estrogen prevents differentiation of osteoclast precursors into osteoclasts; and increases osteoclast apoptosis. This results in prevention of bone resorption by the osteoclasts.

• ***Carcinogenicity***: Estrogens are carcinogenic in animals, and are implicated in the genesis of cancers of the endometrium, breast, liver and vagina (see later).

• ***Antiandrogenic action***: Topical application of small amount of estrogen can counter the action of the androgen on capon's comb. Estrogens have been found to be beneficial in prostatic cancer which is probably androgen dependent.

Absorption, fate and excretion: Both the natural and synthetic estrogens can get absorbed through the skin and the mucous membranes and can cause systemic effects. Given orally, estrogens are well absorbed but the natural estrogens are not so effective as they are metabolized during their passage through the liver (first pass). Enterohepatic circulation of estrogens does occur.

About 65% of the dose is excreted in the urine, 20% of which is estradiol and the rest as metabolites. About 10% of the dose is recoverable in feces; the fate of the remaining is unknown. Liver plays an important role in the conjugation of steroidal estrogens. Nonsteroids are not metabolized so easily and hence a large fraction of nonsteroidal estrogens such as diethylstilbestrol is excreted in urine in free state.

Estrogen esters like benzoate and

dipropionate when injected, are absorbed slowly and are effective for several days or weeks.

Bioassay: The crystalline pure estrogenic preparations need no bioassay. The activity of estrogenic substances is bioassayed in rats by the method of Allen and Doisy, which is based upon the observation of typical cornified vaginal smear following estrogen administration. This test is very sensitive, particularly if the agent is applied locally into the vagina of the test animal.

Adverse reactions: The adverse reactions to estrogens can be grouped as those :

(a) **Following physiological doses in hormone replacement therapy (HRT);** and

(b) **Following pharmacological doses in oral contraceptives.**

This section describes the adverse reactions to replacement doses of estrogens; those due to contraceptive doses of estrogens are discussed in Chapter 66.

Nausea, vomiting and anorexia are the commonest adverse effects of HRT and are similar to those occurring in pregnancy. They can be minimised by taking the drug with food or at bedtime. Sodium and water retention can cause edema, and fullness and tenderness of the breasts; they generally indicate excessive dosage. Intermittent vaginal bleeding occurs in some women on HRT. Any active ectopic endometrial tissue (endometriosis) can undergo deterioration during this therapy. Uncontrolled hypertension and migraine may worsen when the patient is on estrogen. Greater cholesterol saturation in the bile predisposes to gall stones. Estrogens can cause an increase in the plasma TG in those with familial tendency to hyper-triglyceridemia.

• ***HRT does not cause a deterioration of glucose tolerance***. It lowers the plasma levels of LDL and of total plasma cholesterol, while increasing those of plasma HDL. It causes only minimal elevation of the binding proteins (thyroxine binding protein, corticosteroid binding protein, sex hormone binding protein and renin substrate). By multiple mechanisms, including their salubrious effects on the lipid profile, estrogens restore the cardioprotective effects in the menopausal women. *The incidence of hypertension is lower* in postmenopausal women who are on HRT than in those who are not. *The clotting factors are not elevated and the risk of thrombophlebitis is not increased in such women.* HRT is not contraindicated in women with diabetes mellitus, controlled hypertension, varicose veins nor in those with cancers, or history of cancers, other than of the endometrium, breast or liver.

• ***Prolonged, unopposed, estrogen therapy* increases the risk of endometrial carcinoma**. Any existing breast carcinoma can undergo exacerbation during estrogen therapy. The administration of diethylstilbestrol to pregnant women caused a variety of genital abnormalities, including vaginal adenosis and vaginal adenocarcinoma, in the female offsprings of such women. The use of 'synthetic' non-steroidal estrogens for other purposes than prostate cancers is now obsolete.

• ***Pharmacological doses of estrogens administered to prepuberal girls*** can cause: (a) premature breast enlargement (thelarche): and precocious puberty ; and (b) stunting of linear growth of the long bones and hence of final height by accelerating the closure of the epiphysial plate.

Preparations and dosage:

• ***Natural estrogens and their esters***

(i) Estradiol, micronized, 1 mg., 2 mg. tablets (Estrace) for oral use. For IM use, it is available as injection 1 mg./ml. in 10 ml. containers.

(ii) Estraderm MX : These are self-adhesive, estradiol patches, releasing 25, 50 or 100 mcg of estradiol per 24 hours for 3-4 days. They should not be applied near the breasts for fear of causing breast cancer. They are very expensive. Gel and metered dose spray of estradiol are also available.

(iii) Estradiol valerate (Progynova, Delestrogen) 1 and 2 mg. tablets.

(iv) Estradiol benzoate injection usually contains 1 mg. per ml. The effect lasts for several days; dose 1 to 5 mg. by intramuscular injection.

(v) Estradiol dipropionate is adminstered IM in the same dose and by the same route as the benzoate. It is given once in 1-2 weeks.

(vi) The long acting IM estrogen preparations are estradiol cypionate, administered every 3-4 weeks in the dose of 1 to 5 mg., estradiol undeconate, given in the dose of 100 mg. every 3 weeks (mainly in prostatic carcinoma) and estradiol valerate (Progynova, Delestrogen), 5 to 20 mg. given at intervals of 2 to 4 weeks.

(vii) Estriol succinate 2 mg. tablets (Evalon) and *vaginal cream* (0.1%, Ovestin).

(viii) Estradiol vaginal tab (Vagifem) 25 mcg.

• ***Semisynthetic steroidal estrogens***

(i) Ethinyl estradiol tablets (Lynoral) 0.01 and 0.05 mg. In the treatment of prostatic cancer the dose recommended is 1-2 mg. daily.

(ii) Mestranol, the 3-methyl ether of ethinyl estradiol, is a prodrug, converted to ethinyl estradiol; it is ½ as potent as the latter (Chapter 64).

• ***Conjugated estrogens*** (Premarin, Conjugase): This preparation is a mixture of numerous water soluble conjugated estrogens, mainly esters of estrone and equilin, obtained from pregnant mares' urine. They are available as 0.625 and 1.25 mg. *tablets*, as an *injection* containing 20 mg. of the drug in 5 ml, and as *vaginal cream* (0.625 in 1g base). The dose for control of excessive menstrual bleeding is 20 mg. by slow intravenous injection.

Cenestin (Synthetic conjugated estrogens A; Duramed): This preparation contains "nine of the ten known conjugated estrogens present in Premarin." They are water soluble, well absorbed in the GI tract and are metabolized in the liver. Their precautions, adverse effects and contraindications are similar to those of other estrogen preparations. The preparation appears to be safe and effective in the dose of one to two 0.625 mg tablets, for short term treatment of vasomotor symptoms of menopause.

• ***Synthetic nonsteroidal estrogens***

(i) Diethylstilbestrol (Stilbestrol) tablet contains 1, 5 and 25 mg. It is the most potent nonsteroidal estrogen.

(ii) Quinestrol 100 mcg tablets. It is a long acting estrogen.

(iii) Dienoestrol *vaginal cream*.

(iv) Chlorotrianesene (TACE) is a synthetic nonsteroid estrogen. It is rarely used.

• ***Cosmetic preparations***: Topical preparations containing physiological amounts of estrogens or natural progesterone have been promoted as cosmetic, rejuvenating creams. There is no evidence that the hormone creams are any more effective than simple emollients in relieving the dryness of the skin or in improving the facial appearance. However, systemic effects may follow their excessive use.

TIBOLONE (Livial) : This synthetic steroid is a prodrug and undergoes tissue-selective conversion to estrogenic, progestogenic and mildly androgenic metabolites. Its precautions, adverse reactions and contraindications are similar to those of the standard estrogenic preparations. In the dose of 2.5 mg (one tablet) daily, it is used in:

(a) The treatment of vasomotor symptoms and prophylaxis of osteoporosis, in menopausal women. It is given continuously and concurrent administration of a progestin is not necessary. It is unsuitable for use in the first 12 months after the last menstrual period as it may cause irregular bleeding; and

(b) The treatment of vasomotor symptoms in premenopausal women who are being treated with a GnRH analongue.

Its superiority over the standard estrogenic preparations is not established. It is expensive.

Phytoestrogens : These are compounds such as isoflavones and lignans present in plants such as soy, flaxseeds, red clover and cohosh; they are converted in the intestines to compounds with 1/10,000th the estrogenic activity of estradiol. Some of them also have antiestrogenic activity. Phytoestrogens have been promoted for use in postmenopausal women for prevention of osteoporosis, breast cancer and ischemic heart disease. The evidence in their favour is largely epidemiological in that women from certain Asian countries whose daily diet contains substantial quantities of soy have a lower prevalence of the above ailments. Their long term effects when used as medication need further evaluation. The commercially available preparations are expensive.

Selective Estrogen Receptor Modulators (SERMs) : Unlike the predominantly estrogenic compounds (the classical steroidal and non-steroidal estrogens) and the purely antiestrogenic compound (clomiphene), SERMs exert pharmacological actions on binding to the two estrogen receptors (ERα and ERβ), and are tissue-selective. *They are partially estrogenic in some tissues with antiestrogenic activity or no activity in others* e.g. **tamoxifen** has antiestrogenic action on the breast but estrogenic action on the bone and the endometrium. **Raloxifene** is more selective and has estrogenic action on the bone, antiestrogenic action on the breast and negligible action on the endometrium (Chaper 68).

Therapeutic uses of estrogens : Parenteral estrogen preparations are now used rarely. The preparations commonly employed clinically are ethinyl estradiol, conjugated estrogen, estriol and estradiol; their therapeutically equipotent doses are shown in Table 65.3.

Low dose estrogen therapy (vaginal cream and oral estriol in the dose of upto 3 mg/day) relieves menopausal hot flushes and genitourinary symptoms but does not offer protection either to the bones or to the heart; low dose therapy does not stimulate the endometrium either; it can be used without concurrent administration of a progestogen.

Table 65.3: Therapeutically equivalent daily doses of estrogens

- Ethinyl estradiol (oral) 5-10 mcg
- Conjugated estrogen (oral) 0.625 mg
- Micronized estradiol (oral) 1 mg
- Estradiol (oral) 2 mg
- Estradiol (transdermal) 50 mcg

- ***Amenorrhoea*:** Amenorrhoea may be (a) **primary,** where failure of establishment of menstruation has occurred; or (b) **secondary,** which occurs after the menstruation is established.

(a) ***Primary amenorrhoea (Replacement therapy)*:** Hypogonadism is diagnosed when a girl without any abnormality of the genital tract does not start menstruating by the age of 18 years. Although delayed menarche may often be constitutional, a girl who does not start menstruating by the age of 15 years needs to be investigated. Undernutrition and systemic disease are common causes of such delay and need to be treated. If the girl shows good development of secondary sex characters, she can be reassured that things will work out well, and she should be encouraged to wait. But, if breast development has not occurred, the possibility of hypogonadism should be considered. An attempt should be made to distinguish between ovarian causes *(primary or hypergonadotrophic hypogonadism)* and pituitary-hypothalamic causes *(secondary or hypogonadotrophic hypogonadism)*. If hypogonadism is the final diagnosis, such patients will need *hormone replacement therapy* (HRT).

The commonest cause of **primary hypogonadism** is gonadal dysgenesis (Turner syndrome) due to a sex chromosome abnormality. Most of such patients are short, in addition to being sexually infantile.

In *patients who are not short*, replacement treatment is started with ethinyl estradiol 10 mcg or conjugated estrogen 0.3 mg per day. This is continued till the first vaginal bleeding (usually spotting) occurs; breast start developing during that period. Then, the patient is prescribed either (a) a low dose combined oral contraceptive pill (see Chapter 64) for 21 days every month; or (b) conjugated estrogen 0.625 mg. daily, without a break, plus a progestin (medroxyprogesterone 10 mg. per day) for 10 days out of every month.

The advantages of adding a progestin are:

(i) Better breast development.

(ii) More complete shedding of the stimulated endometrium every month, so that a build up does not occur; and

(iii) Prevention of endometrial cancer which has been reported in patients who were treated with unopposed estrogen regimen for long periods of time. Such protection is not complete.

In patients with gonadal dysgenesis *who are short*, treatment should begin with ethinyl estradiol (100 ng/kg/day, uninterruptedly) at about the age of 12 years. Such doses have been found to cause stimulation of linear growth without promoting the development of secondary sexual characters. Therapy with larger, feminizing doses (10 mcg and more) of ethinylestrediol should be initiated only after the linear growth comes to a halt.

Patients with **secondary hypogonadism** are treated in an identical manner as those with primary hypogonadism; but they may require replacement therapy with other hormones (thyroxine, a glucocorticoid) as well.

(b) ***Secondary amenorrhoea***: The important causes are : pregnancy; menopause (normal or premature); systemic disease; chronic anovulation (ovarian cause or other endocrine causes); and pituitary-hypothalamic failure (functional or structural disorder). If the patient is **hypoestrogenic**, she needs hormone replacement as described above. If she is **hyperestrogenic**, as in polycystic ovary syndrome, she only needs periodic withdrawal bleeding with a progestin. The cause, if found, needs to be treated in addition to the hormone treatment. If she desires to become pregnant, ovulation inducing drugs may have to be used. *Severe stress such as occurs in competitive sports needs to be kept in mind as a cause of amenorrhoea.*

• ***Menopause***: With age, the ovarian function decreases and finally ceases, resulting in menopause. The menstrual irregularity observed just prior to the menopause is due to anovulatory cycles and can be treated by cyclic administration of progestins. The occurrence of menopause is sometimes followed by such symptoms as hot flushes, fatigue, loss of concentration, muscle cramps, anxiety, insomnia, vertigo, myalgias and arthralgias. Urinary urgency or incontinence may be present, and fainting may occur. The long term complications are : osteoporosis (Chapter 68), increased liability to IHD and symptoms of urogenital atrophy such as dyspareunia, senile vaginitis, kraurosis vulvae and urinary symptoms.

Mild cases need only proper explanation of the natural physiological process, reassurance and perhaps a tranquillizer. Hot flushes respond to oral estriol (Evalon), which has no other estrogenic effects. Patients with symptoms due to urogenital atrophy without systemic symptoms of estrogen deficiency do well with local application of an estrogen cream (Dienestrol 0.01% cream or Conjugase cream) or estradiol vaginal tablets (Vagifem). Estrogen is absorbed from the vaginal mucosa and may produce systemic effects, if used in large quantities. Further, gynecomastia has been reported in the sexual partners of women using such a cream.

Patients with more troublesome symptoms need short term estrogen replacement treatment for 6 months to 3 years.

Prevention and treatment of menopausal osteoporosis: (Chapter 68). It requires HRT for 5-10 years, starting in the perimenopausal period, and must be initiated *with due caution.*

Estrogens are potent inhibitors of osteoclastic bone resorption. They are (a) more effective in the preventing the worsening of bone status than in the management of established osteoporosis; and (b) more effective in Type I osteoporosis (which occurs in the early postmenopausal years) than in Type II osteoporosis (which occurs in late postmenopausal years). *That they reduce fracture rate has not yet been demonstrated by controlled clinical trials. Further, estrogen + progestin HRT doubles the risk of breast cancer and heart disease in the first year of use. It works for symptoms but not for future health.*

Table 65.4: Contraindications to HRT in menopausal women

- Unexplained vaginal bleeding.
- Endometrial or breast carcinoma.
- Family history of carcinoma of breast.
- Active endometriosis (unopposed estrogen).
- Chronic impairment of liver function.
- Familial hypertriglyceridemia; serum triglyceride above 250 mg/dl.
- Uncontrolled hypertension.
- Any evidence of cardiovascular pathology.
- Seizure disorder.
- Recent thrombophlebitis.
- Unreliable subject.

Hence, its use is restricted to women with severe menopausal symptoms.

Before starting long term HRT (5 years or longer), the patient should be examined carefully for any possible contraindication to such therapy (Table 65.4). She should be told what to expect as a result of the treatment including a possible increase in the chance of developing breast cancer. She is advised to report any untoward symptoms, especially vaginal bleeding. The patient needs regular, periodic monitoring, including breast examination, every 6-12 months while on HRT.

Table 65.5 lists the currently used **HRT regimens in menopausal women;** combined preparations which may be used for the same purpose are: Estradiol valerate 2 mg plus levonorgestrel 75 mcg (Nuvelle), and conjugated estrogen 0.625 mg plus levonorgestrel 75 mcg (Prempak 0.625).

The use of estrogens with the intention of offering cardioprotection is no longer recommended because of increase in morbidity and mortality in those with pre-existing cardiovascular disease.

- ***Vulvo-vaginitis in children***: In this condition, the infection persists because the vaginal pH at this age is alkaline, and the epithelium is columnar and these are not hostile to the growth of pathogens. Following estrogen therapy, the vaginal epithelium cornifies with the deposition of glycogen. The glycogen is converted into lactic acid by the *Doderlein bacilli,* resulting in acidic pH, which prevents growth of bacteria. Ethinyl estradiol in the doses of 0.02-0.05 mg. daily for 6-7 days along with a proper antibiotic is usually recommended. The hormone can also be used topically.

Table 65.5: Current HRT regimens for menopausal women

In women with intact uterus

- Conjugated estrogen 0.625 mg. or an equivalent amount of another estrogen preparation daily for 25 days out of every month *plus* medroxyprogesterone acetate (MPA) 10 mg. daily for the last 10 days of the estrogen cycle.*
- Estrogen (as above) daily, uninterruptedly *plus* MPA (as above) 10 days every month.
  The above two regimens are associated with a return of monthly menstrual bleeding, which is unacceptable to most women.
- Estrogen as above daily *plus* MPA 2.5 mg. or norethisterone 350 mcg. daily, both given without interruption. This regimen causes endometrial atrophy and may be associated with frequent breakthrough bleeding, especially during the first 6 months of therapy.

In women who have had hysterectomy

- Estrogen as above, given continuously.

* Norethisterone 1 mg, levonorgestrel 150-250 mcg, or dehydrogesterone 10-20 mg may be used in place of MPA.

- ***Acute severe dysfunctional uterine bleeding***: Twenty mg of conjugated, equine estrogen (Premarin) given IV every 4 hours for 4-6 doses are occasionally used in this condition. Bleeding usually ceases in 4-24 hours. In patients with an atrophic endometrium, e.g., those on prolonged progestin medication for the treatment of dysfunctional bleeding, concurrent administration of an estrogen preparation is beneficial and may prevent intermittent bleeding from an atrophic endometrium. A progestin such as. norethisterone can also be used to treat DUB (see later)

- ***As post-coital contraceptives***: Chapter 66.
- ***Prostatic cancer***: Chapter 59.
- ***Hirsutism***: Chapter 67.
- ***Miscellaneous uses***: Estrogens can suppress lactation and relieve the engorgement of the breasts; evacuation of the breasts by breast pump is, however, preferred.

Progesterone and Other Progestins

The first effective progestational substance was isolated by Corner and Allen (1930) from the corpus luteum. They also described the 'progestational proliferation' of the endometrium and showed that corpus luteum was necessary for the preparation of the uterus for successful nidation of the fertilized ovum. The hormone, however, could not be used therapeutically because of its short action, ineffectiveness by oral route and short supply. The introduction of new, orally effective, synthetic progestational drugs (progestins) has revolutionized pharmacotherapeutics in gynecologic endocrinology.

Progesterone is naturally secreted by the CL and placenta. It is also synthesized by the adrenals and testes where it acts as a precursor of steroid hormones. (Fig. 65.2)

Physiological functions of progesterone: The important physiological functions are :

- ***Decrease in the estrogen-driven, proliferation of the endometrium (antiestrogen action) and development of secretory endometrium.***
- ***Promotion of the development of the alveolar (acinar) system of the breast;***
- ***Preparation of the endometrium for the implantation of the fertilized ovum*** and to induce ***decidual reaction***;
- ***Induction of changes in the vaginal epithelium and secretion***, characteristic of progestational effect (See below).
- ***Natriuresis,*** especially in pregnancy wherein plasma progesterone levels are high.
- ***Maintenance of pregnancy.***
- ***Metabolic changes*** including the midcycle rise in basal body temperature (BBT) in human females. This rise is correlated with ovulation.

Bioassay of progestational activity: Various procedures now available are based on the technic used originally by Corner and Allen. In this method, an isolated female rabbit in estrous is castrated following the coitus and then given the unknown extract in divided doses for five days. The endometrium is then examined histologically for the degree of secretory changes induced. None of the assay technics, however, can give an unequivocal estimate of the progestational activity of the newer synthetic compounds as some of them have estrogenic and androgenic properties as well.

Classification of progestins:

I **Progesterone.**

II **Derivatives of progesterone:**

- ***Esters of 17-alpha hydroxyprogesterone*** such as caproate or acetate.
- ***C6-substituted 17-alpha hydroxyprogesterone derivatives*** e.g. Medroxyprogesterone acetate (MPA), Megestrol and Chlormadinone acetate.
- ***Dydrogesterone*** or ***dehydrogesterone*** (Duphaston).

III **Derivatives of testosterone,** e.g. Ethisterone and Dimethisterone.

IV **Derivatives of 19-nor testosterone** (testosterone without the 19-methyl group Fig. 65.4), e.g., Norethisterone (Norethindrone), Norethisterone acetate, Norethynodrel, Ethynodiol diacetate, Norgestrel, Lynestrenol, Desogestrel, Norgestimate and Gestodene.

The progestational actions of the

Progesterone Testosterone 19 Nor-testosterone

Fig. 65.4

testosterone derivatives are, in general, similar to those of progesterone except that they are modified by the associated estrogenic and/or androgenic properties of these compounds. Hence, progestins can also be classified as:

I **Pure progestins** e.g. Progesterone, Dehydrogesterone, Esters of 17-alpha hydroxy-progresterone, Chlormadinone and Megestrol.

II **True progestins with possible androgenic effects,** e.g., Medroxy-progesterone, Norgestrel.

III **Progestins with androgenic effects** e.g. Norethisterone.

IV **Progestins with estrogenic effects** e.g. Norethynodrel.

V **Steroids of uncertain status** e.g. Ethynodiol diacetate.

VI **Newer progestins** e.g. Desogestrel, Gestodene, and Norgestimate.

VII **Spironolactone analogue :** Drospirenone.

Pharmacological actions of progestins :

● ***Endometrium***: Progesterone, administered to the properly prepared (estrogen primed) hypogonadal patients, duplicates the changes of secretory phase (luteal phase) of the menstrual cycle. Its continuation prolongs the luteal phase and induces decidual changes, characteristic of early pregnancy. With testosterone derivatives and 19-nor compounds, however, the histological changes are not so classical, on account of their additional estrogenic and/or androgenic actions.

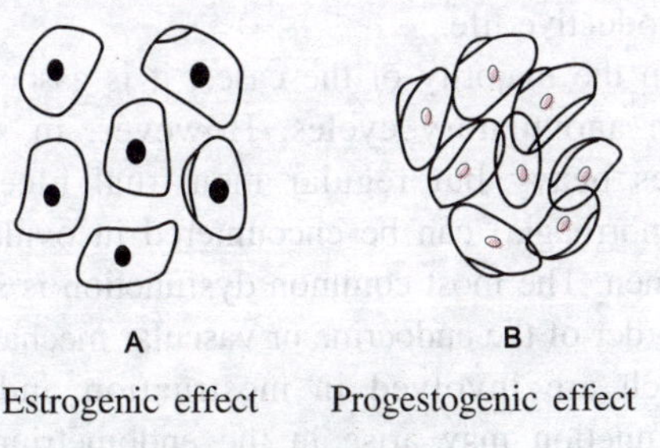

Fig. 65.5 : Vaginal cytology

● ***Vaginal epithelium and secretion***: Progesterone prevents cornification of the vaginal epithelium and brings about increased glycogen deposition. The epithelial cells show increased folding and elongation of nuclei (Fig. 65.5). Complete maturation of cells cannot take place and increased number of cells are desquamated. Thin, watery and profuse vaginal secretion, so characteristic of estrogenic action, becomes thick, viscid and scanty.

● ***Mammary gland***: Exogenous progesterone can promote acinar growth in estrogen primed mammary glands.

● ***Ovulation inhibition***: Progesterone inhibits ovulation only in large doses. *The synthetic 19-nor testosterone derivatives however, are potent gonadotropin and ovulation inhibitors; this could be partly due to their estrogenic activity.*

● ***Metabolic actions***: Exogenous progesterone can raise the BBT similar to that observed during the midcycle. Synthetic progestins such as testosterone derivatives and dehydrogesterone are not thermogenic.

Progesterone causes increase in the basal and postglucose insulin secretion. It promotes glycogen deposition and ketogenesis. It stimulates lipoprotein lipase and causes fat deposition.

Progesterone probably has some catabolic action and has been shown to promote nitrogen loss. It also promotes sodium and chloride loss by competing with aldosterone in the kidney. These actions are prominent in patients with adrenal insufficiency. Synthetic progestins, however, have no such consistent effects. In the doses in which they are used in HRT, MPA and levonorgestrel can cause insulin resistance and impairment of glucose tolerance. Norethisterone seems to be relatively inert in this respect.

• ***Maintenance of pregnancy*:** Natural progesterone probably helps in the maintenance of pregnancy. In *in vitro* studies, progesterone exerts a blocking effect on uterine contractions.

• ***Antineoplastic action*:** There is some evidence to indicate that progesterone can suppress esrogen induced fibromyomata in animals. When added to estrogen as a part the HRT, progestins help to prevent possible development of endometrial carcinoma. Progestins have been used to treat advanced cancer of the breast and the endometrium.

• ***Other actions*:** Progesterone causes mental depression and hypnotic effects. Some of the synthetic progestins have associated estrogenic, androgenic and/or anabolic actions (Table 66.3).

Absorption, fate and excretion: Progesterone is not effective orally, owing to metabolic degradation during its first passage. Further, it has a relatively short biological half-life. Given by injection in oily solution, it is rapidly absorbed and inactivated in the liver. The rate of turnover of progesterone in the body is very rapid. Although other metabolites are also excreted in the urine, estimation of pregnanediol gives valuable information regarding progesterone secretion. The newer progestins are effective orally as they are not easily destroyed during their first pass and have long t½. They are mainly metabolized in the liver.

Adverse reactions: Apart from their pharmacological actions which may modify the menstrual cycle (spotting, breakthrough bleeding) and decrease the flow, progestins, in general, are relatively safe drugs. Derivatives of testosterone and 19-nor testosterone can cause nausea, breast discomfort, headache, fatigue and rarely liver damage.

Some of the synthetic progestins such as norethisterone may cause androgenic actions on developing female foetus and hence, should be avoided during pregnancy. For the same reason, they may cause weight gain, acne and hirsutism.

Preparations and dosage: These are given in Table 65.6. The newer progestins **desogestrel, gestodene** and **norgestimate** are derivatives of norgestrel. As progestins, (1) they are extremely potent inhibitors of ovulation without any androgenic or antiestrogenic effect. (2) In large doses, they have a weaker androgenic and antiestrogenic action than the earlier progestins. (3) They cause fewer changes in lipoprotein metabolism and perhaps in carbohydrate metabolism. Desogestrel and norgestimate are prodrugs. Because of their selectivity of action, they may be preferred in patients with hyperandrogenemia (Chapter 66).

Drospirenone is a spironolactone analogue with progestogenic, anti-mineralocorticoid and antiandrogenic activities. It is a constituent of a combined oral contraceptive pill, Yasmin (Chapter 66). As a spironolactone analogue, drospirenone can cause hyperkalemia.

Therapeutic uses of progestins:

• ***Dysfunctional uterine bleeding (DUB)* :** Primary DUB is not a single entity but a group of diseases. It may be defined as abnormal bleeding from the uterus in the absence of organic disease of the genital tract and extragenital causes. The disorder is common especially at the beginning and the end of reproductive life.

In the majority of the cases, it is associated with anovulatory cycles. However, in some cases heavy but regular menstrual bleeding (menorrhagia) can be encountered in ovulating women. The most common dysfunction is some disorder of the endocrine or vascular mechanism which are involved in mestruation and the dysfunction may arise in the endometrium or hypothalmo-pituitary-ovarian axis. Further,

Table 65.6: Progestins in current use

Preparation	Supplied as	Dosage**	Remarks
Progesterone	Tab. 10, 25 mg. Inj. 25 mg./ml.	Functional uterine bleeding : 5 to 10 mg. I.M. daily; habitual abortion : 1-2 mg. daily; threatened abortion : 5-10 mg. daily.	Mildly catabolic
Derivatives of progesterone :			
Hydroxyprogesterone caproate (Proluton depot)	Inj. 125 and 250 mg./ml.	Threatened and habitual abortion : 125 to 500 mg. weekly I.M.; functional uterine bleeding : same dose.	Mildly catabolic, long acting (8-14 days)
*Medroxyprogesterone acetate (Provera, Farlutal, Modus)	Tab. 5 and 10. mg. Inj. 50 mg.1 ml	Functional uterine bleeding : 5 to 10 mg. daily; threatened and habitual abortion : 10-40 mg. daily orally or 50 to 100 mg. I.M. weekly.	Mildly catabolic.
Dydrogesterone (Duphaston)	Tab. 5 mg.	Dysmenorrhoea : 10 to 25 mg. daily ; same dose also used in threatened abortion and in functional uterine bleeding; in endometriosis : 30 mg. daily.	Does not inhibit ovulation. Mildly catabolic.
Allylestrenol (Gestanin)	Tab. 5 mg.	5-10 mg. daily	
Megestrol		Used in oral contraceptive combination pills.	
Derivatives of testosterone :			
*Dimethisterone	Tab. 5 mg.	15 mg. daily.	Mildly estrogenic
Derivatives of 19 nor-testosterone :			
*Norethisterone (Primolut N)	Tab. 1, 2 and 5 mg.	Primary and secondary amenorrhoea : 5-15 mg. daily; functional uterine bleeding : 10-30 mg. daily; endometriosis : 10-30 mg. daily;	Androgenic and anabolic actions.
*Norethisterone acetate (Regestrone)	Tab. 5 and 10 mg.	2.5 to 15 mg. daily, Indications similar as norethisterone.	Mildly androgenic and anabolic.
*Norethynodrel	Tab. 5 and 10 mg.	Primary and secondary amenorrhoea: 5 to 10 mg. daily ; endometriosis : 20 to 30 mg. daily.	Estrogenic.
Ethynodiol diacetate		Used in combination OC pills:	
Lynestrenol (Orgametril)	Tab. 0.5 mg.	5-10 mg. daily.	
Desogestrel		Used in combination OC pills	

*Also used as oral contraceptive. **For various regimen details, see text. For Progestosert amd Mirena IUCDs, see text.

human endometrium is known to synthesize PGs locally and the local endometrial dysfunction could be related to the excessive formation of PGE_2. Significantly higher amounts of PGE_2 and PGF_2 in mensturual fluid have been reported in patients with menorrhagia, dysmenorrhoea and endometriosis. Diagnosis is usually made by exclusion with curettage or endometrial biopsy and hysteroscopy to rule out organic disease.

The main clinical manifestation, other than menstrual abnormalities, is iron deficiency anemia; infertility is an additional feature in anovulatory women. A detailed history and physical examination help to establish the diagnosis and type (ovulatory or anovulatory) in most women. Counselling of the patient is very helpful, so is correction of anemia with oral iron. Severe cases may require hospitalization.

Symptomatically, a woman with DUB may present with :

(i) **Oligomonorrhoea** - intervals greater than 35 days.

(ii) **Polymenorrhoea** - intervals less than 24 days.

(iii) **Menorrhagia** - regular, normal intervals with excessive flow and duration.

(iv) **Metrorrhagia** - Irregular intervals, excessive flow and duration.

The three major types of bleeding in DUB are:

(a) *Estrogen withdrawal bleeding,* associated with anovulatory cycle; the flow is heavy and usually painful.

(b) *Estrogen break-through bleeding* due to sustained estrogenic, stimulation of the endometrium, not interrupted by cyclic progesterone secretion. This is the most common type of DUB.

(c) *Progestin break-through bleeding* due to abnormal P/E ratio in the blood.

Table 65.7 summarises management of DUB.

Table 65.7: Management of DUB

• ***Specific drug treatment:***		
	Non-hormonal:	NSAID; Tranexamic acid; Ethamsylate
	Hormonal:	Combined OC pill; Norgestrel-releasing IUCD; Progestin; Danazol
• ***Correction of anemia***:		Iron
• ***Non-drug treatment***:		Counselling

PG-synthetase inhibitors such as mefenamic acid and ibuprofen diminish menstrual bleeding in normal as well as DUB women. They are the first line treatment of DUB, particularly in those who are ovulatory but bleed heavily. These drugs are given for 3-4 days, starting with the onset of bleeding. Other non-hormonal agents used are : **tranexamic acid** and **ethamsylate** (Chapter 32). When contraception is desired, a **combined OC pill or a norgestrel releasing IUD** may be preferred. If the DUB is persistant or recurrent despite hormonal therapy, subjects should be investigated to rule out local causes such as submucous myomas or endometrial polyps or a possible coagulation disorder.

Norethisterone given in doses of 5-10 mg. 4-6 hourly will stop the bleeding within 24 hours. It is usually continued in doses of 5 mg. bid 1-2 weeks. The patient should be warned that the first period which follows cessation of the progestin is likely to be heavy. If the uterine bleeding is severe, hospitalization and IM injection of estradiol valerate 10 mg plus hydroxyprogesterone caproate 100 mg usually controls the bleeding. In order to prevent recurrence of excessive bleeding, cyclical progestin should be commenced on 4-5th day of the withdrawal bleeding and continued till the 25th day, for 3 cycles. In patients with endometrial hyperplasia/anaplasia, it is advisable to continue daily progestin for 9-12 months.

Alternatively, a combination low dose OC pill (Chapter 66) may be administered in the dose of 1 pill 4 times a day for 5 days. This is less well tolerated than the progestogen regimen described above. The full course should be given even if the bleeding stops earlier. This is followed by cyclic administration of the same pill once daily from 5th to 25th day of the cycle for 3-6 cycles. Patients in whom combination OCs are contraindicated may be prescribed danazol 200 mg daily on a continuous basis (Chapter 66).

IUCDs incorporating progesterone (**Progestasert**) or levonorgestrel (**Mirena**) are now available. When used, they release the drug slowly. The serum levels achieved are low and suppress the ovarian function. In 90% of the subjects, the cycles are ovulatory. The locally released progestin causes endometrial thinning and atrophy; the cyclical changes related to the menstrual cycle are abolished. Thirtyfive per cent of the women become amenorrhoeic at one year. These changes are, however, reversible and normal menstruation is restored 1-2 months after removal of the device. They can be used to produce endometrial ablation in severe menorrhagia where hysterectomy is contraindicated. They have also been used to control bleeding in uterine fibroids. They are considered highly effective (80-90 %), relatively safe and usually well tolerated.

● ***Dysmenorrhea*:** Some women complain of either discomfort or pain (either dull or colicky) in the lower abdomen before or during menstruation (dysmenorrhea). 'Dysmenorrhea' is only a symptom and not a diagnosis. It is common in the teenagers but also occurs in the older women. *Before starting drug treatment, one should make certain that a local cause such as an intrauterine contraceptive device is not responsible for this symptom.*

The cause of the **primary spasmodic dysmenorrhoea** of the teenager is not known but it generally disappears with increasing age. Most girls with this symptom are helped by physical exercise, explanation, reassurance, and NSAID ± codeine, given either alone or together with an antimuscarinic drug. *Marriage and pregnancy should not be suggested as cures for this condition.* When the symptom is severe and incapacitating, it can be abolished by inhibiting ovulation with a 'combination pill' given daily from 5th to 25th day of the menstrual cycle for 4-6 cycles. While dispensing such pills to unmarried girls, care should be taken not to label the container as 'contraceptive pills'. In most cases the symptom does not recur after stopping the treatment. If inhibition of ovulation is considered undesirable for some reason, oral dehydrogesterone (which is more expensive) may be used from 8th to 25th day of the cycle in the dose of 5-10 mg twice a day.

Patients not responding to the above therapy and all older women with **secondary dysmenorrhea** need careful gynaecological investigation to exclude local lesions such as endometriosis, fibroids and infection. Dysmenorrhoea may be a presenting symptom in pelvic tuberculosis. In all such cases the treatment of the cause is important.

Membranous dysmenorrhea is rare and often familial. The menstrual endometrium is painfully shed in large strips or even as a complete cast. Although the oral pills can be used to treat these cases the results are less rewarding; curettage is also unhelpful. Norethisterone 10 mg. daily given for five, immediately premenstrual days may produce beneficial effects in some patients.

● ***Amenorrhea*:** If a woman presents with amenorrhoea, progestogen withdrawal test is helpful in distinguishing between patients with normal and low circulating estradiol levels. In the former case, administration of medroxy-progesterone or norethisterone (5 mg twice a day) for 5 days is followed by withdrawal bleeding within 7-10 days. Such bleeding, in patients with primary amenorrhoea, also establishes the patency of the lower genital tract. If there is no withdrawal bleeding, the possibilties are either very low estrogen levels or an abnormality of the uterus or vagina. This test is useful but *should be performed only after ruling out pregnancy in sexually active women of the reproductive age.* The same regimen may be used once in 1-2 months in patients with severe oligomenorrhoea due to chronic anovulation from polycystic ovary syndrome (PCO).

● ***Endometriosis*:** Endometriosis is a chronic, estrogen dependent disorder associated with pain and infertility. It is due to the presence of extrauterine, endometrial deposits. The aims of therapy are relief of pain and restoration of

Table 65.8: Drugs used in endometriosis

- Oral Progestins
- Danazol (Chapter 64).
- GnRH analogues (see earlier).
- Combined OC pills (Chapter 64)

fertility. This is done by suppressing ovarian function and limiting growth and activity of the lesions. The drugs (Table 65.8) for this purpose are used for a limited period (generally 6 months) because of unacceptable adverse effects of longer treatment.

Oral progestins, given continuously, are highly effective in this condition. They cause marked regression of the endometrium. Norethisterone can be used daily in doses of 20 mg. increasing by 10 mg. daily if vaginal spotting occurs. Amenorrhoea can be maintained by 40-60 mg. daily dose for 3 to 9 months depending upon the severity of the case. Medroxy-progesterone in the dose of 20 mg. daily is also useful. For use of danazol in endometriosis, see Chapter 66.

- ***Fibrocystic disease of the breast*:** This condition in young women is believed to be associated with excessive estrogen and/or prolactin action on the breast tissue. The clinical features range from mastodynia (painful breasts) through nodularity of the breasts to a large discrete lump that needs to be distinguished from breast cancer. Danazol is the most effective drug for use but it is expensive and may cause undesirable side effects (Chapter 66). A cheaper, though less effective, alternative is one of the progestins given orally. Any of the following may be used in divided, daily doses from 14th to 28th day of the menstrual cycle: medroxyprogesterone, 20 mg; norethisterone, 20 mg; or norethisterone acetate, 10 mg. If the patient has elevated prolactin level, bromocriptine may be tried in the dose of 2.5 mg once to thrice a day. The treatment should generally last for 6 months or longer.
- ***As oral contraceptives*:** (Chapter 66).
- ***Precocious puberty*:** Medroxyprogesterone is useful in treating children with central precocious puberty. It acts by inhibiting the pituitary gonadotropin release and has to be used regularly for several years until the time is opportune to allow the child to mature sexually. Its use has been largely replaced by that of GnRH agonists (see earlier).
- ***Postponement of menstruation*:** Progestins can be used to prolong the luteal phase of the menstrual cycle and thus to postpone the onset of menstruation. Norethisterone orally 5 mg. daily is adequate if the subject comes early in the second half of the menstrual cycle. If, however, she seeks advice only a few days before the due date, higher doses (5-10 mg. tid) are needed. Some women may not tolerate such high doses of norethisterone, orally; in that case, hydroxy-progesterone caproate (250 mg. IM) along with small oral doses of norethisterone may be used.
- ***Endometrial carcinoma*:** Chapter 59.
- ***HRT*:** A progestin is used as a part of the HRT regimen (see earlier).
- ***Male sex offenders*:** Large doses of medroxyprogesterone are used as an adjunct to psychiatric therapy or psychosexual counselling in male sex offenders.
- ***Miscellaneous*:** Progesterone is used to treat short luteal phase. Oral dehydrogesterone 10 mg bid or micronized progesterone 100 mg bid (orally or vaginally) or progesterone IM 25-50 mg daily can be used to provide luteal support when needed. Progestins can be used to treat menopausal hot flushes in women in whom estrogens are contraindicated. Their usefulness in the treatment of threatened and habitual abortion is doubtful.

Antifertility Agents and Ovulation Inducing Drugs

66

World population growth has become a major problem with far reaching con-sequences. According to the United Nations estimate, at the present rate of growth, the world population is expected to doube in 35 years and it would increase eight-fold in a century. If the world resources are considered, this forecasts a disaster for the human race, unless the fertility is controlled. As for India, the equivalent of the entire population of Australia is added every year!

Fertility control is very essential for maintaining satisfactory standards of living and for raising the existing standards in developing countries. Furthermore, it is equally important for family planning which is defined as "the limitation and spacing of births in the best interests of the mother, the child and the rest of the family". The problem is essentially interdisciplinary and can only be tackled by the concerted efforts by biologists, sociologists and educationists; the use of drugs for this purpose is but one aspect of the whole programme.

Physiology of human reproduction: The reproductive cycle in the human, in whom ovulation is a key event, is the result of the interplay of the hypothalamus, the pituitary and the ovaries. With respect to ovulation, the mammalian females can be divided into two groups:

I **Reflex ovulators** e.g. rabbits, cats, ferrets and minks, in whom the sensory stimulus of mating or electrical stimulation of cervix induces ovulation; and

II **Spontaneous ovulators** like cows, monkeys and women, in whom follicular rupture occurs in the absence of any immediate sensory stimulus.

At the time of puberty, the human ovary contains about 3,00,000 immature follicles of which only about 400 mature during the reproductive life of about 30 years. Of these, only a few can get fertilized and lead to successful pregnancies.

Under the influence of pituitary FSH, the ovarian follicle matures and considerable amounts of estrogen are produced. The sudden midcycle spurt of luteinizing hormone (LH) is followed by ovulation, releasing the ovum. Ovulation usually occurs on day 14 (±2) of a 28 day cycle (Fig. 65.1). The oocyte enters the fallopian tube and within 12 hours it reaches the ampullary region where it can be fertilized by the sperm. By 18th day of the cycle, the fertilized ovum is converted into a blastocyst which reaches the cavity of the uterus. By 21st-23rd day of the cycle, the blastocyst begins to get implanted (nidation) beneath the surface of the uterine endometrium. The implantation stage is completed by 35th day from the first day of the last menstrual period; at this time the fetal placental circulation starts developing. This means that pregnancy may be considered as existing only 5 weeks after the onset of last menstrual cycle.

Ovulation may be judged by noting:

- ***Changes in the cervical mucus,***
- ***Vaginal cytology*** (Fig. 66.5):
- ***Serum progesterone level.***
- ***Endometrial biopsy;*** and
- ***Rise in basal body temperature.***

All these changes reflect the production of progesterone by the corpus luteum.

The **cervical mucus** is an alkaline gel, rich in protein and fructose. During the follicular phase it is clear, thin, copious, acellular and somewhat elastic. This property permits the mucus to be stretched into threads from 5 to 15 cm. in length. Because of the presence of abundant sodium and potassium chloride, the mucus assumes a characteristic fern-like pattern when dried on a glass slide. Clinically, ferning and 'thread test' (spinnbarkeit) are utilized to judge the estrogen influence. Just before the ovulation, its consistency is believed to be the most ideal for the transport of sperms into the uterus. Soon after the ovulation, under the influence of progesterone, the cervical mucus becomes tough, viscous and translucent and the sperms may find it difficult to penetrate it. The ferning disappears and it cannot be stretched without breaking. Some women may experience unilateral low abdominal pain at approximately midcycle; this is attributed to the occurence of ovulation.

Although all these parameters are useful clinically, none of them can be considered as a definite evidence of ovulation. The only definite evidence of ovulation is either recovery of the ovum or pregnancy.

Extrahypothalamic regions of the CNS, acting via the hypothalamus, exert a modulating influence on ovulation. The menstrual rhythm and probably ovulation in the human female are influenced by emotional and environmental factors. Thus, irregular menstrual periods are known in nurses on night duty and in air hostesses travelling great distances.

The exact duration of survival of sperms in the vagina is not known but is believed to be about 1-2 hours while they can remain active in the cervix and uterine cavity for about 45-50 hours.

Fertility Control: Apart from the coitus interruptus, theoretically, the fertility control can be achieved by:

- ***Controlling the central mechanisms.***
- ***Modifying other physiological mechanisms of reproduction;*** and
- ***Preventing the union of sperm with ovum*** by using physical or chemical barriers.

Since the hypothalamus is known to play an important role in controlling the secretion of pituitary gonadotropins,emotional factors and certain drugs acting on the hypothalamus can block or induce ovulation by modifying the secretion of GnRH. Thus, lactation amenorrhea due to suckling reflex and amenorrhea in young women due to stress are well known. Tranquilizers like chlorpromazine and reserpine can modify the menstrual cycle in women; and suppression of menses can occur following hypnosis. It has been recognized that conception is delayed in women who breast-feed their babies *fully* probably because of elevated levels of PRL. Breast-feeding thus acts as a natural birth spacer. It is believed that more births are prevented throughout the world by breast feeding than by all other forms of contraception put together!

Birth control by using physical and/or chemical barriers to prevent the union of sperm with ovum is not new. In the Ebers Papyrus of 1550 B.C., the preparation of a tampon treated with a spermicide has been described; and Arabs were using some intrauterine foreign body to prevent the conception in saddled camels for ages. Currently various physical barriers like condoms, pessaries or intraterine devices (IUCD) and chemical barriers in the form of spermicidal gels and foam tablets are used. Such spermicides are simple to use and involve little genital manipulation. Barrier methods, such as use of condoms, have the advantage of reducing the rate of transmission of STD. Most of the spermicides contain the surfactant **nonoxynol 9,** which interferes with sperm motility. These methods, however, are not very reliable and often inconvenient to practise. No doubt, some of these like condoms and IUCD have definite points in favour of their use : (i) they are cheap, safe and readily available, (ii) they require no planned programme as is necessary in the case of oral contraceptives; and (iii) condoms offer protection against STD/HIV.

Fertility can be controlled by using drugs which can act by :

- ***Inhibiting ovulation.***
- ***Modifying the cervical mucus.***
- ***Interfering with the implantation.***
- ***Slowing down the rate of egg transport.***
- ***Preventing the ovum maturation and sperm capacitation.***
- ***Immunological methods;*** and
- ***Inhibiting spermatogenesis in males.***

The drugs which are currently in use act mainly by the first three mechanisms and are discussed below.

Oral contraception is a highly effective and acceptable method. In this method, either an estrogen-progestin combination or a progestin alone is used.

Estrogen-Progestin Combination Pill

Since the first clinical demonstration of usefulness of such an oral combination for contraception by Pincus (1955), several commercial preparations have been available. The following attributes have made these combination pills popular among the educated, higher and middle class women:

- ***Remarkable efficacy.***
- ***Relative safety;*** and
- ***Ease of administration.***

Combination oral contraceptive (COC) pills contain:

(a) Ethinylestradiol or its 3-methyl ether (mestranol) as the estrogen; and

(b) A progestin belonging to 19-nortestosterone group (norethisterone, norgestrel or ethynodiol acetate), one derived from progesterone (megestrol acetate) or a derivative of norgestrel (desogestrel).

Methods of administration:

- ***Fixed dose combination pills*** (Monophasic pills) : The commonest procedure is to administer one pill containing both an estrogen and progestin daily, orally, at bed time, for 21 days, from 5th to 25th day of a 28 day cycle. The next course is started 7 days after the last dose. If the patient forgets to take a 'pill', and she remembers it within 12 hours, she should take the forgotten pill immediately, and then return to the usual schedule. If more than 36 hours have passed between that last (regular) 'pill' taken and the delayed consumption of the missed 'pill', the subject should consider herself unprotected by the pill and use some other method to prevent conception for the next 14 days, in addition to continuing the course of pills. If more than one pill is forgotten, the woman should consider herself similarly unprotected and take other measures to prevent conception.

The pill should be avoided in breast feeding women as it interferes with lactation. If the woman is exclusively breast feeding the baby at regular intervals, including night time (full breast feeding), the pill may be started in the *third post partum month.* If the breastfeeding is partial or not done at all, it can be started in *the third post partum week*; it is not necessary to start it earlier as ovulation is unlikely to occur for 4 weeks after delivery. However, the 'pill' may be started on the very day of an abortion or a medical termination of pregnancy.

When used properly the 'pill' is the most effective (99-100%) contraceptive available.

- ***Biphasic and triphasic combination pills***: These are combination oral contraceptive pills containing varying proportions of an estrogen and a progestin and are designed to simulate the hormonal profile of the normal menstrual cycle. This allows lower doses of both synthetic steroids in the early part of the cycle. Slightly higher doses later in the cycle help to prevent breakthrough bleeding. They are, however, more complex to use, offer little, if any, advantage over the monophasic pills, and are more expensive.

• ***Extended cycle COC:*** (a) A COC pill containing 30 mcg of ethinyl estradiol and 150 mcg of levonorgestrel (Seasonale) is taken daily for 84 days, followed by a placebo pill for 7 days. *This allows withdrawal bleeding once in 3 months i.e. four times a year compared to 13 times during the use of conventional, monthly, COC pills.* Spotting may occur more frequently with this method. The major advantage is that it reduces the number of menses and hence appears to be acceptable to many women.

(b) Another pill available (Lybrel) contains EE 20 mcg and levonorgestrel 90 mcg. It is taken daily, uninterruptedly, for 365 days a year. About 60% of the women develop amennorrhoea within an year. Breakthrough bleeding and spotting are common initially, but decrease subsequently. After stopping the drug, menses resume within 2-3 months in over 90 % of women. The potential long term ADR are not known.

Mechanism of action: The mechanism of the contraceptive action of these agents is complex. The combination type suppresses both FSH rise (due to the estrogen component) and LH peak (due to the progestin component) observed during the normal menstrual cycle, by inhibiting the release of GnRH. *Thus, follicular growth is not initiated and ovulation does not occur.* Although estrogen alone can be effective it is not suitable as it causes profuse, irregular bleeding. The addition of a progestin :

• ***Increases the certainty of the contraceptive effect. In fact, it plays the major role in ovulation inhibition.***

• ***Modifies the cervical mucus, making it thick, tenacious and hostile to the sperms.***

• ***Prevents breakthrough bleeding.***

• ***Ensures predictable withdrawal bleeding after each cycle of treatment;*** and

• ***Reduces the menstrual blood loss.***

The ovulation inhibitory action of progestin is more marked with progestins derived from 19-nortestosterone.

Pharmacological actions of COC pills: These are :

• ***Endometrium*:** The effect produced by the COC pills is similar to that of 'luteal phase'. The full secretory activity of the endometrial glands is achieved within 3-4 days of starting these pills, leading to predecidual changes. Later, the endometrium becomes thin and hypoplastic over a period. The changes are reversed 2-3 months after stoppage of treatment. Continuous administration of a progestin increases the thick cervical mucus, causing a 'cervical barrier' hostile to sperm penetration.

• ***Pituitary-ovarian axis*** **:** Prolonged administration of these drugs does not seem to cause any permanent structural changes in the pituitary or ovary, although during therapy ovaries may appear smaller and their secretion may practically cease. The use of COC pill does not cause permanent infertility.

• ***Metabolic effects*:** Hyperglycemia, glycosuria and mildly impaired glucose tolerance along with a rise in the post-absorptive serum immunoreactive insulin levels have been reported. However, an increased incidence of clinical diabetes mellitus has not been established. The mechanism of these abnormalities is not clearly defined but is believed to be an increased resistance to the peripheral hypoglycemic action of insulin. The incidence of abnormal GTC is related to the dose and potency of progestin. The newer progestins such as desogestrel have little, if any, effect on carbohydrate metabolism.

Increase in cholesterol and low-density lipoprotein (LDL) and lowering of high density lipoprotein (HDL) has been observed following the progestins. Because the estrogen component has an effect opposite to that of the progestin, no significant alterations in the cholesterol level has been observed. The data indicate that the use of COC containing 50 mcg of estrogen by healthy, non-smoking women up to the age of 35 is not associated with an increased risk of serious cardiovascular disease.

The pill also causes a slight increase in plasma triglycerides in some women. Oral contraceptives can accelerate platelet aggregation and adhesion and reduce the activity of the fibrinolytic system. The estrogen component is thought to be responsible for these changes.

• ***Other endocrine glands*** : As in pregnancy, the plasma total thyroxine (T_4) is raised due to a greater concentration of thyroxine binding globulin. There is also an increase in the cortisol binding globulin, transcortin. A slight but definite rise in the free plasma cortisol level and a reduction in the rate of hepatic cortisol metabolism have been reported.

Adverse reactions: *The earlier preparations (in 1970s) contained higher doses of both estrogen and progestin; some of the adverse effects described with those pills may not be relevant to the lower dose pills that came into vogue from the early 1980s and are currently in use.*

• ***General*** : Nausea, anorexia and vomiting are common and are due to the estrogen component. The pill should be taken at bedtime on a full stomach, to minimise them. The estrogen may also be responsible for other effects like breast engorgement, mastalgia, chloasma and increased vaginal secretion (leucorrhea). Excessive estrogen also suppresses lactation.

In certain individuals, the anabolic action of these compounds causes weight gain. In others, the weight gain is due to sodium retention and edema, mostly due to estrogens. Although the compounds from the 19-nortestosterone group have androgenic actions, the latter are rarely evident with therapeutic doses. However, there is a chance of masculinization of a female fetus, if preparations containing 19-norsteroids are taken during pregnancy.

Blurring of vision and mental depression have also been reported; the latter can be serious enough to cause suicidal tendencies and the risk is greater in women with past history of depression.This depression appears to be related to estrogen-induced alteration in vitamin B_6 metabolism and may respond to vitamin B_6 in the dose of 20 mg. twice a day.

Oral contraceptive use increases significantly, though to a small extent, the risk of vaginal infection, particularly candidiasis.

The 'pill' decreases serum levels of pyridoxine, folic acid, vitamin C, calcium and zinc whereas those of vitamin A, copper and iron are elevated.

• ***Bleeding irregularities***: Cycle control is usually excellent. A large proportion of women experience welcome changes in their menstrual cycles. These include regular cycles and relief from dysmenorrhoea, premenstrual tension and excessive menstrual blood loss. Occasionally, however, bleeding similar to that of a normal menstrual period occurs during the course of medication. In such cases, the tablets are stopped and a new course started five days later with a preparation containing larger quantity of progestin. **Spotting** is characterised by intermittent blood-stained trickling during the therapy. Its incidence appears to be higher with low estrogen or no estrogen pills. Occasionally, temporary amenorrhea for 1-2 cycles may occur and is of no significance.

The return of the menstruation following stoppage of the 'pill' may be delayed for 6-8 weeks. Informing the patient about this in advance can spare her many anxious days. Conception may be delayed for 3-4 months after stopping the 'pills'. There is no increased risk of permanent infertility, miscarriage or birth defects.

• ***Thromboembolic phenomena***: There appears to be a definite relationship between the use of COC pill and the incidence of deep vein thrombosis, cerebral thrombosis and pulmonary embolism. This is related to the concentration of the estrogen component. *A dose of 50 mcg. of ethinyl estradiol seems to be the safe upper limit beyond which the risk increases.* The risk is more in women over 35 years of age, especially in those who smoke. The currently used low ethinyl estradiol (30 mcg) pills have considerably reduced this risk. A similar risk is also present in normal pregnancy. In women on the pill, a complaint like persistent headache may be a warning of an impending cerebrovascular accident.

The pill is contraindicated in "patients with thrombophlebitis, thromboembolic disorders, cerebral apoplexy or those with a past history of these conditions". The appearance of any of these or of vascular headaches, leg cramps, visual disturbances or hypertension is an indication for permanent discontinuation of the pill. Oral contraceptives can unmask latent migraine and aggravate existing migrane.

- ***Hypertension***: The reported incidence of hypertension has been as high as 15%. It is reversible within about three months of the discontinuation of the medication and is probably due to the estrogen-induced increase in plasma angiotensinogen. Before treating the hypertension in a female patient, the 'COC pill' as a cause should be ruled out.
- ***Liver***: The hepatic abnormalities induced are usually reversible and are basically alterations in the bile-secreting function of the hepatocytes (cholestatic). Usually, the 'pill' produces no clinical problem, but a substantial number of women have abnormal liver function tests in the absence of symptoms. Only a few women develop clinical cholestatic jaundice. A previous history of jaundice is not a contraindication to oral contraceptives. But, if a woman on the 'pill' develops acute hepatitis the drug should be stopped and should be resumed only after the liver function tests have been normal for at least six months. Rarely, benign vascular hepatomas may occur.
- ***Uterine fibroids***: Uterine fibromyomata can undergo enlargement during therapy with pills, and hence the presence of fibroids is a relative contraindication.
- ***Carcinogenicity***: Although estrogens are carcinogenic, the evidence regarding breast cancer following COC pill use is controversial. However, they should not be used in the presence of estrogen dependent malignancies such as breast cancer, in Hodgkin's disease and in malignant melanoma. *Further, it is a wise precaution to examine the breasts and the cervical smear for malignancy before starting the treatment and then periodically during the therapy.*

Table 66.1 lists the absolute contra-indications to the use of combined COCs.

Table 66.1: Absolute contraindications to combination OC

- Pregnancy.
- Estrogen dependent cancers (endometrium, breast).
- Cardiovascular (CHF, ischemic heart disease, severe uncontrolled systemic hypertension, cardiomyopathy, most types of valvular heart diseases, pulmonary hypertension, vascular malformation of brain, arterial thrombosis, venous thrombosis or known proneness to it).
- Severe or focal migraine,
- Diabetes for 20 years or diabetes with end organ disease
- Hyperlipidemia; and
- Active liver disease.

COC has protective effect against endometrial cancer and epithelial ovarian cancer. Women who use COC for at least a year show a significant protection which persists for at least 15 years after the use of COC ceases.

Drug interactions: See Table 66.2.

Preparations: Table 66.3.

Newer combination OC preparations have been marketed **with shorter hormone-free intervals** than the conventional preparations. The rationale is to reduce the hormone withdrawal symptoms, particularly the withdrawal bleeding, and to decrease the risk of ovulation and unwanted pregnancy. An example

Table 66.2: Drug interactions of combination OC pills

- ***Decreased efficacy of the other drug***: Coumarin anticoagulants; Thyroid hormone; Oral hypoglycemics.
- ***Increased efficacy/toxicity of the other drug***: Theophylline; Imipramine; Cyclosporine; Glucocorticoids (pharmacological doses).
- ***Decreased efficacy of OC pills***: Barbiturates; Antiepileptic drugs; Rifampicin; Griseofulvin; Ampicillin and Tetracyclines.
- ***Increased efficacy of OC pills***: Ascorbic acid 1 g. daily.
- ***Hypercoagulable state***: Aminocaproic acid.

is **Seasonique** with 84 tablets containing levonorgestrel 0.15 mg and EE 30 mcg each, and 10 tablets containing EE 10 mcg each. Other examples are: **Loestrin 24 Fe** and **Yaz,** containing 24 active tablets and 4 inert tablets; the active tablets of both contain EE 20 mcg each. The former contains norethindrone as the progestin whereas the latter contains drospirenone. They appear to have largely served their avowed purposes. But their contraceptive efficacy and liability to cause thromboemolic complications vis-a-vis the conventional preparations is not yet known. With the 20-mcg–EE-containing preparations, breakthrough bleeding and breakthrough ovulation may be a problem. In women chronically taking a preparation containing the mineralocorticoid drospirenone, concurrent use of drugs that increase the serum potassium (ACEI, ARB and NSAID) increases the risk of hyperkalemia.

Table 66.3: Some combination oral contraceptives

Name	Progestin	(mg)
(A) With EE 0.02 mg		
Loestrin 1/20	Norethisterone acetate	1.0
Femilon	Desogestrel	0.15
(B) With EE 0.03 mg		
Eugynon 30	Levonorgestrel	0.25
Microgynon, Ovral L	-Do-	0.15
Triquilar* (Varying E E and levonorgestrel)		
Primovlar 30, Mala D, Choice	Norgestrel	0.30
Novelon	Desogestrel	0.15
Yasmin**	Drospirenone	3.0
(C) With EE 0.05 mg and less progestogenic		
Eugynon 50, Duoluton, Ovral G	Norgestrel	0.5
Ovral, Primovlar 50	Levonorgestrel	0.25
Minovlar Ed,	Norethisterone acetate	1.0
Orlest		1.0
Orthonovin 1/50***	Norethisterone	1.0
(D) With EE 0.05 mg and more progestogenic		
Orgalutin	Lynestrenol	2.5
Norlestrin 2.5/50	Norethisterone acetate	2.5
Gynovlar 21	-Do-	3.0
Anovlar 21	-Do-	4.0

* Triphasic pill.

** Can cause hyperkalemia (Chapter 65).

*** Contains mestranol 0.05 mg and not EE.

Most progestins are derivatives of 19-nortestosterone.

Therapeutic use:

- **As oral contraceptives:** From the therapeutic point of view, the COC can be grouped into those which are **strongly progestogenic** and those which are **weakly progestogenic** in action. Compared on weight basis, the activities of various synthetic progestins differ markedly. Thus, in their progestogenic activity, norethisterone acetate, ethynodiol diacetate and norgestrel are almost twice, 15 times and 30 times as active as norethisterone, respectively. However, in practice, the net pharmacological effect produced by a 'combination pill' probably

Table 66.4: Comparative biologic properties of synthetic progestins in experimental studies

Properties	Norethisterone	Norethisterone acetate	Norgestrel	Lynestrol	Norethynodrel	Ethynodiol diacetate	Desogestrel*
Progestogenic	++	++	++++		++	+++	++++
Estrogenic	—	—	—	+	++	+	—
Antiestrogenic	+	+	++	—	—	+	—
Androgenic	+	++	++	+	—	+	—
Anabolic	+	+	+	+	—	—	—

* Prototype of third generation progestins (the others being gestodene and norgestimate) which are derivatives of norgestrel.

depends upon the relative progestogenic, estrogenic and androgenic properties of its individual constituents (Table 66.4). Since the same combinations are also useful in controlling certain menstrual disorders in a woman with an associated menstrual irregularity, a proper combination can be selected. Thus, premenstrual tension, edema, cyclic weight gain, irregular bleeding and heavy periods suggest an estrogen excess which can be countered by the strongly progestogenic pill (Group D) (Table 66.3) while a patient with excessive acne, hirsuitism, abdominal and leg cramps, and scanty vaginal secretions may benefit from a less progestogenic combination (Group C). *In women with normal menstrual cycles, a combination containing 0.03 mg. or less of ethinyl estradiol with the minimum effective dose of a progestin* (Group A/B) *is preferred.* In patients receiving hepatic microsomal enzyme inducing drugs, pills with 50 μg ethinyl oestradiol are recommended.

In general these pills appear to be safe, highly effective and acceptable. Usually, they do not affect the libido; in fact, the removal of the fear of pregnancy may greatly improve the sexual as well as the marital relationship. Subsequent fertility is not affected. They can be used by women of all ages from menarche to menopause. The non-contraceptive health benefits associated with COC pill are shown in Table 66.5. *Although they may prevent benign breast disease, they should not be prescribed to women with benign breast disease.*

However, the cost and the necessity of following a strict regimen make the acceptance of these drugs as the sole method of contraception difficult. Further, these hormones lack specificity in that they also affect other tissues and alter various metabolic processes.

Before starting the pill, it is essential to go through the personal history and to carry out a detailed examination to exclude any medical contraindication especially cardiovascular risk factors. *Women over 35 years of age who smoke* should be encouraged to seek alternative methods of contraception. However, COC pills

Table 66.5: Non-contraceptive benefits of combination OC pills

- Menstrual benefits such as less menstrual blood loss, less iron-deficiency, lower incidence of menorrhagia, dysmenorrhoea and pre-menstrual syndrome.
- Lowered incidence of benign breast disease, endometrial cancer, ovarian cyst, ovarian cancer and osteopenia.
- Protection against pelvic inflammatory disease; and
- Abolition of the risk of tubal (ectopic) pregnancy because of anovulation.

containing 20 mcg of EE (Loestrin 1/24 and Femilon) (Group A) and those containing 15 mcg of EE + 60 mcg of gestodene are now becoming popular as contraceptives in the older women who are nonsmokers. When the last pill mentioned above is used with *only 4 day pill-free interval*, it seems that ovulation is prevented as effectively as with the conventional OC pills.

After the start of oral contraceptive, the woman should be initially seen during the second or third cycle of medication in order to check that all is well and that she really understands how to take the drug. Thereafter, she may be called after 6 months and still later annually. The observations should include :

(a) Blood pressure and weight.
(b) Liver function and glycosuria.
(c) Cervical and breast abnormalities.
(d) Evidence for thrombophlebitis.
(e) Changes in the retinal blood vessels; and
(f) Mental changes.

Since the pill is capable of causing various systemic effects, *a history of taking the pills should form a part of the routine medical history in women of the child-bearing age* and this information should be made available to any other doctor to whom the case may be referred.

It is advisable to stop the pill for 1 month before any elective surgery, since it increases the vascularity and causes edema of the tissues and elevates the plasma concentration of some clotting factors. As a result, deep vein thrombosis is more common in post-operative period.

Other uses of combination OC pills :

- ***Postcoital contraception*** (see below).
- ***Polycystic ovary syndrome*** (Chapter 67).
- ***Dysfunctional uterine bleeding*** (Chapter 65).
- ***Premature menopause*** (Chapter 65); and
- ***Turner syndrome:*** This is characterised by primary amenorrhoea, lack of secondary sex characters and short stature, with or without certain deformities, due to a chromosomal defect, most commonly an XO karyotype. After initial cautious treatment with small doses of an estrogen (Chapter 65), the patient may be treated with a COC pill. See Chapter 65 for an alternative regimen.

Progestins Alone as Contraceptives

LEVONORGESTREL: This 19,nortestosterone compound possesses very potent progestational activity. In the daily oral dose of 30 mcg. (Microval) continuously, it prevents conception. The drug probably acts by several mechanisms. It reduces the sperm penetrability of the cervical mucus and impairs luteal function. It causes irregular and generally short bleeding intervals and spotting in a high proportion of cases. Other adverse effects are usually mild. ***Norgestrel,*** *a racemic dl mixture, is only half as potent as* ***levonorgestrel*** *(the l-isomer of norgestrel) as the latter isomer alone is active.*

The other **progestin only pills** (POP) are **norgestrel 75 mcg** (Norgest), **norethisterone 350 mcg** (Micronor) and **ethynodiol diacetate 500 mcg** (Femulen). The advantages claimed for such 'minipills' are the lack of the usual estrogen induced adverse effects such as alterations in coagulation factors, suppression of lactation and disturbances in triglyceride metabolism. There is no delay in conception following cessation of POP. They share the disadvantages of the levonorgestrel pill discussed above. Concurrent use of enzyme-inducing drugs such as rifampicin can render POP ineffective.

If not skipping a pill is *important* with the combined pills, it is *critical* with the progestin only pills. If even one pill is forgotten or is delayed by 3 hours or longer by a woman who is not breast feeding, intercourse should be considered as unprotected and an alternative method such as a condom should be used on that day.

The use of progestin alone for contraception is much less reliable than that of COCs and the incidence of annoying adverse effects may be high. Hence, 'progestin-only' pills are currently used only in patients with a specific contraindication to estrogen, in breast-feeding mothers and in those who find other contraceptive measures unacceptable.

The progestin only pill should be started by a breast-feeding mother 6 weeks after childbirth.

Antiestrogenic Agents

LEVORMELOXIFENE (Centchroman, Saheli): This chroman derivative shows weak estrogenicity, potent anti-estrogenicity, and is devoid of progestogenic or androgenic activity.

Given orally, it is well absorbed and is metabolized in the liver. The plasma half life after a single dose of 60 mg is 169 hours. On a weekly schedule of 30-60 mg (once a week pill), it is however, less effective than COC pill and failure rate may be high. The drug appears to be well tolerated. The main side effect is prolongation of the menstrual cycle. It may cause enlargement of ovaries. It should be avoided in polycystic ovarian disease, renal and hepatic disorders, tuberculosis and lactating mothers.

Injectable Contraceptives

Injectable progestational preparations, **depot-medroxyprogesterone acetate** (DMPA, Depot Provera) and **norethisterone enanthate** (NET-EN), are highly effective, long acting and produce reversible effects. They enter the circulation directly without passing through the liver. They do not affect the sex drive nor cause any birth defects. To get the best results the woman must return in time for the next injection. They also have certain disadvantages. The contraindications to the use of these drugs are listed in Table 66.6.

MEDROXYPROGESTERONE ACETATE (MPA) is a potent progestational compound which is effective both orally and parenterally. Unlike 19-norsteroids, it is not metabolized to estrogen in the body. The long acting, slowly absorbed, **depot preparation DMPA** is given IM. It exerts its effect primarily by inhibition of pituitary LH, leading to suppression of ovulation. Its action on the endometrium, the fallopian tubes and the cervical mucus may also contribute to the contraceptive effect. It is excreted in the breast milk but does not suppress lactation.

Repeated injections of DMPA cause prolonged inhibition of ovulation for several months, even after discontinuation.

Adverse reactions: The major drawback is the disruption of the normal menstrual cycle that occurs in two thirds of the recipients. It causes bleeding irregularities, spotting and prolonged amenorrhoea. Severe bleeding, however, is uncommon. Unlike the COC, it has negligible metabolic actions except perhaps on lipids. However, weight gain is common. When it is used in large doses to treat cancer or precocious puberty, adrenal suppression may occur; but this has not been observed during contraceptive usage. It can cause moon face during prolonged use (Chapter 64).

Table 66.6: Contraindications to injectable progestin contraceptives

- The patient has one of the following medical conditions:
  - Likely pregnancy.
  - Unexplained vaginal bleeding suggesting pregnancy or a serious underlying condition.
  - Past or current breast cancer.
  - Severe high blood pressure.
  - Coronary heart disease.
  - Diabetes mellitus with vascular complications.
  - H/O thrombosis, past stroke.
  - Severe liver disease.
- The patient wants to conceive in the next 6 months; or
- The patient does not want weight gain or changes in the pattern of vaginal bleeding.

Table 66.7 : Injectable contraceptives and their doses

Formulation	Brand name	Injection schedule
DMPA 150 mg IM	Depot-Provera	Every 3 months
DMPA 104 mg SC	DMPA–SC	Every 3 months
NET-EN 200 mg IM	Noristerat	Every 2 months
DMPA 25 mg. + estradiol cypionate 5 mg. IM	Cyclofem	Every month
NET-EN 50 mg. + estradiol valerate 5 mg IM	Mesigyna	Every month

NET-EN : This C 18 progestin has properties and mechanism of action similar to DMPA; it, however, has to get hydrolysed to become biologically active. It has a relatively short duration of action. It also causes menstrual disturbances similar to DMPA. Larger doses cause diabetes mellitus in animals, but not in women.

DMPA and NET-EN therapy may be initiated

- Any time the physician is reasonably certain that the patient is not pregnant, e.g., within the first 7 days after the menstrual bleeding starts.
- Immediately after an abortion or after a childbirth if the mother chooses not to breastfeed the baby; it should be delayed by 6 weeks in those planning to breastfeed.

Table 66.7 lists the available injectable contraceptives. Preparations containing E_2 are probably more effective and cause regular vaginal bleeding pattern. Further, fertility returns sooner after stopping these preparations.

LEVONORGESTREL IMPLANT (Norplant): It consists of six, flexible, silastic rods containing levonorgestrel (36 mg per capsule) in crystalline form. The rods are inserted under the skin, usually on the inside of the woman's upper arm. They slowly release norgestrel in progressively diminishing quantities for upto 5 years. The mechanism of action of this preparation is an antiestrogenic action on the endometrium and on the cervical mucus which becomes thick and hostile to sperm penetration. LH peak and ovulation are suppressed in at least half the cycles. Further, even when ovulation occurs, the adverse effect on sperm penetration prevents fertilization. The original Norplant implant is now replaced by a $Norplant_2$ implant containing only 2 rods; it achieves similar blood levels and has similar efficacy.

Adverse reactions : Local infection may occur if the implant is inserted without a proper aseptic technique. About 70% of the users experience irregular bleeding or amenorrhoea. Irregular bleeding is mostly seen during the first year of use. Users have few pregnancies; however, many of them are likely to be ectopic. Other adverse effects are headache, nervousness, nausea, skin rash, acne, hirsutism, breast tenderness, weight gain and enlarged ovarian follicles. It involves an invasive procedure and needs trained personnel and monitoring.

PROGESTIN IUCD : **Progestasert** consists of progesterone micro-crystals in a silicone fluid, surrounded by a release-rate-limiting membrane. The device releases pre-determined, minute quantities of the drug over a period of one year. There is no suppression of ovulation and the menstrual pattern is not disturbed. The incidence of ectopic pregnancy has, however, been reported to be higher than in the general population. A norgestrel-releasing IUCD (Mirena) is not only an effective contraceptive but is also useful in treating menorrhagia (Chapter 65).

Recently, two, new, small, flexible, match-stick sized plastic rod implants have become available. They release a progestin, either levonorgestrel (Jadelle) or etonogestrel (Implanton) slowly in the body. Jadelle is a two rod system (for 5 years), whereas Implanton has a single rod (for 3 years). Their clinical efficacy is similar to that of Norplant, but they are claimed to cause fewer complications. They do not interrupt an existing pregnancy and can be removed any time as per the woman's wish. Long term safety data are not yet available.

Transdermal contraceptive system (TCS): This three layer patch contains norelgestromin and ethinylestradiol. Norelgestromin is the active metabolite of norgestimate. When applied once a week for 3 successive weeks in a month, it delivers the contained hormones continuously and allows withdrawal bleeding. It is as effective as the COC but less so in very obese women.

Antiprogestins

MIFEPRISTONE (RU 486): This derivative of norethisterone has antiprogestin activity.

Pharmacological actions:

• ***Administered to women in early and late luteal phases of the menstrual cycle,*** it shows luteolytic property. It causes inhibition of the uterine glandular secretory activity; and accelerates degenerative vascular changes, leading to menstrual bleeding within 72 hours. These changes are consistent with the withdrawal of progesterone. Hence, it can be used as an emergency contraceptive. Larger doses, however, block the proliferative action of estradiol on the endometrium, leading to endometrial atrophy, suggesting a progestin-like property. Thus, *it acts as a progesterone antagonist in the presence of progesterone, and as an agonist in the absence of progesterone.*

• ***Administered during pregnancy, it*** **:**

(a) Binds the progesterone receptor with high affinity and causes inhibition of transcription resulting in down-regulation of progesterone-dependent genes, with decidual necrosis and detachment of the products of conception.

(b) Damages the endometrial blood vessels.

(c) Inhibits PG dehydrogenase activity thereby increasing the PGE_2 level which stimulates uterine contractility.

(d) Causes cervical dilatation.

• Doses of mifepristone higher than those needed to produce antiprogestin effects block the effects of glucocorticoids at the level of the tissues. Thus, it has been shown to ameliorate the manifestations of hypercortisolism in patients with Cushing's syndrome.

Absorption, fate, excretion: Mifepristone is administered orally or parenterally. Given orally, its plasma level peaks at 1-2 hours. It is metabolized slowly by the liver and is excreted in the bile with an elimination plasma t½ of 20 hours. The plasma level is lower but is sustained longer after intravaginal than after oral administration; It can be used orally in a single dose for terminating a pregnancy. The metabolites also have antiprogestin and antiglucocorticoid activity.

Adverse reactions: Single doses may cause nausea, vomiting, abdominal pain (in > 60%), and sometimes heavy prolonged bleeding. Long term administration of mifepristone can cause fatigue, anemia, weight loss, thinning of hair, menstrual disturbances, decrease in libido and gynecomastia. Mifepristone-prostaglandin combination should be used cautiously in subjects with heart disease.

Therapeutic uses:

• ***Post-coital contraception*****:** Mifepristone in a single dose of 10 mg. is as effective as a combination of 100 mcg of ethinylestradiol and 0.5 mg of levonorgestrel given twice in a day.

• ***Induction of abortion*** (see later)**:** For this purpose, mifepistone is used in a single dose of 600 mg. followed by a vaginal suppository of gemiprostone 48 hours later.

• ***Cervical dilatation*****:** It is useful for preoperative preparation of women for surgical abortion late in the first trimester or in the second trimester. It is as effective as PGs and has fewer side effects.

- ***Induction of labour** in intrauterine fetal* death.

Postcoital Contraception

A possible method of contraception by preventing implantation of the fertilized ovum offers some attractive features. Such a drug need not be taken daily but only after coitus. So far, an ideal anti-implantation drug is not available. The various port-coital contraceptive recommended are given in Table 66.8.

Table 66.8: Various regimens for postcoital contraception

- One levonorgestrel 0.75 mg tablet, as soon as possible (certainly within 72 hours), repeated 12 hours later or 2 tab once.
- Two COC pills containing 50 mcg of EE each (Table 66.3) as soon as possible (certainly within 72 hours) after intercourse, and the same dose 12 hours later.
- Mifepristone 10 mg once within 72-120 hours (see text).
- Copper-containing IUCD (see text).

The emergency oral contraceptives, other than mifepristone, probably act by interfering with tubal transport, preventing implantation, or by causing regression of the corpus luteum. As these drugs are administered within hours of intercourse and implantation occurs only about 7 days after ovulation, *their use is not equivalent to therapeutic abortion.*

The regimen may cause nausea and vomiting and the treatment may fail if the drug is not retained. A pre-existing pregnancy must be ruled out before such treatment is initiated. If such hormonal form of postcoital treatment fails, there is possibility of harm to the embryo and this should be explained to the subject before such therapy. *It does not disrupt an existing pregnancy.* In case of failure, the pregnancy should be terminated by other methods. Although postcoital contraception is safe to use more than once, this method should not be used in place of standard methods of contraception; *it should be used only as an emergency method e.g. following rape.* There is no age bar to using this technique.

Mifeprostone in large doses is the only drug which interrupts pregnancy after implantation has occured (see later).

Copper-containing IUCDs inserted within 5 days from the day of sexual intercourse is also effective as post-coital contraceptive agents. Such IUCDs, therefore, may be preferred if hormonal treatment is contraindicated.

From among the various methods of contraception, in a given patient/situation, one method may be considered better than the others. Hence, it is better to have a 'cafeteria type' approach, where the woman concerned is allowed to choose the method after being adequately informed about the various procedures. Further, "A happy, knowledgeable and communicating couple, especially if they have a sense of humour, can get along with almost any method". Women who cannot be relied upon to take pills regularly should be advised methods such as IUCD or surgical sterilisation.

IUCD is a useful and effective method of contraception for parous women, specially those who want more children or do not wish to undergo sterilization. It is particularly useful for women over the age of 35 years, *in whom the risks associated with the use of COC* and the *effectiveness of IUCD* are both increased. The complications of IUCD are:

- ***Increased menstrual blood loss;***
- ***Increased risk of upper genital infection and pelvic inflammatory disease which can lead to either ectopic pregnancy or infertility;*** and
- ***Rarely, perforation of the uterus.***

For the above reasons, *the use of IUCD is cotraindicated in nulliparous women.*

Male Contraception

In males, spermatogenesis can be inhibited by androgens, estrogens and progestins. Although steroid combinations are being developed which inhibit spermatogenesis experimentally, such hormonal inhibition in a male may cause loss of libidinal drive which, even if psychological, may have damaging effect on the personality of the individual, apart from other adverse effects. *Vasectomy, carried out in properly selected cases, would be the most economical, reliable and relatively safe procedure for the males. It does not affect the libido.*

GOSSYPOL: This is a polyphenolic compound obtained from the cotton seed. In rats, gossypol acetic acid causes dose dependent damage to germinal cells of testes; long term treatment damages spermatogonia leading to sterility. The drug, however, does not damage the Leydig cells. No genetic damage or hormonal disturbances have been observed. Clinical studies from China indicate that gossypol is an effective male antifertility agent. It takes 2-3 months to achieve the desired therapeutic effect. However, its toxicity that includes GI disturbances, fatigue, decreased libido, dizziness, occasional hypokalemic paralysis, and atrophy of seminiferous tubules is not acceptable.

Medical Termination of Pregnancy (MTP)

Although termination of pregnancy has been legalised in many countries it is estimated that 20 million pregnancies are terminated illegally with more than 78,000 deaths, each year. Use of drugs for post-coital contraception is described earlier. Drugs used for medical termination of pregnancy (MTP) during the early part of the first trimester can be classified as:

I **Progesterone synthesis inhibitors,** e.g., Epostane and Trilostane. These drugs act as competitive antagonists of ovarian and placental 3-beta-hydroxysteroid dehydrogenase. They inhibit the synthesis of progesterone from pregnenolone. They are under investigation.

II **Antiprogestins,** eg., Mifepristone (see above).

III **Antiestrogen,** e.g., Tamoxifen.

IV **Trophoblast inhibitors,** eg., Methotrexate.

V **Oxytocics,** eg., Prostaglandins and Oxytocin (Chapter 43).

VI **Miscellaneous,** eg., Ethacridine, Hypertonic saline (Chapter 43).

Although PGs can be given alone to terminate pregnancy with a success rate of 90%, the doses needed cause a high incidence of adverse effects such as nausea, vomiting, diarrhoea, pain and dizziness, requiring supplements of narcotic analgesics. Hence, they are combined with mifepristone or methotrexate. The synthetic PGE compounds **misoprostol** and **gemeprost** are generally preferred. Misoprostol can be stored at room temperature, is relatively inexpensive and is easily available. It is administered orally or vaginally. Gemeprost is more expensive and thermolabile. It is given as vaginal pessary.

Mifepristone in combination with **misoprostol** has been extensively studied and found to be effective almost in 98% of the pregnant women. Mifepristone is given orally as *a single dose of 400-600 mg, (MTP dose, in contrast to 10 mg for emergency contraception,* see earlier) followed 48 hours later by misoprostol 400 mcg or gemeprost 0.5-1.0 mg vaginally. Misoprostol given orally is less effective. The common adverse effects include backache, headache and uterine cramps. They are not dose-related. Severe side effects include prolonged and sometimes excessive vaginal bleeding. Women with severe asthma, adrenal failure and those on long-term glucocorticoid therapy should not be given this combination because of its antiglucocorticoid action. It should be used cautiously in subjects with diabetes mellitus, severe anemia, hemorrhagic disorders and those on anticoagulants.

Methotrexate (Chapter 59), 25-50 mg given orally and followed 3-7 days later by **misoprostol** 800 mcg vaginally, is effective in 85-95% of women with pregnancy of less than 8 weeks duration. The combination may cause nausea, vomiting, pain (due to misoprostol) and stomatitis and oral ulcers (due to methotrexate). This combination treatment is contraindicated in women over 35 years of age and in those with cardiac risk factors, because it can precipitate heart failure.

The advantages of above combinations are:

- ***The termination can be carried out on outpatient basis*** — first dose is given in the clinic and misoprostol is self-administered at home.
- ***Relatively safe, do not require anaesthesia and hence highly acceptable.***
- ***Effective on average in 98% of subjects with less than 8 weeks' pregnancy.*** The treatment failure rate rises with menstrual delay of 35 days or more.

The disadvantages are that they are not 100% effective; further they can sometimes cause prolonged and severe bleeding.

Tamoxifen 20 mg once daily for 4 days, followed by vaginal misoprostol 800 mcg, is also reported to be effective in 90% of women.

Medical termination, however, is more painful and less effective in women with pregnancy of more than 8 weeks duration. In such cases, vaccum extraction is more acceptable.

Ovulation Inducing Drugs

The problem of infertility is a joint one and both the partners need detailed examination. The male should be examined first. This is essential if one decides to treat the female with fertility drugs. The drug therapy of male infertility is, at present, generally disappointing.

The drug therapy of infertility due to ovulatory failure was till recently empirical and disappointing. Various measures such as wedge resection of polycystic ovaries (PCO) and glucocorticoids have been employed with varying success. Before giving credit to any such therapy, it should be remembered that 20-35% of infertile women ovulate spontaneously.

Deficiency of the thyroid hormone is an uncommon cause probably responsible in less than 3% of anovulatory cycles. The results of thyroid medication in euthyroid anovulatory women are not at all convincing.

As mentioned in Chapter 65, estrogens may be responsible in triggering an ovarian signal for midcycle LH release. Estrogen administration has been demonstrated to cause LH release in rodents, monkeys and women, usually after a preceding period of LH suppression. Hence, low dose estrogen may be useful in cases where some follicular activity is present but midcycle LH peak is lacking or corpus luteum is inadequate. An estrogen can be tried along with clomiphene.

Progestins are not useful except perhaps in patients with inadequate corpus luteum and endometriosis.

Dexamethasone in small doses (0.25-0.5 mg daily) induces ovulation in some patients with PCOs, by suppressing the adrenal androgen contribution.

Classification of ovulation inducing drugs:

I **Synthetic GnRH:** Chapter 65.

II **Human menopausal and chorionic gonadotropins** (Chapter 65).

III **Bromergocriptine** (Chapter 65).

IV **Antiestrogenic compound** clomiphene citrate.

CLOMIPHENE CITRATE (Clomid, Fertyl): This is a triphenylethylene compound, with structural resemblance to stilbestrol and chlorotrianisene (Fig. 66.1). It was synthesized during the search for a potent estrogenic compound but was found to possess potent antiestrogenic actions. In rats, it stops the

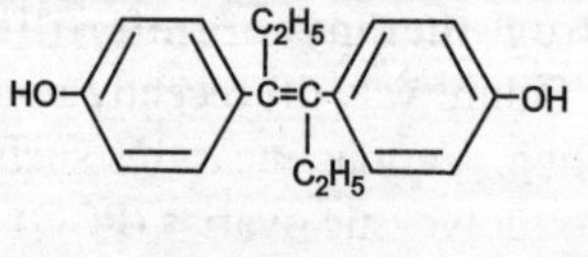

Stilbestrol

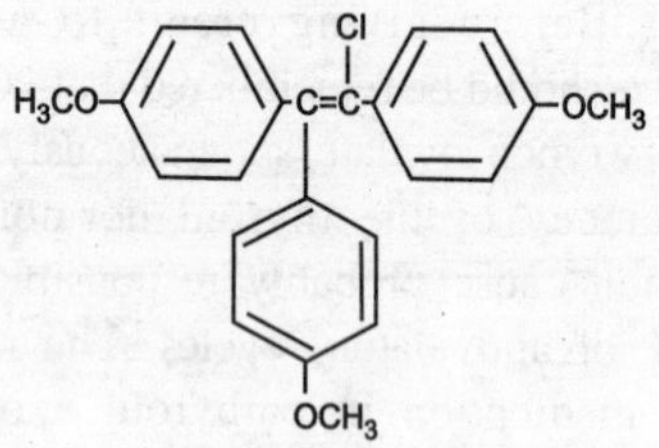

Chlorotrianisene

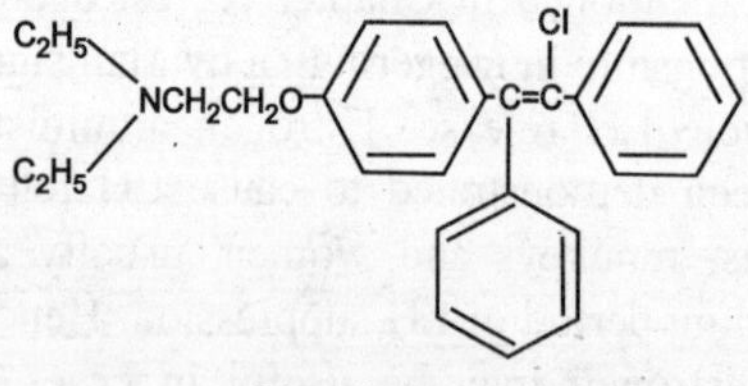

Clomiphene

Fig. 66.1: Structural resemblance between nonsteroidal estrogens and the antiestrogen clomiphene

estrous cycle, decreases the secretion of gonadotropins and reduces the size of the ovaries. However, it is effective in inducing ovulation in women with anovulation.

The available clomiphene preparation contains 'cis' as well as 'trans' forms. It is the 'cis' form which is related structurally to estrogens and is more potent than the racemic form.

Pharmacological actions:

- ***Antiestrogenic action***: Clomiphere acts by competing with the circulating estrogen for receptor sites in the hypothalamus and the pituitary. Being a weak estrogen agonist, its binding to the estrogen receptor result in estrogen antagonist actions (**partial agonist**). This prevents the negative feedback of native estrogen leading to release of FSH and LH by the pituitary and ovulation.

It can produce regression of estrogen induced proliferative endometrium and can counter the keratinization of vaginal epithelium. It can prolong the luteal phase in normally menstruating women and nullify the ovulatory inhibition produced by OC pills.

- ***Miscellaneous actions***: It has a weak estrogenic action, on the bone and endometrium. Given to premenopausal women, it causes hot flushes.

Absorption, fate and excretion: The drug is well absorbed when given orally. It is concentrated in the bile and excreted in the intestines, from where it is reabsorbed. It is mainly excreted in the feces and only a small amount appears in the urine; half of the dose is excreted within 5 days.

Adverse reactions : Commonly, it causes hot flushes. The important drawback is that it causes (1) **ovarian enlargement** and cyst formation due to overstimulation, which may lead to rupture and internal hemorrhage; and (2) it can cause **multiple ovulation**, resulting in multiple pregnancies and fetal wastage. Rarely, it can cause restlessness, blurring of vision; and alopecia.

Therapeutic uses:

- ***Ovulation induction***: Clomiphene is indicated in the treatment of infertility due to chronic anovulation (anovulatory infertility). In such cases, adequate endogenous estrogenic activity is present. Generally, the drug is given in daily doses of 50 mg. for 5-7 days. If there is no response, a second course may be given in the next cycle, with 100 mg. daily for 5-7 days. *Lack of response to clomiphene 150 mg for 3-4 consecutive cycles indicate clomiphene resistance and hence the drug should not be repeated.*

Ovulation usually occurs 2-12 days after completion of the treatment. In case of an amenorrheic patient, the drug can be given at any time but it is customary to start it on the 5th day of withdrawal bleeding after a course of medroxyprogesterone (5 mg. bid for 5 days). In those with regular anovulatory cycles, it is usually started on the 5th day after the onset of menstruation. It must be realised that the response to clomiphene is unpredictable and the dosage effective in one patient may prove inadequate in others. Generally, ovulation occurs in about 70% of women; of these less

Table 66.9: Drugs which impair male and female fertility

Drugs	Male	Female
Cytotoxics, e.g., methotrexate, cyclophosphamide,	Azoospermia	Ovarian failure
Drugs of dependence e.g., alcohol, opioids, marijuana	Decreased testosterone and sperm abnormalities	Menstrual irregularities
Nicotine	—	Premature ovarian failure
Hormones		
Estrogens	Suppression of pituitary and hypothalamus	Menstrual irregularities
Androgens	See 'Abuse of anabolic steroids by athletes'	Anovulation
Prednisolone	Decreased sperm count	—
Levothyroxine	—	Anovulation with large doses
Antipsychotics, e.g., Phenothiazines	Hyperprolactinemia, impotence	Hyperprolactinemia, menstrual irregularities
Metoclopramide	Same as above	Same as above
Miscellaneous		
Cimetidine	Antiandrogen, azoospermia	Menstrual irregularities
Spironolactone	Antiandrogen, decreased testosterone	Menstrual irregularities
Sulphasalazine	Decreased sperm count	—
Phenytoin	Decreased sperm count	—

than 50% may conceive. Possibility of multiple pregnancies is its main disadvantage.

The multiple pregnancy rate of 6% with clomiphene is distinctly lower than that with gonadotropin therapy (20%). The pregnancy wastage rate (20%) is, however, similar with both therapies. As compared to human pituitary gonadotropin, clomiphene is less effective but less hazardous, and is much less expensive. It is claimed that the incidence of abortions can be reduced by using progesterone (micronized 100 mg bid for 14 days) soon after the existence of conception is confirmed.

There is no rationale for the use of clomiphene for 'menstrual regulation' if conception is not desired by the patient, because it can cause dangerous hyperstimulation of the ovaries.

Further, treatment in an individual patient should be limited to 12 cycles in the lifetime because of the reported increase in the incidence of ovarian cancer following longer treatment with clomiphene.

- ***Polycystic ovary syndrome (PCOS)*:** This is characterized by polycystic ovaries associated with anovulation, hyperandrogenism, and infertility. It has a familial basis and many patients show insulin resistance. The current management of PCO includes lifestyle modification; diet control and exercise for weight reduction in obese patients; and cessation of smoking; this treatment often can induce ovulation. **Metformin** can improve insulin resistance, regulate the menstrual cycles and cause ovulation in some patients. It is administered in the dose of 500 mg OD and increased to 500 mg tid. If it is not effective in 3-5 months, **clomiphene may be added** for further 6 months. Metformin should be stopped when pregnancy is confirmed. If the treatment fails after 12 cycles, **gonadotropin therapy** may be considered. *Cauterization of the ovarian cysts may be done only as a last resort.*

- ***Oligospermia***: Clomiphene has also been used in males with low sperm counts with variable results.

Cyclofenil (Ondomid): This compound has a structure similar to clomiphene and is used for similar purposes. It does not exert a peripheral anti-estrogenic effect. Given cyclically in the dose of 200 mg twice a day for 10 days, starting on the third day of menstrual bleeding, it can induce ovulation.

Letrozol: Recently, this aromatase inhibitor has been used for ovulation induction in patients with PCO. It acts by inhibiting aromatase and thus reducing the production of estrogen. Excess estrogen over-suppresses FSH production. By blocking this, aromatase inhibitors promote the development of healthy ovarian follicles and ovulation. The drug is under evaluation.

Table 66.9 lists some drugs which may impair fertility.

Antigonadotropic Compounds

DANAZOL (Danocrine, Ladogal): This is a synthetic derivative of ethisterone.

(a) It has antigonadotropic activity but no estrogenic or progestational properties. Thus, in normal women it eliminates the midcycle LH and FSH surge by acting as selective pituitary gonadotropin inhibitor; and in postmenopausal women it prevents the compensatory increase in FSH and LH.

(b) Peripherally, it binds to androgen, progesterone and glucocorticoid receptors; thus it has some androgenic (partial agonist) and anabolic effects.

(c) It also inhibits directly the ovarian enzymes involved in the estrogen synthesis.

Danazol, thus, induces a hypoestrogenic-hypoprogestational state via hypothalamic-pituitary- ovarian mechanisms. Complete ovarian suppression occurs only with doses of 600 mg or more per day; and at lower doses its other actions may predominate.

Absorption, fate and excretion : It is well absorbed and is extensively metabolized in the liver; the metabolites are excreted in the urine. Its elimination t½ is about 4-5 hours. Therapeutic effect starts only after 4 weeks.

Adverse reactions: These are

- ***General***, such as muscle cramps, rash, benign intracranial hypertension, altered hepatic and lipid metabolism.
- ***Androgenic and anabolic***, such as weight gain, acne, hirsuitism and voice change; and
- ***Hypoestrogenic***, such as hot flushes, atrophic vaginitis and depression.

Therapeutic uses:

- ***Endometriosis***: Danazol is used to treat endometriosis. It reduces ovarian function and causes atrophy of endometrial tissue including that at the ectopic sites, and amenorrhoea. Ovulation and menstruation are re-established promptly on cessation of therapy, and pregnancy may be achieved in the first cycle before menstruation occurs. Therefore, contraception should be practised after stopping danazol treatment if pregnancy is not desired. It is administered orally in the dose of 200-800 mg. daily for 3-9 months. The treatment is initiated during a menstrual period. (Chapter 65).
- ***Benign fibrocystic breast disease.***
- ***Heriditary angioedema***.
- ***Gynecomastia.***
- ***Menorrhagia;*** and
- ***Idiopathic thrombocytopenic purpura***.

Gestrinone (Dimetriose) is an analogue of danazol for the treatment of endometriosis. The dose is 2.5 mg twice a week for 6 months, starting during a menstrual period.

Androgens, Anabolic Steroids and Antiandrogens

67

The early knowledge regarding the relationship between the testes and the secondary sex characters in male was obtained from the studies in castrated animals. It was demonstrated that the typical signs of castration could be reversed by transplantation of gonads. The first pure hormone with androgenic activity—*androsterone*—was isolated from the male urine by Butenandt in 1931. This was followed by the isolation of urinary androgenic steroid, *dehydroepiandrosterone* The active principle of testes, *testosterone,* was isolated in pure form in 1935. The urine contains androsterone and etiocholanolone, the metabolites of testosterone. Steroidogenesis also occurs in the ovary, the adrenal cortex and the placenta.

Physiological actions of androgens: Androgens determine the differentiation of the foetal external genitals in the male direction. Further, in males they prevent the development of the hypothalamic cyclic release of LH. At puberty, testosterone secretion increases markedly and is responsible for transforming a boy into man. The increase in gonadotropin secretion at puberty is due to a reduction in the hypothalamic sensitivity to the circulating androgens. Following this increase, testes enlarge and the testicular activity is initiated.

FSH acts on the seminiferous tubules and is responsible for the growth of the testes. It promotes **spermatogenesis** and stimulates the Sertoli cells. It is thus gametogenic in action. LH (ICSH) stimulates the Leydig cells at puberty, leading to (a) a marked rise in *intratesticular testosterone* which is essential for spermatogenesis and (b) elevated *plasma testosterone* which promotes the development of external genetalia and secondary sexual characters. Thus, both FSH and LH play an important role in initiating and maintaining the normal testicular functions. These are :

- ***Development of male external genitals (penis and scrotum), and secondary sex characters (pubic hair and beard) and change in voice.***
- ***Development of the male internal genitals: seminal vesicles, prostate and epididymis.***
- ***Maintenance of spermatogenesis.***
- ***Development of skeletal musculature and emotional make up of male type***; and
- ***Anabolic and growth promoting effects.***

Failure of the testicular function causes male hypogonadism.

The daily testosterone production by male adults is between 4 and 12 mg. This gives a plasma level of 4-10 ng./ml. A small proportion of the circulating testosterone may arise by extra-adrenal conversion of the weak adrenal androgens dehydroepiandrosterone and androstenedione. In the female, the latter is an important source of plasma testosterone which measures 0.2-0.6 ng./ml.

Testosterone is converted by androgen-responsive tissues to the active metabolites, 5α-dihydrotestosterone and estradiol. Testosterone and dihydrotestosterone bind to a cytoplasmic androgen receptor protein before acting on the nucleus in a similar manner as estrogen. The genetic lack of this receptor results in androgen insensitivity and the syndrome of testicular feminization. About 0.5 per cent of testosterone is converted to estrogen in the body.

Male hypogonadism: Failure of testicular function can be either (a) primary, due to testicular failures or (b) secondary, due to failure of the HP (hypothalamic-pituitary) complex. In primary testicular failure, gonadotropin secretion is increased, producing **hypergonadotropic hypogonadism**, while in HP failure, the gonadotropin secretion does not increase, causing **hypogonadotropic hypogonadism**.

The testicular deficiency could be selectively gametogenic or both gameto- and andro-genic. In the former, the individual is sterile but has normal secondary sex characters; in the second case both the functions are impaired.

Failure of the testes before puberty (pre-puberal hypogonadism) causes infantile penis, feminine distribution of fat (more on buttocks, breast and hips) and arrest of laryngeal and hair growth. The muscles remain soft, skin becomes smooth and there is a lack of sex drive. Intelligence is not affected.

In a patient with *post-puberal hypogonadism*, the general body proportions and size of the penis are not altered. But the body hair become sparse and silky, voice becomes high pitched and libido is greatly reduced. Skeletal muscles become flabby and weak and there is a tendency to develop obesity. However, the life expectancy is not shortened nor is premature senility produced. The volume of semen is markedly decreased and there is a change in the emotional make up, anxiety, fear and inferiority complex replacing self confidence.

TESTOSTERONE: It acts intracellularly in target cells (see earlier). Its biological effects can be considered as:

I **Those which occur via the androgen receptor :**

(a) *Due to testosterone*: Development of the Wolffian duct (epidydimes, vasa differentia and seminal vesicles) during gestation; development of male external genitalia at puberty (penis, scrotum); skeletal muscle; erythropoiesis.

(b) *Due to dihydrotestosterone*: Development of prostate and and masculinization of the male external genitalia in utero; prostatic disease in adulthood; hair follicles of ambisexual and sexual hair in both sexes.

II **Those due to estradiol via the estrogen receptor:** Epiphyseal maturation and fusion in both sexes; negative feedback effect on LH secretion; increased GH secretion in both sexes; and maintenace of bone mass.

Pharmacological actions:

● ***Androgenic action***: Administration of testosterone in pre-puberal hypogonadism reverses most of the changes of hypogonadism. The secondary sex characters develop, muscle strength increases and sex desire and erections occur normally. The testes do not enlarge and spermatogenesis does not occur.

In females, testosterone causes increased libido as well as masculinization, e.g. hirsutism, growth of clitoris and change in voice (male type). The development of proliferative phase of the endometrium may be inhibited and large doses can suppress the ovulation and lactation. During pregnancy, androgenic compounds can masculinize the external genitals of the female foetus.

● ***Anabolic actions***: Protein synthesis (anabolism) and protein breakdown (catabolism) are the important functions of a cell. Adequate supply of nutrient material is necessary for protein synthesis. The anabolic (protein synthetic) action of androgens is demonstrated by the fact that the male is more muscular than the female and that castration in male causes reduction in muscle mass. Testosterone promotes nitrogen retention and increases the appetite, muscle mass and body weight especially in eunuchoid men, in prepuberal boys and in women. It is insignificant in normal healthy male adults. Along with nitrogen, potassium, sulfur and phosphorus are also retained, while the urinary excretion of calcium and creatinine is decreased.

• ***Bones and epiphyses:*** Testosterone in small doses can promote growth of epiphyseal cartilage, particularly in boys with short stature due to hypogonadism. It probably acts by elevating hGH levels in children. *However, large doses testosterone brings about early epiphyseal fusion and reduces the final adult height.*

Androgens may reduce bone resorption and cause beneficial effects in senile osteoporosis.

• ***Effect on pituitary*:** Testosterone exerts a negative feed back effect on LH and a smaller one on FSH. LH and FSH levels rise in primary hypogonadism. The LH- inhibiting action could be due to the small quantities of estrogen to which testosterone is converted in the pituitary. Mesterolone, a testosterone analogue, which is not converted into estrogen, lacks this property.

• ***Miscellaneous actions*:** Androgens increase appetite and cause a feeling of well being. They can cause sodium retention and edema. They also cause growth and increased secretion of the sebaceous glands, clinically manifested as acne. They stimulate erythropoietin secretion by the kidneys, and directly stimulate heme synthesis in the bone marrow. These actions account for the differences in hemoglobin levels between men and women.

These compounds generally antagonize many of the actions of estrogens in females.

Absorption, fate and excretion: Testosterone is well absorbed orally but is largely inactivated by the liver (first pass) and hence, is therapeutically ineffective. Its 17 methyl derivatives methyltestosterone and fluoxymesterone are much less degraded by the liver and are effective orally.

Ninety-eight per cent of plasma testosterone is protein bound and only two per cent is free. Its plasma t½ is about 10-20 minutes. It is largely metabolized in the liver, and excreted in the urine, mostly as androsterone and etiocholanolone, as sulfates and glucuronides. The plasma testosterone levels are a useful indicator of androgen production in the male.

Esters of testosterone with weak organic acids like propionic acid, when injected, produce prolonged action for 2-3 days, while cypionate and enanthate are effective for 1-2 weeks. Pellets of testosterone implanted under the skin are slowly absorbed and their therapeutic effect lasts for 6-8 months.

Assay : For clinical purposes, androgens are individually measured by radiommunoassay. The androgenic activity of a compound can be bioassayed by the measurement of growth of the seminal vesicles or the prostate in castrated rats.

Adverse reactions:

• In large doses, testosterone can cause precocious puberty in boys, and masculinization (deepening of voice, hirsutism, acne, baldness and clitoromegaly) in girls and women. Some of these changes may be irreversible.

• In young children, prolonged use of these drugs in large doses may bring about early closure of the epiphyses and thus stop the growth.

• In pubertal boys, androgens can cause gynecomastia.

• Large doses can suppress spermatogenesis and may even cause degeneration of seminiferous tubules.

• Androgens aggravate a pre-existing cancer of the prostate. They can also aggravate bladder neck obstruction in patients with benign prostatic hypertrophy.

• Large doses can cause retention of sodium and edema.

• Methyl testosterone, fluoxymesterone and many anabolic steroids are potentially hepatotoxic and can cause cholestatic jaundice.

• Hepatic adenocarcinoma has been reported in patients of aplastic anemia receiving 17-alkyl derivatives for prolonged periods.

Preparations and dosage :

● ***Testosterone aqueous* suspension** (Aquaviron) 25 mg./ml. Dose: 50-100 mg. once a fortnight.

● ***Testosterone esters***: Parenteral forms are all 17 ß OH ester derivatives of testosterone.

(a) Testosterone propionate injection. Dose : 10-50 mg. IM three times a week.

(b) Testosterone phenylpropionate 40-60 mg. IM every 7-14 days, usually combined with other testosterone esters.

(c) Testosterone cypionate 100-200 mg. I.M. every 14 days.

(d) Testosterone enanthate (Testoviron depot) 250 mg. IM every 2-3 weeks.

● ***Orally active preparations***: These are 17-alpha methylated (a and b below), 1-methylated (c below) derivatives and 17-beta esters (d below).

(a) Methyl testosterone 5 mg. tablets. Dose : 25 to 50 mg. daily in male.

(b) Fluoxymesterone (Ultandren) 5 mg. tablets. Dose : 5 to 10 mg. daily in hypogonadism.

(c) Mesterolone (Provironum) 25 mg. tablets. Dose 25-100 mg. daily in divided doses. It is not hepatotoxic nor is it converted to estrogen in the body.

(d) Testosterone undecanoate (Restandol) 40 mg per capsule. Dose 120-160 mg /day in divided doses.

● ***Transdermal preparations***: (Testoderm) Testoderm patch and androgel for rubbing are available for application to the scrotal skin daily.

Therapeutic uses : It is used either for its androgenic and antiestrogenic actions or for its anabolic effects. The uses are:

I For replacement therapy:

● ***Hypogonadism***: In primary testicular failure, the treatment should be started at puberty. Full replacement therapy requires at least 10 mg. of testosterone per day; this is met with by giving 25 mg. of the propionate ester IM three times a week, or cypionate or enanthate 200 mg. every 2 weeks. The long acting esters are preferred to the shorter acting ones for sustained effect. The starting dose for the first 6-12 months should be 50-100 mg once a month. Other preparations can also be used but more frequent administration is necessary. Oral preparations are not very effective in initiating sexual development but are often adequate for maintenance therapy.

The diagnosis of hypogonadism in young children should be made cautiously because of marked variations in age of maturation in different individuals. *Testosterone should not be used routinely to hasten the onset of puberty and sexual maturation in otherwise normal boys.*

In post-puberal hypogonadism, only replacement therapy is needed and long acting testosterone preparation is given in the dose of 200 mg. every 2 weeks; some patients need 'low dose' replacement therapy in the form of 50-100 mg of the same preparation(s) IM once every 2 weeks. Oral preparations need to be given daily, some of them more often than once daily.

In men receiving long term testosterone treatment, hematocrit, serum testosterone, lipids and prostate specific antigen should be monitored.

In hypopituitarism in children, the cost of hGH makes it necessary to use small doses of an androgen as a substitute. Hydrocortisone and thyroxine may be added if necessary.

● ***Male climacteric*** (Andropause) : Although there is no such clear-cut parallel to 'female climacteric' in elderly males, testicular function declines as the age advances. This is manifested as muscular weakness and tendency to obesity. In such cases small doses of testosterone may be useful. However, that the criteria for the diagnosis of this condition are very vague.

II For pharmacological therapy:

● ***As anabolic steroid***: To promote anabolism. This is discussed below.

● ***Impotence***: Sexual impotence may be defined as inability for a man to have satisfactory sexual intercouse. This can be due to

(a) Lack of sexual desire (libido),

(b) Inability to achieve or maintain an erection **(erectile dysfunction, ED)**; or

(c) Failure of ejaculation.

The normal erectile response is mediated by a combination of psychogenic (central) and reflexogenic (peripheral) stimuli. The CNS plays an important role by either stimulating or inhibiting the spinal pathways that mediate erectile function and ejaculation. The physiological mechanism of erection involves release of nitric oxide (NO) from the vascular endothelium and the nitrergic nerves into the corpora cavernosa of the penis during sexual stimulation. NO then activates the enzyme guanylate cyclase, which results in increased levels of cyclic guanosine monophosphate (cGMP), producing smooth muscle relaxation in the corpora cavernosa and penile arteries, and allowing inflow of blood. The cGMP is metabolically degraded by the enzyme phosphodisterase-5 (PDE-5) present in the corpora cavernosa. Isoenzymes of PDE are also present in other tissues: PDE-3 in the heart and PDE-6 in the retina. In addition to NO, locally synthesized $PGF_{2\alpha}$ and PGE_2 also contribute to the relaxation of the cavernosal smooth muscle cells.

The **parasympathetic** (cholinergic) input to the penis is pro-erectile, whereas the **sympathetic** (adrenergic) input is anti-erectile. Emission, which is the deposition of the seminal fluid into the posterior urethra, is regulated by activation of the sympathetic system. The pro-erectile afferent stimuli from the perineum and the lower urinary tract to the penis, and the efferent ejaculatory stimuli to the levator ani muscles (which cause rhythmic ejection of the semen out of the penile urethra) are carried through **somatic sacral reflex arc**.

The basic mechanisms involved in ED are:

(a) *Failure to initiate*, due to psychological, endocrinological or neurogenic causes.

(b) *Failure to fill blood into cavernosa,* due to arteriogenic causes; or

(c) *Failure to hold adequate blood volume in the cavernosa* (vaso-occlusive dysfunction).

An organic cause can be found in about 50% of the cases of ED; the rest are either psychogenic in origin or are due to a psychiatric illness such as depression. Systemic disease such as chronic liver or kidney disease and drug addiction are other important causes. Only a few cases are due to androgen deficiency and they alone benefit from treatment with testosterone. The adult replacement dose is 200 mg of a long acting ester of testosterone such as cypionate or enanthate once in 2 weeks or 300 mg once in 3 weeks. Testosterone improves the libido, but not erectile failure in patients with normal libido.

Almost 25-30% of the patients with ED may have drug induced ED. Hence before starting such treatment, drug induced sexual dysfunction should be ruled out (Table 67.1).

Table 67.1: Some drugs causing sexual impotence

Drugs acting on CNS :
- Sedative-hypnotics.
- Antipsychotics.
- Antidepressants.
- Antiparkinson drugs.
- Antihistaminics.
- Opiates.

Anticholinergics

Antihypertensives : including Beta-adrenergic blockers.

Diuretics.

H_1 and H_2 receptor antagonists.

Hormonal agents:
- Estrogens.
- Antiandrogens, Spironolactone
- GnRH agonists.

Fibrates.

Cytotoxic drugs : e.g. Methotrexate

Recreational drugs : e.g. Alcohol, Cocaine, Cannabis.

In many instances, sexual impotence is temporary and situational; and patient, expectant waiting is as good a treatment as any drug.

Table 67.2 shows drugs used in the treatment of sexual impotence. Yohimbine, which acts by

Table 67.2 : Drugs used in the treatment of sexual impotence

Oral: Sildenafil; Tadalafil; Trazodone Bromocriptine; Yohimbine.
Androgen IM: Testosterone.
Intracavernosal injection : Papaverine; Phentolamine; PGE (alprostadil).
Transurethral injection: PGE_1.

blocking central $alpha_2$ adrenergic receptors is no longer recommended.

SILDENAFIL (Viagra, Androz): This methylpiperazine compound inhibits the enzyme PDE-5 in the corpora cavernosa of the penis, thereby prolonging the life of cGMP at that site. This causes relaxation of the smooth muscle of the corpora cavernosa permitting inflow of blood into the sinuses resulting in better erection. The presence of NO is essential for this action. *It does not improve sex desire (libido), orgasm or ejaculation. By itself, it does not bring about erection* but it improves the quality and duration of erection in response to sexual stimulation.

It is not of much value in subject with loss of erection due to spinal or other damage to innervation, and in those who lack libido.

Sildenafil has also been found effective in reducing clinical symptoms as well as pulmonary artery pressure in patients with primary pulmonary hypertension. It can also help women with sexual dysfunction due to antidepressants.

Absorption, fate and excretion : After a single oral dose, peak plasma level is reached in 30-120 minutes. The plasma t½ is 2-4 hours and its clinical effectiveness lasts for 4 hours. It is metabolized in the liver by cytochrome P450 enzymes. It is administered on empty stomach in the dose of 25-50 mg one hour before the intended coitus.

Adverse reactions: Sildenafil causes headache, dyspepsia and nasal congestion. The drug potentiates the hypotensive effects of nitrates, and *hence its administration to persons who are using nitrates in any form is dangerous.* Further, there is some cardiac risk associated with sexual activity, especially in the elderly. As many users of drugs for impotence are likely to be elderly, although such therapy may increase the patients' 'vigour' and make them feel 'younger' it can also increase the risk of morbidity and mortality during sexual activity.

It occasionally causes visual disturbances due to its effect on the PDE-6 in the retina. It is contraindicated in persons with retinal degenerative disorders. The drug has been reported to cause Non-Arteritic-Ischemic Optic Neuritis (NAION), leading to acute loss of vision.

The plasma levels of sildenafil increase in subjects over age 65, those with renal / hepatic impairment and in those who are being concurrently treated with CYP3A4 inhibitors such as erythromycin; its adverse effects are likely to be more frequent in these situations.

Vardenafil, chemically related to sildenafil, has properties and duration of action similar to those of sildenafil; is effective in smaller doses.

TADALAFIL (Cialis; Megalis) : This **long acting drug** is chemically unrelated to sildenafil. Like sildenafil, it selectively inhibits PDE-5; it has less affinity for PDE-6 present in the retina, but greater affinity for PDE-11 present in the skeletal muscle, heart, prostate and kidney. Hence, it is claimed to cause less ocular toxicity.

Food does not interfere with its absorption; and it has a t½ of 17.5 hours, with clinical effect lasting for almost 36 hours. It is metabolized in the liver by CYP3A4. Adverse reactions are similar to those of sildenafil. When given in the dose of 10-20 mg twice a week, its effect is almost continuous and the patient can attempt intercourse any time at will, without planning.

- ***Refractory anemias, particularly aplastic anemia*** : The oral, non-17α-methylated testosterone compound mesterolone is used in this condition.
- ***Suppression of puerperal lactation*** : The preferred therapy of this condition is non-pharmacological such as tight binding of the

beasts. If needed, testosterone propionate 50-100 mg may be injected daily for 2 days, beginning of the day of delivery.

Testosterone is absolutely contraindicated in carcinoma of prostate and breast in males.

Anabolic Steroids

Although testosterone has potent anabolic activity, it cannot be used freely for this purposes because of its potent androgenic action. Hence, various steroids were synthesized with anabolic actions but reduced virilizing effects. The clinically used anabolic steroids are given in Table 67.3. Chemically, these drugs are derivatives of testosterone or methyl testosterone. With the exception of methenolone and nandrolone, they are all C_{17} alkyl substituted steroids. *None of the presently available compounds, however, is selectively anabolic, without an androgenic ADR.*

Pharmacological actions: In therapeutic doses, the anabolic action is predominant. The androgenic effect becomes more apparent during prolonged therapy with larger doses, particularly in females. Androgenic properties are similar to those of testosterone.

- ***Protein anabolism*:** Anabolic steroids promote protein anabolism, as manifested by increase in the muscle mass and the body weight. Protein catabolism or negative nitrogen balance is observed in various disease states such as caloric deficiency, protein deficiency, fever, infections, all forms of stress, prolonged immobilization and following broad spectrum antibiotics. In majority of these conditions correction of the cause and providing adequate calories and nutrients including proteins will accelerate anabolism. *Anabolic steroids are certainly not effective during the acute phase of the illness or continuing stress.* Used during recovery from such conditions, they may stimulate appetite and the sense of wellbeing nonspecifically, and promote weight gain.

What is usually needed for tissue repair following injury and illness is enough protein intake in the diet; the necessary anabolic drive is provided by the body. There is no lack of anabolic drive both in men and women recovering from illness; and the necessity of anabolic steroids in such conditions is highly questionable.

- ***Anticatabolic effects*:** In short term studies, anabolic steroids have been shown to produce positive nitrogen balance in individuals on prolonged glucocorticoid therapy. It is believed, therefore, that anabolic steroids counter the catabolic effects of glucocorticoids.

Use of anabolic steroids routinely with glucocorticoids may be dangerous as ADR due to glucocorticoids such as hypertension, acne, hirsutism and sodium retention may be potentiated by anabolic steroids.

- ***Progestational effects*:** Some of the anabolic steroids like norethandrolone have significant progestational activity.
- ***Miscellaneous actions*:** Like testosterone, anabolic steroids may reduce bone resorption and thus may prevent osteoporosis.

Adverse reactions: These are due to their androgenic action and are similar to those produced by testosterone (hirsutism, hoarse voice and clitoromegaly). The use of anabolic steroids in pregnancy has led to virilization of the foetus and advanced bone age. In addition, the orally active anabolic steroids which have a substituted alkyl group at C_{17} can cause cholestatic jaundice, and death due to liver damage. The hepatotoxicity is probably dose dependent. Prolonged treatment may cause sodium and water retention.

Preparations: See Table 67.3. The pediatric doses of these drugs are: methandienone 0.04 mg./kg./day; ethylestrenol 0.1-0.2 mg./kg./day; oxandrolone 0.1 mg./kg./day.

Therapeutic uses :

- ***Chronic illness*:** They have been used during chronic illness especially HIV coachexia to improve appetite and the sense of well being.
- ***Growth*:** They are used to promote growth in hypogonadal children. Their place in the

Table 67.3 : Anabolic steroids

Generic name (Trade name)	Recommended adult dose
Nandrolone phenyl propionate* (Durabolin)	25-50 mg. every week
Nandrolone decanoate* (Deca-Durabolin)	20-50 mg. every three weeks
Methenolone acetate (Primobolan)	10-20 mg. daily
Oxymetholone (Adroyd)	5-15 mg. daily
Methandienone (Pronabol)	2.5-15 mg. daily
Ethylestrenol (Orabolin)	2-4 mg. daily
Norethandrolone (Nilevar)	20-30 mg. daily
Oxandrolone** (Anavar)	15-30 mg. daily
Oxymesterone (Oranabol)	10-40 mg. daily
Stanozolol (Menabol, Neurabol)	2.5-10 mg daily

* These are given IM; the rest are given orally. The first three are derivatives of testosterone, the rest of methyltestosterone.
** Not converted to estrogen.

treatment of short stature from other causes is very limited. *They should not be used in girls.*

● ***Renal failure***: They are sometimes used in acute or chronic renal failure, along with protein restriction, to reduce blood urea and thus to decrease the nitrogen load on the kidneys.

● ***Anemias***: They are claimed to be effective in certain refractory anemias associated with bone marrow hypoplasia or aplasia.

Contraindications: Anabolic steroids are contraindicated in prostatic and male breast cancer; they should be used cautiously in the presence of cardiac, renal and hepatic diseases and should be avoided during pregnancy.

Causes of failure to gain weight by appa-rently healthy individuals are often undetectable. Use of anabolic steroids to increase the body weight in thin but otherwise healthy children or adults is disappointing; even some of those who appear to benefit lose the weight after the drug is stopped. Anabolic steroids are not tonics and should not be used to treat nonspecific symptoms like anorexia and loss of weight without investigating the cause. They are not useful in the absence of adequate protein intake.

Abuse of anabolic steroids by athletes: Anabolic steroids in large doses are commonly misused by athletes in order to improve their athletic performance. When large doses of these drugs are combined with *intense* athletic training and proper diet, muscles increase in size and strength; the muscle fibres are, however, structurally abnormal. The other perceived benefit is a heightened aggressive tendency ('killer instinct'). The adverse reactions are the well known hepatotoxicity of the orally administered 17 alpha methylated steroids; virilization in women athletes; dimunition in LH and testosterone levels in male athletes; decreased spermatogenesis and testicular size; gynecomastia; insulin resistance and glucose intolerance. Hallucinations, delusions and manic episodes have been reported in athletes who self-administer large doses of anabolic steroids. Puberty may be induced in young boys whose final adult height may be compromised. Hypertension can occur as a result of salt and water retention. Finally, abnormalities of lipid and lipoprotein metabolism, which are potentially atherogenic, can occur in these athletes. Such misuse of anabolic steroids is unfair, illegal and is to be deprecated medically.

Antiandrogens

Any compound which antagonizes or interferes with the action of androgens at the tissue level is referred to as an antiandrogen. Estrogens and potent progestins such as medroxyprogesterone block the synthesis of androgens by their central gonadotropin inhibiting action (Chapter 63). Drugs which act as antiandrogens are :

I **Steroid synthesis inhibitors :** Ketoconazole; relatively toxic in the doses needed and hence not used;

II **5-alpha-Reductase inhibitors :** Finasteride (see below);

III **Non-competitive androgen receptor antagonists :** Cyproterone; and

IV **Competitive androgen receptor antagonists :** Flutamide and Spironolactone.

CYPROTERONE ACETATE (Androcur) : This drug has potent progestogenic, moderately potent antiandrogenic and mild glucocorticoid actions. Its antiandrogenic action is due to interference with the binding of dihydrotestosterone to receptors in the target cells. By its marked progestogenic effect, it reduces the plasma level of gonadotropin and testosterone. Cyproterone, unlike cyproterone acetate, exerts only the peripheral antiandrogenic action.

Cyproterone acetate is used orally in the dose of 50-100 mg. per day to reduce libido and sexual potency in deviant hypersexuality in males. It has been used in precocious puberty in boys; in female hirsutism; and in carcinoma of the prostate as an adjunct to GnRH analogues (Chapter 59)

FLUTAMIDE (Eulexin, Plutamid, Cytomid): This non-steroidal antiandrogen, given orally, is converted to its active metabolite 2-hydroxy flutamide which acts as a competitive antagonist specifically at the androgen receptor. It is used to treat prostatic cancer (Chapter 59). Its use in hirsutism is discussed below.

Bicalutamide and **Nitutamide** are newer analogues of flutamide, used for prostrate cancer. The former has a longer $t^1/_2$ (6 days) and is claimed to be less hepatotoxic.

SPIRONOLACTONE : This aldosterone antagonist (Chapter 38) blocks the binding of androgens to the androgen receptor competitively; in larger doses it also inhibits the synthesis of androgen in the ovaries. It is used in the treatment of hirsutism (see below).

Therapeutic uses of antiandrogen: (1) Hirsutism (see below); (2) Benign prostatic hyperplasia (see below); (3) Prostate cancer (Chapter 59); (4) Acne (Chapter 69); (5) Androgenetic alopecia (Chapter 69).

Management of Hirsutism

The physiology of hair growth is discussed in Chapter 69. **Hirsutism** implies the development of androgen dependent (i.e. sexual) hair in children and adult women due to either inappropriately elevated plasma androgen levels or increased sensitivity of the hair follicles to their normal plasma levels. Hirsutism is commonly accompanied by the occurrence of acne. By contrast, **hypertrichosis** is generalised increase in terminal hair density and may be accompanied by growth of hair in non-androgen-dependent areas. Hypertrichosis can be due to: drugs (phenytoin, diazoxide, glucocorticoids, danazol and minoxidil); hypothyroidism; acromegaly; CNS diseases such as multiple sclerosis and encephalitis; metabolic disorders such as porphyria; or it may accompany congenital conditions such as Hurler's syndrome and trisomy 18.

Hirsutism **in childhood** is always due to inappropriate androgen production or administration, and needs to be investigated thoroughly; the treatment is specific and depends on the cause. *In adult women*, drugs (androgens, anabolic steroids and 19-nor steroidal progestins), adrenal disease (late onset congenital adrenal hyperplasia, Cushing's syndrome and the rare adrenal tumours), and ovarian tumours account for a small proportion of cases. They require cessation of the offending drug, treatment of the cause and cosmetic treatment. The majority of cases in adult women are either idiopathic or due to PCO. Patients with idiopathic hirsutism need treatment with local cosmetic measures, and sometimes

Table 67.4 : Management of hirsutism

- Rule out drugs and neoplasm as cause.
- Reassurance.
- Cosmetic treatment.
- Combined OC.
- Glucocorticoids.
- Spironolactone.
- Bromocriptine.
- Cyproterone acetate (Reverse sequential regimen).
- Flutamide.
- Finasteride; and
- GnRH analogues.

with an antiandrogen such as spironolactone or flutamide. If a woman with PCO desires to conceive, the treatment is ovulation induction with drugs (Chapter 66). If she does not wish to become pregnant, her treatment depends on the degree of hirsutism.

Management: Table 67.4 summarises the principles of management of hirsutism.

● ***In mild cases*** not accompanied by menstrual dysfunction, cosmetic treatment such as shaving, waxing, bleaching, chemical depilation, electrolysis or laser therapy is sufficient. Contrary to popular belief, *shaving does not stimulate faster hair growth.* Cosmetic treatment can also be used in moderate and severe cases.

Eflornithine (Vaniqua): This anti-trypanosomal drug (Chapter 56), applied to the hirsute area of the face as a cream, is effective in inhibiting the growth of hair as long as it is used. It is applied, twice a day, five minutes after hair removal, and is massaged into the skin; it is washed 3-4 hours later. It needs to be applied for several weeks before the result is seen. Hair removal is continued throughout its use. It inhibits the synthesis of the hair cuticle. It is well tolerated generally, but may cause local irritation in some patients.

● ***In moderate cases***, especially when the menses are irregular and acne is troublesome, the treatment of choice is a COC pill taken from day 5 to day 25 of the menstrual cycle, for at least one year. The combined OC pill containing 2 mg of cyproterone acetate (Diane/Dianette/Ginette) is preferred. *A pill containing norgestrel, levonorgestrel, norethisterone or norethisterone acetate should not be used as these drugs have androgenic action* and reduce the plasma level of sex hormone binding protein. A pill containing desogestrel, a third generation progestin (see Chapter 66), e.g., Novelon, would be preferable. Spironolactone, in the dose of 100-200 mg per day may be used to supplement therapy of PCOD with the COC pill; spironolactone has an antiandrogenic action at the level of the hair follicles. As spironolactone is liable to cause irregular vaginal bleeding, it is commonly prescribed together with a COC pill. Further, the COC pill prevents conception in these patients; this is desirable as the antiandrogenic action of spironolactone may cause genital abnormalities should the woman conceives a male fetus.

● ***The severe cases*** need treatment with cyproterone acetate. It is used in the **reverse sequential regimen**. It is administered on days 5 to 15 of the cycle in the dose of 50 to 200 mg. daily, together with ethinylestradiol in the dose of 50 mcg or an OC pill from day 5 to 26 of the cycle; the initial dose should be kept down to 50 mg. in patients with acne as well, as acne may be exacerbated by initial larger doses. Bromoergocriptine is useful when hirsutism is a part of hyperprolactinemia - amenorrhoea syndrome. **Flutamide, finasteride** and **GnRH analogues** are reserved for resistant cases.

Once a hair follicle in an androgen dependent area is stimulated to form terminal hair, it remains sensitive to low levels of androgens throughout its life. Therefore, the response of hirsutism to treatment, even after complete surgical ablation of an androgen producing tumour, is slow and takes many months. The patient should be informed about this at the onset of treatment.

Benign Prostatic Hyperplasia

Benign prostatic hyperplasia (BPH) has two components :

- ***A static component*** that is related to the enlargement of the prostate; and
- ***A dynamic component*** that represents the tone or the degree of contraction of *the smooth muscle within the prostate.*

Alpha$_1$ adrenergic antagonists act on the dynamic component (Chapter 29) and reduce the bladder neck resistance to the urine outflow. They also have additional antihypertensive effect.

The drugs used in treating BPH are listed in Table 67.5. Of these drugs, the alpha$_1$ adrenergic antagonists are more effective and less toxic; further, their action is immediate. GnRH agonists decrease libido and may cause impotence.

Table 67.5: Drugs used in BPH

Non-selective Alpha$_1$ adrenergic antagonists:
(a) *Short acting*-Prazosin; Alfuzosin.
(b) *Long acting*-Terazosin; Doxazosin.
Selective alpha$_{1A}$ adrenergic antagonists :
Tamsulosin; Silodosin.
Androgen antagonists: (a) GnRH agonists;
(b) Antiandrogens; 5-alpha Reductase inhibitor e.g. Finasteride; Dutasteride.

Selective alpha$_{1A}$ antagonists : Tamsulosin (Contiflo) and **Silodosin** rarely cause hypotension and syncope, which may occur following prazosin, terazosin and doxazosin, due to their action on smooth muscle of the vasculature. Tamsulosin may however, cause diminished or retrograde ejaculation.

Alpha$_1$-blockers remain effective for long period of time as tolerance does not develop easily. They are also available as extended release preparation given once daily.

For details of α_1-blockers, see Chapter 29.

Other Uses : As α_1-adrenergic blockers cause relaxation of the ureteric muscle and allow the passage of a stone, tamsulosin has been used to treat patients with ureteral stones measuring less than 1 cm, especially those in the distal ureter. The other drug used for the same purpose is the calcium channel blocker nifedipine (Chapter 28).

FINASTERIDE (Proscar, Fenase): This drug is an inhibitor of the enzyme 5-alpha reductase and blocks the conversion of testosterone to dyhidrotestosterone. *It is effective only in patients with palpably enlarged prostate, in contrast to alpha$_1$ adrenergic antagonists which are effective in patients with and without such enlargement.*

Adverse reactions : It can cause decreased libido, diminution in semen volume and impotence. Women of child bearing age should avoid handling crushed or broken tablets as the drug, after absorption through the skin, can cause abnormalities of the external genitals of a male fetus, should the woman be pregnant. As finasteride is excreted in the semen, the use of a condom is recommended if the sexual partner is pregnant or is likely to become pregnant. It is contraindicated in patients with obstructive uropathy or cancer of the prostate.

Therapeutic uses : It is used in the treatment of benign prostatic hyperplasia. Given orally in the dose of 5 mg daily, it causes 40-50 per cent improvement in about 50% of the patients after several months of use. Finasteride, 1 mg daily, has been used in the treatment of androgenetic alopecia in men. It should generally be avoided in women of the reproductive age.

Dutasteride, an analogue, has similar properties as finasteride. Dose 0.5 mg OD.

Calcium, Phosphorus, Fluoride and Magnesium Metabolism; Parathyroid Hormone and Vitamin D; Treatment of Osteoporosis 68

Calcium, apart from forming an essential constituent of bones, plays an important role in body homeostasis. Disturbances in calcium metabolism are associated with derangement of various cellular functions. Food is the only important source of calcium. Milk and milk products are an excellent source of completely assimilable calcium. Green leafy vegetables and cereals are rich in calcium but their calcium is less well utilized because of the concurrent presence of oxalates and phytates, respectively. Ragi is especially rich and rice (especially highly polished one) very poor in calcium. In certain areas, drinking water contains calcium.

The recommended daily calcium intake is : 500 mg in infants; 600-800 mg in children of age 4-10 year; 1200 mg in children 10-18 years; 1 g in adults including pregnant and lactating women; and 1200 mg in adults over 50 years of age. *Mature foetus* contains about 30 g. of calcium which constitutes 3-4 per cent of the total calcium in the mother. Most of it is deposited during the last trimester of pregnancy; loss of maternal calcium during lactation is even larger, which needs correction by consumption of 1 g. of calcium supplement daily. *A one year old baby* contains about 100 g. of calcium, a gain of 70 g. over the total calcium content at birth; most of this increment is supplied by milk.

The average daily diet of Indians, which is based mainly on milled rice and very little milk, may contain as little as 0.2 to 0.5 g. of calcium.

Body distribution : An adult human body weighing 70 kg. contains about 1.2 to 1.4 kg. of calcium. Ninety-nine per cent of it is present in bones; 1% in the soft tissues, and 0.1% in the body fluids. The bone mineral exists in the form of a complex salt containing calcium, phosphate and carbonate, and it constantly contributes to the maintenance of extracellular levels of calcium and phosphorus by two processes :

- ***Exchange between the newly deposited bone mineral and the extracellular ionic calcium;*** and
- ***Constant and concurrent resorption and formation of bone (remodeling)***, controlled by parathyroid hormone (PTH), calcitonin and vitamin D.

Blood calcium : *Calcium is essentially distributed extracellularly,* its concentration being maintained within narrow limits by :

- ***Intestinal absorption.***
- ***Deposition or release from the bone;*** and
- ***Renal tubular reabsorption.***

Most of the calcium in the blood is present in the plasma. The human plasma contains 9 to 11 mg. of calcium per 100 ml. It is present as:

- ***Ionic calcium*** (65% of total).
- ***Protein bound calcium***; and
- ***Calcium combined with citrate and other organic acids.***

The protein bound fraction is physiologically inactive and is not filtered in the glomeruli. The rest of the plasma calcium is ultra-filterable. Of this, the ionic fraction, 4.5-5.4 mg./100 ml., is diffusible, physiologically active, and exchanges with the bone calcium; it is also the fraction which is affected by bone formation and resorption and which regulates the rates of secretion of the PTH and calcitonin.

Intracellular (cytoplasmic) calcium content is very low, 0.4 to 4.0 mcg%. Most of this is sequestered in the mitochondria and (in the muscles) in the sarcoplasmic reticulum. *Though very low in concentration, it is important in regulating the functions and metabolic processes of cells*, such as stimulus-contraction coupling in the muscles and stimulus-secretion coupling in most exocrine and endocrine glands.

Absorption of calcium: Ingested calcium must be dissolved before it is absorbed. Calcium is absorbed passively, primarily from the distal small bowel, but significant quantities are absorbed actively from the proximal small bowel. This latter is controlled by a calcium binding protein in the cells of the mucosal villi, the level of which is regulated by 1,25 $(OH)_2$ D (calcitriol), the active metabolite of vitamin D. The active absorption is stimulated by low calcium intake (Table 68.1).

Table 68.1: Agents and conditions that stimulate the absorption of calcium

- Low calcium intake.
- Vitamin D.
- PTH. (indirectly)
- Negative calcium balance.
- Acid residue in the intestines.

Absorption of calcium is at best partial. The net calcium absorption on a daily diet containing 1 g. of calcium is about 200-300 mg. However, by virtue of an adaptive mechanism, comprising PTH and 1,25 $(OH)_2D_3$, even in the presence of lower calcium intake of less than 1g., net absorption remains within normal limits. Taking calcium in doses of 500 mg or less with food increases its absorption, particularly in patients with diminished gastric acidity. Calcium absorption declines after puberty, especially in old age. Table 68.2 enumerates substances and conditions that interfere with calcium absorption.

Table 68.2: Agents and conditions that interfere with calcium absorption

- Excess of phosphate, oxalate (from vegetables), phytate (from cereals) and fatty acids* (in malabsorption) in the intestines.
- Deficiency of vitamin D.
- Deficiency of PTH.
- Glucocorticoids.

* Fat does not interfere with calcium absorption in normal subjects.

Human milk contains proportionately less phosphorus (Ca:P=2.2:1) than cow's milk with a Ca:P ratio of 1.1:1. Hence, in infants the calcium absorption from human milk is more efficient than from cow's milk. Mean calcium content of cow's milk, however, is 125 mg. per cent as against 33 mg. per cent in human milk.

Excretion of calcium : Calcium is excreted in feces, urine and sweat. The total amount of calcium secreted into the intestinal tract is about 200 mg. daily, of which 130 mg. is excreted in feces. *Zero dietary calcium intake (as in starvation) and lack of vitamin D will thus cause marked deficiency of calcium as the fecal loss continues.*

Ninety-nine per cent of the calcium filtered by the glomeruli is reabsorbed by the proximal tubules. The absorption of the rest is under the influence of vitamin D and PTH. Calcitonin inhibits proximal tubular reabsorption of calcium and increases its urinary excretion. PTH promotes calcium absorption in the distal tubule. The urine contains 2 to 4 mg. of calcium per kg. body weight per 24 hours. A rise in plasma ionic calcium from any cause (Table 68.5) increases its urinary excretion.

The factors which prevent the precipitation of calcium in normal urine are known incompletely; low calcium concentration and adequate citrate concentration in the urine are two important factors. In alkaline urine, calcium is precipitated as calcium phosphate.

Excretion of calcium in the sweat is negligible in the temperate climate but may be significant in the tropics because of excessive sweating.

The causes of hypercalciuria and hypocalciuria are shown in Tables 68.3 and 68.4, respectively.

Table 68.3: Causes of hypercalciuria

- Hypercalcemia from any cause (primary hyperparathyroidism, malignancy).
- Metabolic acidosis.
- Hyperthyroidism.
- Acromegaly.
- Hyperadrenocorticism.

Table 68.4: Causes of hypocalciuria

- Hypocalcemia from any cause (vitamin D deficiency, hypoparathyroidism).
- Chronic renal failure.
- Metabolic alkalosis.
- Dietary calcium deficiency.

If intestinal absorption and renal tubular reabsorption of calcium are insufficient to maintain the plasma calcium within the normal range, it is mobilized from the bone.

Physiological functions:

- ***Excitability***: Calcium is an important component of the cell membrane and controls its permeability and electrical properties. Calcium ions compete with sodium ions for sites on the membrane. An excess of extracellular calcium reduces the permeability of the membrane to sodium and raises the critical level of depolarization at which sodium permeability is increased and at which the action potential is fired off. This stabilizes the membrane and reduces its excitability. Hypercalcemia thus reduces the excitability of nerves and muscles. Hypocalcemia increases membrane permeability to sodium and reduces its excitation threshold, leading to tetany.

- ***Coupling between excitation and response*** (Second messenger): Calcium is essential as a coupling factor between excitation and contraction in all forms of muscle and between stimulus and secretion in certain endocrine glands, e.g., release of ADH by nerve impulses to the neurohypophysis and of catecholamines from the adrenal medulla by acetylcholine. In mediating these responses, calcium enters the cytoplasm to activate the contractile processes or to cause release of stored hormone from the granules. Further, certain drugs acting on the heart owe their action to promotion (digoxin) or inhibition (CCB) of entry of calcium ions into the cell.

In the visceral smooth muscle, the acetylcholine released upon stimulation of the cholinergic nerves binds to muscarinic receptors, resulting in increased influx of Ca^{++} into the myocytes and their contraction.

- ***Automaticity***: The automaticity of the cardiac pacemaker tissues (nodal and conducting) is dependent predominantly upon the slow, inward calcium current (Chapter 27).

- ***Formation of bone and teeth***: Calcium is essential for proper formation of bone and teeth; calcium deficiency during intra-uterine life and extra-uterine growth period leads to delayed and defective dentition and poor bone formation.

A negative calcium balance leads to **osteoporosis**, in which the bones are normal in chemical composition but the total bone mass is reduced. It also results in stimulation of the parathyroid glands with consequent secondary hyperparathyroidism. Excess PTH, by acting on the liver, increases the metabolic degradation of 25 (OH) D (see later); this seems to be an important mechanism of the occurrence of osteomalacia and rickets in sunny countries such as India. Other mechanisms are vitamin D deficiency, vitamin D resistance and hypophosphatemia.

- ***Coagulation of blood***: Plasma ionic calcium is essential for the conversion of prothrombin to thrombin (see Chapter 32).

- ***Renal concentrating mechanism***: Ability to concentrate the urine maximally is impaired in hypercalcemia and in hypokalemia.

- ***Acting as cofactor to many enzymes.***

Pharmacological actions of calcium: They are best illustrated by a description of the effects of hyper and hypocalcemia.

Hypercalcemia: Table 68.5 shows the common causes of hypercalcemia. The effects of hypercalcemia include lethargy, anorexia, weakness, muscular hypotonia, nausea, vomiting and severe constipation. Kidneys show inability to concentrate the urine, polyuria and dehydration. Heart may show irregularities. Excess calcium gets deposited in tissues (metastatic calcification) such as arteries, cornea, muscles and kidneys. *The development of mental changes indicates severe hypercalcemia (over 15 mg.%) and is a medical emergency.*

Table 68.5: Common causes of hypercalcemia

- Hyperparathyroidism (primary or tertiary).
- Malignancy with or without bone metastases.
- Hypervitaminosis D.

Hypocalcemia: Table 68.6 lists the causes of hypocalcemia. It is characterised by increased neuromuscular irritability with paraesthesiae, tetany, seizures, and laryngeal spasm. Teeth show hypoplasia. Skin and nails may show atrophy. Most of these effects are reversible on treatment.

Table 68.6: Common causes of hypocalcemia

- Vitamin D deficiency.
- Abnormal vitamin D metabolism.
- Vitamin D resistance.
- Chronic renal failure.
- Hypoparathyroidism.

Adverse reactions: Oral calcium supplements are generally well tolerated but may produce constipation, abdominal bloating and rarely intestinal obstruction. Calcium chloride solution is irritating by all routes. Extravasation of calcium salts during IV administration may lead to local sloughing. Rapid IV calcium can cause hypotension, irregular heart beat, nausea, tingling and sweating. Shortening of QT interval can occur. *In digitalized patients IV calcium can cause cardiac arrhythmias and cardiac arrest.*

Preparations and dosage : *The oral preparations* are given in Table 68.7. Calcium carbonate has the highest calcium content (about 40%). It is tasteless and inexpensive and is generally preferred for clinical use. Calcium lactate has a sour taste and is sparingly soluble in water. Calcium citrate is tasteless and water soluble. All calcium salts are poorly absorbed and differ in their absorption; *there is little evidence that any of them is therapeutically superior to others.*

Table 68.7: Calcium content of various calcium salts

Calcium Salts	Ca content mg. per G. of salt	Grams required to provide 1 G. of Ca
Carbonate	400	2.5
Phosphate (dibasic)	230	4.4
Citrate	211	4.7
Glycerophosphate	162	6.2
Lactate	130	7.7
Gluconate	89	11
Heptagluconate	82	12

Calcium compounds for parenteral therapy are:

(i) Calcium gluconate injection 1 g. in 10 ml. Dose : 1 to 2 g. IV.

(ii) Calcium laevulinate injection: given IM or IV as a 10% solution. Its calcium content is 13%.

(iii) Calcium chloride is an ingredient of Ringer-lactate infusion. It is given diluted with saline as a slow infusion.

Therapeutic uses of calcium salts:

- ***To prevent or correct calcium deficiency***, oral supplements of calcium are used. in:

(a) Growing children, pregnant women and lactating mothers.

(b) Individuals with diets deficient in calcium.

(c) Patients with post-menopausal osteoporosis, and osteoporosis due to Cushing's syndrome and long term glucocorticoid therapy.

(d) Patients with vitamin D deficiency rickets and osteomalacia, who are prescribed vitamin D.

(e) Patients who have had removal of a parathyroid adenoma.

- ***In the treatment of hypocalcemic tetany:*** **calcium gluconate IV.**
- ***Osteoporosis*** : See below.
- ***As an antacid*** (Chapter 42).
- ***As phosphate binders in chronic kidney disease (CKD)*** : As the hyperphosphatemia of CKD causes secondary hyperparathyroidism leading to renal osteodystrophy, restraining the former is important. In addition to dietary phosphate restriction, the commonly used drugs are calcium carbonate and acetate. Both are effective but sometimes cause hypercalcemia. In resistant cases and in those with hypercalcemia, **sevelamer** may be used (see later). Aluminium salts are no longer used as their absorption can cause bone disease and toxic encepaloapthy. The carbonate of lanthanum, a rare earth metal, can also control hyperphosphatemia efficiently, but its long term safety is under evaluation.
- ***Lead colic.***
- ***Hypermagnasemia.***
- ***Hyperkalemia*** (Chapter 36).
- ***Cardiac arrest***: Intracardiac injection of calcium in cardiac arrest is for the specialist and should not be attempted outside ICCU; and
- ***Placebo***: Calcium gluconate IV produces a feeling of warmth which spreads as a wave all over the body. In view of its adverse effects, it is no more used as a placebo.

Osteoporosis – Management

Osteoporosis is a multifactorial disease in which there is a diminution in the quantity of trabecular and cortical bone mass, leading to increased frequency of fractures. The common fractures are those of the vertebral bodies, ribs, the neck of femur (hip fracture) and the lower end of radius. The commonest types of osteoporosis are **postmenopausal** (Type I) and **senile** (Type II) (Table 68.8).

Table 68.8: Primary osteoporosis

	Type I	Type II
Age	Postmenopausal	Senile
F:M	6:1	2:1
Calcium deficiency	No	Yes
Bone turnover	High	Low
E_2 deficiency	Yes	No
Functional state	Osteoclastic excess	Osteoblastic deficiency
Type of fracture	Vertebral crush	Vertebral wedge; long bones

The bone mass normally increases upto the age of 30 years, after which there is a gradual but progressive diminution in it, faster in women than in men; to this is added an acceleration of this reduction at menopause in women.

The bone mass is best **estimated** by bone densitometry which measures **Bone Mineral Density (BMD)** and compares it to the mean in a group of healthy young women with peak bone mass. It is expressed as **T score** which stands for its difference in standard deviation from the said mean. The *normal value for T score* is + 1 to -1. **Osteopenia** is said to be present when the T score is between -1.0 and -2.5. A T score of –1 to -2.0 requires only 'general health measures' such as dietary advice, physical exercise, calcium and vitamin D; *these measures should in fact be prescribed for all peri- and post-menopausal women, unless contraindicated.* A T score from -2.0 to -2.5 mandates antiresorptive drug treatment in the presence of one or more risk factors for osteoporosis.

Osteoporosis is diagnosed when the individual has a *non-traumatic, non-*

pathological fracture of the spine *or* when the T score is lower than -2.5 in the hip or the spine. It is an *indication* for anti-resorptive drug treatment to prevent further deterioration.

Table 68.9 outlines the principles of management of postmenopausal osteoporosis.

Table 68.9: Principles of management of postmenopausal osteoporosis

- Risk factor control.
- BMD determination
- Reassurance.
- Lifestyle changes, diet, exercise
- Analgesics as needed.
- Short period of bed rest following a fracture of the spine.
- Calcium and vitamin D.
- Antiresorptive drugs: Estrogen; SERM; Biphosphonate; Calcitonin.
- Anabolic drugs: Parathyroid hormone (PTH).

The **dietary modifications** advised are *reduction in the consumption of* (a) common salt as calcium is co-excreted with sodium in increased quantities in the urine; and (b) animal foods (except milk) as they are acid-ash producing and increase calciuria. The patient is also advised to reduce alcohol consumption and to stop smoking. The **exercises** recommended are walking and resistance exercise (weight lifting), under supervision.

A daily calcium intake of 1200-1500 mg with a vitamin D intake of 800 IU/day and regular physical exercise are recommended in adolescents and in all postmenopausal women in order to retard the osteoclastic bone resorption.

Alendronate, risendronate and **raloxifene** have been used to increase BMD and reduce the incidence of fractures (see later). The use of **HRT** (Chapter 65) is preferred in early menopausal women with menopausal symptoms, whereas the selective estrogen receptor modulator (SERM) **raloxifene** may be preferred in middle and late postmenopause.

RALOXIFENE: This analogue of tamoxifen is a 'selective estrogen receptor modulator' (SERM) with beneficial effects on the bone and CVS. It causes dose-dependent increase in the osteoblastic activity and decrease in the osteoclastic activity. It does not reduce postmenopausal vasomotor symptoms.

Given orally, it undergoes extensive hepatic first-pass metabolism and has low bioavailability. It has an active metabolite. It is used in the dose of 60 mg OD in the prophylaxis of menopausal osteoporosis. Adverse effects include hot flushes, leg cramps and thromboembolic disease.

Intranasal salmon calcitonin in the dose of 200 I U daily is more effective in preventing lamellar bone loss than cortical bone loss in postmenopausal women; it is, however, more effective in relieving severe bone pains.

The above drugs do not truly increase the bone mass though they may increase BMD and reduce fracture rate.

Parathyroid hormone (PTH, Teriparatide): Intermittent (i.e. 20 mcg once daily) SC, h-PTH-1-34 *increases BMD, bone mass and bone strength* by stimulating periosteal and endosteal bone formation. It is the first drug available with **anabolic action** on the bone. Further, it reduces the fracture rate.

Drug-induced osteoporosis: Many drugs can cause/worsen osteoporosis. These include heparin, warfarin, cyclosporine, glucocorticoids, medroxyprogesterone acetate, antiepileptic drugs such as phenobarbitone, phenytoin and carbmazepine, anticancer drugs and thyroid hormones. Caution should be exercised and perhaps BMD monitored during their long term use. For example, minimum effective doses of glucocorticoids and thyroxine should be used; "injectable MPA as a birth control measure should be used longer than 2 years only if other methods are not applicable" (FDA recommendation). Calcium and vitamin D supplements should be routinely prescribed during the use of antiepileptics. In contrast, thiazide diuretics and perhaps statins can minimize bone loss. Hence, a thiazide may be the preferred drug if an osteoporotic patient also has hypertension or nephrolithiasis.

Hypercalcemia – Management :

Mild hypercalcemia can be treated by:

- ***Control of the underlying causative factor.***
- ***Hydration;*** and
- ***Oral administration of a glucocorticoid*** (in granulomatous disorders, lymphoma and myeloma), ***bisphosphonate*** (see later), or ***phosphate.***

Severe hypercalcemia with serum calcium level of 15 mg% or higher requires emergency, intensive management (Table 68.10). The urgent need is to correct dehydration and establish a diuresis with adequate quantities (2-4 litres in the first 24 hours) of **isotonic saline**; this encourages the renal excretion of calcium and reduces the serum calcium. Once diuresis is established, **furosemide**, 20-40 mg. IM 6-12 hourly, further increases the calciuria. *Thiazides should not be used as they cause calcium retention by the kidneys.* Patients with life-threatening hypercalcemia or severe renal insufficiency may need **hemodialysis** or **peritoneal dialysis** to reduce serum calcium.

Table 68.10: Principles of treatment of severe hypercalcemia

Correct dehydration : Isotonic saline IV.

Increase the renal excretion of calcium : Isotonic saline with or without Furosemide.

Inhibit bone resorption : Calcitonin; Plicamycin; Corticosteroids; Biphosphonates; Gallium nitrate.

Reduce the GI absorption of calcium : Reduction in calcium intake; oral Phosphate; Corticosteroids; Cellulose phosphate.

Promote uptake of calcium by bones and other tissues : Phosphate.

Calcitonin inhibits osteoclastic bone resorption and increases the renal excretion of calcium; it has a rapid but short action. **Glucocorticoids** are effective in certain forms of hypercalcemia (see above) but not in primary hyperparathyroidism nor in most malignant solid tumours. **Plicamycin** kills osteoclastic bone cells and may normalize the serum calcium level for several days to weeks; because of its toxicity, however, it is not used as a first line drug. **Bisphosphonates** (pamidronate by IV infusion) are valuable inhibitors of bone reabsorption and are safe and effective in the treatment of mild to moderate hypercalcemia of malignancy. Oral bisphosphonates are less effective than IV pamidronate. **Gallium nitrate** is a potent inhibitor of bone resorption in hypercalcemia of malignancy; it is contraindicated in patients with renal insufficiency and in those receiving other nephrotoxic drugs. **Oral phosphate** (neutral phosphate mixture), is useful in treating mild to moderate hypercalcemia; *IV phosphate is no longer recommended in this condition* because of its liability to cause metastatic calcification.

Reduction of GI absorption of calcium by restriction of calcium intake, oral phosphate, glucocorticoids and cellulose phosphate is often useful in certain forms of hypercalcemia, especially milk-alkali syndrome and hypervitaminosis D. Glucocorticoids have to be used in large doses (prednisolone 40-60 mg/day), are slowly effective (weeks rather than days), and cannot be relied upon in acute hypercalcemia.

Phosphorus Metabolism

Phosphorus is abundantly present in almost all foods: milk, meat, fish, cereals, pulses and nuts. A part of the phosphorus in cereals is present as phytate and is unassimilable.

Dietary requirements : It is estimated at about 0.9 g. in adults. It is higher in growing children, pregnant women and lactating mothers.

Body distribution: The total phosphorus content of the average adult human body is about 500-600 g., 75 per cent of which is in bones and 25 per cent in other tissues. Although most of the body phosphorus is in the organic form, the small amount that is inorganic is the source of ATP.

The RBCs contain far more phosphorus than the plasma; hence, even slight hemolysis gives fallaciously high plasma phosphorus values. The plasma phosphorus is present as :

- ***Inorganic phosphorus*** 3 to 5 mg. per cent.
- ***Ester phosphorus*** 0.1 to 1.7 mg. per cent; and
- ***Lipid phosphorus*** 7 to 15 mg. per cent.

The term 'plasma phosphate' usually means the plasma inorganic phosphate measured as phosphorus. Its plasma concentration varies with age, dietary intake and in relation to meals. It is intimately related to carbohydrate metabolism and falls significantly during glucose utilization. Phosphorus in other tissues is present in the form of nucleoproteins.

Absorption, fate and excretion: Absorption of phosphorus is more complete than that of calcium. Vitamin D stimulates the GI absorption of calcium and phosphorus. About 70 per cent of the dietary phosphorus is absorbed in the small bowel. A high calcium intake and aluminium hydroxide in large doses interfere with its absorption. Phosphorus filtered by glomeruli is largely reabsorbed by proximal tubules and some is secreted by cells of the distal tubules. The excretion increases with increasing levels of plasma inorganic phosphorus. Unlike calcium, the urinary excretion of phosphorus is more intimately related to its dietary intake and is regulated by PTH which diminishes its distal tubular reabsorption.

Physiological functions:

- ***Formation of bone and teeth*** : Along with calcium, phosphorus is essential for the formation of bones and teeth. Phosphorus needed for this is made available 'on site' by the action of alkaline phosphatase on organic phosphates. When the ion product, Ca x P, exceeds a critical level locally, deposition of calcium phosphate as crystals commences.
- ***Phosphorylation***: Phosphorylation of a chemical compound is the transfer to it of a phosphate group from an inorganic or organic phosphate. It is an essential preliminary step in the metabolism of almost all substances in the body including enzyme regulation, energy transformation and storage, and in the regulation of the delivery of oxygen to the tissues.
- ***Buffer***: Phosphates are important intra- and extracellular buffers in the body and regulate the renal excretion of H ions.
- ***Miscellaneous***: Phosphorus forms an integral part of the structure of the nuclei and cytoplasm. Further, chemical energy is stored in the form of 'high energy phosphate bonds'.

Pharmacological actions: *Mild to moderate hypophosphatemia* may occur after severe dietary deprivation of phosphorus, during long-term use of aluminium containing antacids, in primary hyperparathyroidism, in vitamin D deficiency, in patients with phosphaturia (isolated or as a part of deficiency of tubular reabsorption in Fanconi syndrome) and in the rare syndrome of familial hypophosphatemic rickets. The hypophosphatemia interferes with calcification of the osseous matrix, leading to rickets or osteomalacia. The hypo-phosphatemia of primary hyperparathyroidism is without a direct metabolic effect.

Severe hypophosphatemia (serum inorganic phosphorus less than 1 mg.%) can occur in chronic alcoholism, diabetic ketoacidosis and during hyperalimentation without adequate administration of phosphorus. Malnutrition and phosphaturia due to metabolic acidosis act as predisposing factors. Intracellular shift of phosphorus as a result of administration of glucose and/or insulin unmasks the severe hypophosphatemia. *Severe hypophosphatemia is a life threatening condition and* can cause hemolysis, muscular weakness, mental changes, decreased myocardial contractility and respiratory failure.

Hyperphosphatemia is seen in hypoparathyroidism, renal failure and active acromegaly. In renal failure, the elevated plasma phosphorus level depresses that of calcium and causes secondary hyperparathyroidism and metastatic calcification.

Therapeutic uses:

- ***Hypophosphatemia*:** Neutral phosphate solution is used orally to treat familial hypophosphatemic rickets. Its composition is: disodium hydrogen phosphate 3.66 gms, sodium dihydrogen phosphate 1 gm., orange syrup 16 ml., water to make 60 ml. Sixty millilitres of this solution give 1 gm. of phosphorus. Therapy is commenced with small doses such as 5 ml. thrice daily and the dose slowly increased to tolerance but not exceeding 60 ml. three times a day. Larger doses are liable to cause diarrhoea and hyperparathyroidism. Severe hypophosphatemia may be treated by IV neutral phosphate solution.
- ***Hypercalcemia*:** Oral administration of neutral phosphate solution may be used to treat chronic hypercalcemia except in the presence of concurrent hyperphosphatemia.

Sevelamer (RenaGel) is a cationic polymer that binds phosphate through ion exchange. It is as effective as calcium carbonate and acetate in lowering plasma phosphate in patients with chronic renal failure and causes hypercalcemia less frequently. It is very expensive and its use is reserved for resistant cases and those with hypercalcemia.

PARATHORMONE (PTH): This hormone is secreted by the chief cells of the parathyroid glands. It is secreted as an 84 amino acid polypeptide but is cleaved in the plasma. The 'two site' immunoradiometric assay which measures the whole PTH molecule is used in clinical practice.

The secretion of PTH is directly stimulated by a fall and is inhibited by a rise in the plasma ionic calcium level via the calcium sensing membrane receptor in the chief cells. The level of plasma inorganic phosphorus alters the secretion of PTH indirectly through changes in the plasma calcium level. Circulating calcitriol inhibits synthesis of PTH by gene suppression. For **pharmacological suppression** of PTH synthesis by paricalcitol and 22-oxacalcitriol, see later.

Mechanism of action: PTH acts on the cell wall to (a) stimulate the formation of cyclic AMP and (b) increase its permeability to calcium ions which then move intracellularly. In the bone, it stimulates the conversion of mesenchymal cells into osteoclasts; further it inhibits the osteoblasts and hence collagen synthesis.

Physiological and pharmacological actions:

All the actions of PTH are directed towards maintaining the ionic calcium of the plasma and ECF. It probably influences ion movements in other tissues.

- ***Gastrointestinal tract*:** It promotes the active absorption of calcium and phosphorus indirectly, by enhancing the synthesis of 1, 25 $(OH)_2$ vitamin D in the kidneys.
- ***Bones*:** PTH binds to receptors on the osteoblasts which then secrete cytokines that activate the osteoclasts. This initiates bone remodeling, minute zones of osteoclastic resorption followed by osteoblastic bone formation. Such remodeling cycles repeat themselves all over the bone tissue throughout life. After the age of 20, bone formation slightly falls short of bone resorption in each cycle; this is the basis of *age related bone loss in adult life*.

In hyperparathyroidism, there occurs long term exposure to high plasma levels of PTH, resulting in excessive bone loss. On the other hand, controlled, intermittent exposure to mildly elevated levels of PTH appear to stimulate bone formation more than bone resorption (see teriparotide earlier). This process requires a normal vitamin D intake to permit calcification of the matrix laid down during bone formation.

- ***Kidney*:** The effect on the kidney is of more rapid onset than that on the bone.

(a) PTH promotes the calcium reabsorption from the glomerular filtrate by the distal renal tubules. Only when the plasma calcium rises as a result of the action of PTH, the urinary excretion of calcium increases.

(b) It increases the urinary excretion of phosphorus by decreasing its tubular reabsorption.

(c) It increases the urinary excretion of sodium, potassium, bicarbonate and citrate; and decreases the excretion of hydrogen and magnesium; and

(d) It stimulates 1-hydroxylase in the proximal renal tubules which converts circulating calcifediol into calcitriol, the active metabolite of vitamin D.

Absorption, fate and excretion: Given SC, its peak effect is seen in 18 hours and the response lasts upto 36 hours. It is partly degraded by liver and partly excreted in urine.

Adverse reactions: Orthostatic hypotension, hypercalcemia and anaphylactic reactions are the important adverse effects.

Preparation and dosage: rDNA synthetic PTH (Teriparatide). Dose: 20-40 mcg once SC daily.

Therapeutic uses of PTH: Its use to treat postmenopausal osteoporosis with fractures has been described earlier.

CALCITONIN: Calcitonin is a 32 amino acid polypeptide isolated from the mammalian thyroid and from the cells of the ultimobranchial bodies in lower vertebrates. Calcitonins from various animal species including the humans have been characterized; their aminoacid sequences are different.

In the thyroid, it arises from C cells which lie in between the thyroid follicles. In humans, C cells are also present in the parathyroids and thymus. Hence, thyroidectomy has no effect on plasma calcium level. Calcitonin is secreted in response to increased plasma levels of ionic calcium.

In humans, salmon calcitonin has the most potent pharmacological action. Given SC/IM, it rapidly lowers the plasma calcium and phosphorus by blocking the PTH induced bone resorption by direct anti-osteoclastic action. Thus, the calcium from the circulation is shunted to bone. It also increases the urinary excretion of calcium, sodium, potassium and phosphorus. Its action of lowering plasma calcium level is rapid and of short duration. By its central action, it alleviates osteoclastic bone pains.

Preparations and dosage:

(i) Calcitonin (Pork) (Calcitare): Dose SC/IM 80 units three times a week to 4 units/kg daily.

(ii) Salcalcitonin (Salmon calcitonin, Calsynar, Miacalcic): Dose SC/IM 50 units three times a week to 400 units 6-8 hourly.

(iii) Salcalcitonin nasal spray (Miacalcic). Dose 200 units once daily.

Therapeutic uses:

- ***Hypercalcemia***: Pork calcitonin 4 units/kg SC/IM daily or **Salcalcitonin** 5-10 units/kg daily to 400 units 6-8 hourly SC/IM. The latter may also administered by slow IV infusion in the dose of 5-10 units/kg over at least 6 hours.
- ***Paget's disease:*** Pork calcitonin 80 units SC/IM three times a week to 160 units daily or Salcalcitonin 50 units three times a week to 100 units daily. Therapy may be extended to six months in patients with bone pains or nerve compression. (also see later).
- ***Bone pain in neoplastic disease:*** Salcalcitonin 200 units six hourly or 400 units twelve hourly for 48 hours, SC/IM.
- ***Menopausal osteoporosis with unremitting bone pain:*** 100 units SC/IM daily, together with calcium and vitamin D.

VITAMIN D : The term vitamin D is applied to a group of related sterols which have the common property of preventing and curing rickets and osteomalacia.

Chemistry and source: Many sterols develop the antirachitic property on ultraviolet (UV) irradiation. They are fat soluble and have the same general structure. (Fig. 68.1)

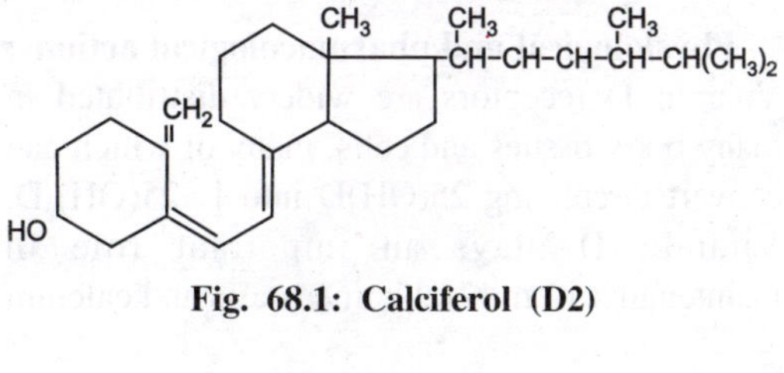

Fig. 68.1: Calciferol (D2)

Solar UV-B irradiation of 7-dehydrocholesterol present in the secretion of sebaceous glands converts it to Vitamin D_3 (cholecalciferol), whereas irradiation of ergosterol present in yeast produces Vitamin D_2 (ergocalciferol).

Vitamin D of animal origin as from fish oil and irradiated milk is D_3.

In human beings D_2 and D_3 have similar actions, qualitatively and quantitatively and hence, both are referred to as vitamin D for discussion.

In the liver, vitamin D is hydroxylated to yield **25-hydroxy vitamin D** (25(OH) D). *Its estimations is used to asses Vitamin D status.* In the kidney, the enzyme 25(OH)D-1-alpha-hydroxylase causes further hydroxylation to produce the active metabolite l-alpha, $25(OH)_2D$, whose biological activity is 500-1000 fold higher than that of the precursor 25 (OH). (Fig. 68.2). Its production is regulated by PTH, and serum calcium and phosphorus levels. The active products of vitamin D are metabolized by 24-hydroxylase to inactive water soluble product calcitroic acid.

The plant *Solanum malacoxylon* contains $1,25\text{-}(OH)_2D_3$ in water soluble form and is responsible for an endemic disease in grazing animals.

Vitamin D may be looked upon both as a vitamin and as a hormone. **As a vitamin**, it prevents:

- ***Rickets and osteomalacia***, by maintaining plasma calcium and inorganic phosphate levels above a certain threshold.
- ***Hypocalcemic tetany***, by maintaining plasma calcium above a certain critical level.
- ***Osteoporosis*** by promoting GI calcium absorption; and
- ***Muscle weakness.***

Physiological and pharmacological actions: Vitamin D receptors are widely distributed in many body tissues and cells, many of which can convert circulating 25(OH)D into 1- $25(OH)_2D$. Vitamin D plays an important role in maintenance of mineral homeostasis and calcium metabolism. In respect of latter, $1,25(OH)_2D_3$, along with PTH and calcitonin, exerts actions on the classic target tissues: bone, kidney and intestine (Fig. 68.2).

(1) **Regulation of calcium metabolism :**

- ***Bone***: Bone tissue undergoes constant remodelling in that the osteoclast-mediated resorption of bone is in approximate equilibrium with osteoblast-mediated re-formation of new bone material. Vitamin D metabolite $1,25(OH)_2D$ in physiological amounts acts as a hormone for the mineralization of new bone. It stimulates bone mineralization (a) by providing mineral for incorporation into bone matrix through increased intestinal absorption of calcium and phosphorus; and (b) by regulating the function of osteoblasts, which possess $1,25(OH)_2D$ receptors. *In vitro,* it modulates the proliferation of, cultured osteoblasts and promotes the synthesis of osteoblast- derived proteins. In large doses, it is a potent bone resorptive agent.

The osteoclast originates from hematopoietic cell of early macrophage lineage. The increase in osteoclasts stimulated by $1,25(OH)_2D$ may indicate a maturational effect of the hormone on myeloid hematopoietic precursor cells, in that these cells are prompted by $1,25(OH)_2D$ to differentiate into functional osteoclasts. Thus, the vitamin D metabolite alters the number but not the function of osteoclasts.

- ***Kidney***: The important actions of $1,25(OH)_2D$ on the kidney are

(a) Inhibition of renal formation of $1,25(OH)_2D$ (negative feedback); and

(b) Stimulation of reabsorption of calcium and phosphorus.

- ***Intestine***: The metabolite $1,25(OH)_2D$ stimulates the intestinal absorption of calcium and phosphate. In the absence of vitamin D, absorption of dietary calcium is about 10-15%, and that of phosphorus is about 60%, which are increased to 30-40 % and 80%, respectively, in response to $1\text{-}25(OH)_2D$. Its deficiency also prevents the adaptive increase in the absorptive capacity of the small intestine for calcium when the dietary calcium supply is low or when the physiological requirements are increased.

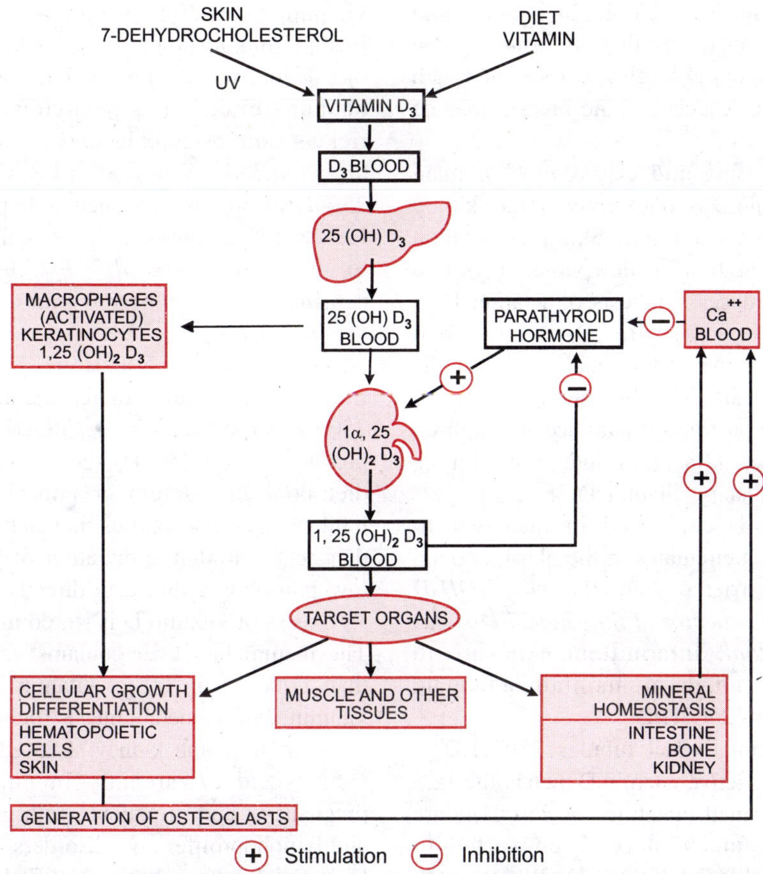

Fig. 68.2 : Actions of Vitamin D

(2) **Muscle:** The uptake of radiocalcium by the sarcoplasmic reticulum is subnormal in vitamin D deficiency; it can be corrected by vitamin D administration. *Clinically, muscle weakness is a prominent feature of vitamin D deficiency; it may be the only manifestation in old persons.*

(3) **Cellular growth and differentiation:** Like the Vitamin A metabolite retinoic acid, $1,25(OH)_2D$, may limit the proliferation and promote the differentiation of several tissues. Under certain conditions, keratinocyte-derived $1,25(OH)_2D$ may induce epidermal differentiation locally and inhibit the proliferation of epithelial cells. Therefore, the active analogue of vitamin D are used topically in the treatment of psoriasis.

$1,25(OH)_2D$ also promotes *in vitro* differentiation of myeloid precursor cells towards cells with the properties of mature macrophages. It has also been associated with functioning of other tissues, not primarily related to calcium metabolism such as pancreas, skeletal and cardiac muscle, thyroid gland and pituitary gland. It promotes cell differentiation and apoptosis, and prevents angiogenesis.

(4) **Immunoregulatory properties:** Receptors for $1,25(OH)_2D$ are expressed in activated, proliferating human B lymphocytes and T lymphocytes, but they cannot be detected in quiescent lymphocytes. It is a potent immunoregulator. People with vitamin D deficiency are more prone to infections such as tuberculosis. Receptors for 1,25 $(OH)_2$ D are also present in a variety of nonleukemic cancer cells.

(5) **Miscellaneous:** 1-25$(OH)_2$D inhibits renin production but increases that of insulin. Very low plasma vitamin D levels are associated with increased risk of cancer of the breast, prostate and colon.

Absorption, fate and excretion: Our main source of vitamin D is that formed in the skin by the action of direct sunshine. Skin pigmentation blocks the penetration of ultra violet rays into the skin and reduces synthesis of vitamin D.

Given orally, vitamin D is absorbed adequately from the distal small bowel in the presence of bile salts. The absorption is defective in patients with obstructive jaundice and in those with steatorrhoea. Mineral oil interferes with the absorption of dietary vitamin D.

Vitamin D is converted in the liver to 25,(OH)D which circulates in the plasma bound to a specific carrier protein. *Plasma 25(OH)D level is a good indicator of the vitamin D status of an individual.* Intermittent exposure to sunshine, is enough to maintain adequate plasma levels of 25(OH)D.

In the proximal renal tubules 25(OH)D is converted to the active vitamin D metabolite 1,25 $(OH)_2$D. Only small quantities of 25(OH)D are so converted; much more is converted to another metabolite 24,25$(OH)_2$D. Whereas the production of 25(OH)D in the liver depends upon the supply of vitamin D to the liver, the production of 1,25$(OH)_2$D is strictly regulated by the demands of the organism. The renal production of 1,25$(OH)_2$D requires the presence of PTH.

The hepatic conversion of cholecalciferol to 25(OH)D is very efficient in the case of vitamin D derived from the skin as the latter is presented to the liver at very slow rates. Vitamin D absorbed from the gut is presented to the liver in relatively larger quantities at a time; as a protective mechanism, the liver degrades it and excretes the metabolites in the bile. *Hence, exposure to natural or artificial sunlight is far more efficient in maintaining plasma 25(OH)D levels than oral administration of vitamin D.*

The metabolic degradation of 25(OH) D in the liver is increased (with resultant depletion of vitamin D) in hyperparathyroidism, primary (parathyroid adenoma) or secondary (deficiency of calcium or vitamin D). The anticonvulsants, phenobarbitone and phenytoin, may cause rickets and osteomalacia *by enhancing this degradation.* Whereas plasma levels of 25(OH)D are low in such patients, levels of 1,25$(OH)_2$D are normal. The anticonvulsants lead to these disorders *also by increasing the resistance of target organs (intestine and bone) to vitamin D.*

The hepatic production of 25(OH)D is inhibited by glucocorticoids and INH; by 25(OH)D itself; and by 1,25$(OH)_2$D. The renal production of 1,25$(OH)_2$ D is stimulated by a diet poor in calcium or phosphorus, and is inhibited by a phosphorus rich diet. Low calcium diet acts through stimulation of PTH release; low phosphorus diet acts directly.

Excess of vitamin D is stored in the body fat. The mammalian liver contains very little (less than 1 mcg. per 100 g.) vitamin D. Very little vitamin D or its metabolites is found in the urine.

Apart from the kidney, 1,25$(OH)_2$D is also synthesized extrarenally in humans during pregnancy, and in patients with granulomatous and lymphoproliferative disorders. Extrarenal 1-hydroxylases have been identified *in vitro* in a variety of tissues including activated macrophages.

Calcium homeostatic mechanism: A tendency to hypocalcemia, as in chronic calcium deficiency, stimulates PTH secretion (secondary hyperparathyroidism). PTH corrects this tendency first by stimulating renal reabsorption of calcium. Continued excess of PTH in continued calcium deficiency stimulates the renal production of 1,25$(OH)_2$D which enhances intestinal absorption of calcium. Increased metabolism of 25(OH) D to 1-25$(OH)_2$ by PTH further aggrevates vitamin D deficiency. High PTH levels also cause phosphaturia and hypophosphatemia.

If increase in intestinal absorption of calcium is not possible, the elevated plasma PTH mobilizes calcium from the bone, and osteoporosis can occur. Persistently very high plasma levels of 1, 25$(OH)_2$D, as in hypervitaminosis D, can cause excessive intestinal calcium absorption and hypercalciuria with or without hypercalcemia.

Assay: An international unit of vitamin D is the specific biological activity of 0.025 μg. of pure calciferol (1 mg. calciferol = 40,000 I.U.). Specific and sensitive immunoassays can measure the plasma levels of 25(OH)D and 1,25$(OH)_2$D; The normal levels are 15-80 ng/ml and 15-60 pg/ml, respectively.

Adverse reactions: Hypervitaminosis D implies the adverse effects of chronic administration of excessive amounts of vitamin D. It is likely to occur in an individual with normal vitamin D sensitivity receiving 50,000 units or more per day for weeks to months. Such doses were used in the past empirically in adults with disorders such as rheumatoid arthritis and cutaneous tuberculosis. They give rise to generalized decalcification of bones, hypercalcemia, hyperphosphatemia, hypercalciuria and metastatic calcification. It does not occur following excessive exposure to sunlight.

Acute 1, 25, $(OH)_2$D toxicity kills rats even before they develop hypercalcemia. The mechanism of this lethal action is probably an inordinate rise in intracellular concentration of 1,25 $(OH)_2$ D, causing generalised cellular poisoning.

Preparations and dosage:

(i) Calciferol contains 40,000 units of antirachitic activity per mg.

(ii) Vitamin D_3 oily injection (Arachitol) 300,000 and 600,000 units of vitamin D_3.

(iii) Shark liver oil contains 6,000 units of vitamin A activity and 1,000 units of antirachitic activity per ml. Dose: 0.5 to 1.5 ml. daily orally.

(iv) For other preparations containing both vitamins A and D, e.g. cod liver oil, and shark liver oil see Chapter 75.

Therapeutic uses: The daily requirement of vitamin D in infants and children is about 400 units (10 mcg). This must be remembered while prescribing vitamin D supplements to infants and children whose 'vitaminized' foods may already be giving them their daily requirement. One teaspoonful (5 ml.) of cod liver oil gives about 650 U (85 U/g.) while 5 ml. halibut liver oil contains 3,000 U of vitamin D. Unfortified cow's milk is a poor source of vitamin D (about 1 mcg. of activity per litre); so is human milk. Some vitamin D is transferred across the placenta and is stored in the fetus, to be utilized in the first few months of extrauterine life. *Vitamin D supplementation of the pregnant mother is thus superior to supplementation of the lactating mother.*

Daily vitamin D requirement is about 800 units in adults, upto the age of 70 years and higher above that age. *Vitamin D supplementation is essential in the elderly in whom both skin synthesis and GI absorption are impaired.*

Deficiency of vitamin D is common, both in children and adults. *The commonest cause of such vitamin D deficiency is a deficient intake or absorption of calcium (because of high phytate and oxalate content of a cereal-vegetables based diet);* this explains why vitamin D deficiency is so common in the tropical countries with abundant sunlight. Further, unlike in the rich western countries, the foods are not fortified with vitamin D. It must be noted that the sun rays which induce vitamin D activity in the skin are in the ultraviolet range and can get absorbed by atmosphere, by glass and by buildings. Vitamin D deficiency can also occur in intestinal malabsorption as in obstructive jaundice; in hepatic cirrhosis, chronic kidney disease, primary hyperparathyroidism and during treatment with anticonvulsants and glucocorticoids. *Generally, a serum level of 25(OH)D below 20ng/ml is considered diagnostic of vitamin D deficiency.*

Vitamin D deficiency leads to rickets in children and osteomalacia in adults, with low plasma inorganic phosphorus, normal or low plasma calcium, hypocalciuria, hyperphosphaturia and aminoaciduria. *Unlike osteoporosis, osteomalacia is accompanced by localized or generalized bone pains, which can be confirmed by pressing the sternum or the anterior tibia.*

The commercially available vitamin D is cholecalciferol (D_3). Its uses are:

• ***For prevention and treatment of vitamin D deficiency***: Unless the pregnant women receive vitamin D supplements, there is hardly any store of vitamin D in the newborn, and its administration is recommended from the first month especially in breast fed infants. If the diet is deficient in older children, the daily requirement can be easily supplied by a teaspoon of cod liver oil. *Excessive administration must be avoided.*

Rickets in children and osteomalacia in adults are best treated with a single oral or IM dose of 300,000-600,000 units (7.5-15 mg.) of calciferol repeated 4-6 weeks later, if the blood chemistry so indicates. Simultaneously, calcium must also be prescribed in order to facilitate the calcification of the osteoid.

Administration of a single IM dose of 600,000 units is desirable in patients with chronic obstructive jaundice.

Routine prophylactic administration of calciferol (600,000 units once in 6 months) may be desirable in patients on long-term therapy with anticonvulsants and glucocorticoids and in elderly people.

For the prevention and treatment of nutritional vitamin D deficiency, the preparation of choice is cholecalciferol. Alphacalcidiol and calcitriol are not appropriate for that purpose (see later).

• ***Vitamin D 'resistant' rickets and osteomalacia***: This term is applied to rickets and osteomalacia not due to vitamin D deficiency but due to chronic renal insufficiency, hereditary hypo-phosphatemic rickets and hypophos-phatasia. Vitamin D in large doses (upto 50,000 U, 1.25 mg., daily) is required to bring about healing of bone lesions in such patients. However, *alfacalcidiol and calcitriol are preferred in these conditions.* Vitamin D requirements for patients with steatorrhoea with bone disease fall midway between those with vitamin D deficiency and those with vitamin D resistant rickets and are 4,000 to 12,000 units per day. Neutral phosphate mixture is also used to treat hereditary hypophosphatemic rickets (see earlier).

• ***In hypoparathyroidism***: Vitamin D together with oral calcium is used in the treatment of hypoparathyroidism. Daily doses of 50,000 to 250,000 units (1.25 to 6.25 mg.) of cholicalciferol are needed. However, *alphacalcidol and calcitriol are preferred in this condition,* at least in the initial days of

Table 68.11: Commonly used compounds with vitamin D activity

Property	Ergocalciferol and cholecalciferol	Calcifediol	Calcitriol	Alfacalcidiol
Physiological dose (mcg/day)*	10	5	0.5-1.0 ☆	0.5-1.0
Pharmacological dose (mcg/day)**	1200	50	0.5-3.0	0.5-3.0
Onset of maximum effect (days)	30	15	2-3	2-3
Duration of toxicity (if it occurs) after cessation of therapy (weeks)	6-18	4-12	0.5-1.0	0.5-1.0
Available as	Variable	20, 50 mcg capsules	0.25, 0.5 mcg tablets	0.5-1.0 mcg tablets

* Will cure nutritional rickets and osteomalacia.
** Used in other conditions listed above.
☆ Dose may be as high as 10 mcg in vitamin D 'dependent' rickets.

treatment till the slower acting cholecalciferol takes effect.

Synthetic vitamin D analogues: 25 $(OH)D_3$ (Calcifediol, Calcidiol, Calderol), 1-alpha (OH) D_3 (Alfacalcidiol, One-alfa) and 1,25 $(OH)_2$ D3 (Calcitriol, Rocaltrol) are the synthetic vitamin D analogues used in therapeutics (Table 68.11). *Unlike calciferol, calcifediol is absorbed from the gut even in patients with fat malabsorption.* It is converted in the kidney to the active metabolite calcitriol. Alfacalcidiol is converted in the liver to calcitriol. Calcitriol supplies the active vitamin D metabolite directly, although all of them have antirachitic activity. However, in contrast to calciferol, which is recommended in treating nutritional rickets and osteomalacia, calcitriol and alfacalcidiol are used primarily in the treatment of:

- ***Hypoparathyroidism.***
- ***Renal osteodystrophy due to chronic renal failure.***
- ***Renal tubular defect with vitamin D 'resistant' rickets and osteomalacia;*** and
- ***Vitamin D 'dependent' rickets.***

Calcipotriol, an analogue of calcitriol suppresses cell proliferation and promotes cell differentiation to the same degree as calcitriol but is 200 times weaker than the latter compound in its action on calcium metabolism. It has proved effective, by topical administration, in the treatment of psoriasis (Chapter 69).

Paricalcitol is a synthetic calcitriol derivative which reduces PTH release without producing hypercalcemia except in overdoses. It is useful in treating secondary hyperthyroidism in patients with chronic renal failure.

22-Oxacalcitriol is another calcitriol derivative which is a potent suppressor of PTH gene, with limited activity on the intestine and the bone. It has been proposed as a treatment for secondary hyperparathyroidism of chronic renal failure, and even for primary hyperparathyroidism.

DIHYDROTACHYSTEROL (DHT): This reduction product of calciferol is also known as A.T. 10 (Anti-tetanic preparation No.10). Its plasma calcium elevating property is similar to that of vitamin D but *its antirachitic property is negligible.* Its action is faster and shorter lived than that of vitamin D. The drug mobilizes calcium from the skeleton, increases the gastrointestinal absorption of calcium and promotes the urinary excretion of calcium and phosphates.

The drug is converted to the active metabolite 25 (OH) DHT which acts directly on the bone and intestine. This is of advantage in patients with advanced chronic renal disease. Its main use is in hypoparathyroidism and renal osteodystrophy, in the dose of 0.2 mg. daily.

Table 68.12 summarises the actions of the 'calcitropic' hormones, calcitriol, PTH and calcitonin.

Miscellaneous :

CINACALCET (Sensipar): This is a *calcimimetic* drug and inhibits PTH secretion by binding to and stimulating the calcium sensing receptor on the parathyroid cells; the latter is rendered more sensitive to serum calcium. Orally, it is well absorbed. It is metabolized by the liver and excreted primarily (85%) in the feces. No dose adjustment is required in chronic renal disease. The adverse reactions are nausea, vomiting and diarrhea. Hypocalcemia can occur and can precipitate seizures in seizure-prone individuals. The drug has been used to treat secondary hyperparathyroidism in chronic kidney disease, and parathyroid carcinoma.

BISPHOSPHONATES: These synthetic pyrophosphate analogues were developed initially as water softners. They are characterized by phosphorus-carbon-phosphorus (P-C-P) bonds. Their potency depends on the length and the structure of the side chain.

Mechanism of action: Bisphosphonates have a strong affinity for the bone apatite; they:

- ***Are effective calcium chelators*** and get deposited in the bone mineral selectively under the oseoclasts. So the their effects are localized.

Table 68.12 : Actions of calcitropic hormones

	Calcitriol	PTH	Calcitonin
Intestinal absorption	Ca^{++} & PO_4^{---} ↑	Ca^{++} & PO_4^{---} ↑ (via calcitriol)	
Kidney	Ca^{++} & PO_4^{---} reabsorption ↑	Ca^{++} reabsorption ↑ PO_4^{---} reabsorption ↓ Calcitriol synthesis ↑	Ca^{++} & PO_4^{---} reabsorption ↓
Bone	Calcification of osteoid*; resorption of bone ↑ in toxic doses	Bone formation > bone resorption on acute administration; Bone resorption > bone formation**	Osteoclastic bone resorption ↓
Plasma values	Ca^{++} & PO_4^{---} ↑ from low to normal	Hypercalcemia and hypophosphatemia	Ca^{++} ↓***
Urinary excretion	Ca^{++} normalizes*; hypercalciuria in toxic doses	Ca^{++} ↑ due to hypercalcemia; PO_4^{---} ↑ by direct tubular action	Ca^{++} & PO_4^{---} ↑

* = In physiological doses. ** = In chronic high concentration. *** = Only in the presence of hypercalcemia.

- ***Inhibit the dissolution of bone crystal;*** and
- ***After ingestion by the osteoclasts,*** are metabolized to toxic compounds that impair the key metabolic pathways of the mature osteoclasts and ***hasten their death by apoptosis***; and
- They also ***block hydroxyapatite crystal growth.***

They are useful for preventing bone resorption and helping to reduce the vertebral and hip fractures in osteoporosis.

They bind to hydroxyapatite, and high doses inhibit bone mineralization. The various drugs used differ in their ability to inhibit bone resorption relative to their ability to inhibit bone mineralization

Absorption, fate and excretion: Given orally, their bioavailablity is low, 1-3% of the ingested dose. Food, iron, calcium, milk, tea, coffee and fruit juices interfere with their absorption. They are rapidly cleared from the plasma, with 50% deposited in the bone where it remains till the bone resorbed; and the remaining excreted in the urine.

They cross the placenta and get deposited in the fetal bone.

Adverse reactions: Bisphosphonates are generally well tolerated. The adverse reactions are nausea, headache, abdominal pain and diarrhoea. Occassionally, they (particularly alendronate) may cuase esophagitis and esophageal ulcers. They can also cause fever, joint pains,myalgia and ocular inflamation. Zolendronate is nephrotoxic. Fractures of the jaw, at the sites of pre-existing infection, can occur during their IV use.

Preparations and dosage: They are listed in Table 68.13.

Table 68.13: Bisphosphonate preparations

Drug	Therapeutic dose
Alendronate*	70 mg once a week
Risendronate	35 mg once a week 75 mg/day for two consecutive days once a month
Ibandronate	150 mg once a month 3 mg IV bolus every 3 months
Zolindronic acid	5 mg, 5 min. IV infusion once a year

Doses are oral unless specified; * preventive dose 35 mg/week

Therapeutic uses:

● ***Osteoporosis:*** Alendronate and risendronate used in combination with calcium and vitamin D reduce the incidence of vertebral and hip fractures (see earlier). Alendronate 70 mg given once a week is as effective and safe as daily administration. The patient should be instructed to take the drug on empty stomach in the morning with 250 ml (a glass) of water, in the erect posture; not to lie down for at least ½ to 1 hour after that; and not to eat or drink anything except water for a similar period.In practice, GI adverse reactions can occur even after following these instructions. He should also be instructed to report any dyspeptic symptoms immediately. Further, a patient with upper GI symptoms should not be prescribed an oral bisphosphanate.

● ***Paget's disease***: Paget's disease of bone (osteitis deformans) is a focal skeletal disorder characterized by : excessive bone resorption followed by excessive bone deposition, that results in structurally disorganized (mosaic) and functionally weak bone, associated local hypervascularity and marrow fibrosis. Its cause is not known. Most patients are asymptomatic, at least initially. Clinically, it causes bone pains, bone deformities, fractures, compressive neurological syndromes and high output heart failure. X'rays show concurrent osteolysis and osteosclerosis side by side. Serum calcium and phosphorus are usually normal; but the serum alkaline phosphatase is commonly elevated. Hypercalciuria and less commonly hypercalcemia may occur. The basic pathogenic feature is increased number, size and resorptive activity of the osteoclasts which erode the bone. Compensatory excessive bone deposition occurs at the sites of resorption.

It is now possible to attack the osteoclasts selectively at one of the stages of their life cycle. The current treatment of Paget's disease includes the use of:

(a) **Bisphosphonates,** especially parenteral zolendronate which circumvents the problem of low oral bioavailability; They act by impairing the key metabolic pathways of mature osteoclasts and disabling them; and perhaps by stabilizing bone against osteoclastic resorption; and

(b) **Osteoprotegerin:** The osteoblasts have on their surface a protein called Receptor Activator of Nf-Kappa B Ligand (RANKL), also called osteoclast differentiation factor (ODF). RANKL initiates osteoclastogenesis by binding to RANK, its receptor, on the surface of bone mesenchymal osteoclast precursors. *Osteoprotegerin is a decoy receptor for RANKL, competes with RANKL for RANK, binds to the latter and disables it, thus inhibiting osteoclastogenesis.* It has not so for demonstrated antigenicity in humans.

The above drugs are administered parenterally and have prolonged action (months to years after a course of therapy). They induce remission; relieve bone pains; prevent fractures and relieve neurocompressive symptoms of Pagets disease. They do not cure the disease, and recurrence can be expected after cessation of treatment. Further, their prolonged biological effects raise the spectre of possible oversuppression of bone resorption (*frozen bone*), leading to inhibition of skeletal metabolic activity and osteonecrosis.

● ***Hypercalcemia of malignancy***: Pamidronate is usually administered by slow IV infusion.

Fluoride

The fluoride ion which is widely distributed in nature is of medical interest because of its toxicity as well as its possible clinical applications. It can enter the human body through edible plants, drinking water, fluorine containing pesticides, contaminated food additives and by inhalation of fluoride dust and gases.

Pharmacological actions: With the exception of its actions on the teeth and bones in very low concentrations, the actions of fluoride are toxic (see below).

Children who drink water containing fluorine (1 part per million) have been shown to develop permanent teeth which are resistant to the development of caries. Topical application of fluoride solution to the teeth after eruption is claimed to reduce the decay.

Fluoride inhibits several enzymes and diminishes tissue respiration and anaerobic glycolysis in excised organs. It is a useful *in vitro* anticoagulant.

Absorption, fate and excretion: Fluoride is absorbed from the GI tract, the lungs and the skin. In the body, fluoride can be detected in all tissues but is preferentially deposited in bones and teeth. It is excreted mainly by the kidneys and in small amounts by the sweat glands, the lactating breast and the GI tract.

Adverse reactions:

- ***Acute poisoning*** : Acute poisoning results from ingestion of insecticides containing fluoride salts. The symptoms are due to irritation of the GI tract (nausea, vomiting, abdominal pain and diarrhoea); hypocalcemia caused by binding of plasma calcium (increased irritability of the central nervous system); and medullary depression (fall of blood pressure and respiratory paralysis). Death is due to respiratory paralysis or cardiac failure. Treatment is symptomatic and consists of stomach wash with lime water, IV fluids, IV calcium and treatment of respiratory and cardiac failure.

- ***Chronic poisoning*** (Fluorosis): Chronic fluoride poisoning is usually reported following drinking contaminated water. It causes two main changes: (1) Osteosclerosis and (2) Mottled enamel. Osteosclerosis consists of an increase in density and calcification of bones and varies greatly in severity. It results in various body deformities. Mottling affects only the developing teeth, teeth which have already erupted being spared.

Therapeutic uses:

- ***Dental caries*** can be defined as " *the localized destruction of susceptible dental hard tissue by acidic byproducts from bacterial fermentation of dietary carbohydrates* ". It is the most common but totally preventable disease in children .

Treated in early stages, the pathological changes can be reversed.

Endogenous microorganisms, mostly mutant streptococci and lactobacillus species present in the biofilms (colonizing the tooth surface) produce weak acid, following fermentation of residual food carbohydrates. The acid decreases the pH and leads to demineralization of tooth tissues. This is naturally prevented by saliva which acts as a buffer and raises the biofilm pH. It can also be reversed by uptake of Ca, P and fluoride. Once the tooth is destroyed, its treatment becomes difficult, and may need maintenance therapy throughout life.

The fluoride ion is one of the micronutrients that has been demonstrated beyond doubt to have a clear effect on dental caries in humans and laboratory animals. The Cochrane review indicated that the use of fluoride tooth paste or gel is highly effective, safe and acceptable. Frequent sipping of sugar containing drinks and eating sugar containing foods such as chocolate, sweets and pastries should be avoided. Replacing such snacks with fruits, vegetables, cheese or nuts is advisable.

Further, rinsing the mouth after eating, and regular brushing of the teeth with fluoride-containing tooth paste at least twice a day after meals is advisable. Decrease or lack of saliva helps the pathological process and should be attended to.

Fluoridation of water supplies is perhaps the most effective procedure for reducing the dental caries in a community. Systemic fluoride is most effective in the reduction of lesions on the incisors and the smooth buccal and lingual surfaces and least effective for the cavities and fissures of the molars. Hence, sealing the cavities and fissures with inert polymer to prevent the start of new lesions is valuable as a complement to water fluoridation. *However, while recommending such procedure, the geographical information regarding the fluoride content of drinking water should be taken into consideration, particularly in the population with anatomic fluorosis.*

The best way to prevent caries is maintaining optimal oral hygiene so as to reduce the causative microbial agents. The teeth should be brushed with a tooth paste and flossed twice a day. Pregnant women should be urged to have all open lesions restored and to follow good dietary practices to reduce the transmission of cariogenic microbes to their infants.

Magnesium Metabolism

Magnesium is an important constituent of the human body. The average amount of body magnesium in an adult weighing 70 kg. is about 2,000 m.Eq. Of this, approximately 50-70 per cent is in bones, 1 per cent is in the ECF and the remaining is intracellular, where it is concentrated mainly in the mitochondria. Bone acts as a magnesium reservoir during depletion. The plasma magnesium levels vary from 1.5 to 2.0 m.Eq./1.; nearly 33 per cent of this is bound to plasma proteins. Cardiac and skeletal muscles, liver, brain and kidneys contain appreciable amounts of magnesium.

Physiological functions and pharmacological actions:

- ***CNS*:** It is a CNS depressant and low magnesium level may evoke increased irritability, confusion and convulsions. Magnesium also possesses local anaesthetic activity and depresses myoneural transmission by reducing the quantal release of acetylcholine and by antagonizing its depolarizing effect at the motor end plates, and by reducing the excitability of muscle cell membrane. Administration of large doses of magnesium resulting in plasma levels over 10 m.Eq./1 can produce fatal respiratory paralysis. The CNS and the myoneural junction depression produced by magnesium can be antagonized by calcium.
- ***CVS*:** The cardiac muscle appears to be less susceptible to the depressant effect of magnesium than the skeletal muscle. However, heart block, prolonged PR interval and widening of QRS complex may result if the plasma level exceed 10 m.Eq./1.

Magnesium causes peripheral vasodilatation. Small doses usually produce flushing while large doses may result in hypotension.

- ***Miscellaneous*:** Magnesium is a co-factor of many vital enzymes like membrane—ATPase. An activating role for magnesium has also been postulated in the uptake and storage of catecholamines within the osmophilic granules of the sympathetic nerve endings and in the activation of ribosomes by the messenger RNA.

Absorption, fate and excretion: Magnesium and calcium probably have common transport mechanisms across the gut and the renal tubules. The daily intake of magnesium in Americans is 20-40 m. Eq. and of this, nearly 1/3rd is absorbed from the GI tract. Low levels of magnesium intake enhance calcium absorption. Magnesium is excreted by the kidney by glomerular filtration. Increased urinary excretion occurs in hyperparathyroidism and in diuresis induced by glucose and by thiazide / loop diuretics. Only 3 to 5 per cent of filtered magnesium appears in urine; the rest is reabsorbed. PTH appears to be essential for both GI (indirect/direct) and renal tubular reabsorption of magnesium. Renal impairment may cause magnesium retention leading to toxicity even with orally administered magnesium containing antacids and purgatives.

Magnesium deficiency: Table 68.14 gives the common causes of hypomagnesemia.

Table 68.14: Common causes of hypomagnesemia

- Severe and continued diarrhoea or fistulous discharge.
- Chronic alcoholism.
- Diabetic ketoacidosis.
- Hyperthyroidism.
- Thiazide/loop diuretic therapy.
- Intestinal malabsorption.
- Hyperparathyroidism.
- Renal tubular acidosis.
- Aldosteronism; and
- During recovery from acute tubular necrosis.

Magnesium deficiency is characterised by weakness and mental disturbances like restlessness, and aggressiveness. Involuntary movements, and rarely tetany may develop. Cardiac arrhythmias of ventricular origin have been reported. The serum magnesium level may be as low as 0.8 m. Eq./1. A low serum level, however, is not necessarily diagnostic of magnesium deficiency.

The urinary output of magnesium is very low and it fails to increase even on magnesium loading. When magnesium deficiency is secondary to excessive renal loss, urinary magnesium levels are obviously above normal.

Magnesium deficiency is usually associated with low level of intracellular potassium, particularly in the skeletal muscle. The plasma potassium levels are usually normal.

Acute hypomagnesemia stimulates PTH secretion; however chronic hypomagnesemia impairs PTH synthesis and release, and causes hypocalcemia. Such patients show symptoms similar to hypoparathyroidism; however, they do not respond till magnesium is given.

Therapeutic uses of magnesium salts:

- ***In magnesium deficiency*:** Magnesium deficiency can be treated by daily administration of approximately 300 m. Eq of magnesium given as magnesium hydroxide mixture. If oral medication is not possible, 4-8 ml. of 50 per cent magnesium sulfate can be given IV slowly.
- ***As antacids and osmotic purgatives*:** See Chapters 42; and 41.
- ***As anticonvulsant*:** Magnesium sulfate is used to control seizures in toxemia of pregnancy where it is considered superior to diazepam and phenytoin. It is administered during labour and for 24 hours afterwards. A 20 per cent solution is usually administered IM or IV for this purpose. In toxemia of pregnancy, parenteral magnesium sulfate also achieves a moderate reduction in blood pressure. Care must be taken to keep a calcium preparation handy to counter excessive central depression with magnesium.
- ***In cardiac arrhythmias*:** Hypomagnesemia is known to occur in the immediate post-myocardial-infarct period and may be associated with cardiac arrhythmias. This responds to IV magnesium sulphate 4 ml, 50% given over 15minutes. It may be repeated if needed.
- ***In raised intracranial tension*:** Concentrated solution of magnesium sulfate is sometimes used rectally to reduce increased intracranial tension.
- ***Local uses*:** Magnesium sulfate in the concentration of 25 to 50 per cent in glycerine is used topically for alleviation of inflammation. It acts by exerting an osmotic effect.

Section XIV
Drugs Used in Common Skin and Eye Disorders

Pharmacotherapy of Common Skin Disorders and Skin Protectives 69

Skin diseases are common in clinical practice, more so in the warm and humid tropical countries. The skin forms a barrier between the organism and its external environment. The skin, the target tissue of drug treatment, is also a route of drug administration. It can function as a drug reservoir. It also acts as a site for drug metabolism. Finally, application of drugs to the skin can alter the function(s) of internal organs.

Anatomy and Physiology of the Skin: Anatomically, the skin consists of three distinct layers (Fig. 69.1):

- ***The epidermis.***
- ***The dermis***; and
- ***The subcutaneous tissue.***

The **epidermis**, consists of a multilayered, keratinizing, stratified, squamous epithelium. The outermost part of the epidermis is the dead **stratum corneum** which prevents water loss from the body. It also protects against noxious agents in the environment.

The **dermis** is a thick, highly vascular layer made up of ground substance, fibroblasts and collagen fibres, together with the appendages of the skin, sweat glands and pilosebaceous

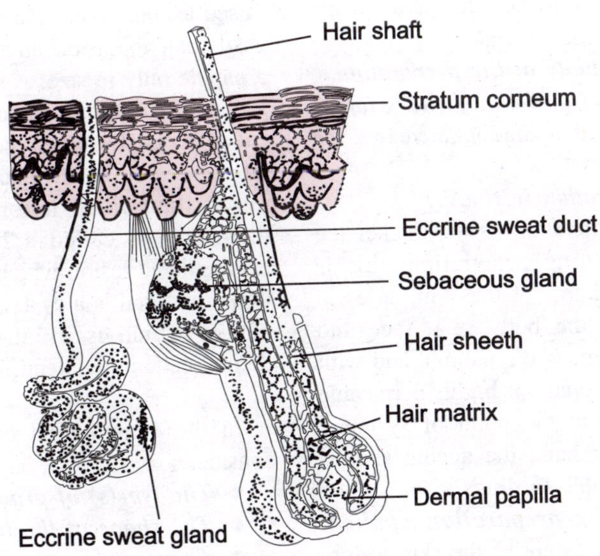

Fig. 69.1: Structure of normal hairy skin

follicles, embedded in it. This layer is richly supplied with nerves. It is metabolically active. The *subcutaneous tissue* is a fibro-fatty layer with varying quantities of adipose tissue in different regions of the body. This layer provides physical and thermal protection to the deeper structures of the body.

The skin is important in regulation of the body temperature.

Principles of Drug Application

To be effective, a drug must enter the skin in adequate concentration. Topical drug treatment aims at providing high concentration of the drug at the site of application with minimal systemic absorption, to avoid systemic adverse effects.

Drugs are applied to the skin in various formulations in pharmacologically inactive *vehicles*. However, the therapeutic effects depend not only on the properties of the drug but also on those of the vehicle. *Occasionally, the vehicle itself may cause local irritation.*

The absorption of drugs into the skin is slow and incomplete. It depends on:

- ***The lipid solubility of the preparation.***
- ***The state of hydration of the srtatum corneum*** — increased hydration increases the drug penetration.
- ***Drug concentration in the vehicle.***
- ***Thickness of the skin*** — the thicker the skin the lower the drug penetration; this is important as the thickness of the skin varies in different regions of the body (e.g. face and intertriginous areas versus the palms), and with age. The skin in the neonates is highly permeable to drugs, sometimes to the point of systemic toxicity; on the other hand the ageing skin is relatively less permeable to drugs.
- ***Quantity of the preparation applied***, which varies with the extent of the skin lesion. Large amounts of 'very potent' glucocorticoids (Chapter 64) can cause serious systemic toxicity. The following quantities of preparations are generally sufficient for one application for the indicated areas in adults: head, face, hand or anogenital area 2 g; an arm, anterior or posterior trunk 3 g; a leg 4 g; the entire body 25-30 g.;
- ***The presence of inflamed skin*** which allows higher penetration of a drug; and
- ***The use of an occlusive dressing*** which increases the penetration of the drug into the skin.

An absorbed drug may be stored in the skin for prolonged periods e.g. *a topical glucocorticoid applied to the skin under occlusion for 24 hours can establish a reservoir lasting for upto 2 weeks.*

To help in the understanding of skin lesions, it is necessary to be acquainted with various descriptive terms used to characterise these lesions. This is important for defining the skin lesions in a given case and also in formulating a differential diagnosis. **Macule** is a flat, coloured lesion, less than 2 cm in diameter, which is not raised above the surface of the surrounding skin. A macule larger than 2 cms is called a **patch. Papule** is a small solid lesion with diameter less than 1 cm, raised above the surface of the surrounding skin, and hence palpable. A raised lesion larger than 1 cm which is firm and easily palpable is called a **nodule.** It differs from a papule only in size. A small fluid-filled lesion less than 1 cm in diameter, often translucent, is called a **vesicle**. When the vescicle is filled with leucocytes, it is designated as a **pustule.** A raised fluid filled lesion more than 1 cm in diameter is called a **bulla.** A soft, raised, encapsulated lesion which contains semisolid or liquid material is **a cyst**. A raised erythematous papule which is usually due to short lived dermal oedema is identified as a **wheal.**

In the examination of the skin, one must consider :

- ***The type(s) of primary lesion(s).***
- ***The shape of the individual lesions(s).***
- ***Their arrangement;*** and
- ***The distribution of the eruption.***

The description of various skin lesions is beyond the scope of this book. However, the pharmacotherapy of some selected, common, dermatological conditions seen in general practice is described below.

As in other areas of medicine, rational therapy in skin disorders depends upon proper diagnosis. Not all skin diseases need urgent treatment. Some, like very localized psoriasis of the elbow, are best left alone. In cases where the diagnosis is not immediately obvious, the prescription of a bland local application such as oily cream (while awaiting specialist opinion) is better than the indiscriminate use of a blunderbuss commercial preparation containing an antibiotic, a glucocorticoid, an antihistamine and perhaps a local anaesthetic, in the hope that 'something will work.' The use of such an irrational preparation can change the morphology of the lesions and make the subsequent diagnosis difficult.

The next step is to choose between local and systemic therapy. Whenever such choice exists, local treatment is always preferable to systemic. However, the local use of some drugs such as antihistaminics and (most) antibiotics is best avoided because of the possibility of inducing allergic dermatitis. While selecting drugs one should take into consideration the physical properties of the formulations and morphology of the skin lesions rather than the etiologic diagnosis. Further, local skin therapy is modified by the changing patterns of the presenting dermatoses.

Intradermal and transdermal drug administration: This is discussed in Chapter 1.

Vehicles and Formulations

Vehicles: Skin therapy is usually symptomatic and topical. Topical preparations consist of two parts: (1) the active ingredient(s), and (2) the base or vehicle. The important vehicles are liquids, powders, oils and ointment/cream bases. Most vehicles have several important functions:

- ***They form a reservoir for the active ingredient.***
- ***They allow local release of suitable amounts of the active drug.***
- ***They provide a reasonably safe infrastructure for practical application; and***
- ***Many vehicles are also useful for their physical actions*** such as soothing, lubricating, cooling, drying, moistening, softening, hydrating or protecting effects.

The factors which influence the choice of a vehicle are listed in Table 69.1.

Table 69.1: Factors determining the choice of a vehicle

- Its hydrating or drying property.
- Its ability to assist in the absorption of the active ingredient.
- Its physical and chemical interactions with the stratum corneum; and
- The stability of the final formulation.

Depending upon the vehicle, the skin preparations can be grouped as powders, wet dressings, lotions, paints, and lubricating preparations such as creams, ointments and pastes.

- ***Powders*** act by their physical property of absorbing moisture. They contain ingredients such as talc, starch, chalk, cellulose, menthol and zinc or magnesium stearate. They can also produce a cooling effect. Finally, they protect the skin by reducing friction especially in the intertriginous areas such as axillae and groins and in the skin folds under the female breasts.
- ***Wet dressings*** are soft dressing material soaked in aqueous solutions containing ingredients such as isotonic saline, aluminium acetate and potassium permanganate. They are used in acute exudative inflammation with marked oozing. *Lotions* are liquid preparations with a viscosity a little higher than that of water and alcohol; e.g. the calamine lotion. Lotions are used to treat subacute inflammation, after the marked exudation has stopped. Evaporation of water from the lotion has a cooling effect

whereas the residual dry powder acts as a protective. However, lotions sometimes cause excessive drying. But, those containing glycerol or propylene glycol, when applied to dry and scaly skin, help to retain water in the epidermis. Addition of alcohol (15%) and menthol (0.25 to 2.0%) enhances the cooling effect. Phenol (0.5 to 1.0%) camphor (1 to 3%), salicylic acid (1 to 2%) and coal tar (1 to 3%) impart an antipruritic and keratolytic action to the lotion.

- ***Lubricating preparations*** (Emolients) include plain oil, liniment, gel, water-in-oil emulsion (*most but not all ointments*), oil-in-water emulsion (*most but not all creams*) and paste. Vegetable oils, liquid, soft and hard paraffin, lard, lanolin and beeswax are important ingredients of lubricating preparations. Emolients soothe, smoothen and hydrate the skin and are indicated for dry or scaling disorders. Ointments and pastes are more hydrating, whereas creams and gels are more drying.

- ***Pastes*** are stiffer than other lubricating preparations, and are made of a finely divided powder incorporated into an ointment base. They protect the skin from external irritants and from sunlight. They also protect it from friction caused by clothing and bandages.

Choice of Preparation

From the therapeutic viewpoint, the skin lesions are divided into (a) oozing and (b) dry types.

- ***An oozing dermatosis*** is associated with dilatation of subepidermal capillaries (erythema), edema and disruption of the epidermis by formation of vesicles. When oozing is copious, folded muslin soaked in a lotion such as an aqueous solution of potassium permanganate (1:5,000 or 1:10,000) is applied half-hourly. Evaporation of water produces surface cooling, capillary constriction and reduces oozing. At that stage, a shake lotion (aqueous suspension) such as calamine lotion is substituted and applied every hour. This formulation, in addition to producing surface cooling, forms an adsorbing layer on the lesion. When oozing is very little, calamine lotion is likely to cake, leading to cracking of the skin due to excessive drying. Such lesions are best treated with a liniment or a cream, e.g. zinc cream which produces an emollient effect. Thus, zinc cream is preferred for keeping the skin soft. When oozing ceases but the lesion still appears moist, a paste is applied. It acts as an adsorbing, protective and splinting agent.

Some dermatoses may be associated with infection as indicated by a seropurulent discharge. In such instances, an appropriate antimicrobial agent such as iodochlorhydroxyquinoline (Vioform), bacitracin, neomycin or hibitane is incorporated into the formulation. Judicious incorporation of a glucocorticoid hastens the subsidence of inflammatory phenomenon. The dangers of local glucocorticoid therapy are discussed in Chapter 64.

- ***Dry skin lesions*** are best treated with an ointment or a paste. An ointment (generally) promotes percutaneous absorption of the incorporated drug, thus allowing an active pharmacologic effect on the skin.

In cases of urticaria and acne vulgaris, a lotion is generally preferred to other forms of applications although the skin lesions are dry.

When penetration of an active drug through the epidermis into the dermis is desired, the base must be chosen with care. In general, penetration of medicaments is better from an aqueous base than from an oily base. Further, raising the local temperature of the skin as by a polyethylene occlusive dressing enhances penetration of the active drug such as a glucocorticoid.

Pruritus: In the management of pruritus, identification and rectification of the underlying cause are important. When pruritus is a skin manifestation of systemic diseases such as drug allergy, obstructive jaundice, Hodgkin's disease and chronic iron deficiency, it responds poorly to antihistaminic drugs. Topical antihistaminics and local anaesthetics are generally marginally effective. Antihistaminics given systemically, however, are useful in itching due to inflammatory or allergic skin diseases. In such cases, these can be combined with topical steroid application. Minor local conditions may respond to calamine lotion and/or 2% menthol in aqueous cream applied locally. Emolients or urea cream may be useful when pruritus is associated with dry skin (Chapter 22).

Keratolytic Agents

Keratolytics are the drugs which, when applied locally, cause a mild peeling of the superficial layers of the skin.

SALICYLIC ACID: In the concentration of 0.5 to 2%, salicylic acid is used to treat acne vulgaris; it causes peeling and comedolysis. A 6% ointment is useful in the treatment of dandruff, seborrheic dermatitis and psoriasis. A 15-25% solution in lactic acid and a 40% plaster are used to treat warts and thick calluses.

PROPYLENE GLYCOL: A 2% aqueous solution of propylene glycol is used as a vehicle. Higher concentrations (upto 70%) affect the keratin and soften the skin, leading to desquamation. It is commonly used in combination with salicylic acid to treat ichthyosis.

UREA: Urea, in the form of cream or ointment, softens the skin and is used in the treatment of psoriasis and atopic dermatitis. It has hydrating, keratolytic and antipruritic actions on the skin. It increases the absorption of hydrocortisone when used in combination.

BENZOYL PEROXIDE: This drug is available as 5-10% cream or lotion and is used for mild to moderate acne. It is effective mainly because of its keratolytic effect although it also has some bacteriostatic activity against acne bacilli. The drug may cause some irritation.

TRETINOIN: It acts on the nuclear retinoid receptors and normalises follicular keratinisation. It is used topically to treat acne vulgaris (see later) and other disorders of keratin. Whatever little is absorbed from the available preparations has not been reported to cause any systemic toxicity, particularly teratogenicity.

Drug Therapy of Bacterial and Viral Skin Infections

Impetigo: This is a common skin condition, characterised by superficial infection by *Staphylococcus aureus* or streptococci. Generally, it is a mixed infection. The primary lesion is a superficial pustule that ruptures and forms a typical yellow brown crust. The lesion may occur on normal skin or may be superimposed upon another skin disease such as pediculosis. The condition usually responds well to topical antibiotic therapy but systemic antibiotics are preferred in certain circumstances. Improvement of personal hygiene is important.

After gentle cleaning and debridement of the adherent crusts, application of an ointment containing neomycin 1%, framycetin 1.5%, bacitracin 1% or mupirocin 2% is recommended. Topical use of antibiotics such as tetracyclin gentamicin, and penicillin should be avoided.

Since glomerulonephritis can develop in children following streptococcal infections of the skin, systemic antibacterial therapy must be considered for impetigo in children between one and eleven years of age. Systemic therapy is also recommended in patients with renal and heart disease, with coexisting eczema and in those on immunosuppressive drugs. In such circumstances, a penicillinase-resistant penicillin like cloxacillin, erythromycin or cotrimoxazole should be given in full doses for 10 to 12 days.

Furuncle or boil: This is an acute infection of the hair follicle commonly caused by staphylococci. In healthy individuals, it responds to fomentation and the use of local antiseptics like povidone iodine and chlorhexidine (Chapter 60). In severe cases and in those with persistent lesions, a cream containing neomycin, framycetin or mupirocin may be applied. Patients who develop boils frequently may require long term treatment with an appropriate antibiotic. *In such cases, an underlying systemic disease like diabetes mellitus or uremia should be excluded.*

Herpes simplex and Herpes zoster: Herpes simplex can be treated by topical application of 5% acylovir or of 1% penciclovir. Both these drugs are applied 4 to 5 times a day. Topical acyclovir is, however, less effective than systemic acyclovir, and it offers no significant clinical advantage in recurrent genital herpes. In severe cases involving the mucosae, it is given orally in the dose of 200 mg. five times a day for 10 to 14 days (Chapter 57).

Infections due to herpes zoster also respond to acyclovir and idoxuridine, but to a lesser extent than herpes simplex. In severe cases of herpes zoster, acyclovir is administered IV in dose of 5 mg/kg every 8 hours for 5 days. Alternatively, vidarabine can be infused IV in the dose of 15 mg/kg once daily, over 12 hours, at a concentration of 0.5 mg/ml. *Use of glucocorticoids in herpes zoster is contraindicated.*

Post-herpetic neuralgia may respond to local application of 2% capsaicin, and to analgesics. Drugs like amitryptyline, gabapentine and carbamazepine are also beneficial. (Chapter 11).

Warts: Warts are human papilloma-virus-induced benign proliferation of the skin and mucosa. Most of the patients do not need any treatment as warts are known to undergo spontaneous regression within 1 to 2 years. Several methods are used to treat warts. These range from cryotherapy and electro-descication to carbon dioxide laser ablation. Warts can also be treated by local application of keratolytic agents like salicylic acid in flexible collodion. Other topical drugs include podophyllin 15 to 25% solution, trichloracetic acid and phenol. Formaldehyde (5% solution) and podophyllin are particularly useful in the management of plantar warts. Silver nitrate in the form of pencil may be used to cauterise the warts. Care must be taken to protect the surrounding skin. (Also see Chapter 51).

Drug Therapy of Fungal Skin Infections

For therapeutic purposes, fungus infections (mycoses) have been classified as *superficial* (affecting the skin, and its appendages hair and nails), *subcutaneous and deep*. The common fungi which cause superficial skin infection are:

- ***The dermatophytes*** (trichophyton, microsporon and epidermophyton) which cause ringworm (dermatophytosis).
- ***The candida species*** which cause mucocutaneous candidiasis; and
- ***Pityrosporon orbiculare, also known as Malassezia furfur,*** which causes tinea versicolor (Chapter 48).

Majority of superficial fungal infections can be treated by local antifungal agents, and **azoles are preferred** because of their wide spectrum and safety (Chapter 48). Only chronic, resistant infections may need systemic antifungal therapy with griseofulvin or an azole. Because tinea infections of the foot are often complicated by bacterial infections and other factors, an ideal antifungal medication for the foot should have antifungal and antibacterial properties and a drying effect. A solution or a cream containing an azole such as clotrimazole or miconazole also covers the candida; it is suited for treating tinea pedis (Chapter 48).

Topically useful antifungal agents are:

BENZOIC ACID AND SALICYLIC ACID: Salicylic acid is a weak antifungal agent but has keratolytic properties. Benzoic acid compound ointment (Whitfield's ointment) contains 6 per cent of benzoic acid and 3 per cent of salicylic acid in an emulsifying ointment. It is effective in

Table 69.2: Azoles for dermal skin infections

For topical use :
Clotrimazole, Miconazole, Econazole, Butaconazole, Oxiconazole, Sulconazole, Ticoconazole.

For systemic use :
Ketoconazole, Itraconazole, Fluconazole, Voriconazole. (These can also be used locally.)

treating dermatophytosis. Sometimes it may cause local irritation.

AZOLES: Various azoles used to treat skin fungal infections are listed in Table 69.2. They are described in detail in Chapter 48.

Imidazoles are now preferred for treating mild to moderate localized lesions. They are used as creams, powders, lotions, and as vaginal tablets or suppositories. Generally, they are safe and do not stain the skin or clothing.

In patients with chronic, extensive infection, infection of the scalp and nails resistant to local therapy and in immunocompomised patients, systemic therapy with itraconazole or fluconazole is indicated. Ketoconazole is not preferred because of its toxicity profile. In all fungal infections, therapy has to be carried out for a few weeks to 3-4 months, depending on the severity, so as to avoid a recurrence. For use of griesofulvin, see Chapter 48.

TERBINAFINE is an allylamine. Applied as 1% cream or solution daily for 1-2 weeks, it is effective in dermatophyte infections. It can also be used orally. **Naftifinene** 1% has similar activity (Chapter 48).

TOLNAFTATE (Tinaderm): This drug, used as 1% solution/cream, is effective in the treatment of superficial fungal infections of the skin caused by trichophyton and epidermophyton though its superiority over the older antifungal preparations is not established. *The drug is not effective against fungal infection of nails and hair,* and relapses are frequent when it is employed in the treatment of *Trichophyton rubrum* of the trunk. It is nonirritating, nonstaining and odourless.

UNDECYLENIC ACID: This drug is applied to the skin in the concentrations of 2 to 15 per cent, sometimes in combination with zinc undecylenate in the treatment of dermatophytoses, particularly tinea pedis.

CICLOPIROX OLAMINE (Loprox, Batrafen): This drug, not related chemically to the imidazoles, is as effective as the imidazoles in the treatment of cutaneous candidiasis and dermatophytoses, as well as in tinea versicolor. It causes minor local but no systemic adverse effects. Its use should be avoided in pregnant and lactating women. It is available as 1% cream.

SELENIUM SULFIDE (Selsun): This drug has been used in the treatment of tinea versicolor, a chronic fungal infection, caused by *Malassezia furfur.* It is also temporarily effective in the treatment of dandruff. It has mild toxicity but possesses unpleasant odour. It is irritant to the eyes. The drug is commonly used as a 2.5% suspension; the preparation is applied once daily for 5 days to the wet skin, lathered in place for 15-20 minutes and then washed thoroughly. After that, one application once a month is continued to prevent re-infection.

ICHTHAMMOL (Ammonium ichthosulfonate): Ichthammol consists of the ammonium salts of the sulfonic acids in an oily substance prepared from the distillate of butiminous schist or shell or from other sources, together with ammonium sulfate and water. It is an almost black, viscid liquid with a strong and a characteristic odour, soluble in water. It is slightly irritant to the skin. Ichthammol is used as 10 per cent cream and ointment in the treatment of resistant dermatomycoses and other chronic skin diseases.

Other topical fungicidal agents include

tincture iodine, iodophors, haloprogin, phenol, oxidising agents e.g. potassium permanganate and dyes like gentian violet. Fungicidal actions of iodochlorhydroxyquinoline 3% and nystatin have already been discussed.

Choice of antifungal therapy: It depends on the site involved and the type of infection. Small localized lesions are best treated with keratolytic agents like salicylic acid (Whitefield's ointment) or topical application of an azole. Systemic antifungal therapy with an azole or griseofulvin is required for extensive lesions, very chronic lesions, tinea capitis, and fungal infections of the nails (Chapter 48).

Tinea versicolor is caused by the fungus *Malassezia furfur,* also known as *Pityrosporon orbiculare.* It causes patches of lesions on the chest, shoulder and back. These patches often appear as hypopigmented areas particularly on a dark skin. Many topical fungicides are effective, but preparations containing salicylic acid 1%, sodium thiosulphate 10%, or selenium sulphide 2.5% are preferred. These preparations have to be used daily for 3-4 weeks and will clear most of the infections. *Repeated infection from the infected clothings must be prevented by proper treatment of clothings.*

It must be emphasized that fungal skin infections and scabies (discussed later) are common among the population from warm and humid climates, particularly in those with unhygienic habits. Simple personal hygiene and environmental control measures usually suffice to limit the infection and hence, preventive measures such as cleanliness and mass education are far more important than any drug.

Dandruff and Seborrhoeic Dermatitis

These conditions are the manifestations of an abnormal immune response to *Pityrospora ovale*, a constituent of the normal skin flora. The lipase in these organisms splits triglycerides into fatty acids, and the latter are thought to be responsible for the dermal irritation. There is often an atopic background. There are several predisposing factors: genetic; winter season; excessive sweating and sebum production; a change in the composition of the sebum; alkalinity of the skin; an emotional component; and a neurological component as in Parkinsonism and other neurological disorders.

Dandruff is scaling and moderate itching of the scalp without inflammation of the skin; the scales are white, dry and loose.

Seborrhoeic dermatitis is an acute, subacute or chronic scaly dermatitis affecting areas of sebaceous activity such as the scalp, hairline, forehead, face (especially the nasolabial folds), retroauricular areas, the external ear canals, the presternal and the interscapular areas. The scales are either dry, gray and flaky, or yellowish and greasy. In severe cases, there may be **seborrhoeic eczema** with or without oozing of the skin. The disease commonly affects the neonates in whom it lasts for about one year and postpuberal persons in whom it is chronic and recurrent in spite of treatment.

The drugs effective in dandruff and seborrhea are listed in Table 69.3. They are usually applied to the scalp as shampooes. It appears that the common denominator in the actions of these

Table 69.3: Drugs effective in dandruff and seborrhoeic dermatitis

- ***Antipityrosporal*:**
  Imidazoles (ketoconazole 2% shampoo, cream or scalp gel)
  Salicylic acid (2% aqueous cream)
- ***Antiinflammatory*:**
  Mild corticosteroid topically
- ***Cytostatic*:**
  Selenium sulfide (2.5% shampoo)*
  Zinc pyrithione (1% shampoo weekly)*
  Sulfur (2% aquous cream)
  Tar (tar B.P.C. 3%)

* Also have antipityrosporal action

drugs is an anti-pityrosporal action, although other actions such as cytostatic, anti-inflammatory and antiseptic may also be contributory.

Topical ketoconazole is the most effective treatment in these conditions. Its high affinity for the keratin of the skin and the hair leaves a prolonged residual anti-pityrosporal activity at the site of application. Therefore, the remission after its use is usually long lasting. Oral ketoconazole is rarely justified because the lesions are generally localised to small areas of the skin and the drug is toxic. Topical corticosteroid treatment (hydrocortisone 1%) is almost as effective as topical ketoconazole but recurrence is invariable after stopping the treatment. The other drugs listed in the table are moderately effective but recurrence is invariable after stopping the treatment. *In view of the chronic and recurrent nature of the illness in adults, the treatment has to continue indefinitely in them.*

In addition to drug therapy, the predisposing causes such as mental tension, excessive sweating and alkalinity of the skin need treatment for good results; the last factor can be taken care of by application of lemon juice to the affected areas of the skin.

Drug Therapy of Scabies and Pediculosis

Scabies: Scabies is caused by the itch mite *Sarcoptes scabiei* var. *hominis.* The female mite burrows into the superficial layers of the skin to form tortuous channels in which the eggs are deposited. Transmission of the mites occurs by close body contact. Away from the human body, the itch mite survives in a moist environment for 1-2 days only. Unhygienic conditions and crowded housing favour the spread of the infection, which is characterised by intense itching, usually worse at night. It is important to note that scabies can give rise to urticarial rash and eczematous lesions, which can be mistaken and wrongly treated with local and even oral steroid therapy. The principles of treatment are:

- All members of the household must receive the treatment simultaneously.
- The medicament is applied to the whole body surface below the lower jaw. Contact with the eyes and the urethral meatus should be avoided carefully for fear of irritation.
- The drug is applied 3-4 times at 12-24 hour intervals, with bathing and scrubbing of the body before and after the complete course.
- Complications are treated either simultaneously or after the basic treatment is over.
- Intimate clothing and bedding used during the previous 48 hours should be disinfected by boiling or by steam, and
- Education regarding personal hygiene.

Drugs used in the treatment of scabies are:

SULFUR : The scabicidal effects of sulfur, the oldest remedy, is probably due to its conversion into hydrogen sulfide and parathionic acid. In addition to its use in scabies, sulfur is also employed in the treatment of other chronic skin conditions like psoriasis and seborrhoea.

Sulfur ointment contains 5 per cent (2.5% in children) of sublimated sulfur in a simple ointment base. Because of its irritant nature, it should not be applied to the face. It stains the clothes and has an unpleasant smell. Though cheap, it needs repeated applications. It is now obsolete.

BENZYL BENZOATE (Ascabiol): Benzyl benzoate is a highly efficient acaricide and is the drug of choice. It is usually applied in the form of benzyl benzoate 25% emulsion. Even after cure of infection, the itching may persist for a few weeks but usually responds to calamine liniment. Children are treated with 12.5 per cent application. Secondary bacterial infection can be successfully treated only after the primary infestation is eradicated. The drug is slightly irritant and has an unpleasant smell.

Although effective in pediculosis, benzyl

benzoate is not recommended in its treatment because of its feeble ovicidal activity and short duration of action.

PERMETHRIN, 5% application, left for 12 hours, is highly effective (see later).

GAMMA BENZENE HEXACHLORIDE (GBH, Gammexane, Lindane): This gamma isomer of hexachlorocyclohexane is an insecticide, larvicide and acaricide. Applied externally, the drug is not so toxic; but when ingested, it can cause convulsions. The drug is excreted slowly from the body. The other serious but rare toxic manifestation is aplastic anaemia.

Fig. 69.2: Gamma benzene hexachloride

A vanishing cream containing 1 per cent of the drug (Lorexane), applied to properly dried skin all over the body in the form of a thin film without preliminary bathing, results in total eradication of scabies. The film is left over for a period of 12 hours following which the patient is given a bath. An average adult requires 25 g. of the cream per treatment. Unlike benzyl benzoate and sulfur, the agent is odourless and non-irritant and can, therefore, be applied safely to the face but care should be taken to prevent contact with eyes and mucus membranes. However, it is neurotoxic, if absorbed. The treatment may be repeated after a week. Not more than two applications should be used during pregnancy.

Because of enhanced skin absorption and the risk of toxicity, gammexane should be avoided in infants and children. At that age, it can cause CNS disturbances and convulsions.

It is also useful in pediculosis.

A 0.1 to 0.5 per cent solution in kerosene is lethal to flies and mosquitoes. It may be combined with other insecticides, such as a pyrethroid (permethrin) to obtain a rapid, lethal effect.

IVERMECTIN: Given orally in a single dose of 200 mcg/kg, ivermectin, an antifilarial drug, (Chapter 58), is highly effective in clearing up scabies. Repetition of the dose after two weeks gives almost 95% cure.

MONOSULPHIRAM (Tetmosol): It is an effective acaricide and is used as 25% solution diluted with 2 to 3 parts of water. It is also incorporated in soap, recommended for the prophylaxis of scabies. The drug may cause mild irritation. Adults using this drug should avoid alcohol because monosulphiram is related chemically to disulfiram (Chapter 6).

CROTAMITON (Eurax, Crotorax): This is available as 10% lotion and as cream. It is applied thrice at 24 hour intervals, followed by a bath.

Pediculosis: Pediculosis, a common condition in tropical countries, is caused by the louse *Pediculus humanus* and usually affects the scalp (capitis), the body (corporis) and pubic area (pubis). It is responsible for intense itching and may cause impetigo and eczematous lesions. Further, during famine and natural calamities, the body louse can act as a vector for typhus, relapsing and trench fevers. Finding of nits or the lice on hair clinches the diagnosis. The drugs used are given in Table 69.4.

Table 69.4: Drugs used in pediculosis
Permethrin 1%
Malathion (Ovide) 0.5%
Dicophane (DDT) 2% (Chapter 60)
Gamma BHC (Lindane) 1% cream, 2% Shampoo
Kerosene oil

PERMETHRIN (Lyclear): This is a synthetic pyrethroid, available as 1% cream or lotion. Applied to clean damp hair, left on for 10 minutes and then rinsed off the hair, it is an effective pediculocide with a residual effect for two weeks. The small quantity absorbed is rapidly metabolized to inactive compounds, and excreted in the urine. It may cause local reactions. It does not have the biological disadvantages of gammexane (Chapter 60), and is usually preferred.

MALATHION (Ovide): This organo-phosphorus compound applied as 0.5% lotion is rapidly pediculocidal and ovicidal in the treatment of head lice, even in patients who are resistant to permethrin. The drug is well tolerated and no systemic adverse effects have been reported. It is usually applied and left in place for 8-12 hours, and the application is repeated 7-9 days later. It is inflammable because of the alcohol base. Care should be taken to keep the lotion away from heat and open flame, and to avoid contact of the lotion with the eyes.

DICOPHANE (DDT): Used as a 10% dusting powder, it is a an effective pediculocide; its prolonged residual effect makes it lethal to the larvae which hatch out later. (See Chapter 60).

For **pediculosis capitis, permethrin** cream/ lotion is preferred for initial treatment. For failures, **malathion**, the fastest-acting and the most ovicidal pediculocide, is recommended. However, it has an objectionable odour. Because it is inflammable, a hair dryer and a curling iron should not be used during the treatment.

In resistant cases, **ivermectin** is safe and highly effective when used as two doses of 200-400 mcg/kg each, a week apart; the second dose is required as the drug is not ovicidal.

The other drugs used are **Gamma BHC, DDT** and **kerosene.** Gamma BHC (lotion, cream 1% or shampoo 2%) and DDT (2% dusting powder) are generally used as two applications, 7-10 days apart. The application of kerosene, though not very pleasant, is the cheapest and effective treatment for head lice. It destroys lice and suffocates nits by covering them with an impervious film. Usually, one tablespoonful of kerosene is rubbed into the whole scalp and the head wrapped in a piece of cloth. Two hours later, it is washed thoroughly with soap and water. Kerosene does not cause irritation and usually, a single application is all that is necessary. *Of course, the individual must keep away from fire.*

In patients with **pediculosis corporis or pubis,** DDT used as 10% dusting powder is highly effective. A single application can give an adequate residual effect against the larvae which hatch out later. **Gamma BHC** is also equally effective. However, its persistence in the environment and its degradation to toxic products makes it undesirable in this condition. Further, lice can develop resistance to all above drugs. Hence, **malathion** or **newer pyrethroids** are preferred. The clothing should be disinfected with heat and all the contacts are treated simultaneously.

Drug Therapy of Acne Vulgaris

Acne vulgaris (pimples) is a very common skin disorder, particularly in teenagers, and it generally regresses with time. However, it can persist for a long time and in some individuals, can cause disfigurement and permanent scarring.

It usually affects the face but can also spread to the trunk. Acne is known to develop frequently in patients with androgen excess. Most patients with acne probably have sebaceous glands that are hyperresponsive to androgens, rather than have over production of androgens.

Pathophysiology: The important features are:

- ***Increased sebum production by the sabeceous glands.***
- ***Hyperkeratinization and excessive desquamation of epithelial cells*** from the walls of the hair follicle, leading to blockade of the follicular openings.
- ***Formation of comedone,*** a fleshy, hyperkeratotic plug blocking the opening of the

pilosebaceous follicle ('Black' and 'White' heads).

- ***Proliferation of locally present Propionibacterium acnes and a few Staphylococci.*** These bacteria split the sebaceous fat to form irritant fatty acids leading to
- ***Local inflammation***

The therapy of acne is, therefore, directed to:

- ***Counteract the excessive production of sebum.***
- ***Prevent the abnormal desquamation of epithelial cells in sebaceous follicles***; and
- ***Treat and control the growth of P.acne.***

Drugs used in the treatment of acne are given in Table 69.5.

Table 69.5: Drugs used in the treatment of acne

- ***Cleansers,*** e.g., Soaps.
- ***Comedolytics,*** e.g., Local tretinoin, Adapalene.
- ***Exfoliants*** (peeling agents), e.g., Salicylic acid.
- ***Sebostatics,*** e.g., Oral Isotretinoin.
- ***Hormones:*** Cyproterone acetate, Estrogen.
- ***Antibacterial drugs:***
  Local- Erythromycin, Clindamycin, Azelaic acid, Benzoyl peroxide.
  Systemic- Tetracyclines, Erythromycin, Minocycline, Cotrimoxazole.

Dietary modifications have not been shown to modify the course of acne vulgaris and undue diet restrictions are unnecessary. Avoiding the application of cosmetic oils and greases to the affected area is helpful; but prolonged and vigorous washing will not resolve the lesions. On the contrary, scrubbing may damage the delicate openings of the hair follicles, and block the flow of sebum, thus worsening the acne.

Comedolytics and exfolients:

TRETINOIN (Trans-retinoic acid, Retin-A) used topically is an effective local comedolytic. It enhances the penetration of other anti-acne agents into the epidermis. Frequent application of this agent, however, produces redness and peeling of the skin. Improved appearance may take as long as two months to develop. It is applied as 0.01 to 0.025% gel, 0.025% lotion or as 0.025% cream. Gels are preferred in hot and humid climate and cream in cold and dry climate. *People using retinoic acid should avoid exposure to sun because of increased susceptibility to sunburns.* Its long term use should be avoided for fear of possible photocarcinogenesis.

Tretinoin is also useful in treating acanthosis nigricans and skin striae such as those of Cushing's syndrome.

ADAPALENE (Differs) : This drug structurally resembles retinoic acid. Used as 0.1% cream, it acts like tretinoin but is claimed to be less irritant.

Salicylic acid has a keratolytic property and is used as 0.5 to 2% hydroalcoholic formulation. All these drugs can be combined with local or systemic antimicrobial agents.

Sebostatics: Sebaceous glands are androgen dependent and therefore, estrogens and antiandrogenic drugs are useful in therapy of acne. Estrogens are usually prescribed as COC pill containing ethinyl estradiol 50 mcg and a nonandrogenic progestin such as desogestrel or cyproterone acetate. The COC pill must be given for 2-4 months before substantial improvement is observed. More prolonged therapy is needed to avoid relapse.

CYPROTERONE ACETETE: A potent antiandrogen, can be used in place of OC pill but is more expensive. **Spironolactone** in the dose of 50-200 mg/day reduces sebum production, but again several months of therapy is required to get maximal benefit. Combination OC pills containing cyproterone acetate 2 mg (Diane, Ginette) are also effective. For obvious reasons *only women should receive the antiandrogen therapy.*

ISOTRETINOIN (13-cis-retinoic acid): This vitamin A metabolite, given orally, as well as applied topically, can cause prolonged remission, permanent in 40%, In fact, oral isotretinoin would be a drug of choice for most patients with acne but for its serious toxic effects and cost. Given orally it causes marked atrophy and inhibition of sebaceous gland activity (**Sebostatic action**) and causes keratinisation of the hair follicle, thus reducing the formation of comedones. It may also suppress inflammation. A dramatic reduction in the oiliness of the skin is apparent within a month of starting treatment. It is usually prescribed at a dose of 0.5-1 mg/kg body weight daily for 3-4 months. Its bioavailability is increased if it is taken during or after meals. The improvement persists even after its stoppage.

Adverse reactions: Common effects include dryness of the skin and mucosae, and itching. Less commonly, it can cause hyperlipidaemia, hypercalcaemia, photosensitivity, hair loss, arthralgia, intracranial hypertension, premature fusion of epiphyses depression and psychosis.

The drug is highly teratogenic and if it is used in women of child-bearing age, oral contraception should be continued for one month after stopping the treatment. There is no risk to male patients treated with this drug. Anyone taking this drug should not donate blood for one month after stopping it. Due to its toxicity and high cost, the drug should be reserved for severe pustular acne not responding to other medications. *This drug is not useful in the treatment of psoriasis.*

Antimicrobial drugs for *P. acnes*: Antibiotics used against *P. acnes* are listed in Table 67.4. Antibiotics, applied locally once or twice daily, exert a beneficial effect both by killing *P. acnes* and indirectly, by inhibiting the production of proinflammatory mediators by the organisms. Combination of **erythromycin** 3% with **benzoyl peroxide** 5% appears to be highly effective topical preparation. Clindamycin is also effective.

Benzoyl peroxide (2.5-10%) as gel or lotion is lipophilic and suppresses the growth of *P.acnes* more effectively than topical antibiotic therapy used alone. Drug resistance does not develop. It has no anti-inflammatory property. It can cause local irritation and allergic dermatitis.

Antibiotics used for the systemic therapy of acne include doxycycline (100-200 mg. daily), minocycline, erythromycin (500-1000 mg daily) and co-trimoxazole. Generally, **doxycycline** is preferred.These drugs need to be given for 4-5 weeks and then tapered off gradually by 10 to 12 weeks. This is followed by topical treatment with tretinon and benzyl peroxide for 6 months.

The suggested therapeutic approach for treating acne is outlined in the Table 69.6.

Table 69.6: Drug therapy of acne vulgaris

• ***Mild cases without inflammation***	Topical : Tretinoin cream/ gel; adapalene 0.1% gel; salicylic acid.
• ***Mild cases with inflammation***	Topical antibiotics, benzoyl peroxide or combination of erythromycin and benzoyl-peroxide for 4 to 5 weeks.
• ***Severe cases with inflammation***	Topical tretinoin plus systemic antibiotic therapy. If response is unsatisfactory, particularly in multinodular cystic lesions, add oral isotretinoin; in women of reproductive age, use OC pill or cyproterone acetate.
To prevent recurrence, topical treatment must continued for 6 months.	

Rarely, severe acne may be associated with fulminating systemic symptomatology such as fever, arthralgia, glomerulonephritis and bone pain. In such case addition of oral glucocorticoids may be useful.

Since acne is a chronic condition, prolonged treatment is required to prevent recurrence.

Various factors can alter and/or exacerbate lesions of acne vulgaris. Thus, friction and trauma may cause rupture and promote inflammatory reaction.

Agents that predispose to the formation of comedones include topical agents such as lanolin, butyl stearate, lauryl alcohol and paraffin in commercial cosmetic and hair preparation. Industrial compounds that contain impure paraffin oil, halogenated hydrocarbons, coal tar and its derivatives can also precipitate or worsen the condition. Glucocorticoids applied topically or administered systemically *for long periods* can also cause acne.

Drug Therapy of Allergic Skin Disorders

Urticaria: See Chapter 22.

Atopic Dermatitis: *Atopy* is defined as a genetically determined tendency to hyper-react to common environmental allergens with the production of IgE and immediate hypersensitivity/allergic (Type I) reaction. Majority of the patients have a family history of asthma or hay fever. Atopic dermatitis is a cutaneous expression of the atopic state. The clinical presentation differs according to the age of the patient. The infantile form is the most common and is characterised by weeping and encrusted inflammatory lesions distributed on the face, neck and extensor surfaces. Itching is prominent. Secondary infection may be present. Atopic dermatitis in infants often resolves spontaneously. The treatment includes:

- ***Avoidance of cutaneous irritants*** like soaps, detergents and hot water.
- ***Adequate cutaneous hydration***; and
- ***Judicious use of mild topical glucocorticoids*** to control itching and inflammation (Chapter 64).

Infection should be treated with systemic antibiotics. Oral antihistaminics may be useful to control the itching. The role of dietary allergens in atopic dermatitis is controversial. However, if such an allergen can be identified, particularly in children, it should be avoided. Severe exacerbations need to be treated with systemic glucocorticoid therapy. Although such treatment will generally clear the skin, the lesion will return after stoppage of therapy.

An antidepressant, **doxepine,** (Chapter 13), 5% cream exhibits significant antipruritic activity in atopic dermatitis. It has some antihistaminic property. It can get absorbed from the skin and may cause drowsiness and anticholinergic effects.

Immunomodulating agents such as **cyclosporine** and **tacrolimus** have been reported to be useful when given orally. They are, however, toxic. Tacrolimus ointment is claimed to be effective (Chapter 76). It does not cause skin atrophy.

Allergic contact dermatitis: This condition is caused by contact of the skin with some offending agents. The commonest type is plant dermatitis caused by members of the Rhus family. It is characterised by erythema, vesciculation, and severe itching at the areas of contact. The other common sensitisers include preservatives in topical preparations, fragrances, formaldehyde, potassium dichromate, rubber curing agents, synthetic paints, plastics and drugs. Chronic and excessive exposure to water and detergents can initiate or aggravate hand dermatitis. This condition is common in housewives and food handlers. However, many times, the offending agent is difficult to identify. The ideal treatment is removal of the offending agent. Symtomatic relief can be achieved by local treatment with high potency fluorinated topical glucocorticoids for about two weeks.

Eczema: Eczema is a common form of inflammation of the skin (dermatitis), with variable clinical and histological features. It may be the common final expression of allergic conditions, such as atopic dermatitis, contact dermatitis, or may accompany seborrheic dermatitis (see earlier). Initial lesions occur as erythematous macules, papules, or vesicles which later coalesce to form patches and plaques. Eczema is associated with itching and may be :

- ***Weeping (oozing);*** or
- ***Dry.***

As in other allergic disorders, attempts should be made to identify the offending agents and eliminate them. These are commonly found in food additives, perfumes, cosmetics, insecticides, mosquito repellents, environmental chemicals, synthetic fibres, plants, flowers and pollen.

Most of the cases of localised eczemas respond well to calamine lotion/liniment or to a mild topical glucocorticoid preparation such as 1-2% hydrocortisone preparation (Chapter 64). Once the eczema is controlled, attempts should be made to reduce the concentration of and finally stop the glucocorticoid therapy.

Due to adverse effects of long term administration of glucocorticoids on the skin, some physicians prefer tar preparations. Other topical preparations which are useful in eczema are potassium permangnate solution used for bringing about drying of weeping lesions; and zinc containing pastes, calamine liniment to counteract excessive dry lesions. A simple emulisifying ointment like rose ointment or a cream containing urea, which acts by increasing the hydration, can also be used for dry lesions. *Systemic glucocorticoid therapy has no place in routine treatment of chronic eczema,* but it can be beneficial in the acute form of the disease. *Antihistaminics should not be used topically because of their propensity to cause contact dermatitis.* In general, antibacterial agents are used only in severe infections.

Various topical glucocorticoid preparations used are described in Chapter 64.

Drug Therapy of Psoriasis

Psoriasis is a common, chronic, inflammatory dermatosis. It is characterised by erythematous, well demarcated plaques, and rounded scales which look like silvery mica. Pruritus may be present. Lesions are usually symmetrical and occur on the extensor surfaces such as the elbows and knees, and on the scalp. About 50% of the patients have involvement of the finger nails and some have psoriatic arthritis. The current therapy only suppresses the disease and recurrence is common. However, the disease may undergo spontaneous remission.

Genetic predisposition to psoriasis is known. Further, drug-induced flares of psoriasis can occur (Table 69.7). Infections, particularly due to streptococci can trigger an attack. The commonest variety of psoriasis is characterised by plaques, which consist of greatly thickened horny layer of the skin (**hyperkeratosis**). Pathologically, they are characterised by hyperproliferation of the epidermal kerotinocytes and inflammation of both the epidermis and the dermis, along with angiogenesis. These changes are due to cytokines released by T-lymphocyte, which initate autoimmune dermal response to unidentified antigenic stimuli (keratinocyte proteins). The affected dermis shows predominance of CD_4 lymphocytes. The activated T cells from the dermis cause the keratocytes to proliferate; the inflammatory changes include infiltration of the epidermis by leucocytes. It is now known that TNF-α is the primary activator of the T-lymphocytes and it also contributes to the maintenence of a complex inflammatory reaction. The permissive role of bacterial superantigens in its pathogenesis is now well established.

Mild cases of psoriasis may not warrant any drug therapy, since the drugs used can produce toxicity. Indications for drug treatment are :

- ***Marked local symptoms*** such as pain and itching.
- ***Prominent hand, leg or facial lesions;*** and
- ***Diminished mobility due to severe lesions.***

The treatment of psoriasis depends on the

Table 69.7: Possible risk factors in psoriasis

- Injury to the skin.
- Infection, particularly streptococcal.
- Some systemic drugs (beta blockers, ACE inhibitors, lithium, indomethacin, chloroquin).
- Psychological stress.

type, the location and the extent of the lesions. The patients are advised to avoid known exacerbating factors (Table 69.7).

Drugs used in the treatment of psoriasis are listed in Table 69.8.

Table 69.8: Drugs used in psoriasis

Topical therapy
- Emollients
- Keratolytic agents: salicylic acid 2-10%.
- Cytostatic agents : coal tar, dithranol
- Glucocorticoids.
- Calcipotriol, Tacalcitol
- Retinoids-Tazaritene (Chapter 68).

Systemic therapy
- Etretinate
- Immunosuppressants: Methotrexate, cyclosporine, mycophenolate mofetil.
- Biological agents
  (a) T cell activation inhibitors – efalizumab, alefacept
  (b) TNF-α inhibitors – Etanercept, infliximab.
- Systemic glucocorticoids.

Phototherapy
- Ultraviolet B irradiation with or without coal tar application.
- Ultraviolet therapy with psoralens.

I Topical Therapy:

Emollients: These act by hydrating and softening the scales. They are used in mild cases. The commonly used emolients are yellow, soft paraffin and aqueous cream. Although greasy emolients are sometimes preferred, they are less well accepted by the patients.

Salicylic acid: This is the most widely used keratolytic agent, used either alone or with coal tar. It is an irritant, and care should be taken to avoid contact with the eyes (see earlier).

Cytostatic agents (dithranol and coal tar) are used, along with UVB phototherapy, in the treatment of psoriasis and other hyperplastic skin disorders. In these conditions they restore a normal rate of epidermal proliferation. In severe cases, systemic therapy with either **etretinate** or **methotrexate**, both of which act as cytostatic agents in the skin, may be needed.

Crude coal tar (3% ointment) **:** This has been used to treat chronic, lichenified lesions. Coal tar, even in low concentration, has an unpleasant odour, and can cause irritation and acneform eruption. Hence it is less acceptable.

DITHRANOL (Anthralin): This synthetic substitute for chrysarobin reduces the epidermal cell DNA synthesis and mitotic activity (antimitotic) of the hyperplastic epidermis. It is an irritant to the skin and the kidney, and should not be applied to the eyes or to tender skin.

The drug is used as an ointment, paste or paint. Since some patients are allergic to this drug, a preliminary test on a patch of skin should be carried out. It is used in the increasing concentrations of 0.05 to 0.5%, along with ultraviolet B light therapy, for 2 to 3 weeks. It stains the skin brown and is not suitable for treatment of lesions on the face.

A commercial preparation, Derobin, contains dithranol 1.15% with salicylic acid and coal tar.

GLUCOCORTICOIDS : (Chapter 64). Topical glucocorticoid preparations of the mild and moderately potent varieties (Chapter 64) are preferred because of their efficacy, high degree of acceptability to the patients and low cost. Once a day application to the lesions is probably as effective as the twice a day regimen and is less liable to cause ADR.

Relapse rate is higher than with other forms of therapy. *The use of potent and very potent, topical, glucocorticoid preparations should be reserved for the specialist.*

CALCIPOTRIOL (Dovonex) : This vitamin D derivative is applied locally to psoriatic lesions in mild to moderate disease. It has minimal effect on calcium metabolism. The drug is as effective as topical, medium potency glucocorticoids but is less toxic. It is applied daily as an ointment containing 50 mcg/g for about 8 weeks. The ointment is colourless, does not stain clothes and docs not have unpleasant smell. It can sometimes cause irritation and hypercalcemia. **Tacalcitol** is another vitamin D analogue which is effective. Combination of a topical vitamin D analogue and phototherapy is a well accepted regimen for psoriasis.

II **Systemic therapy:** Although most patients with psoriasis can be treated effectively with local therapy, about 20% may require systemic therapy. The latter is expensive and more toxic and needs supervision. The drugs used are:

ETRETINATE (Tigason): This vitamin A analogue inhibits keratinization and proliferation, and normalizes differentiation of epithelial tissues. Used alone, it has limited efficacy in psoriasis. It is valuable in generalised psoriasis. It is usually combined with psoralen and UV-A phototherapy in chronic plaque psoriasis. It accumulates in the adipose tissue and the liver. The adverse reactions include dryness, scaly erythema and tenderness. The drug is administered orally in the dose of 0.5-1.0 mg/kg per day. *It is teratogenic* and should not be used in woman of the reproductive age until pregnancy is excluded. Further, *the patient must avoid pregnancy during treatment and for at least 3 years after the treatment is over because of its long half life (about 120 days).* Similarly, anyone taking this drug should not donate blood for 3 years after stopping it. *The drug has no sebostatic action and is of no use in acne vulgaris.*

Acitretin, a metabolite of etretinate, is now preferred to etretinate in therapy. Its limitations are similar to those of etretinate. Topical **tazarotene**, a retenoid applied once daily, is also effective.

METHOTREXATE: This folic acid antagonist acts by blocking DNA synthesis and inhibiting cell proliferation. Methotrexate may also act as an immunosuppressant. It is given orally in 3 doses, usually 2.5-5.0 mg. at 12 hourly, intervals, every week. It is preferred in severe cases, where coal tar-U V therapy has failed. It should be used only in patients with normal hematological, renal and hepatic status. The drug is usually well tolerated in the doses recommended. The main long term dose dependent toxicity is hepatic cirrhosis (Chapter 59).

CYCLOSPORINE : This drug is used as an immunosuppressant and acts by inhibiting the production of IL2, a cytokine necessary for proliferation of activated T cells, and other T cell cytokines (Chapter 24). Cyclosporine is reserved for patients with severe refractory psoriasis. The important adverse effects are hypertension and renal toxicity which may be irreversible.

MYCOPHENOLATE MOFETIL : This immunosuppressant has been reported to be useful in the treatment of psoriasis. Adverse effects reported are mild and dose-dependent. The drug has also been useful to treat pyoderma gangrenosum, pemphigus vulgaris and systemic vasculitis.

Biological agents : Recently, biological agents have been introduced in the treatment of psoriasis (Table 69.7). Given parenterally, they are effective in about 30-70% of patients with moderate to severe psoriasis. They are :

(1) **Alefacept** binds to CD2 on activated T cells and impairs the co-stimulatory signals of leucocyte-function-associated antigen-3 (LFA-3). This decreases the number of T cells.

(2 **Infliximab** inhibits TNF-α functionally.

(3 **Etanercept** is a recombinant human TNF receptor antagonist (Chapter 71).

(4) **Efalizumab**, humanized mAb, blocks T cell migration and interferes with adhesions. *It has been withdrawn because of neuro toxicity.*

Systemic glucocorticoids: Systemic glucocorticoid therapy, though very effective, needs high doses to suppress the disease, and therefore causes ADR. Further, the relapse rate is high. Hence, it should be reserved for patients with erythrodermic psoriasis, who are acutely ill.

Drug Therapy of Alopecia

The skin, except that of the palms and soles, has hair follicles. The hair are of two types: *vellus hair* which are fine, light coloured and straight; and *terminal hair* which are thicker, dark and may be curly. *In the neonate*, terminal hair are present on the scalp and in the regions of eyelashes and eyebrows; these are the androgen independent or *nonsexual hair.* At about the age of 8-10 years, the weak adrenal androgens cause a slight rise in the plasma testosterone level, and terminal hair appear on the forearms and legs in both boys and girls (*ambisexual hair). At puberty*, with the further rise in the plasma testosterone level into the adult female range, terminal hair appear in the pubic and axillary regions; these hair are also ambisexual. Boys with further advanced puberty and adult males develop terminal hair in other regions such as face and trunk *(sexual hair)*.

The circulating testosteropne is converted in the skin into dihydrotesterone (DHT) which acts on the hair follicles and is responsible for the growth of the ambisexual and sexual hair; it is also responsible for the (normal) temporal recession in normal adult males, and for the (abnormal) temporal recession in adult females (see below) and the (abnormal) growth of sexual hair in women and in children of both sexes. Further, it is responsible for the excessive loss of scalp hair in women with elevated plasma androgen levels (see below).

Hair growth is cyclic, with phases of growth (**anagen**), involution (**catagen**) and resting (**telogen**). In the scalp, about 75% of the hair are in anagen (for about 3 years), 5-10% are in catagen (for about 3 weeks) and the rest 20% are in telogen (for about 3 months), after which hair are shed. The growth of scalp hair is asynchronous, with hair in a given area in different phases; there is a balance among **anagen, catagen** and **telogen** hair in all regions of the scalp. A disruption of the balance causes many more hair to enter the telogen phase, and about 3 months later they are shed in bulk causing alopecia; this is called **telogen effluvium**; After that, the hair grow again. Severe stress can cause telogen effluvium; but *as sudden severe hair loss occurs three months after the stressful event*, the latter is likely to be forgotten. Similarly, an abundance of estrogen during pregnancy and COC pills use (Chapter 66) prolongs the anagen of the scalp hair which is responsible for their lush appearance in these women. However, about 3 months after delivery or cessation of COC pills, these hair enter the telogen and are shed, causing alopecia. Some time later, the hair growth returns to normal.

Alopecia is loss of hair in any region of the body. Alopecia of the scalp can be :

I **Scarring** which is associated with inflammation, fibrosis and destruction of the hair follicles due to primary skin disorders such as lichen planus or systemic diseases such as lupus erythematosis. Such alopecia is permanent.

II **Non scarring** in which the hair follicles are preserved, and the alopecia is temporary and reversible. The important causes of non-scarring alopecia are: crash dieting, physical trauma, iron deficiency, hypothyroidism, chronic malnutrition, chronic illness, dandruff, androgen excess and androgenetic alopecia (see below). It can also be caused by drugs (see Table 69.10).

The forms of alopecia of the scalp are:

- ***Androgenic alopecia.***
- ***Androgenetic alopecia*** (male pattern baldness); and
- ***Alopecia areata.***
- ***Drug induced*** (See Table 69.10).

Androgenic alopecia occurs in women and is due to elevated plasma levels of androgens. These women also have other manifestations of hyperandrogenism such as menstrual abnormalities, hirsutism, acne and infertility. The treatment is that of hyperandrogenism (Chapter 67).

Androgenetic alopecia is a hereditary disorder due to excessive conversion of testosterone to DHT in the scalp skin in genetically susceptible men and women. The DHT causes shrinking of the local terminal hair follicles to miniaturised hair follicles. The onset in both sexes is early in life, often in teens. The miniaturised hair of various lengths and diameters are the hallmark of this condition.

In men, the alopecia ranges from bitemporal recession to thinning of the hair in the frontal and vertex regions to complete baldness except in the occipital and temporal regions. **In women**, the thinning is less severe than in men but is maximum in the frontal and parietal regions. Most women with this condition have normal menses, pregnancies and plasma levels of androgens; *endocrine testing is not required if the above described characteristic pattern of hair loss is present, and there in no evidence of hyperandrogenism.* Treatment comprises topical **minoxidil** (see below) in both sexes and oral **finasteride** in men (Chapter 67). The response to finasteride is better in the frontal region of the scalp (which has higher levels of 5-alpha reductase) than in the occipital region (which has higher levels of aromatase).

It must be remembered that androgens cause:

(a) The vellus-hair follicles to be replaced by terminal hair follicles in the region of ambosexual and sexual hair; and

(b) Miniaturization of the terminal hair follicles of the scalp.

As these changes are irresversible, complete reversal of hirsutism (Chapter 67) and of androgenic/androgenetic alopecia is not to be expected.

Alopecia areata (which is non-scarring) causes patches of complete baldness, varying in size, in any region of the body including the scalp. The bald areas may coalesce to produce large areas of baldness. The condition is due to an autoimmune disorder of the hair follicles. The hair tend to regrow on the bald patches but recurrence is common. The treatment comprises topical minoxidil and a topically injected glucocorticoid.

Minoxidil, an antihypertensive agent (see Chapter 29), when applied locally as a 2% solution (Mintop) twice a day over a prolonged period, may produce some hair growth in a few patients. The results are best in mild cases and good to excellent results are seldom seen in more than 30% of patients even after prolonged use. Minoxidil causes an increase in the dermal blood flow; further it causes an elongation and normalization of the hair follicles. New hair follicles are not formed. *Cosmetically acceptable hair growth is uncommon, and the beneficial effect of minoxidil ceases when the treatment is discontinued.* One ml of 2% solution is applied to dry scalp twice daily. The dose of 2 ml. per day should not be exceeded. The therapy is prolonged, expensive and unpredictable.

There is no reliable and safe treatment for irreversible alopecia. Had there been one, many dermatologists themselves would not have been bald.

Drugs Affecting Skin Pigmentation

Drugs can be used :

- ***To decrease localised hyper-pigmentation*** such as freckles and post-inflammatory pigmentation.

- ***To increase pigmentation in acquired, localized, skin disorders with hypopigmentation*** such as vitiligo; and
- ***To treat acanhosis nigricans*** (see later).

Hydroquinone and monobenzone are used as skin bleaching agents whereas the psoralen compounds (trioxsalen and methoxsalen) are used concurrently with exposure to UV light for stimulating melanin synthesis and repigmentation. *These drugs are not recommended below the age of 12 years.*

HYDROQUINONE (Eldoquin): This drug inhibits tyrosinase and hence melanin synthesis in the melanocytes of the skin. It is also toxic to the melanocytes. It is commonly used in the form of a 2-4% cream or lotion in the treatment of freckles, post-inflammatory pigmentation, and melasma of pregnancy and that due to oral contraceptives. Its effect is reversed by sunlight and hence it is used in combination with an opaque sunscreen.

MONOBENZONE (Benoquin): This is a monobenzyl ether of hydroquinone and has similar properties. However, it causes total, irreversible depigmentation. The incidence of skin allergy to this drug is high.

Vitiligo is probably an autoimmune disorder. It may be localised or generalised. The treatment is unsatisfactory. The affected skin can be painted by artificial tanning preparations or with 1-2% dihydroxyacetone in 50 : 50 water and acetone. The concentration should be adjusted to suit the patient.

TRIOXSALEN (Trisoralen): Given orally, it may be effective in the treatment of vitiligo. By increasing the skin pigmentation, it increases the tolerance of the skin to UV light. For large lesions of vitiligo, it is given in the dose of 0.6 mg/kg/day 2-3 times a week 2 hours before exposure to 15-20 minutes of direct, mid-day sunlight. Exposure is increased by 10-20 minutes per day until erythema sets in. If the desired effect is not obtained after 90 minutes of exposure, the dose of the drug is increased gradually upto a maximum of 80 mg daily. Repigmentation is usually evident after 3-4 months of treatment. Blue-grey, plastic sunglasses, opaque to UV rays, and a light-screening lipstick should be used during UV exposure in order to protect the eyes and the lips. The drug sometimes causes cutaneous reaction. It is contraindicated in patients with diseases associated with photosensitivity such as porphyria and systemic lupus erythematosus, and should not be given concurrently with other photosensitizing drugs.

METHOXSALEN (Oxsoralen): This drug is used topically and orally to treat small vitiligenous lesions. Topical application of a 0.1 to 1% lotion is followed by exposure to sunlight or a UV lamp. This causes activation of malanocytes.Topical use can cause acute, vesicular, cutaneous photosensitivity reaction. The drug can also be given orally in the dose of 20 mg/day (single dose), 2-4 hours before exposure to UV light. It can cause gastric discomfort. Precautions similar to those while using trioxsalen should be taken. The risk of severe sunburn is considerable with this drug.

Acanthosis nigricans : This is hyperpigmented, velvety thickening of the skin occuring most commonly on the neck, in the axillae and in the groins. It is believed to be a manifestation of hyperinsulinemia due to insulin resistance. The drugs used locally are : tretinoin 0.025% cream; adapalene 0.1% gel; and calcipotriene 0.005% cream, ointment or gel (see earlier).

Sunscreens and Barrier Preparations

Solar UV radiation that can damage the skin is of three types according to wavelengths: UVA1, UVA2 and UVB. Of these, UVA forms 15% of the total radiation and is mainly responsible for photo-ageing and photo-toxicity. UVB is mostly absorbd in the epidermis and causes sunburn and tanning. UVA2 is also erythemogenic. Both UVA and UVB can damage the DNA, suppress immune mechanisms and can cause skin cancer in animals.

Skin can be protected from solar UV radiation by (1) **Inorganic** preparations such as zinc oxide, calamine and titanium dioxide which are opaque to all wavelengths of light and reflect them (**Reflectant sunscreens**); thus they are physical barriers; and (2) **Organic chemicals** that absorb UVA and UVB at the skin surface (**Absorbent sunscreens**). Examples are aminobenzoates, benzophosphophenones-3 (oxybenzone), methoxycinnamate (octinoxate), a salicylate (octisalate), octocrylone and a dibenzylmethane (avobenzene) (Table 69.9).

Table 69.9: Types of sunscreens

Inorganic (reflectant) sunscreens: UVB, UVA2/1
- Zinc oxide
- Calamine
- Titanium dioxide

Organic (absorbent) sunscreens

UVB
- PABA and PABA derivatives: Octyl dimethyl PABA (Padimat O)
- Cinnamates : Octyl methoxycinnamate, Cinoxate
- Salicylates : Octyl salycilates (Octisalate), Homosalate, Trolamine salycilates
- Octocrylene, Phenylbenzimidazole sulphonic acid (Ensulizole)

UVB, UVA1
- Benzophenones (Oxybenzone, Dioxy-benzone, Sulisobenzone)
- Terephthalydine dicamphor sulphonic acid (Ecamsule)

UVA1
- Butyl methoxydibenzoyl methane (Avobenzone)

UVA2
- Methyl anthranilate (Merdimate)

Since none of these agents give complete protection from solar UV radiation, they are usually combined to increase photostability and to broaden their spectrum. A newer agent, **ecamsule**, has broad protective spectrum.

Barrier preparations: They are used as water repellants to protect the skin against nappy rash. They contain a water repellant such as dimethicone along with zinc oxide. They are used as creams or ointments.

The skin can be protected from solar UV radiation by agents shown in Table 69.9.

Dihydroxyacetone (DHA), a pigment agent, is commonly used for sunless tanning. It binds to stratum corneum and changes the skin colour from white to orange-brown which lasts for 5-7 days.

Cosmetics, Tooth Powders and Dermal Fillers

Various preparations of cosmetic dusting powders contain mainly talc (native magnesium silicate with small amounts of aluminium silicate) which acts as an adsorbent and provides 'slip.' Another substance which also acts as an adsorbent and a mild antiseptic, added to such powders, is zinc stearate, a light, impalpable, amorphous powder. Zinc oxide is commonly used to cover the 'shine', while chalk acts as a colour carrier. However, starch is a better absorbent of moisture than the substances mentioned above. Addition of phenol, menthol and camphor exert a local antipruritic action. To these basic ingredients, various antiseptics like boric acid and salicylic acid may be added. *A powder containing salicylic acid 5g, boric acid 5 g, camphor 5g, starch 30g and talc to 100g can be easily and economically prepared at home.* The powder has absorbent, mild antiseptic and antipruritic properties; it may be applied to the axillae and the groins once or twice daily, with benefit. Application of such powders may cause blocking of the sweat gland pores and hence, after-cleansing is essential. Use of talc on surgical gloves is known to cause granulomatous reaction in wounds.

Baby powder generally contains zinc stearate and talc in the proportion of 1 to 2. There is no evidence that they are superior to good quality regular talc powder. In general, it is better to avoid such medicated powders in babies as they tend to form cake in skin fold causing dermatitis and may also get into the lungs. Similarly there appears to be no need for special 'baby soap' or 'baby oil'. Any non-perfumed quality soft soap and good quality usual oil (e.g. coconut oil) is adequate.

There is no evidence to suggest that medicated cosmetic powders are any better than non-medicated ones for routine use in individuals with healthy skin. Medicated powders are costly and liable to produce skin sensitisation.

Tooth powders contain simple chalk as the basic ingredient, with added white soap, saccharin, colour and flavour. Tooth paste, in addition, has water and glycerin. Various antiseptics and deodorants like clove oil, peppermint oil and lemon oil are added to these basic ingredients. Evidence suggests that non-medicated tooth pastes are as effective as medicated ones and possess the additional advantage of being cheaper and more acceptable. No toothpaste or powder can, however, act as a substitute for simple and repeated cleansing of mouth immediately after eating.

Shampoos are liquid soaps or detergents used to wash the hair and clean the scalp of scales or dandruff. They are expensive cleansers. Toilet soap can be used for the same purposes at a much lower cost. Shampoos are also used as vehicles for applying medicaments to the scalp. Medicated shampoos usually contain various antimicrobial agents such as selenilun sulphide, ketoconazole, povidone, cetrimide, coal tar and salicylic acid.

Most of the commercial cold creams are modifications of a popular emollient preparation, rose water ointment, which contains spermaceti (a waxy substance obtained from the head of the sperm whale), bleached bees wax, almond or prussic oil, rose water and rose oil. Such creams are useful for their soothing effect.

Various injectable **dermal fillers** are used for soft tissue augmentation of facial wrinkles and folds to give an young look. They are used in conjunction with botulinum toxin A. Majority of them consist of hyaluronic acid derived from bacteria or human/bovine collagen. Some contain a biodegradable synthetic polymer. They are used to remove facial wrinkles and lipoatrophy. Their effect lasts for 6-24 months. Usually, they are well tolerated; but sometimes may cause local bleeding, infection or skin discoloration; and rarely necrosis and nodule/granuloma formation. Prior skin testing for allergy is essential.

Anhidrotics and Deodorants

Sweating is common in the tropics and no drug should be used to block this normal physiological response. It could, however, become excessive (hyperhridrosis) particularly during stress. The eccrine sweat glands, although anatomically innervated by sympathetic nerves, are physiologically cholinergic. Anhidrotics (antiperspirants) are the drugs used for controlling hyperhidrosis. They are :

- ***Systemic anhidrotics***: e.g. anticholinergic agents such as belladonna alkaloids and synthetic substitutes like methantheline. These are discussed elsewhere. None of the available systemic anhidrotics, however, has a sufficiently predictable action without adverse effects.
- ***Local anhidrotics***: e.g. aluminium salts like aluminium chlorhydrate, formalin, glutaraldehyde and esters of hyoscine.

Aluminium chlorhydrate acts by local astringent action and blocks the sweat ducts at the skin surface. Formalin acts by forming

Table 69.10: Some dermatological reactions to drugs used systemically and topically

Skin reaction	Examples of implicated drugs
Urticaria	Penicillins, NSAID, sulfonamides, captopril, enalapril
Acne or aggravation of existing acne	Corticosteroids, androgenic and anabolic steroids, phenytoin, oral contraceptives containing androgenic progestogens, iodides, cytotoxic therapy, lithium, danazol, barbiturates, isoniazid
Exfoliative dermatitis	NSAID, sulfonamides, gold salts
Contact dermatitis	Topical antimicrobials like penicillin, chloramphenicol, neomycin; sulfonamides; topical antihitstaminics; cream and lotion preservatives; lanolin cosmetics
Purpura	Corticosteroids, anticoagulants, aspirin, barbiturates, thiazides, sulfonamides, sulfonylureas, cytotoxic drugs
Stevens Johnson syndrome	Sulfonamides, barbiturates, NSAID, phenytoin
SLE like reaction	Hydrallazine, procainamide, phenytoin, isoniazid
Fixed drug eruption	Phenolphthalein, barbiturates, aspirin, sulphonamides, quinine, tetracyclines
Photosensitivity	Tetracyclines (demeclocycline), phenothiazines, griseofulvin, nalidixic acid, sulphonamides, sulphonylureas, thiazides
Alopecia	Cytotoxic drugs, heparin, androgens, carbimazole, valproate, ethionamide, lithium, oral contraceptives, vitamin A (large doses), beta blockers, levodopa, thallium
Hirsutism	See Chapter 67

keratin plugs in the orifices of sweat ducts; its frequent use may cause allergic reactions. Glutaraldehyde is a tanning agent with antibacterial and deodorant activity. Anticholinergic drugs like propantheline bromide and esters of hyoscine are also effective when applied locally in the form of lotions.

Mild hyperhridrosis of the feet is easily managed by foot-baths with **potassium permanganate**, 1:10,000, and simple talcum powder. Individuals should be instructed to avoid nylon socks and rubber footwear and to use open sandals. Where an emotional factor is suspected, small doses of an anxiolytic agent may help.

Undesirable body odour results from the action of bacteria on the organic substances in the apocrine sweat. Excess eccrine sweat promotes this process by increasing wetness, which encourages bacterial growth. Anhidrotics, by virtue of their drying action, also act as deodorants. The other drugs used as deodorants are:

- ***Cleansers*** such as Sodium carbonate 20% in talc.
- ***Aluminium salts,*** e.g., Aluminium chloride hexahydrate.
- ***Antibacterials*** which retard bacterial decomposition of the apocrine sweat e.g. Hexachlorophane, Tetrachlorosalicylanilide, Trichlocarbon, Thiram and Bithionol; and
- ***Masking perfumes.***

Some of these agents can cause irritation, allergy, contact dermatitis and photosensitivity reactions.

It may be noted that there is a great demand for deodorants in today's society and it is estimated that an affluent country like the USA spends more than half a billion dollars a year on being 'nice to be near.' Most of us do not really smell as much as we are made to believe by the advertisers, and simple measures like personal cleanliness, shaving of axillae, daily bath with ordinary soft soap, and applying, if required, a simple adsorbent like talcum powder will provide similar good results as any expensive spray with much less risk of deodorant allergy.

Drug-Induced Skin Disorders

Adverse skin reactions to drugs are frequent in clinical practice (Table 69.10). The most common morphologic patterns are exanthematous reactions (rashes) and urticaria. Other relatively rare reactions are erythema multiforme, Stevens Johnson syndrome, exfoliative dermatitis and toxic epidermal necrolysis. A few of these reactions have an immunological basis.

Urticaria can be produced by allergic mechanism by several drugs such as ampicillin and antisera; and by drugs which liberate autocoids such as histamine. Urticaria can be dangerous if accompanied by angioedema of the larynx (Chapter 22).

The **photosensitivity** disorders of the skin can occur following topical as well systemic administration of drugs. They may be either phototoxic or photoallergic in nature. **Phototoxicity** is a nonimmunologic reaction, usually occurring as erythema that desquamates or 'peels' within several days; edema and vesicles may appear. **Photoallergy** is an immunologic cell mediated process and usually manifests as intensely pruritic, eczematous dermatitis, which later leads to local, thickened, 'leathery' changes in sun-exposed areas.

The treatment of drug-induced skin reactions includes:

- ***Stoppage of the offending agent.***
- ***Systemic antihistaminic therapy***; and
- ***Use of glucocorticoids and SC adrenaline*** in severe cases.

Exfoliative dermatitis, Stevens-Johnson syndrome, and allergic vasculitis are serious drug reactions and will need systemic glucocorticoid therapy. *With the first occurrence of an allergic drug reaction, the patient should be informed that he/she is allergic to the particular drug, so that its future administration may be avoided.*

Ocular Pharmacology

70

Eye problems are common in general practice and some of them, if neglected, can lead to blindness. The eye is readily accessible to observation, and the diagnosis of several eye diseases can be made easily. The drug treatment of eye problems is largely concerned with alleviation of inflammation, control of infection and reduction in intraocular pressure.

Anatomy and Physiology of the Eye: Figure 70.1 depicts the various parts of the eyeball. The human eyeball is composed of three concentric layers from without inwards: (a) the cornea and sclera; (b) the iris, ciliary body and choroid; and the lens; and (c) the retina.

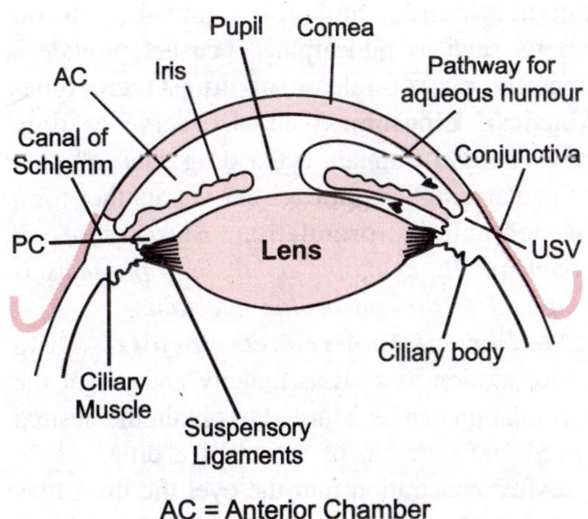

Fig. 70.1 : Anatomy of the eye and pathway for secretion and drainge of aqueous humour in the anterior chamber. USV = Uvea scleral vasculature

The **cornea** is an almost avascular, transparent structure which acts as an important barrier to foreign matter, including drugs. Drug absorption accross the cornea involves penetration through its multiple layers. The **sclera** is the outermost, dense, imperfectly elastic, opaque, supporting coat of the eyeball; its forward continuation is the cornea.

The **conjunctiva** is a modified mucous membrane that lines the outer surface of the anteriormost part of the sclera and the inner surface of the eyelids. The conjunctival epithelium is continuous with the corneal epithelium.

The **iris, ciliary body and choroid** form the uveal tract. The iris is a free, circular diaphragm hanging in front of the lens. The pupillary size is controlled by two types of muscle fibres: (1) *radial,* innervated by the sympathetic nerve fibres, causing dilatation of the pupil (mydiasis); and (2) *circular,* innervated by the parasympathetic nerve fibres, causing constrictioin of the pupil (miosis). The ciliary body is made up of unstriated muscle fibres (ciliary muscle) and epithelial cells; the latter secrete aqueous humor into the posterior chamber; that fluid passes through the pupil into the anterior chamber, and from there drains into the canal of Schlemm. When the ciliary muscle contracts, the zonules which suspend the lens relax, and the lens becomes more convex and is drawn slightly forward. This process is known as accommodation and allows focusing on near objects.

Pharmacokinetics of topically administered ocular drugs: Most drugs in ophthalmic practice are administered topically in the form of eye drops or ointments. The time-course of drug delivery from eye drops into the eyeball follows first order kinetics (Chapter 1). For majority of drugs, 1% or less of an applied dose is absorbed across the cornea to reach the anterior chamber. Table 70.1 summarises the factors affecting the penetration of ocular drugs. The classical pharmacokinetic theory based on systemic drug administration (Chapter 1) *does not apply fullly* to all ocular drugs.

Table 70.1: Factors influencing penetration of ocular drugs

- ***Drug-related:*** Chemical nature, lipid solubility, dissociation constant and route of administration.
- ***Vehicle-related:*** Chemical nature, physical state (liquid or solid) and viscocity; and
- ***Formulation-related:*** Drug concentration, osmolality, tonicity and pH

- ***Drug-related factors***: These are similar to those that govern the classical pharmacokinetics. Topically administered drugs can be absorbed through the cornea, conjunctiva and sclera. Drugs injected subconjunctivally and under the Tenon's capsule as well those injected into the retrobulbar space diffuse through the sclera and the cornea into the anterior and posterior chambers and into the vitreous humour. Systemically administered drugs have to cross the blood-eye barrier, which resembles the blood-brain barrier (Chapter 1), to enter the eye. Hence, drugs with large molecular size such as penicillin, administered systemically, penetrate the normal, uninflamed eye poorly but do so better if the drug is highly lipid-soluble e.g. chloramphenicol or if the eye is severely inflamed. Lipid soluble drugs pass readily through the corneal epithelium and endothelium, whereas the water soluble agents penetrate through the stroma. Therefore, drugs which have polar as well non-polar groups penetrate the cornea more freely than the purely polar or purely non-polar compounds.
- ***Vehicle and ocular drug delivery***: Most of the ophthalmic drugs are administered in aqueous solution. Since the aqueous solutions are liable to be carried away by the tears, their repeated administration is necessary to maintain their local concentration. Ointment bases act as reservoir for drugs, release them slowly and ensure higher penetration as well as prolonged action. Petrolatum and lanolin are viscous vehicles commonly used as bases in ophthalmic ointments. Other bases used to enhance drug penetration into the eye are a gel-forming base for timolol, and 0.5% hydroxycellulose for dorzolamide. Polymers are also used to increase the penetration of drugs; these are cellulose-ether, polyvinyl alcohol, carbopol, polyacrylamide, and poloxamer-407. Solid inserts such as pilocarpine **ocusert** provide a constant rate of release of drugs (zero order kinetics). **Liposomes** can also serve as drug reservoir and maintain better drug concentration of ocular drugs. **Applicaps** are yet another form of ophthalmic formulation. *Sterility of all commercially available ophithalmic products is essential to prevent ocular infection.*
- ***Formulation-related factors***: Drug concentration as well as tonicity and pH of the formulation can be adjusted to obtain the desired speed and duration of action of a drug.

After penetration into the eye, the drug may be washed out rapidly from the inflamed eye because of hyperemia. On the other hand, it may accumulate in an ocular tissue e.g. a-adrenergic receptor agonists bind to and accumulate in the melanin pigment in the iris. This has therapeutic and toxicological implications. Sometimes, the drug may be biotransformed locally into an active compound. Thus **dipivefrin** is a prodrug for adrenaline, and **lanatoprost** is a prodrug for $PGF_{2\alpha}$ The local toxicity may be due to either the active drug or some other ingredient such as the preservative in the formulation.

Since all ophthalmic medications are liable to be absorbed into the systemic circulation, they can cause systemic toxicity. This is particularly true of drugs reaching the nasal cavity through the nasolacrymal duct; it is more likely to happen with eye drops than with ointments. The final disposal of the ocular drugs may often take place after absorption into systemic circulation.

Systemic administration of drugs: Certain ocular disorders require systemic drug therapy e.g. carbonic anhydrase inhibitors in glaucoma; glucocorticoids in uveitis; and analgesics for ocular pain; antibiotics for deep ocular infections; and antihistaminics for ocular allergy.

General principles of local eye therapy: The selection of the drug(s) depends upon accurate diagnosis, although symptomatic treatment may at times be necessary.

I **Nonpharmacological modalities :** These include: eye rest; bed rest; proper lighting; protection from strong light, infection and trauma; hot or cold compresses; eye exercises; and nutritional management.

II **Pharmacological treatment :**

- Apart from the diagnosis, choice of the drug depends upon an assessment of the potential/actual threat to vision. Further, the presence of a local condition or a systemic disease that might worsen with the use of a particular drug should be looked for. For example, beta-adrenergic receptor blocker eye drops can aggravate bronchial asthma. Persons with a family history of open angle glaucoma are more likely to develop glaucoma during glucocorticoid therapy. For other problems with topical glucocorticoids, see later.
- The health-care-giver and the patient should observe hygienic and aseptic practices strictly while applying the medication to the eye.
- The ophthalmic formulation should be used as purchased and no attempt should be made to dilute it or otherwise modify it.
- The remnant after the patient gets well should not be stored for future use.
- Eye drops are convenient for ambulatory patients who are well enough to continue working. Their main disadvantage is their short duration of action and hence the necessity of frequent instillation. *Only one drop should be instilled into an eye at one time because that is the capacity of the conjunctival sac.* The patient should then lie down with the eye(s) closed. If a drop of another medication needs to be instilled at the same time, then 5 minutes should be allowed to elapse before adding the second drop. Ointments act as reservoir of the drug whose action is, therefore, prolonged. However, apart from being messy, they may cause blurring of vision.
- Associated conditions such as diabetes mellitus and hypertension should be treated.
- Systemic drug therapy may have to be employed in serious ocular conditions and in those which have failed to respond to topical drug therapy.
- Corneal ulcers and keratitis require specialist treatment.

Classification of drugs used in the eye :

I **Antimicrobials:** Antibacterials; Antivirals; Antifungals; Antiprotozoals.

II **Anti-inflammatory agents** such as NSAIDs.

III **Glucocorticoids.**

IV **Antihistaminics and mast cell stabilizers.**

V **Mydriatics and Miotics.**

VI **Drugs for glaucoma.**

VII **Immunomodulatory drugs** such as Immunosuppressives, VEGF antibodies and Antimitotic agents.

VIII **Local anaesthetics.**

IX **Diagnostic agents** such as Fluorescin and Rose bengal.; and

X **Miscellaneous drugs** such as Tear substitutes and Zinc preparations.

Antimicrobial Agents

Eye infections can be caused by bacteria, viruses, fungi and protozoa. Many antimicrobial agents are used topically. Drugs with limited solubility are administered as suspensions, whereas ointments are preferred when prolonged contact with medication is desired. The choice of the appropriate antibiotic depends on clinical diagnosis, the suspected infective agent and its predicted antibiotic sensitivity.

The common eye infections are blepharitis, hordeolum, acute conjunctivitis, infective corneal ulcers, ophthalmia neonatorum, and iridocyclitis. Table 70.2 lists the anti-infective preparations used in eye infections. All fluroquinolones are active against most Gram negative organisms associated with conjunctivitis. They are, however, not effective against MRSA. Trimethoprim has a broad spectrum of activity including against MRSA. Bacitracin and erythromycin are not effective against Gram-negative organisms.

Table 70.2: Anti-infective drugs used in the eye

Antibacterial :
Chloramphenicol 0.5% S, 1% O
Ciprofloxacin 0.3% S
Norfloxacin 0.3% S,O
Ofloxacin 0.3% S,O
Gatifloxacin 0.3% S,O
Erythromycin 0.5% O
Gentamicin / Tobramycin 0.3% S,O
Sulfacetamide 10 % S
Tetracycline 1% S
Combination :
Bacitracin + Polymyxin B
Trimethoprim + Polymyxin B
Antiviral :
Acyclovir 3% O; 400-800 tab
Ganciclovir
Foscarnet IV, Intravitreal
Idoxiuridine 0.1% S
Vidarabine 3% O
Trifluridine 1% S
Antifungal :
Amphoterecin B 0.1-0.5% S; 0.8-1.0 mg subconjun. ; 5 mcg intravitreal
Natamycin 5% S
Fluconazole oral
Ketoconazole oral
Miconazole 5-10 mg subconjuntival
S = Solution as eye drops. O = Ointment

Antibacterial agents:

Acute blepharitis may be caused by staphylococci or by parasites such as the head lice. Since eye drops do not penetrate well into the eyelids, ointments are the mainstay of treatment, accompanied by removal of the crusts. Staphylococcal infection is best treated with topical erythromycin or sulfacetamide. Recurrent disease may need additional treatment with a topical glucocorticoid. **Chronic blepharitis** is due to a combination of staphylococcal infection and seborrhea. It requires additional anti-seborrhoeic treatment (Chapter 69). Angular blepharitis is mainly caused by the gram-ve Morax Axenfield bacilli. It responds to the topical application of sulfacetamide, gentamicin or zinc sulfate. For allergic blepharitis, see later.

Hordeolum (stye) is staphylococcal infection of sebaceous glands of the eyelids and is usually self limiting. The treatment comprises hot moist compresses, removal of the eyelashes to facilitate the drainage and antibacterial ointments. Repeated styes possibly indicate uncorrected refractive error.

Acute conjunctivitis and **bacterial corneal ulcers** can be treated with one of the preparations shown in Table 70.2. The bacteria commonly encountered are staphylococci, streptococci, pneumococci and Hemophilus species. **Ophthalmia neonatorum**, caused by chlamydia, gonococci or other organisms, needs more aggressive treatment. Gonococcal illness needs systemic and local therapy (Chapter 51). Chlamydial infection (trachoma) is best treated with topical tetracycline or sulfacetamide *plus* oral erythromycin. Tetracycline or erythromycin ointment may be applied to the conjunctivae prophylactically in neonates at risk. For **herpetic ophthalmia neonatorum** see below.

Antiviral agents: The common viral infections of the eye are conjunctivitis, keratitis, iridocyclitis and retinitis. They are due to herpes simplex virus, herpes zoster virus and cytomegalovirus.

Table 70.2 lists the antiviral preparation commonly used in the eye.

Viral keratitis is either (a) epithelial which responds to topical treatment with antiviral dugs; or (b) stromal and requires administration of the same drugs orally. **Herpes zoster ophthalmicus** is more serious and needs systemic acyclovir in addition to local antiviral therapy. **Viral retinitis** requires prolonged treatment with antiviral drugs, by either intravitreal or IV route.

Antifungal agents: Fungal infections of the eye are rare.The important ones are keratitis, scleritis, endophthalmitis and canaliculitis. They are best left to the specialists. The antifungal agents commonly used in ocular fungal infections are shown in Table 70.2.

Antiprotozoal agents: The protozoa causing eye infections are *Toxoplasma gondii* and Acanthamoeba. Ocular toxoplasmosis is the ocular manifestation of a systemic infection (Chapter 56). Acanthamoeba causes deep eye infections which occur more commonly in contact lens users than in others. They require a combination of topical and systemic multi-drug therapy.

Oncocerciasis caused by *Onchocerca volvulus* is one of the major causes of blindness. Its treatment is described in Chapter 58.

Anti-inflammatory Drugs

The drugs belonging to this group are the NSAIDs such as **diclofenac** (0.1% eye drops), **flurbiprofen** (0.03% eye drops) and **ketorolac** (0.5% eye drops). They are commonly used topically during and following *ocular surgery* such as cataract extraction, for prevention of intraoperative miosis and postoperative inflammation (Chapter 11).

Glucocorticoids in the Eye

Topical glucocorticoids (Table 70.3) are used for treating anterior uveitis and for reducing postoperative inflammation following eye operations. Posterior uveitis needs to be treated with oral or parenteral glucocorticoids or with sub-Tenon's-capsular injections of a glucocorticoid. Optic neuritis is treated with parenteral administration, followed by tapering oral doses of glucocorticoids.

Table 70.3: Glucocorticoid ocular preparations

Preparation
Betamethasone 0.1% S, O
Dexamethasone 0.1% S, O
Hydrocortisone 1% S, 0.5% O
Prednisolone 1% S
S = Solution as eye drops. O = Ointment

The main ocular adverse effects of glucocorticoids are posterior subcapsular cataract (*steroid cataract*), open angle glaucoma (*steroid glaucoma*) and secondary infection. *Undiagnosed Red Eye may be due to Herpes simplex infection and glucocorticoids may aggrevate the condition, leading to corneal ulceration and loss vision. Routine use of a combination of a glucocorticoid with an anti-infective agent is not justified.*

Topical glucocorticoids are *contraindicated* in herpetic epithelial keratitis due to active viral replication, fungal disease of the eye, other viral diseases of the cornea and conjunctiva, ocular tuberculosis, hypersensitivity, and after removal of a superficial corneal foreign body.

Antihistaminics and Mast Cell Stabilisers

Allergic conjunctivitis can be treated with topical antihistaminics such as antazoline 0.05%, emedastine 0.05% and levocabastine 0.05%.

Mast cell stabilizers such as cromolyn sodium 4%, ketotifen 0.025%, nedocromil 2% and epinastin 0.05% can also be used to treat allergic and vernal conjunctivitis.

Mydriatics and Miotics

Mydriatics: These drugs produce pupillary dilatation.They are of two types:

- ***Muscarinic antagonists***, atropine and atropine substitutes, which also cause paralysis of the iris and ciliary body and lead to cycloplegia (paralysis of accommodation) by blocking the muscarinic receptors.

The main drawback of atropine is its long duration of action so that the cycloplegia lasts for 7-10 days. Atropine substitutes which have a shorter duration of action and produce minimal cycloplegia are preferred.

- ***α-Adrenergic Agonists*** (sympathomimetic agents) which directly stimulate the adrenergic receptors in the radial muscle fibres of the iris, and do not lead to cycloplegia.

Mydriasis is required for:

(1) Determination of refractive error.

(2) Fundoscopic examination of the eyes.

(3) Treatment of iridocyclitis, an inflammation of the iris and the ciliary body in which there is severe pain due to spasm of these muscles; atropine paralyses these muscles and relieves the pain; and

(4) Breaking the adhesions between the lens and the ciliary body, by alternating mydriatics with miotics.

Miotics: These are drugs which produce constriction of the pupils by acting as muscarinic agonists (pilocarpine), or as anticholinesterases (physostigmine) on the circular fibres of the iris. They also constrict the ciliary muscle, thus improving trabecular pathway. They are used in the treatment of glaucoma (see below). Their adverse effects include headache, browache, vascular congestion, conjunctival congestion, burning and blurred vision. Prolonged use may cause myopia and vitreous hemorrhage.

Miotics are contraindicated in acute iritis and acute uveitis. They should be avoided in acute inflammatory diseases of the anterior segment.

Table 70.4 lists the mydriatics and miotics in common use (Chapters 18, 19).

Table 70.4: Mydriatics and Miotics

Mydriatics
Antimuscarinic
Atropine 0.5-2% drops
Homatropine 2-5% drops
Eucatropine 2-5% drops
Cyclopentolate 0.5-2% drops
Tropicamide 0.5-2% drops
Sympathomimetic
Phenylephrine 0.12-10% drops
Miotics
Cholinomimetic
Pilocarpine 0.5% drops;ocusert
Cholinesterase inhibitors
Physostigmine 1% drops

Drug Therapy of Glaucoma

Glaucoma, the second most frequent cause of blindness in the world, is a disease of unknown origin. It is characterized by progressive degeneration of retinal ganglion cells and optic nerve fibers, and is usually accompanied by, but not always, increased intraocular pressure (IOP).

If untreated, it leads to optic neuropathy with loss of optic nerve tissue and excavation or 'cupping' of the ophthalmoscopically visible optic nerve head. This may be accompanied by loss of vision. *Most forms of glaucoma are painless initially and the loss of vision is insidious.* If diagnosed and treated early, most patients retain good vision. Reduction in IOP may protect against damage to the optic nerve head.

Glaucoma is classified into : (a) open angle, (b) closed angle, (c) congenital, and (d) drug induced. The condition may be either primary or secondary. The etiology of **primary glaucoma** is not known. The common causes of **secondary glaucoma** include inflammation, neovascularisation, pigment dispersion syndrome and drugs.

Fig. 70.1 shows the pathways for secretion and drainage of aqueous humour in the anterior chamber of the eye.

Elevated IOP may be reduced by:

- ***Increasing the outflow of aqueous humor*** through :

(1) The trabecular meshwork (cholinergic agonists and cholinesterase inhibitors),

(2) The uveoscleral pathway (PG analogues) or

(3) A surgically created pathway; and/or

- ***Decreasing the production of aqueous humor by the ciliary body*** (Table 70.5).

Drugs used in the treatment of glaucoma are classified in Table 70.5. *Before starting the treatment, drugs as a cause of increased IOP should be ruled out.*

In acute (narrow angle) congestive glaucoma, the iris probably blocks the entrance to the trabecular space at the canal of Schlemm. This blockade causes a precipitous increase in IOP and severe pain, nausea and often loss of vision due to optic atrophy. The reversible anticholinesterases are invaluable for reducing the increased IOP. The contraction of sphincter of iris induced by the anticholinesterases removes the iris blockade and facilitates the drainage of the intraocular fluid. Acute congestive glaucoma is a medical emergency and a combination of pilocarpine nitrate (4%), timolol and **aproclonidine** is the preferred treatment. Adjuvants such as acetazolamide (a carbonic anhydrase inhibitor) are also employed (Chapter 38). In an emergency, 20% mannitol (maximum 500 ml.) may be infused IV to lower the IOP. Once the acute attack is controlled, definitive surgery is advised. Even after surgery,

Table 70.5: Drugs used in glaucoma

I **Those which increase the outflow of aqueous humor**

- ***Cholinergic agonists (Miotics)***
  - * Pilocarpine drops 0.25-4.0% (Pilocar)
    Pilocarpine ocusert
- ***Cholinesterase inhibitors (Miotics)***
  - ** Physostigmine (Eserine) 0.25% ointment
    Demecarium (Humorsol) 0.125 - 0.25% drops.
  - ** Echothiophate 0.03-0.25% drops
- ***Prostaglandin analogues***
  Latanoprost 0.005% (Xalatan) drops
  Bimatoprast 0.03%
  Unoprostone 0.15 %

II **Those which decrease the production of aqueous humor by the ciliary body**

- ***Non selective beta adrenergic blocking agents***
  Timolol (Timoptic) 0.25-0.5 % drops
- ***Selective beta$_1$ adrenergic blocking agents***
  Betaxolol (Betoptic) 0.5% drops
- ***Non selective adrenergic agonists***
  Adrenaline hydrochloride 0.1 - 2.0 % drops
- ***Selective alpha$_2$ adrenergic agonists***
  Apraclonidine (Iopidine) 0.5-1% drops
  Brimonidine (Sephogan) 0.2% drops
- ***Carbonic anhydrase inhibitors***
  (a) Topical : Brinzolamide (Azopt) 1% suspension
  Dorzolamide (Trusopt) 2%
  (b) Systemic: Acetazolamide (Diamox) 250 mg qid; Methazolamide (Neptazane) 25 mg bid.

* = For details, see Chaper 16
** = Now used rarely
All eyedrops except PG analogues are generally used twice daily; PG analogues are used once daily in the evening.

continuation of drug therapy may be required.

Chronic (wide angle)simple glaucoma has an insidious onset and needs lifelong drug therapy. The cause of raised IOP is not known. Because the decline in vision is gradual, the diagnosis is often delayed. The mechanism of reduction of tension in chronic wide (open) angle glaucoma by drugs is not definitely understood as there is no physical obstruction in this condition.

The major goals of therapy are:

(1) To maintain an IOP below which further optic nerve damage is unlikely to occur (target IOP); (2) to reset the IOP to a lower level if deterioration occurs; (3) to minimise the local and systemic side effects of the drugs, and to improve the quality of life; (4) to educate the patient about his/her disease and emphasize the importance of compliance.

In general, the initial aim is to achieve a 20-50% reduction in the IOP at diagnosis, with the least amount of medication. The PG analogues eg. **latanoprost** are usually the drugs of choice to start with because of their once-a-day dosage, fewer systemic effects and good therapeutic efficacy. However, *they are very expensive*. Alternatively, a beta adrenergic blocker **timolol** may be used. The α_2 adrenergic agonists appear to be less effective than the above two. *Brimonidine should be avoided in children* for fear of respiratory arrest.

Topical carbonic anhydrase inhibitor preparations, **dorzolamide** and **brinzolamide**, cause less systemic toxicity and are preferred to oral acetazolamide. The latter is used in resistant cases in the dose of 0.25-1.0 g daily, in 3-4 divided doses.

Reversible anticholinesterases give fairly satisfactory results in glaucoma following cataract surgery. They avoided in patients with cataract because they may impair vision further; the long acting miotics may exacerbate cataract and increase the risk of complications (retinal detachment) during and after cataract surgery. *Sufficient transconjunctival absorption of anti-ChE drugs can occur following their repeated instillation and can cause systemic adverse effects.* Absorption can be minimised by digital compression of the inner canthus of the eye during and after instillation.

Pilocarpine is now less often used because of its short duration of action and ADR.

Beta adrenergic blockers may cause cardiovascular and respiratory adverse effects. PG agonists may cause increase in growth of eyelashes, irreversible darkening of the iris and rarely macular edema.

Finally, it is important to remember that lowering of IOP may not necessarily halt the progression of the disease and damage to the optic nerve in all cases of glaucoma.

Immunosuppressives and Antimitotic Drugs

Fluorouracil and mitomicin-C are used in ophthalmic practice (a) to limit scarring after certain types of surgical procedures; and (b) in certain systemic diseases such as

Wegner's granulomatosis and Behcet's disease with life threatening ocular manifestations.

The anti-VEGF monoclonal antibodies bevacizumab and ranizumab are used in the treatment of age-related, wet, macular degeneration (AMD) (off-label use).

Bevacizumab (Avastin) : This angiogenesis inhibitor (Chapter 59) has successfully prevented further loss of vision in many patients. It is administered *intravitreally*, once a month for three months initially, and then as required. It has become the treatment of choice in wet AMD. It is expensive.

Ranibizumab (Lucentis) : This derivative of bevacizumab, specially tailored for intraocular use, is also an angiogenesis inhibitor. It does the same thing as the parent drug in AMD, but at a very high cost. It is under evaluation.

Local Anaesthetics

These agents are used topically to anaesthetize the ocular surface :

(a) To remove foreign bodies from the cornea and conjunctiva.

(b) Prior to tonometry.

(c) For pre-operative preparation.

(d) In the manipulation of the nasolacrymal system.

Proparcaine and **tetracaine** are used in a, b and c.

(e) During the use of Eximer laser for surgery for refractive errors (tetracaine), and

(f) For infiltration and retrobulbar block anaesthesia (**lidocaine** and **bupivacaine;** Chapter 15).

Local anaesthetics should never be used for management of ocular pain.

Diagnostic Agents

The dyes fluorescein and rose Bengal are the most commonly used diagnostic agents for anterior and external lesions of the eye. Both are available as 2% alkaline solutions and as impregnated paper strips.

Fluorescein is preferred for detecting epithelial defects in the cornea and the conjunctiva, and leakage of aqueous humor that may occur after trauma or surgery. It is also used to test the patency of the nasolacrymal system.

Rose bengal stains devitalized tissue of the cornea and the conjunctiva, and helps to detect tears in those structures.

In the posterior segment of the eye, fluorescein and **indocyanine green** are used for retinal angiography. They may cause nausea and may precipitate severe allergic reactions.

Miscellaneous Agents

Wetting agents and **tear substitutes:** Many systemic and local diseases damage/disrupt the precorneal tear film, leading to 'dry eyes'. The discomfort may be relieved symptomatically by using either (a) artificial tears which are aqueous, hypotonic or isotonic solutions containing sodium chloride and hydroxymethyl cellulose; or (b) ophthalmic lubricants which are complex, viscous formulations, including ointments. Appropriate treatment of any systemic, causative disease is important.

Drug Induced Ocular Toxicity

Some drugs used in therapeutics (Table 70.6) can cause ocular toxicity as their adverse effects.

Table 70.6: Drugs causing ocular toxicity

Drug	Ocular toxicity
Ethambutol	Optic neuritis
Chloroquine	Retinopathy
Chlorpromazine	Retinal pigmentation
Chloramphenicol	Retinal pigmentation
Aminoglycosides	Optic neuritis
Sildenafil	Blue vision
Antimuscarinics	Glaucoma
Vigabatrine	Visual field constriction
Tamoxifen	Visual field constriction; cataract
Digoxin	Scotoma
Alendronate	Conjunctivitis; iritis

It must be remembered that the three major causes of blindness in developing countries are: vitamin A deficiency; trachoma and oncocerciasis, all of which are preventable. They are discussed elsewhere.

Section XV
Miscellaneous

Pharmacotherapy of Gout, Rheumatoid Arthritis and Osteoarthritis

71

The generic term gout is used for the microcrystal-induced acute or chronic arthritis or periarthritis. The important microcrystals identified include monosodium urate (MSU), calcium pyrophosphate dihydrate (CPPD), calcium hydroxyapatite (HA) and calcium oxalate. Inspite of differences in composition, the deposition of these crystals in the joints causes clinically indistinguishable arthropathies. The definitive diagnosis of the type of arthritis can only be made by aspiration-analysis of the synovial effusion for the type of microcrystals. They have similar clinical picture.

Monosodium urate gout is a metabolic disorder comprising:

- ***Arthritis due to a reaction to the deposition of urate crystals in the joint.*** It is acute, recurrent, monoarticular, at least in the initial years, and usually involves a peripheral joint in the lower limbs.
- ***Painless deposition of urate crystals in the soft tissues such as cartilage, bursae and tendons.***
- ***The development of 'tophi'*** in the latter after many years of recurring gouty arthritis; and
- ***Renal calculi and nephropathy***

The first episode of acute MSU gouty arthritis many times begins at night with dramatic joint pain and swelling which mimic cellulitis. Less commonly, the arthritis may be less severe and more indolent, and involve more than one joint at one time.

The diagnosis of MSU gout depends upon:

- ***A characteristic clinical arthritis.***
- ***Tophi***; and
- ***The presence of typical urate crystals*** in the joint fluid and the tophi.

The disease largely affects middle aged to elderly men and only 5-15% of women.

The incidence of gout rises with the serum uric acid level and the duration of hyperuricemia; however *hyperuricemia per se does not confirm or exclude the diagnosis of gout.* Hyperuricemia is necessary but not sufficient for the development of gout; only about 5% of patients with hyperuricemia, in fact, ever develop gout. Thus, other unknown factors are necessary forthe development of gout.

Hyperuricemia may be primary; or secondary to (a) renal impairment; (b) drugs (Table 71.3); or (c) massive lysis of cells during cancer chemotherapy.

Only about 10% of patients with primary gout overproduce urate; others have diminished fractional renal clearance of urate in spite of normal overall renal function. In lower primates, uric acid is oxidised by uricase to allantoin, a highly soluble substance. In humans who genetically lack uricase, urate which is less soluble circulates as such in the plasma. The plasma urate level rises with age.

Asymptomatic hyperuricemia upto 12 mg/dl does not warrant drug treatment. However, the *correction of reversible risk factors such as obesity, hyperlipidemia, excess alcohol consumption, high purine diet (meat and fish) and drugs known to cause hyperuricemia is wise.*

Table 71.1 outlines the principles of diet in prevention and treatment of hyperuricemia and gout.

Table 71.1: Diet in prevention and treatment of hyperuricemia and gout

- ***Avoid/minimise consumption*** of fatty meats (animal flesh and organ meats such as liver and kidney); fish; and fats.
- ***Consume regularly*** cereals; pulses; fruits; vegetables; nuts in moderation; and low fat milk and milk products.
- ***Purine-rich fruits, beans and legumes have not been shown to be a risk factor in gout.*** Consumption of eggs is not a risk factor but they have high cholesterol content. Tea, coffee and spices pose no risk. Salt and pickles are not a risk factor in gout but an excess salt consumption is a risk factor in hypertension, and in hypercalciuria ± renal calculi.
- ***Carbonated beverages may contain added phosphoric acid and their regular consumption may be a risk factor for calcium oxalate renal calculi.***

Patients with clinical MSU gout need drug therapy (Table 71.2).

Table 71.2: Drugs used in gout

I **To treat acute gouty arthritis**

Colchicine: Specific; slow acting; adverse effects.

NSAID (short acting such as ibuprofen and indomethacin) **:** Non-specific; rapid; better tolerated.

Corticosteroids : Effective intraarticularly and systemically; potential for rebound inflammation and adverse effects.

II **To prevent acute attacks :**

Colchicine : Effective in a dose adjusted not to cause diarrhoea.

NSAID : Less well tolerated for this purpose but may be used if colchicine alone is not sufficient to prevent frequent acute attacks.

III **To lower serum urate levels**

Probenecid: Well tolerated; interferes with excretion of many drugs; risk of urolithiasis. Uricosuria is reversed by salicylates.

Allopurinol: Inhibits uric acid synthesis; once a day dosage increases convenience; excretion impaired in renal insufficiency.

Sulfinpyrazone and benzbromarone are less commonly used drugs.

Drugs Used During Acute Stage

COLCHICINE is an alkaloid obtained from *Autumn crocus* (colchicum). It is a highly effective and specific for the treatment and prevention of acute gouty arthritis.

Mechanism of action: Sodium urate crystals in joints are coated by either anti-urate IgG antibody or lipoprotein containing apolipoprotein B and then ingested by granulocytes; the latter then release a glycoprotein which amplifies neutrophil infiltration into the joint. By binding to tubulin, colchicine damages the microtubules in the granulocytes and inhibits their migration into an inflamed area. It does not prevent phagocytosis of urate crystals but prevents the production or release of the glycoprotein by the granulocytes. Thus, it prevents the intra-articular release of mediators of inflammation by neutrophils.

Adverse reactions: Commonly, it produces GI upset and diarrhoea. Occasionally, it may cause anemia, alopecia, leucopenia and agranulocytosis. Prolonged therapy may rarely cause myopathy (proximal muscle weakness). Because of the troublesome diarrhoea, some workers prefer indomethacin to colchicine in the treatment of acute gouty arthritis.

Cimetidine and erythromycin reduce the metabolism of colchicine and therefore increase its toxicity. Colchicine is rapidly degraded by exposure to light and loses its therapeutic efficacy.

Therapeutic uses:

- ***Treatment of acute attacks of gouty arthritis*:** The drug is administered orally in doses of 1 mg., followed by 0.5 mg. every two hours until pain is relieved or diarrhoea starts. It relieves pain in most cases within 24-48 hours. If taken early in the attack, it can relieve the attack within a few hours or even abort it. The total amount of colchicine required generally varies between 4 to 8 mg. IV colchicine, though more reliable, can be more toxic, sometimes even lethal. Colchicine may be used for a therapeutic trial when the diagnosis of gouty arthritis is in doubt, because the response to colchicine is specific to gout. Once the nature of the acute attacks is established, indomethacin may be preferred in future attacks. As colchicine does not cause fluid retention, it is valuable in patients in heart failure. Further, it can be given to patients receiving anticoagulants.
- ***Prevention of acute attacks of gouty arthritis*** : Prophylactically administered in small doses of 0.5 mg. once or twice daily, it can reduce the frequency of attacks and hence, it can also be used in maintenance therapy along with uricosuric drugs. For chronic use in small doses, it is better tolerated than NSAID. Precipitation of an acute attack by a surgical procedure or by initiation of hypouricemic drug therapy can also be prevented by prophylactic colchicine therapy.
- ***Primary biliary cirrhosis*** : Colchicine (0.5 mg twice daily) 5 days a week has been reported to be useful in the treatment of primary biliary cirrhosis, wherein it prevents extracellular collagen deposition. It causes an improvement in the liver function tests but not in the clinical features.
- ***Prevention of attacks of familial Mediterranean fever*** (familial paroxysmal polyserositis.)

INDOMETHACIN: This NSAID, in the dose of 25-50 mg. tid for 5-7 days, can promptly relieve pain. However, the incidence of gastric intolerance is high. The drug can also be administered as 100 mg. suppositories. Ibuprofen is equally effective and less toxic (see Chapter 11).

GLUCOCORTICOIDS: Glucocorticoids can be used in very severe cases, refractory to colchicine and NSAID. Their action is not specific and the relapse rate is very high following the withdrawal. Prednisolone is given in the dose of 30-40 mg. on the first day and the dose is progressively reduced by 5-10 mg. every day. When a large joint such as the knee joint is affected, aspiration and intra-articular injection of hydrocortisone acetate may give dramatic relief.

Miscellaneous drugs: In severe cases with excruciating pain, an opioid analgesic such as pethidine 100 mg. IM may be necessary until pain is relieved by other agents. Addiction liability of such drugs, however, prevents their repeated use.

Drugs Used in Long Term Therapy of Gout

These drugs act by reducing the plasma urate levels. Although they do not prevent the acute attacks, they decrease the frequency of such attacks and may diminish the incidence of renal damage and other complications due to urate deposition. Reduction of plasma urate level to less than 6 mg% is required to prevent acute gouty arthritis and less than 5 mg% for reabsorption of tophi. The drugs are :

I **Uricosuric drugs;** and
II **Xanthine oxidase (Uric acid synthesis) inhibitors.**

Such therapy to reduce plasma urate level should be started only after the subsidence of acute joint inflammation as otherwise it may delay recovery from the acute attack. However, *pre-existing therapy with plasma urate lowering drugs should not be stopped in case of an acute attack.* If started in the interval between acute attacks, it should be preceded by prophylactic treatment with colchicine as otherwise, an acute attack of gouty arthritis may be precipitated. Such prophylactic doses of colchicine should be continued for one year after the plasma urate level has returned to the target level.

Correction of hyperuricemia by altering the lifestyle has already been discussed. Purine content of the diet contributes to at the most 1.0 mg% of the plasma urate concentration; nevertheless, reduction in excessive purine consumption is desirable. Table 71.1 lists foods which a patient with gout may avoid.

Indications for plasma urate lowering drugs: Drugs which lower the plasma urate level are indicated when *all* the following criteria are fulfilled:

- ***The cause of hyperuricemia cannot be corrected*** or such correction does not lower the plasma urate to less than 7 mg%.
- ***The patient has had at least two definite attacks of acute gouty arthritis or has tophi;***
- ***The patient agrees to take the medication regularly and lifelong;*** and
- ***Acute attacks with serum uric acid level of 9 mg% or higher.***

Uricosuric Drugs

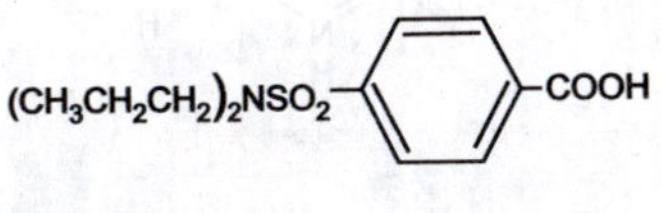

$(CH_3CH_2CH_2)_2NSO_2-C_6H_4-COOH$

Fig. 71.1 : Probenecid

PROBENECID (Benemid): This uricosuric agent is given orally, initially in doses of 0.5 g. once daily, gradually increasing to three times daily. *In low doses, it causes a decrease in distal tubular secretion of uric acid but in larger therapeutic doses, it increases its excretion, by blocking tubular reabsorption.* After treatment for some months, the serum uric acid may return to normal levels together with significant mobilization of gouty tophi.

Adverse reactions: The drug is relatively non-toxic and is well tolerated. Occasionally, it causes dyspepsia, skin rashes and deposition of urate crystals in the renal tubules/pelvis; this risk can be minimised by maintaining a high volume of alkaline urine (give 1g of sodium bicarbonate orally 3-4 times a day or 250 mg of acetazolamide at bed time daily). If the patient takes the drug intermittently, the risk of crystalluria recurs with each fresh starting of drug therapy. The drug inhibits the renal excretion of drugs such as penicillin, indomethacin and dapsone. It also impairs heparin metabolism thus reducing the dose of heparin necessary for anticoagulation.

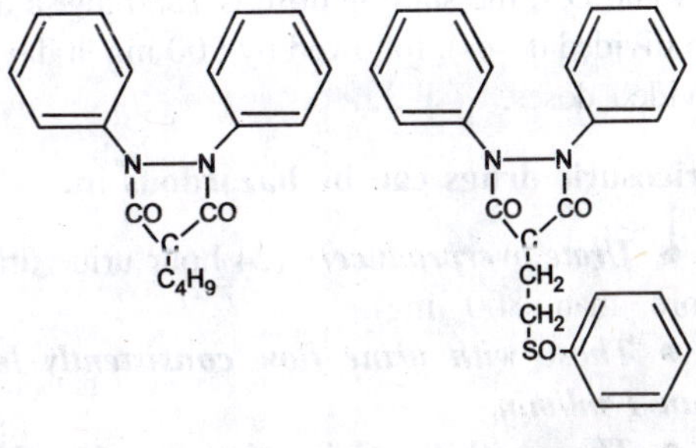

Fig. 71.2 : Phenylbutazone **Sulfhinpyrazone**

SULFINPYRAZONE (Anturan): This is a sulfoxide derivative of phenylbutazone with some anti-inflammatory activity but marked uricosuric property. It is administered orally in doses of 100-200 mg. thrice daily. The daily dose should not exceed 600 mg. In general, it is well tolerated.

The common toxicity includes vomiting, upper abdominal discomfort and skin rashes. Rarely, it can aggravate an existing peptic ulcer and may produce bone marrow depression. Sulfinpyrazone inhibits platelet aggregation.

Neither probenecid nor sulfinpyrazone is effective in the presence of impaired renal function. (creatinine clearance less than 50 ml/ minute).

Benzbromarone, a benzofuran compound, is another uricosuric drug. It is potent and is claimed to be effective even when the GFR is reduced to 25-50 % of normal.

AZAPROPAZONE (Apazone): It is a potent uricosuric agent and is useful for the treatment of acute gout. It has weak analgesic, antipyretic and antiflammatory actions; it is a weak inhibitor of cyclooxygenase. The drug is rapidly and almost completely absorbed from the gut and is well tolerated; the adverse reactions comprise mild GI effects and headache. The dose in acute gout is 600 mg. four times on the first day, followed by 1800 mg. a day in divided doses until the acute attack has subsided; the daily maintenance dose is 1200 mg. a day in divided doses. It has also been used for the treatment of RA and OA; the starting dose is 1200 mg. a day (in divided doses), followed by 900 mg. a day in divided doses.

Uricosuric drugs can be hazardous in:

- ***Urate overproducers*** (24 hour urine urate more than 800 mg).
- ***Those with urine flow consistently less than 1 ml/min.***
- ***Those with creatinine clearance less than 50 ml/min***; and
- ***Those with history of renal calculi.***

Aspirin, an analgesic, relieves joint pains (Chapter 11). Although it has a uricosuric action, the dose required for persistent uricosuria is large, which is unsuitable for the treatment of gout. In smaller doses aspirin acts as anti-uricosuric and also blocks the uricosuric effect of other drugs. *Salicylates, therefore, should be avoided in gout.*

Xanthine Oxidase Inhibitors

ALLOPURINOL (Zyloric): It is 4-hydroxy-pyrazolo 3, 4 d-pyrimidine and is a very useful long term agent in the management of gout.

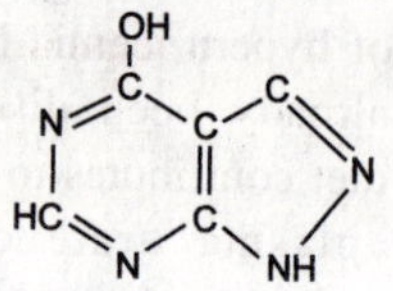

Fig. 71.3: Allopurinol

Mechanism of action: During purine metabolism, the purine nucleotides are degraded to hypoxanthine and xanthine. These purine bases are then oxidised to uric acid by the action of xanthine oxidase. Allopurinol and its degradation product alloxanthine, are potent inhibitors of xanthine oxidase (Fig. 71.4) and hence, they:

- ***Inhibit the oxidation of hypoxanthine and xanthine to uric acid.***
- ***Lower serum and urine uric acid;*** and
- ***Increase the excretion of hypoxanthine and xanthine in the urine.*** Both these oxypurine compounds are cleared rapidly by the kidney and

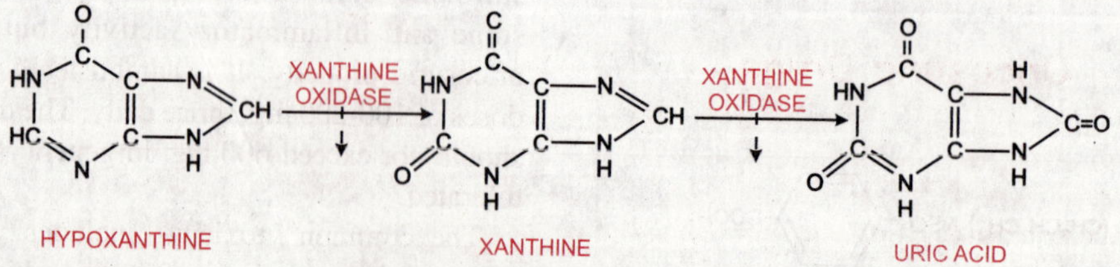

HYPOXANTHINE → XANTHINE OXIDASE → XANTHINE → XANTHINE OXIDASE → URIC ACID

Fig. 71.4 : Synthesis of uric acid

hence, there is less hazard of their crystallization in the kidneys. This is an advantage over uricosuric agents.

Adverse reactions: The incidence of adverse reactions is 15%-20%. The most common are allergic skin rash, nausea, vomiting, diarrhoea. Leucopenia and hepatic damage can occur. Haemosiderosis is a rare but serious complication. The other severe ADR are toxic epidermal necrolysis, bone marrow suppression and ototoxicity.

Preparation and dosage: It is supplied as 100 mg. tablets. It is *started in a dose of* 50-100 mg. per day and *increased gradually* in 2-3 weeks upto 300 to 600 mg. daily, in a single dose, as the half life of the active metabolite, oxypurinol, is about 20 hours. The dose of allopurinol should be reduced in the same proportion as GFR in chronic renal failure.

Therapeutic uses:

- ***Gout***: Allopurinol is used for controlling hyperuricemia in patients who produce large quantities of uric acid as shown by the urinary excretion of over 800 mg. per day. It is particularly useful in patients with gouty tophi or uric acid calculi and in those with renal failure which renders uricosuric drugs less effective. In contrast, uricosuric drugs are indicated in patients with hyperuricemia who excrete less than 800 mg. of uric acid per day but have normal renal function. Allopurinol may be combined with uricosuric drugs.

With the use of these agents in the treatment of MSU gout, rigid dietary control is rarely necessary though the control of risk factors, especially obesity, is essential.

- ***Secondary hyperuricemia***: This occurs following the use of cytotoxic drugs in the treatment of leukemia and lymphoma. Therefore, allopurinol is started before starting chemotherapy. Inhibition of xanthine oxidase which metabolises 6-mercaptopurine markedly prolongs its t½; hence its dose is reduced to 1/3 rd or ¼ th of the usual dose to avoid serious toxicity.

Febuxostat : This orally active, nonpurine analogue acts as an inhibtor of xanthine oxidase. It is well tolerated and can be used in patients allergic to or intolerant of allopuriol. The daily dose is 80-120 mg. It is mainly metabolized in the liver. Mild to moderate renal insufficiency does not alter its serum uric acid lowering ability. Its ADR include liver function abnormalities, headache and nausea.

Other measures in gout: With the uricosuric drugs used in between the attacks, a fluid intake sufficient to yield daily urinary output of at least 2 litres and the maintenance of a neutral or slightly alkaline urine pH are desirable to prevent any possible renal damage. This is particularly important during hot weather and in the tropics.

Drugs which can cause hyperuricemia are listed in Table 71.3.

Table 71.3: Drugs causing hyperuricemia

- Alcohol
- Thiazides, Bumetanide
- Cytotoxic drugs
- Amiloride, Ethacrynic acid
- Isotretinoin
- Ethambutol, Pyrazinamide
- Salicylates in low doses
- Cyclosporine
- Levodopa
- Niacin

Other crystal-induced arthropathies : Acute CPPD arthritis was formerly known as pseudogout because of its similarities with MSU gout. Definitive diagnosis needs synovial fluid analysis for the typical crystals. There is no effective therapy to remove the synovial deposits, and the treatment is symptomatic viz. NSAID, colchicine and intra-articular glucocorticoid injections.

The treatment of HA arthritis and calcium oxalate arthritis is also symptomatic.

Pharmacotherapy of Rheumatoid Arthritis (RA)

Rheumatoid arthritis (RA) is a chronic, systemic, inflammatory disease predominantly affecting joints, and periarticular tissues. Of all the rheumatoid disorders, RA still remains a formidable disease, being capable of producing severe crippling deformities and functional disabilities. The exact etiology of RA is still unknown although genetic susceptibility to RA has been demonstrated and infection as the initial trigger has been suspected.

Current evidence indicates that RA is an **autoimmune disease**. Autoantibodies to the FC portion of IgG antibody are produced by B lymphocytes in the blood and synovial tissues in 80% of RA patients. High titres of serum RA factor (RF), typically of the IgM isotype, is associated with more severe joint disease with extra-articular manifestations.

Pathophysiology of RA : Although *RA is classified as an autoimmune, inflammatory arthritis,* the disease comprises three basic interrelated pathological processes:

- ***Inflammation.***
- ***Synovial proliferation;*** and
- ***Joint tissue destruction.***

The focus of RA is the synovial lining. RA factor-containing immune-complexes found in the joints activate the pathological process. Tumour necrosis factor (TNF alpha), the product of macrophages, has been demonstrated to play an important role in the pathogenesis of RA. It exerts powerful effects on the immune system, including induction of pro-inflammatory mediators such as interleukin 1, nitric oxide, PGs, metalloproteases and adhesive molecules.

The earliest lesion is vasculitis, an inflammation of small blood vessels. The inflammation causes edema of the synovium and infiltration with mononuclear cells, macrophages, lymphocytes and plasma cells. There is intense local production of IgG by the plasma cells. The activated macrophages, lymphocytes and fibroblasts produce a variety of cytokines that promote further synovial proliferation and inflammation. Synovial fluid in RA contains PGs (mainly PGE_2), leukotriene B_4, TNF-alpha, interleukins and other cytokines. It is now believed that the monokines IL1 and IL6, and TNF alpha are the central mediators of active rheumatoid process.

Joint damage occurs early in the course of RA. The cartilage degranulation is now considered to be due to release of factor(s) capable of stimulating chondrocytes to degrade their own extracellular matrix. This factor from the synovial lining has characteristics similar to interleukin-1 (IL-1). Interleukin 1 has been shown to stimulate release of lytic enzymes and PGE_2 from chondrocyte monolayer and inhibit synthesis of proteoglycans by articular cartilage. Thus IL-1 could contribute to cartilage and bone destruction, and to the fibrosis.

Rheumatoid vasculitis, which can affect any organ system, is seen in patients with severe RA and high circulating levels of RA factor.

The principles of management of RA are given in Table 71.4.

Table 71.4: Principles of management of RA

- Rest to acutely inflamed joints.
- Relief of pain and stiffness.
- Reduction of inflammation by use of antiinflammatory drugs.
- Prevention of articular damage by use of drugs modifying the disease course (DMARD).
- Preservation of joint function and muscle strength: use of graded exercises, and physiotherapy.
- To treat comorbid conditions such as infections and osteoporosis; and
- Modification of the diet, using more omega-3 fatty acids in place of omega-9 fatty acids; in this respect, vegetarian diet may be beneficial.

Classification of drugs used in RA:

I **Antiinflammatory-analgesic drugs:** Aspirin and other NSAID (Chapter 11).

II **Antiinflammatory drugs with indirect analgesic action:** Glucocorticoids (Chapter 64).

These two groups act rapidly, relieve pain and control inflammation; they thus help to improve and maintain joint function and to prevent deformities. However, they do not halt the underlying destructive process in the joints.

III **Disease Modifying Antirheumatic Drugs, (DMARD):** They have no analgesic or immediate anti-inflammatory effect and begin to act after 6-12 weeks. They remain in the body for a long time and probably modulate immune function. They arrest the basic destructive process in the joints, modify the course of the disease, and hence the name. They may even induce remission e.g. Methotrexate, Sulfasalazine, Chloroquine, Penicillamine, Gold salts, and Leflunomide.

IV **Biological agents :**

(a) ***TNF-alpha blockers*** : Infliximab, Adalimumab and Etanercept.

(b) ***Interleukin-1 receptor antagonist*** – Anakinra.

(c) ***T cell activation inhibitors*** – Abatacept.

(d) ***Anti B-lymphocyte antibody*** – Rituximab.

V **Immunosuppressants:** Azathioprine and Cyclosporine. These may be life saving when vasculitis complicates the clinical picture and threatens life.

Although none of the drugs available at present can induce permanent remission, they are of great value in achieving symptomatic relief and functional improvement of the joints.

I **Anti-inflammatory analgesics:** Detailed pharmacology of NSAID is discussed in Chapter 11. These drugs act symptomatically, relieve pain, decrease the swelling and help to improve the joint movements. No NSAID is consistently more effective than any other, but some patients may not tolerate a particular drug. Aspirin still remains a useful drug; however in high doses in which it is effective, it causes GI adverse reactions. It is usually given in the dose of 3-5 g. daily to maintain therapeutic blood levels of 20 to 30 mg%. Enteric coated aspirin causes less gastric irritation and may be preferred. However, it should be avoided in the elderly. Aspirin and indomethacin can be given as rectal suppositories so as to avoid gastric irritation.

The NSAIDs used are ibuprofen (200-400 mg. thrice daily), diclofenac 75-100 mg twice daily, naproxen (250 mg. twice daily) and ketoprofen (50 mg. thrice daily), given with food. A single dose of naproxen 500 mg. taken at bedtime may also be effective. Ibuprofen is perhaps the best tolerated among the NSAIDs. Since piroxicam and diclofenac have prolonged action, a single dose at bed-time often may be effective for relieving the night pain and the early morning stiffness. (Chapter 11). However, both can cause severe gastric irritation.

II **Glucocorticoids:** These drugs have potent anti-inflammatory action; given orally, they produce dramatic symptomatic relief which lasts as long as they are used. In moderate to severe cases, prednisolone is started in the dose of 1 mg/kg/day, and then tapered gradually to a maintenance dose of 7.5 mg/day. The small maintenance dose is continued as needed, to minimise adverse effects.

Glucocorticoids are not used as monotherapy and low doses of prednisolone (5-10 mg/day) may be combined with DMARD. Larger doses are required to control severe systemic manifestations of RA such as pericarditis and vasculitis. *The newer synthetic 'supersteroids' do not offer any advantages over prednisolone.* Their major drawback is their toxicity; further, once glucocorticoids are started, few patients with RA are willing to discontinue them. (Chapter 64).

III **DMARDs:**

Gold salts: Water soluble gold preparations like **sodium aurothiomalate**, aurothiosulfate and aurothioglucose have been shown to produce some beneficial effect in RA. The drug gets deposited in synovial macrophages in actively inflamed joints and inhibits their function. They produce marginal but definite clinical improvement accompanied by lower titres in the RA test. Sodium aurothiomalate (Myocrisin) is the usually employed drug. It is given in the dose of 10-25 mg. IM weekly for prolonged periods or 50 mg. IM weekly for 20 injections.

Absorption, fate and excretion: Sodium aurothiomalate given IM is rapidly absorbed and gets distributed in the kidney, liver, spleen and other tissues including syncytial lining cells. The drug is excreted in urine, about 15-25 per cent being excreted during the first week. Gold salts are cumulative and the metal remains in the kidney for many years after injection.

Adverse reactions : Like other heavy metals, gold salts can cause various toxic manifestations. The important effects are dermatitis, nephropathy, oral ulceration, bone marrow depression and liver damage. The incidence of toxicity is fairly high and regular clinical and hematological supervision is mandatory. Gold toxicity is treated with prednisolone (10-20 mg. daily) and dimercaprol.

Auranofin, a gold compound, is effective orally. Though it is better tolerated and less toxic than the injectable gold salts, it is much less effective and is not commonly used.

Chloroquine and Hydroxychloroquine: These antimalarials produce moderate benefit in active RA. Chloroquine phosphate is administered in the dose of 250 mg. (maximum 4 mg/kg) daily. The improvement is usually seen after 3 months of therapy and prolonged treatment (6-12 months) is necessary for full benefit. *After good relief has been obtained, the frequency of administration of the same daily dose may be progressively reduced to once a week; but the drug may have to be continued in that dose perhaps indefinitely,* as the activity of the disease is likely to recur on stopping the drug. The dose of hydroxychloroquine sulfate is 400 mg/day; the maintenance dose is 200-400 mg (maximum of 6.5 mg/kg/day, not exceeding 400 mg/day); after good relief is obtained, the frequency of administration may be reduced in the same manner as with chloroquine. These drugs also have mild anti-inflammatory action and probably act as immunomodulators. They are taken up by macrophages and lymphocytes. They inhibit phagocytosis.

They are perhaps the best tolerated and relatively safe DMARD. Long term therapy may rarely cause retinopathy and irreversible visual impairment. It is advisable to carry out periodic ophthalmic examination during chloroquine therapy (Chapter 54).

d-Penicillamine: This is a sulphur containing amino acid used as a chelating agent (Chapter 72). Apart from chelation, it causes a split in the rheumatoid factor and also selectively reduces the serum levels of certain immunoglobulins. The drug induces some relief in the patients with RA. *Unfortunately, the incidence of adverse reactions is high, making the withdrawal of the drug necessary in 30 per cent of the patients.* It is now rarely used.

Methotrexate: This folic acid antagonist, given intermittently, appears to be highly effective and less toxic. The initial dose of methotrexate is usually 5-7.5 mg orally, taken as a single dose once a week. In these small doses, methotrexate has anti-inflammatory action but no immunosuppressant action. Clinical response is usually seen in 4-8 weeks. Its action is probably related to inhibition of aminoimidazole carboxamide (AICAR) transformylase and thymidylate synthetase, thereby preventing neutrophil chemotaxis (Chapter 59).

If no response is seen after 8 weeks of therapy, the dose may be increased by 2.5 mg every other week to a maximum of 15-20 mg once weekly and maintained until improvement occurs. After improvement sets in, it is given at the lowest effective dose indefinitely, as relapse occurs following discontinuation of therapy. The toxicity is dose-related. *In the dose recommended (7.5 mg or less per week), the drug appears to be well tolerated and risk of toxicity is small.* However, long term use is suspected to cause cirrhosis of the liver. Hence, most physicians would not prescribe methotrexate for patients with pre-existing liver disease nor to chronic alcoholics. Since methotrexate is teratogenic, it should not be used during pregnancy. Men should not take the drug for three months, and women for one menstrual cycle, before a planned pregnancy. It should also be avoided in patients with significant renal dysfunction. Folic acid supplements, 1-4 mg/day, may reduce the toxicity of methotrexate without impairing its beneficial effects in RA.

Sulfasalazine: This drug, used in the treatment of ulcerative colitis, is discussed in Chapter 44. It has been found to be useful and much safer than gold salts in the treatment of RA. The dose required (1-2 gm/ per day) is larger than that required to treat ulcerative colitis. With this dosage, adverse reactions are common and include nausea, vomiting and headache. Rarely, neutropenia, hemolytic anemia and thrombocytopenia may occur.

Leflunomide, a pyrimidine synthesis inhibitor, in short term studies, is as effective as sulfasalazine in decreasing signs and symptoms, and slowing the radiological progression of RA. After absorption, it is converted to its active metabolite which inhibits RNA synthesis and cell growth; it also prevents T cell proliferation. It remains in the body for a long time (up to 2 years). The advers effects are diarrhoea, reversible alopecia, skin rash and hepatic damage. Anaphylaxis and Stevens-Johnson syndrome have been reported. The drug is carcinogenic and teratogenic. Hence, it is advisable for a woman to postpone conception and for a man to postpone fathering a child for at least two years after stopping treatment. The dose is 100 mg daily for three days, followed by maintenance dose of 10-20 mg per day.

IV **Biological agents**

(a) **TNF-alpha blockers :**

INFLIXIMAB (Remicade): This is a chimeric, monoclonal anti TNF antibody that is 75% human protein and 25% mouse protein. The cytokine TNF alpha is actively produced at the synovial sites in RA. Infliximab binds to the TNF alpha with high affinity, avidity and specificity. Given by IV infusion it causes dose-dependent neutralisation of human TNF alpha. It is distributed mostly in the vascular compartment with a terminal half-life of 8-12 days. Being a protein, it is not metabolised by the hepatic cytochrome P450 enzymes. It can cause consistent and sustained benefit in patients with RA, even those who are resistant to DMARD, and methotrexate. The clinical improvement is associated with decrease in C reactive protein.

The antibody is well tolerated in the doses used. The most common adverse reactions are headache, nausea, rash and coughing. It may precipitate upper respiratory tract infection. The recipient can develop antibodies to infliximab.

Infliximab has been used in the treatment of Crohn's disease, psoriasis and aukylosing spondylitis.

ADALIMUMAB: This is a recombinant, human-anti-TNF monoclonal antibody. It is given SC and has t½ of 9-14 days. It has similar actions as infliximab.

ETANERCEPT: This is a dimer consisting of TNF receptor joined to Fc domain of human IgG molecule. Like infliximab, it binds to TNF alpha. In addition, it also binds to *the cytokine lymphotoxin alpha (TNF beta).* It is given SC 25 mg twice a week, whereas infliximab is given by IV infusion once in 2 months. The drug has been found to be useful in RA, including juvenile RA where infliximab is less effective.

The TNFα inhibitors should be avoided in the presence of infections, particularly tuberculosis and viral hepatitis, as well as in the presence of a demyelinating disease or CHF. Live virus vaccines are contraindicated in patients receiving a TNFα inhibitor.

(b) **Interlukin-1 receptor antagonist :**

ANAKINRA (Kineret) is recombinant human

IL-1 receptor antagonist and is given SC. It is used in combination with methotrexate in methotrexate-resistant cases. Close monitoring is required. The drug is under evaluation.

(c) **T cell activation inhibitors :**

ABATACEPT: This is a fusion protein of cytotoxic T-lymphocyte antigen-4 linked to IgG-1. It prevents T-cell activation and lowers the serum concentration of inflammatory cytokines in RA. It is given IV, slowly, on day one and repeated at two and four weeks thereafter. Its mean t ½ is 13 days. It appears to be well tolerated and has been used to treat RA not responding to DMARDs. Abatacept can be combined with DMARDs but not with TNFá inhibitors or anakinra. The patient should be tested for tuberculosis before starting the treatment, and should be watched for any infection. The drug needs long term evaluation.

(d) **Anti–B–lymphocytic antibody :**

RITUXIMAB is a monoclonal antibody which selectively depletes the CD20+ B-lymphocytes which play a role in the autoimmune response and in the chronic synovitis associated with RA. It is claimed to be useful in RA which has proved resistant to TNFα blockers.

V **Immunosuppressive agents** (Chapter 76): Various alkylating agents like azathioprine, cyclosporine, cyclophosphamide have been used to induce remission in RA. This is because RA is an autoimmune disease and these drugs act as suppressors of B and T lymphocytes. However, all these agents are toxic.

Choice of drug therapy: Patients with confirmed diagnosis of RA have a lifelong disease which persists, spreads and causes damage throughout its course. Although the inflammation associated with it may be reversible, the cytokine-induced damage is not. Bone loss has been shown to occur rapidly at the onset of the clinical disease. Unfortunately, the prediction of which patients will have a rapidly downhill course and which will not is as yet not possible. The current goals of therapy of RA are to arrest the disease progression or at least induce and maintain a long-lasting remission. There is now convincing evidence that *early treatment with DMARD has the potential to improve the quality of life and long term outcome in patients with RA.*

In all cases aspirin/NSAID in adequate doses should be given initially for quick symptomatic relief. However, these drugs do not cause a change in the cytokine-mediated acute phase reactants such as ESR and C reactive protein. The current recommendation for optimum treatment is to start the treatment in new cases with a *combination* of an NSAID and a DMARD (methotrexate, hydroxychloroquine or sulfasalazine) in order to achieve quick relief of symptoms and remission of the disease process. Such combination treatment has been shown to delay bone damage. In severe cases, a glucocorticoid, in large initial doses, may be added at the onset, and then tapered to a maintenance dose.

Methotrexate and sulfasalazine in the recommended doses appear to be relatively safe, whereas gold salts are more toxic and difficult to handle.

Although there is no definite evidence pointing to any particular DMARD as the drug of first choice, *weekly methotrexate is currently favoured because of its relatively rapid onset of action, long term benefit, acceptable toxicity and low cost.* The maximum improvement usually occurs after 6 months of therapy. The drug may be supplemented by folic acid which may counter some of its toxicity without compromising its efficacy. Patients who do not respond to one DMARD may respond to another or to a combination of DMARDs — methotrexate, sulfasalazine and hydroxy-chloroquine.

The TNFα inhibitors appear to be superior to methotrexate and other DMARDs in halting the joint destruction; but their long term safety is not clear. Hence, they should be used only in RA resistant to conventional DMARDs. They are also expensive. The combination of TNFα with anakinra or abatacept is not recommended as that increases the risk of serious infections.

Local intra-articular injection of a glucocorticoid is useful in controlling inflammation. Indications for local glucocorticoid therapy are:

- ***One or two joints that are 'resistant' in the patient, otherwise well controlled on medical therapy;*** and
- ***Patients with one active joint in whom oral NSAID are contraindicated.***

Usually, hydrocortisone acetate suspension is given in the dose of 25-50 mg. for big joints and 5-10 mg. for small joints. The number of injections depends upon the response; but it is advisable to avoid injection into a joint more often than once in 3 months. The drug may also be injected extra-articularly into painful ligaments, tendons and inflamed bursae with beneficial results. The duration of relief obtained varies from a few days to a few weeks.

Supportive therapy: Rheumatoid arthritis being a chronic disease, general supportive therapy including good nutrition and attention to psychological aspect is as important as drug therapy. Both physical and mental rest is essential. During the acute stage the rest must be complete, along with proper splinting of affected joints. A firm mattress with only one firm, low pillow should be allowed at bed-time. Antianxiety and antidepressant drugs may be necessary along with analgesics to control anxiety and insomnia. In most patients with active disease, bed rest for 4 weeks followed by 2-6 weeks of planned rehabilitation is advisable. Immobilization of inflamed joints is carried out for 4 weeks followed by active exercises. Light exercises should also be prescribed during complete rest, to be carried out in the recumbent position for improving circulation and correcting faulty posture. *Proper exercises and physiotherapy during the recovery stage are essential for achieving maximum benefit.*

Use of warm baths and hot packs helps to loosen joints and relieve the stiffness. Exercise following heat helps to maintain the mobility of joints. Although definite infection such as tuberculosis must be treated promptly, removal of "suspected teeth or tonsils" will not help; on the contrary, removal of teeth will affect the nutrition and the mental get up of the patient.

Anemia may respond to iron therapy. Other co-morbid states such as osteoporosis and CV disorders should be treated. Patients may also need help to combat the serious social and economic problems that are usually associated with such a chronic and disabling ailment.

Since the definitions of terms 'active disease', 'improvement' and 'remission' are imprecise, caution is advocated before accepting any new remedy claimed to 'benefit many patients' RA.

Osteoarthritis (OA)

Osteoarthritis is a common disease in the ageing population and results from a complex interplay of genetic, metabolic, biochemical and biomechanical factors with secondary local inflammation. The process involves the interaction of degradation and repair of the articular cartilage, bone and synovium. The most important cells in the entire disease process are the chondrocytes.

The initiating event in OA seems to be injury to the chondrocytes from a single macrotrauma or repeated microtraumas to the joint. The chondrocytes react by proliferation and release of enzymes which degrade the articular cartilage. The products of degradation, released into the synovial fluid, evoke the formation and release of mediators of inflammation by the synovial macrophages; the latter cause further damage to the cartilage. The cartilage also responds by misplaced attempts at repair with the formation of osteophytes at the edge of the cartilage.

OA is not an invariable and natural accompaniment of ageing; several other risk factors are involved in its pathogenesis e.g. obesity, lack of exercise, and occupational as well as sports trauma to the joints.

Early OA may be clinically silent. The important symptoms, when they occur, are pain, tenderness, movement limitation, disability and deformity. Muscle wasting is common and contributes to the disease process. Acute effusion occurs in large joints such as the knee in response to acute trauma. Unlike in RA, there are generally no systemic symptoms, and blood indicators of inflammation such as elevated ESR are generally absent. In most patients, the disease stabilizes after initial progression.

Management: *No treatment available at present can halt the degradation of the cartilage or stimulate its fresh synthesis nor reverse the pathological changes of OA.* All treatment is aimed at (a) pain relief; and (b) increasing the range of joint mobility.

I **Non-pharmacological treatment:** This includes physical therapy (heat, cold and transcutaneous electrical nerve stimulation); and exercise. Proper posture and weight reduction are important. Intermittent rest during the day, use of a walking stick and properly cushioned shoes are helpful; a properly fitting brace can relieve backache.

II **Pharmacological treatment:** Local application of methylsalicylate ointment containing additional capsaicin may bring relief in mild cases. When oral therapy is required, preference should be given to paracetamol in the dose of 2-3 g/day in divided doses; this relieves the pain in most patients. A mild NSAID such as ibuprofen may be added to paracetamol in the presence of joint stiffness or swelling, or pain which interferes with work or sleep. Stronger NSAID should be avoided. This is especially important in the elderly who are particularly liable to the adverse effects of NSAID; they should be prescribed in the smallest possible dose for the shortest possible period. COX-2 inhibitors are being promoted as 'stomach-friendly' but they can cause cardiovascular adverse effects. (Chapter 11). Their routine use in all patients is not recommended.

The use of intra-articular glucocorticoids at three monthly intervals should be limited to patients with severe pain, especially with an effusion. Intra-articular injection of hyaluronic acid has been claimed to relieve pain. *Systemic glucocorticoids have no place in the treatment of OA.*

Glucosamine (Rejoint) is derived from marine shells or is synthetic. It is the sulfate or hydrochloride of aminomonosaccharide glucosamine, a normal constituent of glycosaminoglycan in the cartilage. Given orally in the dose of 1500 mg daily in divided doses for long periods (2-3 years), it is claimed to slow down the progression of OA. However, the current evidence about the usefulness of glucosamine and **chondroitin sulfate,** given individually or in combination, for the treatment of knee pain, is equivocal.

There is no evidence at present that these supplements prevent OA in healthy persons or in patients with knee pain but normal X'rays. The drugs are well tolerated. Their usefulness as a DMARD in OA and their long term safety evaluation need confirmation.

Surgical treatment: Joint replacement can help patients with advanced OA and unbearable pain.

Metals and Their Antagonists 72

The heavy metals are of great interest mainly from the toxicological point of view. It is, therefore, proposed to discuss briefly their toxicity and its treatment.

Pharmacological actions: The organic and the inorganic salts of heavy metals possess astringent, corrosive and caustic properties on local application. They also act as general protoplasmic poisons, interfering with various enzymes and altering cell membranes, thus impairing cell function. The heavy metal salts, in very small quantities, are lethal to several Gram-positive and Gram-negative organisms.

Heavy metals exert their toxic effects by combining with one or more reacting groups such as the SH groups, essential for normal physiological functions. The heavy metal antagonists (chelating agents) compete with these groups for the metals and spare the former; they prevent or reverse the toxic effects and enhance the excretion of the metals.

Adverse reactions: All the heavy metals are cumulative and potentially toxic. They cause damage to various organs like the liver, the kidney and the gut. Rapidly proliferating tissues such as the bone marrow, the gastrointestinal mucosa and other delicate cells such as neurons and renal tubular cells are also affected.

The **major treatment** of metal toxicity is to prevent or terminate exposure to them. Chelating agents are used to bind metals into stable cyclic compounds of low toxicity (see later). **Activated charcoal does not bind metals** and hence is not useful in acute metal poisoning.

Many herbomineral products available over the counter (OTC) may contribute to heavy metal toxicity.

ARSENIC: Arsenic, though ordinarily presumed to be a metal, is in fact a metalloid. Very minute quantities of arsenic have been detected in majority of the vertebrates. The physiological role of such minute amounts is, however, not known. It is a notorious poison since ancient times. Arsenical compounds can be divided into:

- ***Inorganic arsenicals***, used mainly as rodenticides, herbicides and insecticides and
- ***Organic arsenicals***, used in the chemotherapy of trypanosomiasis. They were once mainstay of treatment of syphilis.

The organic arsenicals can be further subdivided into trivalent and pentavalent compounds. The pentavalent compounds, which are anionic in character in body fluids, probably penetrate the host cells less readily than the trivalent compounds and consequently, have a higher therapeutic index than the latter. Although it is claimed that the therapeutic activity of pentavalent compounds is partly due to their reduction into trivalent forms *in vivo*, trivalent compounds as such are not used in therapeutics because of their high toxicity. Recently, arsenic trioxide has been introduced for the treatment of acute myeloblastic leukemia.

Absorption, fate and excretion: Soluble arsenical salts are rapidly absorbed from the gut. Absorption also occurs through the skin. Arsenic is stored mainly in the gut, liver, spleen, kidney and lung, small amounts are also present in the brain and the skeletal muscle. It also accumulates in bones and hair. Arsenic is mainly excreted in urine and feces. Urinary excretion usually starts within 2 to 8 hours after oral administration and continues for 8 to 10 days. Cumulative poisoning can thus occur on repeated ingestion of small amounts. Small amounts also appear in sweat and in saliva. Arsenic deposited in hair and bones is retained for years.

Arsenic poisoning: Arsenic poisoning is usually homicidal but occasionally, may occur accidentally, particularly in children, following ingestion of arsenical herbicides or insecticides. Ground water in some areas of the world (parts of West Bengal in India) contains high concentrations of arsenic, and is responsible for chronic poisoning.

- ***Acute arsenical poisoning*** is characterised by severe GI irritation, vomiting, diarrhoea, circulatory collapse and renal failure. The GI symptoms usually begin within 1 hour after ingestion of the arsenical compound but may occasionally be delayed upto 12 hours. The symptomatology closely resembles that seen in cholera and a careful distinction is essential before institution of treatment. In severe poisoning, death may occur within 24 hours.

Treatment consists of correction of fluid and electrolyte imbalance and administration of the specific antidote, dimercaprol. Prophylactic antibiotic therapy is advocated to prevent secondary infection. Hemodialysis may be necessary in the event of renal shutdown.

- ***Chronic arsenic poisoning***: Chronic arsenic poisoning has a relatively insidious onset and this is the main reason for its use as a poison for homicidal purposes. The early symptoms are weight loss, anorexia, fatigue and diarrhoea or constipation. Later manifestations are edema, particularly of eyelids and ankles, hyperpigmentation of the skin, especially the eyelids, neck, nipples and the axillae, and dermatitis including exfoliative, and inflammatory lesions of the mucous membranes. There may be loss of hair; finger nails become brittle and may eventually drop off. The breath has a garlic odour. Late manifestations of arsenic poisoning include jaundice, aplastic anemia and peripheral neuropathy leading to numbness, paraesthesiae, wrist and foot drop. Necrosis and degeneration of renal tubules and liver cirrhosis may develop. Arsenical encephalopathy has also been reported. Hyperkeratosis of palms and soles may undergo malignant change in the form of basal cell carcinoma. Chemical analysis of hair and bones is often helpful in establishing the diagnosis.

Treatment of chronic arsenic poisoning consists of prolonged administration of dimercaprol. (see later). However, arsenical aplastic anemia and jaundice usually do not respond, while arsenical encephalopathy is relieved only partially even if the therapy is instituted promptly.

Preparations: The organic arsenical compounds used in the therapeutics are discussed in Chapters 55 and 56.

LEAD: Lead compounds have hardly any therapeutic use. They are, however, used in various industries such as paint and plumbing fixtures and are responsible for causing chronic lead poisoning in workers. Poisoning may also occur from lead projectiles, particularly lead shots embedded in the skin or the muscle.

Absorption, fate and excretion: Children absorb upto 50% of the ingested lead whereas adults absorb about 10-20%. Diets poor in calcium, iron and zinc promote its absorption. It can also be absorbed from the respiratory mucous membrane. Respiratory absorption of lead is more dangerous than its GI absorption where the liver acts as a barrier. Organic lead compounds like tetraethyl and tetramethyl lead are absorbed more rapidly by the respiratory mucosa than the inorganic compounds. In addition, they can also be absorbed from the unbroken skin.

Following absorption, inorganic lead is mainly associated with erythrocytes. High concentrations are initially present in liver and kidneys. Subsequently, it is mobilised from these sites and deposited in bones in the form of insoluble tertiary lead phosphate, mainly in epiphyseal regions of growing long bones, where it can be detected radiologically. High phosphate intake and vitamin D favour the deposition of lead into bones whereas a high calcium and low phosphate intake, parathyroid hormone, dihydrotachysterol and iodides cause mobilization of lead from the bones. Lead deposited in bones does not contribute to the toxicity. A small amount is also present in hair, nails, sweat and excrement. The t½ of lead is 25 days in the blood, 40 days in soft tissues and more than 25 years in the non-labile bone.

Lead deposited in soft tissues and in bones is excreted very slowly mainly by the kidneys, within a few weeks to years. A small amount is present in milk and sweat.

Toxicity of lead is due to its affinity for the cell membrane and mitochondria. It impairs the activity of calcium-dependent intracellular messengers and of brain protein kinases.

Lead poisoning can be acute or chronic.

- ***Acute lead poisoning*:** Acute lead poisoning is a rare entity, usually secondary to ingestion of soluble lead compounds like lead acetate. It is characterised by a metallic taste in mouth, GI irritation and occasionally, acute nervous system symptoms like paraesthesiae, muscle cramps and weakness. The stools have a dark colour owing to the presence of lead sulfide. An acute hemolytic crisis resulting in severe anemia and hemoglobinuria may occur and usually proves fatal.

Treatment of acute lead poisoning consists of prompt gastric lavage and administration of laxatives like magnesium sulfate to hasten the evacuation of lead from the gut and use of calcium and phosphate salts and chelating agents for its elimination from the circulation. Anticholinergics like atropine are used to relieve the intestinal colic while parenteral fluids and vasopressor agents are employed to treat the shock, and diazepam for seizures.

- ***Chronic lead poisoning*:** Chronic lead poisoning is commonly seen in young children from sucking lead paint or lead toys, in workers engaged in printing and paint industries, and in petroleum industry where organic lead compounds like tetraethyl lead and tetramethyl lead are added to petrol as anti-knock remedies. The manifestations of chronic poisoning are:

Gastrointestinal tract: The commonest symptoms are a persistent metallic taste in mouth, anorexia, constipation and abdominal pain due to intestinal colic, termed 'lead colic'. Chronic constipation due to lead poisoning is often ignored and itself enhances the absorption of lead from the GI tract. A diagnostic feature of importance is the grayish *lead line* which appears along the gingival margin and is due to periodontal deposition of lead sulfide; this may not be seen in the presence of good dental hygiene.

Skeletal muscles: Muscle weakness and increased fatiguability leading subsequently to paralysis is described as 'lead palsy'. The paralysis may cause unilateral wrist drop, and less commonly, foot drop. The extraocular muscles are also occasionally involved. Long standing paralysis may produce atrophy or contractures. Degenerative changes in the motor-neurones and their axons, and impairment of high energy phosphate metabolism of the affected muscles have been incriminated.

Haemopoietic system: Punctate basophilic stippling of erythrocytes is regarded as a cardinal manifestation of chronic lead poisoning. However, that stippling upto a limit of 800 to 1000 per million erythrocytes is physiological and it is only when this count exceeds 35,000 per million erythrocytes that the suspicion of lead poisoning should be entertained. Further, absence of stippling does not rule out lead intoxication.

Other hemopoietic disturbances are a microcytic hypochromic anemia, jaundice secondary to increased hemolysis, and excretion of abnormal products of porphyrin metabolism in urine, which is attributed to defective hemoglobin synthesis.

Central nervous system: Central nervous system toxicity is commoner in children than in adults and is described as **lead encephalopathy**. It is manifested by increased irritability, headache, restlessness and tremors, followed by delirium and convulsions or by lethargy and coma. Visual disturbances may occur and stippling of the retina adjacent to the optic disc is claimed to be an early diagnostic sign. Lead encephalopathy has a mortality of 25 per cent and nearly 1/4th of the survivors develop permanent mental deficiency.

Organic lead compounds produce acute CNS toxicity in adults, with similar manifestations.

Kidney: It may cause interstitial nephritis, tubular damage, hyperuricemia and renal failure.

Treatment : The drug of choice in chronic lead poisoning is the chelating agent, **calcium disodium edetate** (see later). Dimercaptosuccinic acid (Succimer) is a chelating agent useful in lead poisoning. Less useful agents are penicillamine and dimercaprol. A combination of dimercprol and calcium disordium edetate is claimed to be more efficious. Lead colic can be controlled by the administration of antispasmodics and calcium gluconate 2 g. I.V. Convulsions are best treated with diazepam. Increased intracranial tension can be relieved by mannitol or by lumbar puncture.

ANTIMONY: This metal resembles arsenic in chemical and biological properties. Antimony, however, is more irritant locally and certain antimony salts like antimony potassium tartrate possess a powerful emetic activity.

The trivalent and pentavalent compounds are absorbed slowly from the gut. The trivalent compounds are more firmly bound to erythrocytes than pentavalent compounds and exhibit slower renal excretion than the latter.

The toxic effects of antimonials resemble those of arsenic. Dimercaprol is protective against the toxic effect of organic forms but its efficacy against the inorganic antimony compounds is doubtful. (For uses, see Chapters 55 and 58).

BISMUTH: Compounds such as carbonate, subsalicylate, subgallate and subnitrate are used to treat diarrhoea because of their mild astringent and mechanical coating effects. Bismuth subgallate is used orally to control fecal odour in an ileostomy. Bismuth subsalicylate is used to treat *H.pylori* infections in patients with peptic ulcer disease (Chapter 42).

Intoxication due to bismuth is rare. Chronic poisoning may lead to fever, GI disturbances, stomatitis, urticaria, nephritis and nephrosis. A metal line on the gums is often seen. Dimercaprol is an effective antidote.

MERCURY: The mercury compounds are sometimes used as antiseptics, preservatives, and spermicides and in industry. Organic mercurials are lipid soluble and readily cross the blood brain barrier and the placenta. They accumulate in the kidney and the brain, and their t½ is almost 70 days. Fish, particularly tuna and sword-fish, can concentrate large amounts of methyl mercury.

- ***Acute mercury poisoning*** is usually due to accidental ingestion of mercuric chloride (corrosive sublimate) and other readily ionizable mercury salts. It is characterised by severe GI irritation, diarrhoea, electrolyte disturbances and circulatory collapse. The patient complains of a metallic taste in mouth; there is excessive salivation and inflammation of gums. Arrhythmias may develop due to its toxic effect on the myocardium. Marked renal impairment leading to death occurs due to its nephrotoxic action. Secretion of mercuric ion into the gut and its reabsorption prolong the toxic effects.

Treatment is directed towards removal of mercuric ions from the GI tract and towards its quick renal elimination. The former is achieved by administration of proteins in the form of raw eggs or milk, which form non-toxic proteinates and by giving medicinal charcoal in suspension. This is followed by gastric lavage, though it is of doubtful value after the first 15 minutes or so, since mercury is rapidly absorbed by the mucous membrane of the alimentary tract. Sodium formaldehyde sulfoxylate which reduces the mercuric ion to the less soluble mercurous form may also be used. About 200 to 250 ml of 5 per cent solution is employed for gastric lavage and an equal volume is left in the stomach.

Dimercaprol is an effective antidote for countering the toxicity. However, to be maximally effective, it must be injected within first hour or two after poisoning. It is ineffective in the event of extensive renal damage for which hemodialysis is indicated. **Acetyl penicillamine** and **succimer** have also been used. Supportive treatment with IV fluids, treatment of shock and prophylactic antibiotics to prevent secondary infection are also instituted.

- ***Chronic mercury poisoning*** is manifested by increased irritability, tremors, headache, easy fatiguability, stomatitis, colitis, increased salivation and dermatitis. Electrolyte imbalance, neurotoxity, hepatotoxicity and renal damage are also seen. **Minamata disease**, reported from Japan was found to be due to consumption of fish from waters contaminated by methyl mercury from the industry. It was characterized by birth defects and neurological damage. Succimer is the treatment of choice for chronic poisoning.

An allergic manifestation seen in children, due to systemic absorption of topically applied mercurial antiseptics is termed *Pink disease* or acrodynia. Its manifestations include marked swelling and erythema of the extremities with sweating, itching and polyarthritis. It responds to therapy with acetyl penicillamine. Fever and skin rashes of various types have also been reported in adults using mercurial antiseptics.

GOLD: Chapter 71.

CADMIUM: This metal is employed in a wide range of manufacturing processes. Acute cadmium poisoning, when due to ingestion, is characterised by severe GI irritation and circulatory collapse; acute poisoning due to inhalation of cadmium fumes results in cough, sore throat, vertigo, dyspnoea, cyanosis and bronchopneumonia. Chronic cadmium poisoning causes a characteristic yellow pigmentation of teeth (the yellow ring of cadmium), anosmia, emphysema and proteinuria. Calcium gluconate, administered IV in the early stages, is claimed to be of some value. *Both dimercaprol and EDTA are not recommended for treatment as they may further aggravate the kidney damage caused by cadmium.*

THALLIUM: This metal was employed as the acetate for depilation. When ingested or inhalcd, it is, however, highly toxic and may lead to marked neurological disturbances on systemic absorption. Treatment is symptomatic, including hemodialysis.

Heavy Metal Antagonists

The toxicity of the heavy metals is attributed to their ability to form complexes with important biological radicals like the sulfhydryl, the hydroxyl, the carboxyl, the amino and the imidazole. Affinity for sulfhydryl group leads to inhibition of vital SH-containing enzymes. Inhibition of various enzymes leads to the toxic effects. Attempts were, therefore, made to develop organic compounds which would have a high affinity for the metallic ions. Such drugs would combine with the metallic ions to produce relatively nontoxic and easily water-soluble complexes which are subsequently eliminated by the kidneys. The process by which these organic compounds combine with the metals to form relatively stable nonionized ring complexes is called *chelation* (chele=claw), the compounds being designated as **Chelating agents**. (Table 72.1).

DIMERCAPROL (BAL): Dimercaprol, or British Anti-Lewisite, was synthesized by Stocken and Thompson during the World War II to ensure protection against poisoning by the arsenical war gases such as Lewisite. Chemically, it is a dithiol having two SH groups (Fig. 72.1).

Table 72.1: Metal-chelating agents used in therapy

Drug	Used against
$CaNa_2$ EDTA*	Lead
Dimercaprol*	Arsenic, copper
Succimer	Lead, arsenic, mercury
Penicillamine	Copper, mercury, lead
Trientine	Copper
Deferrioxamine	Iron
Deferiprone*	Iron

* Given by injection. Others are effective orally.

Pharmacological actions: Dimercaprol forms poorly dissociable complexes with arsenic, mercury and cadmium ions and thus protects the sulfhydryl (SH) enzymes. In case of mercury and cadmium, the dimercaprol-metal complex further reacts with another molecule of dimercaprol to form a still more stable, inactive complex.

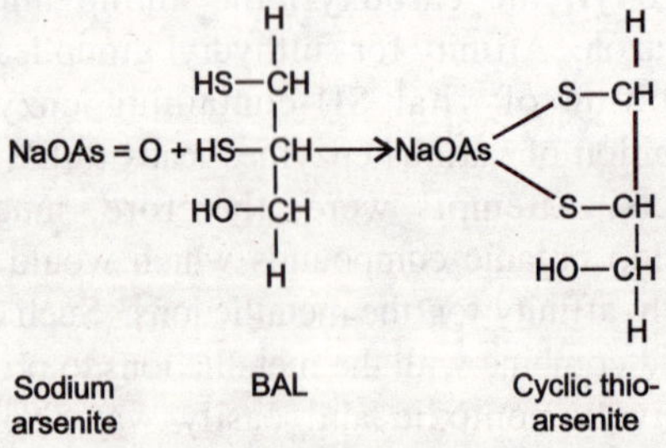

Fig. 72.1: Mode of action of BAL

Even though the dimercaprol-metal complexes are poorly dissociable, some amount of dissociation does occur *in vivo*, causing the release of the toxic metal in the active form. To overcome this drawback, the dosage schedule of dimercaprol is adjusted in such a way that an excess of free drug is always present in the body to bind the free metal released as a result of dissociation. Dimercaprol also reactivates the inhibited enzymes. However, its ability to achieve reactivation is limited by the amount of the metallic ion present in circulation, and by the duration of poisoning. Thus, dimercaprol fails to protect or reactivate the sulfhydryl enzymes if administered late or in the presence of overwhelming amounts of the metal.

Dimercaprol itself inhibits enzymes peroxidase, catalase and carbonic anhydrase in which the heavy metals constitute prosthetic groups.

Absorption, fate and excretion: Following the IM administration, the peak plasma levels are reached in about 2 hours and the drug is entirely metabolized within 6 to 24 hours. A part is excreted as a glucuronide in urine.

Adverse reactions: Injection of BAL is painful and can cause sterile abscesses and drug fever. Doses of dimercaprol in the range of 4 to 5 mg per kg body weight produce a variety of ADR in approximately 50 per cent of patients. These include nausea, vomiting, headache, burning sensation in the mouth and eyes, lachrimation, sialorrhoea, paraesthesiae of the extremities, muscle pain and muscle spasm. It can also cause anginal pain, tachycardia and hypertension.

Dimercaprol-metal complex dissociates more readily in an acidic medium. The urine, therefore, should be made alkaline during dimercaprol therapy to protect the kidneys from the toxic effects of the released free metal.

The use of dimercaprol is contraindicated in the presence of hepatic damage and in iron poisoning, as it forms a toxic complex with iron. Dimercaprol increases the urinary excretion of cadmium but the kidneys are likely to be damaged by the metallic ion. It should be used with caution in hypertensive individuals.

Preparation: Dimercaprol injection 50 mg per ml is a solution of dimercaprol in a mixture of benzyl benzoate and arachis oil. It has a strong characteristic smell.

Therapeutic uses:

- ***Acute poisoning*** due to arsenic, mercury, gold, antimony, bismuth and thallium.

In severe cases of arsenical and gold poisoning, 3 mg per kg. is given deep IM, at 4 hourly intervals for the first 2 days, at 6 hourly intervals on the third day, and twice daily for the next 10 days or until the recovery is complete. In case of gold poisoning, the maintenance dose may have to be administered for as long as 3 months.

Dimercaprol is effective in protecting the eyes from the effects of accidental contamination by arsenical vesicants. Complete recovery is usually achieved if 5 to 10 per cent oily solution of dimercaprol is instilled into the conjunctival sac within 5 minutes of contamination.

In acute mercurial poisoning, dimercaprol is administered initially in the dose of 5 mg. per kg. followed by 2 or 3 injections of 2.5 mg per kg during the next 12 hours, or until recovery is assured.

- ***Wilson's disease***: In patients with Wilson's disease allergic to penicillamine, dimercaprol is given I.M. in the dose of 2.5 mg per kg twice daily for first 2 days, followed by 2 days rest; and this course may be repeated as often as necessary. The drug causes a moderate increase in the urinary excretion of copper in this condition.
- ***Lead poisoning :*** Already discussed.

SUCCIMER (2,3 – Dimercaptosuccinic acid): This chemical, a water soluble analogue of dimercaprol, is effective orally. After absorption, it is biotransformed to a mixed disulfide with cysteine. It is an effective chelator of lead, arsenic, cadmium and mercury, but does not significantly mobilize essential metals such as zinc, copper and iron. Adverse effects are nausea, vomiting, diarrhoea, loss of appetite and skin rash. It is recommended for children with lead poisoning.

d-PENICILLAMINE: This compound, a monothiol (containing one SH group), is prepared by alkaline hydrolysis of benzyl penicillin. Chemically, it is beta dimethylcysteine.

Pharmacological actions: Penicillamine forms a water soluble complex with copper, mercury and lead ions and thus facilitates their excretion in urine. Like dimercaprol, it inhibits a number of enzymes, including transaminase and desulfhydrase which have one of these metals as the prosthetic group.

Penicillamine is well absorbed on oral administration and rapidly excreted in urine.

Adverse reactions: Penicillamine is a toxic drug. It causes :

- ***General toxicity*** such as headache, sore throat, fever, rash, nausea lymphadenopathy, and ecchymosis; loss or impairment of sense of taste can be very upsetting, neuritis.
- ***Haematologic toxicity***: Leucopenia, thrombocytopenia, aggranulocytosis and aplastic anemia.
- ***Renal toxicity***: Proteinuria, reversible nephrotic syndrome, hematuria.
- ***Autoimmune Syndrome***: Myasthenia like syndrome, diabetes, polymyositis and SLE.

Allergic reactions occur occasionally and patients who are sensitive to penicillin may have a similar reaction to penicillamine. Long term use may cause a myasthenia-like syndrome, iron and pyridoxine deficiency. Optic neuritis responding to pyridoxine has been reported.

Preparation: d-Penicillamine is available in capsules containing 250 mg. of the base equivalent to 300 mg. of the hydrochloride.

Therapeutic uses:

- ***Hepatolenticular degeneration*** (Wilson's disease): Wilson's disease is a rare, hereditary disease of abnormal copper metabolism characterised by degenerative changes in the basal ganglia and cirrhosis of the liver. The copper content of the liver, brain, kidneys and other tissues is grossly increased, the total serum copper and ceruloplasmin copper content are reduced and the urinary excretion of copper is enhanced. The Kayser-Fleischer ring, brownish pigmented ring at the corneal margin, is diagnostic of this condition.

Treatment is directed towards reducing the total body copper. This is achieved by administration of penicillamine or trientine, given in conjunction with a high protein, low copper diet with potassium disulfide (20 mg. thrice daily with meals). The latter precipitates dietary copper and thereby reduces its absorption. Zinc acetate and zinc sulfate 50 mg tid also reduce copper absorption.

Penicillamine is administered in the dose of 1-2 g (base) daily, in divided doses, before food. Depending on the urinary levels of copper, the dose may be subsequently increased to 4 to 5 g. daily and continued indefinitely.

Foods rich in copper (shell fish, nuts, chocolates, mushrooms and organ meats) should be avoided.

Clinical improvement in response to penicillamine therapy varies considerably despite a significant increase in the urinary excretion of copper. The response, therefore, probably depends upon the degree of irreversible structural damage.

- ***Rheumatoid arthritis (adjunctive treatment)***, (Chapter 71).
- ***Cystinuria;*** and
- ***Copper, arsenic and gold poisoning. Oral succimer is preferred in lead and mercury poisoning.***

ACETYL d-PENICIILLAMINE: This drug, a less toxic but weaker chelating agent than d-penicillamine, has been shown to be particularly effective in mercury poisoning. It is administered in the dose of 1 g. daily in 3 or 4 divided portions, for 10 days. The course may be repeated after a week's interval.

TRIENTINE (Triethylene tetramine): Given in doses of 400-800 mg. thrice daily on empty stomach, it is as effective as penicillamine in reversing the neurological lesions of Wilson's disease. It appears to be less toxic than penicillamine and may cause less iron deficiency.

DISODIUM CALCIUM EDETATE AND DISODIUM EDETATE : The calcium-disodium and the disodium salts of ethylene diamine tetraacetic acid (EDTA) form stable and highly water soluble complexes with many divalent and trivalent metallic ions and owe their therapeutic application to this chelating property (Fig. 72.2).

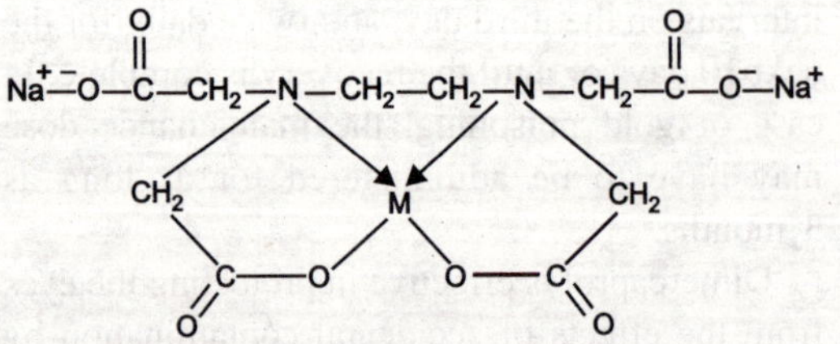

Fig. 72.2: Mode of action of disodium edetate. 'M' stands for chelated metal.

The calcium sodium salt has a high affinity for lead, while the disodium salt exhibits a high affinity for calcium. The affinity for other metals like sodium, magnesium and potassium is much less and this permits their selective use in the treatment of lead poisoning and hypercalcemia respectively.

Absorption, fate and excretion: Both the salts are poorly absorbed from the GI tract and are given IV or IM routes. The latter is very painful. They are excreted almost completely within 24 hours, both by glomerular filtration and tubular secretion.

Adverse reactions: Besides thrombophlebitis, these agents cause nausea, diarrhoea and toxic nephrosis. Oliguria and renal failure have been reported but generally, the damage is reversible following the cessation of drug therapy. Renal damage has been attributed to the free metallic ion released as a result of dissociation of the metal-chelate complex.

A febrile reaction, followed by myalgia, nausea, vomiting, histamine like reaction with rhinorrhoea, lacrimation and dermatitis are the other adverse effects reported, particularly with the disodium salt. The disodium salt may also cause hypocalcemic tetany due to excessive chelation of calcium.

Preparations: (i) Sodium calcium edetate (Ledclair) injection is a sterile 20 per cent w/v solution (5 ml per ampoule) of anhydrous sodium calcium edetate in water. It should be diluted with normal saline or 5 per cent dextrose before IV administration.

(ii) Disodium edetate injection 20 ml. ampoules containing 3 g. of the drug.

Therapeutic uses:

- ***Lead poisoning*:** Disodium calcium edetate is used in the treatment of acute and chronic lead poisoning. It acts by exchanging its calcium for lead in the blood to form a stable, nonionisable, water-soluble lead compound which is rapidly eliminated in urine. This exchange between lead and calcium is selective because other metals such as mercury, iron, copper and cobalt are more strongly bound to tissue proteins and hence, not available for exchange.

In acute lead poisoning, the agent is given by slow IV infusion in the dose of 40 mg. per kg. in two divided doses/day, as a 0.5 to 3 per cent solution in 0.9 per cent saline or 5 per cent dextrose, for a maximum period of 5 days. The course may then be repeated after an interval of 2 to 3 days. Smaller doses are recommended in the presence of encephalopathy and increased intracranial pressure. In children, the dose should not be larger than 55 mg. per kg. This should be divided into two portions and given by IV drip. It is necessary to monitor urine output as the chelator-lead complex is nephrotoxic.

The salt can also be used as a diagnostic test for lead poisoning. A total dose of 75 mg. per kg. divided into 3 doses, is administered as 20 per cent solution by deep IM injection with 1.5 per cent procaine. If the excretion of lead is more than 500 mcg. per 24 hours, the ingestion of lead is concluded to be excessive.

Disodium calcium edetate has also been used in the treatment of porphyria and in poisoning with iron, cadmium and plutonium.

There is no evidence that repeated IV infusion of EDTA (Chelation therapy) is beneficial in any form of atherosclerotic cardiovascular disease.

DITHIOCARB: This agent, administered orally in the dose of 2 g. daily for 7 days, preceded by an initial dose of 200 mg. IV, has been found useful in the treatment of nickel carbonyl poisoning and also to some extent in acute thallium poisoning and in Wilson's disease. The toxicity reported in animals includes visual disturbance and blindness.

DESFERRIOXAMINE and other iron-chelating agents are discussed in Chapter 33.

73 Gases: Therapeutic and Toxic

Apart from the anaesthetic gases, other gases of therapeutic importance are oxygen, carbon dioxide and nitric oxide. Helium, an inert gas present in the atmosphere in minute amounts, has also found therapeutic applications.

Some gases and organic solvent vapours exist as environmental pollutants and are of toxicological concern, e.g., carbon monoxide, sulfur dioxide and ozone.

Therapeutic Gases

OXYGEN: Inspired air contains 21 per cent of oxygen. It is carried in the body largely in combination with hemoglobin and a small quantity is transported in physical solution in plasma. With an increase in the ambient pressure, the amount of oxygen carried in the form of physical solution progressively increases.

Effects of oxygen administration: Inhalation of 100 per cent oxygen in a normal subject produces the following effects:

- ***Ventilation:*** Oxygen at atmospheric pressure initially depresses and later mildly stimulates the ventilation; the depressor effect is probably indirect, due to inhibition of the chemoreceptor activity. Oxygen also directly decreases the sensitivity of the respiratory centre to carbon dioxide. This effect is particularly apparent when the gas is given under more than one atmospheric pressure.
- ***Cardiovascular system:*** In normal individuals, oxygen produces a slight reduction in the heart rate and a moderate decrease in the cardiac output. The coronary and the cerebral blood flow are probably reduced, while the pulmonary vessels are dilated. It does not modify the blood pressure significantly.
- ***Nitrogen concentration:*** Inhalation of oxygen leads to a reduction in the partial pressure of nitrogen within the pulmonary alveoli, with its subsequent diffusion from the body cavities and blood into alveoli from where it is eliminated.

Methods of administration: Two types of equipment are available for administering oxygen.

- ***Those that aim at ensuring the highest concentration of oxygen in the inspired air:*** These include the oxygen tent and the various types of closely fitting aero-nasal masks with a non-return valve and either a reservoir bag or a demand valve on the oxygen supply line. The tents are cumbersome and require careful vigilance particularly against fire. Masks are particularly useful at high altitudes and in the treatment of bronchial asthma, pulmonary edema and chronic pulmonary diseases. Because of the irritant effect of oxygen on the respiratory tract, oxygen in high concentration is humidified by passing it through either a humidifier or a nebulizer. The widely followed method of bubbling the oxygen through a Wolff's bottle containing cold water has been shown to be valueless.

• ***Those that aim at achieving a steady concentration, less than 60 per cent in the inspired air:*** These include such simple devices as the nasal cannula and the nasal catheter (inserted through the nostril into the nasopharynx) and the more sophisticated equipment such as the Ventimask. This latter operates according to Bernoulli's principle: the pressure of a flowing gas is least where the rate of flow is greatest. If one injects oxygen through a small orifice, it attains great velocity but its pressure falls; it, therefore, sucks the room air from the surroundings and thus gets diluted. A flow of 1 to 6 litres of oxygen per minute through a cannula or a catheter ensures an oxygen concentration of 24 to 44 per cent in the inspired air. *Larger flow rates of oxygen flow do not achieve higher concentrations of oxygen and are, therefore, wasteful.* The Ventimask is available in different models designed to deliver oxygen at fixed concentrations.

Adverse reactions:

(a) **Due to formation of reactive O_2 species:**

• ***Respiratory tract:*** Inhalation of oxygen in the concentration of 60 per cent or more for 36 hours or longer may damage the pulmonary epithelium and inactivate a substance (surfactant) secreted by the alveoli and which helps to keep the alveoli patent by reducing the surface tension within them; consequently, extensive pulmonary atelectasis may occur. This is especially likely to occur when high concentration is used along with assisted mechanical ventilation and the arterial oxygen tension is allowed to remain above 150 mm. Hg. for prolonged periods. Administration of oxygen at a pressure greater than 1 atmosphere may cause respiratory distress in neonates, particularly in premature ones.

• ***Central nervous system:*** Inhalation of pure oxygen at pressures greater than 2 atmospheres may lead to paraesthesiae, mental disturbances, twitching, loss of consciousness and generalised convulsions. Convulsions may develop within a few minutes or several hours after inhalation of the gas.

• ***Retrolental fibroplasia:*** High arterial oxygen tension (over 100 mm. Hg.) interferes with the retinal blood supply and produces an occlusive proliferative retinal disease termed retrolental fibroplasia. This is observed mainly in premature infants. Retinal changes appear within 3rd to 6th week of life and may either regress or progress to blindness.

(b) **Others :**

• ***Hyperoxia*** can reduce coronary blood flow.

• ***Carbon dioxide narcosis:*** In patients with COPD, status asthmaticus, weakness of the respiratory muscles (from polyneuritis, poliomyelitis or myasthenia gravis), and in those with central respiratory depression (from narcotic poisoning, head injury or raised intracranial tension), the alveolar ventilation is inadequate to prevent a rise in the arterial carbon dioxide tension ($PaCO_2$). With increasing hypercapnea (raised $PaCO_2$), the respiratory centre becomes progressively more tolerant of CO_2 and its activity is solely maintained by the stimulus of hypoxemia (hypoxemic drive) reflexly through the carotid and aortic bodies. A removal of this stimulus by oxygen administration reduces the ventilation still further with a consequent rise in $PaCO_2$. This gives rise to the syndrome of carbon dioxide narcosis with raised intracranial tension and clinically manifested by sweating, twitchings, drowsiness, convulsions, papilledema and coma. It is a potentially lethal condition.

• ***Fire hazard:*** Every oxygen appliance is a potential fire hazard and no naked flame, lighted cigarette or electric switch should be brought near a patient receiving oxygen.

Preparations: Oxygen is dispensed in a compressed state in cylinders painted black with a white shoulder. Cylinders of oxygen mixed with carbon dioxide are also painted black but have grey and white quarterings on neck and shoulder.

Therapeutic uses:

(a) **Correction of hypoxia:** The primary indication of oxygen therapy is hypoxia. Hypoxia may be defined as inadequate tissue oxygenation. "Hypoxia" said Haldane "not only stops the machinery but also wrecks the machine". The brain is the organ most sensitive to hypoxia, and irreversible damage usually results within 3 to 4 minutes of its onset. Hypoxic damage to the kidney, liver and heart is also seen.

Types of hypoxia are shown in Table 73.1.

Table 73.1: Types of hypoxia

I **Hypoxic,** characterised by hypoxemia.

II **Anemic,** due to deficiency of hemoglobin as in anemia or due to inability of the altered hemoglobin to take up oxygen as in methemoglobinemia, and carbon monoxide poisoning. In this variety, the oxygen tension in the arterial blood is normal but the 'oxygen content' is reduced.

III **Stagnant,** due to excessive slowing of blood supply to the peripheral tissues e.g., in shock.

IV **Histotoxic,** due to increase in metabolic oxygen demand of the tissues as in thyrotoxicosis, and/or the tissue may be unable to utilise the available oxygen either as a result of paralysis of essential enzyme systems (cyanide poisoning) or due to a mechanical barrier (tissue edema).

A healthy person at rest, breathing room air with 21 per cent oxygen at a partial pressure of 160 mm. Hg., maintains the partial pressure of oxygen in the pulmonary alveoli (PAO2) at 100 mm. Hg. The oxygen in the alveoli equilibrates with the blood in the pulmonary capillaries and produces in the arterial blood a partial pressure of oxygen dissolved in the plasma (arterial oxygen tension, PaO2) of 80-100 mm. Hg. and an oxygen saturation (SaO2) of over 95 per cent. A reduction in the arterial oxygen tension is called **hypoxemia**. This must be distinguished from **hypoxia** which means inadequate tissue oxygenation. Hypoxemia generally (but not always) leads to hypoxia; on the other hand, hypoxia can arise from other causes than hypoxemia.

The carotid and the aortic bodies are the chemoreceptors which sense hypoxemia and stimulate breathing (mechanical ventilation) and the heart reflexly so that the hypoxemia tends to be corrected. In this process, the additional breathing effort and cardiac work increase the oxygen requirement of the body. At a certain stage, the body finds the increased ventilation and cardiac work uneconomical in terms of oxygen consumption and settles for a lower level of mechanical ventilation (breathing) even at the risk of continued hypoxemia. This is what commonly happens when a patient with COPD gets an acute chest infection and starts hyperventilating in order to compensate for the increase in the hypoxemia.

Hypoxemia can arise in several ways and can be detected by measurement of PaO_2. Our understanding of hypoxemia and its treatment is incomplete without an understanding of CO_2 transport and disposal in the body. Carbon dioxide is one of the final metabolic waste products in the body and enters the blood through the peripheral tissue capillaries. In the blood, it is carried (1) dissolved in the plasma; it is this CO_2 which accounts for the partial pressure of CO_2 (CO_2 tension or PCO_2); (2) as carboxyhemoglobin in the red blood cells; and (3) as bicarbonate to which it is rapidly converted in the red blood cells with the help of enzyme carbonic anhydrase. In the lungs, it diffuses rapidly across the alveolocapillary barrier into the pulmonary alveoli. The rate of washing out of carbon dioxide from the alveoli and hence from the blood, at a given rate of CO_2 production (i.e. at a given metabolic rate), is determined solely by the adequacy of alveolar ventilation. When more CO_2 is produced as a result of increased metabolic rate (as in fever), the ventilation (i.e. breathing) increases proportionately to wash out the excess of CO_2 and maintain the carbon dioxide tension in the alveoli ($PaCO_2$) and in the arterial blood ($PaCO_2$) at the normal level of 30-50 mm. Hg. Whenever ventilation fails to increase proportionately to the rise in CO_2 production, $PaCO_2$ is elevated above 50 mm. Hg. In any situation of hyperventilation, $PaCO_2$ falls below 30 mm. Hg. Thus, the $PaCO_2$ level faithfully reflects the adequacy or otherwise of alveolar ventilation. This has important implications in oxygen therapy. In any cardio-pulmonary disease where $PaCO_2$ is low or normal, it is safe to administer oxygen in high concentration without special precautions. In any condition accompanied by elevated $PaCO_2$, oxygen in high concentration tends to precipitate carbon dioxide narcosis. These patients are, however, badly in need of oxygen which should not be withheld from them. Only, it should be administered in low concentration so that the hypoxemia is only partly corrected, unless they can also be given mechanical assistance to ventilation. Administration of sedatives and hypnotics makes patients drowsy and abolishes their voluntary ventilatory drive, leading to CO_2 narcosis. So can the administration of depressants of the respiratory centre such as morphine.

The clinical recognition of 'hypoxia' is largely inferential. Hypoxia cannot be measured but has to be surmised by the presence of

- ***A clinical situation known to produce hypoxia;*** and
- ***Hypoxemia which can be detected by measurement of PaO_2.***

In acute lung disease, hypoxemia can be clinically diagnosed by the presence of central cyanosis. Cyanosis is difficult to make out in anemic patients. In patients with chronic hypoxemia due to COPD, it is difficult to clinically make out an increase in the hypoxemia such as occurs in a super-added acute chest infection. These patients then show signs of carbon dioxide narcosis or of right sided cardiac failure which should be taken as indications of increased hypoxemia. The other parameters useful in assessing a hypoxemic patient are (a) the clincial assessment of cardiac, circulatory and neurological status of the patient; and (b) laboratory measurement of hemoglobin, $PaCO_2$, acid-base and electrolyte status (Chapter 36).

The results of oxygen administration are the best in situations where there is deficiency of oxygen in the inspired air as at high altitude, where breathing 100% oxygen is beneficial.

In cardiopulmonary disorders, the conditions maximally helped by oxygen therapy are those associated with alveolar hypoventilation due to any cause, venous admixture as in COPD and alveolo-capillary block as in interstitial lung disease. Those in which $PaCO_2$ is elevated should be treated with oxygen in low concentration and the effect on the patient's clinical condition (and on the $PaCO_2$ if possible) should be watched carefully. Others can be safely treated with high concentration oxygen therapy.

Conditions with an intrapulmonary shunt can be safely treated with and benefit from oxygen in high concentration. Conditions with ventilation in excess of perfusion e.g. pulmonary emphysema are likely to show less benefit.

Administration of oxygen in high concentration to patients in shock increases the amount of dissolved oxygen in the plasma; though it may be small, it may be sufficient to tip the scales in patient's favour in this critical condition. Besides, it can relieve the pain of MI, an important cause of shock.

In severe anemia, oxygen in high concentration does the same thing that it does in shock viz. that it adds that little extra dissolved oxygen which helps the critically ill patient.

In a cyanotic, congenital heart disease such as Fallot's tetralogy, the patient has hypoxemia and reduced arterial oxygen content despite the compensatory polycythemia. These patients tolerate their hypoxemia very well in the ordinary circumstances but need oxygen in high concentration during a chest infection and during surgery.

(b) **Reduction in the partial pressure of an inert gas:** Oxygen is used by workers in pressurised spaces to reduce the inhaled nitrogen concentration and thus to prevent the decompression sickness. It is also commonly used during anaesthesia with the gaseous and the volatile general anaesthetic agents.

(c) **Oxygen as a diluent:** Oxygen is used as a diluent for anaesthetic gases. In this setting, oxygen also serves to cater to the metabolic demands, as the anaesthetic agents commonly depress the ventilation and circulation.

HYPERBARIC OXYGEN: According to Henry's law, the volume of a gas dissolved in a solution depends upon its partial pressure. Thus, the amount of oxygen dissolved in the plasma can be increased by breathing oxygen at an absolute atmospheric pressure greater than one. The larger amount of oxygen present in physical solution in the plasma enables better tissue oxygenation. Hyperbaric Oxygen (HBO) Therapy is defined as " a mode of treatment in which the patient is entirely immersed in a pressure chamber and breathes oxygen at a pressure greater than 1 atmosphere absolute (ATA)". One ATA is equal to 760 mm Hg at sea level. HBO is administered by using a special chamber which is pressurized by either (a) 100 % oxygen at 2-3 ATA, which the patient breathes; or (b) compressed air, with the patient breathing 100 % oxygen at 2-3 ATA through special masks or oxygen hoods. At these pressures, the amount of oxygen dissolved in the plasma rises from 0.3 ml % at 1 ATA to 4.4 ml % at 2 ATA and 6.8 ml % at 3 ATA, respectively (hyperoxygenation). The chamber may house a single patient with a chronic, stable condition (monoplace chamber); or many acutely ill patients needing the presence of attendants (multiplace chamber).

Pharmacological actions: HBO exerts several beneficial actions in the body.

(1) **Mechanical:**

- ***Reduction in the size of the gas (mainly nitrogen) bubbles*** in the circulation and the tissues in patients with decompression sickness and air/gas embolism, leading to amelioration of the symptoms of the former and improvement in the circulation in the latter.

(2) **Hyperoxygenation:**

- ***Displacement of carbon monoxide (CO) from carboxyhemoglobin*** in carbon monoxide poisoning and smoke inhalation.
- ***Peripheral vasoconstriction in tissues, with, nonetheless, increased oxygen delivery to the tissues.*** This helps to restore oxygenation of the ischemic tissues and to clear edema surrounding an abscess, especially in the brain and spinal cord. The heart is slowed and the cardiac output is reduced. The effect on blood pressure is variable.
- ***Increased neovascularisation in hypoxic areas.***
- ***Direct bactericidal action on anaerobic organisms.***
- ***Killing of other pathogens by stimulating the immune system*** by way of restoring and enhancing the phagocytic and bactericidal functions of the leucocytes.
- ***Promoting wound healing in radiation-damaged tissues*** e.g. osteonecrosis, cystitis, enteritis and so on.

Adverse reactions : Upto 3 ATA, HBO is safe. Yet, adverse effects and accidents can occur:

(a) **In the patient**

- ***Claustrophobia***
- ***Damage to the ear drums*** (otic barotrauma).
- ***Barotrauma to the lungs*** resulting in pneumothorax or air embolism.
- ***Pulmonary and neurological toxicity*** from oxygen free radicals.
- ***Retrolental fibroplesia.***
- ***Hypersesitivity to oxygen.***

(b) **In the attendants** in the multiplace chambers, who may suffer from **decompression sickness** if the chamber is decompressed rapidly.

(c) **Fire hazard** is a real but avoidable risk.

Therapeutic uses :

(1) **Metabolic :** Carbon monoxide poisoning, smoke inhalation and cyanide poisoning. Exceptional blood loss with severe anemia.

(2) **Mechanical:** Decompression sickness and air/gas embolism.

(3) **Ischemic conditions :** Acute traumatic ischemia and crush injuries; retinal artery thrombosis.

(4) **Infective conditions:** Clostridial infections (gas gangrene). Other severe/refractory tissue infections such as chronic osteomyelitis and brain abscess.

(5) **Wound healing problems :** Non-healing ulcers and wounds; compromised skin grafts, thermal burns.

(6) **Early and late radiation damage** to bone (radio-osteonecrosis) and soft tissues (e.g. cystitis and enteritis).

CARBON DIOXIDE: Normally it is produced in the body during tissue and food metabolism. The inspired atmospheric air contains 0.04 per cent of carbon dioxide. Carbon dioxide has marked effects on the CNS, the respiration and circulation.

Effects of carbon dioxide inhalation:

- ***Respiration:*** Carbon dioxide stimulates respiration by its direct action on the brain stem areas and to a smaller extent by action on the peripheral arterial chemoreceptors. It increases both the rate and the tidal volume of respiration. This effect is seen with inhalation of even 2 per cent carbon dioxide. The respiratory response to CO_2 is considerably enhanced when the PaO_2 is lowered.
- ***Circulation:*** Carbon dioxide, by a direct action, tends to decrease the heart rate and the myocardiac force of contraction. It also relaxes the vascular smooth muscle, tending to cause vasodilatation.

The direct circulatory effects are antagonised by the sympathetic activation induced by it, causing an increase in the peripheral release of the catecholamines. The total circulatory response, therefore, is the outcome of two opposite actions. Thus, inhalation of carbon dioxide in a normal man increases the heart rate, the cardiac output, the systolic and the diastolic blood pressures and the pulse pressure. Cerebral and coronary vessels, which are devoid of a significant sympathetic control, dilate after carbon dioxide inhalation and so do the splanchnic and the skeletal muscle blood vessels. *Carbon dioxide is probably the most potent cerebral vasodilator studied so far.*

- ***CNS:*** Carbon dioxide, inhaled in low concentration, stimulates the cerebral cortex and reduces seizure threshold. Higher concentrations depress the cortex, while activating the subcortical areas that have cortical projections.

Adverse reactions : Above a concentration of 7 per cent in inhaled air, carbon dioxide gives rise to headache, dizziness, mental confusion, palpitation, dyspnoea and an increase in BP. Loss of consciousness occurs when its concentration exceeds 10 per cent. Withdrawal of carbon dioxide after prolonged inhalation often leads to pallor, hypotension, dizziness, nausea and vomiting. These effects can be minimised by its tapered withdrawal. Carbon dioxide narcosis has already been discussed earlier.

Preparations :

(i) Carbon dioxide is marketed in steel cylinders painted grey, usually in a liquid form, under a pressure of 58 to 72 atmospheres.

(ii) Combinations of oxygen and 5-10% carbon dioxide are marketed as 'carbogen'.

(iii) Solid carbon dioxide is available in two forms : dry ice and carbon dioxide snow.

Therapeutic uses :

- ***Hiccups:*** Hiccup represents the sound produced by the sudden contraction of inspiratory muscles terminated by abrupt closure of the glottis. It is a common disorder due to a wide variety of causes including gastric distension, alcohol ingestion, excessive smoking, psychogenic disorders, disorders of the cns, toxic-metabolic causes, irritation of the diaphragm, drugs and so on. Hiccups appear to serve no useful purpose. Usually it is self limited and harmless; but, sometimes it is an indicator of a serious disease and may last for many days. Inhalation of 10 to 25 per cent of carbon dioxide may be used in the treatment of intractable hiccups. Rebreathing into a paper bag is a household method of achieving the same effect. The other measures tried are:

(a) **Non-pharmacological :** Stimulation of the uvula or the nasopharynx (touching the uvula with a spoon; sipping iced water; sucking hard candy; swallowing dry, granulated sugar; inhalation of ammonia); valsalva manoeuvre; sneezing; breath holding; phrenic nerve block.

(b) **Pharmacological :** A variety of drugs have been used to treat hiccups with variable results. Chlorpromazine; Haloperidol; Metoclopramide; Carbamazepine orally; Phenytoin IV; Magnesium sulfate IM.

Benzodiazepines are not useful in hiccups.

- ***Neuropsychiatry:*** Inhalation of 30 per cent of carbon dioxide with 70 per cent oxygen has been employed for the treatment of anxiety neurosis and personality maladjustments. Its therapeutic value is not well established.
- ***Local uses:*** Carbon dioxide snow, which has a temperature of -800 C is used to destroy warts and naevi by local application for 5 to 6 seconds. The procedure is almost painless and scarring is minimum. The surrounding tissue should be protected with soft paraffin.
- ***Miscellaneous :*** Supersaturated solution of carbon dioxide or aerated waters possess a mild rubefacient action and are believed to increase the secretion of gastric juice particularly hydrochloric acid. They are often used as carminatives and for masking unpleasant taste of saline purgatives.

HELIUM: This inert gas, in the concentration of 80 per cent along with 20 per cent oxygen, is used by intermittent inhalation for treating prolonged asthmatic attacks resistant to other forms of therapy. Because of its lower density, it minimises the breathing effort. It is also employed prophylactically for prevention of Caisson disease, and in the treatment of edema and spasm of larynx.

NITRIC OXIDE (NO): (Chapter 28) It has selective vasodilatory effect on the pulmonary circulation when it is inhaled. It is used to improve oxygenation in hypoxic respiratory failure with pulmonary hypertension in term and near-term neonates; and in adults with various types of pulmonary hypertension, including primary pulmonary hypertension, and in adult respiratory distress syndrome (ARDS). The outcome is less satisfactory in adults than in the neonates. It is administered by inhalation in the concentration of 10-80 ppm. Higher concentrations can be toxic because of its metabolic degradation to NO_2 and because of methemoglobinemia. Experience (particularly long-term) with nitric oxide is still limited.

Water vapour: Inspired water is administered either as a vapour (from a humidifier) or in particulate form (from a nebulizer) in patients with respiratory infection/irritation. It decreases crusting of the respiratory mucosa, liquefies thick secretions, promotes mucociliary drainage, limits loss of body water and conserves body heat by reducing the evaporation in the airway (Chapter 25). It is also useful in patients whose airways are chronically intubated. Aerosol are used to deliver drugs such as bronchodilators and mucolytics to the airways.

Toxic Gases

In the pursuit of making life more and more comfortable and with increasing urbanization, environmental pollution has become a major health problem in modern life. People are exposed to various pollutants in the air, which enter the body not only through the lungs but also through skin and eyes, and cause local and systemic toxicity. The major air pollutants are shown in Table 73.2.

CARBON MONOXIDE (CO): This is a colourless, odourless, non-irritating gas which constitutes almost 50% of the air-pollutants.

Table 73.2: Major gaseous air pollutants

- Carbon monoxide (CO).
- Sulfur dioxide (SO_2).
- Nitrogen dioxide (NO_2).
- Hydrocarbon vapours; and
- Glycols (Chapter 6).

CO is responsible for many accidental deaths every year. The automobile is the largest source of CO.

It is also generated by incomplete combustion of organic matter as well as from smoking.

Actions: Carbon monoxide combines with hemoglobin to form carboxyhemoglobin (COHb) which cannot carry oxygen, thus reducing the oxygen delivery to the issues. The affinity of CO for hemoglobin is more than 200 times that of O_2. CO interferes with feroproteins such as myoglobin and cytochrome oxidase.

The signs and symptoms of acute CO poisoning are those of hypoxia. Acute CO poisoning causes headache, weakness, dizziness, nausea, vomiting, coma and intermittent convulsions. The patient is cyanosed. Sudden exposure to very high concentrations of CO can cause immediate death without any warning symptoms. Following recovery, neuro psychiatric effects may be observed. Cherry-red colour of the blood is highly suggestive of the diagnosis, which is confirmed by spectroscopy of the blood.

Early symptoms of poisoning are flu-like and may be wrongly diagnosed.

Chronic exposure to low concentrations of CO facilitates the development of atherosclerosis, cardiac disease, neurological damage and parkinsonism.

Treatment of acute CO poisoning: COHb is fully dissociable and CO is rapidly excreted through the lungs. Treatment, therefore, consists of transport to an open space with fresh air, rapid administration of 100% oxygen with a tight fitting mask, and supportive therapy to correct hypotension and acidosis in severe cases. Recovery is almost complete if the patient is treated early. It can also be treated with hyperbaric oxygen (see earlier).

SULFUR DIOXIDE (SO_2): This gas is primarily generated during burning of fossil fuels that contain sulfur. Though it rarely causes death, it is a respiratory irritant, leads to the production of thick mucus and causes bronchoconstriction. Chronic exposure results in abnormal pulmonary function and can predispose to chronic respiratory disease. A part of the atmospheric sulfur is converted to sulfuric acid and particulate sulfates. Sulfuric acid in the atmosphere causes further damage to the respiratory passages, increases airway resistance and predisposes to chronic respiratory diseases. Sulfuric acid also dissolves in rain water and returns to the earth as ‘acid rain’ which can cause extensive damage. The treatment is essentially symptomatic.

OZONE (O_3): This gas is formed from a complex reaction of a major atmospheric pollutant NO2 with UV light. Thus:

$$NO_2 \longrightarrow NO + O$$
$$O + O_2 \longrightarrow O_3$$

Ozone is a respiratory irritant and can cause pulmonary edema and death. It is a potent oxidant, and pulmonary injury may be due to the formation of highly reactive free radical intermediates. Chronic exposure to ozone may cause chronic bronchitis, emphysema and pulmonary fibrosis. It increases the sensitivity of the lung to other bronchoconstrictors such as histamine, acetylcholine and to allergens. The treatment of the toxicity is symptomatic. Antioxidants such as vitamin C and vitamin E may be useful.

NITROGEN DIOXIDE (NO_2): This pollutant gas is also a pulmonary irritant and, like ozone, causes pulmonary edema and changes in pulmonary function.

ORGANIC SOLVENT VAPOURS: In addition

to the above pollutant gases, we are constantly exposed to organic solvent vapours such as petrol, crude oil, aerosol sprays and floor cleaners. Some of these solvents and hydrocarbons cause pleasant sensations when inhaled, and are frequently abused. The common hazardous solvents are shown in Table 73.3.

Table 73.3: Common hazardous organic solvents

- ***Aliphatic hydrocarbons:*** Methane, Ethane, n-Hexane.
- ***Aromatic hydrocarbons:*** Benzene, Toluene.
- ***Halogenated hydrocarbons:*** Carbon Tetrachloride, Tetrachlorethylene.

Kerosene and **petroleum** products contain a variety of hydrocarbons. Petroleum vapours, when inhaled, cause sensitization of the myocardium to noradrenaline and may precipitate ventricular arrhythmias. Ingestion of kerosene causes symptoms like ethyl alcohol poisoning and pulmonary edema.

Many of the hydrocarbons cause GI disturbances, CNS depression, neurological damage, polyneuropathy and aplastic anemia. They are also carcinogenic.

CYANIDE: This is one of the deadliest of all poisons causing death within a matter of minutes. It acts by forming a complex with cytochrome C oxidase, thereby inhibiting cellular O2 use. Cyanide normally present in the body is biotransformed to the much less toxic thiocyanate; this reaction is catalysed by an intracellular enzyme rhodanase which requires thiosulfate or colloidal sulfur as a substrate. As the availability of this substrate is limited, rhodanase is unable to biotransform large amounts of cyanide.

Treatment: *The treatment must be instituted immediately to prevent the fatal outcome.* Initially, methemoglobinemia is produced by amyl nitrite inhalation for 30 seconds every 2 minutes, along with IV administration of 300 to 500 mg. of sodium nitrite dissolved in 10 to 15 ml. of water over 3 minutes. Methemoglobin competes with cytochrome C oxidase for cyanide, to form cyanmethemoglobin and thus protects the enzyme. This is followed by administration of sodium thiosulfate slowly, IV, in the dose of 25 ml of 5.0% solution (containing 1.25 g of sodium thiosulfate) over a period of 10 minutes. This results in the formation of relatively non-toxic thiocyanate which is excreted in urine.

Hyperbaric oxygen and IV methylene blue as 1 per cent solution in the dose of 1 to 4 mg. per kg. are the other measures employed.

Dicobalt edetate (Kelocyanor), a chelating agent, is also used to treat cyanide poisoning. It is given IV in the dose of 300 mg (one 20 ml ampoule) over one minute followed by 50 ml of 50% glucose by IV infusion. Both may be repeated once or twice as necessary. The drug is toxic and can cause severe hypotension, particularly in those subjects who are suspected but in fact are not suffering from cyanide poisoning.

Owing to its toxicity, the use of this drug must be limited to a patient who is tending to lose, or has lost, consciousness; it should not be used as a precautionary measure.

74 Enzymes in Therapy

Enzymes being extremely potent substances, the possibility of their therapeutic application is attractive. However, majority of these substances have to be administered parenterally as they are inactivated within the gastrointestinal tract. In addition, because of their proteinic nature, they are likely to evoke allergic reactions and because of their high potency, their careless use may result in alarming adverse effects. Lastly, because of the complicated method of their preparation, the cost of such therapy is likely to be high.

Enzymes such as pancreatin, diastase, pepsin and papain, used in the treatment of certain GI disturbances have been described in Chapter 39. The enzymes fibrinolysin, thromboplastin, urokinase and arvin involved in the process of blood coagulation are discussed in Chapter 32. The therapeutic application of pancreatic dornase is discussed in Chapter 25 and the use of asparaginase in Chapter 59.

The other enzymes used therapeutically are:

HYALURONIDASE (Hyalase, Rondase): This enzyme, prepared from mammalian testes acts by de-polymerizing hyaluronic acid, an essential component of the intercellular ground substances which determines the permeability of the tissues. Thus, hyaluronidase, administered SC, increases the tissue permeability or exhibits 'spreading activity'. Certain snake-venoms and bee-venoms also contain hyaluronidase. Similarly, certain virulent organisms also liberate hyaluronidase.

Hyaluronidase is an odourless, fluffy powder containing not less than 300 units of activity per mg. Therapeutically, hyaluronidase is employed to promote the rapid absorption of drugs and fluids given SC or IM. The agent is particularly useful in aiding the absorption of relatively large quantities of fluids, administered SC in infants and young children, in whom IV injection may be difficult. For hypodermoclysis 1500 units are added to each litre of fluid to be administered.

Substances used in radiography are rapidly absorbed on IM injection with the aid of hyaluronidase, thus providing an alternative to their IV administration. The agent has also been used to promote the absorption of blood and fluid in traumatic or post-operative edema or hematoma. Sodium hyaluronate in highly purified form is used in a number of ophthalmic surgical procedures. It should not be applied directly to the cornea and should not be used to reduce the swelling of bites and stings.

Hyaluronidase is antigenic and may occasionally produce allergic reactions. Because of the danger of spreading the infection, the enzyme should not be injected into or around an infected area. Malignancy is also considered a contraindication for hyaluronidase for similar reasons.

STREPTOKINASE AND STREPTODORNASE (Varidase): **Streptokinase,** a non-enzyme protein produced by certain strains of beta hemolytic streptococci, causes fibrinolysis and dissolution of clot mainly by converting the intrinsic plasminogen present in the fibrin clot to its active form plasmin. In addition, it is also capable of activating the plasminogen in the body fluids (extrinsic plasminogen) to plasmin; but this mechanism is probably of secondary importance in its clot-dissolving effect. Its maximum activity is seen between pH 7.3 to 7.6 (Chapter 32).

Streptodornase is not a single enzyme but a group of rapidly acting enzymes which promote the depolymerization of the complex nucleoproteins derived from degenerated leucocytes and injured tissue cells. They act directly and not through plasminogen activation. Their action results in a rapid conversion of thick, viscous and purulent material to thin, easy flowing fluid. The enzymes do not attack the nucleoproteins of living cells. Their optimum activity is observed between the pH 7.0 and 8.5 and requires the presence of magnesium ions.

Both these are stable for several months in desiccated form but solutions at room temperature deteriorate rapidly.

Adverse reactions : As with other enzymes, the use of streptokinase-streptodornase may occasionally result in allergic reactions like urticaria, rash, fever and anaphylaxis. A febrile reaction may occur. Streptokinase-streptodornase should not be employed in the presence of acute cellulitis and inflammation, as it may encourage the spread of localised infection. Since these substances are bacterial antigens, therapy with them results in rapid antibody formation rendering further treatment ineffective.

Preparations and dosage: Powder for topical application (Varidase) containing 100,000 units of streptokinase and 25,000 units of streptodornase, buffered with sodium phosphate to pH 7.5.

Therapeutic uses: Streptokinase streptodornase is used topically, for debridement of chronic ulcers.

It is no longer used for intracavitary instillation as in empyema of the pleural cavity; some physicians use streptokinase instead, for that purpose.

The use of streptokinase for lysing intravascular thrombi is discussed in Chapter 32.

TRYPSIN: This enzyme is obtained from an extract of the ox pancreas. It is available as a white powder soluble in water. The enzyme is active at a pH range of 5 to 8 with optimum activity at pH 7. Trypsin directly hydrolyzes natural proteins, including the respiratory mucins.

Adverse reactions: These are similar to those of streptokinase-streptodornase. Application of the dry powder to surface lesions may cause a severe burning sensation. Intramuscular injection may be followed by pain and induration at the site of injection and occasionally by fever, leucocytosis, angioneurotic edema and urticaria.

Contraindications and precautions for the use of trypsin are similar to those with streptokinase-streptodornase. The agent should be used cautiously in the presence of renal damage and be avoided in individuals with hepatic insufficieny. It should never be given intravenously.

Therapeutic uses: Trypsin has therapeutic applications similar to streptokinase streptodornase. For infiltration or by instillation, it is used as a solution containing 3 to 5 mg. of the enzyme per ml. The dry powder may be applied every 15 to 30 minutes to small areas and every 3 hours to large areas; wet dressings and irrigations should be repeated 3 hourly. Small gelatin capsules containing the enzyme may be inserted into inirrigable sinuses and fistulae. An aerosol of trypsin has been used to liquefy excessive bronchial secretions but its irritant nature makes it of doubtful value.

Proteolytic enzymes from *Carica papaya* (papase) and concentrated protease (bromelains) obtained from pineapple plant have the same indications as trypsin. They act by depoly-merizing the soft fibrin deposits in the inflamed areas and by facilitating the drainage of fluids. Their therapeutic use is not well established.

CHYMOTRYPSIN: This is a proteolytic enzyme obtained from the bovine pancreas. It is available as tablets containing 50,000 units of the enzyme per tablet. Tablets containing trypsin and chymotrypsin (Chymoral) are also available.

Chymotrypsin is proposed for use as an adjunct to the conventional treatment of traumatically induced inflammation and edema of soft tissues. It is applied locally or given orally. However, its usefulness is doubtful. Its oral toxicity is mild.

ALPHA-CHYMOTRYPSIN: This pro-teolytic enzyme is mainly used in ophthalmology for dissolving the suspensory ligament of the lens to facilitate the dissection of the lens during intracapsular extraction of cataract. The procedure is called zonulolysis. It is used as 0.2 to 0.5 ml. of a freshly prepared 1:5000 solution injected slowly behind the lens into the posterior chamber. The adverse effects include transient glaucoma, wound disruption, loss of vitreous and rarely retinal damage, if it penetrates the vitreous. It can aslo be applied locally.

COLLAGENASE : This enzyme is derived from fermentation of Cl. histolyticum. It acts on both denatured and undenatured collagen. Newly formed collagen and healthy tissue collagen are not attacked. The activity is optimal at pH 6-8. Adverse effects are uncommon. It is used for debridement of dermal ulcers and in severe burns. It is applied in the form of an ointment once daily.

Deoxyribonuclease : DNA released from neutrophils forms long fibrils that contribute to the viscosity of sputum in cystic fibrosis. Inhaled recombinant human deoxyribonuclease which cleaves DNA has been tried in patients with cystic fibrosis who have purulent sputum and airway obstruction.

Serratiopeptidase: This proteolytic enzyme, administered orally, is claimed to be useful for 'digesting' necrotic tissue, cell debris, cellular exudate and coagulated blood. It is promoted in combination with other active agents for the oral treatment of inflammatory edema and hematoma. Present evidence, however, is very inadequate to substantiate this claim.

Vitamins and Antioxidants 75

A vitamin is an organic substance that is found in food, is not made in the body, and is required in small quantities, usually as a cofactor for enzymes. Some of the vitamins such as vitamin K, pantothenic acid, folic acid and cyanocobalamin are also synthesized by the intestinal bacterial flora. Vitamins form components of important enzyme systems which catalyse the reactions by which the body metabolizes carbohydrates, proteins and fats. It is beyond the scope of this book to discuss in detail the physiological aspects of vitamins. The discussion is, therefore, limited to the pharmacological aspects when vitamins are employed as drugs for therapeutic purposes.

The only source of vitamins that can be regarded as natural is food. A normal individual ingesting a well balanced diet, containing a wide variety of foods, gets adequate supply of vitamins and needs no supplements. Vitamin deficiency, however, can arise in various ways:

- ***Deficient dietary intake :*** Undernutrition from any cause including food fads.
- ***Inadequate absorption from the gastrointestinal tract:*** Chronic diarrhoea, malabsorption syndrome, obstructive jaundice, interference with the function of the intestinal flora by oral antibiotics and interference with absorption by drugs like liquid paraffin.
- ***Interference with utilization*** usually by drugs e.g. pyrimethamine, trimethoprim and methotrexate which interfere with folic acid utilization; INH prevents the conversion of pyridoxal to pyridoxal phosphate.
- ***Increased demand:*** During growth, in pregnancy, during lactation, under stress, in fevers and other catabolic conditions such as hyperthyroidism.

Vitamins are classified as :

I **Fat soluble** vitamins such as A, D, E and K; and

II **Water soluble** vitamins such as B complex and C.

The former are stored in the body and cannot be excreted easily; hence, excessive administration of these can cause serious toxicity. Water soluble vitamins, on the other hand, are rapidly excreted in the urine following excessive administration.

Recommended daily allowances of vitamins exceed the nutrient requirement and they acknowledge the range of nutrient requirements in healthy individuals. They do not allow for such factors as illness and interaction with drugs. However, short illnesses where the normal eating pattern is resumed early are unlikely to lead to vitamin deficiency. Clinical manifestations of deficiency of B vitamins are often not specific e.g. glossitis may be due to a deficiency of riboflavin, niacin, pyridoxine, folic acid or vitamin B_{12}. Vitamin deficieny may occur when large doses of certain vitamins (Vitamin C and pyridoxine) are reduced abruptly. Vitamin deficiency can occur, unless specifically prevented by supplements, during total parenteral nutrition therapy.

Groups vulnerable to develop vitamin deficiency, other than those already mentioned above, are socioeconomically disadvantaged persons; institutionalized persons; elderly persons on medications; heavy smokers who often lose interest in eating; women of childbearing age; infants (especially premature infants); and food faddists. Oral contraceptive pills reduce the serum levels of vitamin B_6, folic acid and vitamin C, but raise that of vitamin A.

A diet that is deficient in one vitamin is likely to be deficient in others as well. In general, vitamin supplements should be used only when a dietary solution cannot be found. However, in advanced vitamin deficiency, it may be worth replenishing body stores with single nutrients, the deficiency of which may be the principal problem. Lastly, using food as the source of vitamins is the best safeguard against vitamin toxicity; the only exception to this rule is the livers of certain marine and arctic animals which are very rich in vitamin A.

Fat Soluble Vitamins

VITAMIN A: Vitamin A is available from the diet either

- ***As preformed vitamin, retinol***, which is a complex, primary alcohol; or
- ***Esters of retinol in the form of carotenoid pigments*** (particularly beta carotene) which can be considered as provitamin A.

Sources: Carotene is present in green and yellow vegetables and fruits: leafy vegetables, carrots, papaya, mango etc. Retinol is present in animal foods: eggs, milk, milk products and meat. Animal liver (cod, halibut and mammals) is a rich source of retinol.

The daily requirements of vitamin A is about 5000 U in adults and older children and about 3000 U in children below 5 years. About 35 g. of dark leafy vegetables or 100 g. of mango will supply the daily dietary requirements of children. Small fish, eaten whole (with their livers), are a good supplementary source of vitamin A in diet. Human milk supplies sufficient vitamin A for infants unless the mother's diet is grossly inadequate; in the latter instance, enough vitamin A should be given during the first six months after birth to provide about 1500 U daily to normal-birth-weight infants and 2000-2500 U daily to premature infants.

Vitamin A and the carotenes are stable to moderate heat in the absence of oxidising agents. The ordinary cooking processes do not destroy the vitamin A in vegetables. Prolonged, high temperature cooking, exposure to light and rancidity of fat hasten vitamin A destruction but frozen foods retain their vitamin A content for a long time.

Physiological functions : Vitamin A plays a vital role in the phenomenon of dark adaptation where it is essential for the synthesis of rhodopsin, the photosensitive pigment of rods. Rhodopsin decomposes when light strikes the rod, thus initiating the nerve impulse. The vitamin is also essential for the integrity of epithelial cells, maintenance of CMI, morphogenetic signals in embryogenesis, and for somatic growth.

Deficiency of vitamin A has been shown to affect the immune system at multiple sites. It affects certain subsets of T lymphocytes, natural killer (NK) cells, cytotoxic activity and the antibody response to bacterial polypeptides. Mortality from infectious diseases, which accompany xerophthalmia, can be reduced by intermittent, massive vitamin A therapy. The vitamin may be involved in the antioxidant processes against oxidation by free radical attack.

Clinical vitamin A deficiency is characterized in early stages by *night blindness, xerosis of conjunctivae (manifested as Bitot's spots) and xerophthalmic or "dry eye"*. This may be associated with squamous metaplasia of the mucosal surface of the upper respiratory tract and the periodontal tissues, *follicular hyperkeratosis of the skin* (also termed toad skin), and in increased incidence of renal calculi. Similar changes may occur in the intestinal epithelium leading to diarrhoea. In advanced stages, true keratomalacia may occur, leading to blindness. The manifestations of this condition are necrosis, ulceration and finally, perforation of the cornea and panophthalmitis. *Vitamin A deficiency is one of the major preventable causes of blindness in children in developing countries.*

Absorption, fate and excretion: Retinol is readily absorbed from the GI tract but requires the presence of dietary protein. The absorption is reduced in the presence of biliary obstruction or liver disease; however, this is not due to bile deficiency as externally administered bile salts are unable to promote the absorption of vitamin A. It is likely that specialised enzymatic processes concerned with intestinal absorption of the vitamin from the small intestine are deficient in hepatic insufficiency.

Following absorption, vitamin A is stored in the Kupffer cells of the liver as **retinyl ester** and following hepatic saturation, it is released into the plasma as **free alcohol (retinol)** in combination with specific proteins. Liver disease, therefore, may be associated with low plasma vitamin A levels. In kwashiorkor, plasma vitamin A levels are low, probably owing to the deficiency of the carrier protein.

As opposed to vitamin A, GI absorption of carotene is slow and requires the presence of bile and absorbable fat. Carotene is converted to vitamin A in the intestinal wall and is subsequently stored in the liver. However, only about 30% of the dietary carotene is converted to retinol and is available as vitamin A activity. In the event of large dietary intake of carotene, some of it may escape into the circulation, leading to carotenemia, which causes a characteristic yellow discoloration of the skin.

Vitamin A is metabolized in the body to:

- ***Esters*** which are stored in the liver.
- ***The aldehyde retinal*** which is the active element of the visual pigment; and
- ***Retinoic acid,*** an intracellular messenger that modulates cell differentiation.

Normal human urine does not contain any vitamin A.

Adverse reactions: Both acute and chronic intoxication with vitamin A have been reported.

- ***Acute intoxication:*** Consumption of the liver of polar bear (vitamin A content, 10,000 to 34,000 I.U./g.) leads to anorexia, nausea, vomiting, abdominal pain, headache, papilloedema, diplopia, convulsions, delirium and coma. Several of these effects are similar to those of a brain tumour. Bulging of fontanelles and vomiting have also been reported in infants given a single, large dose of 300,000 I.U. of vitamin A.
- ***Chronic intoxication*** usually develops following the administration of large doses of vitamin A (over 33,000 units daily) for prolonged periods. The usual symptoms are anorexia, dry itching skin (hyperkeratosis), loss of weight, increased irritability, low grade fever, alopecia, dependent edema with erythema and ecchymosis, bleeding, fissuring, refractory skin ulcer, anemia and hepatosplenomegaly. Headache and visual upsets are often encountered. Subcutaneous swellings, tenderness over long bones and bony exostoses are other notable features. X-ray studies have revealed premature closure of epiphyses and consequent retardation of growth in children. The symptoms usually appear after a latent period of 6 to 15 months. The characteristic skin desquamation is a major diagnostic point to hypervitaminosis A.

Large doses (more than 20,000 IU/day) of vitamin A should not be used during pregnancy; similarly, large amounts of liver in the diet should be avoided.

Preparations and dosage:

(i) Concentrated vitamin A solution contains not less than 50,000 units/ml. of vitamin A activity. Dose : 0.06 to 0.6 ml.

(ii) Vitamin A tablet : Contains 50,000 units of vitamin A (Arovit). Dose: 1 to 2 tablets daily.

(iii) Vitamin A injection : Contains 100,000 units per ml. (Arovit). Dose: 1 ml. IM once or twice a week.

Synthetic and natural preparations

containing both vitamin A and vitamin D are:

(i) Vitamin A and D capsule or tablet Contains 4000 units of vitamin A and 400 units of antirachitic activity. Dose: 1-2 capsules daily.

(ii) Shark liver oil is obtained from the fresh or carefully preserved livers of the shark and allied species. It contains not less than 6,000 units of vitamin A activity in 1 g. Dose: 0.2 to 1 ml. orally, approximately equivalent to 1,500 to 7,500 units of vitamin A.

(iii) Halibut liver oil is extracted from the fresh or suitably preserved liver of halibut species belonging to the genus *Hippoglosus*. It contains not less than 30,000 units of vitamin A activity and 2,500 to 3,500 units of antirachitic activity per g. Dose: 0.2 to 0.5 ml. daily.

Therapeutic uses: As vitamin A deficiency is a preventable cause of blindness, prophylactic use of this vitamin is important in the high risk, malnourished populations. Further, even mild degree of vitamin A deficiency is associated with increased morbidity and mortality in children, largely as a result of vulnerability to diarrhoea and repeated infections.

Vitamin A supplements are not required in adults eating a well balanced diet. The prophylactic schedule recommended by the W.H.O. is shown in Table 75.1.

Table 75.1: W.H.O. recommended prophylactic, oral vitamin A doses (in units)

• **At birth (neonate)**	50,000 (single dose)
• **Upto 1 yr.**	1,00,000 once in 4-6 months
• **Children above 1 yr.**	2,00,000 once in 4-6 months
• **Immediately after delivery (mother)**	3,00,000 (single dose)
• **Pregnant and lactating women**	5,000 daily

In the treatment of nightblindness and xerophthalmia, vitamin A is administered in the dose of 1,00,000 units by IM injection. This condition rarely responds completely to vitamin A therapy except in the early stages. Severe cases may need repeated doses. Improvement begins within a week after administration but several months are required for complete healing.

Measles can precipitate acute, severe vitamin A deficiency by depleting the hepatic stores of vitamin A. WHO/UNICEF have, in a joint statement, recommended that "High dosage of vitamin A supplementation should be provided to all children diagnosed with measles in communities in which vitamin A deficiency is a recognized problem". The recommended dose, to be administered as soon as measles is diagnosed, is 100,000 units in children under the age of 12 months and 200,000 units in children over that age. If any eye sign of vitamin A deficiency is present, repeat the same dose the next day and again after one to four weeks.

Deficiency of vitamin A is also seen in coeliac disease, sprue, and with excessive use of liquid paraffin. This generally responds to the treatment outlined above.

Synthetic analogues of vitamin A: Vitamin A has the important antikeratinizing property. Retinol, to be effective, must be administered in doses that cause hypervitaminosis A. Synthetic analogues of retinol are useful in a variety of skin disorders in doses that do not cause hypervitaminosis A. The analogues are:

(1) **Tretinoin** (Vitamin A acid, 13-transretinoic acid, Retin-A) which is used locally as a comedolytic in the treatment of acne vulgaris (Chapter 69).

(2) **Isotretinoin** (13-c is retinoic acid, Roaccutane) which is used locally and orally as a sebostatic in the treatment of severe acne vulgaris (Chapter 69).

(3) **Etretinate** (a derivative of tretinoin, Tigason) and **acetretin** (a metabolite of

etretinate, Neotigason) which are used orally as inhibitors of keratinization and of cell proliferation in the treatment of psoriasis (Chapter 69). They have also been used in the prevention and treatment of skin tumours in certain groups of people with high genetic predisposition to such tumours. Finally, they have been used to treat mycosis fungoides, basal cell carcinoma of the skin, oral leukoplakia and superficial bladder tumours.

VITAMIN D: Chapter 68.

VITAMIN E (Alpha tocopherol): This vitamin is present in soya bean oil, wheat germ oil, rice germ oil and in green leaves of lettuce. Natural vitamin E is d-alpha tocopherol in contrast to the synthetic vitamin E which dl-alpha tocopherol. The former is more bioavailable and is retained longer than the latter. The daily requirement of vitamin E is 3-15 mg.

In lower animals such as rats its prolonged deprivation leads to sterility in the male and abortion and foetal resorption in the female. In gunieapigs, vitamin E deficiency gives rise to dystrophy of the cardiac and the skeletal muscle. Some experimental evidence indicates that vitamin E is important in maintaining the integrity and the stability of biological membranes. Thus, it is essential for the maintenance of normal structure and function of the nervous system. Vitamin E deficiency is characterised by low serum levels and increased fragility of RBCs to hydrogen peroxide. These may occur particularly in low birth weight infants and in patients with prolonged malabsorption of fats from various causes such as cystic fibrosis and obstructive jaundice. Infants fed commercial formula milk high in polyunsaturated fatty acids (PUFA) can develop vitamin E deficiency and need supplementation.

Although vitamin E has antioxidant properties, its therapeutic usefulness in preventing cancer or cardiovascular disease is not established.

VITAMIN K : Chapter 32.

Water Soluble Vitamins

Vitamin B Complex group includes thiamine, riboflavine, nicotinic acid, pyridoxine, pantothenic acid, inositol, biotin, methionine, folic acid and cyanocobalamin.

THIAMINE (Aneurine, vitamin B1): This was the first member of the B complex series identified chemically, and hence the designation, vitamin B1. It can withstand boiling but is easily destroyed by an alkaline solution. Peas, beans, oatmeal, the outer germ layer of the cereal grains, peanuts and mammalian organ meat are rich sources of thiamine. In addition, appreciable amounts are also present in vegetables and fruits.

Physiological functions: Thiamine pyrophosphate, the physiologically active form of vitamin, constitutes the prosthetic group of the decarboxylases involved in the metabolism of pyruvic and alpha-ketoglutaric acids and thus plays an important role in the intermediary carbohydrate metabolism. The daily thiamine requirement is believed to be between 1 to 2 mg.

Thiamine deficiency produces a symptom complex with characteristic neuropathy termed beriberi. Beriberi occurs in three main forms :

- ***Wet beriberi*** characterised by dependent edema and high output cardiac failure;
- ***Infantile beriberi*** which occurs within the first few months of life, with a high output failure, cyanosis, tachycardia, convulsions, anorexia, vomiting, greenish stools and sometimes sudden death as the noteworthy features; and
- ***Dry beriberi,*** which is usually seen in adults and in which peripheral neuritis and muscular atrophy are predominant.

Even though neuropathy in some form is common to all the three varieties, it is the most important manifestation in dry beriberi, while nervousness, increased irritability and depression may occur in all the three types. In addition to beriberi, **Wernicke's**

encephalopathy, characterised by confusion, ophthalmoplegia, nystagamus, tremors and often peripheral neuropathy, is looked upon as a manifestation of severe thiamine deficiency; Korsakoff's psychosis encountered in chronic alcoholics may owe some of its symptoms to the lack of this vitamin and so may the neuritis encountered in pregnancy and pellagra.

Vague symptoms like epigastric pain, anorexia, flatulence, constipation and lethargy or easy fatiguability are also attributed to thiamine deficiency.

Absorption, fate and excretion: Thiamine is incompletely absorbed from the GI tract mainly from the duodenum and the small intestine. It is distributed in all tissues. Approximately 1 mg. of the vitamin is degraded in the tissues per day. Thiamine appears in urine only when the minimal requirements are satisfied and the stores (liver, heart, brain, kidney) are saturated.

Adverse reactions: Thiamine administered orally usually does not evoke any adverse effects. Administration of large dose by IM / IV route, however, may result in anaphylactoid shock. Large doses may also interfere with the metabolism of other members of B complex group. Except in the initial treatment of acute wet beriberi, there is no justification for exceeding the dose of 100 mg. daily, parenterally.

Preparations and dosage:

(i) Thiamine hydrochloride tablet contains 5 to 50 mg. of the drug. Dose: prophylactic, 2 to 5 mg. daily; therapeutic 25 to 100 mg daily.

(ii) Thiamine hydrochloride injection. Dose: 25-100 mg. SC or IM.

Therapeutic uses: Thiamine deficiency can be prevented by improvement in the dietary intake and by preventing overmilling of cereals, particularly rice. Acute wet beriberi responds dramatically to oral or parenteral administration of thiamine. Treatment is initiated with 20 to 50 mg. of thiamine, given parenterally. A maintenance dose of 5 to 10 mg. is given subsequently by mouth. Within a few hours of thiamine therapy, diuresis starts and most of the edema fluid is eliminated within 48 to 72 hours.

In dry beriberi, it is advisable to use thiamine with other members of vitamin B complex. Alcoholic and pregnancy neuritis respond well to the oral administration of 5 to 10 mg. of thiamine daily. In Wernicke's encephalopathy, a dose of 50 mg. is usually advocated; improvement is rapid, particularly in ophthalmoplegia. In contrast, the neuritis of Korsakoff's psychosis may respond slowly.

RIBOFLAVINE (Vitamin B2): Riboflavine occurs as yellow or orange yellow crystals; it is heat stable.

It is present in the liver, kidney, meat, eggs, milk, yeast and green vegetables. In plants, it is present as a greenish fluorescent pigment. The daily riboflavine requirement in an adult is 1.5 to 3 mg. and in a child 0.6 to 2 mg.

Physiological functions : The physiologically active form of riboflavine is formed by phosphorylation. The two coenzymes flavin mononucleotide (FMN) and flavine adenine dinucleotide (FAD), which contain this active form, play an important role in transfer of hydrogen and in oxidation of carbohydrates, amino acids and other products of metabolism.

Riboflavine deficiency in man is characterised by angular stomatitis, glossitis, a peculiar magenta pigmentation of the tongue and cheilosis (loss of epithelium at the mucocutaneous junction of lips resulting in reddened, shiny and denuded lips); the other features are seborrheic follicular keratosis of the nasolabial folds, nose and forehead, dermatitis of the ano-gential region and 'burning feet'. Certain ocular manifestations such as conjunctivitis, blepharospasm, photophobia, burning, lacrimation and vascularization of the cornea leading to diminution in visual acuity are seen in some cases.

Absorption, fate and excretion : Riboflavine is synthesized in the large intestine, but whether it is available for absorption is uncertain.

Riboflavine and FMN are readily absorbed

from the gut. Phosphorylation of riboflavine to the active form occurs in the intestinal wall, liver and erythrocytes. Excess of vitamin B2 is stored in liver and kidneys. Only 9 per cent of the orally administered dose appears in urine; the metabolic fate of the remainder is not known. Riboflavine administered by oral or parenteral route, does not produce any significant toxic effects. Excess of riboflavine imparts yellow colour and fluorescence to the urine.

Preparations and dosage:

(i) Riboflavine tablet contains 2 mg. of the vitamin. Dose: prophylactic, 1 to 4 mg. daily; therapeutic, 5 to 10 mg. daily.

(ii) Riboflavine injection 10 mg. of riboflavine per ml. Dose: 2-5 mg. daily SC or IM.

Therapeutic uses : In the treatment of ariboflavinosis, the vitamin is given daily in the dose of 2 to 10 mg., in combination with other members of vitamin B group.

NICOTINIC ACID AND NICOTINAMIDE

(Vitamin B_3): This vitamin, also termed as pellagra preventing factor (PPF), is a simple organic acid. Its amide, nicotinamide, is also equally effective in the treatment of pellagra. Nicotinic acid is present in large quantities in rice polishings, liver, milk, eggs and lean meat, and to a smaller extent in potatoes and in vegetables. It is also synthesized from tryptophan in the intestines and in the tissues. The normal daily requirement is 15-20 mg.

Physiological functions and pharmacological actions: Nicotinic acid as nicotinamide adenine dinucleotide (NAD) and its phosphate (NADP) is the constituent of a number of coenzymes involved in the metabolism of proteins necessary for cellular respiration.

• ***Pellagra,*** a symptom complex due to deficiency of nicotinic acid, occurs endemically in individuals subsisting mainly on a diet of maize. The latter has poor nicotinic acid and tryptophan content. Non-endemic pellagra occurs in chronic alcoholism, malabsorption syndrome, carcinoid syndrome, liver cirrhosis, poorly controlled diabetes mellitus, and in cachexia secondary to malignancy.

The characteristic features are dermatitis and pigmentation of the skin, especially in regions exposed to sunlight and at various pressure points, anorexia, lethargy, stomatitis, glossitis, diarrhoea, mental confusion (dementia) and a megaloblastic anemia. Hallucinations and other mental abnormalities may occur and spinal cord degeneration leading to spastic paraplegia rarely develops as a complication.

Nicotinic acid deficiency is the major cause of pellagra. Folic acid deficiency is probably responsible for the megaloblastic anemia. Deficiency of riboflavine which is necessary for the conversion of tryptophan into nicotinic acid, and of pyridoxine; may account for the cheilosis, stomatitis, dermatitis, vaginitis and proctitis.

• ***Vascular smooth muscle actions:*** Nicotinic acid, causes peripheral vasodilatation by direct relaxation of the vascular smooth muscle and causes flushing. This may be accompanied by pruritus.

• ***Serum lipids:*** Large doses of nicotinic acid lower the serum cholesterol and trigyceride levels and activate fibrinolysis (Chapter 39). Nicotinamide is devoid of these effects.

Absorption, fate and excretion: Both nicotinic acid and nicotinamide are readily absorbed from the GI tract and from parenteral sites. They are distributed to all the tissues. Inactivation occurs mainly by N-methylation and to some extent by conjugation, and the products are eliminated in the urine. The vitamin may appear in urine in the active form if large doses are given orally.

Adverse reactions: Besides flushing, urticaria and pruritus, **large doses** may cause furunculosis and other skin lesions, malaise, GI disturbances, activation of peptic ulcer, amblyopia, impairment of liver function and jaundice, decrease in glucose tolerance and hyperuricemia. Nicotinic acid may potentiate the action of vasodilator drugs.

Preparations and dosage:

(i) Nicotinic acid tablet 50 mg. Dose: prophylactic 15 to 30 mg. daily; therapeutic, 50 to 250 mg. daily.

(ii) Nicotinamide tablet 50 mg. Dose: similar to nicotinic acid.

Therapeutic uses:

● ***Pellagra:*** Nicotinic acid or its amide is used in the treatment of pellagra in the daily dose of 50 to 500 mg. Usually, nicotinamide is preferred because of its lack of adverse effects. If the patient is unable to accept oral medication, nicotinamide may be administered parenterally. Therapy with the vitamin produces a striking improvement in the mental, dermal and alimentary manifestations within 24 hours. The neuropathy and the lesions of face and lips, however, may need adjuvant treatment with riboflavine.

● ***As a vasodilator:*** Nicotinic acid, in the dose of 100 to 300 mg. by subcutaneous or oral route, has been employed as a vasodilator in the treatment of Meniere's disease and in peripheral vascular disorders including chilblains and frostbite.

● ***Hyperlipidemia:*** Large doses of the vitamin (3 to 6 g. daily) lower blood lipids (Chapter 39).

PYRIDOXINE (Vitamin B_6): Pyridoxine, pyridoxal and pyridoxamine are collectively called as vitamin B_6. It is present in yeast, cereals, legumes, milk, meat etc. All the three forms are converted in the body to pyridoxal phosphate which is the physiologically active form. The daily requirement is estimated at 1-2 mg.

Physiological functions: Pyridoxal phosphate acts as a coenzyme for amino acid decarboxylases and transaminases. It is thus intimately involved in the synthesis and degradation of biogenic amines like the catecholamines, 5-HT and other important compounds like GABA.

A syndrome in infants secondary to ingestion of proprietary milk preparation deficient in pyridoxine has been described. The characteristic features include irritability, abdominal distension, twitching, failure to gain weight, hypochromic microcytic anemia and convulsions. The anemia is probably due to inadequate utilization of iron for erythropoiesis. Pyridoxine deficiency in adults may lead to lesions of the skin and mouth resembling those seen in ariboflavinosis and pellagra, to peripheral neuritis and to mental changes. Convulsions and hypochromic microcytic anemia have also been observed.

Vitamin B_6 deficiency may cause abnormal GTT.

Absorption, fate and excretion: All the three forms of the vitamin are readily absorbed from the GI tract. The end product of metabolism, 4-pyridoxic acid, is eliminated in urine.

Adverse reactions : Pyridoxine, administered in physiological doses, does not produce any adverse effects. Administration of large doses has been reported to cause peripheral sensory neuropathy and ataxia. Pyridoxine interferes with therapeutic effect of levodopa (Chapter 14).

Preparations and dosage:

(i) Pyridoxine tablet 5 mg.. Dose: 5 to 10 mg. daily.

(ii) Pyridoxine injection. Dose: 25-100 mg. IM or IV.

Therapeutic uses:

● ***Convulsions due to pyridoxine deficiency in infants:*** 4 mg/kg/day for short periods.

● ***Anemia due to pyridoxine deficiency :*** 50-150 mg/ day in divided doses.

● ***Pellagra:*** As an adjuvant in the dose of 5-10 mg/day.

● ***Vomiting of pregnancy, post irradiation vomiting*** (Chapter 40).

● ***Mental depression during oral contraceptive therapy*** (Chapter 66).

● ***INH and alcohol induced peripheral neuritis*** (Chapter 52 and 6).

● ***Penicillamine induced optic neuritis.***

PANTOTHENIC ACID (Vitamin B_7): This is an organic acid which serves its physiological function by being converted into coenzyme A. Yeast, wheat, peanuts, cereals, milk and liver contain large amounts of pantothenic acid. The daily human requirement of pantothenic acid is estimated to be below 5 mg.

Physiological actions: Coenzyme A is involved in several fundamental biological reactions. In general, all the acetylation reactions are influenced by this enzyme.

Pantothenic acid deficiency in human beings under normal circumstances is not known. In animals, deficiency of the vitamin results in keratitis, dermatitis, arrest of growth, depigmentation of hair, neuromuscular degeneration and fatal bilateral adrenal hemorrhage. Artificial deficiency produced in human volunteers by administration of a low vitamin diet containing a pantothenic acid antagonist is characterised by fatigue, malaise, headache, somnolence, paraesthesiae, nausea, occasional vomiting, abdominal cramps and flatulence.

Absorption, fate and excretion: The vitamin remains stable in foodstuffs for long periods and little is destroyed during cooking. Pantothenic acid is rapidly absorbed from the gut and is concentrated in liver, heart and kidneys. It is mainly excreted in the urine.

Pantothenic acid is non-toxic and does not possess any other known pharmacological actions.

Preparations and dosage:

(i) Calcium pantothenate: 10 mg. tablets. Dose: 10 to 50 mg.

(ii) Dexpanthenol: This analogue of pantothenic acid is readily converted to the parent compound on administration. It is given by IM or IV injection in the dose of 250 to 500 mg. For topical application, 2 to 5% cream/ ointment are available.

Therapeutic uses: Calcium pantothenate has been employed in post-operative paralytic ileus and as a nutritional supplement along with other members of the B-complex group. Dexpanthenol has been employed systemically for the prevention and treatment of post-operative intestinal atony and topically for various skin lesions including burns, wounds and ulcers; their utility in these conditions, however, is doubtful.

BIOTIN: Biotin is an organic acid which functions as a coenzyme for numerous carboxylation reactions. Biotin deficiency is not encountered naturally in humans but has been produced in human volunteers by administering a diet containing large amounts of raw egg white or avidin. It is characterised by seborrheic dermatitis, lassitude, anorexia and paraesthesiae. The daily human requirement of the vitamin is unknown. The vitamin is synthesized by the intestinal flora. As a clinical deficiency syndrome has not been demonstrated clearly so far, the vitamin does not have any rational therapeutic application.

Miscellaneous: These include **inositol, choline, methionine** and **para-aminobenzoic acid (PABA).** Choline and methionine, the so called "lipotropic factors", have been used in the treatment of liver cirrhosis; inositol has been used in the management of diseases associated with the metabolism of fat. This is based on the observation that experimental deficiency of these substances in animals causes fatty livers. Their efficacy in human conditions is, however, equivocal. Methionine is used to treat acute paracetamol poisoning when acetyl cysteine is not available (Chapter 11).

For **folic acid** and **vitamin B_{12}**, see Chapter 34.

ASCORBIC ACID (Vitamin C): The dietary sources of ascorbic acid include citrus fruits, tomatoes, plants, potatoes and green vegetables. One ml. of lemon juice contains about 0.5 mg. of this vitamin. Lemon juice as a sole source of this vitamin is not reliable and was the cause of an outbreak of scurvy in thc North Pole Expedition of 1875. Although cereals and other seeds are devoid of vitamin C, they produce it on germination. Levo compound is more active. Vitamin C is unstable and is destroyed by boiling and by alkali.

Physiological actions: Ascorbic acid, along with its oxidation product dehydroascorbic acid, is intimately involved in biological oxidation-reduction reactions and in cellular respiration. Ascorbic acid is essential for the functional integrity of sulfhydryl group of enzymes and also for the formation of collagen and intercellular matrix, and hence, for the development of cartilage, bone and teeth and for healing of wounds. It influences the formation of hemoglobin, erythrocyte maturation, certain immunological reactions of the body and the conversion of folic acid to tetrahydrofolate.

Ascorbic acid is involved in carbohydrate metabolism and in the oxidation of phenylalanine and tyrosine. Scorbutic animals exhibit hyperglycemia, lowered glucose tolerance and resistance to insulin.

Ascorbic acid deficiency leads to the development of scurvy. The characteristic features in adults are perifollicular hemorrhages, petechiae, ecchymoses, particularly in "saddle areas" and posterior thighs, hemorrhages in subcutaneous tissues, muscles and joints; swollen, inflamed, bleeding and spongy gums and normocytic or microcytic anemia. In infants, loss of appetite, listlessness and subperiosteal hemorrhages leading to tenderness and restriction of limb movements are the cardinal features. Ecchymoses and gum changes similar to adult scurvy may also be seen. Infantile scurvy is usually seen in bottle-fed babies as human milk contains appreciable amounts of ascorbic acid.

Patients suffering from extensive burns and those suffering from malabsorption syndrome may also develop ascorbic acid deficiency.

Absorption, fate and excretion: Ascorbic acid is synthesized in the liver by majority of the animals except man and guineapigs and hence, deficiency of ascorbic acid can be produced in these two species.

The minimum daily requirement of ascorbic acid for an adult is about 30 mg. and for infants, 5 mg. per kg. of body weight.

Ascorbic acid is readily absorbed from the gastrointestinal tract. After absorption, it circulates in the plasma and is concentrated in the glandular tissues. The leucocyte and the platelet levels of ascorbic acid are higher than the corresponding plasma levels.

Ascorbic acid is partly metabolized and excreted in urine as oxalate and a part is eliminated in the free form. Urinary excretion depends upon saturation of body stores and in individuals with ascorbic acid deficiency, the vitamin may not appear in urine even on administration of large doses.

In ordinary doses, ascorbic acid is essentially non-toxic. Vitamin C in urine gives a false positive test for sugar while using Benedict's test and a false negative test while using glucose oxidase test.

Preparations and dosage:

(i) Ascorbic acid tablet contains 50 mg. Dose: Prophylactic, 25 to 75 mg. daily; therapeutic 200 to 500 mg. daily.

(ii) Ascorbic acid injection: 0.1-1 g. IM/IV

Adverse reactions: Prolonged ingestion of large quantities of vitamin C is known to lead to increased urinary excretion of oxalate with stone formation and kidney damage. Rebound scurvy may occur in the offspring of mothers taking high doses; and similar phenomenon is observed when a person habitually taking large amounts of vitamin C suddenly stops taking it.

Therapeutic uses:

- ***Scurvy:*** In the treatment of scurvy, ascorbic acid is administered in the dose of 100 to 500 mg. per day. As a prophylactic measure, it is important to ensure adequate Vitamin C intake in infancy and old age. Infantile scurvy can be prevented by adding 5 mg. of the vitamin to the feeds of bottle-fed infants. For prophylactic purposes, a daily dose of 50-100 mg. is advocated in adults. Ascorbic acid increases the absorption of iron from the GI tract by facilitating the conversion of ferric into ferrous form.

• ***Methemoglobinemia:*** Because of its ability to function as a reducing agent, ascorbic acid in the daily dose of 300 to 600 mg is used in the treatment of methemoglobinemia; it is, however, less effective than methylene blue.

The vitamin is also used as an antioxidant in emulsions of fats and oils, in certain injections and eye drops, and as a preservative.

Its use in large doses in the prevention and treatment of common cold has not been substantiated. It has been used empirically in a wide variety of conditions including nonspecific hemorrhagic states, anemia and dental infections, without clear benefit.

Multivitamin Combinations: *Prophylactic multivitamin preparations* should contain from one-half to one and one-half times the recommended dietary allowances (Table 75.2) except for vitamin D which should not exceed the daily recommended dietary allowance. Larger doses of ascorbic acid and B-complex in such preparations are wasteful, though not harmful. *Multivamin pills may be useful in old people, who for some reasons cannot get adequate nutrition*, and during recovery from acute illnesses.

Table 75.2: Recommended dietary allowances (RDA) of various vitamins per day for adults

Vitamins	Recommended by *ICMR (for Indians)	Recommended by WHO/FAO Expert Group
Thiamine	1.2-2.0mg	1.0-1.5mg
Riboflavin	1.3-2.2mg	1.3-2.1mg
Pyridoxine	--	1.5-2.0mg
Niacin	16-26mg	---
Vitamin B_{12}	1 µg	2 µg
Folate	100µg	200µg
VitaminC	50mg	30mg
VitaminA	750µg	750µg
VitaminD	5 µg (200 I.U.)	2.5µg (100 I.U.)

*ICMR--Indian Council of Medical Research

Routine prophylactic supplementation of vitamin D should be avoided in young, healthy persons.

Multivitamin preparations for therapeutic uses may contain 4-5 times the recommended dietary allowances. Selective deficiency of a single vitamin B factor occurs less commonly and hence, combined B-complex therapy is commonly employed prophylactically as well as therapeutically in the management of generalised avitaminosis. Multivitamin therapeutic preparations should be used only for deficiency states and during periods of increased vitamin requirement. Used indiscriminately as dietary supplements to 'keep up the energy and strength', they act no better than placebos, are wasteful and may even be harmful. Further, some of these preparations are quite expensive as they contain large doses of water soluble vitamins most of which are washed out in the urine within 24 hours.

Vitamins A, C and E, and many carotenoids have been shown to be effective antioxidants, and experimentally some of these have been shown to *scavenge free radicals* when used in pharmacological doses. However, *their therapeutic role in preventing diseases such as cancer, atherosclerosis and diabetes mellitus in humans has not yet been established.*

Megavitamin therapy is the administration of doses which are several fold the amounts required for normal body metabolism. Such therapy has been advocated in a variety of disorders; as yet, there is no evidence that, except in a few well defined inherited metabolic diseases, such megavitamin therapy is of benefit. Patients may take abnormal doses of vitamins as a pathological feature of a psychiatric disorder (perhaps an eating disorder) or they may take them in a misguided attempt to treat a psychiatric illness. In either case, the toxicity of the vitamin may exacerbate the psychiatric illness. In some countries, injectable and oral combinations of large doses of vitamins B_1, B_6 and B_{12} are promoted; their use is irrational.

Antioxidants

Chemically, oxidation is the removal of electrons and reduction is the gain of electrons; oxidation is always coupled with reduction. Many biological oxidations can take place without the participation of molecular oxygen, e.g., dehydrogenations. Further, molecular oxygen has very little capability to oxidize other chemicals. Instead, it must first be converted to an 'active' form called reactive species of oxygen (an oxidant). Many of the reactive oxygen species are free radicals but all are not e.g. singlet oxygen and hydrogen peroxide are not free radicals. A free radical is an atom or a molecule with one or more unpaired electrons. Its tendency to acquire electron(s) from other substances makes it highly reactive. Table 75.3 lists the reactive oxygen species in the animal body.

Table 75.3: Reactive oxygen species

Symbol	Name
$^1O_2$	Singlet oxygen
$O^•$	Superoxide free radical
$OH^•$	Hydroxyl free radical
$RO^•$	Alkoxyl free radical
$ROO^•$	Peroxyl free radical
H_2O_2	Hydrogen peroxide
LOOH	Lipid peroxide.

These oxidants (reactive oxygen species) are generated during the normal metabolic reactions in the body. For example, when molecular oxygen is reduced to water by cytochrome oxidase, four electrons are acquired, one at a time (univalent reductions); the intermediates in that process are highly reactive oxygen species. The other sources of free radicals and other oxidants in the animal body are shown in Table 75.4.

Table 75.4: Sources of oxidants in the body

- ***Cyclooxygenation.***
- ***Lipooxygenation.***
- ***Lipid peroxidation*** (auto-oxidation on exposure to oxygen).
- ***Neutrophils*** stimulated by exposure to microbes.
- ***Re-perfusion of ischemic organs.***
- ***Metabolism of xenobiotics*** (foreign chemicals) including alcohol, cigarette smoke and motor car exhaust; and
- ***Ultraviolet and ionizing radiation damage.***

Small amounts of reactive oxygen species are continually formed in the cell membrane and close to the cell organelles. They act where they are generated. Hence, they can damage most cell structures including membrane lipids, proteins, enzymes and nucleic acids. However the body has inbuilt mechanisms to mop up the small amounts of oxidants normally formed during metabolic reactions (Table 75.5).

Reactive species formed in controlled amounts by neutrophil leucocytes on exposure

Table 75.5: Body defences against oxidants

- ***Intracellular enzymes*** (catalases, superoxide dismutases, glutathione peroxidases) which dispose of the oxidants.
- ***Antioxidants obtained along with nutrients***

  Vitamins A, C, E.

  Trace elements: selenium.

  Flavinoids and polyphenolic substances present in plant foods (fruits, vegetables, amla, tea, garlic and others).

  Others present in spices such as coriander, clove, cardamom and so on.

to microbes are beneficial to the body in that they participate in destroying the microbes. Excess of oxidants, however, can be harmful to the body. In fact, it has been proposed from epidemiological studies that free radicals and other oxidants may be involved in the pathogenesis of diseases such as cancer, diabetes mellitus, cardiovascular and neurological diseases. Attempts have been made to make a case for supplementation of human diet with antioxidants given as pharmacological agents. *Currently, there is no pharmacological antioxidant agent available which has been convincingly shown to be useful in prevention or treatment of disease in humans.* Hence, the **current recommendation** is to increase the consumption of cereals, pulses, nuts, fruits and vegetables, all of which are good sources of antioxidants. There is some evidence to indicate that increased fruit and vegetable intake raises plasma concentration of α and β carotene, lycopene, b cryptoxanthine and ascorbic acid and decreases both diastolic and systolic blood pressure. For vitamin E, see earlier.

Coenzyme Q10 (Ubiquinone) : This is a fat-soluble antioxidant, currently sold as a dietary supplement. The humans synthesize as well as obtain it from dietary sources. It is present in the mitochondria of human cells, and high concentrations are found in the heart, liver, kidney and skeletal muscle. Tissue concentrations decline with age. Coenzyme Q10 is involved in ATP generation. The usual dose is 100-200 mg/day in divided doses. It has been reported to be of some benefit in many conditions including Parkinson's disease and CHF. The drug is well tolerated and the adverse reactions are mild, comprising nausea, vomiting and abdominal discomfort. It may decrease response to warfarin. Its place in therapeutics needs further substantiation

Spirulina: This product, obtained from the marine algae, has been promoted as the "most powerful food on earth." It is claimed to contain 70% by weight of protein and many micronutrients. The daily dose recommended by the manufacturer is 2 tablets (each containing 500 mg of spirulina). This dose contains only 700 mg of protein and miniscule quantities of micronutrients, much below their Recommended Daily Allowance (RDA). Hence, the claim of the manufacturer is unjustified, and this expensive product cannot be recommended.

Immunotherapy, Immunosuppressants and Immunostimulants

76

Whereas the 'fight or flight' response by an animal to external danger preserves its integrity at the macro level, its safety from bodily invasion (external, by microbes; or internal, by errant cancer cells) at the micro level and survival depends upon the immune system. The science of immunology is all about the response of an animal's body to invading 'foreign' antigens and consequences (usually beneficial but occasionally detrimental) of that response. New knowledge and technology have helped the science of immunology to expand its original scope, preventive inoculation, to other areas such as diagnostics, allergy, autoimmunity, organ transplantation and therapeutics including that of cancer.

Antigens may be classified, from the point of view of an animal, as 'self' and 'non-self or foreign;" antigens in 'dysregulated' tissues (tumours) can also be regarded as foreign. **Immunity** may be defined as the ability of an animal's body to react to a foreign antigen and eliminate it, in the interest of safety of the animal. As described in Chapter 2, immunity is of two types: (a) innate or natural; and (b) adaptive or acquired. Both work closely together and are mediated by cells which constitute the Immune System. **Innate immunity** is not dependent upon prior antigen exposure (priming), is primitive and of relatively low affinity, but is broadly reactive. The **effectors** of innate immunity are: complement, granulocytes, monocytes/ macrophages, natural killer (NK) cells, mast cells and basophils. By contrast, **adaptive immunity** is antigen-specific, depends on antigen priming, and can be of very high affinity. Its **mediators** are the lymphocytes, T and B types. The innate immune system is most active early in an immune response whereas the adaptive immunity becomes progressively dominant over time. The immune cells learn at an early stage in fetal life how to discriminate between self and foreign antigens, and do not attack the former. Serious consequences may follow if that ability is impaired or lost at any time in life so that the immune cells attack and damage the animal's own tissues (**autoimmune disease**); however it is actively and beneficially suppressed during pregnancy, so that the fetus, a mass of foreign antigens, is not rejected.

Immunological agents, which produce immunity, are used to prevent or modify certain infectious diseases. That some of these agents have been spectacularly successful is attested by the remarkable decline of diseases such as small-pox, cholera, and poliomyelitis.

Immunity is subdivided into:

I **Active immunity;** and

II **Passive immunity.**

Active immunity : This type of immunity is due to the development of antibodies by the individual himself. It can be natural and species specific e.g. the relative immunity of horses, dogs and rats to tuberculosis, or it can be acquired by introduction of an antigen.

Passive immunity: Immunity acquired by the transfer of antibodies from a donor to a recipient, is called passive immunity. It can be acquired naturally e.g., by a foetus receiving maternal antibodies across the placenta, or artificially by the administration of antisera containing **immunoglobulin** (Ig) antibodies.

The various preparations employed for conferring immunity are :

- ***Vaccines:*** Vaccines are suspensions of dead microorganisms (inactivated vaccines) or attenuated but live microorganisms (live vaccines) which stimulate the immune system of the receipient, resulting in the development of either CMI e.g. BCG vaccine or humoral immunity from protective antibodies e.g. typhoid vaccine. Vaccines are employed prophylactically and are of no value if administered during the incubation period or in the active stage of a disease. In general, live, attenuated vaccines are antigenically more potent than the inactivated vaccines. Live vaccines generally achieve almost lifelong immunity with a single dose (but multiple doses are required with polio vaccine and typhoid vaccine). Inactivated vaccines require a 'primary course' of doses, followed by repeated booster doses. Viral vaccines are either live or inactivated. BCG vaccine (against tuberculosis) is the only live bacterial vaccine; all other bacterial vaccines are either inactivated vaccines or toxoids.

The antibody response occurs after 7-10 days. Initially, antibodies are usually of IgM type, followed later by IgG antibodies. IgG antibodies are produced in high concentrations, and are mainly responsible for resistance to infection.

Many viral vaccines contain traces of antibiotics used in their preparation. Such vaccines may have to be withheld from individuals known to be allergic to the antibiotic concerned. Further, they should be avoided in individuals on corticosteroid therapy or immunosuppressive drugs and in those with impaired immune responses.

- ***Toxoids:*** Toxoids are produced by addition of formalin to the toxins of microorganisms and incubating them at 37ºC for 3 to 4 weeks. This results in loss of toxicity without reduction of the antigenicity. Toxoids are more immunogenic if adsorbed onto an adjuvant.

- ***Nucleic acid vaccines :*** Recently, nucleic acid vaccines, mainly DNA-vaccines have been developed. They have many advantages — they are safer, stable and heat-resistant. They all are genetically engineered and induce both humoral immunity and CMI including cytotoxic T cells. The immunity persists for prolonged periods.

- ***Immune animal serum*** (antiserum) : This is the serum obtained from animals like horse and rabbit which have been injected with a vaccine, either a toxin or a toxoid. The sera of such animals contain antibodies either against the microorganisms or their toxins.

Antisera containing antibodies against the toxins of C. diphtheriae, Cl. tetani and Cl. welchii are used widely.

- ***Immune human sera:*** These are derived from convalescent, immune or hyperimmunized adults, eg, human, hyperimmune antitetanus serum.

- **Immunoglobulin Ig** (Human): Formerly termed as gamma globulin, this agent is a refined product prepared from pooled human blood plasma having a high antibody titre. Placentae of mothers immunized by the administration of a toxoid a few weeks before delivery have also been used as a source.

- ***Monoclonal antibodies*** (see later).

Active Immunization

This may be primary or secondary.

- ***Primary immunization*** is commonly carried out in infants and in children to induce primary immunity and consists of administering two or more doses of the vaccine or the toxoid at suitable intervals. A mixture of 2 or more agents e.g., vaccine-toxoid mixtures such as diphtheria and tetanus toxoid with whooping cough vaccine, is employed commonly for primary immunization.

- ***Secondary immunization*** is carried out to reinforce the primary immunity by giving a single 'booster' or 'recall' dose of the antigen.

All vaccines and antisera should be stored at temperature recommended by the manufacturer. Otherwise, the preparation may become denatured and ineffective. Refrigerator storage at 2-8°C is usually necessary. Multi-dose vials without any preservative, once opened, should be used within 1 hour and those with a preservative within 3 hours.

Adverse reactions to vaccines are generally mild and consists of local tenderness, erythema, induration, fever, arthralgia and malaise. Allergic reactions are not common but can occur particularly if the organisms are grown on foreign protein material. Any vaccine produced from the organisms grown in chick embryo culture is contraindicated in patients allergic to eggs, chicken or chicken feathers. Allergic reactions can also occur due to other components of the vaccine such as preservatives, antibotics and stabilizers such as gelatin.

Generally, vaccines (particularly those containing live organisms) are not administered in the presence of a severe acute illness, in patients with debilitating diseases or agammaglobulinemia and in patients receiving immunosuppressive agents or radiotherapy. Corticosteroids may induce immunosuppression that reduces the ability to respond to a killed vaccine or enhance the susceptibility to live vaccines which could result in disseminated disease. Live virus vaccines are usually avoided during pregnancy for fear of infecting the fetus; however, such risk has not been substantiated.

Although vaccination may be avoided during severe acute illnesses, mild upper and lower respiratory tract infections and other mild illnesses are no more considered as contraindications. In fact, it is now recommended that children with minor illnesses should be vaccinated regardless of the degree of fever. Prematurity does not increase the incidence of vaccine-induced adverse reactions.

The vaccines and toxoids employed for active immunization are listed in Table 76.1 and 76.2. Dosage schedules recommended by the manufacturer should be followed.

BCG VACCINE: Discussed in Chapter 52.

MMR VACCINE (Tresivac) : The contraindications to MMR vaccine include children with altered immunity and those on high doses of corticosteroids or immunosuppressants. It is avoided in children who have received another live virus by injection within the past three weeks. If it is given to an adult woman, pregnancy should be avoided for a month; the vaccine should not be given within 3 months of an immunoglobulin injection.

POLIOMYELITIS VACCINES: **The Salk vaccine** induces only limited resistance to growth of the virus in the intestine and thus, does not affect the carrier state (excretion of the virus in feces). The vaccine is given by SC or IM injection, 3 doses each of 0.5 ml., at an interval of 4 to 6 weeks between the 1st and the 2nd dose, and 12 months between the 2nd and the 3rd. Adverse effects are usually mild and consist of local pain, induration and fever.

The **Sabin vaccine** (OPV), in addition to systemic immunity, provides a local resistance (intestinal immunity) to reinfection by the poliovirus by inducing mucosal secretion of IgA antibodies. This leads to stoppage of fecal excretion of the virus and consequent elimination of the carrier state.

In contrast to the situation in the West, three doses of OPV do not provide immunity, especially to poliovirus type 3, in 100% of infants, in the developing countries including India. Further, the median age of poliomyelitis in India is from 12 to 18 months; this means that about half the cases occur between about 6 and 12-18 months of age. It is thus important to complete the primary immunisation before the age for greatest risk of poliomyelitis. Hence, the

Table 76.1: Bacterial vaccines and toxoids

Vaccine /Toxoid	Immunizing agent	Route	Adverse reactions	Efficacy and remarks
		Bacterial vaccines		
BCG	Live attenuated M. bovis	ID	Fever; regional adenitis	75-80% against military and meningeal TB; controversial in other forms
Pertussis	(a) Inactivated bacterial antigen (b) Acellular	IM	Local reaction	80-90%. Combined with diphtheria and tetanus vaccines – DPT
Typhoid	Whole cell, killed bacteria*	IM	Fever; local swelling	50-70%; short lived
Typhoid oral (Typhoral)	Live mutant bacilli TY2IA	Oral	Mild GI disturbance; fever	50-70%
Typhoid (Vi)	Vi capsular polysaccharide	IM; SC	Local reaction	70-75%; single dose per course
Cholera	Inactivated bacteria	SC; IM	Fever; swelling	50%; short lived;3-4 months
Cholera (oral)	Do. (El tor strain)	Oral	None	50%; protection 3 years
Plague	Inactivated bacteria	IM	Fever; swelling	90% antibody response; efficacy variable
Anthrax	Inactivated, avirulent bacteria	SC	No serious reaction	90% antibody response; efficacy variable
		Bacterial toxoids		
Diphtheria	Inactivated toxins	IM	Local reactions	95%-98% } Can be combined
Tetanus	Inactivated toxins	IM	Local reactions	95%-98%
H. influenzae type B (Hib)	Bacterial polysaccharide	IM; SC	Local reaction	90%; not beyond 6th birthday
Meningococci A,C,Y,W135	Bacterial polysaccharide	SC	Local reaction	90%; given after 2nd birthday
Pneumococci, 7-valent	Bacterial polysaccharide	IM; SC	Local reaction	60-80%
		Rickettsial vaccine		
Typhus vaccine	Killed organisms	SC	Allergic reactions	High

ID= Intradermal. SC = Subcutaneous. IM = Intramuscular * = *Not available*

Table 76.2: Viral and rickettsial vaccines

Vaccine /Toxoid	Immunizing agent	Route	Adverse reactions	Efficacy and remarks
Viral vaccines				
Varicella (Chicken pox)	Live attenuated virus	IM	Local reaction	95%; CMI lasts longer
Measles	Live attenuated virus	SC	? Encephalopathy	95% } Usually given as MMR (Trevisac)
Mumps	Live attenuated virus	SC	Parotitis	90%
Rubella	Live attenuated virus	SC	Arthralgia	95%
Poliomyelitis:				
Sabin (Trival-ent, oral OPV)	Live attenuated virus	Oral	Rare, vaccine associated polio	95%; ,may eliminate carrier state
Salk (IPV)	Inactivated virus	SC	Local reaction	95%; does not affect carrier state
Rabies:				
(a) **Semple vaccine**	Inactivated virus	SC	Local reaction; neurological	60-70% response; short lived immunity; multiple complications doses
(b) **Human diploid vaccine**	Inactivated virus	IM; ID	Local reaction; arthritis; angioedema	> 95%; safer
(c) **Purified chick embryo vaccine** (Rabipur)	Inactivated virus	IM	Local reaction; fever; allergy; arthralgia	95%; safer
Hepatitis B (Harvix)	Inactivated viral antigen	IM	Arthralgia	80-95%
Hepatitis B rDNA	rDNA antigen	IM	None	80-95%
Hepatitis A	Killed virus	IM	Fever; arthralgia	95%
Yellow fever	Live attenuated virus	SC	Encephalitis	High; 6-8 years
Japanese B encephalitis	Inactivated virus	SC	Allergic reactions	80-90%
Influenza	Inactivated virus; or virus component	IM	? Neurological	40-60%; efficacy varies due to changes in the infective strain
Rotavirus	Pentavalent	Oral	Diarrhoea	95%
HPV	Multivalent	IM	–	Under evaluation

ID = Intradermal. SC = Subcutaneous. IM = Intramuscular.

current recommendation is to give the first dose of OPV (along with BCG) at birth, and to follow it up with three more doses (along with Triple i.e. DPT antigen) at 6,10 and 14 weeks of age. A booster dose of OPV is given 12-15 months after the last dose of primary immunisation, and another at the time of school entry. Repeated **mass vaccination with OPV** upto the age of 5 years is also recommended (**Pulse Polio Immunization**). Such simultaneous administration of OPV to all susceptible infants and children blocks the circulation of wild poliovirus in the community and can eradicate poliomyelitis.

ROTAVIRUS VACCINE (Rotateq): Rotavirus infects the intestines of virtually all children by the age of 3 years. Public health measures and personal hygiene are unable to prevent the gastroenteritis caused by it. A pentavalent, human-bovine reassortant rotavirus vaccine is now available. It is effective and safe. The oral vaccine is administered in three, monthly doses from the age of 6-12 weeks to the age of 32 weeks. It may cause mild diarrhea or vomiting in some children. It may be given concurrently with other vaccines.

HUMAN PAPILLOMA VIRUS VACCINE (HPV): This virus causes carcinoma of the uterine cervix and genital warts in women. A reassortant vaccine (Gardasil), now available, effectively protects against four HPV types and is safe. It is administered IM to girls/women between the ages of 9 and 26 years in three doses, the second and the third being given 2 and 6 months after the first dose.

RABIES VACCINES: Rabies occurs commonly after the bite of an infected animal such as a dog. Rabies virus can be found in the saliva for upto 7 days before the appearance of signs of illness. Rabies infection can also occur without direct animal contact by inhalation of the virus in bat infested caves or in the laboratory. Although the usual incubation period is 4-6 weeks, a range of 5 days to more than 1 year has been reported.

In endemic areas, it must be emphasized that a bite is not necessary for transmission of the virus and that children must be guarded against contact with unknown animals.

In unvaccinated patients, the mortality from rabies is almost 100%. Although it is never too late to vaccinate, the effect of vaccination decreases sharply with delay in excess of 2 weeks. Immunosuppression by drugs, HIV or chronic liver disease such as cirrhosis could prove rapidly fatal. All rabies vaccines can be used prophylactically in persons suspected to be bitten by a rabid animal. The treatment is started immediately after the bite. *The course may be discontinued if it is proven that the animal is still alive and healthy 10 days after the bite.*

It has been demonstrated that thorough washing of the suspected wound with soap and water alone increases the survival by almost 50%. Local dressing with povidone iodine, ethyl alcohol/methylated spirit is recommended.

The rabies vaccines available are:

1 **Nerve tissue vaccines :**

- ***Semple vaccine:*** This is a sterile suspension of sheep brain substance containing fixed virus of rabies, inactivated by the addition of phenol. The vaccine is given SC into the cellular tissue on the side of the abdominal wall below the costal margin. Immunity conferred by it lasts only for about 3 months, is incomplete and unpredictable.

W.H.O. recommends the dose of 2 ml SC on the lower abdominal wall daily, for 14 consecutive days, with booster doses on days 21, 28 and 91. The dose for a child less than 12 years of age is half or three quarters that of the adult. The Semple vaccine, however, offers protection only in 60-70% of cases even when it is started on the day of the bite. Further, serious neurological complications such as polyneuritis, myelitis and encephalomyelitis can occur occasionally.

2 **Tissue culture vaccines :**

- Purified chick embryo cell rabies vaccine (PCECV1, Rabipur): This vaccine is obtained by

Table 76.3 : Suggested regimens for various rabies vaccines

Vaccine type	Pre-exposure treatment	Post-exposure treatment
1 Semple vaccine (Sheep brain)	See text	See text
2 HDCV (Imovax rabies) 1 ml vial	Three, 1 ml doses IM in deltoid on 0, 7, and 21 or 28 days. Booster after 1year OR 0.1 ml ID for three doses as above	Five doses IM on 0, 3, 7, 14, and 28 days. Use anterolateral thigh in children OR 1 ml in divided doses ID at eight sites (about 0.1 ml per site) on day zero; 0.1 ml at four sites on day 7; and 0.1 ml at one site on days 28 and 91
3 PCECV (Rabipur, Rab-Avort) 1 ml vial	Doses as above	Doses as above
4 PVRV (Verorab) 0.5 ml vial	—	Five, 0.5 ml doses IM, similar to HDCV OR 0.1 ml intradermally at two sites on day 0, 3, 7, and single ID dose given on day 28 and 91. Similar schedule may be used as for HDCV and PCECV using 0.2 ml of PVRV instead of 0.1 ml.

HDCV = human diploid cell vaccine PCECV = Purified chicken embryo cell vaccine
PVRV = Purified Verocell vaccine ID = Intradermal

growing the virus in primary cultures of chick fibroblasts.

- ***Human diploid cell inactivated vaccine*** (HDCV) (Imovax Rabies): This is obtained from human fibroblast culture.
- ***Purified Verocell vaccine,*** (PVRV) (Verorab) grown in verocell line.

Tissue culture vaccines give a better antibody response than the older vaccines. Further, the immunity lasts longer and the vaccine is free from serious adverse reactions. Hence, they are now considered the vaccines of choice. Various vaccine regimens recommended are given in Table 76.3.

All severely bitten persons should be given rabies immunoglobulin (IgG). Human rabies immunoglobulin is safer than the antiserum but is more expensive.

Staff in attendance on a patient who is highly suspected of, or known to be suffering, from rabies should be offered immunisation. Four intradermal doses of 0.1 ml of HDCV given on the same day at different sites is the suggested regimen. *There is no specific contraindication to HDC rabies vaccine.*

HEPATITIS B VACCINE (Engerix B, Shanvac, HB Vac): This vaccine contains

Table 76.4 : Immunization Schedule

Age	Vaccine
Birth	BCG, OPV_0, Hepatitis B_1
6 weeks	DTP_1, OPV_1, Hepatitis B_2, Hib_1 *Pneumococcal Conjugate $Vaccine_1$*
10 weeks	DTP_2, OPV_2 Hib_2 *Pneumococcal Conjugate $Vaccine_2$*
14 weeks	DTP_3, OPV_3, Hepatitis B_3, Hib_3 *Pneumococcal Conjugate $Vaccine_3$*
9 months	Measles
15-18 months	$DTPB_1$, $OPVB_1$, Hib B_1, MMR *Pneumococcal Conjugate Vaccine B* *Hepatitis A Vaccine (after 18 mths)* *Varicella Vaccine (after 15 mths)[$]*
2 years	Typhoid[#] (Only Vi polysaccharide vaccine available in India)
5 years	DTP B_2, $OPVB_2$
10 years	Td_Δ /TT
16 years	Td_Δ /TT

Vaccines in italics = Voluntary B = booster
Hepatitis B_3 can be given at 6 months
Hepatitis A Vaccine 2nd dose after 6-12 months,
[$] If started 13 years and above give 2 doses 4-8 weeks apart
[#] Revaccination every 3 years till 12 years of age
Δ Td preferred to TT; Pregnant women given 2 doses 1 mth. apart
OPV = Oral Polio Vaccine; DTP = Diphtheria, Pertussis, Tetanus Toxoid
Td = Tetanus, Diphtheria; TT = Tetanus Toxoid; Hib = Hemphilus influenzae B
MMR = Mumps, Measles, Rubella
Ref. IAP Guidebook on Immunization 2007 (4th Ed.)

inactivated hepatitis B virus surface antigen (HBsAg). It is now prepared biosynthetically using recombinant DNA technology. Adequate immunity against the infection develops after 6 months and is believed to last for 5-7 years. Immunisation of infants is expected to provide long lasting immunity.

TETANUS TOXOID : After the full course of seven doses (Table 76.4), booster doses need to be given every 10 years only.

During pregnancy, two doses of adsorbed toxoid are administered at 6 weeks interval, in the second trimester, to women not previously immunized; this prevents neonatal tetanus. A single dose is enough in previously immunized pregnant women.

Hypersensitivity reactions are known to occur due to high concentrations of the antibody in persons given too frequent booster doses.

Active immunization programme: A majority of the serious infections with high mortality and morbidity rates can now be successfully prevented by prophylactic immunization. Combined prophylaxis reduces the number of visits, the incidence of adverse reactions and the cost (Table 76.4).

The neonate is naturally immune to a majority of infections because of maternal antibodies; such immunity, however, may last for only the first 6 to 10 months. The newborn does not have any immunity against tuberculosis. Immunoprophylaxis is recommended right from birth so as to build up a substantial active immunity against a number of viral and bacterial infections, within the first few months of life. Ideally, the aim should be to achieve the goal of > 90% vaccination coverage by the 2 years of age. Subsequently, the antibody titre can be maintained/augmented by the 'booster doses' of antigens at regular intervals. The principles of active immunization are given in Table 76.5.

Simultaneous active and passive immunization may be necessary because of imminent exposure to disease. There is little interaction between IgG and inactivated or non-live vaccines e.g. HIV and hepatitis B IgG. *With live virus vaccines e.g. measles vaccine immunity may be compromised by IgG administration;* so vaccination should be repeated after 3 months, unless specific antibodies are demonstrable on serological testing. However, OPV and yellow fever vaccines are not affected by IgG administration at any time.

Table 76.5: Principles of active immunization

- Use only a properly stored vaccine.
- *Avoid all vaccines* in the first trimester.
- *Avoid live virus vaccines* in women who are pregnant or are likely to become pregnant within three months.
- Killed or live vaccines do not affect the safety of breast feeding.
- *Avoid live vaccines* also in immunocompromised persons. They may be administered 3 months after stopping corticosteroids and 6 months after stopping cancer chemotherapy.
- In infants, immunization should not be postponed because of mild respiratory infections, diarrhoea or low grade fever.
- In premature infants, vaccination should be carried out as per the usual schedule.
- Healthcare workers should be immunized against hepatitis B, measles, rubella, influenza and varicella.
- If a vaccine and Ig are to be administered concurrently, each should be administered at a separate site.
- Many vaccines can be safely and effectively given simultaneously e.g. pneumococcal polysaccharide vaccine with whole virus influenza vaccine. But, two different vaccines should not be mixed in a syringe for administration. Use premixed vaccine, if available.
- If two live virus vaccines are to be given, they should be given on the same day, or at least 30 days apart. The response to tuberculin test may be hampered by live virus vaccines.
- A vaccine should be injected IM into the lateral aspect of the thigh in infants.

Passive Immunization

Passive immunization involves the administration of antibodies in the form of serum, plasma or Ig to a person who is exposed to infection but in whom the disease has not yet developed. It provides readymade antibodies against the organisms; such immunity, however, is short lived. In addition, passive immunization is often associated with unpleasant allergic reactions including fatal anaphylaxis, particularly when a heterologous serum is used. Some authorities use adrenaline, glucocorticoids and an antihistaminic prophylactically with the hope of preventing such serious reactions. The current trend, however, is to use homologous antibody preparations and concentrated immuno globulins. Immunoglobulins for passive immunization are now prepared by hybridoma technique.

It is advisable to determine the sensitivity of the patient before giving an injection of an antiserum regardless of whether or not he has previously received an injection of serum.

The intradermal test dose is 0.01 ml. of a 1:100 dilution of the serum, injected intradermally. In subjects with a history of allergy it should be reduced to 0.02 ml. of a 1:1,000 dilution. The test is considered as positive if a wheal develops within 30 minutes. In the scratch test, one drop of a 1 : 100 dilution of the test serum in saline is applied to a superficial scratch on the skin. A positive reaction consists of erythema and wheal formation. For the conjunctival (eye) test, one drop of a 1:10 dilution of serum in normal saline solution is put into one eye; one drop of normal saline alone is instilled into the other eye as a control. The patient is considered as allergic if the treated eye shows lacrimation and conjunctivitis within 30 minutes. The intradermal skin test is performed if the conjunctival or scratch test is negative. Intradermal skin tests have rarely resulted in fatalities but eye and scratch tests have not.

A patient who is allergic but needs the antiserum can be desensitized by injecting small, graded doses of the antiserum. Thus, the following doses are injected either SC or IM generally at 15 minutes intervals, the next dose being injected if there is no reaction to the previous one:

0.05 ml of 1 : 20 dilution, SC
0.1 ml of 1 : 10 dilution, SC
0.3 ml of 1 : 10 dilution, SC
0.1 ml of undiluted serum, SC
0.2 ml of undiluted serum, IM
0.5 ml of undiluted serum, IM

Finally, the entire remaining dose is injected IM. In case of anaphylaxis 0.5 ml. of adrenaline 1:1,000 is injected IM (less dose in children) and repeated if necessary. For details see Chapter 22.

The important antisera available are:

DIPHTHERIA ANTITOXIN: This is a serum preparation from the horse, actively immunized against C. diphtheriae. It contains the antitoxin globulins. It neutralizes the diphtheria toxin at the site of infection and also that circulating in the blood. However, it is probably ineffective in neutralising the toxin fixed to the tissues.

An IM injection of at least 4,000 units should be given immediately to all suspected cases even before taking throat swabs. The physician should then judge the severity of the case clinically and administer the additional dose without waiting for the results of investigations.

The dosage range of antitoxin is still controversial, but in mild diphtheria confined only to the nasal or laryngeal regions, a dose of 8,000 units by IM injection is usually adequate. Moderately severe cases require 10,000 to 30,000 units. *In all severe cases, a portion of the dose is given IM, followed 1½ to 2 hours later by the bulk of the dose IV.* The IM injection should be given in the lateral aspect of the thigh. *In no case should the IV administration precede the IM dose,* nor should it be resorted to in individuals with an allergic diathesis or a family history of allergic disorders.

The use of penicillin and erythromycin in diphtheria is discussed in Chapter 45.

TETANUS ANTITOXIN: This is a serum preparation from the horse, actively immunized against the toxins of Cl. tetani. It contains the antitoxin globulins.

The prophylactic dose of the antitoxin is 3,000-5,000 units, administered by SC or IM injection, after preliminary testing. The immunity conferred wears off within 1 to 3 weeks. The utility of this procedure is not clearly proven. In areas where tetanus is almost endemic, severely contaminated or deep penetrating wounds should be treated with wound toilet, ATS and a course of an antibiotic to give the maximum protection. Clean wounds or small abrasions or lacerations should be treated without ATS. *A second dose of ATS, in a patient who has received ATS once before, is very rapidly eliminated and hence, is ineffective.* In such cases, active immunization should be started at once. Due to possible severe allergic reactions to ATS, tetanus human immunoglobulin is preferred to ATS.

Of course, the ideal thing to do is to immunize everyone in the country by pre-exposure tetanus toxoid injections. In such individuals, post-exposure prophylaxis is also with tetanus toxoid.

TETANUS IMMUNOGLOBULIN (Human): This preparation contains specific gamma globulin prepared from human plasma having a high titre of tetanus antitoxin. Such plasma is obtained from blood of hyperimmunized subjects, or from placentas from mothers who have received tetanus booster inoculations a few weeks before delivery. The preparation is less prone to cause serious allergic reactions.

The half life of human immune globulin is between 3 to 4 weeks. Its prophylactic dose is 250-500 IU, IM. Active immunization with tetanus toxoid should be carried out simultaneously. It is also used in proven or suspected cases in the dose of 500-10000 units given IV. Serious adverse effects are rare.

GAS GANGRENE ANTITOXIN: Antitoxin is not so useful and is no longer recommended. The treatment of this condition consists of high dose IV penicillin G, surgical debridement of the lesion and hyperbaric oxygen (when available).

BOTULINUM ANTITOXIN: This is a horse serum preparation, containing the antitoxin globulins which neutralise the toxins formed by *Cl. botulinum*, types A, B and E.

For effective treatment, the polyvalent antitoxin must be administered in the very early stage of botulism. The antitoxin is administered for prophylaxis in the dose of 2-10 ml IM as soon as possible after exposure. For therapy, 10-20 ml is administered by slow IV infusion, followed by 10 ml 2 and 4 hours later; further doses at intervals of 12-24 hours may have to be adminstered by the same route if needed.

RABIES ANTISERUM: This is a hyperimmune, horse serum containing the globulins that have the specific power of neutralising the rabies virus. It is usually given along with rabies vaccine in patients who have received severe bites. For this purpose, not less than 400 units are infiltrated around the wound and at the same time, a dose of 40 units per kg. is given IM, simultaneously with rabies vaccine. Due to possible severe allergic reactions to the rabies horse antiserum, rabies immune globulin is to be preferred.

A highly purified immunoglobulin prepared from plasma of hyperimmunized horses (Pasteur antirabies serum) is now available.

RABIES IMMUNE GLOBULIN (Berlrab) prepared from plasma of donors hyperimmunized with the rabies vaccine is available. It is indicated for all persons with known or suspected severe exposure to rabies virus and is given in conjunction with rabies vaccine. The dose is 20 IU/kg; one half of the dose should be infiltrated around the wound if feasible. It is expensive.

HEPATITIS B GLOBULIN (HBIG): This is immune globulin prepared from the pooled plasma of donors with high titres of antibody to the surface antigen but not containing the surface antigen (HBsAg). It is indicated for post-exposure prophylaxis in susceptible individuals. The adverse reactions consist of local pain and tenderness and angioedema. The injected antibodies persist for three months.

ANTI-D (Rho) IMMUNOGLOBULIN (Human) : This is prepared from pooled plasma of naturally immunized women with high titre of anti-D antibodies or from the serum of suitably immunized males. A highly purified preparation (RhoGAM) is also available.

In an Rh negative woman with an Rh positive husband, if the foetus is Rh positive, the foetal erythrocytes may escape into the maternal circulation across the placenta, commonly during delivery but rarely even during pregnancy. In order to neutralize this antigen before it causes maternal rhesus immunization and to prevent erythroblastosis foetalis in subsequent pregnancies, it is necessary to give a dose of Rho (D) Ig, 500 units within 72 hours of delivery. Antenatal dose at 28 weeks of pregnancy is now recommended.

Rho (D) immunoglobulin is contraindicated in Rh positive women and in Rh negative women who develop Rh antibodies because of a previous conception or transfusion of Rh positive blood. *The preparation is to be given to the post partum mother and not to the neonate*. It is also used after abortion, whether spontaneous or induced. Adverse reactions are usually mild.

ANTI-SNAKE – VENOM SERUM: The poisonous snakes belong to three families:

- ***Viperidae*** (phoorsa, rattle snake, daboia),
- ***Elapidae*** (cobra, krait, mamba) and
- ***Hydrophiidae*** (sea-snakes).

The viper venom commonly kills by its action on the cardio-vascular system, though some venoms contain a neurotoxin as well. The elapid venom contains mainly a neurotoxin which causes muscle paralysis by its neuromuscular blocking action. Such paralysis is not always reversible with the antivenom, particularly in case of krait bite. *However, it is spontaneously reversible after about two days. Hence, management involves general support such as artificial respiration, intragastric feeding and maintaining vital parameters.*

The dangers of poisonous snakebite in human victims appear to be greatly exaggerated. Nearly half of the people bitten by poisonous snakes such as cobra and vipers develop no significant systemic poisoning because of very low dose of the venom injected. Obviously, such patients need no antivenom therapy. Hence, in doubtful cases it is better to wait and watch the patient carefully for clear clinical evidence of systemic poisoning such as ptosis, limb and neck muscle paresis, blood stained sputum and failure of the blood to clot, before giving antivenom. *However, such patients must be hospitalised and examined at 15 minute intervals.* Since antivenom can sometimes cause severe reactions e.g. anaphylaxis, sensitivity tests must be performed prior to its administration.

Polyvalent, anti-snake-venom serum (antivenin) obtained from immunized horses contains the purified antitoxin globulins that have the power of neutralising the venom of cobra, krait, Russell's viper and saw-scaled viper. It is reconstituted by adding 10 ml. of distilled water. A sensitivity test is performed by injecting 0.02-0.1 ml. of 1:10 diluted antivenom SC. If no reaction occurs within 30 min., 20-40 ml. is injected IV, very slowly (0.5-1 ml./min.) as the first dose and repeated thereafter, if necessary, every 3-4 hours upto a total of 100 ml., depending upon the severity of the case. In case of viper bite, some serum is injected around the site of the bite to prevent the development of gangrene. The serum may also be given IM or SC though the IV route is preferred.

The presence of allergy demands desensitization and administration of the antiserum in small, multiple doses. Allergic reactions and anaphylaxis may occur and they should be treated by the conventional methods. Antivenin is probably not effective against the toxin fixed to the tissues, nor can it reverse the damage already caused by the toxin. In a serious case, one may not wait for the sensitivity test but give the serum immediately. In such circumstances, it is advisable to use prophylactic adrenaline, an antihistaminic and a glucocorticoid simultaneously, and repeat them later, if needed, to protect the patient against allergic reactions. For the use of **cholinesterase inhibitor, edrophonium,** for antagonizing neuromuscular blockade in the treatment of snake bite, see Chapter 18.

Immunoglobulins

Antibody molecule (immunoglobulin, Ig) consists of two light and two heavy chains composed of different domains (1) Fab fragment and (2) Fc fragment (Fig. 76.1).

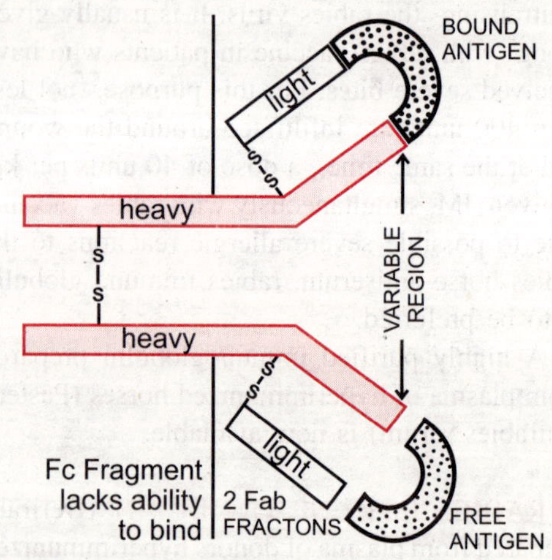

Fig. 76.1 : Basic structure of an immunoglobulin molecule. Two heavy and two light chains of amino acids are linked by disulfide (S-S) bridges. At one end of the molecule, the three dimensional stearic configuration (idiotypic determinant) of each arm allows only one antigenic determinant to have best fit status. The Fab fractions are variable and have antibody activity; and the other fraction is relatively constant (Fc). The amino acid sequence of the Fc fraction determines the main functional activity of the molecule.

The **Fab fraction** serves as the antigen binding site. The specific antigen-binding properties of an IgG molecule are conferred by the three dimensional stearic arrangement inherent in the amino acid sequence of the variable region of the light and the heavy chains of the molecule. This portion of the IgG molecule is called the *idiotypic determinant.* Only one antigenic determinant can have a 'best fit' with this arrangement. Apart from the idiotypic region, the remainder of the Ig G molecule viz, the **Fc fragment** is relatively constant and determines the effector function of the antibody. The Fc domain is necessary for interaction with the effector cells and for activating the complement cascade.

'HUMAN NORMAL IMMUNOGLOBULIN' (HNI): (Histafine, Histaglobulin): Roughly, plasma protein can be fractionated into four important components, viz. albumin and the alpha, beta and gamma globulins. The gamma globulin carries antibodies.

Immunoglobulin (Ig) is a sterile serum protein solution (15-18%) containing antibodies from human blood, which is derived from pooled human serum; it consists primarily of IgG (95%) and small amounts of other Igs (IgM and IgA) and other serum proteins (Chapter 1).

The Ig obtained from pooled, human, adult blood is known as **immune serum.** More selective type of gamma globulin against a particular infection can be obtained from the blood of individuals convalescing from that disease or from the blood of subjects recently immunised against that disease. This is called **Hyperimmune Serum** or **Human Specific Ig.**

Ig can be used both for prophylactic and therapeutic purposes. *It is administered IM.*

Adverse reactions: Ig can cause pain at the site of injection. Allergic reactions can occur. It may give rise to fever, flushing, shivering, joint pain and nausea. Severe bronchospasm, hypotension and collapse, however, are rare and occur mostly following IV therapy. Human Ig preparations are contraindicated in patients with class specific antibodies to IgA.

Therapeutic uses:

- ***Hypogammaglobulinemia:*** Normally, the total gamma globulins in the plasma vary between 600 and 1500 mg. per 100 ml. Total serum gamma globulins in normal Indians are much higher than those in Western people. Patients with serum gamma globulin concentration of 200 mg. or less are considered to be suffering from hypogamma-globulinemia. HNI is usually given in dose of 0.025 to 0.05 g. per kg. body weight, at weekly intervals. Usually, very prolonged therapy is necessary along with prophylactic antibiotics.

- ***Measles and rubella prophylaxis:*** HNI will attenuate or prevent the symptoms of measles if given early in the incubation period. The doses recommended are: for attenuation, 250 mg. at all ages; for prevention 250 mg. below one year, 500 mg. at 1-2 years and 750 mg. at 3 years and above. The effect lasts only for a few weeks. In pregnant women exposed to rubella, the dose recommended is 1 g.

- ***Infective hepatitis:*** Gamma globulin can suppress the clinical symptoms and if they occur, they are usually mild. The dose of HNI recommended is 750 mg. given prophylactically in contacts. The effect lasts for 6 months. *It is not effective in preventing serum hepatitis.*

- ***Mumps and poliomyelitis:*** Immune gamma globulin has been claimed to be useful in preventing the complications of mumps and in reducing the incidence of paralytic poliomyelitis.

- ***Diphtheria:*** Hyperimmune specific serum can be used both prophylactically and therapeutically.

Specific immunoglobulins are available for hepatitis B, rabies and tetanus. (See earlier).

It is currently thought that with the exception of primary and secondary immunodeficiency states, inadequate immunoregulation is the fundamental cause of immunopathology. Thus, IgG appears to be involved in the regulation of both allergic and autoimmune reactions i.e. disease-inducing reactions to foreignness and self, respectively. Although allergy is commonly equated with IgE mediated immediate hypersensitivity reaction (Chapter 2), there is increasing recognition that the undisciplined and even chronic release of cytokines represents a form of allergy that may produce disease analogous to diseases caused by the undisciplined release of histamine-like agents from the basophils and mast cells. Cytokines such as IL1, IL6, interferons a and b and TNF a have an effect both on the cells of the immune system and on many other cells and body systems from the CNS to the liver.

We all constantly make small amounts of antibodies to our own tissue proteins and in turn also make anti-idiotypic antibodies to these auto-antibodies. This latter manoeuvre is designed to prevent any important immunologic attack on self. Highly concentrated IgG preparations are now available for IV use. It follows that such preparations will contain a vast "library of antibodies" capable of reacting with thousands of determinants because of the diversity of the experience of the thousands of donors contributing to the pool. Among such antibodies will be many with anti-idiotypic specificities.

IV IMMUNOGLOBULIN-G (IVIG) : The various, purified IVIG preparations commercially available differ to some extent with regard to their content of so dium and sugar, a stabilizing agent, and traces of IgA. They are supplied in liquid or lyophilized form.

Adverse reactions: They can cause acute reactions such as headache, fever, myalgia and nausea. Rarely anaphylaxis, aseptic meningitis, thromboembolic events or renal tubular necrosis can occur.

Therapeutic uses: In addition to primary and secondary immunodeficiency states, it is recommended for treating idiopathic thrombocytopenic purpura, Kawasaki syndrome and pediatric HIV. It has been found useful in chronic inflammatory, demyelinating polyneuropathy, Guillain-Barre syndrome, multifocal motor neuropathy, dermatomyositis, SLE and renal transplant rejection. Doses vary according to the disease. It is usually given in the dose of 0.5-1.0 g/kg /d for 5days. For primary immunodeficiency, it is given in the dose of 300-600 mg/kg every 3-4 weeks. It is very expensive.

Monoclonal Antibodies (mAb) in Therapeutics

The first Nobel Prize in Medicine was awarded to immunologist Emil von Behring in 1901 for his work on serum therapy against infections like diphtheria. This showed a new mode of treating diseases apart from drugs. Later, two other Nobel laureates, Rodney Porter and Gerald Edelman, in 1959 discovered the structure of antibodies, immunoglobulins. However, the greatest impetus to the development of immunology came from the discovery of the **hybridoma technique** for producing **monoclonal antibodies** (mAb) by George Kohler and Cesar Milstein in 1975. This helped to produce several mAbs for specific binding sites. They were awarded Nobel Prize in 1984.

Monoclonal antibodies (mAb) are antibodies produced by a single clone of B cells. Compared to polyclonal antibodies, mAb are monospecific and homogenous. Such antibodies are now being used for diagnostic procedures and therapeutic purposes.

Structure of mAb and its functions are described earlier (Fig. 76.1). Recently developed humanised antibodies are less immunogenic and more efficient than the earlier introduced mouse mAb. Further, they remain in circulation for a longer time and are now preferred.

Mechanism of action : They specifically block the characteristic of the targeted antigen, its function, its cell surface density and tissue distribution. Their action is directed against T lymphocytes. B lymphocytes, TNF and interleukins. Addition of active compounds to mAb to produce immuno-conjugates can provide targeting specificity to cytotoxic actions. Thus, mAb can be conjugated with catalytic toxins, radioisotopes and chemotherapeutic agents, and can be used as therapeutic missiles to target specific tissues with cytotoxic payload.

Epidermal Growth Factor Receptor (EGFR) is a cell surface receptor involved in regulation of cell proliferation and survival. Some antibodies e.g. cetuximab act as EGFR inhibitor.

Absorption fate and excretion: mAb are used IV and they remain essentially intravascular, the volume of distribution is small and tissue penetration is limited. Depending on their nature, they remain in human circulation for 2 days to 2 weeks.

The currently available mAb are listed in Table 76.6. They are all expensive.

Adverse reactions

- ***Hypersensitivity reactions*** are rare. However, sometimes the first injection may induce an influenza like syndrome causing fever, headache, chills, tachycardia, vomiting, arthralgia and hypotension. The reaction is not life-threatening and is reversible. It is believed to be due to massive systemic release of cytokines, following activation of T lymphocytes.
- ***Suppression of physiologic function*** may occur depending on specificity of tissues targeted; thus, anti-lymphocytic mAb causes immunosuppression.
- ***Activation of inflammatory cells;*** and
- ***Increased risk of infection and cancer*** (the latter has not been observed so far).

Therapeutic uses of mAb :

- As immunosuppressants, e.g., to prevent the rejection of renal transplant
- In autoimmune disease, e.g., infliximab in RA (Chapter 71)
- As antiplatelet agents (Chapter 32)
- In cancer; and
- As antiviral agent in treatment of

Table 76.6: Monoclonal antibodies for clinical use

Generic name	Brand name	Target	Indications
Muromonab	Orthodone; OKT3	CD3 (T cell)	Graft rejection
Basilliximab	Simalect	CD25 (IL2–receptor)	Do.
Daclizumab	Zenepax	CD25 (IL–2 receptor)	Do.
Alemtuzumab	Campath-1H	CD52	Graft rejection; CLL
Infliximab	Remicade	TNF alpha	RA; Crohn's disease
Adalimumab	Humira	TNF alpha	Do.
Trastuzumab	Herceptin	HER2/neu	Breast cancer
Rituximab	Rituxan	CD20 (B cell)	Lymphoma; CLL
Abciximab	Reopro	GpIIb/IIIa	Antiplatelet
Palivizumab	Synagis	Fusion Protein	Anti Resp. syncitial virus
Gemtuzumab	Mylotong	CD 33	AML
Cetuximab	Erbitux	EGFR	Colorectal cancer; NSCLC
Panitumumab	Vectirix	EGFR	Do
Efalizumab	Raptiva	$CD11_a$ (LFA-1)	Psoriasis
Bevacizumab	Avastin	VEGF	Colorectal cancer; AMD
Ranibizumab	Lucentis	VEGF	AMD
Eculizumab	Soliris	Complement protein C5	Paroxymal nocturnal hemoglobinuria
Omalizumab	Xolair	IgE receptor	Bronchial asthma
Natalizumab	Tysabri	Integrin	Crohn's disease; MS
Certolizumab	Cimzia	TNF alpha	Crohn's disease

respiratory syncitial virus infection in infants (see later).

Diagnostic uses of mAb : They are extensively used in immunoassay and other procedures in the laboratory.

Immunosuppressants

Drugs which are used to suppress the immunity are called immunosuppressants. Since immunity confers resistance to disease, the use of drugs for deliberately suppressing it appears odd at first sight. However, according to present concept, the ability of the body to recognize self from not-self or foreign, which is the basis of immunity, is liable to cause disorders due to failure to recognize and tolerate antigens produced by its own tissues. This may cause exacerbation of an existing disease process or even produce new ones called **auto-immune diseases** e.g. rheumatoid arthritis and SLE.

Immunosupressive drugs are useful in: (1) treating autoimmune diseases; and (2) preventing immunorejection of organ transplants. They can be classified as shown in Table 76.7.

Table 76.7: Immunosuppresants

(1) **Calcinurine inhibitors:**	Cyclosporine Tacrolimus
(2) **Glucocorticoids**	Prednisolone
(3) **Cytotoxic/antiproliferative agents**	Azathioprine Mycophenolate Sirolimus
(4) **Antibodies**	
(a) T cell depleting antibodies	Muromonab Antilymphocytic antibodies Antithymocytic antibodies
(b) Anti CD25 antibodies	Basilliximab Daclizumab

(1) **Calcineurine inhibitors:**

CYCLOSPORINE (Sandimmune) : The drug, formerly known as cyclosporin A, is a cyclic undecapeptide (11 amino acid peptide) produced by the fungus *Beauveria nivea.*

It has now been synthesized. Its action is largely selective and differs from that of the older immunosuppressant drugs.

Mechanism of action : It acts as an immunosuppressant by blocking an early stage in the activation of cytotoxic T lymphocytes after the recipient is exposed to the antigen. Within the T lymphocytes, it binds to cyclophilin, an intracellular protein; the complex then binds to and inhibits calcineurin. Calcineurin-induced dephosphorylation is required for induction of a T cell specific transcription factor involved in synthesis of cytokines by activated T cells.

Absorption, fate and excretion : Its bioavailability after oral administration is 20 - 50%. In the circulation, 50% is bound to erythrocytes, 10% to leucocytes and 40% to lipoproteins in the plasma. It is almost completely metabolized.

Adverse reactions: The major toxic manifestations of cyclosporine are nephrotoxicity, hypertension and hyperlipidemia; the others are hypertrichosis, gum hypertrophy, increased susceptibility to infection, leucopenia thromboytopenia and development of lymphomas caused by Epstein- Barr virus.

Preparations : Cyclosporine is available as 25, 50 and 100 mg capsules; as 100 mg/ml oily solution for oral use and as a 50 mg/ml solution for IV administration.

Therapeutic uses: It is mainly used for prophylaxis and treatment of organ rejection in transplantation surgery. In recipients of renal transplants, the renal function is not as good in those treated with cyclosporine as in those treated with azathropine plus glucocorticoids. However, cyclosporine is the preferred drug in 'high risk' recipients of renal transplants viz. the elderly and the recipients of second and third grafts. It is used together with a glucocorticoid. Its other attempted therapeutic use is autoimmune diseases such as RA.

TACROLIMUS (Prograt): It is a macrolide antibiotic isolated from *Streptomyces tsukubaensis*. It acts by inhibiting T cell activation and proliferation by binding to an immunophilin which inhibits calcineurin. This results in inhibition of lymphokine expression, apoptosis and degranulation. Tacrolimus is 100 times more potent than cyclosporine as an immunosuppresant.

Given orally, its bioavailability is variable, ranging from 6% to 56%. The drug is extensively metabolized in the liver and less than 1% is excreted unchanged. It can also be given IV.

Adverse reactions: These are similar to those of cyclosporine, with nephrotoxicity being the major toxic manifestation. Other adverse reactions include nausea, diarrhoea, neurotoxicity, hypertension, hypomagnesenia, hyperkalemia and hyperglycemia.

Therapeutic uses: The therapeutic uses of tacrolimus are similar to those of cyclosporine

(2) GLUCOCORTICOIDS are potent immuno-suppressants and are used to prevent organ transplant rejection. They also possess anti-inflammatory action (Chapter 64).

(3) **Cytotoxic/antiproliferative agents:** These are cytotoxic drugs which act on the dividing cells. An immune response is associated with division of lymphoid cells and these drugs act by interfering with the dividing lymphoid cells in the body. They, however, are not specific and produce toxicity as they also affect the other rapidly dividing cells, (Chapter 59).

AZATHIOPRINE: (Imuran) and METHOTREXATE are the most commonly employed compounds. Continuous, prolonged immunosuppression with cytotoxic agents is associated with a number of hazards particularly increased susceptibility to infection and hence, is to be recommended only in special circumstances e.g. organ transplants.

MYCOPHENOLATE MOFETIL: This prodrug, given orally, is rapidly hydrolysed to the active compound, mycophenolic acid. The latter inhibits purine synthesis and has a potent cytostatic effect on both B and T lymphocytes. This results in inhibition of lymphocyte proliferation and antibody formation. Mycophenolic acid is metabolized in the liver. Its adverse effects include GI and urinary disturbances and bone marrow suppression, which are predominantly dose-dependent. The drug is used for the prophylaxis of allograft rejection and in the treatment of psoriasis, pemphigus vulgaris and systemic vasculitis.

Sirolimus (Rapamune) though structurally related to tacrolimus, differs in its mechanism of action. It forms a complex with immunophilin *but does not inhibit calcineurine.* Instead, the complex binds to inhibitors of a specific kinase essential for cell-cycle progression.

(4) **Monoclonal Antibodies** (See Table 76.7)

For specific T cell depleting antibody muromonab, and anti CD25 antibodies, see earlier

Antilymphocytic serum (ALS): The serum or semipurified antilymphocytic globulin is obtained from horses immunized against human thymus, lymph node and spleen cells (lymphoid tissue).

Specific antithymocytic globulin is obtained by injecting into horses, T cells from the thymus glands of children undergoing open heart surgery. The T cells are more vulnerable to ALS which depletes the thymus dependent areas of lymphoid tissue, the lymphocytes being replaced by histiocytes.

When administered IM in the dose of 1000 units per kg (1 to 5 ml. of the serum), along with other immunosuppressants like azathioprine and corticosteroids, in patients undergoing renal homotransplantation, ALS enables a considerable reduction in the dose of the other immuno-suppressants. It, however, is not a substitute for these drugs.

ALS is of benefit during bone marrow

transplantation and in the treatment of rejection crises after renal transplantation.

Adverse reactions reported include pain and induration at the site of injection, fever, occasionally anaphylactic response and thrombocytopenia. An increased incidence of malignant tumors like lymphomas has been reported in patients receiving it IV, repeatedly.

Immunostimulants and Immunomodulators

The use of a variety of agents to enhance immunological and nonspecific host defences and thus to modify the defences favourably is an exciting development in immunopharmacology. Such agents may act by:

- ***Increasing the humoral antibody responses,***
- ***Enhancing the phagocytic activity of macrophages,*** or
- ***Modifying the cell-mediated immune responses.***

Drugs like **amantadine** and **tilorane** stimulate the humoral immune system. The role of **BCG** vaccine in strengthening the immune defence mechanisms is discussed in Chapter 52. Nonspecific immunostimulation with BCG has been used along with the conventional therapy in the treatment of leukemias, melanoma and lung and bladder carcinoma with some beneficial results.

THALIDOMIDE (Thalomid) : This drug, chemically related to barbiturates, and introduced as a hypnotic and antiemetic, was found to be teratogenic and hence rejected. It has now staged a comeback in therapeutics as an **immunomodulator.**

Mechanism of action : It inhibits the production of TNF a and interferon, and has stimulatory effects on IGF1 and IL6. It also inhibits the induction of COX2 and the biosynthesis of PGE2 needed for angiogenesis. It reduces phagocytosis by neutrophils and enhances CMI by interacting with T cells. Thus, it exerts anti-inflammatory, immunomodulatory and antiangiogenesis actions.

Given orally, it is well absorbed and is metabolized to several metabolites. 5-Hydroxy thalidomide is an active metabolite. It is administered in the dose of 100-800 mg daily.

Adverse reactions: It can cause sedation, dizziness, constipation, tremors, mood changes, rash and rarely, peripheral neuropathy and hypothyroidism. *It is highly teratogenic* (see art plate).

Therapeutic uses:

- ***Drug of choice in symptomatic treatment of moderate to severe ENL*** (Chapter 53).
- ***Refractory cutaneous lupus lesions.***
- ***Crohn's disease.***
- ***Treatment of cachexia and weight loss in HIV and that due to TNF-α in cancer patients.***
- ***Multiple myeloma, refractory to other treatments.***
- ***In advanced prostatic cancer, as an immunomodulator.***
- ***Treatment of nausea, vomiting and anorexia due to TNF-α in cancer patients.***

For use of monoclonal antibodies, see earlier.

Levamisole, an anthelmintic drug, also possesses immunotropic properties and has been claimed to help in restoring the efficiency of host defence mechanisms (Chapter 58). It probably acts by modulating cell mediated immune responses. It enhances T cell-mediated immunity. It restores or augments cutaneous-delayed hyper-sensitive reactions in anergic (state of immunologic deficiency) patients with cancer. Like BCG and **clofazimine,** (Chapter 53) its effect is associated with enhanced phagocytic activity of the macrophages. The drug may cause GI disturbances, headache, dizziness, insomnia, thrombocytopenia and agranulocytosis.

Interferons are naturally occurring proteins

with complex effects on immunity. They may act directly on normal cells and induce enzymes that attack viral RNA; or indirectly by stimulating the immune system. Interferons have been shown to produce some beneficial effect on certain human lymphoreticular and other cancers, in muliple selerosis and in hepatitis B. (Chapter 59).

GLATIRAMER ACETATE: This is a synthetic co-polymer with some immunological similarity to myelin basic protein, one of the major components of myelin. Given SC, it is claimed to reduce the relapse rate in relapsing - remitting multiple selerosis. It probably acts as an immunomodulator.

Drug Therapy of Scorpion Sting

This is a hazardous and potentially lethal condition caused by the sting of poisonous scorpions including the Indian red scorpion (*Mesobuthus tamulus*). The scorpion venom is a potent ANS stimulant. In addition to intense pain at the site of the sting, there is initially transient cholinergic stimulation followed by a prolonged sympathetic storm, due to release of massive amounts of catecholamines. The initial manifestations are vomiting, sweating, excessive salivation, hypotension, priapism, bradycardia and ventricular ectopy. The later manifestations are hypertension with either bradycardia or tachycardia, cardiogenic, pulmonary oedema, arrhythmias, hyperglycemia and peripheral circulatory failure.

Without adequate treatement the mortality may be as high as 30%. Temporary relief of local pain can be obtained by infiltrating with a local anaesthetic agent without adrenaline. Longer relief is given by a local injection of 0.1 to 0.2 ml of dehydroemetine 0.03%. As the systemic manifestations are due to sympathetic overactivity, the rational treatment is to counter the same. This is particualry important as specific antivenom may not be readily available.

The drug of choice is **prazosin** (Chapter 29) in the dose of 0.25 to 0.5 mg (adult dose) orally, repeated six hourly till improvement occurs. The initial dose must be administered with patient lying down to prevent the first dose effect. In life threatening pulmonary oedema, sodium nitroprusside by IV infusion under careful monitoring has been recommended. Aminophylline IV can also help in the management of pulmonary edema. Although sublingual nifedipine can reduce the BP and afterload, given rapidly, the negative intropic action of nifedipine can precipitate or worsen pulmonary edema.

At present, antivenom serum against the Indian red scorpion, manufactured by Haffkine Biopharmaceuticals, Mumbai, is available and is being evaluated.

The following drugs should be used with care or avoided in victims of scorpion sting as they are likely to worsen the clinical condition: atropine, antihistamines, glucocorticoids, digoxin, diuretics, dopamine and dobutamine.

77 Drugs, Pregnancy and the Infant

Drugs are likely to be self administered or prescribed by the physician during pregnancy. Intelligent use of drugs during pregnancy requires that the physician understands the interaction between drugs and pregnancy so as to avoid indiscriminate use of drugs with disastrous consequences as illustrated by the thalidomide tragedy. At the same time, over-cautious timidity on the part of the physician casts the pregnant mother in the role of a therapeutic orphan. It must be remembered that most of the drugs prescribed during pregnancy are given for the benefit of the mother and that we must not deny her adequate treatment for a serious illness.

In addition to drugs, the pregnant woman is likely to be exposed to a variety of environmental, nontherapeutic or illicit agents which can affect the fetal health.

Pharmacokinetics During Pregnancy

Most of the available information on **pharmacokinetics** of drugs during pregnancy has been obtained from animal experiments and may not be directly applicable to humans. Although pregnant women do not differ qualitatively from the non-pregnant ones in their response to drugs, certain quantitative differences do occur because of physiological changes during pregnancy, with consequent alterations in pharmacokinetics of drugs. Further, the fetus has its own pharmacokinetic peculiarities.

Drug absorption : High circulating levels of progesterone slow the gastric emptying as well as gut motility, thus increasing the intestinal transit time. One might expect slower drug absorption during pregnancy for that reason. However, this does not occur except *at term when parenteral drug administration is preferred* in order to obtain a quick response. Administration of iron and antacids may also interfere with the absorption of certain drugs. Drug compliance may be poor during pregnancy because of nausea and fear of possible adverse effects.

Drug distribution: Pregnancy is accompanied by an increase in total body water by upto 8 litres and a 30% increase in plasma volume, with consequent decrease (0.5 - 1.0 g%) in plasma albumin due to hemodilution. Drugs which have low lipid solubility and are also highly plasma protein bound (e.g. warfarin, benzodiazepines) have a low apparent volume of distribution (Vd). The Vd of such drugs increases markedly during pregnancy. The protein bound fraction of the drug in the plasma diminishes and so does the concentration of the total drug in the plasma. Although the fraction of unbound drug increases, a greater pharmacodynamic effect is prevented by more rapid elimination of the drug by metabolism and/or excretion (see below). The therapeutic range for drugs whose use is monitored by measurement of total plasma concentration (e.g. phenytoin) must be adjusted downwards to make allowance for the above mentioned changes, if their plasma protein binding changes during pregnancy.

Drug metabolism: Hepatic drug metabolizing enzymes are induced during pregnancy, probably by the high concentrations of circulating progesterone. This can lead to more rapid metabolic degradation, especially of the highly lipid soluble drugs. However, this is of little clinical consequence because the meta-bolism of most such drugs is ordinarily so fast that their clearance is limited only by hepatic blood flow, which does not change appreciably during pregnancy. The contribution of the placenta and the fetal liver to the clearance of drugs from the maternal body is thought to be small.

Drug excretion: During pregnancy, the renal plasma flow increases by 100% and the glomerular filtration rate by 70%. Add to this the increase in the unbound fraction of the drug in the plasma. Hence, drugs which depend for their elimination mainly on the kidney are eliminated more rapidly than in the non-pregnant state. Examples are ampicillin, aminoglycosides, cephalexin and digoxin.

The conventional dose of ampicillin needs to be doubled during pregnancy if it is used for a systemic infection in the mother, but not if it is used for a urinary tract infection. An increase in the dose of cefuroxime and lithium is needed for similar reasons. In the case of phenytoin (whose unbound plasma level diminishes due to more rapid metabolism, in addition to total plasma level), an increase in the daily dose by 25 - 100 mg may be required to maintain good seizure control; a similar increase is also required in the dose of phenobarbitone and carbamazepine. In spite of pharmacokinetic alterations, the doses of benzodiazepines, aspirin, propranolol, sulfafurazole and metronidazole do not require alterations during pregnancy. The pharmacokinetics of furosemide do not alter during pregnancy and no dose adjustment is required.

Drugs, the Fetus and the Newborn

Placental transfer of drugs: The placenta acts as an intravenous portal for entry of drugs into the fetus. Such entry of drugs is governed by several considerations. As pregnancy progresses and the placenta develops, the surface available for transfer between the maternal and fetal circulations increases; at the same time, the placento-fetal barrier becomes progressively thinner. Transfer across this barrier is governed by the same properties of drugs which regulate the transfer across other biological membranes: unbound, non-ionized, lipid-soluble molecules of low molecular weight cross the barrier more easily than those which do not possess these attributes; most of the drugs in use fulfil these criteria and are able to cross the placental barrier. However, because of the differences in the plasma protein concentration and the pH between maternal and fetal blood, the concentration of drugs in the two circulations, even at equilibrium, may differ considerably. Add to this, the differences in pharamacokinetics between the mother and the fetus. Further, the placenta is capable of metabolising drugs; this is of little relevance to the mother but can protect the fetus from the entry of many drugs. For example, prednisolone and hydrocortisone, which are metabolized by the placenta to inactive compounds prednisone and cortisone, are safer for the fetus than dexamethasone and betamethasone, which are not so metabolized.

The method of drug administration to the mother may also decide the fetal concentration. For example, at term, antibiotics given by intermittent intravenous infusion can achieve higher concentrations in the fetal blood and amniotic fluid than when the same total dose is given by continuous infusion; this may be important in the treatment of intrauterine infections.

In spite of above considerations, the fetal: maternal ratio of unbound drug concentration is generally close to unity. Further, the placenta is always available to the fetus as a route of drug elimination. After birth, the placental route of drug elimination is no longer available and the neonate is on its own.

Compared to adults, both fetus and infants differ in their handling of drugs, as related to pharmacokinetics as well as pharmacodynamics.

Fetal/Neonatal pharmacokinetics : Human growth is not a linear phenomenon. Age-related changes in body composition and organ function are dynamic and can be discordant during the first decade of life. *Hence, the simplified dosage approaches calculated by standard formulae may not be adequate for individualizing drug doses across the span of infancy and childhood.*

During the neonatal period, intragastric pH is relatively higher (>7.4). Hence, orally administered drugs such as penicilln G have greater broavailability in neonates than in adults. On the other hand, weak acids such as phenobarbitone need higher doses in the young children. Generally, the rate at which majority of drugs are absorbed is slower in the neonates than in the older children. Further, developmental differences in the activity of intestinal drug metabolizing enzymes and changes in the intestinal microflora may also affect the plasma levels of drugs.

Compared to adults, neonates and infants have relatively larger extracellular and total body water spaces. This, along with the adipose tissue stores that have a higher lipid/water ratio, leads to lower EC concentrations when drugs are given on weight basis. Distribution of highly protein bound drugs is also modified by the amount of circulating plasma albumin and 1-acidglycoprotein.

In infants and young children, the ratio of total body surface area (BSA) to body mass far exceeds that in adults. Hence, the relative systemic exposure of infants to topically applied drugs such as glucocorticoids may exceed that in adults, leading to adverse systemic effects.

Delayed maturation of hepatic drug metabolising enzymes in infants can cause increased drug toxicity.

The expression of Phase I metabolising enzymes such as cytochrome P-450 undergoes marked changes during development of neonates.This affects the hepatic clearance of various drugs metabolised by the isoforms of these enzymes. The clearance of carbamazepine is greater in children than in adults. In the case of phenytoin, its t½ is about 75 hours in preterm infants, which decreases to about 20 hours during the first week of life and to 8 hours after the second week of life. The plasma clearance of morphine is known to quadruple between 27th and 40th weeks of gestatenal age, thus requiring corresponding increase in the dose of morphine for effective analgesia.

Because of significant developmental changes during the neonatal period, drugs such as methylxanthines morphine, captopril and third generation cephalosporins need age-appropriate dosage regimens.

In view of the above problems, it is safer to consult worked-out dosage tables for neonates and infants than to use formulae based on body weight and/or BSA.

Various developmental changes in the kidney function during infancy can alter the plasma clearance of drugs that are primarily excreted by th kidney, e.g. aminoglycosides, famotidine, ceftazidime, digoxin, chlorpropamide, penicillin, salicylic acid, indomethacin and paracetamol. This obviously will need age-appropriate selection of dosage regimen.

Fetal-neonatal pharmacodynamics: Age-dependent differences in the interaction of the drugs with specific receptors does probably exist but the data are limited. This may modify the safety and efficacy of drugs in the neonates and infants. For a given plasma concentration, the response of the fetal tissues to most drugs is equal to or less than that of maternal tissues. There are some notable exceptions. Certain drugs given in the second and third trimesters produce either exaggerated effects or effects that are unique to the fetus. For example, tetracyclines get deposited in the fetal teeth and bones and retard their growth; coumarins can cause fetal and neonatal hemorrhages. Salicylates given at term can cause neonatal hemorrhage. PG synthetase inhibitors given near term can induce premature closure of ductus arteriosus and pulmonary hypertension in the fetus. Antithyroid drugs can inhibit fetal thyroxine synthesis and can cause goitre formation. Opiates and barbiturates (given to mother) achieve very high concentrations in the fetal brain and can cause respiratory depression at birth. Phenothiazines given to the mother can cause extrapyramidal signs in the neonate which may persist for several months. (Also see Chapter 13).

Effects of Drugs on Pregnancy

Effective treatment of maternal illness with drugs such as insulin, thyroxine, antibiotics and antihypertensives may be said to have a beneficial effect on the course of pregnancy.

On the other hand, in certain situations drugs can cause harm to the conceptus. These harmful effects depend upon the nature of the drug and its dose and route of administration; the stage of pregnancy at which the drug is used; and the genetic constitution and susceptibility of the fetus, which in turn, depend upon the age, nutritional status and health of the mother. Gestation may be divided into four major stages.

- ***Pre-implantation*** stage (blastocyst formation) which lasts about 16 days from conception to implantation. Exposure to harmful drugs (such as anticancer drugs) can kill the embryo or else the damaged cells are replaced by undifferentiated cells which have the potential to develop normally. This is an all-or-none effect.
- ***Period of organogenesis*** from 17th to 56th day. Pre-implantation stage and the stage of organogenesis together constitute the first trimester. Exposure to harmful drugs (and other environmental influences) during the period of organogenesis can cause congenital malformations (**teratogenicity**) or abortion.
- ***The second and third trimesters*** are periods during which considerable growth and development occur in teeth, bones and in central nervous, endocrine, genital and immune systems. During this period drugs can cause either teratogenesis or a variety of other effects such as retardation of physical or brain growth, behavioral teratogenicity, premature labour, neonatal toxicity and even late post natal effects such as cancer(s).
- ***A short labour-delivery stage:*** Drug administration during this period is mainly fraught with the danger of toxicity in the neonatal period for reasons already discussed.

Teratogenicity

This word was originally used in the sense of congenital malformations grossly visible at birth and caused by exposure to exogenous agents **(teratogens)** in the first trimester. The definition has now been broadened to include any birth defect (morphological, biochemical or behavioral) induced at any stage of pregnancy and detected at birth or later in life. *Birth defects are known to occur in 2 - 4% of all births in the population. Out of all birth defects,* the cause is unknown in 65 - 70% ; 25% can be attributed to genetic defects and 3% to chromosomal aberrations. *Only about 3% can be ascribed to environmental factors* including maternal infection, radiation and drug administration. The overall incidence of congenital malformations does not appear to have increased in the last 30 years in spite of the dramatic increase in the number of drugs available.

Teratogenesis includes restricted growth of the fetus, malformations, carcinogenesis and behavioral teratogenicity (see later). It should be

Table 77.1: Drug with proven teratogenic effects in humans

Drug	Teratogenic effect
Methotrexate	CNS and limb malformations
ACE inhibitors	Prolonged renal failure in the neonate, renal tubular dysgenesis, decreased skull ossification.
Anticholinergic drugs	Neonatal meconium ileus
Antithyroid drugs	Fetal and neonatal goitre and hypothyroidism, aplasia cutis (with methimazole)
Carbamazepine	Neural tube defects
Cyclophosphamide	CNS malformations, secondary cancer
Danazol and other androgenic drugs	Masculinization of female fetus
Diethylstilbestrol*	Vaginal carcinoma and other genitourinary defects in female and male offspring
Lithium	Ebstein's anomaly
Misoprostol	Moebius sequence
NSAID	Constriction of the ductus arteriosus, necrotizing enterocolitis
Oral hypoglycemic drugs	Neonatal hypoglycemia
Phenytoin	Growth retardation, CNS defects
Psychoactive drugs	Neonatal withdrawl syndrome when drug is taken in late pregnancy
Systemic retinoids (isotretinoin, etretinate)	CNS, craniofacial, cardiovascular and other defects
Tetracycline	Anomalies of teeth and bones
Thalidomide	Limb-shortening, internal organ defects
Trimethadone	Malformed ears, cleft palate, cardiac, urogenital and skeletal defects
Valproic acid	Neural tube defects
Warfarin	Skeletal and CNS defects, Dandy-Walker syndrome

Modified from: Koren G., Pastukzak A. and Ito S.: Drugs in Pregnancy, NEJM, 338: 1128, April 16, 1998

noted that fewer than 30 drugs have been proved to be teratogenic in humans when used in clinically effective doses. Many of the commonly used drugs, once thought to be teratogenic, have been shown by subsequent studies to be safe; they include salicylates, glucocorticoids, diazepam, combination oral contraceptive pills and spermicides. Much of the information on teratogenicity of drugs has been obtained from animal experiments and mishaps in clinical practice. Because of species variability and the high doses used in these experiments, such data are not directly applicable to humans; but they have a high positive predictive value. Almost every drug that has been found to be teratogenic in humans has caused similar teratogenicity in animals. However, there are drugs that have caused teratogenic effects in animals in large doses that are not teratogenic in humans in clinically effective doses. Individual case reports and limited epidemiological surveys provide the information available about teratogenicity of drugs in humans.

FDA ratings for drug use in pregnancy are shown in Table 77.2.

Table 77.2: Drugs used in Pregnancy, FDA categories

FDA Rating	Conditions	Examples
A	Controlled human studies show no risk	Folic acid
B	No confirmatory evidence of risk in humans	Metronidazole
C	Risk cannot be ruled out	Most drugs
D	Positive evidence of risk exists	Antiepileptics (Table 77.1)
X	Absolutely contraindcated.	Cytotoxics, Etretinate (Tablc 77.1)

Except in a few instances, congenital malformations produced by drugs are not unique. In animal experiments, a given drug may produce different congenital abnormalities whereas a given congenital abnormality may be produced by several drugs. Most drugs currently suspected of being teratogenic in humans are, in fact, weak teratogens and probably increase the frequency of congenital malformations only 2 - 3 fold. In fact, smoking and alcohol are more harmful to the fetus than most drugs. Table 77.1 lists the drugs which are known or suspected to be teratogenic in humans. *Absence of a drug from the list should not be interpreted to mean that it is necessarily safe during pregnancy.*

The teratogenic effects of thalidomide have been described in Chapter 1; those of alcohol in Chapter 6; tetracycline in Chapter 48 and retinoic acid derivatives in Chapter 69.

Patient is advised to delay pregnancy for certain periods of time after completing the course of certain drugs: one month after isotretinoin (Chapter 69); three months after mefloquine (Chapter 54); one year after cytotoxic drugs (methotrexate, cyclophosphamide); and three years after etretinate (Chapter 69) in order to allow the elimination of the drug. However, azathioprine following renal transplantation has not been found to pose an excess risk of congenital malformations in succeeding pregnancies.

Testosterone and its derivatives, including progestogens derived from 19 - nortestosterone, can masculinize the external genitals of a female fetus. Estrogens and progestins, on the other hand, are known to induce defective masculinization of the external genitals of a male fetus. However, inadvertent continuation of a COC pill during the first month of gestation has not been found to be harmful to the fetus. Diethylstilbestrol administration during pregnancy has been associated with the development of congenital anomalies of external genitals in fetuses of both sexes, and with the development of vaginal adenosis and vaginal adenocarcinoma in girls whose mothers had received the drug.

The use of coumarin anticoagulants is associated with congenital malformations and high incidence of fetal loss from abortion, retroplacental and intracerebral fetal bleeding.

Consumption of even one drink (10 g of alcohol) per day is associated with fetal growth retardation and an increased incidence of abortion. Consumption of large quantities (40 g per day) is associated with 'fetal alcohol syndrome'.

Behavioral teratogenicity: Apart from the structural teratogenicity discussed above, drugs

Table 77.3: Points to remember while prescribing drugs to a woman of reproductive age

- Enquire whether she is pregnant or is likely to become pregnant in near future.
- Ask her if she is having unprotected, sexual intercourse. If yes, tell her that if she has an unplanned pregnancy she runs the risk of exposing her fetus to a drug or drugs she may be taking, even before she knows that she is pregnant.
- Advise her to avoid conception for specified periods of time after completing therapy with certain drugs (see text).
- If a known or potentially teratogenic drug must be prescribed, she may be asked to sign a consent form that she agrees to use two effective methods of contraception.
- Further, inform her of the availability, efficacy and safety of long acting injectable contraceptives and postcoital contraceptives.
- The patient should be encouraged to participate in decision making about whether the drug is necessary and which drug to use.

can also cause behavioral teratogenicity i.e. abnormal behaviour in the newborn. Such effects have been observed in animal models when drugs such as reserpine, phenothiazines, barbiturates, amphetamine and cannabis were administered during pregnancy. So far, behavioral teratogenicity has been observed in human newborns of mothers who were exposed to methylmercury by eating contaminated fish and those who smoked during pregnancy. Animal studies indicate that the developing CNS is highly susceptible to the effects of psychoactive drugs. In humans, the brain development extends into early infancy and hence, the extended vulnerability of the brain in humans to the effects of such drugs.

Table 77.3 lists points to remember while prescribing drugs to women who are of the reproductive age and sexually active.

Drug Prescribing During Pregnancy

Table 77.4 summarises the precautions to be taken while prescribing drugs to a pregnant woman.

Nausea and vomiting of pregnancy can be treated without drugs in most women. Reassurance and high carbohydrate diet will help them. If required, an antihistaminic-antiemetic (cyclizine, meclizine, diphenhydramine, dimenhydrinate) may be prescribed. Metoclopramide is safe in the third trimester of pregnancy and may be prescribed in resistant cases.

Table 77.4: Precautions while prescribing drugs to a pregnant woman

- Treat minor ailments without drugs.
- If a drug must be prescribed, it should be one which is known to be safe during pregnancy.
- Prefer a drug which has been in use for long periods of time to a newly introduced drug as the safety of the latter for the fetus is not likely to be *known* completely.
- Adjust the dose of the drug to the pregnant state; with most drugs, it is generally at the lower end of the therapeutic range. However, because of pharmacokinetic factors (increased body weight and more rapid clearace), the dose of certain drugs such as lithium, digoxin and phenytoin is likely to be higher than in the non-pregnant state in some women.
- Discourage the patient from self-administering OTC drugs.
- Advise the patient that absolute safety of the fetus cannot be guaranteed even by not prescribing *any* drug to women between the ages of 15 and 45. Therefore, do not sacrifice the mother's interest for the sake of the fetus.

Heartburn is very common in pregnancy and is relieved by a small carbohydrate meal; by avoiding fatty food, smoking and alcohol; and by maintenance of upright posture. Consumption of aerated lemonade 2-3 times a day is also effective. Non-systemic antacids and metoclopramide may be needed in some cases. Anticholinergics usually worsen the heartburn by relaxing the lower esophageal sphincter.

Peptic ulcer should be treated with dietary modification and non-systemic antacids. Sucralfate which is not absorbed, H_2 receptor blockers and bismuth subsalicylate are safe during pregnancy. H_2 receptor blockers can also be used to treat GERD.

Constipation generally responds to high fibre diet, plenty of liquids and a mild laxative such as milk of magnesia, docusate sodium, glycerin, mineral oil or bisacodyl.

Antimicrobial drugs: Betalactam antibiotics (penicillins and most of the cephalosporins) are safe during pregnancy. Ampicillin achieves very high concentrations in the fetal circulation and amniotic fluid and is very suitable for treatment of uterine infections during pregnancy. Erythromycin base is safe but erythromycin estolate should be avoided for fear or hepatotoxicity. Nitrofurantoin and methanamine mandelate are safe during pregnancy. So are nystatin and miconazole; but ketoconazole and 5-flucytosine should be avoided.

Aminoglycosides are ototoxic to the fetus and should be avoided; if one is needed to treat a serious systemic infection in the mother, gentamicin or tobramycin should be preferred. Tetracyclines damage the fetal teeth and bones and should be avoided. High doses of tetracycline intravenously have been associated with serious hepatotoxicity in the mother. Chloramphenicol is absolutely contraindicated during pregnancy; it can cause fetal bone marrow toxicity and 'grey baby syndrome' in the neonate. Co-trimoxazole should be avoided especially in the first trimester (because of its trimethoprim content) and the third (because of its sulfonamide content). Griseofulvin and nalidixic acid are embryotoxic and should be avoided. The use of sulfonamides at term can cause kernicterus in the neonate by displacing bilirubin from binding with albumin; the other drugs which displace bilirubin from albumin are aspirin, and water soluble vitamin K analogues.

Tuberculosis: Isoniazid and ethambutol are safe during pregnancy. Rifampicin should be avoided as far as possible but may be used if a third drug is required. While using rifampicin, its hepatatoxicity should be kept in mind. *Streptomycin is ototoxic to the fetus and should never be used in pregnant women.*

Parasitic diseases: Amoebiasis should be treated with the usual drugs: metronidazole, diodoquin and diloxanide. However, large dose, short term therapy (such as single daily doses of 30 mg/kg) with metronidazole should be avoided.

Primaquine, pyrimethamine and mefloquine are contraindicated. Chronic suppressive use of chloroquine and its use to treat acute attacks of malaria during pregnancy are safe. Quinine may be used to treat acute attacks of chloroquine-resistant malaria.

Piperazine, bephenium and pyrantel are safe for use during pregnancy. Most people consider mebendazole unsafe during pregnancy. Unless the parasite load is heavy, the treatment of intestinal parasitic infections is best postponed till after delivery.

NSAID: Aspirin is not teratogenic but high dose aspirin treatment during the last six months is associated with increased gestation time, higher incidence of postmaturity and increased duration of labour. Further, it can also cause severe post-partum haemorrhage, bleeding in the neonate and premature closure of ductus arteriosus with pulmonary hypertension in the fetus and the newborn. Aspirin and other NSAID are, therefore, best avoided during pregnancy. Paracetamol in the usual doses is safe during pregnancy.

Glucocorticoids: Chapter 64.

Antihypertensives : Methyl-dopa is usually safe and preferred. Beta blockers in the second and third trimesters can cause general retardation, whereas ACEI and ARB-A can cause fetal abnormalities Labetalol IV may be used when rapid reduction in BP is desired. of renal function and skull development. These drugs probably interefere with the maturation of specific organ systems (Chapter 29).

Heart disease: This is treated as in non-pregnant women. Digoxin clearance by the kidney increases during pregnancy. If the dosage remains unchanged by the end of pregnancy, the serum concentration will have fallen to about half the value before pregnancy.

At the therapeutic concentration, quinidine appears to be safe and the drug has only mild oxytocic activity. Quinidine is normally 80% bound to plasma protein. Changes in plasma protein concentration during pregnancy cause total plasma quinidine concentrations to fall and free concentration to be underestimated. After delivery, total concentration of quinidine increases by about half.

Vasopressor agents (noradrenaline, dopamine and dobutamine) all decrease the uterine blood flow and may stimulate uterine contractions. Their use in pregnancy is justified only if the mother's survival is at stake.

Anticoagulants: Warfarin is best avoided in pregnant women, except those who have an artificial heart valve; in these latter subjects, heparin does not give adequate anticoagulant cover. In other patients, subcutaneous heparin should be used if anticoagulation is required. One dose of heparin should be omitted when labour is imminent, so as to avoid post-partum hemorrhage.

Deep vein thrombosis may be treated with heparin. The use of streptokinase is associated with the risk of bleeding.

Allergic rhinitis: This may be treated either locally (with glucocorticoids or decongestants) or systemically with antihistaminics (diphenhydramine, dimenhydrinate, tripelenamine).

Cough: Diphenhydramine, codeine and dextromethorphan may be used safely to treat cough during pregnancy.

Pruritus: This may be treated locally (with topical moisturizing creams or lotions, calamine lotion, zinc oxide cream or ointment or glucocorticoids) or systemically (with hydroxyzine, diphenhydramine or glucocorticoids)

Bronchial asthma is treated with inhaled beta adrenergic agonists, inhaled glucocorticoids, or with aminophyllin. However, IV Salbutamal used to delay labour is known to cause pulmonary edema especially (a) in individuals with mitral stenosis and (b) when corticosteroids are administered concurrently to promote fetal lung maturation (with death in some cases). This therapy should not be used in hypertensive subjects. Further, in diabetic subjects IV salbutamol can cause severe hyperglycemia and ketoacidosis, resistant even to aggressive insulin therapy.

Headache may be treated with paracetamol, codeine and benzodiazepines. Aspirin and NSAID may be used in the first and second but not in the third trimesters.

Migraine may be treated with analgesics, propranolol, dimenhydrinate and amitryptiline.

Diabetes mellitus should be treated with dietary restriction and insulin, if required; the use of oral hypoglycemic agents is not recommended. In insulin dependent diabetics who become pregnant, the insulin requirement drops somewhat during the first trimester (owing to nausea and poor food intake), then rises progressively to 2-3 times the pre-pregnancy level upto 36 weeks, and then drops again upto term. After delivery, insulin requirement dives dramatically to pre-pregnancy level.

Thyrotoxicosis: Thioamides are the therapy of choice for thyrotoxicosis during pregnancy; propylthiouracil is preferred to carbimazole. The dose should be kept as low as possible. Stable iodine and radioactive iodine are contraindicated.

Epilepsy: Adequate seizure control is important during pregnancy as convulsions themselves are harmful to the fetus. Phenobarbitone, phenytoin and carbamazepine may be used during pregnancy; as discussed carlier, their doses may have to be increased slightly in order to maintain seizure control. *All pregnant women on antiepileptic drugs should be prescribed folic acid 5 mg per day throughout pregnancy.* Vitamin K_1 should be administered to such patients routinely for 3 weeks before delivery and to their newborn babies at birth. The use of valproic acid is contraindicated during pregnancy.

Drugs acting on the CNS: Barbiturates, benzodiazepines and antidepressants have not been shown to have any significant teratogenic effects. Lithium has been reported to be teratogenic and also to be deleterious to the fetus in the last trimester.

The use of CNS depressants such as diazepam, antidepressants, phenothiazines and opioids at term and specially during labour, exposes the neonate to the risk of serious CNS depression.

Benzodiazepines are best avoided towards the end of pregnancy.

Phenothiazines and tricyclic antidepressants can be continued during pregnancy in minimum possible doses. Antiparkinsonian drugs, commonly prescribed together with phenothiazine, should not be used during the first trimester. *MAO inhibitors are contraindicated during pregnancy.* Further, it is desirable to taper and omit tricyclic antidepressants in the last few weeks of pregnancy and to restart them after delivery.

Breast Feeding and Drugs

Nearly all agents received by the mother are likely to be found in her milk and could theoretically harm the infant. However, the data on excretion of drugs in milk and its possible harmful effects on the newborn are scanty.

Breast feeding is important not only from nutritional point of view but it also supplies IgA and IgM immunoglobulins which afford protection against gastroenteritis. More and more women are now electing to breast feed their babies. Although several drugs are known to increase prolactin secretion, no suitable drug is available at present, which could consistently augment the milk production in the human female. Thyrotropin releasing hormone (TRH) and metoclopramide have been shown to increase milk production in some studies. However, it appears that determination on the mother's part is more important than prolactin-inducing drugs. Lactation will stop if the breast is not suckled. Suckling stimulates the release of prolactin.

Most of the lipid soluble drugs get into breast milk, though not necessarily in concentrations that can adversely affect the infant. Milk is slightly more acidic (pH 7.0) than plasma and hence, weak bases that become more ionized with decrease in pH will have equal or higher concentrations in milk than in plasma. Nonelectrolytes like alcohol (ethanol) can readily enter into the milk independently of the pH. Majority of the drugs get into the milk by passive diffusion although active transport may occur in a few cases e.g. iodide. The amount of a drug transferred into the milk depends on various factors. The maternal volume of distribution for lipid soluble drugs is larger than for water soluble drugs; this results in low plasma levels relative to the dose. Further, only the unbound drug in the plasma is able to diffuse into the milk. Drugs like warfarin which are highly protein bound (over 95%) cannot be detected in breast milk. Even for a lipid soluble, poorly protein bound, basic drug the milk to plasma ratio does not exceed four. Hence, drug toxicity based on the principal pharmacological action of the drug is considered unlikely in breast fed infant. However, toxicity based on idiosyncrasy or a particular sensitivity of the infant to very low doses of a drug may occur.

The available data suggest that the net transfer of most drugs in breast milk is too small to produce significant adverse effect in the breast fed infant. However, in view of such a possibility, drugs, particularly the newer ones, must not be prescribed during parturition unless essential. It must be remembered that the elimination rate for most drugs is slower in neonates than in the adults and this may lead to accumulation of the drug in neonates, particularly when it is taken for long courses by the mother.

Table 77.5: Drugs not recommended for use in breast feeding women

- **Radionuclides and radiopharmaceutical.**
- **Antibacterials:** Sulfonamides, Tetracyclines Chloramphenicol, Nalidixic acid, Isoniazid, Erythromycin estolate.
- **Analgesics:** Indomethacin, Phenylbutazone, Aspirin (in large doses for long periods), Opioids (regular use of large doses).
- **Psychoactive drugs:** Diazepam, Lithium.
- **Antihypertensives:** Reserpine, Clonidine.
- **Antithyroid drugs :** Thioamides
- **Antineoplastic drugs**
- **Miscellaneous:** Amantadine, Phenindione, Cimetidine, Anthraquinones, Amiodarone, Ephedrine, Aminophylline, Ergotamine, Vitamin D (prolonged use of large doses).

Fortunately, majority of the drugs appear to cause no adverse effects on breast fed babies. Table 77.5 gives a list of the drugs not recommended during breast feeding. Aspirin and paracetamol have been used extensively in the puerperium without apparent ill effects on the infant. Heparin and warfarin are not detected in the milk. There is no contraindication to thyroxine treatment for hypothyroidism during breast feeding. But, breast feeding should be discouraged in women taking antithyroid drugs. Radioiodine is absolutely contra-indicated during breast feeding. Since most of the antibiotics pass into breast milk, it may be advisable to avoid drugs like chloramphenicol, tetracycline and sulfonamides in breast-feeding women. Penicillins, erythromycin, lincomycin, quinine and chloroquine appear to be safe for the treatment of nursing mothers. Aminoglycoside antibiotics, though they appear in breast milk, are not considered dangerous as they are not absorbed from the gut. Metronidazole is considered quite safe during breast feeding but may make the milk taste bitter. Beta-blockers, thiazide diuretics, captopril and digoxin levels achieved in breast milk are probably too low to have any significant effect on the breast fed infants. All centrally acting drugs, being lipid soluble, have a high volume of distribution. Hence, the total amount of drug available for concentration in the milk is likely to be small. Opiate analgesics, phenothiazines, chloral hydrate and antiepileptics may, therefore, be used safely by the mothers, if necessary. However lithium has a high milk to plasma ratio and the dose available to breast fed infant is likely to be similar to that of the mother. Hence, it should be avoided during breast-feeding. Regular use of opioids in high doses by the mother may lead to dependence and withdrawal in the neonate. Ergotamine may lead to ergotism and chloroquine in the treatment of rheumatoid arthritis may cause retinal damage in the newborn infant. Amiodarone is present in the milk in significant quantities; it is best avoided because of the possible effects of the released iodine on the neonatal thyroid. The neonate has been reported to become irritable when the breast feeding mother is taking ephedrine, or 200 mg or more of aminophylline every 6 hours; slow release preparations of aminophylline are probably safe. High levels in breast milk have been reported for the H_2-blocker, cimetidine. *Cytotoxic drugs, in general, are absolutely contraindicated in mothers who are breast feeding.*

It should be realized that certain chemicals like DDT or methyl mercury acquired environmentally, could appear in milk and cause chronic toxicity in breast fed babies. *Finally, if a drug is used therapeutically in the neonatal period, one may use it safely in breast feeding women.*

APPENDIX: Guide to Further Reading

Only a selected list for further reference and reading is given below. This, obviously, does not detract from the extensive and high-quality references available on the various topics.

Alpers D.H., Stenso W.F. Bier D. M : *Manual of Nutritional Therapeutics*, 5th Ed., 2008, Lippincott, Philadelphia.

Bennett P. N. and Brown M. J., *Clinical Pharmacology*, 10th Ed., 2008; Churchill-Livingstone, London.

Schaefer C., Paul W. J., *Drugs During Pregnancy and Lactation*, 2nd Ed., 2007, Academic Press, London

British National Formulary 57, March 2009, British Medical Association.

Brunton L. B., Lazo J. S., Parker K. L. (ED): Goodman & Gilman's *The Pharmacological Basis of Therapeutics.* 11th EDtion. 2006, Mc Graw-Hill. New York

Cooper D.H., Krainik A.J., and Lubner S.J. (Ed) 2007. *The Washington Manual of Medical Therapeutics, 32nd* Edition, 2007 W. B. Saunders & Co., Philadelphia

Feinstein A.R.: *Clinical Biostatistics*, 1977, The C.V. Mosby Co., St Louis.

Goldman L. and Ausiello D. (Ed); *Cecil Textbook of Medicine*, 23nd Ed., 2008, W. B. Saunders & Co., Philadelphia.

Kasper D.,Kasper D.,Fauci A. S, Braunwald E., Kasper D., et al. (Ed), *Harrison's Principles of Internal Medicine*, 17th Ed., 2008, Mc-Gtaw-Hill Inc., NY.

Katzung B. G. (Ed); *Basic and Clinical Pharmacology*; 11 th Ed.; 2009, Mc Graw-Hill, New York.

Kim R. B.: *The Medical Letter Handbook of Adverse Drug Interactions*, 2001, The Medical Letter Inc., N.Y. Krantz J.C.: Historical Medical Classics Involving New Drugs 1974, William & Wilkins Co., U.S.A.

Male D., Brostoff J., Roth D., Roitt I.,S.: *Immunology*, 5th Edition, 1998, Mosby, St. Louis.

Opie L.H., Gersh B. J. (Ed.): Drugs for the Heart, 7th Ed., 2008, W.B. Saunders Co. Philadelphia.

Pratt W.B., and Taylor P.: *Principles of Drug Action*, 3rd Ed. 1990, Churchill Livingstone, London.

Raddle I.C., MacLeod S.M.: *Pediatric Pharmacology and Therapeutics*, 2nd Ed., 1993 Mosby, St. Louis.

Rakel R. E. (Ed) *Conn's Current Therapy*, 60 th Ed 2008, W. B. Saunders & Co., Philadelphia.

Rang H.P., Dale M.M., Ritter J.M.: *Pharmacology, 6th Edition, 2007*, Churchill Livingstone, Edinburgh.

The Essentials of Contraceptive Technology: A Handbook for Clinic Staff, 1997, The Johns Hopkins School of Public Health, Baltimore.

The Medical Letter, Vol. 43 (2001), 44 (2002), 45 (2003), 46 (2004), 47 (2005), 48 (2006); 49 (2007); 50 (2008) The Medical Letter Inc., NY.

Students may also refer to the following journals for interesting articles, reviews, and symposia: Ann. Int. Medicine, New Eng. J. Medicine, British Medical Journal, The Lancet, Clinical Pharmacology and Therapeutics, Ann. Rev. Pharmacology, W.H.O. Technical Reports, Pharmacological Review, Drugs, British J. Pharmacology and Brit. J. Clin. Pharmacology.

INDEX